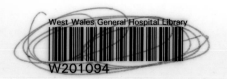

Levin *and* O'Neal's
The
Diabetic
Foot

Levin *and* O'Neal's
The
Diabetic
Foot

John H. Bowker, MD

Professor Emeritus
Department of Orthopaedics
Miller School of Medicine
University of Miami;
Co-Director, Diabetic Foot and Amputation Clinics
Jackson Memorial Medical Center
Miami, Florida

Michael A. Pfeifer, MD, CDE, FACE

Senior Director and Franchise Development Leader
Metabolic Diseases
Pharmaceutical Research and Development
Johnson and Johnson
Raritan, New Jersey

SEVENTH EDITION

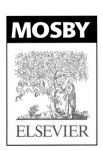

MOSBY

ELSEVIER

1600 John F. Kennedy Blvd.
Ste 1800
Philadelphia, PA 19103-2899

LEVIN AND O'NEAL'S THE DIABETIC FOOT   ISBN: 978-0-323-04145-4

Previous Editions Copyrighted

Library of Congress Cataloging-in-Publication Data

Levin and O'Neal's the diabetic foot. — 7th ed. / [edited by] John H. Bowker, Michael Pfeifer.
  p. ; cm.
  Includes bibliographical references and index.
  ISBN 978-0-323-04145-4
  1. Foot—Diseases. 2. Diabetes—Complications. 3. Foot—Surgery. I. Levin, Marvin E., 1924- II. O'Neal, Lawrence W., 1923- III. Bowker, John H. IV. Pfeifer, Michael A. V. Title: Diabetic foot.
  [DNLM: 1. Diabetic Foot. WK 835 L6645 2008]
  RC951.D53 2008
  617.5'85—dc22

                                        2007018659

Acquisitions Editor: Emily Christie
Developmental Editor: Karen Carter
Senior Project Manager: David Saltzberg
Design Direction: Lou Forgione

Printed in China

Last digit is the print number: 9 8 7 6 5 4 3 2 1

DEDICATION

This volume is respectfully dedicated
to the memory of

Paul Wilson Brand, MB, BS, MD, FRCS, CBE,

pioneering investigator and healer for those who have lost
"the gift of pain."

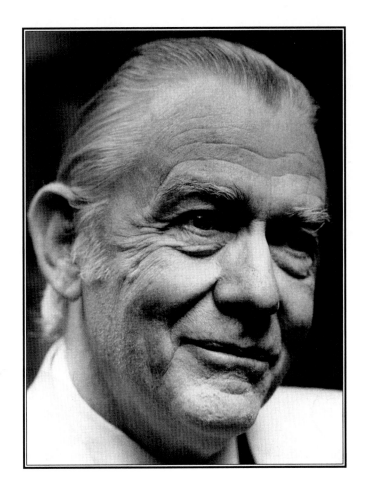

CONTRIBUTORS

Andrew J.M. Boulton, MD, FRCP
Professor of Medicine
University of Manchester;
Consultant Physician
Manchester Royal Infirmary
Manchester, United Kingdom;
Professor of Medicine
Department of Endocrinology and
    Diabetes
University of Miami
Miami, Florida

John H. Bowker, MD
Professor Emeritus
Department of Orthopaedics
Miller School of Medicine
University of Miami;
Co-Director, Diabetic Foot and Amputation
    Clinics
Jackson Memorial Medical Center
Miami, Florida

James W. Brodsky, MD
Clinical Professor of Orthopaedic Surgery
University of Texas Southwestern Medical
    School;
Director, Foot and Ankle Surgery
    Fellowship Training Program
Baylor University Medical Center and
    University of Texas Southwestern
    Medical School
Dallas, Texas

Peter R. Cavanagh, PhD, DSc
Chairman
Department of Biomedical Engineering
Lerner Research Institute
Cleveland Clinic
Cleveland, Ohio

Paul Cianci, MD
Clinical Professor of Medicine Emeritus
University of California, Davis
Davis, California;
Medical Director
Department of Hyperbaric Medicine

Doctors Medical Center
San Pablo, California;
Medical Director
Department of Hyperbaric Medicine
John Muir Medical Center
Walnut Creek, California;
Medical Director
Department of Hyperbaric Medicine
Saint Francis Memorial Hospital
San Francisco, California

Curtis R. Clark, PT
Assistant Chief Physical Therapist
Medical/Surgical Unit
Jackson Memorial Hospital Rehabilitation
    Center
Jackson Health Systems
Miami, Florida

William Coleman, DPM
Ochsner Medical Center
New Orleans, Louisiana

John A. Colwell, MD, PhD
Professor
Department of Medicine
Medical College of South Carolina;
Professor
Department of Medicine
Medical University Hospital
Charleston, South Carolina

Kevin P. Conway, MD
Surgical Resident
Wound Healing Research Unit
Cardiff University
Cardiff, Wales, United Kingdom

Kenrick J. Dennis, DPM
Fallbrook Crossing Medical Center
Houston, Texas

Peter D. Donofrio, MD
Professor of Neurology
Chief of the Neuromuscular Center
Vanderbilt University Medical Center
Nashville, Tennessee

**Dorothy B. Doughty, MN, RN, CWOCN,
FNP, FAAN**
Emory University Wound, Ostomy, and
    Continence Nursing Education Center
Department of Surgery
Emory University School of Medicine
Atlanta, Georgia

Michelle Draznin, MD
Department of Dermatology
University of California, Davis
Davis, California

Robert Eison, MD
Department of Internal Medicine
University of California, Davis
Davis, California

Robert G. Frykberg, DPM, MPH
Adjunct Associate Professor
Department of Podiatric Medicine
Midwestern University
Glendale, Arizona;
Chief, Podiatry
Department of Surgery
Carl T. Hayden VA Medical Center
Phoenix, Arizona

Robert S. Gailey, PhD, PT
Associate Professor
Department of Physical Therapy
Miller School of Medicine
University of Miami
Coral Gables, Florida;
Health Science Researcher
Department of Research
Miami Veterans Affairs Health Services
Miami, Florida

Ignacio A. Gaunaurd, MSPT
Health Science Researcher
Department of Research
Miami Veterans Affairs Health Services
Miami, Florida

Jeffrey S. Gonzalez, PhD
Behavioral Medicine
Harvard Medical School/Massachusetts
    General Hospital;
Department of Psychiatry
Massachusetts General Hospital
Boston, Massachusetts

Linda Haas, PhC, RN, CDE
Endocrinology Clinical Nurse Specialist
VA Puget Sound Health Care System
    Seattle Division;
Clinical Assistant Professor of Nursing
University of Washington
Seattle, Washington

Allen D. Hamdan, MD, FACS
Assistant Program Director
BIDMC General Surgery and Vascular
    Surgery Residency;
Director
Clinical Research Vascular Surgery,
    BIDMC;
Director
HMFP Vascular Laboratory
Boston, Massachusetts

K. G. Harding, MB, ChB, FRCS, FRCGP
Staff in Medicine
Wound Healing Research Unit
Cardiff University
Cardiff, Wales, United Kingdom

Lawrence B. Harkless, DPM
Professor
Department of Orthopaedics
Louis T. Bogy Professor of Podiatric
    Medicine and Surgery
Department of Orthopaedics/Podiatry
    Division
The University of Texas Health Science
    Center at San Antonio
San Antonio, Texas

Irl B. Hirsch, MD
Professor
Department of Medicine
University of Washington School of
    Medicine;
Medical Director
Diabetes Care Center
University of Washington Medical Center
Seattle, Washington

Hanno Hoppe, MD
Clinical Fellow
Dotter Interventional Institute
Oregon Health and Science University
Portland, Oregon

Thomas K. Hunt, MD
Department of Surgery
University of California–San Francisco
San Francisco, Califonia

Arthur Huntley, MD
Associate Professor
Department of Dermatology
University of California, Davis
Davis, California

Joseph J. Hurley, MD
General and Vascular Surgeon
St John's Mercy Medical Center
Creve Coeur, Missouri

Dennis J. Janisse, CPed
Clinical Assistant Professor
Physical Medicine and Rehabilitation
Medical College of Wisconsin;
Froedtart Memorial Lutheran Hospital;
President and CEO
National Pedorthic Services, Inc.
Milwaukee, Wisconsin

Jeffrey E. Johnson, MD
Associate Professor
Department of Orthopaedic Surgery
Washington University School of
    Medicine;
Chief
Foot and Ankle Service
Department of Orthopaedic Surgery
Barnes-Jewish Hospital at Washington
    University School of Medicine
St. Louis, Missouri

Rudolf J. Jokl, MD
Assistant Professor
Department of Medicine
Medical University of South Carolina
Charleston, South Carolina

John A. Kaufman, MD
Dotter Interventional Institute,
Oregon Health & Science University,
Portland, Oregon

Janet L. Kelly, PharmD, BC-ADM
Outcomes and Cost Management
    Pharmacist
Department of Pharmacy
University of Washington Medical Center;
Clinical Associate Professor
School of Pharmacy
University of Washington
Seattle, Washington

Richard L. Klein, PhD
Assistant Professor
Medical University of South Carolina
Division of Endocrinology, Diabetes and
    Medical Genetics
Charleston, South Carolina

Shelley H. Leinicke, JD
Wicker, Smith, O'Hara, McCoy, Graham &
    Ford, PA
Fort Lauderdale, Florida

Steven Y. Leinicke, JD
Wicker, Smith, O'Hara, McCoy, Graham &
    Ford, PA
Fort Lauderdale, Florida

Joseph W. LeMaster, MD, MPH
Assistant Professor
Department of Family and Community
    Medicine
University of Missouri–Columbia
Columbia, Missouri

Benjamin A. Lipsky, MD, FACP, FIDSA
Professor of Medicine
University of Washington;
Director, Antibiotic Research
General Internal Medicine Clinic
VA Puget Sound Health Care System
Seattle, Washington

Mary D. Litchford, PhD, RD, LDN
President
CASE Software
Greensboro, North Carolina

Maria E. Lopes-Virella, MD, PhD
Professor
Departments of Microbiology and
    Immunology, Bioengineering,
    Endocrinology, Diabetes, and Medical
    Genetics;
Co-Director
Cholesterol Clinic
Endocrinology, Diabetes and Medical
    Genetics
Medical University of South Carolina;
Chief, Nutrition Support Team
Chief, Clinical Chemistry, Immunology and
    Serology, and Microbiology;
Co-Director, Cholesterol and Lipid Clinics
Ralph H. Johnson VA Medical Center
Charleston, South Carolina

Timothy J. Lyons, MD
Medical Director
Diabetes Center of Excellence
University of Oklahoma Health Sciences
    Center
Oklahoma City, Oklahoma

Emanual Maverakis,
Department of Dermatology
University of California, Davis
Davis, California

Donald E. McMillan, MD, AB
Research Professor of Engineering
Professor Emeritus of Internal Medicine
Professor Emeritus of Physiology
University of South Florida;
Staff Physician, Family Health Center
Tampa, Florida

Michael J. Mueller, PT, PhD, FAPTA
Associate Professor
Program in Physical Therapy
Washington University School of Medicine
St. Louis, Missouri

Lawrence W. O'Neal, MD, FACS
Emeritus Professor
Department of Surgery
St. Louis University School of Medicine
St. Louis, Missouri;
Emeritus Chairman
Department of Surgery
St. John's Mercy Medical Center
Creve Coeur, Missouri

Walter J. Pedowitz, MD
Clinical Professor of Orthopaedic Surgery
Columbia University College of Physicians
  and Surgeons;
Private Practice
Union County Orthopedic Group
Linden, New Jersey;
Member, Coding Committee
American Academy of Orthopaedic
  Surgeons;
Member, Coding Committee
American Orthopaedic Foot and Ankle
  Society;
Advisor on Current Procedural
  Terminology to the American Medical
  Association

Michael A. Pfeifer, MD, CDE, FACE
Senior Director and Franchise
  Development Leader
Metabolic Diseases
Pharmaceutical Research and
  Development
Johnson and Johnson
Raritan, New Jersey

Jeffrey M. Pitcher, MD
Faculty
Office of Graduate Medical Education
Indiana University School of Medicine
Indianapolis, Indiana

Frank B. Pomposelli, Jr., MD
Associate Professor
Department of Surgery
Harvard Medical School
Beth Israel Deaconess Medical Center
New England Baptist Hospital
Boston, Massachusetts

Gayle E. Reiber, MPH, PhD
VA Career Scientist
VA Puget Sound Health Care System;

Professor
Departments of Health Services and
  Epidemiology
University of Washington
Seattle, Washington

Lee J. Sanders, MD
Chief
Podiatry Service
VA Medical Center
Lebanon, Pennsylvania

V. Kathleen Satterfield, DPM
Assistant Professor
Department of Orthopaedics
Director of Podiatric Research
Department of Orthopaedics/Podiatric
  Service
The University of Texas Health Science
  Center at San Antonio
San Antonio, Texas

David R. Sinacore, PhD, PT, FAPTA
Associate Professor
Internal Medicine and Physical Therapy
Washington University School of Medicine
St. Louis, Missouri

Jay S. Skyler, MD, MACP
Professor
Division of Endocrinology, Diabetes, and
  Metabolism
Associate Director
Diabetes Research Institute
Miller School of Medicine
University of Miami;
Chairman
NIDDK Type 1 Diabetes TrialNet
Miami, Florida

Robert J. Tanenberg, MD, FACP
Professor of Medicine
Director, Diabetes Fellowship
Division of Endocrinology

Brody School of Medicine;
Director, Diabetes and Obesity Center
East Carolina University
Greenville, North Carolina

Andrew Brian Thomson, MD
Fellow
Department of Orthopaedic Surgery
Washington University School of Medicine
Barnes-Jewish Hospital at Washington
  University School of Medicine
St. Louis, Missouri

Jan S. Ulbrecht, MB, BS
Associate Professor
Department of Biobehavioral Health
Pennsylvania State University
University Park, Pennsylvania

Loretta Vileikyte, MD, PhD
Honorary Lecturer
Department of Medicine
University of Manchester
Manchester, United Kingdom;
Visiting Research Assistant Professor
Division of Endocrinology, Diabetes and
  Metabolism
University of Miami
Miami, Florida;
Visiting Research Assistant Professor
Institute for Health, Healthcare Policy and
  Aging Research
Rutgers, The State University of New Jersey
New Brunswick, New Jersey

William A. Wooden, MD, FACS
Vice Chairman
Department of Surgery
Professor of Surgery
Division of Plastic Surgery
IUPUI School of Medicine
Indianapolis, Indiana

FOREWORD

Karel Bakker, MD, PhD

More than 200 million people in the world have diabetes mellitus. Foot problems are a threat to every person with this condition. Worldwide, more than a million lower limb amputations are performed each year as a consequence of diabetes, which means that every thirty seconds a lower limb is lost to diabetes. This figure is unacceptably high. The treatment and subsequent care of people with diabetic foot problems have a significant impact on health care budgets and a potentially devastating impact on the lives of affected individuals and their family members.

Recently, initiatives and programs have been developed to direct and improve diabetic foot care and address the lack of awareness of foot problems in diabetic patients among health care professionals and those with or at risk of diabetes. In order to improve outcomes for people with diabetic foot ulcers, effective communication and collaboration are required between the many professionals directly involved in diabetic foot care and those in a position to decide health care policy and provide funding. Such communication and collaboration have been encouraged by the formation of the International Working Group on the Diabetic Foot (IWGDF) in 1996 and by the establishment of international definitions and guidelines on the prevention and management of diabetic foot complications.

As a result, the *International Consensus on the Diabetic Foot* and the *Practical Guidelines on the Management and Prevention of the Diabetic Foot* were launched during the 3rd International Symposium on the Diabetic Foot in Noordwijkerhout, The Netherlands, in 1999. At the present time, these concise, compact and clinically useful documents have been translated into 26 languages. Supplements were added on CD-ROM in 2003. New and updated consensus items were introduced at the 5th International Symposium on the Diabetic Foot in May 2007. IWGDF now counts members from over 80 countries and has distributed more than 80,000 copies of the *International Consensus on the Diabetic Foot/Guidelines*. Both the printed and CD-ROM formats are available through the IDF website: www.idf.org/bookshop for a modest fee.

The mission of the International Diabetes Federation (IDF), which represents 145 countries, is to promote diabetes care, prevention, and cure worldwide. It has maintained official relations with the World Health Organization (WHO) for more than 50 years. IDF has developed various activities to achieve its objectives, such as the World Diabetes Day global awareness campaign. The year 2005 was proclaimed the Year of the Diabetic Foot. That year IDF and IWGDF's year-long awareness campaign on diabetes and foot care culminated in World Diabetes Day on 14 November, reaching its largest audience ever, numbered in the millions.

With the growth in professional and academic interest has come increased political awareness. This provides a solid foundation on which the future can be built. It is the structural and financial support that health care policy- and decision-makers put in place that will define the future for many people living with and at future risk of diabetic foot complications.

In the field of research into the diabetic foot, more preclinical randomized, controlled trials are underway and will continue into the future. These studies will stress the importance of identifying the missing links between the outcome of diabetic foot problems and the descriptive variables found in earlier studies.

Over the past 10 years, standards of diabetic foot care have improved considerably. Each year, an increasing number of articles appear in leading journals and a growing number of local, national, and international meetings are held, either directly addressing or including themes related to the diabetic foot. In 2003, more than 400 articles appeared in internationally renowned journals—a fourfold increase over the previous decade. It is particularly encouraging that there is a noticeable increase in the diversity of countries from which the articles originate. All of this drives improvements in the delivery of foot care for people with diabetes and unifies the professional community. In the field of diabetic foot care, the view that care is best delivered when health care professionals from different disciplines come together is now widely held.

Surely the most important message is a positive one: the current situation can be changed. It is possible to reduce amputation rates by between 49% and 85% through preventive initiatives, the interdisciplinary treatment of foot ulcers, and appropriate education of not only people with diabetes but also of health care providers. A solid knowledge of pathophysiology and the management of the diabetic foot are mandatory for all professionals in the field.

This beautiful seventh edition of Levin and O'Neal's gold standard book, so marvelously edited again by John Bowker and Michael Pfeifer, is an indispensable tool in acquiring the up-to-date knowledge so necessary for all of us. Most chapters are totally rewritten and reorganized and several new authors have been added. A nice feature is the placement of boxes at the end of most chapters containing "Pearls and Pitfalls"—a very helpful instrument to highlight the critical points.

I heartily congratulate the authors, on behalf of many, on the publication of this splendid new edition.

KAREL BAKKER, MD, PhD
CHAIR, CONSULTATIVE SECTION ON THE DIABETIC FOOT
INTERNATIONAL DIABETES FEDERATION
CHAIR, INTERNATIONAL WORKING GROUP ON THE
DIABETIC FOOT

FOREWORD

Marvin E. Levin, MD
Lawrence W. O'Neal, MD, FACS

Of the many complications affecting the person with diabetes mellitus, none are more devastating than those involving the foot. These include peripheral arterial disease, peripheral neuropathy, ulceration, infection, and amputation. As the number of persons with diabetes increases, we will see more and more foot problems, and that is why this textbook has been published and updated periodically.

In the United States there are currently 21 million diabetic persons, with 42 million diabetic feet and 210 million diabetic toes—less those lost to amputation. It is estimated that in any given year between 3% and 18% of the 21 million Americans with diabetes will experience a foot ulcer, and that 15% will develop a foot ulcer at some point during their lifetime. Many of these people will require hospitalization and amputation. The cost per month for treating a foot ulcer is approximately $1,200.00; the cost of treating all foot ulcerations in the United States exceeds one billion dollars annually.

To understand what the feet endure during a lifetime, simply look at the statistics associated with everyday activities. The average person takes between 8,000 and 10,000 steps a day, equal to walking 115,000 miles in a lifetime, more than four times around the earth. If the person taking these steps is diabetic, has peripheral neuropathy with loss of protective sensation and peripheral arterial disease, it is not surprising that his or her feet develop ulceration and infection, all too frequently resulting in amputation.

The escalating number of foot problems is due not only to the increasing diabetic population but to the fact that people with diabetes are living long enough to develop foot complications. Despite the many treatment modalities available today, the number of amputations, including toes to midthigh, is increasing. In fact, every thirty seconds a lower limb is lost worldwide as a consequence of diabetes (*Lancet*, November 2005).

The Centers for Disease Control and Prevention (CDC) noted that approximately one third of persons with diabetes are at high risk for lower-limb amputation. The exact number of amputations in the United States due to diabetes is unknown. In 1995, the number reported was 77,112, and in 1996, 85,530. We predict that by 2007 the number will be close to 100,000. However, with patient education (see Appendix I: Patients' Instructions for the Care of the Diabetic Foot) and aggressive treatment, this number can be significantly reduced.

Beginning in the 1960s and up to the 1970s, medical textbooks contained very little information about the diabetic foot. A review of five major medical textbooks of that period revealed that there was anywhere from zero to all of one and one half pages devoted to the diabetic foot. In those days, if one wanted a complete evaluation of the problems and treatment of the diabetic foot, it was necessary to consult at least ten different textbooks, mostly surgical. Their abbreviated coverage consisted primarily of hygienic care of the foot. In the late 1960s, Dr. O'Neal and I came to the conclusion that what was lacking in the literature was a complete and concise textbook on the care and problems of the diabetic foot. The lack of information, we believed, resulted in excessive amputations, with their monetary and emotional costs.

Therefore, in 1973 we published the first edition of *The Diabetic Foot*, feeling at the time that it was a complete book on the treatment of the diabetic foot, which, of course, was not quite true. That first edition consisted of 262 pages, divided into ten chapters with twelve contributing authors.

The seventh edition of *Levin and O'Neal's The Diabetic Foot*, by contrast, consists of more than 600 pages divided into 33 chapters, written by 58 authors. The purpose of this text is to bring to all who care for the diabetic patient the latest information on the pathophysiology of diabetic foot lesions, their treatment, and the prevention of amputation. Unfortunately, all too often the treatment of the diabetic foot falls below the standard of care, which can lead to litigation. Therefore, an important chapter in this edition is on the medical legal aspects of caring for the diabetic foot.

Beginning with the sixth edition, Dr. O'Neal and I turned the editorship of *Levin and O'Neal's The Diabetic Foot* over to Drs. John Bowker and Michael Pfeifer. Because of their vast experience and expertise in the management of the diabetic foot, they have compiled in this seventh edition the very latest information and techniques useful in caring for diabetic foot complications.

MARVIN E. LEVIN, MD
LAWRENCE W. O'NEAL, MD, FACS
EMERITUS EDITORS, *THE DIABETIC FOOT*

With the seventh edition of this work, the present editors are renewing a commitment made by Drs. Levin and O'Neal 34 years ago when they published a brief monograph entitled *The Diabetic Foot.* Their goal was to help decrease the appalling incidence of lower-limb amputations in diabetic persons by gathering, into a single volume, authoritative discussions of the many factors that may lead to loss of the foot in this condition. The first edition had just ten chapters written by twelve authors from various medical disciplines for a total of 262 pages. With each succeeding edition, updated subject matter has been added from each field of endeavor that has some bearing on preventive and therapeutic foot care for the person with diabetes. Using this format, over the years, the book has become an ever more valuable reference work for all members of the diabetic foot care team.

To help clinicians keep abreast of the advances in this rapidly changing field, 23 chapters have been completely updated by their previous authors while eight have entirely new authorship. Three chapters, those dealing with off-loading techniques, psychological aspects, and medical-legal pitfalls, respectively, have been considerably expanded. Because of the real or perceived difficulty of receiving adequate compensation for the care of these complex, chronic patients, a chapter on diagnostic and procedural coding has been added. Altogether, this latest edition has 33 chapters, 58 contributors, and more than 600 pages. Two appendices have been added. The first, prepared by Drs. Levin and O'Neal, is a comprehensive list of foot care instructions to be provided to each diabetic patient. The second appendix lists relevant web sites that will allow the reader to obtain continually updated material to keep abreast of this expanding area of medical care.

This edition has been reorganized into six sections. The first explores the foundations of diabetic foot care beginning with the epidemiology and economic impact of foot ulcers and amputations, followed by an update on diabetes management, neuropathic problems of the lower limb, the pathogenesis of vascular disease, diabetic foot biomechanics, and dermatologic and nutritional issues.

The second section presents evaluation techniques, including the classification of foot lesions by their depth and vascularity, radiologic imaging, noninvasive vascular testing, and an in-depth discussion of Charcot neuroarthropathy. The third section covers nonsurgical approaches such as weight redistribution to assist the healing of foot lesions, radiologic intervention in peripheral vascular disease, continuing with comprehensive discussions of the principles of wound healing, the indications for hyperbaric oxygen therapy in the management of problem wounds, and the control of infection.

The fourth section is devoted to the surgical aspects of care, starting with surgical pathology of the foot and followed by perioperative medical management specifically related to diabetic patients, the present role of the vascular surgeon in salvage of the diabetic foot, soft-tissue reconstruction by the plastic surgeon, and a reasoned appraisal of the indications for foot surgery in Charcot neuroarthropathy. The section ends with an expanded chapter on minor and major lower-limb amputation.

The fifth section covers interdisciplinary team management, opening with a survey of approaches to diabetic foot care in various regions of the world. Next, an overview of the organization and day-to-day operation of one such interdisciplinary clinic is presented as an example. Succeeding chapters contain discussions of the roles of the podiatrist, wound care nurse, pedorthist, physical therapist, diabetes educator, and psychologist as diabetic foot team members.

The sixth and last section deals with two subjects, one faced on a daily basis and the second, ideally, rarely encountered. The first chapter explains the nuances and pitfalls inherent in diagnostic and procedural coding used for reimbursement of diabetic foot care by third-party payers. The second is a review of the medical–legal problems associated with the care of diabetic patients with foot disease, liberally illustrated with actual cases and their legal outcome. As patients and attorneys become more knowledgeable about the potentially disastrous results of inappropriate foot care, it becomes essential that caregivers fully understand both their own scope of responsibility in the prevention and management of foot problems and that which is assignable to the patient.

With the kind collaboration of the International Working Group on the Diabetic Foot (IWGDF), a Consultative Section of the International Diabetes Federation, each copy of this book includes a lagniappe (New Orleans Creole for an extra unexpected benefit) consisting of a comprehensive interactive DVD developed by the IWGDF in 2007 entitled *International Consensus on the Diabetic Foot*. The editors wish to thank Elsevier for this unique opportunity to further spread the vital message of the IWGDF throughout the world by the inclusion of their DVD with each book.

The editors and contributors hope that the information presented in this seventh edition will assist caregivers as well as patients and their families, working as a team, to drastically reduce the alarming rate of major lower-limb amputation associated with the diagnosis of diabetes mellitus.

JOHN H. BOWKER, MD
MICHAEL A. PFEIFER, MD, CDE, FACE

CONTENTS

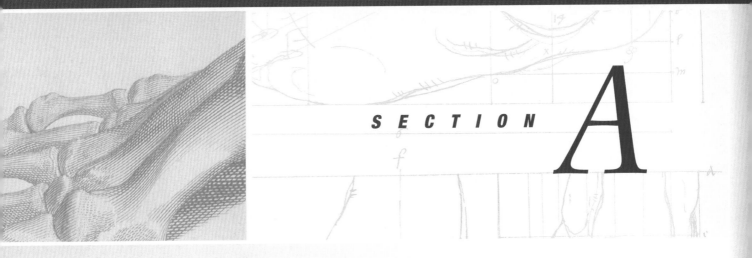

THE FOUNDATIONS OF DIABETIC FOOT MANAGEMENT

A

SECTION

THE FOUNDATIONS OF
DIABETIC FOOT
MANAGEMENT

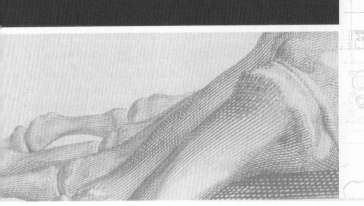

EPIDEMIOLOGY AND ECONOMIC IMPACT OF FOOT ULCERS AND AMPUTATIONS IN PEOPLE WITH DIABETES

GAYLE E. REIBER AND JOSEPH W. LEMASTER ∎

The global burden of diabetes is projected to increase from the current 246 million people to over 380 million people by the year 2025.[1] Many people with diabetes develop complications that seriously affect their quality and length of life. Lower-limb complications are common, particularly foot ulcers and amputations, and show striking global variation in annual incidence, prevalence, and economic impact. Development of these complications is attributed to individual risk factors, poverty, racial and ethnic differences, and quality of local and national health care systems. The wide variation noted suggests that "best practices" in the low-incidence areas could be adapted to higher-incidence areas to reduce the frequency and burden of ulcers and amputations. In this chapter, the incidence, prevalence, and risk factors for ulcers and amputations in people with diabetes are reviewed, using English-language population-based, analytic and experimental studies. The chapter concludes with a discussion of the economic impact of foot ulcers and amputations.

Historical Perspective

In the 1920s, Elliott Joslin and his colleagues in Boston began to investigate new medical and surgical strategies to save feet and legs from amputation due to complica-
tions of diabetes. In 1934, Joslin's paper, published in the *New England Journal of Medicine*, indicated that gangrene was not heaven-sent but earth-born. He described how a team approach to diabetes care could prevent or minimize limb loss. His message was not widely implemented.

In the 1970s, Kelly West, considered the father of diabetes epidemiology in the United States, identified gangrene as one of the most important and distressing manifestations of diabetes.[2] He indicated that it was not generally appreciated that among populations of people with diabetes, there were very great differences in susceptibility to this dreaded complication and suggested excellent opportunities for elucidation and prevention through epidemiologic approaches. Dr. West indicated little had been learned previously concerning the epidemiology of gangrene and other disorders secondary to diabetes-related peripheral vascular disease and described the status of data in this field is an epidemiologist's nightmare.[2] "Methods and standardization are poorly developed. Except in Scandinavia, few studies have been performed in representative samples of diabetics or nondiabetics. Controls have been few and suboptimal in character. The relationship between diabetes and peripheral vascular disease is so strong that little need has been perceived for investigation. To most Western clinicians this suggested an inevitability of association, and tended to stifle incentives to look for preventative measures."[2]

Today, advances are occurring in accurately documenting and understanding the epidemiology of lower-limb complications in people with diabetes. However, the reader will note that the prevention of lower-limb complications in global health care systems, as described by Joslin and West, remains somewhat elusive.

Epidemiologic Considerations: Definitions, Numerators, Denominators, and Search Strategies

In population-based studies using administrative databases, people with diabetes, ulcers, and amputations are often identified from registries or codes using the International Classification of Disease, Versions 9 and 10. While the codes for nontraumatic lower-limb amputation are straightforward, there is considerable misclassification in the coding for foot ulcers. Pressure ulcers, surgical wounds, puncture injuries, sequelae of vasculitis, and dermatologic conditions such as pyoderma gangrenosum are not foot ulcers but are among the conditions that are frequently misdiagnosed and coded as foot ulcers.

The definitions and ulcer classification systems used in studies reported in this chapter vary by study, thus basic criteria for inclusion follow:

Diabetes: One or more occurrences of ICD code(s) 250.xx in hospital or clinic settings.

Foot ulcer: A full-thickness wound below the ankle, irrespective of duration.[3]

Ulcer episode: The interval from ulcer identification to healing. Multiple ulcers occurring on the same day on the same foot (often the results of minor trauma) are defined as a single episode. Other ulcer episodes are numbered consecutively.

Nontraumatic lower-limb amputation: The removal of a terminal, nonviable portion of a limb.

Ulcer-free survival: A foot ulcer outcome measure that reflects effective foot ulcer management and allows across-sites comparison.[4]

Ulcer severity classification: There is no uniformly accepted foot ulcer classification system for patients with diabetes to quantify ulcer severity. Several foot ulcer classifications are used, including the Wagner system, which specifies ulcer depth, presence of osteomyelitis and/or gangrene on the following five-grade continuum: [5]

Grade 0   Preulcerative lesion
Grade 1   Partial-thickness wound up to but not through the dermis
Grade 2   Full-thickness wound extending to tendons or deeper subcutaneous tissue but without bony involvement or osteomyelitis
Grade 3   Full-thickness wound extending to and involving bone
Grade 4   Localized gangrene
Grade 5   Gangrene of the whole foot

University of Texas System classification additions to Wagner system:
Stage A   Clean wounds
Stage B   Nonischemic infected wounds
Stage C   Ischemic, noninfected wounds
Stage D   Ischemic, infected wounds[6]

The S(AD) SAD system from researchers in the Department of Diabetes and Endocrinology at the University of Nottingham, U.K., adds to the University of Texas system:
a) Cross-sectional ulcer area
b) Presence or absence of peripheral neuropathies[7]

Global awareness of lower-limb complications is leading to studies on the incidence (new onset) and prevalence (history) of diabetic foot ulcers and amputations in many countries. To identify these studies, a literature review was conducted by using the Ovid Information Service, which includes Medline, the Cumulative Index to Nursing and Allied Health Literature, the Cochrane Controlled Trials register, and Current Contents. We searched for articles published between January 1964 and April 2006 that used the following terms: *diabetes* or *diabetic, incidence, prevalence, foot ulcer, foot, feet,* and *amputation.* We also searched the bibliography of identified articles. The published studies that we reviewed include population-based cohort studies, large randomized controlled trials used to report foot ulcer incidence in the comparison group, and clinic-based studies. We excluded studies that reported only lower-limb ulceration (without specifying foot ulcers),[8,9] studies that did not specify a foot ulcer or amputation definition of any sort,[10–12] and studies that described a series of foot ulcers or amputation patients without clearly specifying a population base, since that would preclude accurately estimating incidence and prevalence.[13–16]

Several methodologic considerations influence the precision of incidence and prevalence computations. The numerator is those who develop a new ulcer or amputation during the interval according to a prior definition. The study population denominator is optimally based on a registry of people with diabetes living in a defined geographic area or enrolled in a large managed health care system. When the focus is specifically on foot ulcers and amputations, their occurrence is underestimated if more severe presentations (e.g., involving cellulitis or gangrene) are not counted as foot ulcers when the episode begins as a foot ulcer. In one survey of 1654 diabetes patients hospitalized with foot problems in the Congo, only 1.2% of the cases were classified as foot ulcers, while 70.4% were reported with local abscess or wet gangrene.[17]

Foot ulcer and amputation prevalence is underestimated if care is not taken to include patients with new onset diabetes as well as previously diagnosed diabetes, since a proportion of patients are diagnosed with diabetes at the time when they present to clinics with their foot ulcer or amputation. In the Congolese survey cited, Monabeka and colleagues found that diabetes was first diagnosed in 2.8% of patients admitted for diabetic foot problems,[17] while in the United Kingdom, 15% of patients admitted for amputation were first diagnosed with diabetes on admission to the hospital.[18] Those foot ulcer and amputation cases for whom diabetes is diagnosed at the time of foot ulcer detection are optimally included in the numerator and the denominator in calculating incidence or prevalence.

A number of Asian, African, and South American studies have been published that use foot ulcers or amputations as the numerator and hospitalized patients as the denominator. This may incorrectly estimate both the incidence and prevalence without data for the entire population of reference. A number of clinic-based studies have attempted to estimate the population prevalence (and in some cases the incidence) of diabetic foot ulcers and amputations for a geographic area.[12,17,19–32] Clinic-based studies make use of accessible patients. Some of these studies may be well-conducted and require substantial coordination across health care systems. For example, in France, a cross-sectional survey was conducted on one day in May 2001 involving all patients attending outpatient clinics or admitted by 16 hospital departments.[30] However, as a measure of foot ulcer incidence or prevalence in a defined geographic area of community-dwelling people with diabetes, this information may be biased because not all those with diabetes attend clinics, and those who do attend are more likely to have complications such as diabetic foot problems when they attend. Cross-sectional surveys of clinic attendees that select a random or consecutive sample of clinic attendees are more likely to sample patients with more severe disease, since these patients attend the clinic more often.

Reported foot ulcers (either by patients in surveys or by providers and clinics) should be corroborated by direct examination by investigators to avoid possible misclassification. Self-reports of amputation are relatively accurate. Routine administrative or clinical billing data are subject to reporting bias, because health professionals might fail to enter the correct diagnostic code or might assign codes to maximize reimbursement. Reimbursement and administrative systems are not well suited to tracking clinical information such as ulcer episodes, including those resulting in amputation. The method of subject ascertainment also influences data precision. For example, Kumar and colleagues used direct examination for foot ulcers and found a 5.3% diabetic foot ulcer prevalence, whereas the Behavioral Risk Factor Surveillance System used a self-report measure for foot ulcers and reported an 11.8% prevalence.[33,34]

Although randomized, controlled trial cohorts allow for careful ascertainment of foot ulcer and lower-limb amputation incidence, they might be unsuitable to estimate the population-based incidence in the region where the study was conducted. Even in controls or in studies in which the intervention was not successful, application of results from a highly skewed study population do not represent population-based findings. In one recent clinical trial sample that was used to estimate the incidence of foot ulcers, participants' inclusion criteria were age 18 to 70 years; being a man or a nonpregnant woman; a vibration perception threshold (VPT) of > 25 volts or more on at least one foot; and no prior foot ulceration or lower-limb amputation, nondiabetic causes of neuropathy, history of alcohol abuse, previous treatment with radiotherapy or cytotoxic agents, uncontrolled hypertension, or any renal disease.[35] These criteria make it impossible to generalize results from such a study to estimate foot ulcer incidence in the general population of people with diabetes.

Epidemiology of Foot Ulcers in People with Diabetes

The annual population-based incidence of foot ulcers in people with type 1 or 2 diabetes shown in Table 1-1 is from 1.9% to 2.2%.[10,22,33–40] Reported foot ulcer prevalence ranges from a low of 1.8% in South Asians living in a defined geographic area in the United Kingdom to 11.8% based on self-report from a stratified sample of U.S. residents with telephones.[33,34] The lifetime risk for foot ulcers in people with diabetes is estimated to be 15%.[41]

Foot Ulcer Location, Outcomes, and Time to Outcome

The anatomic site of foot ulcers has both etiologic and treatment implications and varies according to the population from which the patients are drawn. Table 1-2 presents data from three prospective studies that reported foot ulcer site. The most common sites were the toes (dorsal or plantar surface), followed by the plantar metatarsal heads and the heel.[42,43] Ulcer severity may be more important than ulcer site in determining the final ulcer outcome.[42] Although foot ulcers reepithelialized in the majority of patients in these three studies, amputations occurred in 14% to 24% of the patients. In the research by Oyibo and colleagues, 8% of ulcers were unhealed at the conclusion of 6 to 18 months follow-up.[44] A small percentage of patients in each study died. Only one death in one study was related to foot ulcer (septicemia).[45] Other deaths were attributed to age and other comorbidity.[43–45]

Studies show that time to ulcer outcome is influenced by several factors. A number of studies report delayed ulcer healing, despite similar care, ulcer surface area, and ulcer duration prior to the start of treatment.[11,44,46–48] In a study in which 194 ulcers were examined weekly for 6 to 18 months, Oyibo and colleagues found that ulcer surface area differed strongly and significantly between ulcers that healed, did not heal, or proceeded to amputation (larger ulcers having worse outcomes and taking longer to heal). Patient gender, age, diabetes duration, and ulcer site did not affect time to healing. Neuroischemic ulcers took longer to heal (20 weeks versus 9 weeks) and were three times more likely to lead to amputation.[44] Margolis and colleagues found, after pooling data from the control arms of five related randomized studies investigating new ulcer-healing therapies, that neuropathic wounds were more likely to heal within 20 weeks if they were smaller (<2 cm^2), if they had existed for a shorter period before they were treated (<6 months), or if the patients were of nonwhite ethnicity.[11] Gender, age, and glycosylated hemoglobin (HbAIC) level had no impact on healing in their multivariable regression model. In an analysis that utilized medical records from 150 wound care facilities in 38 U.S. states, these investigators

TABLE 1-1 Selected Population-based Studies Estimating Incidence and Prevalence of Diabetic Foot Ulcers

Study (Country)	Population Base	N	Annual Incidence (%)	Prevalence (%)	Ulcer Definition	Method of Ulcer Ascertainment
Abbott et al.[49] (United Kingdom)	Registered type 1 and type 2 diabetes patients in six U.K. districts	15,692	—	5.5% White European 1.8% South Asian 2.7% African Caribbean	Wagner grade ≥ 1 foot lesion	Clinical examination (plus chart review)
Centers for Disease Control and Prevention[34] (United States)	U.S. BRFSS* respondents with diabetes, 2000–2002	NS	—	11.8%	Foot sore that did not heal for > 4 weeks	Random-digit-dialed telephone interview
Kumar et al.[33] (United Kingdom)	Type 2 diabetes patients registered in three U.K. cities	811	—	5.3%	Wagner grade ≥ 1 foot lesion	Direct exam by trained observers (current), and structured interview (history of ulcer)
Moss et al.[10] (United States)	Population-based sample of persons with diabetes	1834	2.2%	10.6%	N/A	Medical history questionnaire administered at baseline and 4 years later
Muller et al.[40] (Netherlands)	Registered type 2 diabetes patients (1993–1998)	3827 person-years	2.1%	—	Full-thickness skin loss on the foot	Abstracted medical records
Ramsey et al.[38] (United States)	Registered adult type 1 or 2 diabetes patients in a large HMO (1992–1995)	8905	1.9%	—	ICD codes: 707.1 (ulcer of lower leg)	Medical billing record audit and clinical exam
Walters et al.[37] (United Kingdom)	Registered patients with diabetes from ten U.K. general practices	1077	—	7.4%	Wagner grade ≥ 1 foot lesion	Direct examination and structured interview

* BRFSS, Behavioral Risk Factor Surveillance Survey; N/A, not applicable.

TABLE 1-2 Anatomic Location of Diabetic Foot Ulcers in Three Prospective Studies

	All Ulcers[a] (%) (N = 314)	Most Severe Ulcer[b] (N = 302)	All Ulcers Followed 6–18 Months[c] (N = 194)
Ulcer Site			
Toes (dorsal and plantar surface)	51	52	
Plantar metatarsal heads, midfoot, and heel	28	37	
Dorsum of foot	14	11	
Multiple ulcers	7	NA	
Forefoot			78
Midfoot			12
Hindfoot			10
Total	100	100	
Ulcer Outcome			
Unhealed			16
Reepithelialization/primary healing	63	81	65
Amputation at any level	24	14	15
Death	13*	5	3.5
Total	100	100	100

[a] Apelqvist et al.[42] included consecutive patients whose lesions were characterized according to Wagner criteria from superficial nonnecrotic to major gangrene.

[b] Reiber et al.[43] patients were enrolled with a lesion through the dermis extending to deeper tissue.

[c] Oyibo et al.[45] patients scored ≥ Grade 1 in the S(AD) SAD foot classification system.

*Includes eight amputees who had not yet met the 6-month healing criterion.

confirmed that among 72,525 diabetic foot wounds in 31,106 patients, wounds that were older, larger, and deeper in grade (especially Wagner grade ≥3) were more likely to take more than 20 weeks to heal, after adjustment for gender and age.[46] Pecoraro and colleagues described the importance of a 4-week reduction in ulcer volume and reported that low levels of periwound $TcPO_2$ and CO_2 were significantly associated with initial rate of healing, while an average periwound $TcPO_2$ lower than 20 mm Hg was associated with a 39-fold increased risk of early healing failure.[48] Later Sheehan and colleagues reported that among 276 patients with Wagner grade 1 or greater diabetic foot ulcers of 30 days' duration, a decrease in ulcer area within 4 weeks of treatment onset strongly predicted complete wound healing by 12 weeks.[47] Patients in each of the above studies received similar ulcer care, including off-loading, wound debridement, and moist wound healing.[11,45–48]

Risk Factors for Foot Ulcers in People with Diabetes

Studies that met our search criteria identified categories of independent risk factors for diabetic foot ulcers, including demographic, foot findings, health findings and history, and health care and education.

Demographic Variables

Demographic variables were identified from the nationwide Behavioral Risk Factor Surveillance System (BRFSS) 2000–2002 for people with diabetes and foot ulcers.[34] In this population-based study of noninstitutionalized adults over age 18 years, the self-reported foot ulcer prevalence was highest (13.7%) in people ages 18 to 44 years, followed by 13.4% for ages 45 to 64, 9.6% for ages 65 to 74, and 9% for those over age 75. The prevalence of foot ulcers was similar in men and in women (11.8% versus 11.9%) and increased with duration of diabetes, from 9% in those with a duration less than 6 years to 19% in those with a duration over 21 years.

Using BRFSS data from 2001, relative odds of foot ulcer were compared across ethnic groups using Asians as the reference group. Compared to Asians (1.0), the odds and 95% confidence levels for foot ulcer were 1.5 (CI: 0.6 to 3.6) in African Americans, 2.8 (CI: 1.2 to 6.9) in Hispanic individuals, 4.2 (CI: 1.4 to 12.8) in Native Americans, 7.4 (CI: 1.3 to 41.2) in Pacific Islanders, and 1.8 (CI: 0.8 to 4.2) in Whites.[49] Abbott and colleagues identified ethnic differences in age-standardized foot ulcer prevalence rates were also reported comparing Europeans (5.5%), South Asians (1.9%), and African Caribbeans (2.7%) with diabetes and foot ulcers residing in the Manchester, U.K., area. Asian men and women had similarly low foot ulcer rates; fewer were treated with insulin; and significantly fewer Asians had ever smoked.[50]

Foot Risk Factors

Foot risk factors include peripheral neuropathy, peripheral arterial disease, and foot deformities. Several semiquantitative and quantitative measures of peripheral neuropathy or neurologic summary scores were used to describe associations between peripheral neuropathy and foot ulcers (Table 1-3). In a randomized clinical trial using a VPT of 25 or greater as an entry criterion, Abbott and colleagues determined that both baseline VPT and a combined score of reflexes and muscle strength were significant predictors of incident ulcers.[35] In a later cohort study of 6619 people with diabetes, Abbott and colleagues reported similar neuropathy findings.[39] Boyko

and colleagues identified increased relative risk of ulcer 2.03 (CI: 1.50 to 2.76) in patients who were unable to detect the 5.07 (10-g) Semmes-Weinstein monofilament, a semiquantitative measure of light touch.[22,51] Carrington and colleagues' study reported that even after controlling for sensory neuropathy, peroneal motor nerve conduction velocity was strongly associated with foot ulcer risk.[27] In Kastenbauer and colleagues' cohort study, patients with type 2 diabetes were followed for 3 years on average. The authors report that elevated VPT greater than 24 volts significantly predicted foot ulcers.[25] The only study from Table 1-3 that did not report a significant association between peripheral neuropathy and foot ulcer was the study by Moss and colleagues, which did not include any physical lower-limb measures.[10] In summary, aberrations in various sensory modalities and the presence of motor neuropathy independently predict increased foot ulcer risk in people with diabetes.

Abbott and colleagues measured peripheral arterial function by using absent pulses (dorsalis pedis and/or posterior tibial arteries) and ankle-arm index (AAI). In their study, "peripheral vascular status was assessed by palpation of the dorsalis pedis and posterior tibial pulses on both feet. Presence of two or less of the four pedal pulses, either with or without the presence of oedema, indicated PVD."[39] Kumar and colleagues defined peripheral arterial involvement as the absence of two or more foot pulses or a history of prior peripheral arterial revascularization and found a significant association between these variables and foot ulcers.[33] Walters and colleagues reported that an absent pedal pulse was associated with a 6.3-fold increased risk of foot ulcers.[37] In the most recent study published by Boyko and colleagues, peripheral pulses and AAI were not reported in the analysis.[51]

Peripheral neuropathies and peripheral arterial disease commonly coexist in patients with diabetes and foot ulcers. Kumar and colleagues reported that among the foot ulcer patients studied, both neuropathy and peripheral arterial disease were present in 30%, neuropathy alone in 46%, ischemia alone in 12%, and neither risk factor in 12%.[33] Findings from Walters and colleagues in the United Kingdom and from Nyamu and colleagues in a clinic-based study in Kenya report that the greatest proportion of ulcers are neuropathic in origin, followed by neuroischemic and then ischemic alone.[37,28] These two studies reported that about half the foot ulcers they studied included an ischemic component. Using the Wagner Classification System, Morbach reported variation in the frequency of peripheral arterial disease and foot ulcers across countries. Arterial disease was present in 48% of foot ulcers in Germany but only 11% in Tanzania and 10% in India.[52]

Foot deformity was reported as significantly associated with foot ulcer in only one selected study.[39] In Abbott and colleagues' cohort study, a six-point composite measure of foot deformity was developed by dichotomizing the following variables: small muscle wasting, hammertoes or

TABLE 1-3   Risk Factors for Foot Ulcers in Patients with Diabetes Mellitus from Final Analysis Models of Select Studies

Author, Type of Analysis	Study Design, Diabetes Type	Foot Findings: Neuropathy (Monofilament, Reflex, Vibration, or Neurologic Summary Score)	Low AAI or Absent Pulses	Deformity	Health and Health History Findings: Long Duration	High HbA1C	Smoking	Ulcer	LEA
Abbott et al.[35], Cox regression analysis	RCT, patients with VPT ≥ 25 (U.S., U.K., Canada) type 1 = 255 type 2 = 780	0 Monofilament + VPT + Reflex		Exclusion criteria	0		Exclusion criteria	Exclusion criteria	
Abbott et al., Cox regression analysis[39]	Cohort, U.K. registered DM patients from 6 Health Districts, type 1, 2 = 6613	0 VPT + Monofilament + NDS + Reflex	+	+	0		0	+	
Boyko et al.[51], Cox proportional hazards	Cohort, 1285 veterans	+	Data not included	0	0	+	0	+	+
Carrington et al.[27], Cox regression	Cohort, single U.K. clinic; type 1 = 83, type 2 = 86, no DM = 22	+ Motor neuropathy 0 VPT 0 Pressure 0 Thermal	Exclusion criteria		0	0		0	Exclusion criteria
Kastenbauer et al.[25]	Cohort, type 2 N = 187	0 Monofilament + VPT	Exclusion criteria	0	0	0	0	Exclusion criteria	Exclusion criteria
Kumar et al.[33] Logistic regression	Cross-sectional 811 type 2 from U.K. general practices	+ NDS	+		+		0	0	+
Litzelman et al.[53], GEE	RCT, type 2 patients, 352	+ Monofilament		0	0	0		+	Exclusion criteria
Moss et al.[10], Logistic regression	Cohort, 2990 patients with early- and late-onset diabetes				+	+	Young		
Rith-Najarian et al.[36], Chi square analysis	Cohort 358 type 2 Chippewa Indians	+ Monofilament		0	+				
Walters et al.[37], Logistic regression	Cohort, 10 U.K. general practices 1077 type 1, 2	+ Absent light touch + Impaired pain perception 0 VPT	+ Absent pulses 0 Doppler		+	0			

AAI, ankle-arm index; DM, diabetes; HbA1C, hemoglobin A1C; LEA, lower-limb amputation; NDS, neuropathy disability score; RCT, randomized controlled trial; $TcPo_2$, transcutaneous oxygen tension; VPT, vibration perception threshold.
Blank cell, not studied; +, statistically significant finding; 0, no statistically significant finding.

clawed toes, bony prominences, prominent metatarsal heads, Charcot arthropathy, and limited joint mobility.[39] No other study combined diverse foot characteristics to create a composite measure of deformity, and the studies reporting on single foot deformities found no statistically significant associations.[25,36,51,53]

Health Findings and History Factors

Health and history factors include long duration of diagnosed diabetes, high HbA1C, smoking, prior ulcer, and prior amputation. A connection between diabetes duration and development of foot ulcer was a significant finding in four studies.[10,33,36,37] A number of recent studies have not identified this association, perhaps in part because of the improved ability to control for confounding variables in the analysis.[25,27,35,39,51,53]

Elevated levels of HbA1C were significantly associated with development of foot ulcers in studies by Moss and colleagues[10] and Boyko and colleagues.[51] Moss and colleagues reported an odds ratio of 1.6 (CI: 1.3 to 2.0) for every 2% deterioration in HbA1C.[10] Boyko and colleagues reported an odds ratio of 1.10 (CI: 1.06 to 1.15) for every 1% increase in HbA1C level.[51] No significant associations were reported in other studies that measured this variable.[25,27,53]

Smoking was significantly associated with foot ulcer only in the cohort study by Moss and colleagues,[10] while five studies found no statistically significant association.[25,33,39,51,54] The distal proximity of the smoking exposure to foot ulcer development might partially account for this finding.

The risk associated with a prior history of foot ulcers and amputations was assessed in five studies. Studies by Abbott and colleagues,[39] Boyko and colleagues,[51] and Litzelman and colleagues[53] all reported a significant association between prior and future foot ulcers. Boyko and colleagues' study reported the odds for subsequent ulcers given a prior amputation at 2.57 (CI: 1.60 to 4.12),[51] and Kumar and colleagues reported an odds ratio of 12.7 for subsequent amputation.[33] Other independent risk factors for foot ulcer reported in the study by Boyko and colleagues include onychomycosis and history of impaired vision.[51]

Health Care and Education Variables

Health care and education variables have been reported as risk factors for foot ulcers. Litzelman and colleagues conducted a U.S. randomized trial in patients served by a county hospital.[53] Patients were randomized to education, behavioral contracts, and reminders, while their providers received special education and chart prompts. The study controls received usual care and education. After 1 year, patients in the intervention group developed fewer serious foot lesions, including ulcers, than did those in the control group; they were also more likely to report appropriate foot self-care behaviors, including inspection of feet and shoes, washing of feet, and drying between toes.[53] There was no significant difference between groups in testing bathwater temperature and reporting foot problems.[53] In a community-based cohort, Abbott showed that prior attendance at podiatry clinic conveyed an elevated risk of 2.19 (CI: 1.5 to 3.2).[39] This variable is a likely intermediary in the pathway to foot ulcer and a proxy for other conditions that would increase the likelihood of these patients being served by podiatrists.

Foot Ulcer Recurrence

Foot ulcer recurrence was addressed in several studies. In a study by Mantey and colleagues, diabetic patients with an initial foot ulcer and two ulcer recurrences were compared with diabetic patients who had only one ulcer and no recurrences over a 2-year interval.[55] The authors reported greater peripheral sensory neuropathy and poorer diabetes control in the ulcer recurrence group. Members of the ulcer recurrence group also had higher HbA1C levels, waited longer after observing a serious

foot problem to seek care, and consumed more alcohol than did the group without ulcer recurrences. Connor and Mahdi reported on findings from 83 patients who were followed from 2 to 10 years after their initial foot ulcer. Their rate of ulcer recurrence was 37% (3.5 or more ulcers per foot per 10 years).[56] Problems with reulceration were attributed to patients with neuroarthopathy, who were more likely to wear unsafe footwear and have problems with footwear or orthoses, and those without neuroarthropathy who attended clinic irregularly. Glycemic control was poorer in patients in both groups compared to patients without ulcer recurrence.[56] Muller and colleagues performed a study in primary care patients in the Netherlands and reported that 25% of type 2 patients who developed foot ulcers had two or more subsequent ulcer recurrences during the 6-year study interval.[40]

Epidemiology of Lower-Limb Amputation

Incidence, Prevalence, and Amputation Level

Amputation rates differ widely across geographic regions within countries as well as between countries. Figure 1-1 illustrates this point showing U.S. Medicare data from Wrobel and colleagues. There is an 8.6-fold difference in age-adjusted nontraumatic major amputation incidence rates across the 306 geographically defined U.S. Hospital Referral Regions.[57]

The Global Lower Extremity Amputation Study Group reported rates for incident (first ever) and all amputations occurring in 10 study centers over a 2-year interval. Sources of numerator data were from hospital discharges, operating room records, rehabilitation and limb-fitting centers, and prescribing physicians. The denominator reflected total population, not just individuals with diabetes. The authors reported that the lowest 2-year population-based amputation incidence rate was in Madrid, Spain (2.8 per 100,000 person-years total population), while the highest rate was in the Navajo population (43.9 per 100,000 person-years total population).[58]

Figure 1-2 shows the reduction in U.S. hospital discharge rates for people with diabetes and nontraumatic amputations in U.S. short-stay nonfederal hospitals. This decline is mirrored by a decrease in the numbers of hospitalizations for diabetic nontraumatic amputations from a high of 84,000 in 1997 to 75,000 in 2003.

Annual amputation incidence rates for many populations with diabetes are shown in Table 1-4. Rates range from 0.7 per 1000 in East Asian populations to 31.0 per 1000 in U.S. Pima Indians.[54,59–66] This variation is provocative and suggests that "best practices" in the low-incidence areas could be examined and considered for implementation in high-incidence areas.

Frequency of amputation differs between people with and without diabetes. Population-based amputation

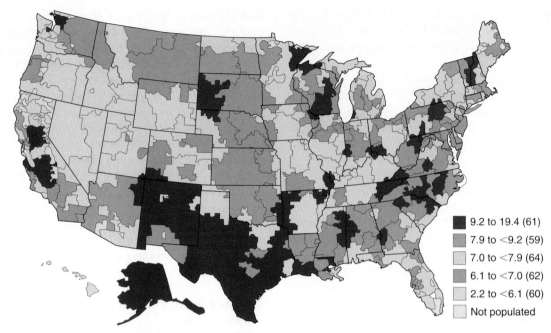

Figure 1–1 Major amputation rates per 1000 diabetic Medicare enrollees (1996–1997). *(Redrawn from Wrobel JS, Mayfield JA, Reiber GE: Geographic variations of lower extremity major amputation in individuals with and without diabetes in the Medicare population. Diabetes Care 24: 860–864, 2001.)*

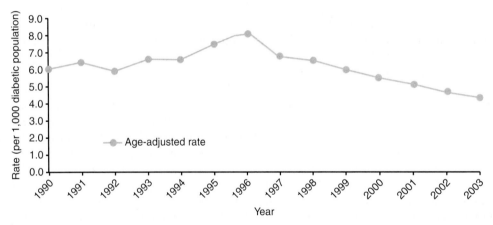

Figure 1–2 U.S. age-adjusted hospital discharge rates for nontraumatic lower-limb amputation per 1000 diabetic population, United States, 1990–2003. *(Redrawn from U.S. Centers for Disease Control and Prevention.)*

prevalence data are available from the U.S. National Health Interview Survey for people with and without diabetes. Individuals with diabetes had a tenfold higher overall amputation prevalence than did people without diabetes: 2.8% versus 0.29%.[67]

When amputation data were analyzed by site, more distal amputations were performed in people with diabetes than in people without diabetes (data not shown). Figure 1-3 presents 2002 U.S. nontraumatic amputation levels for people with diabetes from the U.S. Hospital Discharge Survey using 3-year averages to improve the precision of annual estimates. Excluded are minor amputations occurring in podiatry offices and short-stay surgery facilities and those from federal facilities. Hospital discharge rates for amputations increased with advancing age across all amputation levels, the transtibial

(below knee) and transfemoral (above knee) rates showing the greatest increases.

An important trend is the decline in amputation rates in developed countries that have relatively homogeneous racial and ethnic populations. Holstein and colleagues report a decreased amputation rate based on 15 years of clinical records from Bispebjerg Hospital, Copenhagen, from 27.2 to 6.9 per 100,000 total population.[68] Van Houtum and colleagues, reporting on data from the Dutch National Medical Register, identified a decrease in amputations between 1991 and 2002 from 55.0 to 36.3 per 10,000 patients with diabetes.[69] Trautner and colleagues examined amputation rates from three hospitals in the German city of Leverkusen from 1990 to 1998 and reported data on the 76% of amputees with diabetes and the 24% without diabetes. In this population, there was

TABLE 1-4 Age-Adjusted Population-Based Amputation Incidence Rates* among Patients with Diabetes from Select Studies

Author	Population Studied	Annual Incidence Rate//1000
Chaturvedi et al.[75]	*Type 1 Diabetes:*	
	American Indian (Pima, Oklahoma Indians)	31.0
	Cuban	8.2
	European	3.5
	East Asian	1.0
	Type 2 Diabetes:	
	American Indian (Pima, Oklahoma Indians)	9.7
	Cuban	2.0
	European	2.5
	East Asian	0.7
Humphrey et al.[59]	Nauru	7.6
Humphrey et al.[60]	Rochester, MN, United States	3.8
Letho et al.[61]	East and West Finland	8.0
Morris et al.[62]	Tayside, Scotland	2.5
Moss et al.[54]	Wisconsin, United States	
	Younger onset diabetes	5.1
	Older onset diabetes	7.1
Muller et al.[40]	Type 2, primary care, the Netherlands	6.0
Nelson et al.[63]	Pima Indians, United States	13.7
Siitonen et al.[64]	Incident LEA	3.4 men
	East Finland	2.4 women
Trautner et al.[65]	Leverkusen, Germany	2.1
Van Houtum and Lavery[66]	California, United States	4.9
	The Netherlands	3.6

* Rates are for any amputation, unless incident amputation is specified.

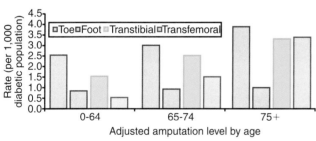

Figure 1–3 Hospital discharge rate for nontraumatic lower-limb amputation per 1000 diabetic population, by level of amputation and age, United States, 2002. *(Redrawn from U.S. Centers for Disease Control and Prevention.)*

a modest decrease in amputation rates among people with diabetes, from 5.49 to 4.66 per 1000, but no difference in people without diabetes.[70] Eskelinen and colleagues reported a decrease in amputations in Helsinki, Finland, from 1990 to 2002. While the reduction was 23% in people with diabetes (0.95 to 0.73 per 1000), it was 40% in people without diabetes (0.89 to 0.53 per 1000).[71] Many of these studies report that foot care interventions were initiated between the first and final

measures of amputation rates. In addition to provision of improved foot care, other explanations for the decrease in amputation rates include greater use of peripheral vascular bypass procedures, percutaneous transluminal angioplasty, reductions in risk factors associated with vascular disease and peripheral neuropathy, and, in the United States, a change in the methodology used to compute amputation rates, which greatly expanded the denominator.[72,73]

Risk Factors for Nontraumatic Lower-Limb Amputations in People with Diabetes

A population-based analysis of diabetic individuals with nontraumatic amputations from the U.S. Hospital Discharge Survey demonstrates three well-known demographic risk factors: age, gender, and nonwhite racial status. Amputation risk increases with advancing age are displayed in Figure 1-4. The 2003 amputation rates for those age 75+ are nearly twofold higher than the rates for people younger than age 64. Figure 1-5 shows age-adjusted amputation rates by gender, with hospital discharge rates consistently higher in males than in females. Figure 1-6 shows that black individuals experienced higher hospital amputation discharge rates than did the combined group of white and Hispanic Americans. The importance of access to care, quality of care, and socioeconomic status needs to be considered in assessing racial and ethnic differences and rates for amputations in people with diabetes. Many authors have described widely varying amputation rates by ethnic and racial category.[21,74–78] The central nonbiologic risk factor for amputation identified by Wachtel and colleagues was family poverty. In this study, amputation rates in age 50+ African Americans, Hispanic Americans, and others were attributed to family poverty.[79] In contrast, in a setting in which 3 million members were enrolled in a prepaid managed care organization (Kaiser Permanente Medical Care Program), amputation risk was not significantly different by ethnic and racial group. Similarly, in a case-controlled study among veterans having equal access to care, after controlling for socioeconomic factors, there were no differences in amputation rates among black, white, and Latino subjects.[80–82]

Foot Findings

An array of measures was used to quantify peripheral neuropathy associated with amputation risk. These included insensitivity to the 10-g Semmes-Weinstein monofilament, motor nerve conduction velocity of the deep peroneal nerve, sensory nerve conduction velocity of the sural nerve, VPT, absent or diminished bilateral vibration sensation, and absent Achilles tendon and patellar reflexes. Table 1-5 shows the eight studies that reported a statistically significant association between one or more measures of peripheral neuropathy and

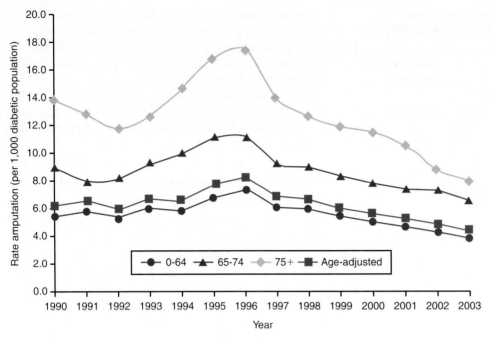

Figure 1–4 Hospital discharge rates for nontraumatic lower-limb amputation per 1000 diabetic population, by age, United States, 1990–2003. *(Redrawn from U.S. Centers for Disease Control and Prevention.)*

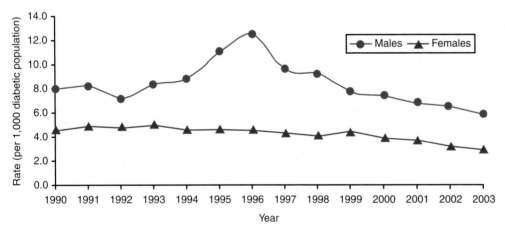

Figure 1–5 Age-adjusted hospital discharge rates for nontraumatic lower-limb amputation per 1000 diabetic population, by sex, United States, 1990–2003. *(Redrawn from U.S. Centers for Disease Control and Prevention.)*

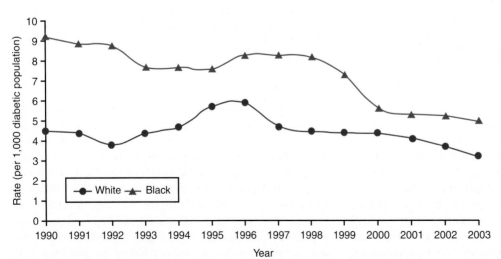

Figure 1–6 Age-adjusted hospital discharge rates for nontraumatic lower-limb amputation per 1000 diabetic population, by race, United States, 1990–2003. *(Redrawn from U.S. Centers for Disease Control and Prevention.)*

TABLE 1-5   Risk Factors for Nontraumatic Lower-Limb Amputation in Patients with Diabetes Mellitus from Final Analysis Models of Select Studies

Author, Type of Analysis	Study Design, Diabetes Type	Foot Findings			Health and Health History Findings				
		Neuropathy (Monofilament, Vibration, Reflex, NCV)	PAD AAI, MAC, TcPO$_2$, Pulses	HBP	Duration	High HbA1C FPG	Smoking	Ulcer	Retinopathy
Adler et al.[83], Multivariate proportional hazards	Cohort, 776 type 1 and 2 veterans	+	+		0	0	0	+	
Hamalainen et al.[84], Logistic regression	Nested, case control, 100, Finland	+	+	0	+	0			+
Hennis et al.[88], Logistic regression	Case control, 309, Barbados	+	+	0	0	+	0	0	
Lee et al.[87], Cox regression	Cohort, 875 type 2 Oklahoma Indians			+SBP ♂ +DBP ♀	+	+ ♂	0	0	+
Lehto et al.[61], Cox regression	Cohort, 1044 type 2, Finland	+	+	0	+	+	0		+
Mayfield et al.[86], Logistic regression	Retrospective case-control, 246 type 2 Pima Indians	+	+	0	+	+	0	+	+
Moss et al.[54], Logistic regression	Cohort, 2990 early and late onset, S. WI			+DBP	+	+	+Younger	+	+
Nelson et al.[63], Stratified	Cohort, 4399 Pima Indians, AZ, United States	+	+	0	+	+	0		+
Reiber et al.[80], Logistic regression	Prospective case-control, 316 type 1, 2 veterans	+	+	0	Control variable	+	0		+
Resnick et al.[131], Logistic regression	Cohort		+ ABI > 1.4	OK = + Pima = 0	+	+	0		
Selby and Zhang[81], Logistic regression	Nested retrospective case-control, 428 type 1, 2, HMO	+		+SBP	+	+	0		+

AAI, ankle-arm index; DBP, diastolic blood pressure; FPG, fasting plasma glucose; HbA1C, hemoglobin A1C; HBP, high blood pressure; MAC, medial arterial calcification; NCV, nerve conduction velocity; Pt Ed, patient outpatient education; PVD, peripheral vascular disease; SBP, systolic blood pressure; TcPO$_2$, transcutaneous oxygen tension. Blank cell, not studied; +, statistically significant finding; 0, no statistically significant finding.

amputation.[61,63,80,81,83–86,88] In the three studies that did not report this association, peripheral neuropathy was not measured directly.[87,54,131]

Hamalainen and colleagues measured nerve conduction velocities and VPT in addition to grading neuropathic symptoms and signs. In their final logistic regression model, they report the odds ratio for VPT and risk of amputation as 14.5 (CI: 3.6 to 57.8).[84] In the study by Hennis and colleagues, in the multivariate model, there was a significant association between VPT and minor amputation; however, the association between VPT and major amputation did not achieve statistical significance.[88] In the cohort study by Lehto and colleagues, two measures of peripheral neuropathy were significantly

associated with amputation: bilateral absence of Achilles tendon reflexes, with a relative risk of 4.3 (CI: 2.5 to 7.3), and bilateral absence of vibration sense, with a relative risk of 2.7 (CI: 1.6 to 4.7).[61]

The importance of peripheral arterial function, as measured by low TcPO$_2$, low AAI, and absent or diminished dorsalis pedis and posterior tibialis pulses as well as medial arterial calcification and its relationship to amputation, was directly assessed in eight studies and found to independently predict amputation in each.[61,63,80,83,84,86,88,131] Studies using AAI established cut points on both ends of the spectrum. The cut points for low AAI were 0.8 and 0.9, and the cut points indicating incompressible vessels were AAI greater than 1.3 and 1.4.[83,84,131]

In the cohort study by Adler and colleagues, three models were presented using three different measures of peripheral arterial disease: AAI, TcPO$_2$, and pulses. In each analysis, the relative risk was approximately 3.0, and the 95% confidence intervals were tight and excluded 1.[83] Lehto's cohort study, using the Cox regression model, identified the absence of two or more peripheral artery pulses, femoral artery bruit, and bilateral absence of Achilles tendon reflexes as significantly associated with amputation.[61]

In the cohort study by Nelson and colleagues, the presence of medial arterial calcification was based on radiographic examination of the feet obtained during biennial examinations. Medial arterial calcification was a significant risk factor for amputation, with a relative risk of 4.9 (CI: 2.9 to 8.1).[63] Reiber and colleagues measured both TcPO$_2$ and AAI and identified both as significantly associated with amputation in a prospective case-control study of veterans.[80] Clinicians are increasingly able to distinguish the importance and adequacy of cutaneous circulation, measured by using TcPO$_2$, and major arterial circulation. Both parameters are important in preventing and healing amputations. Cutaneous perfusion not only depends on the underlying arterial circulation, but also may be critically influenced by other factors, including skin integrity, mechanical effects of repetitive pressure, and tissue edema.

Palumbo reported that major symptoms of lower-limb arterial disease include intermittent claudication, absent peripheral pulses, and rest pain. In a defined population, the incidence of lower-limb arterial disease was 8% at diabetes diagnosis, 15% at 10 years, and 45% at 29 years.[41] Intermittent claudication, a fairly benign condition, progressed to rest pain or gangrene in only 1.6% and 1.8% of men and women, respectively, over 10 years.[89] In the Framingham Study, intermittent claudication was 3.8 and 6.5 times more common in diabetic than nondiabetic males and females, respectively.[90]

Health and Health History Findings

High blood pressure was an independent predictor of amputation in four analytic studies.[54,81,87,132] Two of these studies included no direct measure of peripheral arterial function.[54,87] Six other analytic studies assessed this measure and reported no statistically significant association between blood pressure and amputation in the final model.[61,63,80,84,86,88] Lee and colleagues reported that elevated systolic blood pressure was a significant risk factor only for men, while elevated diastolic blood pressure was a significant predictor only for women.[87]

Long duration of diagnosed diabetes was found to be significantly associated with lower-limb amputation in eight studies.[54,61,63,81,84,86–88,131] In the study by Hennis and colleagues, however, although the average duration of diabetes was 18 years in their cases and 12 years in the controls, duration was not a predictor of amputation in the final multivariate model.[88]

Poor glycemic control as measured by elevated HbA1C or plasma glucose was associated with an increased risk of amputation in nine analytic studies presented in Table 1-5.[54,61,63,80,81,86–88,131] Lehto and colleagues modeled high plasma glucose (>13.4 mmol/L), controlling for different groups of demographic and health variables. In each of three models, the relative risk was between 2.2 and 2.5, and the tight confidence intervals excluded 1.[61] In the two studies not reporting HbA1C associations with amputation, Hamalainen and colleagues used blood glucose findings,[84] while Adler used a categorical variable glycated hemoglobin.[83] The initial Diabetes Control and Complications Trial randomized patients with type 1 diabetes to either the intensive blood glucose control group or a conventional control group. The intensively treated group achieved nearly normal blood glucose levels compared to the control group, whose blood glucose values remained in the conventional range. The intensively treated group had a 69% reduction in subclinical neuropathy, a 57% reduction in clinical neuropathy, and fewer peripheral vascular events than the control group. In the striking 16-year follow-up to this study, the Epidemiology of Diabetes Interventions and Complications, the authors report the metabolic memory associated with prior intensive and conventional control and establish the role of intensive therapy and chronic glycemia with regard to atherosclerosis.[91]

Major alterable risk factors for development of atherosclerosis in nondiabetic people are cigarette smoking, lipoprotein abnormalities, and high blood pressure. These factors are assumed to be similarly atherogenic in diabetic individuals. Smoking was a risk factor, however, in only one study among people with younger onset diabetes.[54] There are several possible explanations. Smoking was reported as an infrequent exposure by several authors. Other measures of peripheral arterial disease, more proximal in time to the amputation, such as TcPO$_2$, AAI, or peripheral pulses, might better capture this domain in a multivariate analysis. An interesting association reported by Moss and colleagues was the protective effect of aspirin on lower-limb arteries in younger onset patients. This trend was not significant in older onset patients.[54] Aspirin has long been used as a preventive agent for cardiovascular disease.

History of a prior foot ulcer was an independent predictor in three studies.[54,83,86] Foot ulcers preceded approximately 85% of nontraumatic lower-limb amputations in two clinical epidemiology studies.[92,93] In studies by Boulton[94] in the United Kingdom and Reiber and colleagues[43] in the United States, 45% to 60% of patients with new-onset ulcers reported a prior history of foot ulcer.

History of retinopathy was assessed in eight studies shown in Table 1-5. There was a statistically significant association between retinopathy and lower-limb amputation in each study.[54,61,63,80,81,84,86,87] Moss and colleagues report in their logistic regression model that each step increase in retinopathy was associated with an odds ratio of 1.15 (CI: 1.07 to 1.23).[54] Retinopathy might reflect the extent of microvascular disease and might also be a proxy for diabetes severity.

Health Care and Education

Health care system modifications, patient self-management education, and subsequent self-care behaviors were linked to a decreased amputation risk in several studies. Rith-Najarian and colleagues' prospective intervention in a U.S. population of Native Americans showed substantially lowered rates of amputation with changes in health care delivery system.[95,96] Following a needs assessment of diabetic residents in a reservation community in Minnesota, amputation was identified as the most common diabetes complication. Subsequently, a registry was established to follow 639 diabetic individuals through four phases spanning 14 years.[95,96] During the first 4 years (1986 to 1989), no change was made to the organization of care, and the observed amputation rate was 29 per 1000 person-years. During the second 4-year period (1990 to 1993), the delivery system was strategically changed, with modifications in self-management support, patient education, prophylactic foot care, and footwear for those who were at highest risk. The amputation rate during this phase was 21 per 1000 person-years. During the next 3 years, further refinements (access to a multidisciplinary foot-care team in primary care, better communication and coordination, therapeutic targets, treatment options, and improved foot care monitoring) were undertaken within the Staged Diabetes Management framework, and the amputation rate fell to 15 per 1000 person-years.[95] During the final 3 years (1997 to 1999), the introduction of an outreach wound care clinic and the extension of foot care services to dialysis patients resulted in amputation rates falling to 7 per 1000 person-years.[97]

Veterans with high-risk foot conditions were randomized to "usual education" or a 1-hour lecture showing pictures of ulcers and amputations and a one-page instruction sheet. After a 1-year follow-up, those who had received the special educational session had a threefold decrease in ulceration ($p < .005$) and amputation rates ($p < .0025$).[98] A prospective case-control study, also in veterans, reported a strong protective effect comparing patients who did and did not receive outpatient education.[80] Several foot care intervention programs reported decreases in amputations, reduced days of hospitalizations, and decreased costs. Their descriptive interventions consisted of patient and professional education and structural changes in the organization of foot care services. Given the multidimensional nature of these interventions, there were many components that could have contributed to their reported success.[99–101]

In 1999, Driver and colleagues established a limb preservation program in a multidisciplinary foot care clinic at a regional referral hospital for patients with diabetes. Patients were followed for 5 years, with specific management plans stratified by patient risk category. The incidence of nontraumatic lower amputations fell from 9.9 per 1000 to 1.8 per 1000.[102]

Although foot examinations take minimal time to complete, national surveys reported that only about 50% of patients with diabetes reported a foot examination from their health care provider within the past 6 months. Foot examination frequency was lowest in type 2 patients on insulin, of whom only 41% had been examined.[67] The frequency of foot examinations increased when there were chart reminders or clinician prompts or when the nurse removed the patient's shoes and stockings before the clinician entered the room.

Davis and colleagues described lower-limb amputation in patients with diabetes from a rehabilitation perspective. He suggested that rather than being considered a failure in patient care, amputation should be viewed as a chance for patients to improve their quality of life through the removal of a sometimes painful and nonfunctional limb. With modern prosthetic technology and input from rehabilitation specialists, there is a real possibility that some patients can improve their level of ambulation.[103]

Subsequent Amputations

Subsequent amputations on the same side (ipsilateral) or opposite side (contralateral) are common in people with diabetes and amputations. Table 1-6 displays the frequency of these subsequent amputations from eight studies by year since amputation. Dillingham and colleagues examined subsequent amputation in Medicare beneficiaries.[104] Statewide hospital discharge data from two separate states indicated that 1 year following amputation, 9% to 13% of amputees experienced a new same-side or contralateral amputation.[105,106] Denmark has an amputation registry for surveillance purposes (which excludes toe amputations). This registry includes 27% of people who reported diabetes and 73% who did not have a diabetes diagnosis.[107] According to Danish Registry reports, 19% of all patients undergoing a major amputation for arteriosclerosis and gangrene had another same-side amputation within 6 months. This percentage increased to only 23% by 48 months following amputation, suggesting that most same-side amputations above the toe level would be performed within 6 months of the initial amputation.[107]

The study by Braddeley and colleagues reported that 12% of diabetic individuals had a contralateral amputation at 1 year, 23% at 3 years, and 28% at 5 years.[108] According to the available descriptive findings, subsequent contralateral limb amputations occurred in people with diabetes in 23% to 30% at 3 years and in 28% to 51% at 5 years.[108–110] The notable exception was the study from Newcastle upon Tyne, where the 3-year ipsilateral amputation frequency was 6% and contralateral amputation frequency was 3%. However, this study did report a 50% 3-year mortality rate.[18] A recent study by Izumi and

TABLE 1-6   Percent of Diabetic Individuals with Amputation from Select Studies Undergoing Subsequent Ipsilateral and Contralateral Amputation by Time Interval

Author	Population	1 Year			3 Years			5 Years		
		Ipsilateral	Both	Contralateral	Ipsilateral	Both	Contralateral	Ipsilateral	Both	Contralateral
Braddeley and Fulford[108]				12			23			28
Deerochanawong et al.[18]	Newcastle, United Kingdom				6		3			
Dillingham[104]	Medicare, U.S.	Toe 37 Foot 40		39						
Izumi et al.[111]	San Antonio, TX	Toe 23 Ray 29 Midfoot 19 Major 5		Toe 4 Ray 9 Midfoot 9 Major 12	Toe 40 Ray 41 Midfoot 33 Major 12		Toe 19 Ray 22 Midfoot 19 Major 44	Toe 52 Ray 50 Midfoot 43 Major 13		Toe 30 Ray 29 Midfoot 33 Major 53
Larsson[109]	Lund, Sweden		14			30			49	
Miller et al.[105]	State of New Jersey	9								
Silbert[110]	New York				30		51			
Wright and Kaplan[106]	State of California	13								

TABLE 1-7   Percent Mortality in Diabetic Amputees from Select Studies by Time Interval

Author	Population	Perioperative (28 days)	1 Year	3 Years	5 Years
Braddeley and Fulford[108]	Birmingham, United Kingdom		16%	35%	
Chaturvedi et al.[75]	Type 1: European				24%
	American Indian				44%
	Cuban				38%
	Type 2: European				16%
	American Indian				23%
	Cuban				42%
Deerochanawong et al.[18]	Newcastle, United Kingdom	10%	40%	50%	
Dillingham[104]	U.S. Medicare				
	Toe		23%		
	Foot, ankle		27%		
	Transtibial		34%		
	Transfemoral		50%		
	Bilateral		46%		
Ebskov and Josephsen[107]	Denmark* excludes toe amputations	32%	55%		72%
Izumi[111]	University of Texas, San Antonio				34%
Larsson et al.[92]	Lund, Sweden		15%	38%	68%
Lee et al.[87]	Oklahoma Indians, United States			40%	60%
Mayfield et al.[86]	U.S. veterans	10%	13%	41%	65%
Nelson et al.[63]	Pima Indians				39%
Pohjolainem and Alaranta[118]	S. Finland		38%	65%	80%
Reiber et al.[67]	U.S. National Hospital Discharge	5.8%			
Subramaniam[114]	Beth Israel Deaconess Medical Center	7%		50%	
Tenttolouris[115]	Manchester Royal Infirmary		17%	37%	44%

* 27% of individuals in Danish Registry have diabetes.[107]

colleagues in San Antonio examined 277 people with incident amputations between 1993 and 1997.[111] The authors suggest that subsequent ipsilateral amputations were significantly more common than contralateral amputations. Part of the variation in the frequency of ipsilateral and contralateral amputations reported in these studies is related to the age structure of the study population.

Subsequent Mortality

The cause of death among amputees is rarely attributable to amputation and is usually related to concurrent comorbid conditions such as cardiac or renal disease.

Mortality following amputation has been examined by interval: 28 days (perioperative) and 1, 3, and 5 years. Table 1-7 presents amputation mortality data from 14 select studies.

U.S. perioperative mortality from the National Hospital Discharge Survey is less than 6%.[112] Perioperative mortality was 10% in both the Newcastle study and studies of diabetic amputees in the Department of Veterans Affairs in 1998.[18,113–117] Reports indicate that the 1-year mortality rate in diabetic amputees approaches 50% in select older populations, while the 3-year mortality rate approaches 65% in a Swedish study, and the 5-year mortality rate approaches 80%.[18,63,67,87,92,107,108,113,118] In Statewide California Hospital Discharge data, the age-adjusted amputation mortality rates were 1.6% among Hispanics, 2.7% among non-Hispanic whites, and 5.7% among African Americans.[119]

Economic Considerations for Foot Ulcers and Amputations

Episodes of care for foot ulcers and amputations are costly for patients, providers, and payers. A number of studies were identified with relevant cost information on the cost for foot ulcers. A study of patients with type 2 diabetes determined that costs for "chronic skin ulcers" (excluding peripheral neuropathy, peripheral arterial disease, and amputation) accounted for $150 million of the $11.6 billion of direct diabetes patient care costs.[120] A subsequent study by Harrington and colleagues used the 1995 Medicare claims database standard analytic sample file to estimate U.S. costs for ulcer episodes. They reported that ulcer episodes cost Medicare $1.5 billion.[121] Stockl and colleagues analyzed outpatient, inpatient, medical, skilled nursing facility, pharmacy, and home therapy costs in a population of 2.7 million from January 2000 until December 2001. They report the average costs per foot ulcer episode in people with diabetes stratified by severity level 1 through 4/5. Reported costs by level range from $1892 to $27,721. In this study, 30% of ulcer episodes required subsequent amputation.[122]

Three studies comparing the cost of foot ulcers are presented in Table 1-8. The study by Apelqvist followed 314 patients through their ulcer episode.[123] Healing was achieved in less than 2 months in 54% of patients, in 3 to 4 months in 19% of patients, and in 5 or more months in 27% of patients. Sixty-three percent of patients healed without surgery at an average cost of $6664; 24% of patients required lower-limb amputation at an average cost of $44,790. Patients who died prior to final ulcer resolution (13%) were excluded from this analysis. The proportion of all costs that were related to hospitalization was 39% among ulcer patients and 82% among amputees.[123]

Ramsey conducted a nested case-control study in a large health maintenance organization involving 8905 patients with diabetes. In this group, 514 diabetic indi-viduals developed one or more foot ulcers, and 11% of these patients required amputation. Costs were computed for the year prior to the ulcer and the 2 years following the ulcer for both cases and controls. The excess costs attributed to foot ulcers and their sequelae were $27,987 per patient for the 2-year period following ulcer presentation.[38]

Holzer and colleagues obtained direct cost data on private insurance patients from the MEDSTAT Group, a large U.S. integrated administrative claims system affiliated with private health insurance plans. Study enrollment criteria were ages 18 to 64 years, employed and not on Medicare, and in this system during 1991 to 1992. Ulcer claims were submitted for 5.1% of diabetic patients. These 3013 patients had 3524 ulcer episodes costing an average of $4595 per episode. When ulcers were categorized by outcome, the costs were $1929 for ulcers that healed without complications, $3980 for those complicated with osteomyelitis, and $15,792 for patients whose ulcers were complicated with gangrene and required amputation. In this study, over 70% of total costs were from hospital settings.[124]

There were several studies comparing costs between people with and without diabetes. Jacobs and colleagues analyzed hospitalization for late complications of diabetes in the United States and compared 1987 hospital discharge data for diabetic and age- and sex-matched nondiabetic individuals. They found that the relative risk for skin ulcer/gangrene comparing people with and without diabetes was 21.8 (95% CI: 21.6 to 22.0).[125] A similar study was conducted in Wales by Currie using National Health Service data to examine differences in admissions, length of stay, and costs between diabetic and nondiabetic individuals. The relative risk for a foot ulcer comparing diabetic to nondiabetic individuals was 21.1 (95% CI: 16.6 to 26.9).[126] The authors conclude that 20% of inpatient costs were used by the 2% of their population with diabetes.

In people with and without diabetes, Diagnostic Related Groups (DRG) hospital reimbursement is available for patients with private insurance and those with Medicare. Table 1-9 shows that in 2005, under DRG reimbursement for code 271 (skin ulcer), patients with

TABLE 1-8   Direct Cost for Diabetic Foot Ulcers in Three Studies

Author	Number of Patients/Study Type	Outcome	Average Episode Cost (U.S. $)	Inpatient Cost	Outpatient Cost
Apelqvist et al.[123]	Prospective 314 general internal medicine patients	Primary healing, 63%	$6,664	61%	39%
		Healed after amputation, 24%	$44,790		
Holtzer et al.[124]	Retrospective, administrative records of 3013 patients, and 3524 episodes	Primary healing, 52%	$1,929	23%	77%
		Osteomyelitis, 33%	$3,980	23%	77%
		Gangrene/amputation, 14%	$15,792	12%	88%
Ramsey et al.[38]	Nested case-control study in HMO of 8905 type 1, 2	Primary healing, 84%	$27,987 total attributable cost	18%	82%
		Amputation, 16%			

TABLE 1-9   Lower-Limb Complications and Lower-Limb Amputation Reimbursement to Hospitals for Patients with and Without Diabetes, 2005

		Medstat (Private)[128]		Medicare[127]	
DRG	Condition	Length of Stay	Average $ Reimbursement	Length of Stay	Average $ Reimbursement
Ulcer-Related					
18	Peripheral neuropathy with complications	4.9	9398	5.2	5220
19	Peripheral neuropathy without complications	3.8	6978	3.4	3521
271	Skin ulcers	11.0	13,328	6.8	5460
238	Osteomyelitis	7.0	10,981	8.1	7822
277	Cellulitis > age 17 with complications	5.0	7508	5.4	4405
278	Cellulitis > age 17 without complications	3.3	4668	4.0	2394
263	Skin graft/debridement/complications	11.6	24,232	10.5	11,713
264	Skin graft/debridement/no complications	5.3	10,322	6.2	5494
287	Skin graft/debridement/endocrine	8.5	18,081	9.5	10,662
Lower-Limb Amputation					
113	Lower-limb amputation except toes	13.3	30,433	12.6	16,136
114	Toe and upper-limb amputation	NA	NA	8.4	9597
285	Endocrine amputation	7.3	17,131	9.8	11,729

DRG, Diagnostic Related Group.

Source: Medstat Group, Thompson Corporation, 2006; Centers for Medicare and Medicaid Services, 2006

TABLE 1-10   Twelve-Month Service Use and Medical Care Costs Among Medicare Beneficiaries with Diabetes Undergoing Dysvascular Amputations in 1996[104]

	Average Cost by Setting (U.S. $)						
Initial Amputation Level	Acute Care Hospital Costs	Inpatient Rehabilitation	Physician/ Outpatient Care	Skilled Nursing Facility	Home Health Care	Prostheses, Footwear, Assistive Devices	Average Total Cost
People with Diabetes							
Toe	35,673	1153	4729	2440	2073	1518	45,513
Foot and/or ankle	36,636	3314	22,020	9348	11,541	4161	75,479
Transtibial	38,830	6552	18,928	10,851	7447	7496	82,657
Transfemoral	26,100	2816	13,956	9106	5461	5739	57,717

private insurance reimbursed hospitals on average $13,328 for an average 11-day length of stay, while hospitals with Medicare recipients were reimbursed an average of $5,460 (41%) for an average 6.8-day length of stay.[127,128] Payment for the health care provider and subsequent outpatient care and rehabilitation is in addition to these figures.

Amputation reimbursement is also shown in Table 1-9. In 2005, the average reimbursement to private hospitals for DRG 113, a lower-limb amputation in people with and without diabetes, was $30,422 for an average 13.3-day hospitalization compared to $16,136 (53%) for an average 12.6-day hospital stay for Medicare patients. Again, physician, related outpatient, rehabilitation, and other follow-up costs of care would have to be added to compute the costs for an episode of care resulting in an amputation.

Dillingham and colleagues prepared episode costs for dysvascular amputations in people with diabetes on Medicare, as shown in Table 1-10. Included were costs for inpatient and outpatient care, inpatient rehabilitation, skilled nursing facilities, home health care and prostheses, footwear, and assistive devices. The annual amputation episode costs were lowest for a toe amputation ($45,513) and highest for a transtibial amputation ($82,657). There were significant differences by level of amputation between amputees who did and did not have diabetes (data not shown).[104]

In 2004, people who were hospitalized with diabetes and lower-limb amputations showed striking differences in amputation rates by expected source of payment as shown in Figure 1-7. The number of amputations per 1000 hospital stays for was twice as high among the uninsured (12.7), compared to hospital stays covered by Medicare (5.7), private insurance (6.2), and Medicaid (6.7).[129]

The discharge status of diabetic amputees has been monitored in several populations. In Colorado, the percentage of patients discharged to home or self-care after amputation gradually declined from 66% for those age 45 years or younger to 23% for those age 75+. Conversely, as age increased, an increasing proportion required relocation from home or self-care settings to other acute, skilled, and intermediate care facilities for inpatient care.[130] In Larsson and colleagues' cohort in Sweden, 93% of patients living independently before their minor index amputation were able to return to

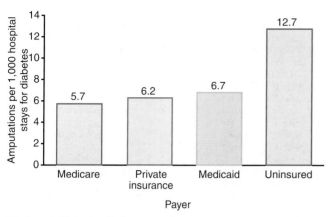

Figure 1–7 Lower-limb amputations among patients hospitalized with diabetes, by payer, 2004. *(Redrawn from AHRQ, Healthcare Cost and Utilization Project, Statistical Brief 17, 2006.)*

living independently compared to 61% of patients after a major amputation.[92] Lavery and colleagues reported that while only 2.3% of amputees in south Texas were admitted from an institutional care facility, over 25% were discharged to one following amputation.[119]

Summary

Ulcers and amputations are an important and costly problem for people with diabetes. Hospital amputation discharge rates in several developed countries are showing encouraging reductions. Many of the independent risk

factors for ulcers and amputations have been identified from population-based, analytic, and experimental studies and are similar. Many risk factors have the potential for modification by patients and their health care providers. Subsequent chapters will discuss the self-management and health care strategies that are available.

Once an individual has an ulcer, the risk of reulceration is high. Similarly, once an individual has had an amputation, the likelihood of a subsequent amputation is high at 5 years. Mortality following amputation rises steadily but is largely related to age and comorbid conditions.

ACKNOWLEDGMENTS

This research was supported by the Department of Veterans Affairs, Veterans Health Administration, Health Services Research and Development.

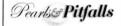

Pearls

- Greater attention is needed to correctly diagnose and classify wounds on the foot of a patient with diabetes.
- "Best practices" used to achieve success in low-incidence areas can be considered for implementation in high-incidence areas to reduce ulcer and amputation rates.
- Ulcer-free survival is an excellent outcome measure that combines health care quality and patient self-management.
- Diabetes mortality in people with amputations is almost exclusively related to their age and comorbid conditions, not amputation.

Pitfalls

- Lesions such as pressure ulcers, surgical wounds, puncture injuries, sequelae of vasculitis, and dermatologic conditions are not foot ulcers yet are frequently coded as such.
- Methodologic issues will influence the precision of incidence and prevalence computations.
- Involving an epidemiologist or biostatistician at the outset of a project involving data collection for incidence and prevalence will help in avoiding common pitfalls.
- A growing body of evidence suggests that disparities in quality of care among people with amputations from different racial and ethnic groups can be attributed to issues related to poverty and health care access.

References

1. "Facts & Figures: Did You Know?" International Diabetes Federation. Available at http://www.idf.org.
2. West KM: Atherosclerosis and Related Disorders: Epidemiology of Diabetes and Its Vascular Lesions. New York, Elsevier North-Holland, 1978, p 391.
3. IWGDF: International Consensus on the Diabetic Foot. Amsterdam, International Working Group on the Diabetic Foot, 1999.
4. Pound N, Chipchase S, Treece K, et al: Ulcer-free survival following management of foot ulcers in diabetes. Diabet Med 22:1306–1309, 2005.
5. Wagner FW Jr: The dysvascular foot: A system for diagnosis and treatment. Foot Ankle 2(2):64–122, 1981.
6. Lavery LA, Armstrong DG, Harkless LB: Classification of diabetic foot wounds. J Foot Ankle Surg 35(6):528–531, 1996.
7. Treece K, Macfarlane R, Pound N, et al: Validation of a New System of Foot Ulcer Classification in Diabetes Mellitus. Nottingham, UK: Department of Diabetes and Endocrinology, City Hospital, 2005.
8. Wong I: Measuring the incidence of lower limb ulceration in the Chinese population in Hong Kong. J Wound Care 11(10): 377–379, 2002.
9. Andersson E, Hansson C, Swanbeck G: Leg and foot ulcer prevalence and investigation of the peripheral arterial and venous circulation in a randomised elderly population: An epidemiological survey and clinical investigation. Acta Derm Venereol 73(1):57–61, 1993.
10. Moss SE, Klein R, Klein BEK: The prevalence and incidence of lower extremity amputation in a diabetic population. Arch Intern Med 152:610–616, 1992.
11. Margolis DJ, Kantor J, Santanna J, et al: Risk factors for delayed healing of neuropathic diabetic foot ulcers: A pooled analysis. Arch Dermatol 136(12):1531–1535, 2000.
12. Tseng CH: Prevalence and risk factors of diabetic foot problems in Taiwan: A cross-sectional survey of non-type 1 diabetic patients from a nationally representative sample. Diabetes Care 26(12): 3351, 2003.
13. Gulam-Abbas Z, Lutale JK, Morbach S, Archibald LK: Clinical outcome of diabetes patients hospitalized with foot ulcers, Dar es Salaam, Tanzania. Diabet Med 19(7):575–579, 2002.
14. Yalamanchi H, Yalamanchi S: Profile of diabetic foot infections in a semiurban area of a developing country. Diabetologia 40(suppl 1): A468, 1997.
15. Akanji AO, Adetuyidi A: The pattern of presentation of foot lesions in Nigerian diabetic patients. West Afr J Med 9(1):1–5, 1990.
16. Benotmane A, Mohammedi F, Ayad F, et al: Diabetic foot lesions: Etiologic and prognostic factors. Diabetes Metab 26(2):113–117, 2000.

17. Monabeka HG, Nsakala-Kibangou N: Epidemiological and clinical aspects of the diabetic foot at the Central University Hospital of Brazzaville. Bull Soc Pathol Exot 94(3):246–248, 2001.

18. Deerochanawong C, Home PD, Alberti KGMM: A survey of lower limb amputation in diabetic patients. Diabet Med 9:942–946, 1992.

19. Holewski JJ, Moss KM, Stess RM, et al: Prevalence of foot pathology and lower extremity complications in a diabetic outpatient clinic. J Rehabil Res Dev 26(3):35–44, 1989.

20. Wikblad K, Smide B, Bergstrom A, et al: Outcome of clinical foot examination in relation to self-perceived health and glycaemic control in a group of urban Tanzanian diabetic patients. Diabetes Res Clin Pract 37(3):185–192, 1997.

21. Nielsen JV: Peripheral neuropathy, hypertension, foot ulcers and amputations among Saudi Arabian patients with type 2 diabetes. Diabetes Res Clin Pract 41(1):63–69, 1998.

22. Boyko EJ, Ahroni JH, Stensel V, et al: A prospective study of risk factors for diabetic foot ulcer: The Seattle Diabetic Foot Study. Diabetes Care 22(7):1036–1042, 1999.

23. Vijay V, Narasimham DV, Seena R, et al: Clinical profile of diabetic foot infections in south India: A retrospective study. Diabet Med 17(3):215–218, 2000.

24. Pham H, Armstrong DG, Harvey C, et al: Screening techniques to identify people at high risk for diabetic foot ulceration: A prospective multicenter trial. Diabetes Care 23(5):606–611, 2000.

25. Kastenbauer T, Sauseng S, Sokol G, et al: A prospective study of predictors for foot ulceration in type 2 diabetes. J American Podiat Med Assoc 91(7):343–350, 2001.

26. Gulliford MC, Mahabir D: Diabetic foot disease and foot care in a Caribbean community. Diabet Res Clin Pract 56(1):35–40, 2002.

27. Carrington AL, Shaw JE, van Schie CH, et al: Can motor nerve conduction velocity predict foot problems in diabetic subjects over a 6-year outcome period? Diabetes Care 25(11):2010–2015, 2002.

28. Nyamu PN, Otieno CF, Amayo EO, McLigeyo SO: Risk factors and prevalence of diabetic foot ulcers at Kenyatta National Hospital, Nairobi. East Afr Med J 80(1):36–43, 2003.

29. Stein H, Yaacobi E, Steinberg R: The diabetic foot: Update on a common clinical syndrome. Orthopedics 26(11):1127–1130, 2003.

30. Malgrange D, Richard JL, Leymarie F, French Working Group on the Diabetic Foot: Screening diabetic patients at risk for foot ulceration: A multi-centre hospital-based study in France. Diabetes Metab 29(3):261–268, 2003.

31. Lavery LA, Armstrong DG, Wunderlich RP, et al: Predictive value of foot pressure assessment as part of a population-based diabetes disease management program. Diabetes Care 26(4):1069–1073, 2002.

32. Lavery LA, Armstrong DG, Wunderlich RP, et al: Diabetic foot syndrome: Evaluating the prevalence and incidence of foot pathology in Mexican Americans and non-Hispanic whites from a diabetes disease management cohort. Diabetes Care 26(5):1435–1438, 2003.

33. Kumar S, Ashe HA, Parnell LN, et al: The prevalence of foot ulceration and its correlates in type 2 diabetic patients: A population-based study. Diabet Med 11(5):480–484, 1994.

34. Centers for Disease Control and Prevention: History of foot ulcer among persons with diabetes: United States, 2000–2002. MMWR Morb Mortal Wkly Rep 52(45):1098–1102, 2003.

35. Abbott CA, Vileikyte L, Williamson S, et al: Multicenter study of the incidence of and predictive risk factors for diabetic neuropathic foot ulceration. Diabetes Care 21:1071–1075, 1998.

36. Rith-Najarian SJ, Stolusky T, Gohdes DM: Identifying diabetic patients at high risk for lower-extremity amputation in a primary health care setting: A prospective evaluation of simple screening criteria. Diabetes Care 15(10):1386–1389, 1992.

37. Walters DP, Gatling W, Mullee MA, Hill RD: The distribution and severity of diabetic foot disease: A community study with comparison to a non-diabetic group. Diabet Med 9:354–358, 1992.

38. Ramsey SD, Newton K, Blough D, et al: Incidence, outcomes, and cost of foot ulcers in patients with diabetes. Diabetes Care 22(3):382–387, 1999.

39. Abbott CA, Carrington AL, Ashe H, et al: The North-West Diabetes Foot Care Study: Incidence of, and risk factors for, new diabetic foot ulceration in a community-based patient cohort. Diabet Med 19(5):377–384, 2002.

40. Muller IS, de Grauw WJ, van Gerwen WH, et al: Foot ulceration and lower limb amputation in type 2 diabetic patients in Dutch primary health care. Diabetes Care 25(3):570–574, 2002.

41. Palumbo PJ, Melton LJI: Peripheral vascular disease and diabetes. In National Diabetes Data Group (ed): Diabetes In America, 2nd ed (NIH publ. no. 495-1468). Washington, DC, U.S. Government Printing Office, 1995, pp 401–408.

42. Apelqvist J, Castenfors J, Larsson J: Wound classification is more important than site of ulceration in the outcome of diabetic foot ulcers. Diabet Med 6:526–530, 1989.

43. Reiber GE, Lipsky BA, Gibbons GW: The burden of diabetic foot ulcers. Am J Surg 176(2A):5S–10S, 1998.

44. Oyibo SO, Jude EB, Tarawneh I, et al: The effects of ulcer size and site, patient's age, sex and type and duration of diabetes on the outcome of diabetic foot ulcers. Diabet Med 18(2):133–138, 2001.

45. Apelqvist J, Larsson J, Agard C: Long term prognosis for diabetic patients with foot ulcers. J Int Med 233:485–491, 1993.

46. Margolis DJ, Allen-Taylor L, Hoffstad O, Berlin JA: Diabetic neuropathic foot ulcers: The association of wound size, wound duration, and wound grade on healing. Diabetes Care 25(10):1835–1839, 2002.

47. Sheehan P, Jones P, Caselli A, et al: Percent change in wound area of diabetic foot ulcers over a 4-week period is a robust predictor of complete healing in a 12-week prospective trial. Diabetes Care 26(6):1879–1882, 2003.

48. Pecoraro RE, Ahroni JH, Boyko EJ, Stensel VL: Chronology and determinants of tissue repair in diabetic lower-extremity ulcers. Diabetes Care 40:1305–1313, 1991.

49. McNeely MJ, Boyko EJ: Diabetes-related comorbidities in Asian Americans: Results of a national health survey. J Diabetes Complications 19(2):101–106, 2005.

50. Abbott CA, Garrow AP, Carrington AL, et al: Foot ulcer risk is lower in South-Asian and African-Caribbean compared with European diabetic patients in the U.K.: The North-West Diabetes Foot Care Study. Diabetes Care 28(8):1869–1875, 2005.

51. Boyko EJ, Ahroni JH, Cohen V, et al: Prediction of diabetic foot ulcer occurrence using commonly available clinical information: The Seattle Diabetic Foot Study. Diabetes Care 29(6):1202–1207, 2006.

52. Morbach S, Lutale JK, Viswanathan V, et al: Regional differences in risk factors and clinical presentation of diabetic foot lesions. Diabet Med 21(1):91–95, 2004.

53. Litzelman DK, Slemenda CW, Langefeld CD, et al: Reduction of lower extremity clinical abnormalities in patients with non-insulin-dependent diabetes mellitus: A randomized, controlled trial. Ann Intern Med 119(1):36–41, 1993.

54. Moss SE, Klein R, Klein BE: The 14-year incidence of lower-extremity amputations in a diabetic population: The Wisconsin Epidemiologic Study of Diabetic Retinopathy. Diabetes Care 22(6):951–959, 1999.

55. Mantey I, Foster AV, Spencer S, Edmonds ME: Why do foot ulcers recur in diabetic patients? Diabet Med 16(3):245–249, 1999.

56. Connor H, Mahdi OZ: Repetitive ulceration in neuropathic patients. Diabetes Metab Res Rev 20(suppl 1):S23–S28, 2004.

57. Wrobel JS, Mayfield JA, Reiber GE: Geographic variation of lower-extremity major amputation in individuals with and without diabetes in the Medicare population. Diabetes Care 24(5):860–864, 2001.

58. The Global Lower Extremity Amputation Study Group: Epidemiology of lower extremity amputation in centres in Europe, North America and East Asia. Br J Surg 87(3):328–337, 2000.

59. Humphrey A, Dowse G, Thoma K, Zimmet P: Diabetes and non-traumatic lower extremity amputation: incidence, risk factors and prevention: A 12 year follow-up study in Nauru. Diabetes Care 19(7):710–714, 1996.

60. Humphrey L, Palumbo P, Butters M, et al: The contribution of non-insulin dependent diabetes to lower extremity amputation in the community. Arch Intern Med 154:885–892, 1994.

61. Lehto S, Pyorala K, Ronnemaa T, Laakso M: Risk factors predicting lower extremity amputations in patients with NIDDM. Diabetes Care 19(6):607–612, 1996.

62. Morris AD, McAlpine R, Steinke D, et al: Diabetes and lower-limb amputations in the community. Diabetes Care 21:738–743, 1998.

63. Nelson R, Gohdes D, Everhart J, et al: Lower-extremity amputations in NIDDM: 12-yr follow-up study in Pima Indians. Diabetes Care 11:8–16, 1988.

64. Siitonen OL, Niskanen LK, Laakso M, et al: Lower extremity amputations in diabetic and nondiabetic patients. Diabetes Care 16:16–20, 1993.
65. Trautner C, Haastert B, Giani G, Berger M: Incidence of lower limb amputations and diabetes. Diabetes Care 19(9):1006–1009, 1996.
66. van Houtum W, Lavery LA: Outcomes associated with diabetes-related amputations in the Netherlands and in the state of California. J Int Med 240:227–231, 1996.
67. Reiber GE, Boyko EJ, Smith DG: Lower extremity foot ulcers and amputations in diabetes. In National Diabetes Data Group (ed): Diabetes in America, 2nd ed (NIH publ. no. 95-1468). Washington, DC, U.S. Government Printing Office, 1995, pp 409–428.
68. Holstein P, Ellitsgaard N, Olsen BB, Ellitsgaard V: Decreasing incidence of major amputations in people with diabetes. Diabetologia 43(7):844–847, 2000.
69. van Houtum WH, Rauwerda JA, Ruwaard D, et al: Reduction in diabetes-related lower-extremity amputations in the Netherlands: 1991–2000. Diabetes Care 27:1042–1046, 2004.
70. Trautner C, Haastert B, Spraul M, et al: Unchanged incidence of lower-limb amputations in a German city, 1990–1998. Diabetes Care 24(5):855–859, 2001.
71. Eskelinen E, Eskelinen A, Alback A, Lepantalo M: Major amputation incidence decreases both in non-diabetic and in diabetic patients in Helsinki. Scand J Surg 95(3):185–189, 2006.
72. Botman SL, Moore TF, Moriarity CL, Parsons VL: Design and estimation for the National Health Interview Survey, 1995–2004. Vital Health Stat 2 130:1–31, 2000.
73. National Center for Health Statistics: National Health Interview Survey (NHIS): Survey Description. Washington, DC, National Center for Health Statistics, 1997.
74. Resnick HE, Valsania P, Phillips CL: Diabetes mellitus and nontraumatic lower extremity amputation in black and white Americans: The national health and nutrition examination survey epidemiologic follow-up study, 1971–1992. Arch Intern Med 159:2470–2475, 1999.
75. Chaturvedi N, Stevens LK, Fuller JH, et al: Risk factors, ethnic differences and mortality associated with lower-extremity gangrene and amputation in diabetes: The WHO Multinational Study of Vascular Disease in Diabetes. Diabetologia 44(suppl 2):S65–S71, 2001.
76. Leggetter S, Chaturvedi N, Fuller JH, Edmonds ME: Ethnicity and risk of diabetes-related lower extremity amputation: A population-based, case-control study of African Caribbeans and Europeans in the United kingdom. Arch Intern Med 162(1):73–78, 2002.
77. Chaturvedi N, Abbott CA, Whalley A, et al: Risk of diabetes-related amputation in South Asians vs. Europeans in the UK. Diabet Med 19(2):99–104, 2002.
78. Abbas ZG, Archibald LK: Epidemiology of the diabetic foot in Africa. Med Sci Monit 11(8):RA262–RA270, 2005.
79. Wachtel MS: Family poverty accounts for differences in lower-extremity amputation rates of minorities 50 years old or more with diabetes. J Nat Med Assoc 97(3):334–338, 2005.
80. Reiber GE, Pecoraro RE, Koepsell TD: Risk factors for amputation in patients with diabetes mellitus. Ann Intern Med 117(2):97–105, 1992.
81. Selby JV, Zhang D: Risk factors for lower extremity amputation in persons with diabetes. Diabetes Care 18(4):509–516, 1995.
82. Karter AJ, Ferrara A, Liu JY, et al: Ethnic disparities in diabetic complications in an insured population. JAMA 287(19):2519–2527, 2002.
83. Adler AL, Boyko EJ, Ahroni JH, Smith DG: Lower-extremity amputation in diabetes: The independent effects of peripheral vascular disease, sensory neuropathy, and foot ulcers. Diabetes Care 22:1029–1035, 1999.
84. Hamalainen H, Ronnemma T, Halonen JP, Toikka T: Factors predicting lower extremity amputations in patients with type 1 or type 2 diabetes mellitus: A population-based 7-year follow-up study. J Int Med 246:97–103, 1999.
85. Selby JV, Karter AJ, Ackerson LM, et al: Developing a prediction rule from automated clinical databases to identify high-risk patients in a large population with diabetes. Diabetes Care 24(9):1547–1555, 2001.
86. Mayfield JA, Reiber GE, Nelson RG, Greene T: A foot risk classification system to predict diabetic amputation in Pima Indians. Diabetes Care 19(7):704–709, 1996.
87. Lee J, Lu M, Lee V, et al: Lower extremity amputation: Incidence, risk factors, and mortality in the Oklahoma Indian Diabetes Study. Diabetes 42:876–882, 1993.
88. Hennis AJJ, Fraser HS, Jonnalagadda R, et al: Explanations for the high risk of diabetes-related amputation in a Caribbean population of black African descent and potential for prevention. Diabetes Care 27(11):2636–2641, 2004.
89. Palumbo P, Melton L: Peripheral Vascular Disease and Diabetes (NIH Publ 85–1468). Washington, DC, U.S. Government Printing Office, 1985.
90. Kannel WB, McGee DL: Diabetes and cardiovascular disease: The Framingham Study. J Am Med Assoc 241(19):2035–2038, 1979.
91. Nathan DM, Cleary PA, Backlund JY, et al: Intensive diabetes treatment and cardiovascular disease in patients with type 1 diabetes. N Engl J Med 353(25):2643–2653, 2005.
92. Larsson J, Agardh CD, Apelqvist J, Stenstrom A: Long term prognosis after healed amputations in patients with diabetes. Clin Orthop Rel Res 350:149–158, 1998.
93. Pecoraro RE, Reiber GE, Burgess EM: Pathways to diabetic limb amputation: Basis for prevention. Diabetes Care 13:513–521, 1990.
94. Boulton AJM: Diabetic Neuropathy. Carnforth, Lancashire, UK, Marius Press, 1997.
95. Rith-Najarian S, Branchaud C, Beaulieu O, et al: Reducing lower-extremity amputations due to diabetes: Application of the staged diabetes management approach in a primary care setting. J Fam Pract 47(2):127–132, 1998.
96. Rith-Najarian S, Gohdes D: Preventing amputations among patients with diabetes on dialysis [letter]. Diabetes Care 23(9):1445–1446, 2000.
97. Mazze R, Strock E, Simonson G, et al: Staged Diabetes Management: Decision Paths, 2nd ed. Minneapolis, International Diabetes Center, 1998.
98. Malone JM, Snyder M, Anderson G, et al: Prevention of amputation by diabetic education. Am J Surg 158(6):520–524, 1989.
99. Davidson JK, Alogna M, Goldsmith M: Assessment of program effectiveness at Grady Memorial Hospital, Atlanta. In Steiner G, Lawrence PA (eds): Educating Diabetic Patients. New York, Springer-Verlag, 1981.
100. Miller LV: Evaluation of patient education: Los Angeles County Hospital experience. Report of National Commission on Diabetes, Vol 3. 1975.
101. Runyon J: The Memphis chronic disease program. JAMA 231:264–267, 1975.
102. Driver VR, Madsen J, Goodman RA: Reducing amputation rates in patients with diabetes at a military medical center: The limb preservation service model. Diabetes Care 28(2):248–253, 2005.
103. Davis BL, Kuznicki J, Praveen SS, Sferra JJ: Lower-extremity amputations in patients with diabetes: pre- and post-surgical decisions related to successful rehabilitation. Diabetes Metab Res Rev 20(suppl 1):S45–S50, 2004.
104. Dillingham TR, Pezzin LE, Shore AD: Reamputation, mortality, and health care costs among persons with dysvascular lower-limb amputations. Arch Phys Med Rehabil 86(3):480–486, 2005.
105. Miller AE, Van Buskirk A, Verhoek W, Miller ER: Diabetes related lower extremity amputations in New Jersey, 1979–1981. J Med Society NJ 82:723–726, 1985.
106. Wright WE, Kaplan GA: Trends in lower extremity amputations, California, 1983–1987 (California Chronic and Sentinel Diseases Surveillance Program Resource Document). Sacramento, California Department of Health Services, 1989.
107. Ebskov B, Josephsen P: Incidence of reamputation and death after gangrene of the lower extremity. Prosthet Orthot Int 4:77–80, 1980.
108. Braddeley RM, Fulford JC: A trial of conservative amputations for lesions of the feet in diabetes mellitus. Br J Surg 52:38–43, 1965.
109. Larsson J: Lower extremity amputation in diabetic patients [doctoral dissertation], Lund, Sweden, Lund University, 1994.
110. Silbert S: Amputation of the lower extremity in diabetes mellitus. Diabetes 1:297–299, 1952.
111. Izumi Y, Satterfield K, Lee S, Harkless LB: Risk of reamputation in diabetic patients stratified by limb and level of amputation: A 10-year observation. Diabetes Care 29(3):566–570, 2006.
112. Preston SD, Reiber GE, Koepsell TD: Lower extremity amputations and inpatient mortality in hospitalized persons with diabetes: National population risk factors and associations [thesis]. Seattle, University of Washington, 1993.

113. Mayfield JA, Reiber GE, Maynard C, et al: Trends in lower limb amputation in the Veterans Health Administration, 1989–1998. J Rehabil Res Dev 37(1):23–30, 2000.

114. Subramaniam B, Pomposelli F, Talmor D, Park KW: Perioperative and long-term morbidity and mortality after above-knee and below-knee amputations in diabetics and nondiabetics. Anesth Analg 100(5):1241–1247, 2005.

115. Tentolouris N, Al-Sabbagh S, Walker MG, et al: Mortality in diabetic and nondiabetic patients after amputations performed from 1990 to 1995. Diabetes Care 27(7):1598–1604, 2004.

116. Lavery LA, van Houtum WH, Armstrong DG, et al: Mortality following lower extremity amputation in minorities with diabetes mellitus. Diabetes Res Clin Pract 37:41–47, 1997.

117. Moulik PK, Mtonga R, Gill GV: Amputation and mortality in new-onset diabetic foot ulcers stratified by etiology. Diabetes Care 26(2):491–494, 2003.

118. Pohjolainen T, Alaranta H: Ten-year survival of Finnish lower limb amputees. Prosthet Orthot Int 22:10–16, 1998.

119. Lavery LA, Ashry HR, van Houtum W, et al: Variation in the incidence and proportion of diabetes-related amputations in minorities. Diabetes Care 19(1):48–52, 1996.

120. Huse DM, Oster G, Killen AR, et al: The economic costs of non-insulin-dependent diabetes mellitus. J Am Med Assoc 262(19): 2708–2713, 1989.

121. Harrington C, Zagari MJ, Corea J, Klitenic J: A costs analysis of diabetic lower-extremity ulcers. Diabetes Care 23(9):1333–1338, 2000.

122. Stockl K, Vanderplas A, Tafesse E, Chang E: Costs of lower-extremity ulcers among patients with diabetes. Diabetes Care 27(9):2129–2134, 2004.

123. Apelqvist J, Ragnarson-Tennvall G, Persson U, Larsson J: Diabetic foot ulcers in a multidisciplinary setting: An economic analysis of primary healing and healing with amputation. J Int Med 235(5): 463–471, 1994.

124. Holzer SE, Camerota A, Martens L, et al: Costs and duration of care for lower extremity ulcers in patients with diabetes. Clin Ther 20(1):169–181, 1998.

125. Jacobs J, Sena M, Fox N: The cost of hospitalization for the late complications of diabetes in the United States. Diabet Med 8(symposium):S23–S29, 1991.

126. Currie CJ, Morgan CL, Peters JR: The epidemiology and cost of inpatient care for peripheral vascular disease, infection, neuropathy, and ulceration in diabetes. Diabetes Care 21:42–48, 1998.

127. CMS: DRG Inpatient Billing Data, 2005. Washington, DC, Bureau of Data Strategy and Management, 2006.

128. MEDSTAT: DRG Guide Descriptions and Normative Values. Ann Arbor, MI, Thomson Healthcare, 2006.

129. Russo CA, Jiang HJ: Hospital Stays Among Patients with Diabetes, 2004 (HCUP Statistical Brief 17). Agency for Healthcare Research and Quality (AHRQ). Available at http://www.ahrq.gov/data/hcup/.

130. Colorado State Department of Health: Diabetes Prevalence and Morbidity in Colorado Residents, 1980–1991. Colorado State Department of Health, 1993.

131. Resnick HE, Carter EA, Sosenko JM, et al: Incidence of lower-extremity amputation in American Indians: The Strong Heart Study. Diabetes Care 27(8):1885–1891, 2004.

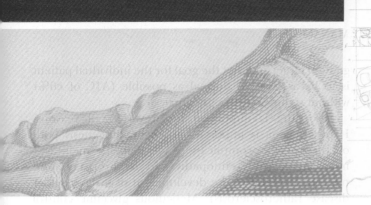

2

DIABETES MELLITUS: OLD ASSUMPTIONS AND NEW REALITIES

JAY S. SKYLER ∎

Nearly 21 million Americans, approximately 7% of the population, suffer from diabetes mellitus.[1] Unfortunately, 6.2 million of these people are unaware that they have diabetes. Each year, approximately 1.5 million Americans develop diabetes. The cost of caring for diabetes now exceeds $132 billion per year, approximately one of every seven health care dollars, including 30% of the Medicare budget. Each year, 224,000 deaths are linked to diabetes, 73,000 of those deaths being directly attributable to diabetes.[1] Yet the human burden of diabetes is a consequence of the devastating chronic complications of the disease. In the United States, diabetes remains the leading cause of new blindness in adults; 24,000 individuals become legally blind every year because of diabetes. Diabetes now accounts for 44% of patients entering dialysis or transplantation, making it by far the leading cause of end-stage renal disease.[1] Compared to the nondiabetic population, people with diabetes are twofold to fourfold more likely to have heart disease or a stroke. Diabetes results in a 15- to 40-fold increased risk of amputations and thus is the nation's leading cause of nontraumatic lower-limb amputations, 60% of which occur in people with diabetes.[1] Each year, an estimated 82,000 limbs are lost owing to diabetes.

The impact of diabetes is staggering. In the decades ahead, this need not be. Future development of blindness, kidney failure, amputation, and heart disease can be markedly lessened by scrupulous attention to therapies and preventive approaches that have been demon-strated to be effective. This includes attainment of meticulous glycemic control, aggressive blood pressure control, careful attention to lipid abnormalities, and the use of aspirin and other preventive therapies, coupled with appropriate use of proven therapies and technologies such as laser photocoagulation, early introduction of angiotensin-converting enzyme inhibitors or angiotensin receptor blockers, and routine foot care.

Randomized, controlled clinical trials that have been completed over the last several years have clearly and unambiguously demonstrated the benefits to diabetic patients of meticulous glycemic control, aggressive blood pressure control, lowering of low-density lipoprotein cholesterol (LDL-C), and use of aspirin therapy. There can no longer be any excuse for ignoring these important risk factors.

New Diabetes Criteria and Clinical Implications

The American Diabetes Association (ADA) Expert Committee on the Diagnosis and Classification of Diabetes Mellitus released its report in 1997[2] and revised it in 2003.[3] They recommended moving toward an etiopathogenetic classification of diabetes that emphasizes the two principal types and also recommended that the classification terminology of diabetes be changed. The official names for the two principal types became "type 1 diabetes" and "type 2 diabetes" (using Arabic numerals 1 and 2) while "IDDM" and "NIDDM" were deleted.

More important, the Expert Committee recommended a major shift in the way diabetes is diagnosed. The previous criteria were based on evidence that there is increased retinopathy risk when an oral glucose tolerance test (OGTT) 2-hour value exceeds 200 mg/dL (11.1 mmol/L). The older data implied that retinopathy risk increased when fasting plasma glucose (FPG) exceeded 140 mg/dL (7.8 mmol/L). Newer data suggest that this FPG cut point is too high. The Expert Committee also noted that an estimated 30% to 35% of people with diabetes in the United States are undiagnosed. One of the reasons they are undiagnosed is that the OGTT is not routinely performed in clinical practice. As a consequence, the default criterion for diagnosis has been an FPG of less than or equal to 140 mg/dL (7.8 mmol/L). The Expert Committee found that by lowering this FPG cut point to 126 mg/dL (7.0 mmol/L) or lower, two things would happen. First, it would acknowledge that retinopathy risk begins at a lower FPG than is now used for diagnosis. Second, most people with undiagnosed diabetes would become recognized without very much risk of a false-positive diagnosis. Thus, 126 mg/dL (7.0 mmol/L) becomes a surrogate for an OGTT 2-hour value of 200 mg/dL (11.1 mmol/L). This change really does not increase the number of people with diabetes. Rather, it increases the number of people with *known* diabetes. That is why it is a crucial public health measure.

The old criteria used an FPG of less than 115 mg/dL (6.4 mmol/L) for normal. In contrast, the 1997 ADA criteria initially used an FPG of less than 110 mg/dL (6.1 mmol/L) for normal,[2] but in 2003, ADA lowered this further to 100 mg/dL (5.5 mmol/L).[3] Individuals having FPG levels of 100 to 125 mg/dL (5.5 to 6.9 mmol/L), too high to be considered altogether normal, are now defined as having "impaired fasting glucose" (IFG). This group (IFG) is considered to be at increased risk of diabetes, similar to those with impaired glucose tolerance, who have OGTT 2-hour values of 140 to 199 mg/dL (7.8 to 11.0 mmol/L).

Glycated hemoglobin (HbA$_{1c}$ or A1C) is not currently recommended for diagnosis of diabetes, although some studies have shown that the frequency distributions for A1C have characteristics similar to those of the FPG and the 2-hour OGGT plasma glucose. However, both A1C and FPG (in type 2 diabetes) have become the measurements of choice in monitoring the treatment of diabetes, and decisions on when and how to implement therapy are often made on the basis of A1C. The revised criteria are for diagnosis and are not treatment criteria or goals of therapy. Rather, current glycemic targets from the ADA include fasting and preprandial plasma glucose of 70 to 130 mg/dL (3.9 to 7.2 mmol/L), plasma glucose less than 180 mg/dL (10 mmol/L) 1 to 2 hours after eating, and particularly a target A1C of <7%.[4] However, it should be noted that this A1C recommendation is a

general target and that the goal for the individual patient is to be as close to normal as possible (A1C of <6%) without significant hypoglycemia.

Screening is important for a variety of reasons. Hyperglycemia is important in the pathogenesis both of the specific complications of diabetes mellitus—microangiopathy (retinopathy and nephropathy) and neuropathy—and in the development of macrovascular disease (atherosclerosis). Meticulous glycemic control slows the course of development of diabetic complications. Prolongation of normoglycemia reduces the risk of diabetic complications. Undetected type 2 diabetes is common; it is estimated that 30% to 35% of individuals with type 2 diabetes are unaware that they have the disease and that undiagnosed diabetes exists for 4 to 7 years prior to clinical recognition.[5] Studies suggest that interventions such as diet and exercise may forestall the evolution of type 2 diabetes.[6,7] Screening for type 2 diabetes is now easy; only a simple FPG is required. The more cumbersome OGTT is no longer the primary screening tool. Screening and early diagnosis of type 2 diabetes should be highly cost-effective. All adults over age 45 should be screened every 3 years. All individuals at higher risk (based on obesity, ethnicity, etc.) should be screened annually, starting at an earlier age.

Glycemic Control

The debate over the role of careful glycemic control in the evolution of complications has ended, thanks in particular to the *Diabetes Control and Complications Trial* (DCCT), which studied patients with type 1 diabetes, and the *United Kingdom Prospective Diabetes Study* (UKPDS), which focused on patients with type 2 diabetes. Yet the evidence that hyperglycemia is important had been accumulating from many other epidemiologic studies and small randomized controlled clinical trials, all of which suggested a significant relationship between glycemia and complications.[8]

One of the longest, largest, and most carefully conducted epidemiologic studies is the *Wisconsin Epidemiologic Study of Diabetic Retinopathy* (WESDR), which, although named for retinopathy, examined a whole array of complications.[9–12] The Wisconsin study was a population-based study among diabetic patients receiving community care in 11 counties in southern Wisconsin. The sample included a "younger onset cohort" of all diabetic subjects with onset less than age 30 years ($n = 1210$), presumably mostly with type 1 diabetes, and an "older onset cohort" of a probability sample of those with onset greater than age 30 years ($n = 1780$ of 5431 patients with a confirmed diagnosis of diabetes). For many analyses, the older onset cohort was divided into those not treated with insulin (53.7% of the original sample), presumably with type 2 diabetes, and those treated with insulin (46.3% of the original sample), most likely a mixed group with most having type 2 diabetes. These individuals underwent baseline evaluation in 1980 to 1982, with follow-up evaluations performed after 4, 10, and 14 years. Evaluations were conducted in a van and included historical data, blood pressure, visual acuity, seven-field fundus photography, and measurement of A1C and urine protein.

Data from the WESDR demonstrated a strong consistent relationship between hyperglycemia and the incidence and/or progression of microvascular (diabetic retinopathy, loss of vision, and nephropathy), neurologic (loss of tactile sensation or temperature sensitivity), and macrovascular (amputation and cardiovascular disease mortality) complications in people with type 1 and type 2 diabetes.

Epidemiologic studies, however, cannot demonstrate a treatment effect. A number of randomized, controlled clinical trials have shown that meticulous control of blood glucose dramatically reduces the frequency and progression of diabetic complications.

The DCCT, a randomized, multicenter controlled clinical trial, demonstrated that intensive treatment of type 1 diabetes, with the goal of meticulous glycemic control, reduced the frequency and severity of retinopathy, nephropathy, and neuropathy.[13] The DCCT was conducted in 29 centers across North America (26 in the United States and three in Canada) and included 1441 subjects with type 1 diabetes. Of the subjects enrolled, 726 were in a primary prevention cohort, with less than 5 years' duration of diabetes, normal albumin excretion, and no retinopathy at baseline. Another 715 subjects were in a secondary intervention cohort, with less than 15 years' duration of diabetes and at baseline having mild to moderate background retinopathy and either normal albumin excretion or microalbuminuria. Subjects were randomly assigned either to intensive therapy or to conventional therapy. Intensive therapy consisted of insulin administered either by continuous subcutaneous insulin infusion with an external insulin pump or by multiple daily insulin injections (three or more injections per day) guided by frequent self-monitoring of blood glucose three to four times daily, with additional specified samples including a weekly overnight sample, as well as meticulous attention to diet, with monthly visits to the treating clinic. Conventional therapy consisted of no more than two daily insulin injections, urine glucose monitoring or self-monitoring of blood glucose no more than twice daily, periodic diet review, and clinic visits every 2 to 3 months.

The intensive group achieved a median A1C of 7.2% versus 9.1% for the conventional group ($p < .001$). Mean blood glucose was 155 mg/dL (8.6 mmol/L) in the intensive group and 230 mg/dL (12.8 mmol/L) in the conventional group. Glycemic separation was maintained for 4 to 9 years, with mean duration of follow-up of 6.5 years, for a total of approximately 9300 patient-years of observation. Of 1430 subjects who were alive at the end of the study, 1422 came for evaluation of outcomes.

Risk reductions for microvascular and neurologic end points in the DCCT were dramatic: over 70% for clinically important sustained retinopathy, 56% for laser photocoagulation, 60% for sustained microalbuminuria, 54% for clinical grade nephropathy, and 64% for confirmed clinical neuropathy. Macrovascular end points demonstrated a trend in risk reduction (42%), which did not quite reach statistical significance. In the DCCT, there was a continuous exponential relationship between prevailing glycemia and complications, without evidence of a glycemic threshold.[14]

At the end of the DCCT, although the care of all patients was transferred to their own physicians, most were enrolled in the *Epidemiology of Diabetes Interventions and Complications* (EDIC) study, an observational study to assess the long-term outcomes in subjects who had participated in the DCCT. During EDIC follow-up,[15,16] the difference in median A1C narrowed, and by year 6, both groups had A1C levels of 8.1%. Nevertheless, during 8 years of follow-up, a smaller proportion of patients in the previous intensive group, compared to those in the previous conventional group, had worsening of retinopathy or nephropathy. Although the EDIC follow-up demonstrated narrowing of the differences between the groups in terms of median A1C, differences between the groups persisted, with continued lower risk of retinopathy, nephropathy, and neuropathy in the previous intensive therapy group. There is no way to distinguish whether the differences that were noted are related to continuing effects from some self-perpetuating process initiated by hyperglycemia or whether they also demonstrate, to some extent, a sustained effect of intensive control, perhaps below a threshold.

Most important, after 11 years of EDIC follow-up and a mean of 17 years of total observation, an impact on macrovascular disease could be demonstrated.[17] Intensive treatment reduced the risk of any cardiovascular disease event by 42% ($p = .02$) and the risk of nonfatal myocardial infarction, stroke, or death from cardiovascular disease by 57% ($p = .02$). The decrease in A1C values during the DCCT was significantly associated with most of the positive effects of intensive treatment on the risk of cardiovascular disease.

The UKPDS, a randomized, multicenter, controlled clinical trial, demonstrated that an intensive treatment policy in type 2 diabetes, with the goal of meticulous glycemic control, could decrease clinical diabetic complications.[18,19] The UKPDS was conducted in 23 centers and included 5102 subjects with newly diagnosed type 2 diabetes, 25 to 63 years of age at entry (median: 53 years). Subjects were randomly assigned to either intensive treatment policy or conventional treatment policy. Intensive policy aimed at achieving fasting plasma glucose of 108 mg/dL, using various pharmacologic agents. Conventional policy attempted control with diet alone, adding pharmacologic therapy only when symptoms developed or when FPG exceeded 270 mg/dL (15.0 mmol/L).

The intensive policy group achieved a median A1C of 7.0% compared to 7.9% in the conventional policy group ($p < .001$). Although there was a progressive deterioration in glycemia over time, a degree of glycemic separation was maintained for 6 to 20 years, with a median duration of follow-up of 11 years. The primary outcome measures in the UKPDS were three aggregate end points: "any diabetes-related end point," "diabetes-related death," and "all-cause mortality." Of these, only "any diabetes-related end point" was significantly affected, with a 12% risk reduction. In addition, risk reductions were seen for other end points. Patients assigned to intensive policy had a significant 25% risk reduction in microvascular end points compared with conventional policy, most of which was due to fewer cases of retinal photocoagulation, for which there was a 29% risk reduction. There was also a decreased risk of cataract extraction (24%), deterioration in retinopathy (21% reduction at 12 years' follow-up), and microalbuminuria (33% reduction at 12 years' follow-up). A decrease in microvascular complications was seen regardless of the primary treatment modality for intensive therapy, that is, insulin, sulfonylureas, or metformin. Thus, improved glycemic control was the principal factor. The only macrovascular end point that demonstrated a trend on risk reduction in the main analysis was myocardial infarction (16%), which did not quite reach statistical significance. However, with longer poststudy follow-up of UKPDS subjects, a beneficial impact on cardiovascular disease also emerged,[20] similar to what was seen in the EDIC follow-up of DCCT.

In the metformin subgroup analysis within the original UKPDS, however, there were significant risk reductions in diabetes-related deaths (42%), any diabetes-related end point (32%), and myocardial infarction (39%).[19] A combined analysis of all macrovascular end points (myocardial infarction, sudden death, angina, stroke, and peripheral vascular disease) showed a risk reduction of 30% over the conventional therapy group.

The beneficial effects and impact of effective glycemic control were also seen in a small study reported from Kumamoto University in Japan that involved 110 nonobese patients with type 2 diabetes.[21] This study contrasted intensive insulin therapy (multiple daily injections, preprandial regular and bedtime intermediate acting insulin) with conventional insulin therapy (once- or twice-daily intermediate acting insulin) in two cohorts, a "primary prevention cohort" and a "secondary intervention cohort." Over 6 years of follow-up, glycemic outcomes and risk reductions were almost identical to those found in the DCCT. The intensive therapy group achieved a mean A1C over the 6 years of the study of 7.1% versus a value in the conventional therapy group of 9.4% ($p < 0.001$). Mean fasting blood glucose was 157 mg/dL (8.7 mmol/L) in the intensive group and 221 mg/dL (12.3 mmol/L) in the conventional group. Retinopathy progression was reduced by 69%, nephropathy progres-

sion by 70%, while motor and sensory nerve conduction velocities and vibration thresholds were better in the intensive group than in the conventional group.

Thus, there are consistent and substantial beneficial effects of improved glycemic control in both type 1 and type 2 diabetes, affecting the entire array of diabetic complications. The current glycemic recommendations of the ADA appear in their *Standards of Medical Care for Patients with Diabetes Mellitus.*[4] The goal is, ideally, fasting plasma glucose (FPG) 90 to 130 mg/dL (5.0 to 7.2 mmol/L), peak postprandial glucose less than 180 mg/dL (10.0 mmol/L), and A1C below 7% (normal range: ~3.0% to 6.0%) for patients in general, namely, any group of patients. However, beginning in 2006, the ADA also asserts that "The A1C goal for the individual patient is an A1C as close to normal (<6%) as possible without significant hypoglycemia." In the view of the author, an additional category should be "unacceptable" glycemic control when FPG is consistently more than 140 mg/dL (7.8 mmol/L) or A1C is above 8%.

Contemporary diabetes management is based on the concept of targeted glycemic control. Therapy, based on glycemic goals, utilizes progressive stepwise additions of whatever treatment modality is necessary to achieve those goals. Medical nutritional therapy and promotion of physical activity are fundamental and needed for all patients, as is basic diabetes education.

Intensive insulin therapy is mandatory in type 1 diabetes. This is accomplished, as in the DCCT, with insulin administered either by continuous subcutaneous insulin infusion with a pump or by multiple daily insulin injections; frequent self-monitoring of blood glucose; and meticulous attention to balancing insulin dose, food intake, and energy expenditure.[22] Better postprandial glycemic control may be achieved with the addition of the amylin analogue pramlintide before meals.[23]

In type 2 diabetes, progressive pharmacologic therapy is required; the specific choice based on disease severity and glycemic targets.[24,25] A growing number of classes of pharmacologic agents are available to control glycemia. These include insulin secretagogues (e.g., sulfonylureas and glinides), which stimulate insulin production; insulin sensitizers (e.g., biguanides and thiazolidinediones), which enhance muscle glucose uptake and decrease hepatic glucose production; α-glucosidase inhibitors, which retard carbohydrate absorption; incretin mimetics (e.g., exenatide), which restore islet sensitivity to glucose and modulate carbohydrate absorption; incretin enhancers (also known as DPP4 inhibitors), which prolong activity of circulating incretins; and replacement of insulin deficiency with insulin or insulin analogues. The availability of agents with differing and complementary mechanisms of action allows them to be used in various combinations, thus increasing the likelihood that satisfactory glycemic control can be achieved in any given patient.

Blood Pressure Control

Several clinical trials have addressed the influence of blood pressure control in diabetes. The *Hypertension in Diabetes Study* (HDS) was embedded in the UKPDS by using a factorial design.[26,27] HDS was conducted in 20 centers among 1148 patients with type 2 diabetes and coexisting hypertension. The design was a randomized controlled trial comparing tight control of blood pressure aiming at a blood pressure of less than 150/85 mm Hg with less tight control aiming at a blood pressure of less than 180/105 mm Hg. Median follow-up was 8.4 years. The tight control group achieved a mean blood pressure of 144/82 mm Hg versus 154/87 mm Hg in the less tight control group ($p < .0001$).

Risk reductions in the HDS were substantial. Patients assigned tight control had a 24% risk reduction for any diabetes-related end point, a 32% risk reduction for diabetes-related deaths, 56% risk reduction for heart failure, a 44% risk reduction for stroke, and a 37% risk reduction for microvascular disease, compared to the less tight control group. After 7.5 years of follow-up, the group assigned to tight control also had a 34% reduction in risk of deterioration of retinopathy and a 47% reduced risk of deterioration in visual acuity.

The *Hypertension Optimal Treatment* (HOT) *study* was a randomized multinational trial involving 18,790 hypertensive patients, aged 50 to 80 years (mean: 61.5 years) with diastolic blood pressure of 100 to 115 mm Hg, including 1501 patients with diabetes at baseline.[28] They were randomly assigned to three different target diastolic blood pressure groups: less than or equal to 90 mm Hg, less than or equal to 85 mm Hg, and less than or equal to 80 mm Hg. Felodipine was given as baseline therapy with the addition of other agents, according to a five-step regimen.

In the patients with diabetes in HOT, with the lowest target blood pressure (≤80 mm Hg), there was a decline in the rate of major cardiovascular events, cardiovascular mortality, and total mortality. In the group that was randomized to 80 mm Hg or lower, the risk of major cardiovascular events was halved in comparison with that of the target group (≤90 mm Hg). This change was attenuated but remained significant when silent myocardial infarctions were included. The approximate halving of the risk was also observed for all myocardial infarctions, although it was not significant. Stroke also showed a declining rate with lower target blood pressure groups.

The *Systolic Hypertension in Europe* (Syst-Eur) *trial* included a post hoc analysis of the data in this trial to determine the effects on long-term outcome in diabetic versus nondiabetic patients with hypertension.[29] In Syst-Eur, 4695 patients (≥60 years of age), including 492 (10.5%) with diabetes, who had systolic blood pressure of 160 to 219 mm Hg and diastolic pressure below

95 mm Hg, were randomly assigned to receive either active treatment or placebo. Active treatment consisted of nitrendipine, with the possible addition or substitution of enalapril or hydrochlorothiazide or both, titrated to reduce the systolic blood pressure by at least 20 mm Hg and to less than 150 mm Hg. In the control group, matching placebo tablets were administered similarly. Among the diabetic patients, after a median follow-up of 2 years, the systolic and diastolic blood pressures in the two treatment groups differed by 8.6 and 3.9 mm Hg, respectively. Active treatment of the diabetic patients reduced their overall mortality by 55%, mortality from cardiovascular disease by 76%, all cardiovascular events combined by 69%, fatal and nonfatal strokes by 73%, and all cardiac events combined by 63%.

The *Antihypertensive and Lipid-Lowering Treatment to Prevent Heart Attack Trial* (ALLHAT) studied whether treatment with a calcium channel blocker or an angiotensin-converting enzyme inhibitor decreases clinical complications compared with treatment with a thiazide-type diuretic in 13,101 subjects with type 2 diabetes.[30] It found that there was no fundamental difference in cardiovascular outcomes for treatment with any of these agents as first-step antihypertensive therapy.

Thus, there are consistent and substantial beneficial effects of improved blood pressure control in diabetic patients, affecting various complications of diabetes. In patients with diabetes, current blood pressure recommendations of the American Diabetes Association appear in their *Position Statement on Treatment of Hypertension in Diabetes*,[31] which is based on a technical review on the same subject.[32] Similar recommendations are contained in the *Seventh Report of the Joint National Committee on Detection, Evaluation, and Treatment of High Blood Pressure*[33] and in the guidelines developed by the European Society of Hypertension and European Society of Cardiology.[34]

The primary goal of therapy for nonpregnant adults (>18 years of age) with diabetes is to decrease blood pressure to, and maintain it at, less than 130 mm Hg systolic and less than 85 mm Hg diastolic. In children, blood pressure should be decreased to the corresponding age-adjusted 90th percentile values. It should be noted, however, that in the general population, the risks for end-organ damage appear to be lowest when the systolic blood pressure is less than 120 mm Hg and the diastolic blood pressure is less than 70 mm Hg. For patients with an isolated systolic hypertension of greater than 180 mm Hg, the initial goal of treatment is to reduce the systolic blood pressure to less than 160 mm Hg. For those with systolic blood pressure of 160 to 179, the goal is a reduction of 20 mm Hg. If these aims are achieved and well tolerated, further lowering to less than 140 mm Hg may be appropriate. An approach for achieving such control has been reviewed.[35]

Control of Lipids

The *Scandinavian Simvastatin Survival Study (4S)* was a randomized, multinational trial involving 4444 patients, aged 35 to 70 years (mean: 58.9 years) with known coronary heart disease (CHD) manifested by angina pectoris or previous myocardial infarction, who had serum cholesterol levels of 5.5 to 8.0 mmol/L (213 to 310 mg/dL) while on a lipid-lowering diet.[36] The study included 202 diabetic patients. In 4S, patients were randomly assigned to receive either active treatment with simvastatin 20 mg/day (with masked dosage titration up to 40 mg/day, according to cholesterol response during the first 6 to 18 weeks) or placebo. Over the 5.4-year median follow-up period, simvastatin produced mean changes in total cholesterol, LDL-C, and high-density lipoprotein cholesterol (HDL-C) of –25%, –35%, and +8%, respectively.

The investigators performed a post hoc subgroup analysis comparing the diabetic and nondiabetic patients.[37] Mean changes in serum lipids in diabetic patients were similar to those observed in nondiabetic patients. The results strongly suggest that lowering cholesterol improves the prognosis of diabetic patients with CHD. Among the diabetic patients, active treatment reduced total mortality by 43%, major cardiovascular events combined by 55%, and any atherosclerotic event by 37%. The corresponding risk reductions in nondiabetic patients were less, such that the investigators asserted that the absolute clinical benefit achieved by cholesterol lowering might be greater in diabetic than in nondiabetic patients with CHD because diabetic patients have a higher absolute risk of recurrent CHD events and other atherosclerotic events.

The *Cholesterol and Recurrent Events* (CARE) *trial* was a randomized, multicenter trial involving 4159 patients with myocardial infarction who had plasma total cholesterol levels below 240 mg/dL (mean: 209) and LDL-C levels of 115 to 174 mg/dL (mean: 139).[38] The study included 586 patients (14.1%) with a clinical diagnosis of diabetes and 342 patients with IFG at entry,[39] as defined by the 1997 American Diabetes Association criteria, that is, 110 to 125 mg/dL.[2] In CARE, patients were randomly assigned to receive active treatment with pravastatin 40 mg daily or placebo for 5 years. The primary end point was a fatal coronary event or a nonfatal myocardial infarction. The investigators performed a post hoc subgroup analysis comparing the diabetic and nondiabetic patients.[39] Mean LDL-C reduction was similar (27% and 28%) in the diabetic and nondiabetic groups, respectively. As in 4S, in the placebo group, the diabetic patients suffered more recurrent coronary events (CHD death, nonfatal myocardial infarction, coronary bypass surgery, and coronary angioplasty) than did the nondiabetic patients (37% versus 25%). Pravastatin treatment reduced the absolute risk of coronary events for the diabetic and nondiabetic patients by 8.1% and 5.2%

and the relative risk by 25% and 23%, respectively. For the diabetic patients, the relative risk for revascularization procedures was reduced by 32%. Patients with IFG had a higher rate of recurrent coronary events than did those with normal fasting glucose, but the recurrence rates for nonfatal myocardial infarction in IFG patients were reduced by 50%.

The *Heart Protection Study* (HPS) was a randomized, multicenter trial involving 5963 diabetic patients and 14,973 nondiabetic patients with coronary disease or other occlusive arterial disease who had total cholesterol concentrations of at least 135 mg/dL (3.5 mmol/L).[40,41] In HPS, patients were randomly assigned to receive either active treatment with simvastatin 40 mg daily or placebo for 5 years. The primary outcomes were mortality and fatal or nonfatal vascular events. The average difference in LDL-C was 39 mg/dL (1.0 mmol/L). Among the diabetic patients, treatment with simvastatin reduced major coronary events, strokes and revascularizations, with a 22% reduction in the first event rate of these ($p < .0001$). The beneficial effects were seen among both the 2912 diabetic participants who did not have any diagnosed occlusive arterial disease at entry (reduction of 33%, $p = .0003$), and among the 2426 diabetic participants whose pretreatment LDL-C concentration was 116 mg/dL (<3.0 mmol/L) (reduction of 27%, $p = .0007$). Thus, the HPS provides direct evidence that statin therapy is beneficial for people with diabetes even if they do not already have manifest coronary disease or high cholesterol concentrations.

The *Collaborative Atorvastatin Diabetes Study* (CARDS) was a randomized, multicenter trial involving 2838 patients with type 2 diabetes without either raised cholesterol levels (average baseline LDL-C: 118 mg/dL or 3.1 mmol/L), or prior clinical history of coronary, cerebrovascular or peripheral vascular disease.[42] Thus, this was a primary prevention study. Patients were randomly assigned to receive either active treatment with low-dose atorvastatin 10 mg daily or placebo. The study was terminated early after a median follow-up of 3.9 years. The primary end point was time to first occurrence of acute coronary heart disease events, coronary revascularization, or stroke. Treatment with low-dose atorvastatin resulted in a 37% risk reduction for the primary end point, including a 36% risk reduction for acute coronary events and a 48% risk reduction for strokes. The CARDS investigators concluded that it might be that all persons with diabetes warrant statin treatment.

The *Anglo-Scandinavian Cardiac Outcomes Trial-Lipid Lowering Arm* (ASCOT-LLA) was a randomized, multicenter trial involving 10,305 hypertensive patients with at least three other cardiovascular risk factors, with total cholesterol concentrations less than 252 mg/dL (6.5 mmol/L).[43] The study included 2532 diabetic patients. Although treatment with low-dose atorvastatin reduced total cardiovascular events, total coronary events, and strokes by 36%, the relative reduction was less (only 16%) for the primary end point among patients with diabetes than among those without and did not reach statistical significance.

The *Pravastatin or Atorvastatin Evaluation and Infection Therapy-Thrombolysis in Myocardial Infarction* (PROVE-IT) trial was a randomized, multicenter trial involving 4162 people who had been hospitalized for an acute coronary syndrome within the preceding 10 days. This trial compared pravastatin standard therapy (40 mg/day) with atorvastatin high-dose intensive therapy (80 mg/day).[44] The study included 734 diabetic patients. The primary end point was a composite of death from any cause or a major cardiovascular event (myocardial infarction, documented unstable angina requiring rehospitalization, revascularization, or stroke). The median LDL-C level achieved was 95 mg/dL (2.46 mmol/L) in the pravastatin group and 62 mg/dL (1.60 mmol/L) in the atorvastatin group ($p < .001$). Overall, intensive therapy showed a 16% risk reduction ($p = .005$) in the primary end point. Among the relatively small proportion of subjects with diabetes, the risk reduction was 17%, which did not reach statistical significance.

The *Fenofibrate Intervention and Event Lowering in Diabetes* (FIELD) study was a randomized, multicenter trial involving 9795 patients with type 2 diabetes not taking statin therapy at study entry, designed to assess the effect of micronized fenofibrate 200 mg daily or matched placebo on cardiovascular disease events.[45] The primary outcomes were coronary events (coronary heart disease death or nonfatal myocardial infarction). After a median 5 years of follow-up, there was a reduction of 11% in the risk for the primary end point, but this did not reach statistical significance ($p = 0.16$). Although some secondary end points were significant, the FIELD study did not provide evidence to warrant a recommendation for fibrate use in patients with diabetes.

Collectively, these studies unambiguously demonstrate the beneficial effects of lipid-lowering therapy with statins for people with diabetes. The benefits are seen across the spectrum of baseline levels of cholesterol, whether or not there are other cardiovascular risk factors.

Thus, careful control of lipids has consistent and substantial beneficial effects; specifically, LDL-C in diabetic patients, affecting recurrent coronary disease. Although this was not directly examined in these studies, it is probably a reasonable assumption that such lipid lowering will reduce the risk from peripheral vascular disease as well.

In patients with diabetes, current lipid treatment recommendations of the American Diabetes Association appear in their *Standards of Medical Care for Patients with Diabetes Mellitus*[4] and in a position statement on management of dyslipidemia in adults with diabetes,[46] which is based on a technical review on the same subject.[47] The National Cholesterol Education Program Expert Panel on Detection, Evaluation, and Treatment of High Blood Cholesterol in Adults (Adult Treatment Panel III) identified diabetes as a high-risk condition.[48] More recently,

these recommendations have been updated, taking into account the recent studies cited above.[49] Thus, patients with the combination of diabetes and cardiovascular disease deserve intensive lipid-lowering therapy. In high-risk individuals, the recommended goal is LDL-C less than 100 mg/dL (2.6 mmol/L), but when risk is very high, an LDL-C goal of <70 mg/dL (1.8 mmol/L) is a reasonable clinical strategy, on the basis of available clinical trial evidence. For patients with diabetes plus cardiovascular disease, it is reasonable to attempt to achieve a very low LDL-C level, <70 mg/dL (1.8 mmol/L). On the basis of the HPS, the presence of this combination appears to support initiation of statin therapy regardless of baseline LDL-C levels. This therapeutic option extends also to patients at very high risk who have a baseline LDL-C less than 100 mg/dL (<2.6 mmol/L).

Target levels for HDL-C are >40 mg/dL (1.02 mmol/L); and target triglyceride levels are <150 mg/dL (1.7 mmol/L). In women, who tend to have higher HDL-C levels than men, an HDL-C goal that is 10 mg/dL higher may be appropriate. Moreover, when a diabetic patient, particularly one with high risk, has high triglycerides or low HDL-C, consideration can be given to combining a fibrate or nicotinic acid along with an LDL-C-lowering drug.

Aspirin and Other Antiplatelet Therapy

The *Physicians' Health Study* was a randomized trial involving 22,071 healthy U.S. male physicians aged 40 to 84, designed to determine whether low-dose aspirin (325 mg every other day) decreases cardiovascular mortality.[50] The aspirin component was terminated earlier than scheduled after an average follow-up time of 60.2 months, owing to the dramatic results. There was a 44% reduction in the risk of occurrence of a first myocardial infarction ($p < .00001$) in the aspirin group. Subgroup analyses in the diabetic physicians revealed a reduction in myocardial infarction from 10.1% (placebo) to 4.0% (aspirin), yielding a risk reduction of 61% for the diabetic men on aspirin therapy. This supports the use of aspirin therapy for primary prevention in patients with diabetes. In addition, there was a 46% reduction in the risk of peripheral artery surgery in the aspirin group ($p = .03$).[51]

The *Early Treatment Diabetic Retinopathy Study* (ETDRS) was a randomized trial involving 3711 type 1 and type 2 diabetic men and women, about 48% of whom had a history of cardiovascular disease.[52] The study therefore may be viewed as a mixed primary and secondary prevention trial. Patients were randomly assigned to aspirin or placebo (two 325-mg tablets once per day). The risk reduction for myocardial infarction in the first 5 years in those who were randomized to aspirin therapy was 28%. In the HOT study mentioned earlier, aspirin reduced major cardiovascular events by 15% and all myocardial infarctions by 36%.[28] The effect was seen in both diabetic and nondiabetic patients.

The *Department of Veterans Affairs Cooperative Study on Antiplatelet Agents in Diabetic Patients After Amputation for Gangrene* was a small multicenter, randomized trial on the effects of aspirin plus dipyridamole versus placebo on major vascular end points in 231 diabetic men with either a recent amputation for gangrene or active gangrene.[53] Survival curve analyses revealed little difference between groups for major vascular end points, total mortality, all amputations, or myocardial infarctions. However, the overall rate of atherosclerotic deaths was 20.3%, and the overall rate of opposite-side amputations was 22.1%. This suggests that the subjects might have had such advanced disease that any effect of antiplatelet therapy was precluded.

An analysis of antiplatelet therapy, particularly with aspirin, has been published.[54] The analysis considered 174 randomized trials involving approximately 100,000 patients. In each of four main high-risk categories (patients with acute myocardial infarction, patients with a past history of myocardial infarction, patients with a past history of stroke or transient ischemic attack, and patients with some other relevant medical history [unstable angina, stable angina, vascular surgery, angioplasty, atrial fibrillation, valvular disease, peripheral vascular disease, etc.]), antiplatelet therapy was definitely protective. Reductions in vascular events were about one quarter in each of these four main categories and were separately statistically significant in middle age and old age, in men and women, in hypertensive and normotensive patients, and in diabetic and nondiabetic patients. Taking all high-risk patients together showed reductions of about one third in nonfatal myocardial infarction, about one third in nonfatal stroke, and about one third in vascular death. It was estimated that 38 ± 12 vascular events per 1000 diabetic patients would be prevented if they were treated with aspirin as a secondary prevention strategy. The most widely tested regimen was medium-dose (75 to 325 mg/day) aspirin. Doses throughout this range seemed similarly effective. There was no appreciable evidence that either a higher aspirin dose or any other antiplatelet regimen was more effective than medium-dose aspirin in preventing vascular events. Among low-risk recipients of primary prevention, a significant reduction of one third in nonfatal myocardial infarction was, however, accompanied by a nonsignificant increase in stroke.

Thus, there are beneficial effects of antiplatelet therapy, particularly with aspirin, in diabetic patients, affecting various diabetic complications. In patients with diabetes, current recommendations of the American Diabetes Association appear in their *Standards of Medical Care for Patients with Diabetes Mellitus*[4] and in a position statement, "*Aspirin Therapy in Diabetes*,"[55] which is based on a technical review on the same subject.[56] The ADA specifically advocates the use of aspirin therapy as a secondary prevention strategy in diabetic men and women who have evidence of large vessel disease, including a history of myocardial infarction, vascular bypass procedure, stroke or transient ischemic attack, peripheral vascular disease, claudication, and/or angina. The ADA also recommends considering aspirin therapy as a primary prevention strategy in high-risk men and women with type 1 or type 2 diabetes. The U.S. Preventive Services Task Force has recommended aspirin as a primary and secondary therapy to prevent cardiovascular events in diabetic and nondiabetic individuals.[57,58] Clopidogrel has been demonstrated to reduce cardiovascular disease rates in diabetic individuals.[59] Adjunctive therapy with clopidogrel should be considered in very high risk patients or as alternative therapy in those who are aspirin-intolerant.

Smoking

Issues of smoking in diabetes are reviewed in detail in the ADA technical review[60] and position statement[61] on smoking cessation. A large body of evidence from epidemiologic, case-control, and cohort studies provides convincing documentation of the causal link between cigarette smoking and health risks. Cigarette smoking contributes to one of every five deaths in the United States and is the most important modifiable cause of premature death. On the other hand, although cigarette smoking is a major risk factor for peripheral vascular disease and amputation in nondiabetic people, among people with diabetes, the evidence for a relationship between tobacco and ulcers or amputation is variable. In the WESDR mentioned earlier, in type 1 diabetes, there was an association between foot ulcers and either being a current smoker or having a 10+ pack-year history of smoking.[62] However, no increased risk was found for smokers with type 2 diabetes in the same population. Most other studies have failed to show an association between cigarette smoking and an increased risk of macrovascular disease, peripheral vascular disease, diabetic foot ulcers, or amputation in diabetic individuals, as was recently discussed in an American Diabetes Association *Technical Review on Foot Problems in Diabetes*.[63] Only a few studies show a weak relationship between smoking and peripheral vascular disease, ulcers, or amputation risk. On the other hand, in people with diabetes, tobacco use has been associated with both microvascular disease (i.e., retinopathy, nephropathy) and cardiovascular disease. As a consequence, smoking cessation should be recommended to all individuals with diabetes, and that recommendation should be continually reinforced.

Concluding Remarks

The American Diabetes Association annually publishes its *Clinical Practice Recommendations*,[64] including its *Standards of Medical Care for Patients with Diabetes*

Mellitus.[4] These are contained in a supplement to *Diabetes Care* and are available on the World Wide Web at *www.diabetes.org.* Patients with diabetes mellitus have long suffered from the devastating complications that threaten their lives. The challenge for all health care providers caring for diabetic patients is to recognize that there is a growing body of evidence, based on controlled clinical trials, demonstrating that the impact of this dreaded disease can be dramatically lessened. To benefit from recent advances, patients with diabetes must understand the treatment goals and must strive to attain excellent glycemic control, aggressive control of blood pressure, and normalization of lipids. A combination approach that stresses all of these variables has proven to be particularly beneficial.[65–67] Patients also should avoid cigarette smoking, use prophylactic aspirin therapy, take excellent care of their feet, have regular medical examinations, and avail themselves of appropriate interventions as needed. When this occurs on a regular basis, it should be possible to reduce the risk of complications and lessen the burden of diabetes.

References

1. Centers for Disease Control and Prevention: National diabetes fact sheet 2005. Available at *http://www.cdc.gov/diabetes/pubs/ estimates05.htm#prev.*
2. American Diabetes Association: Report of the Expert Committee on the Diagnosis and Classification of Diabetes Mellitus. Diabetes Care 20:1183–1197, 1997.
3. American Diabetes Association: Report of the Expert Committee on the Diagnosis and Classification of Diabetes Mellitus. Diabetes Care 26:3160–3167, 2003.
4. American Diabetes Association: Standards of medical care for patients with diabetes mellitus. Diabetes Care 30(suppl 1):S4–S41, 2007.
5. Harris MI, Klein R, Welborn TA, Knuiman MW: Onset of NIDDM occurs at least 4–7 years before clinical diagnosis. Diabetes Care 15:815–819, 1992.
6. Finnish Diabetes Prevention Study Group: Prevention of type 2 diabetes mellitus by changes in lifestyle among subjects with impaired glucose tolerance. N Engl J Med 344:1343–1350, 2001.
7. Diabetes Prevention Program Research Group: Reduction in the incidence of type 2 diabetes with lifestyle intervention or metformin. N Engl J Med 346:393–403, 2002.
8. Skyler JS: Diabetic complications: Glucose control is important. Endocrinol Metab Clin North Am 25:243–254, 1996.
9. Klein R, Klein BEK, Moss SE, et al: Glycosylated hemoglobin predicts the incidence and progression of diabetic retinopathy. JAMA 260:2864–2871, 1988.
10. Klein R, Klein BEK, Moss SE, Cruickshanks KJ: Relationship of hyperglycemia to the long-term incidence and progression of diabetic retinopathy. Arch Intern Med 154:2169–2178, 1994.
11. Klein R: Hyperglycemia and microvascular and macrovascular disease in diabetes. Diabetes Care 18:258–268, 1995.
12. Klein R, Klein BEK, Moss SE: Relation of glycemic control to diabetic microvascular complications in diabetes mellitus. Ann Intern Med 124:90–96, 1996.
13. Diabetes Control and Complications Trial Research Group: The effect of intensive treatment of diabetes on the development and progression of long-term complications in insulin-dependent diabetes mellitus. N Engl J Med 329:683–689, 1993.
14. Diabetes Control and Complications Trial Research Group: The relationship of glycemic exposure (HbA$_{1c}$) to the risk of development and progression of retinopathy in the Diabetes Control and Complications Trial. Diabetes 44:968–993, 1995.
15. The Diabetes Control and Complications Trial/Epidemiology of Diabetes Interventions and Complications Research Group: Effect of intensive therapy on the microvascular complications of type 1 diabetes mellitus. JAMA 287:2563–2569, 2002.
16. The Diabetes Control and Complications Trial/Epidemiology of Diabetes Interventions and Complications (DCCT/EDIC) Study Research Group: Sustained effect of intensive treatment of type 1 diabetes mellitus on development and progression of diabetic nephropathy: The Epidemiology of Diabetes Interventions and Complications (EDIC) study. JAMA 290:2159–2167, 2003.
17. The Diabetes Control and Complications Trial/Epidemiology of Diabetes Interventions and Complications (DCCT/EDIC) Study Research Group: Intensive diabetes treatment and cardiovascular disease in patients with type 1 diabetes. N Engl J Med 353: 2643–2653, 2005.
18. UK Prospective Diabetes Study Group: Intensive blood-glucose control with sulfonylureas or insulin compared with conventional treatment and risk of complications in patients with type 2 diabetes (UKPDS 33). Lancet 352:837–853, 1998.
19. UK Prospective Diabetes Study Group: Effect of intensive blood-glucose control with metformin on complications in overweight patients with type 2 diabetes (UKPDS 34). Lancet 352:854–865, 1998.
20. Holman RR: UKPDS update. Presented at International Diabetes Federation, Paris, France, 2003.
21. Ohkubo Y, Kishikawa H, Araki E, et al: Intensive insulin therapy prevents the progression of diabetic microvascular complications in Japanese patients with non-insulin-dependent diabetes mellitus: A randomized prospective 6-year study. Diabetes Res Clin Pract 28:103–117, 1995.
22. Hirsch IB: Intensive treatment of type 1 diabetes. Med Clin North Am 82:689–719, 1998.
23. Ratner RE, Dickey R, Fineman M, et al: Amylin replacement with pramlintide as an adjunct to insulin therapy improves long-term glycaemic and weight control in type 1 diabetes mellitus: A 1-year, randomized controlled trial. Diabet Med 21:1204–1212, 2004.
24. Skyler JS: Diabetes mellitus: Pathogenesis and treatment strategies. J Med Chem 47:4113–4117, 2004.
25. Nathan DM, Buse JB, Davidson MB, et al: Management of hyperglycaemia in type 2 diabetes: A consensus algorithm for the initiation and adjustment of therapy. A consensus statement from the American Diabetes Association and the European Association for the Study of Diabetes. Diabetologia 49:1711–1721, 2006; Diabetes Care 29:1963–1972, 2006.
26. UK Prospective Diabetes Study Group: Tight blood pressure control and risk of macrovascular and microvascular complications in type 2 diabetes: UKPDS 38. BMJ 317:703–713, 1998.
27. UK Prospective Diabetes Study Group: Efficacy of atenolol and captopril in reducing risk of macrovascular and microvascular complications in type 2 diabetes: UKPDS 39. BMJ 317:713–720, 1998.
28. Hansson L, Zanchetti A, Carruthers SG, et al: Effects of intensive blood-pressure lowering and low-dose aspirin in patients with hypertension: Principal results of the Hypertension Optimal Treatment (HOT) randomised trial. Lancet 351:1755–1762, 1998.
29. Tuomilehto J, Rastenyte D, Birkenhager WH, et al: Effects of calcium-channel blockade in older patients with diabetes and systolic hypertension. N Engl J Med 340:677–684, 1999.
30. Whelton PK, Barzilay J, Cushman WC, et al: Clinical outcomes in antihypertensive treatment of type 2 diabetes, impaired concentration, and normoglycemia: Antihypertensive and Lipid-Lowering Treatment to Prevent Heart Attack Trial (ALLHAT). Arch Intern Med 165:1401–1409, 2005.
31. American Diabetes Association: Position statement: Hypertension management in adults with diabetes. Diabetes Care 27(suppl 1): S65–S67, 2004.
32. Arauz-Pacheco C, Parrott MA, Raskin P: The treatment of hypertension in adult patients with diabetes. Diabetes Care 25:134–147, 2002.
33. Chobanian AV, Bakris GL, Black HR, et al: The seventh report of the Joint National Committee on Prevention, Detection, Evaluation, and Treatment of High Blood Pressure: The JNC 7 report. JAMA 289:2560–2572, 2003.
34. Guidelines Committee: 2003 European Society of Hypertension-European Society of Cardiology guidelines for the management of arterial hypertension. J Hypertens 21:1011–1053, 2003.

35. Marks JB, Raskin P: Nephropathy and hypertension in diabetes. Med Clin North Am 82:877–907, 1998.

36. Scandinavian Simvastatin Survival Study Group: Randomised trial of cholesterol lowering in 4444 patients with coronary heart disease: The Scandinavian Simvastatin Survival Study (4S). Lancet 344:1383–1389, 1994.

37. Pyorala K, Pedersen TR, Kjekshus J, et al: Cholesterol lowering with simvastatin improves prognosis of diabetic patients with coronary heart disease: A subgroup analysis of the Scandinavian Simvastatin Survival Study (4S). Diabetes Care 20:614–620, 1997.

38. Sacks FM, Pfeffer MA, Moye LA, et al: The effect of pravastatin on coronary events after myocardial infarction in patients with average cholesterol levels: Cholesterol and Recurrent Events Trial investigators. N Engl J Med 335:1001–1009, 1996.

39. Goldberg RB, Mellies MJ, Sacks FM, et al: Cardiovascular events and their reduction with pravastatin in diabetic and glucose-intolerant myocardial infarction survivors with average cholesterol levels: Subgroup analyses in the Cholesterol and Recurrent Events (CARE) trial. Circulation 23:2513–2519, 1998.

40. Heart Protection Study Collaborative Group: MRC/BHF Heart Protection Study of cholesterol lowering with simvastatin in 20,536 high-risk individuals: A randomised placebo controlled trial. Lancet 360:7–22, 2002.

41. Heart Protection Study Collaborative Group: MRC/BHF Heart Protection Study of cholesterol-lowering with simvastatin in 5963 people with diabetes: A randomised placebo-controlled trial. Lancet 361:2005–2016, 2003.

42. Colhoun HM, Betteridge DJ, Durrington PN, et al: Primary prevention of cardiovascular disease with atorvastatin in type 2 diabetes in the Collaborative Atorvastatin Diabetes Study (CARDS): Multicentre randomised placebo-controlled trial. Lancet 364:685–696, 2004.

43. Sever PS, Dahlof B, Poulter NR, et al: Prevention of coronary and stroke events with atorvastatin in hypertensive patients who have average or lower-than-average cholesterol concentrations, in the Anglo-Scandinavian Cardiac Outcomes Trial-Lipid Lowering Arm (ASCOT-LLA): A multicentre randomised controlled trial. Lancet 361:1149–1158, 2003.

44. Cannon CP, Braunwald E, McCabe CH, et al: Intensive versus moderate lipid lowering with statins after acute coronary syndromes. N Engl J Med 350:1495–1504, 2004.

45. The FIELD study investigators: Effects of long-term fenofibrate therapy on cardiovascular events in 9795 people with type 2 diabetes mellitus (the FIELD study): Randomised controlled trial. Lancet 366:1849–1861, 2005.

46. American Diabetes Association: Position statement: Dyslipidemia management in adults with diabetes. Diabetes Care 27(suppl 1):S68–S71, 2004.

47. Haffner SM: Management of dyslipidemia in adults with diabetes. Diabetes Care 21:160–178, 1998.

48. National Cholesterol Education Program Expert Panel on Detection, Evaluation, and Treatment of High Blood Cholesterol in Adults (Adult Treatment Panel III): Third Report of the National Cholesterol Education Program (NCEP) Expert Panel on Detection, Evaluation, and Treatment of High Blood Cholesterol in Adults (Adult Treatment Panel III) Final Report. Circulation 106:3145–3421, 2002.

49. Grundy SM, Cleeman JI, Merz CN, et al: Implications of recent clinical trials for the National Cholesterol Education Program Adult Treatment Panel III guidelines. Circulation 110:227–239, 2004.

50. Steering Committee of the Physicians' Health Study Research Group: Final report on the aspirin component of the ongoing Physicians' Health Study. N Engl J Med 321:129–135, 1989.

51. Goldhaber SZ, Manson JE, Stampfer MJ, et al: Low-dose aspirin and subsequent peripheral arterial surgery in the Physicians' Health Study. Lancet 340:143–145, 1992.

52. ETDRS Investigators: Aspirin effects on mortality and morbidity in patients with diabetes mellitus: Early Treatment Diabetic Retinopathy Study Report 14. JAMA 268:1292–1300, 1992.

53. Colwell JA, Bingham SF, Abraira C, et al: Veterans Administration Cooperative Study on antiplatelet agents in diabetic patients after amputation for gangrene: II. Effects of aspirin and dipyridamole on atherosclerotic vascular disease rates. Diabetes Care 9:140–148, 1986.

54. Antiplatelet Trialists' Collaboration: Collaborative overview of randomised trials of antiplatelet therapy: I. Prevention of death, myocardial infarction, and stroke by prolonged antiplatelet therapy in various categories of patients. BMJ 308:81–106, 1994.

55. American Diabetes Association: Aspirin therapy in diabetes (position statement). Diabetes Care 27 (suppl 1):S72–S73, 2004.

56. Colwell JA: Aspirin therapy in diabetes. Diabetes Care 20:1767–1771, 1997.

57. Hayden M, Pignone M, Phillips C, Mulrow C: Aspirin for the primary prevention of cardiovascular events: A summary of the evidence for the U.S. Preventive Services Task Force. Ann Intern Med 136:161–172, 2002.

58. US Preventive Services Task Force: Aspirin for the primary prevention of cardiovascular events: Recommendation and rationale. Ann Intern Med 136:157–160, 2002.

59. Bhatt DL, Marso SP, Hirsch AT, et al: Amplified benefit of clopidogrel versus aspirin in patients with diabetes mellitus. Am J Cardiol 90:625–628, 2002.

60. Haire-Joshu D, Glasgow RE, Tibbs TL: Smoking and diabetes. Diabetes Care 22:1887–1898, 1999.

61. American Diabetes Asociation: Smoking and diabetes (position statement). Diabetes Care 27(suppl 1):S74–S75, 2004.

62. Moss SE, Klein R, Klein BE: The prevalence and incidence of lower extremity amputation in a diabetic population. Arch Intern Med 152:610–616, 1992.

63. Mayfield JA, Reiber GE, Sanders LJ, et al: Preventive foot care in people with diabetes (technical review). Diabetes Care 21:2161–2177, 1998.

64. American Diabetes Association: Clinical practice recommendations 2007. Diabetes Care 30(suppl 1): 2007:S1–S103.

65. Gæde P, Vedel P, Parving HH, Pedersen O: Intensified multifactorial intervention in patients with type 2 diabetes mellitus and microalbuminuria: The Steno type 2 randomised study. Lancet 353:617–622, 1999.

66. Gæde P, Vedel P, Larsen N, et al: Multifactorial intervention and cardiovascular disease in patients with type 2 diabetes. N Engl J Med 2003;348:383–393.

67. Gæde P, Pedersen O: Intensive integrated therapy of type 2 diabetes: Implications for long-term prognosis. Diabetes 53(suppl 3): S39–S47, 2004.

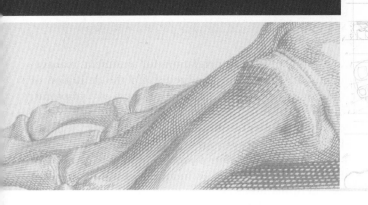

CHAPTER

3

NEUROPATHIC PROBLEMS OF THE LOWER LIMBS IN DIABETIC PATIENTS

ROBERT J. TANENBERG AND PETER D. DONOFRIO ∎

Introduction

This chapter defines diabetic neuropathy and reviews the pivotal role this complication plays in lower-limb disease and disability. Although diabetic peripheral neuropathy (DPN) is common and a frequent cause of morbidity and disability, early assessment and management of diabetic neuropathy are often overlooked or forgotten. The American Diabetes Association (ADA) has been recommending a neurologic examination on the initial patient visit for over 10 years and currently recommends annual screening for DPN in all patients with diabetes.[1,2] Unfortunately, neuropathy screening has not become a universal standard of care in the United States, as is illustrated by its exclusion in the 2002 Health Employer Data and Information Set criteria for diabetes management for U.S. health plans.

A 2005 study of 20 health plans found two thirds of health care providers in compliance with all six of their diabetes management criteria (e.g., measuring hemoglobin A1C, lipids, and microalbuminuria and referring patients for dilated retina exams).[3] In contradistinction, a recent study of over 2000 primary care providers in the United States found that these practitioners were able to correctly identify the presence of mild to moderate neuropathy in only 31% of their patients.[4] This study (The Underdiagnosis of Peripheral Neuropathy in Type 2 Diabetes) also found that one third of patients with

severe DPN (defined as the inability to sense a 5.07 monofilament) were not identified by this same group of primary care providers.

Either a disinterest in the condition or an inability of health care providers to diagnose DPN is reflected in a similar lack of appreciation of the condition by patients with diabetes. A recent ADA telephone survey of over 8000 respondents who claimed to have diabetes (ADA Diabetic Neuropathy Campaign) confirms a general lack of recognition of the term *neuropathy* and the cause of their neuropathic symptoms.[5] The key findings of this survey included the following:

1. Only 42% of the two thirds of survey respondents who experience symptoms of DPN had been told by their doctor that diabetes was the cause.
2. Only 25% of survey respondents who experience symptoms of DPN had been diagnosed with the condition.
3. Fewer than 50% of those with DPN symptoms were aware of the term *diabetic neuropathy*.

This widespread failure by both patients and physicians to understand and appreciate the importance of DPN is not without consequence. Furthermore, the common omission of a neurologic exam of the lower limbs in the physician's office or at the bedside often leads to a failure to diagnose DPN. When the DPN is not diagnosed in the early stages, a window of opportunity is missed to ameliorate symptoms and prevent the development of the major clinical neuropathic endpoints of the lower limb: the chronic painful foot, the insensate foot, the Charcot foot, and the neuropathic ulcer.

This chapter reviews the epidemiology, pathogenesis, and classification of DPN. The evidence base supporting "tight" glycemic control to prevent or delay the onset or progression of DPN is presented. The chapter presents a practical approach to the evaluation and treatment of the patient with DPN for the clinician. The approach focuses on the lower limb and includes (1) neurologic history, (2) neurologic examination, (3) use of ancillary testing, (4) pharmacologic treatment of the patient with painful neuropathy, and (5) office management of the insensate foot. The authors' goal for this chapter is to improve the reader's understanding of DPN as a critical cause of the lower-limb morbidity that, when detected and addressed in the early stages, can reduce pain and suffering and improve the lives of patients with diabetes.

Definition, Pain Overview and Stages of Diabetic Neuropathy

Definition

In 2005, the American Diabetes Association published a statement on diabetic neuropathies that reviewed accepted definitions, classification, diagnostic criteria, epi-demiology, and recommendations for treatment, manage-ment, and screening.[6] They reiterated the definition of diabetic neuropathy as "the presence of symptoms, and/or signs of peripheral nerve dysfunction in people with diabetes after the exclusion of other causes."[7] Clinical diabetic neuropathy requires the presence of an abnormal neurologic examination done by a physician skilled in the proper examination technique and the finding that the abnormal neurologic exam is consistent with nerve damage from diabetes.

Confirmed clinical neuropathy is defined as clinical neuropathy plus confirmation by abnormal quantitative neurologic function tests (e.g., electrophysiologic tests, quantitative sensory testing, or autonomic function tests) in two or more nerves. "Subclinical diabetic neuropathy" is the presence of abnormal quantitative neurologic function tests with little or no evidence of clinical neu-ropathy by exam.[8] There are sensory nerves (controlling sensation), motor nerves (controlling the musculature), and autonomic nerves (controlling functions such as sweating, vascular flow, heart rate, gastric emptying, and other visceral organs).

Illustrations of the major types of diabetic neuropathy are depicted in Figure 3-1. Sensory neuropathy can result in abnormal sensations, such as pain or lack of sensation (numbness), typically in the glove and stocking distribu-tion (Fig. 3-2).

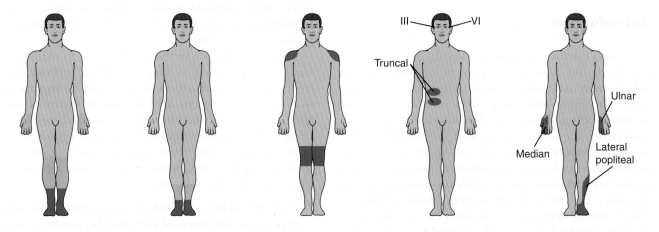

Large-Fiber neuropathy	Small-Fiber neuropathy	Proximal Motor neuropathy	Acute Mono-neuropathies	Pressure palsies
Sensory loss: 0 → +++ (touch, vibration) Pain: + → +++ Tendon reflex: N → ↓↓↓ Motor deficit: 0 → +++	Sensory loss: 0 → + (thermal, allodynia) Pain: + → +++ Tendon reflex: N → ↓ Motor deficit: 0	Sensory loss: 0 → + Pain: + → +++ Tendon reflex: ↓↓ Proximal motor deficit: + → +++	Sensory loss: 0 → + Pain: + → +++ Tendon reflex: N Motor deficit: + → +++	Sensory loss in nerve distribution: + → +++ Pain: + → ++ Tendon reflex: N Motor deficit: + → +++

Figure 3–1   Five clinical presentations of DPN. Schematic representation of five different clinical presentations of peripheral diabetic neuropathy with both sensory and motor components. DPN may predominantly affect large fibers or small fibers (see text). Proximal motor deficits in diabetic patients may be from another etiology and will require a full neurologic evaluation. Proximal diabetic neuropathy, also known as diabetic amyotrophy, may be associated with weight loss and a progressive disability. Mononeuropathies may be acute or chronic, are generally unilateral, and can involve various peripheral nerves, such as the median (carpal tunnel), ulnar, truncal, and lateral popliteal nerves. *(Redrawn from Vinik AI, Mehrabyan A: Diabetic neuropathies. Med Clin N Am 88:947–999, 2004.)*

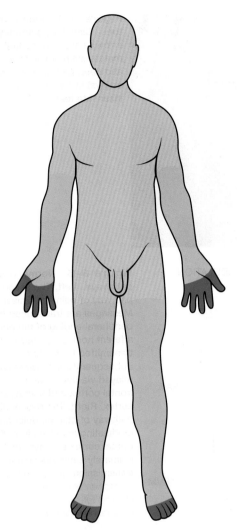

Figure 3–2 Stocking-and-glove distribution. Stocking-and-glove distribution of diabetic distal symmetrical polyneuropathy. Diabetic distal symmetrical polyneuropathy involves both sides relatively equally, involves feet more than hands, is distal rather than proximal, and involves multiple nerves. There is a distal dying of the nerve fiber. This results in a dying-back clinical picture. Thus, the involvement of hands and feet presents as a stocking-and-glove pattern.

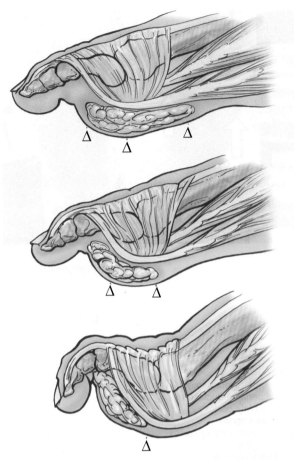

Figure 3–3 Development of claw toe deformity. As the flexor muscles of the foot become weakened disproportionately to the extensor muscles, the toes are pulled into a claw deformity. This action pulls the fat pad off the metatarsal heads of the foot. The pressure is no longer distributed along a wide base but rather at a narrow point beneath the metatarsal heads, which no longer have any fat padding. The plantar surface of the metatarsal heads, the cocked-up toe knuckle (more likely to hit the top of the toe box), and the tip of the toe are at increased risk for ulceration with this common deformity.

Motor neuropathy can result in muscle atrophy. This may lead to imbalances between muscle groups in the foot. These imbalances can result in foot deformities. A common example is the claw toe deformity, which is caused by the constant flexion of the toes (Figs. 3-3, 3-4). Autonomic neuropathy may lead to decreased sudomotor function and dry feet or abnormal blood flow in the soles of the feet.

Pain Overview

In 1931, Charles Mayo once remarked that "of all the symptoms for which physicians are consulted, pain in one form or another, is the most common and most urgent."[9] In 1995, the American Pain Society created the phrase "Pain: The 5th Vital Sign"™ to emphasize the importance of pain and the need for providers to ask about it at every patient encounter.[10] It is important that physicians and other health care providers understand that diabetic neuropathy can occur with no pain or with an insensate foot or may present with pain in the form of dysesthesias and paresthesias as described below (see the section entitled "Epidemiology and Risk Factors"). It is estimated that 15% of individuals with diabetes will present with painful DPN.[11] The most recent data from the Centers for Disease Control and Prevention give the prevalence for diabetes as approximately 22 million people, which would translate to over 3 million people in the United States suffering from painful neuropathy.[12] However, patients may have nonneuropathic or nociceptive pain or conditions with both elements. Nociceptive pain arises from a stimulus outside the nervous system and is proportionate to receptor stimulation. When nociceptive pain is acute, it serves as a protective function.

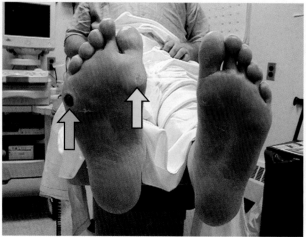

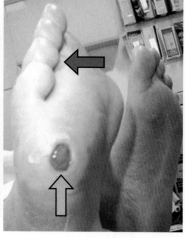

Figure 3–4 **Photos of claw toes.** Claw foot deformity (*green arrow*), callus on the first metatarsal head (*yellow arrows*), and neuropathic ulcer (*orange arrows*) in a patient with insensate feet.

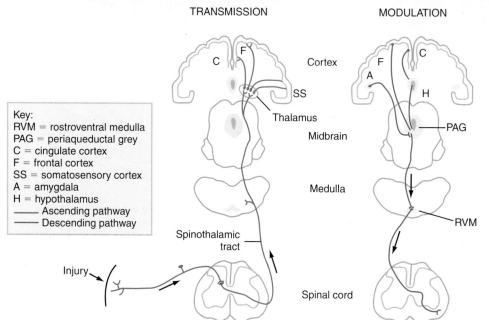

Figure 3–5 **Normal pain pathways. Left,** The ascending pathway of pain transmission. Messages are transduced by the peripheral ending of the primary afferent nociceptor and then transmitted to the spinal cord. Subsequently, messages are relayed via the thalamus to the frontal cortex and somatosensory cortex. **Right,** The descending pathway of pain modulation. Pain-modulating impulses from the frontal cortex and hypothalamus ultimately suppress spinal pain transmission. *(Adapted with permission of the publisher, from The Placebo Effect: An Interdisciplinary Exploration, edited by A. Harrington, p.106, Cambridge, Mass: Harvard University Press. Copyright © 1997 by the President and Fellows of Harvard College.)*

Examples of nociceptive pain include arthritis, sports injuries, postoperative pain, and mechanical low back pain. These pains fit the official definition of the International Association for the Study of Pain. They have defined pain as "an unpleasant sensory and emotional experience associated with actual or potential tissue damage or described in terms of such damage."[13] In contradistinction, neuropathic pain arises from a primary lesion or dysfunction in the nervous system and is disproportionate to receptor stimulation.[14] Neuropathic pain does not require nociceptive stimulation, and there is often other evidence of nerve damage. In addition to DPN, other examples of neuropathic pain include postherpetic neuralgia, trigeminal neuralgia, neuropathic low back pain, complex regional pain syndrome, and distal HIV polyneuropathy. Clinical entities with both nociceptive and neuropathic pain include fibromyalgia, certain cancer pain, and various neck and back pains.

Our understanding of neuropathic pain was greatly enhanced with neurobiological models described by

Fields. In Figure 3-5, the diagram on the left demonstrates the normal ascending pathway of pain transmissions described by Fields. Messages are transduced by the peripheral ending of the primary afferent nociceptor and then transmitted to the spinal cord and then relayed through the thalamus to the frontal and the somatosensory cortex.[15] The diagram on the right of Figure 3-5 illustrates the normal descending pathway of pain modulation. In this case, pain-modulating impulses from the frontal cortex and hypothalamus ultimately suppress spinal pain transmission.[16] These paradigms are invaluable to clinicians in improving their understanding of pain transmission in neuropathies such as DPN.

Stages

A useful staging method is the one described by the Mayo Clinic.[17] Stage 0 is no evidence of neuropathy. Stage 1 is subclinical neuropathy defined as no signs or symptoms of neuropathic problems but abnormal quan-

TABLE 3-1   Stages of Diabetic Neuropathy

Stage	Description	Signs or Symptoms	Abnormal Quantitative Tests
0	No neuropathy	No	No
1	Subclinical neuropathy	No	Yes
2	Clinically evident neuropathy	Yes	Yes
3	Debilitating neuropathy	Yes	Yes

titative neurologic function tests. Stage 2 is clinical neuropathy (i.e., findings of signs and symptoms consistent with diabetic neuropathy). Usually, this can be confirmed by evaluating quantitative neurologic function tests. Stage 3 is end-stage, debilitating neuropathy. Typically, people with stage 3 neuropathy have an abnormal gait, cannot walk on their heels, or have had a foot ulcer. Table 3-1 summarizes these stages.

Classification of Diabetic Neuropathy

Diabetic neuropathy can be classified in several ways: clinical presentation (symmetrical, focal, or multifocal or painful, paralytic, and ataxic), predominant type of fibers affected (motor, sensory, autonomic), or painful or nonpainful.

The classification by P. K. Thomas was the first attempt to separate diabetic neuropathy into symmetrical, focal, or multifocal. Symmetric neuropathies were sensory or sensorimotor, acute or subacute, or autonomic. Focal or multifocal neuropathies were cranial, trunk or limb, or proximal.[18] A popular classification is the one created by Dyck and colleagues in 1987; it groups neuropathies by the predominant clinical presentation (Box 3-1). It can be appreciated as a modification of the classification proposed by P. K. Thomas earlier. Neuropathies are grouped as symmetrical, asymmetrical, or both.[19] Box 3-2 briefly describes the various types of neuropathy in terms of their onset, symmetry, and clinical course.

A symmetrical distal neuropathy is the most common presentation of diabetic neuropathy. It can be symptomatic in a patient complaining of numbness, tingling, and burning in the feet and lower shins or it can be asymptomatic, first detected on neurologic examination or electrophysiologic testing. The symmetrical proximal neuropathies are extremely rare and are typically observed in the setting of a distal symmetrical neuropathy. The asymmetrical neuropathies are clustered together, each with its unique presentation of ocular involvement, pain over the chest or abdomen, lumbosacral distribution of weakness and pain, or a mononeuropathy at a common entrapment site or in the setting of severe prolonged ischemia. The final term in Dyck's classification describes the common occurrence of an asymmetrical neuropathy and the common symmetrical distal neuropathy, for example, diabetic amyotrophy superimposed on a patient

---

BOX 3-1   Classification of Diabetic Neuropathy

I.   Symmetrical distal neuropathy
II.   Symmetrical proximal neuropathy
III. Asymmetrical proximal neuropathy
    A. Cranial
    B. Trunk radiculopathy or mononeuropathy
    C. Limb plexus or mononeuropathy
    D. Multiple mononeuropathy
    E. Entrapment neuropathy
    F. Ischemic nerve injury from acute arterial occlusion
IV.   Asymmetrical neuropathy and symmetrical distal neuropathy

From Dyck PJ, Kratz KM, Karnes JL, et al: The prevalence by staged severity of various types of diabetic neuropathy, retinopathy, and nephropathy in a population-based cohort: The Rochester Diabetic Neuropathy Study. Neurology 43:817–824, 1993.

BOX 3-2   Types of Diabetic Neuropathy

I.   **Focal neuropathies**
    A. Ischemic neuropathies
      1. Sudden onset
      2. Asymmetrical
      3. Ischemic etiology
      4. Self-limited
      5. Examples
        a. Mononeuropathies
        b. Femoral neuropathies
        c. Radiculopathies
        d. Plexopathies
        e. Cranial neuropathies
    B. Entrapment neuropathies
      1. Gradual onset
      2. Usually asymmetrical but can be bilateral
      3. Compression etiology
      4. Waxing and waning progressive course without spontaneous recovery
      5. Examples
        a. Carpal tunnel syndrome
        b. Ulnar entrapment (tennis elbow)
        c. Lateral cutaneous femoral nerve entrapment
        d. Tarsal tunnel syndrome

II. **Diffuse neuropathies**
    A. Insidious onset
    B. Symmetrical
    C. Abnormalities secondary to vascular, metabolic, structural, and autoimmune aberrations
    D. Progressive without spontaneous recovery
    E. Examples
      1. Distal-symmetrical polyneuropathy
      2. Autonomic neuropathies

---

with a symmetrical distal neuropathy. In Dyck's classification, autonomic involvement would be grouped with the symmetrical distal neuropathy.

The Consensus Panel Report and Recommendations of the San Antonio Conference on Diabetic Neuropathy in 1988 grouped neuropathies into symptomatic and asymptomatic and whether the patient had signs of neuropathy or only symptoms. Feldman adapted this classification so that class I or subclinical neuropathies were subgrouped into those that had abnormal nerve conduction results, abnormal quantitative sensory testing, or abnormal autonomic testing. Class II or clinical neuropathies were divided into diffuse and focal neuropathies. Diffuse neuropathies were grouped again into the predominant fiber type abnormality (small, large, or mixed fibers) or the type of autonomic neuropathy. Focal neuropathies were mononeuropathies, mononeuropathy multiplex, cranial neuropathies, plexopathies, or polyradiculopathy.[20] Focal neuropathies can also be divided into ischemic and entrapment neuropathies.

Focal ischemic neuropathies are believed to be due to an acute ischemic event to a nerve, a plexus of nerves, or a nerve root. As a result, this type of neuropathy tends to have a sudden onset, to be asymmetrical in distribution, and to have a self-limiting course. Examples of acute ischemic focal neuropathies include mononeuropathies, femoral neuropathies, radiculopathies, plexopathies, and cranial neuropathies. Diagnosis is typically via clinical examination and symptoms. Therapy relates to time. Cranial neuropathies (e.g., third-nerve palsy) may improve in days to a few weeks, whereas femoral neuropathies may take months to a year and a half to improve. No known therapy has been proven to shorten the time to recovery.

Focal Entrapment Neuropathies (Tarsal Tunnel Syndrome)

Focal entrapment neuropathies occur when a nerve is compressed in a specific body compartment. They tend to have a gradual onset, to occur in an asymmetrical distribution (but can occur bilaterally), and often have a progressive course. Examples include carpal tunnel syndrome, ulnar entrapment, and tarsal tunnel syndrome. Tarsal tunnel syndrome occurs when the tibial nerve becomes entrapped in the tarsal tunnel. The tarsal tunnel is located on the medial surface and just below the medial malleolus. As the tibial nerve traverses into the foot, it splits into two branches, one to the heel and the other to the remainder of the foot. The split of the tibial nerve can occur before or within the tarsal tunnel (Fig. 3-6). Thus, people with tarsal tunnel syndrome may have a variety of symptoms. Symptoms may include paresthesias or numbness in the distal foot with the heel spared, or the heel may be involved as well. Pain from tarsal tunnel entrapment generally worsens throughout the day, as there is increased pain with activity. Thus, the pain is typically worse at the end of the day and improves on resting the foot. This pain scenario is very different from the pain associated with distal symmetrical polyneuropathy.

Examination findings of the tarsal tunnel syndrome include an abnormal two-point discrimination test, abnormal vibratory sensation, and weakness and wasting of foot muscles and a positive Tinel's sign. To perform the Tinel's test, one taps posterior to the medial epi-

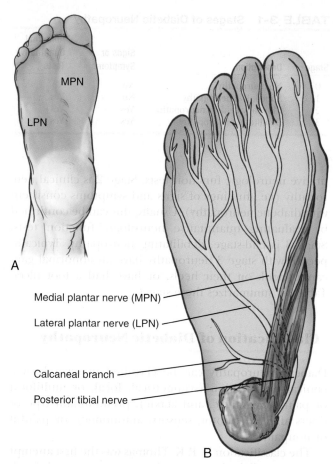

Figure 3–6 Tarsal tunnel. Compression of either the posterior tibial nerve at the tarsal tunnel or the plantar nerves causes a combination of sensory impairment of the sole and intrinsic weakness of the pedal musculature. *(Adapted from Aguayo AJ: Neuropathy due to compression and entrapment. In Dyck PJ, Thomas PK, Lambert EH (eds): Peripheral Neuropathy. Philadelphia, W.B. Saunders, 1975.)*

condyle of the ankle as you would tap for a carpal tunnel Tinel's sign at the wrist. If the test is positive, the patient notes a tingling in the sole of the foot. In addition, there may be loss of flexibility of the metatarsophalangeal joint (inability to hold a pencil with toes or inability to grab a handkerchief placed flat on the floor with the toes). A gait disturbance is occasionally observed. The diagnosis of the tarsal tunnel syndrome is made via appropriate signs and symptoms and confirmed by electrodiagnostic measures above and below the tarsal tunnel. Therapy may include surgery or steroid injections (see the Surgery section later in this chapter).

Epidemiology and Risk Factors

Epidemiologic Perspective

Only a few studies have addressed the prevalence of diabetic neuropathy, with varying results. Some of the best information on the prevalence of diabetic neuropathy is from the population-based Rochester Diabetic Neuropathy Study conducted by epidemiologists from the Mayo Clinic in Rochester, Minnesota.[21] This study noted that between 60% and 65% of patients with either type 1 or type 2 diabetes had some (any) neuropathy. Forty percent to 45% had symmetrical distal polyneuropathy (see the definition of this type of diabetic neuropathy below). Approximately 30% had carpal tunnel syndrome. Six percent had autonomic neuropathy. Fewer than 5% had "other" neuropathies (including plexopathies, mononeuropathies, cranial neuropathies, and radiculopathies). There was no statistically significant difference in the prevalence of neuropathy between the two types of diabetes mellitus.

In a household-based population survey of neuropathic symptoms in 2400 subjects, Harris and coworkers with the NIH estimated the prevalence of neuropathic symptoms to be about 30% in patients with type 1 diabetes. In respondents with type 2 diabetes, they estimated a prevalence of 36% for men and 40% for women compared to 10% to 12% in a control group of matched nondiabetic men and women.[22] In addition, the prevalence of neuropathic symptoms increased twofold with the duration of diabetes over 20 years compared to subjects at 0 to 4 years since diagnosis. This finding confirms previous results published by Pirart, who analyzed the findings of a large population of patients with diabetes over many years.[23] He found an increase in the prevalence of neuropathy with both increased duration of diabetes and worse glycemic control.

In a longitudinal study from Finland, Partenen and colleagues performed nerve conduction testing in 133 patients with newly diagnosed type 2 diabetes.[24] The baseline prevalence of definite or probable DPN was 8.3% versus 2.1% in a control group. The prevalence of DPN in the group with diabetes increased to 16.7% after 5 years and 41.9% after 10 years. The prevalence of DPN was increased in patients with higher fasting glucose and A1C values and lower fasting plasma insulin concentrations. A cross-sectional study from Turkey evaluated 866 patients with type 2 diabetes for a mean duration of 8.5 years.[25] These investigators defined neuropathy as the presence of (a) abnormal neurologic symptom scale, (b) abnormal neurologic disability score, (c) abnormal sensory or motor signs and symptoms, and (d) decreased toe vibration perception. The prevalence of DPN in their patients according to these criteria was 60%. The part of the world reporting the highest prevalence of DPN is South India. Mohan and colleagues, defining neuropathy as bilateral absence of ankle jerks and/or vibratory loss using biothesiometry, reported a 69.8% prevalence of DPN in 726 patients with type 2 diabetes of over 25 years' duration.[26] Unfortunately, this trend toward a higher prevalence of DPN will most likely continue. As the worldwide prevalence of diabetes increases from an estimated 200 million people in 2005 to 333 million people by 2025, epidemiologists have already predicted a corresponding increase in all complications, including diabetic neuropathy.[27,28]

Risk Factors

There are both modifiable and nonmodifiable risk factors for the development of diabetic neuropathy (Box 3-3). Only hyperglycemia has been proven to be a risk factor via prospective, randomized, multicenter, parallel design clinical trials.[1] The other factors are considered to be risk factors via retrospective or cross-sectional data analysis. Nonmodifiable risk factors include older age, longer duration of diabetes, HLA DR 3/4 genotype, and height. Many studies have found that men are at greater risk for neuropathy than are females, but reanalysis of these data shows it to be height rather than gender that is significant. It is hypothesized that longer nerves are more prone to nerve damage.[29,30]

Age, duration of diabetes, and the DR 3/4 genotype are also risk factors for the other two microvascular complications of diabetes: retinopathy and nephropathy. Genetic investigations into the polymorphisms of the aldose reductase gene have revealed various susceptibilities to microvascular complications including neuropathy. Initial work on the Z-2 gene was promising, but at this time, one can only conclude that more work is necessary to further define the role of the polymorphisms of the aldose reductase gene and their role in the pathogenesis of diabetic neuropathy.[31]

Hyperglycemia

Modifiable risk factors include hyperglycemia, hypertension, elevated cholesterol, smoking, and heavy alcohol use. The Diabetes Control and Complications Trial (DCCT) and the United Kingdom Prospective Diabetes Study have demonstrated conclusively that better glucose control prevents or slows the progression of diabetic neuropathy[8,32,33] (Table 3-2). The recent EDIC Study confirms that this effect persists in slowing the progression of microvascular disease, including diabetic neuropathy, even after the improved glycemic control is no longer present ("metabolic memory")[34,35] (Fig. 3-7).

BOX 3–3 Risk Factors for Diabetic Neuropathy

Nonmodifiable risk factors
    Older age
    Longer duration of diabetes
    HLA DR 3/4 genotype
    Greater height
Modifiable risk factors
    Hyperglycemia
    Hypertension
    Elevated cholesterol levels
    Smoking
    Heavy alcohol use

TABLE 3-2   DCCT and UKPDS Landmark Clinical Trials of Glucose Control

	DCCT	UKPDS
Type of diabetic patients	1	2
Number of patients	1441	4209
Length of study (years)	10	20
Average length of patient follow-up (years)	5	10
Average HbA1C (%)		
Standard therapy	8.9	7.9
Intensive therapy	7.1	7.0
Average glucose level (mg/dL)		
Standard therapy	231	177
Intensive therapy	155	147
Reduction in retinopathy (%)	76	21
Reduction in nephropathy (%)	56	34
Reduction in neuropathy (%)	60	25

DCCT, Diabetes Control and Complications Trial; UKPDS, United Kingdom Prospective Diabetes Study; HbA1C, glycosylated hemoglobin.

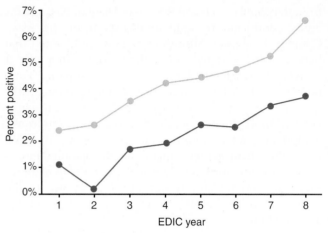

Figure 3-7   EDIC study. Frequency of neuropathy-positive questionnaires across 8 years of the EDIC among former DCCT conventional therapy (*yellow dots*) and intensive therapy (*blue dots*) without confirmed DPN at the end of the DCCT. (*p* <.0001 on average for all EDIC years combined.) *(Redrawn with permission from Martin C, Albers J, Herman W, et al: Neuropathy among the Diabetes Control and Complications Trial cohort 8 years after trial completion. Diabetes Care 29:340–344, 2006.)*

The EDIC Study also recently demonstrated a statistical reduction in the number of foot or leg ulcers in the DCCT intensive versus the conventional therapy group (4 versus 11, *p* = .01).[36] The authors of this prospective epidemiologic trial call for "the implementation of intensive therapy as early as is safely possible and the maintenance of such therapy for as long as possible, with the expectation that a prolonged period of nearly normal blood glucose levels will result in an even greater reduction in the risk of complications in patients with type 1 diabetes."[37] Since the etiology of DPN in type 2 diabetes is presumably the same as that in type 1 diabetes, early intensive glycemic control with a target A1C of 6.5% should be the goal of clinicians who treat these patients. The same target A1C of 6.5% is recommended by the investigators of the Kumamoto Study.[38] In this 10-year prospective study, 110 patients with type 2 diabetes were randomly assigned to one of two groups: a multiple insulin injection therapy group or a conventional insulin injection therapy group. The multiple-injection therapy group maintained a 64% risk reduction in diabetic neuropathy as defined by significant improvement in nerve conduction velocity and vibration threshold.[39]

Vascular Risk Factors

A recent publication of a large prospective study of patients with type 1 diabetes, the EURODAIB IDDM Complications Study, has expanded our understanding of the role of vascular risk factors in diabetic neuropathy.[40] In this prospective multicenter study, new-onset neuropathy developed in 276 of 1172 patients with type 1 diabetes during an average follow-up of 7.3 years. As expected, the development of DPN was highly correlated with both the duration of diabetes and the level of the hemoglobin A1C. Using a multivariate logistic-regression model to adjust for duration of diabetes and glycemic control, these investigators noted the following risk factors to be statistically significant for the development of DPN: total cholesterol, low-density lipoprotein cholesterol, triglycerides, body mass index, a history of smoking, hypertension, the presence of microalbuminuria, and cardiovascular disease. Noting that only aggressive medical treatment to control glucose has been demonstrated to reduce the progression of neuropathy, the authors of this study propose clinical trials to "confirm the efficacy of antihypertensive agents and possibly other strategies for cardiovascular risk reduction in slowing progression of neuropathy."[24]

Alcoholism, Uremia, and Organ Transplantation

Alcoholism, a common cause of polyneuropathy in non-diabetic individuals, is, like DPN, often associated with prominent neuropathic pain.[41] Alcoholic neuropathy is considered to result from a direct neurotoxic effect of ethanol independent of thiamine deficiency.[42] Therefore, listing it as an independent risk factor for the development of diabetic neuropathy is problematic.[43,44] It would be reasonable to postulate that the increased incidence of neuropathy in diabetic patients who are heavy alcohol users is no more than a combination of two neuropathies occurring in the same individual. In an individual patient, it can be very difficult if not impossible to determine which condition is responsible for the clinical findings. It is of interest to note that a reversal of alcoholic neuropathy has been described in patients with end-stage liver disease following successful liver transplantation.[45]

The situation of mixed etiologies for neuropathy with ethanol is similar to patients with diabetes who develop end-stage renal failure. Uremic polyneuropathy "occurs in about half of patients undergoing dialysis and is characterized by axonal degeneration with secondary segmental demyelination."[46] Diabetic patients with renal failure are more likely to have greater sensory involvement with uremia than are nondiabetic individuals, and diabetic patients are less likely to respond to newer treatments such as erythropoietin therapy.[47]

Hemodialysis or peritoneal dialysis typically halts the progress of polyneuropathy but usually does not bring improvement. However, clinical improvement in DPN and overall prognosis in both patients with diabetes and patients without diabetes is much greater with successful renal transplantation than with either hemodialysis or peritoneal dialysis.[48]

The most dramatic change in uremic and diabetic neuropathy in patients with diabetes occurs after successful simultaneous pancreas and kidney transplantation. Numerous studies have demonstrated that restoration of normoglycemia with successful pancreas transplantation is not only able to halt the progression of diabetic polyneuropathy but also may lead to objective improvement.[49,50]

Pathogenesis

Much information as to the etiology of the diffuse neuropathies has been established in the last 30 years. After reviewing the risk factors, it would be of interest to ask four important questions about neuropathy that have stymied clinicians for years:

1. How do the various pathogenic mechanisms of diabetic complications explain the link between hyperglycemia and neuropathy?
2. Why do patients develop neuropathy with only minimal hyperglycemia, for example, impaired glucose tolerance?
3. Why do neuropathic symptoms often become exacerbated after glycemic control is improved?
4. Why do some individuals seem less likely to develop neuropathy than others despite worse glycemic control?

Clearly, these questions would apply to all the microvascular complications, not just to diabetic neuropathy. At this time, at least theoretical answers to these elusive questions are finally appearing in the medical literature. The authors will attempt to answer these four questions in this section on the pathogenesis of diabetic neuropathy.

Hyperglycemia

As with most diabetic complications, insulin deficiency and hyperglycemia are considered the initiating factors. Although there are multiple retrospective studies that support this hypothesis, the results of the DCCT[51] and the United Kingdom Prospective Diabetes Study[18,19] are the strongest evidence supporting this mechanism in both type 1 and type 2 diabetic patients (see Table 3-2).

Both these trials were prospective randomized studies comparing groups utilizing intensive versus conventional therapy to achieve "tighter" glycemic control. In both of these trials, patients who were randomized to the intensive control group had better nerve conduction velocity tests. Furthermore, the DCCT demonstrated better autonomic nervous tests and less "confirmed clinical" neuropathy in patients with better glucose control. As was previously noted, long-term follow-up of the DCCT patients has finally demonstrated that 5 years of better glucose control early in the course of diabetes results in fewer neuropathic foot ulcers.[22]

Neuropathy Associated with Prediabetes

In 1997, the ADA changed the diagnostic criteria for diabetes, lowering the fasting glucose from 140 mg/dL (7.8 mmol/L) to 126 mg/dL (7.0 mmol/L).[52] They also created new categories called *impaired fasting glucose* (plasma glucose fasting 110 to 125 mg/dL) and *impaired glucose tolerance* (IGT), defined as patients with a 2-hour postprandial glucose between 140 and 199 mg/dL.[53] More recently, the ADA cutoff for the fasting glucose has been lowered to 100 mg/dL for impaired fasting glucose, and this group and the IGT group are now sometimes lumped together under the term *prediabetes*.[54,55]

The clinician needs to be cognizant that neuropathy can frequently be the presenting symptom of these patients who are not diabetic but meet the diagnostic criteria of IGT or prediabetes.[56] These patients may present with a "length-dependent polyneuropathy that typically is sensory predominant and painful."[57] Typical symptoms of this condition include paresthesias and dysesthesia of the toes and fingers in which the only objective findings are neurologic signs limited to those of small-caliber sensory nerve fiber involvement: reduced distal pinprick sensation. However, vibratory sensation and reflexes (which require large fibers) are intact. Although nerve conduction velocity (NCV) studies will be normal, distal leg skin biopsies show loss of small-caliber nerve fibers.[58]

Most patients with neuropathy associated with prediabetes are typical of people with the metabolic syndrome. They are obese with a preponderance of visceral fat; exhibit the classic metabolic manifestations of insulin resistance, including diabetes or prediabetes, dyslipidemia, and hypertension; and have an increased risk for premature cardiovascular disease.[59] In general, neuropathy associated with prediabetes is thought to be less severe and more likely to be reversible than is the classic neuropathy occurring in patients with diabetes.[43] Thus, early diagnosis will be important for the physician to institute treatment for neuropathic pain and to address the manifestations of metabolic syndrome by treating obesity, postprandial hyperglycemia, dyslipidemia, and associated hypertension. A final caveat for clinicians is to consider the diagnosis of prediabetes in patients presenting with a painful distal symmetrical polyneuropathy of no obvious etiology.

If the fasting glucose is between 100 and 125 mg/dL, a simple 2-hour oral glucose tolerance test will confirm the diagnosis of IGT or prediabetes. If no other etiology of the DPN is found, the patient can be presumed to have neuropathy associated with prediabetes.[43]

A recent publication from Germany has given new insight into the possible etiology of neuropathy associated with prediabetes in these patients who are only minimally hyperglycemic.[60] In a pilot study, sural nerve biopsies were found to stain positively for the receptor for advanced glycation end-products (RAGE) in the perineurium, in the epineurial vessels, and in part in endoneurial vessels. Control patients with another neurologic disorder had no significant staining for this antigen. These investigators believe that their preliminary data "suggest that activation of the RAGE pathway may be one of the first steps in the pathogenesis of diabetic polyneuropathy even before chronic hyperglycemia occurs."[60]

Vasa Nervorum

It has been proposed that an abnormal vasa nervorum causing local nerve ischemia will lead to poor nerve function (NCV, nerve conduction amplitude, quantitative sensory tests, and abnormal autonomic function tests) and nerve morphometry.

This concept is illustrated in a medical cartoon comparing healthy and normal nerves and vessels (Fig. 3-8). Several studies lend credence to these mechanisms.[61–63] One study demonstrated that treatment with a prostaglandin I_2 analogue (beraprost sodium) resulted in improved nerve function by theoretically inducing relaxation of vascular smooth muscle and reducing nerve ischemia.[64] Furthermore, lisinopril, an angiotensin-converting enzyme inhibitor, has shown an improvement in nerve conduction velocity (NCV) both in experimental studies with rats and in individuals with DPN. The improvement of NCV by lisinopril was hypothesized to be secondary to vasodilatation secondary to increase in nitric oxide.[65–67]

Other work has suggested that the increased aldose reductase activity secondary to hyperglycemia competes with nitric oxide synthetase for NADPH, resulting in decreased nitric oxide. The reduction in nitric oxide reduces nerve blood flow, resulting in nerve ischemia. In experimental diabetic animals, a nitric oxide synthetase inhibitor was able to block the beneficial effect of sorbinil (an aldose reductase inhibitor [ARI]) on NCV.[68,69] This implies that the beneficial effects on DPN of sorbinil and other experimental drugs in this class (ARIs) seen in diabetic animals and humans might be secondary to their vascular effects on the nerve. Sural nerve biopsies from patients with DPN consistently demonstrate defects in the endoneurial vessels, including thickening of the basement membrane, endothelial cell proliferation, and hypertrophy that often closes the vessels[70] (Fig. 3-9).

Using a sophisticated experimental technique of fluorescein angiography and nerve photography, a group of investigators in Britain was able to demonstrate abnormal epineural vessel (vaso nervorum) anatomy and arteriovenous shunting in subjects with chronic sensory motor neuropathy.[71] A more recent work from this group has demonstrated arteriovenous shunting and proliferating new vessels in so-called insulin neuritis.[72] This is an uncommon disorder of acute neuropathic pain that is seen in patients shortly after rapid improvement of glycemic control (usually with the initial institution of insulin therapy). Using their nerve photography-fluorescein angiography technique, these investigators were able to demonstrate proliferation of new leaky epineural vessels analogous to those seen fundoscopically with proliferative diabetic retinopathy. The authors postulate the epineural new vessel "lead to a 'steal' effect rendering the endoneurium ischemic."[59]

Protein Kinase C Pathway Activation

The diacylglycerol–protein kinase C (PKC) pathway activation has been proposed to explain some of the complications of diabetes and might help to explain the

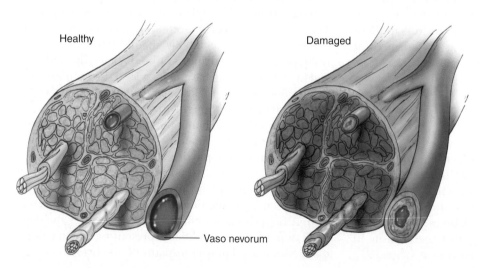

Healthy   Damaged

— Vaso nevorum

Figure 3-8 Normal and damaged nerves. Examination of tissues from patients with diabetes reveals capillary damage, neovascularization, and occlusion in the vasa nervorum. Reduced blood supply to the neural tissue results in impairments in neurotransmission that affect both sensory and motor conduction. *(References: Cameron NE, et al: Diabetologia 44:1973–1988, 2001. Dyck PJ, Giannini C: J Neuropathol Exp Neurol 55:1181–1193, 1996. Copyright 2005 International Medical Press.)*

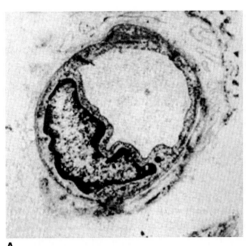

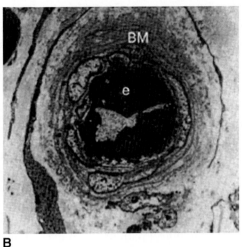

A   **B**

Figure 3–9   Photomicrographs of endoneurial capillaries. Photomicrographs of endoneurial capillaries from sural nerve biopsies showing **(A)** a normal capillary from a diabetic subject without neuropathy and **(B)** a closed capillary from a subject with diabetic neuropathy with basement membrane (*BM*) thickening and endothelial cell (e) proliferation. *(Courtesy of RA Malik, University of Manchester, Manchester, U.K. Reprinted with permission from Cameron NE, Eaton SE, Cotter MA, et al: Vascular factors and metabolic interactions in the pathogenesis of diabetic neuropathy. Diabetologia 44:1973–1988, 2001.)*

above findings in a unified hypothesis. Hyperglycemia increases the formation and the metabolism of diacylglycerol, which in turn activates PKC.[73] In addition, hyperglycemia activates the polyol pathway, which in turn decreases *myo*-inositol (see below).[74] The altered inositol phospholipid metabolism also increases PKC activity.[75] PKC mediates a vascular response to hyperglycemia that involves both the endothelium and smooth muscle tissue. PKC regulates vascular permeability, contractility, basement membrane synthesis, and cellular proliferation.[76–79] Inhibition of the β form of PKC with LY333531 appears to decrease vascular endothelial growth factor in the retina and transforming growth factor beta (TGF-β) in the kidney.[80,81] Vascular endothelial growth factor and TGF-β are believed to play pivotal roles in the development of diabetic retinopathy and nephropathy, respectively.[82,83] Recent clinical trials of protein kinase inhibitor LY333531 (now know as ruboxistaurin) for diabetic microvascular complications, including DPN, are currently under way.[84]

Abnormal Fatty Acid Metabolism

Linoleic acid is converted to γ-linolenic acid, which is converted to dihomo-γ-linolenic acid. Dihomo-γ-linolenic acid will eventually be converted (through several more steps) to arachidonic acid, which helps to dilate blood vessels. In diabetes, the δ-6-desaturation of linoleic acid to γ-linolenic acid is impaired. This forces prostaglandin metabolism down an alternative pathway, leading to a decrease in nerve function either directly or indirectly via nerve ischemia as a result of altered prostaglandin metabolism (see above).[85,86] When patients were given evening primrose oil, which is high in γ-linolenic acid, in a double-blind, placebo-controlled, randomized, multicenter study, both peroneal and median motor NCV and thermal perception threshold improved in the patients who were randomized to γ-linolenic acid treatment compared to the control patients.[87] However, clinical signs and symptoms were unchanged. A more detailed discus-

sion of evening primrose oil and α-lipoic acid will follow in the section on treatment of painful DPN.

Polyol Pathway

The polyol pathway consists of converting glucose to sorbitol via aldose reductase and then converting sorbitol to fructose via sorbitol dehydrogenase. The pathway is relatively dormant at normal glucose levels and activated during hyperglycemia owing to the K_m of the aldose reductase enzyme. Besides the competitive consumption of NADPH and the theoretical decrease in nitric oxide synthetase activity, the increased activity of the polyol pathway also decreases nerve *myo*-inositol through mechanisms that are not well understood.[88–90]

Shunting of glucose into the polyol pathway leads to an accumulation of fructose and sorbitol and an increase in intracellular osmolality. As cells accommodate to maintain osmotic balance, there may be a compensatory depletion of other intracellular compounds such as endoneurial *myo*-inositol and taurine. The decrease in nerve *myo*-inositol may also lead to a decrease in nerve function (i.e., NCV) and to abnormal morphometry.[91] The role of taurine in neuropathy and other diabetic complications is currently under investigation.[92]

Clinical studies with ARIs have documented improved morphometry and an improvement in NCV.[93] Only one study using an ARI has attempted to prevent the development of diabetic neuropathy. In this double-blind, randomized, placebo-controlled, multicenter study, results showed an improvement in peroneal motor, median motor, and median sensory NCV, but prevention of confirmed clinical neuropathy was not statistically different between the ARI group and the placebo group.[94] However, the statistical power of the study was noted to be inadequate. In a small, single-center, longitudinal study, long-term treatment with the ARI sorbinil prevented the deterioration of tactile and thermal perception threshold.[95]

In summary, therapy with an ARI is associated with both an improvement of NCV and morphometry, presumably via a restoration of nerve *myo*-inositol concentration and improved nerve blood flow. However, clinical efficacy of this class of medicines has not been established. This may be due to clinical trial design rather than lack of efficacy.

Investigators are still interested in this area of research, and one group has recently stated that "renewed efforts to develop aldose reductase inhibitors for the treatment and prevention of diabetic complications are warranted."[96]

Myo-inositol

Hyperglycemia, per se, competitively inhibits neural uptake of *myo*-inositol (in addition to the polyol pathway decreasing nerve *myo*-inositol). It is hypothesized that Na^+-K^+-ATPase activity is decreased by lower *myo*-inositol concentrations and thus presumably slows NCV.[97] In some studies, patients and animals placed on a high-*myo*-inositol diet showed improvement in NCV, but in other studies, the results were contradictory.[98–100] Improvement in nerve morphometry and autonomic neuropathy has been shown in animals placed on high-*myo*-inositol diets.[101–104]

Advanced Glycated End-Products

Increased levels of glycosylated neural proteins have also been attributed to hyperglycemia. The first step in glycosylation of proteins is bonding of glucose to a free amino group. Subsequent glycosylated neural protein can crosslink, leading to the formation of advanced glycosylated end-products (AGEs). Cross-linking changes the three-dimensional configuration of the proteins, and the proteins may become dysfunctional. This might account for the slowing of axonal transport that is observed in diabetic neuropathy. Aminoguanidine prevents this crosslinking from occurring. Future studies might show that aminoguanidine or similar products may be useful in the prevention of the development of diabetic neuropathy. In addition, aminoguanidine appears to have ARI properties and effects on nitric oxide and vascular flow in animal models of diabetes.[105,106] However, these latter effects of aminoguanidine have not been confirmed by other studies.

Antibodies to Neural Tissue

Although antibodies to nerve tissue are associated with the presence of neuropathy in both type 1 and type 2 diabetic patients, it is not clear that these antibodies play an initial etiologic role. These antibodies could simply be a response by the immune system to damaged nerves. However, once the autoantibodies have been produced, it is certainly feasible that they might further impair nerve integrity and function.[107–109] Clinical trials of immune suppression therapy for diabetic neuropathy have not been conducted. In a recent review, Vinik and colleagues present a strong case for the importance of neural antibodies in diabetic autonomic neuropathy but admit that evidence for an etiologic role of antibodies in somatic neuropathy has not yet been convincingly demonstrated.[110]

Nerve Growth Factors

Distal dying back of nerves is a common morphometric finding in patients with diabetic neuropathy. Efforts to reverse this process with nerve growth factor and gangliosides have been attempted in clinical trials. Both nerve growth factor and ganglioside treatment result in axonal sprouting and could theoretically improve nerve function, especially in small nerve fibers. To date, results of these trials have been inconsistent and disappointing.[111,112]

One of the neurotrophic factors is nerve growth factor (NGF). In a recent review of the subject, Pittenger and Vinik state that "there is increasing evidence that there is a deficiency of NGF in diabetes, as well as the dependent neuropeptides substance P (SP) and calcitonin gene-related peptide (CGRP) that may also contribute to the clinical symptoms resulting from small fiber dysfunction."[113]

Delineating the Etiologies

It is clear that many etiologies can lead to the common clinical manifestation of diabetic neuropathy (Fig. 3-10). Although all the pathways are feasible and appear to be valid in animal studies, confirmation in human clinical trials, with the exception of hyperglycemia, is generally lacking. In a recent review article, Cameron and colleagues note that although "it is clear that impaired blood flow and endoneurial hypoxia play a major role in causing diabetic neuropathy in human and animal models," the "link between vascular dysfunction and long-term degenerative changes is not entirely clear and merits future attention."[114]

Clinical trials of the chronic complications of diabetes require demonstrating that the progression of the specific complications can be slowed or prevented. This requires adequate time for the control group to develop the complication or demonstrate a worsening of the condition. In diabetic individuals with stage 0 or 1 neuropathy, the rate of progression is very slow. It has been estimated that NCV (one of the most reliable and precise measurements) deteriorates at a rate of 0.5 m/sec/yr. This would imply that the minimum worsening in NCV that would be considered clinically significant (2 to 3 m/sec) in the control group would take 4 to 6 years. This is compounded by the fact that physiologic changes in NCV can be as much as 2 to 3 m/sec. For instance, one study showed that an improvement in plasma glucose levels via a 20-minute intravenous insulin infusion can improve NCV by 2 m/sec.[115,116] Furthermore, there appear

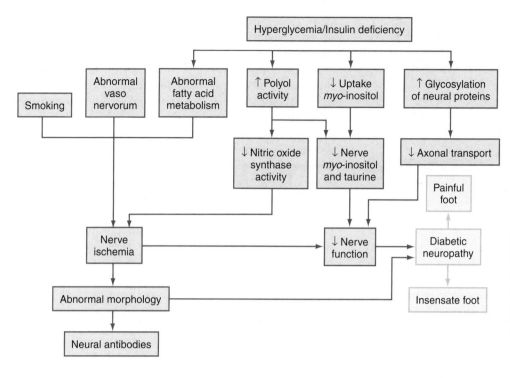

Figure 3-10 Proposed etiologies of diffuse diabetic neuropathy. Abnormal vasa nervorum, insulin deficiency, hyperglycemia, abnormal fatty acid metabolism, increased polyol activity, decreased nerve *myo*-inositol, increased glycosylation of neural proteins, and neural autoantibodies have all been suggested as etiologies of diabetic neuropathy. There appears to be a common end result: confirmed clinical neuropathy. In a single individual, one or more of these pathways may be prominent. In another individual, other pathways may play a more predominant role. *(Redrawn with permission from Pfeifer MA, Schumer MP: Clinical trials of diabetic neuropathy: Past, present and future. Diabetes 44:1355–1361, 1995.)*

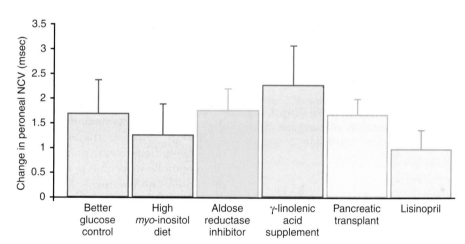

Figure 3-11   Change in peroneal NCV. Change in peroneal NCV in human diabetic individuals in various clinical trials. Better glucose control, a high-*myo*-inositol diet, use of an aldose reductase inhibitor, γ-linolenic acid oral supplementation, pancreatic transplant, and use of an angiotensin-converting enzyme inhibitor (lisinopril) have been evaluated in human clinical trials. Interestingly, the change in peroneal nerve conduction velocity has been very similar (an increase of 1 to 2 m/sec) in all these well-done, controlled clinical trials. Therefore, it would not appear that one of the etiologic pathways plays a consistently dominant role. Combined-therapies clinical trials have not been done. *(References: Reja A, Tesfaye S, Harris ND, Ward JD: Is ACE inhibition with lisinopril helpful in diabetic neuropathy? Diabet Med 12:307–309, 1995. The γ-Linolenic Acid Multicenter Trial Group: Treatment of diabetic neuropathy with γ-linolenic acid. Diabetes Care 16:8–15, 1993. Obrosova I, Faller A, Burgan J, et al: Glycolytic pathway, redox state of NAD (P)-couples and energy metabolism in lens in galactose-fed rats: Effect of an aldose reductase inhibitor. Curr Eye Res 16:34–43, 1997.)*

to be a metabolic component and a structural component to diabetic neuropathy. The metabolic component could be the result of any of the proposed etiologies listed above.

Theoretically, this component is reversible if the underlying abnormality is corrected. In fact, many of the clinical trials that test the various hypothesized pathogenic mechanisms demonstrate a small (1 to 2 m/sec) statistical but not clinically meaningful improvement in NCV. Figure 3-11 compares change in NCV in various clinical trials.[67,87,90,118–121]

It is interesting that this improvement is very consistent among the various trials and methods. This implies that most, if not all, of the proposed mechanisms play a similar contributing role or that they interplay in a single common pathogenic mechanism. The most likely common mechanism might be the vascular component. The structural component does not appear to be

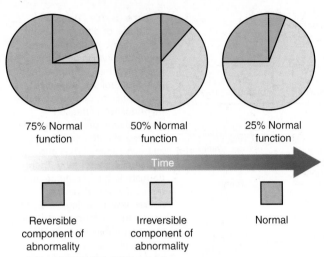

75% Normal function

50% Normal function

25% Normal function

Time

Reversible component of abnormality

Irreversible component of abnormality

Normal

Figure 3–12 Reversible and irreversible components of DPN. Reversible and irreversible components of diabetic neuropathy as a function of time. There appear to be both a reversible (metabolic) and an irreversible (structural) component to diabetic neuropathy. The reversible component appears to play a greater role earlier in the natural history of diabetic neuropathy. In contrast, the irreversible component appears to play a greater role later. The response of any treatment modality would be limited to the reversible component. Thus, early prevention and consistent treatment of the reversible components appear to be the only practical approach for the therapy of diabetic neuropathy. It is unlikely that reversibility of advanced neuropathy is any more likely than is reversibility of the other chronic complications of diabetes (retinopathy or nephropathy). By controlling blood glucose level, the DCCT (see text) was able to prevent the development of diabetic neuropathy in patients without neuropathy at the beginning of the trial. However, some patients already had neuropathy at the beginning of the DCCT, and there was no difference in the reversibility of neuropathy in these patients with better glucose control compared to the less well-controlled patients.

reversible and might represent a greater portion of the sum total nerve abnormality and damage over time (Fig. 3-12). Therefore, even small reversibility of late stage 2 or 3 neuropathy is probably not feasible.

Delineation of etiologies also requires clear-cut end points. However, with the exception of the DCCT, clinical trials of diabetic neuropathy have been too short, underpowered, and conducted in patients with advanced disease and without clear-cut demonstrable end points. In the future, further delineation of the causes of diabetic neuropathy will be possible only by meeting this requirement.

A Unifying Hypothesis of Diabetic Complications

In the 2004 Banting Lecture, Brownlee proposed that the four major pathogenic mechanisms of hyperglycemic damage may result from a single mechanism.[122] The four known mechanisms are (1) increased polyol pathway flux, (2) increased intracellular formation of AGEs, (3) activation of protein kinase C and (4) increased hexosamine pathway flux. All of these mechanisms "seem to reflect a

single hyperglycemia-induced process of overproduction of superoxide by mitochondrial electron-transport chain."[107] Furthermore, Brownlee speculates that the phenomenon of hyperglycemia-induced mitochondrial superoxide production may provide an explanation for the "metabolic memory" phenomenon described in the EDIC trial, that is, the development or exacerbation of diabetic complications during years of improved glycemic control after years of poor control. In the same Banting lecture, Brownlee also suggests a potential answer to the question posed about individual susceptibility to neuropathy at the beginning of this section.[107] He describes familial clustering of microvascular and macrovascular complications, although most of these reports from clinical trials have been described for retinopathy and nephropathy.

A further link between the four mechanisms of hyperglycemic complications noted by Brownlee and DPN is suggested in a recent review titled "Neural Redox Stress and Remodeling in Metabolic Syndrome, Type 2 Diabetes Mellitus, and Diabetic Neuropathy."[123] The authors review the data indicating that a compromise of antioxidant reserve and toxicities from excessive glucose, free fatty acids, amylin, AGEs, homocysteine, and other metabolic substrates are associated with an abundance of reactive oxygen species (ROS). They note that elevated tension of redox stress and ROS have been reported to lead to an increase in matrix metalloproteinase (MMP) activity.[124] They postulate that a key link to DPN would be a proposed "robust activation of MMP-9," which could result in a "complete disconnection of the neuronal microvascular cells within the neuronal unit."[109] These associations might help to explain the proclivity of patients with the metabolic syndrome to develop DPN before they are diagnosed with overt type 2 diabetes.

Documentation of Neuropathy

Clinical Presentation

Symptoms of a distal diabetic polyneuropathy vary from patient to patient, but common complaints are numbness, tingling, and pain beginning in the toes and soles of the feet, progressing over months to years to affect the top of the feet, ankles, and lower shins. Patients often volunteer a variety of other descriptions including a dead feeling in the feet, burning sensation, and pins and needles in the feet (paresthesias). Some patients state their feet feel as if immersed in cold water or a block of ice. In addition to a baseline burning pain or discomfort, superimposed shock-like, electric, or ice-pick pains frequently complicate the lives of patients with diabetic neuropathy and commonly are the most concerning complaints during an office visit. Other descriptors used by patients include jabbing, icy cold, formication (sensation of bugs crawling on the skin), cramping, sunburn, frostbite, intense itching, and the perception of walking on broken glass. Sensory symptoms are commonly worse at night, particularly when the patient is trying to fall asleep. Often, patients with diabetic neuropathy state that movement, walking, or standing lessens the pain, a characteristic that is unusual in patients with nociceptive pain such as osteoarthritis of the feet or plantar fasciitis. Unclear is the explanation for the seemingly paradoxical worsening of pain at night. It might relate to the absence of distractibility, which is present during the day but not when one is trying to fall asleep.

Types of Pain

Three types of pain have been described in patients with painful diabetic neuropathy: According to the pain model developed by David Ross, the three categories are dysesthesia, paresthesia, and muscular pain[125] (Table 3-3, Fig. 3-13). Dysesthetic pain has been attributed to a cutaneous or subcutaneous distribution and may be attributable to increased firing of damaged or abnormally excitable nociceptive fibers, particularly sprouting regenerating fibers. The pain descriptors that a patient

may use with this type of pain are "burning sensation," "sunburn-like," "skin tingles," or "painful sensation when something touches me" that normally would not hurt, such as bed sheets or stockings.

Paresthesic pain is thought to occur from several possible etiologies: (1) spontaneous activity and increased mechanosensitivity near the cell body of damaged afferent axons in the dorsal root ganglion; (2) loss of segmental

TABLE 3-3   Descriptors of Different Types of Neuropathic Pain

Dysesthesia	Paresthesia	Muscular Pain
Burning sensation	Pins and needles	Dull ache
Sunburn-like	Electric-like	Night cramps
Skin tingles	Numb but achy	Band-like sensation
Painful sensation when something touches me that normally would not hurt (e.g., bedsheets or stockings)	Like feet in ice water	Drawing sensation
	Knife-like	Deep aches
	Shooting pain	Spasms
	Lancinating pain	Toothache-like

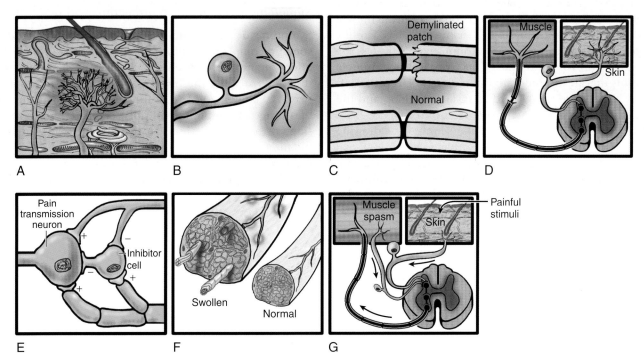

Figure 3–13   Three types of pain. The proposed etiologies of the different types. **A,** Dysesthesia pain. Increases firing of damaged or abnormally excited nociceptive fibers, particularly sprouting regenerating fibers in the cutaneous tissue. **B,** Paresthesia pain. Spontaneous activity and increased mechanosensitivity near the cell body of damaged afferents in the dorsal root ganglion. **C,** Paresthesia pain. Ectopic impulses generated from demyelinated patches of myelinated axons. **D,** Muscular pain. Ectopic impulses to the muscle generated from demyelinated patches resulting in muscle spasms and pain. **E,** Paresthesia pain. Loss of large myelinated fibers on the effects of the small unmyelinated fibers (modified gate control hypothesis). Pain signals are transmitted from the spinal cord pain transmission neuron as a result of the input from the unmyelinated, myelinated, and inhibitor cells. **F,** Paresthesia pain. Increased firing of endings of nociceptive afferents that innervate the nerve sheaths themselves (nervi nervorum). The endoneurial swelling is secondary to endoneurial sodium accumulation and marked nerve hydration. **G,** Muscular pain. Reflex loop (Livingston's vicious cycle) involving a nociceptive input that activates the motor neuron within the spinal cord causing muscle spasms that in turn activate the muscle nociceptors and feeds back to the spinal cord to sustain the spasm. *(Redrawn with permission from Pfeifer MA, Ross D, Schrage J, et al: A highly successful and novel model for the treatment of chronic painful diabetic peripheral neuropathy. Diabetes Care 16:1103–1115, 1993.)*

inhibition of large myelinated fibers on small unmyelinated fibers (modified gate control in which pain signals are transmitted from the spinal cord transmission neuron as a result of the input from the unmyelinated, myelinated, and inhibitor cells); (3) ectopic impulses generated from demyelinated patches of myelinated axons; or (4) increased firing caused by physiologic stimulation of endings of nociceptive afferents that innervate the nerve sheaths themselves (nervi nervorum). Morphologic changes in affected nerves include nerve fiber loss, axonal atrophy, nodal swelling, and endoneurial swelling.[126] These abnormalities may lead to other structural changes (e.g., axonal degeneration, myelin wrinkling, and Wallerian degeneration). The endoneurial swelling may be secondary to endoneurial sodium accumulation and marked increase in nerve hydration. The pain descriptors that are used to describe paresthesia include "pins and needles," "electric-like," "numb," "aching feet," "feel as if my feet have been in ice water," "knife-like," "shooting pains," or "lancinating pains."

The third type of pain is muscular pain. This is believed to be secondary to injury to the motor neurons (e.g., demyelinated patches) or "Livingston's vicious cycle."[127] Ectopic neural impulses to the muscle may be generated from the demyelinated patches in motor nerves. These ectopic impulses would result in muscle spasms and pain. Livingston's "vicious cycle" is a reflex loop involving a nociceptive input that activates the motor neuron within the spinal cord causing muscle spasms that in turn activate the muscle nociceptors and feed back to the spinal cord to sustain the loop and the spasms and pain. Muscular pain descriptors include "dull ache," "night cramps," "band-like sensation," "drawing sensation," "spasms," and "toothache-like." Physical examination often reveals tight, contracted foot extensors and gastrocnemius muscles. Treatment for muscular pain includes lower-limb stretching exercises twice a day and proper footwear, including custom shoes and metatarsal bars where necessary. Patients are encouraged to avoid high heels because they cause undue strain on the gastrocnemius muscles. If the muscular pain continues after 2 weeks of exercise, a muscle relaxant should be considered. Alternatively, a nonsteroidal anti-inflammatory drug could be used to break "Livingston's vicious cycle."

Motor Signs and Symptoms

Imbalance of walking is a commonly elicited complaint even if not volunteered by the patient initially. It often begins with difficulty maintaining balance in the shower when washing hair and the feet are close together. The patient may have gait ataxia walking in the dark yet no ataxia during the day. This symptom relates to the loss of proprioception in the toes and ankles, a sign that is commonly confirmed on testing of joint position sense in the feet.

Leg weakness is typically a late feature of diabetic neuropathy, as patients usually do not complain of toe weakness, the first body region affected by weakness in most people with diabetic neuropathy. Ankle weakness or foot drop is typically the first motor symptom of diabetic neuropathy noted by patients. Intuitively, one would predict that the weakness or foot drop would be symmetrical, but commonly, it presents in one leg before the other. Not infrequently, the foot drop also affects foot eversion, a clinical presentation that is more in keeping with a common peroneal palsy, one of the common compression mononeuropathies observed in diabetic neuropathy. Over time, the asymmetrical foot drop spreads to the contralateral foot. When the weakness moves to the hands, patients often complain about dropping of objects, deteriorating handwriting, and loss of muscle mass in the hands. Entrapment neuropathies are common in diabetic neuropathy. Patients with a superimposed carpal tunnel syndrome will have complaints that are unique to that diagnosis, such as atrophy and weakness of thumb abduction, numbness and pain in the distribution of the median nerve, and worsening hand pain at night.

Symptoms of Autonomic Neuropathy

Symptoms of autonomic neuropathy frequently parallel somatic complaints. Autonomic neuropathy in diabetes affects many organ systems, including the skin, the conduction system of the heart, gastric and bowel motility, urinary bladder, and sexual function. Patients complain of a range of symptoms from dry, cracked, and mottled skin, orthostatic dizziness, and syncope to abdominal bloating after eating, diarrhea or constipation, urinary retention or incontinence, and penile erection and ejaculation impairment. The most common cardiac complaint is orthostatic hypotension, yet it is well known that resting tachycardia and silent myocardial infarction are common in diabetic patients, reflecting underlying autonomic system disease.

Neurologic Examination

Overview

The physical examination of a patient with diabetic neuropathy often begins with the vital signs and the need for pulse and blood pressure measurements in several positions (supine, sitting, and standing) to assess for orthostasis and pulse change. Patients with symptoms that are suggestive of orthostatic hypotension should be tested supine, sitting, and standing, delaying measurements until at least 1 minute after the position change. In the setting of profound orthostasis, patients with autonomic neuropathy might have little or no change in pulse, reflecting sinoatrial node disease and the inability to generate a tachycardia during position changes and stress. In contradistinction, patients with hypovolemia and normal cardiac function should have a rise of pulse of 20 to 30 when the patient changes position.

Observation of the lower limbs and particularly the feet often gives clues to abnormalities betraying an underlying neuropathy. Patients often have dry and cracked skin, nail changes, and skin discoloration, raising the possibility of autonomic disease. Feet are most often cold to touch, yet at other times, they may be warm. Even though patients and physicians often attribute excessive coldness to "poor circulation," foot pulses are often easily palpated, since the underlying mechanism is autonomic impairment and not large vessel disease.

In mild diabetic distal neuropathy, the two most prominent changes on neurologic examination will be a reduced or lost ankle reflex and a distal gradient loss of large and small sensory fiber modalities; the latter is often referred to as "stocking-and-glove" sensory loss. Examination with a 128-Hz tuning fork is the most practical way to check for the presence or absence of vibratory sensation in the feet (Fig. 3-14). Most often, patients show deficits in vibration perception at the great toe. Over time, the deficits move proximally to the metatarsalphalangeal joints, dorsum of the foot, ankle, and the mid-shin region. In typical cases, patients have similar but less severe abnormalities in the fingers by the time deficits are found at the mid-shin or knee. A similar distal

gradient loss is detected to cold perception in patients with small sensory fiber involvement. This writer has found with experience that a cold perception gradient loss is easier to define than is loss of pin and pain perception. Loss of joint position sense (proprioception) is usually the last sensory modality to become abnormal in a distal gradient loss neuropathy but is commonly detected in patients with long-standing diabetic neuropathy.

Sense of Touch: Monofilament Testing

Performing monofilament testing on the plantar surface of the great toe and the pulp of the index finger bilaterally can assess the sense of touch. They are often used as screening devices for determining whether patients have neuropathy or have lost their protective sensation, rendering them much more prone to ulceration. The currently available instruments are known as the Semmes-Weinstein monofilaments. They are usually made of fine nylon and designed so that the amount of pressure administered to the plantar surface is a function of the instrument and not the examiner. Each of the 24 available nylon monofilaments is calibrated to deliver a different bowing force (buckling stress). Each monofilament is marked with a number that represents the decimal log of 10 times the force in milligrams ranging from 1.65 (000.45 g) to 6.65 (447 g) of linear force (Fig. 3-15). The various sites for monofilament testing on the plantar surface of the feet are illustrated in Figure 3-16.

In examining the foot, a series of monofilaments that range in size from 2.83 to 6.65 are typically used. The tip of the monofilament is gently placed perpendicularly on the surface until the monofilament buckles (Fig. 3-17). The approach, skin contact, and departure of the monofilament should be approximately 1.5 seconds. Examiners should not allow the filament to slide across the skin or make repetitive contact to the site. Examiners should also be sure to avoid callused areas. The patient should be able to sense the monofilament by the time the monofilament buckles. The thicker (higher the number) the monofilament, the more force is required to cause the buckle. Patients without neuropathy should be able to sense the 3.61 monofilament (equivalent to 0.4 gram of linear force). The inability to sense monofilaments of 4.17 (equivalent of 1 gram of linear pressure) or higher is considered consistent with neuropathy (large fiber modality). Inability to sense a monofilament of 5.07 (equivalent to 10 grams of linear force) is consistent with severe neuropathy and loss of protective sensation (see Fig. 3-17). Custom footwear is indicated for diabetic people who cannot feel the 5.07 monofilament.

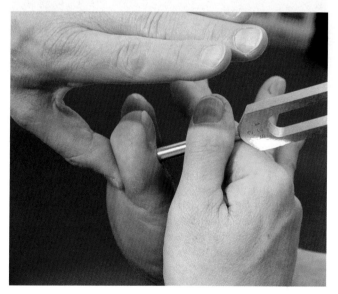

Figure 3–14 Vibration sense. It is difficult to establish a quantitative assessment, so a 128-Hz tuning fork is commonly used. Have the patient close his or her eyes. Demonstrate the feeling to be expected to the patient by touching his/her jaw with the vibrating tuning fork. Make the tuning fork vibrate by hitting it close to the base of the tines with the heel of your hand. Place the tuning fork at the base of the great toenail for at least 10 seconds. The response should be present or absent. The test is repeated in the other foot and at the base of both thumbnails. The inability to feel the tuning fork at the base of the great toenail carries the same significance as the inability to feel a 5.07 monofilament, and the patient should be referred for custom footwear. This is considered to be a large nerve fiber function.

Deep Tendon Reflexes

Documentation of the presence or absence of the knee and ankle (Achilles) reflexes are an essential part of the physical examination in the patient with known or

Evaluator size		Target force in grams	Plantar thresholds
1.65		0.008	Normal
2.36		0.02	
2.44		0.04	
2.83	✪	0.07	
3.22		0.16	
3.61	✪	**0.4**	
3.84		0.6	Diminished light touch
4.08		1	
4.17		1.4	
4.31	✪	2	
4.56	✪	4	Diminished protective sensation
4.74		6	
4.93		8	
5.07	✪	10	Loss of protective sensation
5.18		15	
5.46		26	
5.88		60	
6.10		100	
6.45		180	
6.65	✪	300	Deep pressure sensation only

Figure 3–15   Monofilament Table. This table lists 20 of the 24 Semmes-Weinstein monofilaments by size and grams of linear force. The most important calibrations: 3.61, 431, 4.56, 5.07 and 6.65 are marked (✪). Commercially available kits of six typically include these plus the 2.83 evaluator size.

Patients who are able to sense the 3.61 size (0.4 grams of force) are presumed not to have small fiber neuropathy. Patients who are able to sense the 5.07 monofilament (10 grams target force) have retained protective sensation even if they have may have mild small fiber neuropathy. Inability to sense the 5.07 size is: (1) consistent with severe neuropathy, (2) greatly increases the possibility of a neuropathic ulcer and (3) is one of the five indications for custom insoles/footwear for the diabetic patient (ses text and *Pearls*).

Monofilaments with an evaluator size smaller than the 3.61 are primarily utilized for the evaluation of the hands. Evaluation of sensation of the hands requires different thresholds than those illustrated for the foot (plantar).

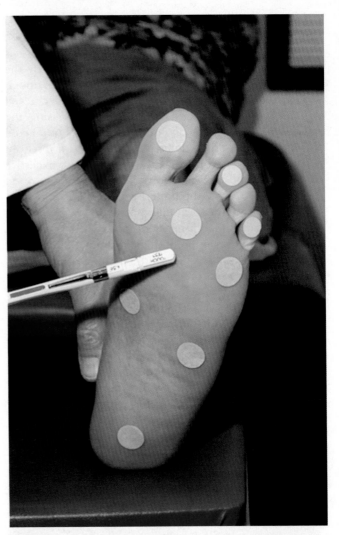

Figure 3–16   Monofilament sites on plantar surface. The photo demonstrates various sites on the plantar surface of the foot that have been standardized for examination with the Semmes-Weinstein monofilaments (see text).

suspected peripheral neuropathy (Fig. 3-18). Deep tendon or muscle stretch reflexes are reduced or absent in a length-dependent pattern such that the ankle reflex is typically lost first followed by the knee reflex. Upper-limb reflexes are usually preserved in early diabetic neuropathy yet become reduced or absent as the disease progresses. It is common for patients with diabetes for 15 to 20 years to be areflexic. If a patient with recent-onset diabetes and a rapidly progressive peripheral neuropathy is areflexic in the arms and legs, the neuropathy is likely to arise from another cause. The leading consideration would be chronic inflammatory demyelinating polyneuropathy (CIDP), a chronic inflammatory polyneuropathy that bears some resemblance to Guillain-Barré syndrome in pathogenesis and pathophysiology.[128] The recognition of CIDP in a diabetic patient is crucial, since treatment differs from the usual approach of diet control, exercise, and glycemic control. CIDP can be treated with a variety of agents from corticosteroids to other immunosuppressant agents, plasma exchange, and intravenous immunoglobulins. CIDP is estimated to be 11 times more common in patients with type 2 diabetes than in nondiabetic individuals.[129]

Motor Function

Loss of motor function most commonly follows the changes in sensation and reflexes. Many patients will have no demonstrable weakness in the lower limbs on formal strength testing after years of diabetic neuropathy. Typically, weakness will first be detected in the toe extensors followed by the toe flexors, a pattern that follows the length-dependent nature of diabetic neuropathy. As the disease progresses, patients develop weakness of ankle

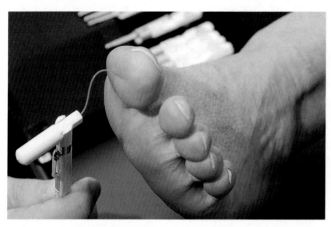

Figure 3–17   Monofilament on the great toe. This photo demonstrates the correct usage of the Semmes-Weinstein monofilament to detect the presence or absence of neuropathy and the retention or loss of protective sensation The latter is measured with the 5.07 monofilament (as shown here). The patient should be comfortable and have his or her eyes closed. Note that the monofilament buckles when the 10 grams of linear force are applied by the examiner for about 10 seconds. Note that this patient has early claw toe deformities. He was insensate to the 5.07 and even the 6.65 monofilament.

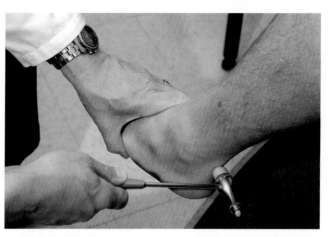

Figure 3–18   Ankle jerk. Have the patient kneel on the edge of a high-backed, stable chair with his or her back toward you. Gently apply pressure on the sole of the foot (causing some dorsiflexion and muscle stretching). Strike the Achilles tendon. Observe plantar flexion of the foot via muscle contraction of the gastrocnemius and soleus muscles. Alternatively, the patient can be examined while sitting on the exam table or at the bedside (as illustrated). Patients who are hospitalized or who are disabled and cannot sit up can be examined while lying on their back with their head at about 45 degrees for maximum comfort. The examiner holds the foot just off the bed as he or she strikes the Achilles tendon. Note that the photograph illustrates the Traumner reflex hammer. This is an excellent hammer because of its ideal weight and shape. It also has a smaller head, which is very useful for the upper-limb deep tendon reflexes or with children.

dorsiflexion and eversion before ankle plantar flexion and inversion, deficits that are explainable by the relatively smaller muscle mass of the tibialis anterior and peroneal longus muscles compared to the posterior tibial and gastrocnemius group. Proximal muscles of the legs are often spared unless the diabetic neuropathy is unusually long-standing, for example, 25 to 30 years, if it is rapidly progressive, or if another illness is superimposed. If proximal weakness is observed in one leg and the patient complains of pain in the same region, the examiner should consider diabetic amyotrophy, one of the focal diabetic neuropathies that affect the lumbosacral roots or plexus, or multiple proximal mononeuropathies.

Once diabetic neuropathy advances to the level of the knee, patients begin to complain of hand weakness, and the examination often confirms the deficits. In most cases, the examiner will find weakness of the dorsal and ventral interossei muscles and the abductor digiti minimi. Over time, weakness will progress to the thumb abductors and finger extensors.

Electrophysiologic Testing

Electrophysiologic testing plays a major role in the evaluation of patients with both suspected distal symmetrical neuropathy and well-documented neuropathy, using motor and sensory nerve conduction studies, the needle examination, and autonomic testing. Electrophysiologic testing can document that the neuropathy is present, define the fibers that are affected (motor, sensory, and autonomic), render a gross estimate of the duration of the neuropathy, and even give insight into the prognosis.

It can assess whether a superimposed process is present, such as a mononeuropathy, mononeuritis multiplex, brachial or lumbosacral plexopathy, or a polyradiculopathy. Common mononeuropathies that are observed in diabetic patients are median mononeuropathy at the wrist (carpal tunnel syndrome), ulnar neuropathy at the elbow or cubital tunnel, facial mononeuropathy (Bell's palsy), and common peroneal palsy.

Much information can be gleaned from the testing of a few nerves that are carefully chosen by clinical examination. As is true in most neuropathies, the sensory nerves will be more affected than will motor nerves. Little information is gained from the testing of severely affected nerves such as the sural, peroneal, or tibial nerves in a patient with long-standing diabetic neuropathy. In that situation, the action potentials are usually unrecordable, so the electromyographer cannot determine whether the primary process is axon loss or demyelination. A rule of thumb is to test lower-limb nerves in a patient who is thought to have a mild neuropathy and to focus testing on upper-limb nerves in a patient with a suspected severe neuropathy. The amplitude of the motor compound muscle action potentials and the sensory nerve action potentials can be used to estimate the number of intact motor and sensory nerve fibers, respectively, unless a demyelinating process is present between the point of stimulation and the recording electrode. A good correlation exists between the severity and number of the nerve conduction study abnormalities and the severity of the clinical neuropathy. Nerve conduction studies primarily measure the function of large myelinated fibers, so it is possible for a diabetic patient to have a painful small fiber neuropathy and to have a normal nerve conduction study. It is estimated that approximately 5% of patients with neuropathy will have normal nerve conduction studies.

Electromyography (EMG) can be a useful examination in diabetic neuropathy to detect denervation and to decipher chronicity, the latter by analyzing the morphology of motor units. Electromyography can detect active or chronic denervation in patients with diabetes who have normal nerve conduction studies and thus verify the diagnosis. The needle examination can test for superimposed processes such as a brachial plexopathy, lumbosacral plexopathy (diabetic amyotrophy), thoracolumbar radiculopathy, or motor neuron disease such as amyotrophic lateral sclerosis or progressive muscular atrophy.

Nerve conduction studies are often abnormal in diabetic patients who clinically do not have a neuropathy. Hendriksen and colleagues studied 88 diabetic patients for subclinical neuropathy who had no clinical evidence for polyneuropathy using nerve conduction studies, papillary latency and diameter testing, and single fiber electromyography. Of the group, 52 patients had type 1 diabetes and 36 had type 2 diabetes. The authors found a high percentage of abnormalities. The tibial nerve and the tibial H-reflex were abnormal in 69% to 81% of patients, the sural nerve was abnormal in 56% to 64% of patients, the ulnar sensory nerve in 33% to 40%, and the ulnar motor nerve in 9% to 31% of patients. Pupil constriction latency and pupil diameter percentage was abnormal in 62% to 69% of patients. The severity of the polyneuropathy electrophysiologically was equal in patients with type 1 diabetes and those with type 2 diabetes when the results were corrected for age, height, and duration of the illness.[130]

The results of nerve conduction studies can be used to monitor the course of diabetic patients treated with insulin or oral hypoglycemic agents, treated with intensive insulin therapy, or enrolled in clinical trials. In the DCCT, velocities of the sural and median sensory nerves increased modestly in the first year of therapy in patients in the primary convention cohort who received intensive therapy, and the median sensory velocities returned to baseline by year 5. In the motor nerves, conduction velocities remained steady or increased slightly in the intensive therapy group compared to the conventional therapy group where motor nerve conduction velocities consistently decreased. Amplitudes of the motor and sensory nerves did not change significantly in the two treatment groups. Changes favoring the intensive therapy group were also recorded in autonomic testing. The intensive therapy group experienced slower worsening of the R-R variation, reflecting some delay in the progression of cardiac autonomic neuropathy.[131]

Extensive testing and retesting are usually not necessary; the repeated measurement of one or two nerves often suffices.[132] Reeves and colleagues studied the medial plantar sensory nerve in 10 diabetic patients who underwent a 6-month program of intensification of therapy to treat diabetes. Near normalization of glucose levels led to a return of the sensory nerve action potentials in 7 of 10 patients and a normalization of the sensory distal latency in all patients.[133]

Prevention and Treatment

Pain Management

Pain is a common complication of diabetic neuropathy. From a clinical and pathologic standpoint, pain can be divided into nociceptive and neuropathic pain. The former arises from the presence of a pathologic process that produces continuing tissue damage. Examples include osteoarthritis, cholecystitis, phlebitis, cellulitis, and abscess. Conversely, neuropathic pain stems from injury to the peripheral nerve or central somatosensory pathways. Neuropathic pain is commonly constant and associated with paroxysms of pain that do not follow a specific pattern. Pain is experienced by over 10% of patients with diabetic polyneuropathy, and management of this pain can be a challenge for even the most skilled physician.

Once it has been determined that the pain is secondary to distal symmetrical polyneuropathy, the pain is classified as acute or chronic painful neuropathy (Table 3-4). Acute painful neuropathy lasts less than 12 months and is mostly attributable to metabolic abnormalities rather than to structural abnormalities. Proposed etiologies include decreased nerve taurine concentration and endoneurial swelling. The typical scenario is the newly diagnosed diabetic patient who has just been started on insulin. Acute, painful diabetic neuropathy is self-limited. The patient often responds well to analgesic therapy with nonsteroidal anti-inflammatory drugs.

Chronic, painful diabetic neuropathy typically occurs in patients with intermediate duration (8 to 12 years) of diabetes. It has a gradual and insidious onset, and the pain typically lasts more than 12 months. There are structural abnormalities (see below). The pain may persist for years, and relapses occur. Treatment of chronic, painful diabetic neuropathy requires a more complex

TABLE 3-4 Compendium of Treatments for Neuropathic Pain

NSAIDs	Transdermal clonidine
Tricyclic antidepressants	Tramadol hydrochloride
SSRIs	Antiarrhythmics
Anticonvulsants	Antispasticity medications
Topical capsaicin	Narcotics
Lidocaine cream	α-Lipoic acid
	Epidural spinal cord stimulation

approach but can be greatly or moderately successful in patients who do not have motives for treatment failure (e.g., sympathy-seeking behavior, narcotic-seeking behavior, wishing to gain or maintain disability).

Although improved glycemic control is advocated for all patients with DPN, the pain response might not correlate with achievement of an ideal A1C level. An interesting paradox is the exacerbation of pain in some patients as better glucose control is achieved.

Figure 3-19 demonstrates the relationship between nerve function and painful neuropathic symptoms. As nerve function worsens, the pain threshold may be exceeded. Once this occurs, the pain continues until the nerve becomes so dysfunctional that pain signals are not easily transmitted to the central nervous system. Eventually, nerve function worsens and sensation decreases to the point that the foot becomes numb. Some individuals get numb or insensate feet without ever breaching the pain threshold (see Fig. 3-19).

Depending on the location of the patient on the pain curve, an improvement in nerve function could either cause the pain to drop below the pain threshold or increase pain. Glucose control can improve nerve function enough to cause such changes. This would explain the decreased pain in some patients (located on the left side of the curve) and increased pain in other patients (located on the right side of the curve) with better glucose control. Regardless of the change in pain symptoms, glucose control is still desirable and should be initiated in all patients.

To understand the use of a vast array of treatments for neuropathic pain, a fundamental understanding of pain pathways within the peripheral and central nervous system is necessary. Pain is carried primarily by unmyelinated C-fibers within the peripheral sensory axons.

Those fibers enter the dorsal root and synapse in laminae I and II within the dorsal horn of the spinal cord. Many of the fine afferents terminating in the dorsal horn contain neuropeptides such as substance P, cholecystokinin, and somatostatin. Opiate receptors are also found on the terminals of the primary afferents and dorsal horn neurons. Consequently, both presynaptic and postsynaptic mechanisms are important in the analgesic effect of opiates at the spinal level.

To comprehend the effect of drugs that reduce norepinephrine and serotonin reuptake on pain, one needs to understand the two major descending pathways for pain modulation. The first is the reticulospinal tract that originates in the periaqueductal gray region and gives rise to serotonergic fibers that synapse on the dorsal horn. The second descending pathways begin in the locus coeruleus of the medulla oblongata and send noradrenergic fibers to the dorsal horn. The periaqueductal gray region of the midbrain, the raphe nuclei of the medulla, and the dorsal horn contain a high density of endogenous opiate peptides and receptors. In animals, stimulation of the periaqueductal gray region inhibits the discharge of nociceptive neurons at spinal levels. At the level of the spinal cord, the descending tracks from the periaqueductal gray region and raphe nuclei directly inhibit pain-responsive neurons, some of which contain endogenous opioid transmitters.

Current knowledge suggests that both central and peripheral mechanisms play a role in initiating and perpetuating neuropathic pain. Peripheral mechanisms include sensitization and abnormal ectopic discharges; both phenomena are thought to result from an increase in the number of sodium channels that develop on peripheral nerves after trauma or toxic or metabolic derangement to a nerve. Peripheral sensitization refers to an increased sensitivity of the peripheral nociceptors to stimuli and a lower threshold of the nociceptors to fire. Ectopic pacemakers arise in injured peripheral nerves and fire spontaneously to a broad series of physical, chemical, and metabolic stimuli. Central sensitization refers to the phenomenon by which peripheral nerve injury causes release of various neurotransmitters at the dorsal horn region, which in turn leads to increased calcium influx into a cell, an activation of nitric oxide synthase, an expression of early genes, and activation of phosphatases. The latter results in a lower threshold for depolarization and spontaneous discharges of the spinal cord dorsal horns. Consequently, the spinal cord becomes hypersensitive to afferent fibers. An understanding of the central and peripheral mechanism for neuropathic pain gives relevance to why different classes of drugs can be beneficial for treating neuropathic pain.

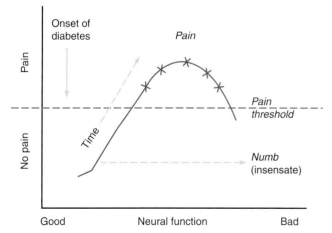

Figure 3–19   Neural functions. This figure demonstrates the relationship between nerve function and painful neuropathic symptoms. As nerve function worsens, the pain threshold may be exceeded. Once this occurs, the pain continues until the nerve becomes so dysfunctional that pain signals are not easily transmitted to the central nervous system. Eventually, nerve function worsens such that sensation decreases to the point that the foot becomes numb. Some individuals get numb or insensate feet without ever breaching the pain threshold.

*From Dwight C. McGoon: Ecstasy, a basis for meaning in the world. In Huth EJ, Murray TJ (eds): Medicine Quotations: Views of Health and Disease Through the Ages:. Philadelphia: American College of Physicians, 2000.

Treatment of Neuropathic Pain

The authors strongly recommend that physicians and other health care providers who are entrusted to relieve the pain and suffering of patients with painful neuropathy should abide by two important dictums: *Primum non nocere* ("First, do no harm") and "Your compassion for your patients—trying to do the best for them—must be the major motivating force in your effort to remain competent."* The authors are of the opinion that clinicians who follow these principles will have a greater chance of success while they garner the respect of both their patients and their colleagues.

The treatment of neuropathic pain includes pharmacologic and psychological approaches. The clinician should understand the difficulty in completely eliminating pain associated with diabetic neuropathy. Some patients respond poorly to these drugs; others develop adverse effects even at the lowest dosages. In some patients, a reduction of pain of 30% to 40% is appreciated and is considered a good response. In most instances, the drugs listed below are started slowly and titrated upward until satisfactory pain relief is achieved or side effects develop.[134]

Figure 3-20 is an algorithm that the authors have found effective for providing guidance to clinicians who are neither specialists in pain management nor familiar with treatment of this condition. This algorithm condenses and simplifies a practical approach to the management of patients utilizing one or more of the agents described in this section. A recent study by Gilron and associates underscores patients' attitudes toward the treatment of neuropathy and the relative undertreatment of their condition. In a study of 151 patients with neuropathic pain, of whom more than half had painful diabetic neuropathy, 72.8% complained of inadequate pain control, and more than 25% had never been treated with a drug whose mechanism was directed at neuropathic pain. The mean daily pain score was 7.6 on a 10-point scale. New agents, such as gabapentin, had been prescribed for only 16.6% of patients. Opioids, tricyclic antidepressants, and anticonvulsants had never been prescribed for 41% of patients. Approximately 32% of patients expressed fear of addiction and adverse effect from medications prescribed.[135] Data that are often reported in studies of painful diabetic neuropathy are the number of patients needed to treat (NNT) to achieve a beneficial effect and the number needed to treat before an adverse event or harm results (NNH). An ideal medication has a low NNT and a high NNH.[136] Table 3-4 overviews a compendium of treatments for neuropathic pain.

Nonsteroidal Anti-Inflammatory Drugs

In 1987, Cohen and associates published a single-blind study of 18 patients with DPN who were treated with placebo, ibuprofen, or sulindac.[137] They showed that the response to both ibuprofen and sulindac was better than that to placebo for the entire group. Within the group, eight patients were particularly good responders to the nonsteroidal anti-inflammatory agents. During the course of the study, there was no change in glucose control or renal function that might have influenced the results. Although not helpful for many patients with neuropathic pain, anti-inflammatory agents may be useful in a small group and should be considered for initial therapy if renal function is normal.

Tricyclic Antidepressants

Tricyclic antidepressant (TCA) medications serve as a mainstay of treatment for neuropathic pain. They can be divided into secondary and tertiary amine agents. The secondary amines nortriptyline, desipramine, and maprotiline are selective inhibitors of norepinephrine, whereas the tertiary amines amitriptyline, imipramine, and clomipramine block the reuptake of both serotonin and norepinephrine. The most effective agents are those that inhibit the reuptake of both norepinephrine and serotonin yet have a good adverse effect profile. Many studies have demonstrated the efficacy of these agents for the treatment of painful diabetic neuropathy.[138] The therapeutic dosage range is 25 to 150 mg per day with most or all of the drug taken at night. It is best to start with a low dosage in treating elderly patients and to advance in weekly increments of 10 to 25 mg. Relief of pain might not occur until several weeks after the treatment with TCAs is initiated.

The efficacy of antidepressants for the management of neuropathic pain is separate from its antidepressive effect.[139] Commonly observed side effects include drowsiness, dry eyes and mouth, increased appetite, weight gain, urinary retention, and constipation. In the elderly, moderate doses of antidepressants may cause disorientation, confusion, and excessive sleepiness. An understanding of the different types of antidepressants and their side effect profiles allows selection of an agent that has an either greater or lesser effect on norepinephrine and serotonin reuptake as well as a minimal tendency to produce anticholinergic side effects. TCAs should be used with caution in patients with a history of coronary artery disease and cardiac conduction defects, as TCAs can incite cardiac arrhythmias or heart block.

Mitchel Max and colleagues showed that amitriptyline and desipramine provided moderate to good relief of pain in 61% to 71% of patients with painful diabetic neuropathy.[140] Amitriptyline and desipramine were as effective in nondepressed patients as in depressed patients. The authors identified a linear relationship between pain relief and dosage of the antidepressive agent.

Little information from human studies is available comparing the analgesic potency of one antidepressant to that of another. In animal studies using response to a painful stimulus, amitriptyline was more potent than nortriptyline, imipramine, and desipramine. Amitriptyline was judged to be approximately 70 times more potent than aspirin as an analgesic.[141]

Algorithm for treatment of painful DPN ①

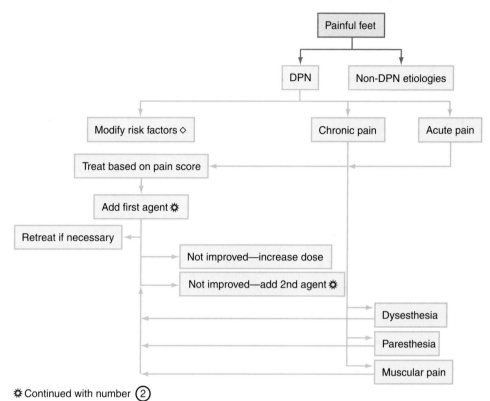

☀ Continued with number ②

A ◇ Risk factors: hyperglycemia, hypertension, hyperlipidemia, smoking, ethanol intake

Algorithm for treatment of painful DPN ②

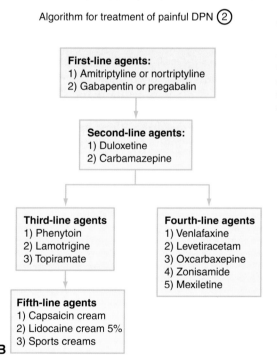

B

Figure 3–20 **Algorithm for the treatment of painful diabetic neuropathy.** This algorithm has proven to be successful in a prospective clinical trial. It requires the health care professional to query the patient as to the type of neuropathic pain. Therapy is then directed toward the specific type of pain (dysesthesia, paresthesia, muscular pain, or combinations of the three). *(Redrawn with permission from Pfeifer MA, Ross D, Schrage J, et al: A highly successful and novel model for the treatment of chronic painful diabetic peripheral neuropathy. Diabetes Care 16:1103–1115, 1993.)*

Selective Serotonin Reuptake Inhibitors

The neurologic literature supports marginal benefit from using selective serotonin reuptake inhibitors (SSRIs) to treat neuropathic pain. Although better tolerated than TCAs, in a study of fluoxetine compared to placebo, amitriptyline, and desipramine, fluoxetine was no better than placebo in relieving the pain associated with diabetic neuropathy. SSRIs may play a greater role in treating the depression of patients with painful neuropathies. Common adverse effects of SSRIs are sweating, insomnia, dizziness, headache, visual disturbances, and

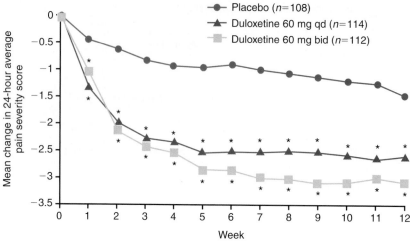

*p < .001 vs. placebo.

Figure 3–21 **Duloxetine graph.** In a recent 12-week study, patients with diabetic neuropathic pain and without comorbid depression were randomized to treatment with duloxetine 60 mg four times a day (n = 114), duloxetine 60 mg twice a day (n = 112), or placebo (n = 108). The primary outcome in this study was the weekly mean score of 24-hour average pain severity on the 11-point Likert scale. Both dosages of duloxetine were superior to placebo in reducing pain as measured by the weekly 24-hour average pain severity score, with statistically significant separation from placebo occurring at week 1 and continuing throughout the 12-week period (p < .001). Duloxetine was also superior to placebo for almost all secondary outcomes (e.g., Brief Pain Inventory severity scores), with no significant differences between the two dosages. *(Redrawn with permission from Wernicke J, Lu Y, D'Souza D, Waninger A, Tran P: Duloxetine at doses of 60 mg QD and 60 mg BID is effective in treatment of diabetic neuropathic pain (DNP) [abstract]. J Pain 5(suppl 1):48, 2004.)*

sexual dysfunction. SSRIs can be used with TCAs only with great caution, as both paroxetine and fluoxetine block the cytochrome P450 2D isoenzyme that is integral to the metabolism of TCAs. Blood levels of TCAs can rise as much as sevenfold when used in the setting of SSRIs.

The efficacy and safety of venlafaxine was studied in a 6-week trial in a multicenter, double-blind, randomized, placebo-controlled study of 244 patients with diabetic neuropathy. Patients received either the 75-mg ER or the 150- to 225-mg ER tablets. The reduction of the visual analogue scale for pain intensity statistically favored the groups that received the active drug. The visual analogue scale for pain relief was statistically better than placebo for the 150- to 225-mg dosing. The number needed to treat (NNT) for the higher dose of venlafaxine was comparable to those of tricyclic antidepressants and gabapentin.[142]

Duloxetine is the newest compound in this group of reuptake inhibitors. It is considered a balanced selective serotonin and norepinephrine reuptake inhibitor and is approved for use in the treatment of painful DPN. The half-life of the drug is 12 hours, and the maximum plasma concentration is reached in 6 hours.[143] In a 12-week, multicenter, double-blind study of 457 patients with DPN pain randomized to duloxetine 20, 60, or 120 mg per day or placebo, Goldstein and colleagues showed benefit in the groups receiving the two highest doses. Statistically significant improvement was observed in the primary efficacy measure of the 24-hour average pain score and in nearly all the secondary measures including the health-related outcome measures. Fewer

than 20% of patients discontinued duloxetine because of adverse events.[144] Figure 3-21 illustrates the pain score response to duloxetine in a double-blind randomized clinical trial.[145]

Anticonvulsants

Many anticonvulsants have been shown to be effective in the management of neuropathic pain (Table 3-5). Although the exact mechanism of their benefit remains unknown for some of the drugs, these agents probably work by modulating sodium channels, stabilizing nerve

TABLE 3-5 **Anticonvulsants for Neuropathic Pain**

Generic Name	Trade Name	
First-Generation		
Phenytoin	Dilantin	√
Phenobarbital		
Primidone	Mysoline	
Ethosuximide	Zarontin	
Carbamazepine	Tegretol	√√
Valproic acid	Depakote	
Second-Generation		
Gabapentin	Neurontin	√√√√
Pregabalin	Lyrica	√√ ☺
Lamotrigine	Lamictal	√
Topiramate	Topamax	√√
Tiagabine	Gabitrol	
Levetiracetam	Keppra	
Oxcarbazepine	Trileptal	√
Zonisamide	Zanegran	
Felbamate	Felbatol	

√, clinically prescribed or studied for painful DPN; ☺, FDA approved for DPN.

fiber membranes, and suppressing ectopic discharges that give rise to the paroxysms of pain. Phenytoin, carbamazepine, gabapentin, pregabalin, lamotrigine, valproic acid, and topiramate have been studied in uncontrolled and controlled patient populations.

Phenytoin

The response rate to phenytoin has been reported to be as high as 68% in patients taking 100 mg three times per day for 2 weeks.[146,147] When successful, the response usually occurs within 1 to 4 days after the initiation of therapy. In another study of only 12 patients, using a study design in which patients received either active drug or placebo on alternate weeks for a total of 4 weeks, no statistical significance was found between the group that was prescribed 300 mg daily and placebo. The results were confounded by the observation that blood glucose levels were elevated in the diabetic patients taking phenytoin.[148] Phenytoin can be an attractive choice to treat neuropathic pain because of its low cost, well-known side effect profile, and ease of use (nighttime dosing), but in this author's opinion, it rarely leads to impressive pain relief in most patients with painful diabetic neuropathy.

Carbamazepine

In a double-blind-crossover study of carbamazepine compared to placebo in the treatment of painful diabetic neuropathy, Rull and colleagues recorded symptomatic improvement in 28 of 30 patients taking 200 mg three times per day.[149] Adverse effects were recorded in over 50% of patients, but those effects were often mild and transient. Mean improvement in pain varied between 56% and 75%. In another crossover study conducted over 2 weeks, Wilton and colleagues showed that carbamazepine was effective in relieving pain by the second week of treatment in 40 patients with painful diabetic neuropathy. No benefit was observed in the reversal of numbness or improvement in sleep.[150]

Carbamazepine is most effective in relieving the sharp, lancinating component of neuropathic pain rather than the dull, constant pain. Although it is well tolerated initially, approximately 30% to 40% of patients discontinue carbamazepine within 1 year because of side effects. Common adverse effects include dizziness, drowsiness, diplopia, unsteady gait, impaired cognition, nausea, and vomiting. A rash occurs in 10% to 15% of patients who take carbamazepine. In prescribing carbamazepine, a complete blood count (CBC) with differential, serum sodium, and liver function tests should be drawn at the onset of treatment and at 3 and 6 months to screen for the rare complications of aplastic anemia, hepatitis, and the syndrome of inappropriate antidiuretic hormone secretion (SIADH). Approximately 3 weeks after beginning therapy, carbamazepine tends to induce its own metabolism, often necessitating an increase in drug dosing.

Oxcarbazepine

Oxcarbazepine is a metabolite of carbamazepine and shares many of the antiepileptic properties of the drug. In a 9-week, open-label trial of oxcarbazepine in the treatment of painful diabetic neuropathy, Beydoun and colleagues studied 30 patients. The drug was initiated at a dose of 150 mg per day and titrated up to 1200 mg per day or maximum tolerated dose. The mean daily dose taken was 814 mg. The mean visual analogue scale drop was 66.3 during the screening phase to 34.3 at the end of the trial for a mean reduction of 48.3%. Significant improvement was also observed in the total pain score and present pain intensity.[151] In a multicenter, randomized placebo-controlled 16 week trial of oxcarbazepine in patients with painful diabetic neuropathy, significant improvement was observed in the average change in the visual analogue score, the number of patients experiencing a greater than 50% reduction in pain, and global assessment of therapeutic effect. Most adverse effects were mild to moderate and transient.[152]

Gabapentin

Gabapentin is related structurally to the inhibitory amino acid γ-aminobutyric acid, yet the mechanism of its effect on modulating neuropathic pain is not completely understood. Recently, Gu and Huang showed that gabapentin's action on the N-methyl-D-aspartate receptor is protein kinase C–dependent. This response indirectly suggests a possible inflammatory component at the dorsal horn, since in inflammation, endogenous PKC is elevated.[153] Although gabapentin has been used to treat neuropathic pain for years, the first controlled study of gabapentin in diabetic neuropathy was published in December 1998.[154] In that protocol, 165 patients were tested, 84 receiving gabapentin and 81 receiving placebo. As tolerated, patients were titrated up to a daily dose of 3600 mg during the first 4 weeks of the study and maintained on the achieved dose for 4 additional weeks. The authors reported statistically significant lower daily pain scores (primary efficacy measure) and improved secondary measures of efficacy in the group taking gabapentin. At the end of the trial, the mean reduction of pain scores was 39% in the gabapentin-treated group compared to 22% in the group taking placebo ($p < .001$). Patients who received gabapentin but not placebo reported improved sleep and quality of life. All secondary measures of pain showed statistical significance. The most frequently recorded adverse effects to gabapentin were dizziness and somnolence.

Gorson and colleagues reported their results in 40 patients using a placebo-controlled, double-blind, crossover trial. The maximum dose of gabapentin prescribed was 900 mg per day. Statistical improvement was observed only in one of four end points, the McGill Pain Questionnaire, between the initial and final study visits. The most common adverse effects were drowsiness, fatigue, and imbalance. The authors concluded that gabapentin at a dose of 900 mg per day was ineffective or only minimally effective for the treatment of painful diabetic neuropathy.[155]

In 2003, Backonja and Glanzman reviewed the data on the efficacy and tolerability of gabapentin for the treatment of neuropathic pain and to determine the optimal dosing. They accepted only randomized controlled studies of more than 100 patients per treatment arm. Gabapentin was effective in the treatment of painful diabetic neuropathy, postherpetic neuralgia, and other pain syndromes, relieving symptoms of shooting pain, burning pain, allodynia, and hyperesthesia. Most adverse effects abated after 10 days of treatment. The authors advocated starting gabapentin at a dosage of 900 mg per day in three divided doses and titrating the dose upward to 1800 mg per day. Some patients needed doses as high as 3600 mg per day for good pain relief.[156]

Dallocchio and colleagues compared the efficacy of gabapentin to that of amitriptyline in 25 patients with painful diabetic neuropathy in an open-label, prospective, randomized trial. Greater pain and paresthesia relief and fewer side effects were achieved in the group receiving gabapentin compared to the amitriptyline group.[157] In a similar small but randomized prospective, double-blind, double-dummy, crossover study in 28 patients, Morello and colleagues reported moderate or greater pain relief after treatment with gabapentin or amitriptyline and no statistical difference between the two groups.[158]

Treatment with gabapentin should begin with a bedtime dose of 300 mg. The dose can be increased by 300 mg every 3 to 5 days with the eventual goal of achieving a thrice-daily dosing schedule. Many patients respond to a total dosage of 900 to 1200 mg per day, whereas others need 3600 or 4800 mg per day for good pain relief. An attractive feature of gabapentin is its lack of interaction with other medications.

Pregabalin

Pregabalin is an analogue of the neurotransmitter γ-aminobutyric acid, which possesses anticonvulsant, anxiolytic activity, and analgesic properties. It interacts with the α2-delta protein subunit of the voltage-gated calcium channel. The latter characteristic makes it attractive for treating neuropathic pain, particularly for central sensitization pain. Peak plasma levels occur 1 hour after an oral dose; the half-life is 6 hours. Pregabalin is usually excreted unchanged in the urine.[159] Rosenstock and colleagues studied its effect on painful diabetic polyneuropathy in 146 patients in a randomized, double-blind, placebo-controlled, parallel-group study. At a dosage of 300 mg per day, pregabalin produced clinically significant improvement compared to placebo in the primary efficacy measure of the mean pain score as well as secondary efficacy measures of sleep interference, mood

disturbance, and several McGill Pain Questionnaires. Pregabalin was well tolerated. The most common adverse effects were dizziness and somnolence, which were judged to be mild to moderate in severity.[160]

In a review of three randomized clinical trials of 5 to 8 weeks' duration and two clinical trials of 12 weeks' duration, pregabalin at fixed dosages of 300 and 600 mg per day produced superior pain relief and improved pain-related sleep disturbance. The most common side effects associated with the medication were dizziness, somnolence, and peripheral edema.[161] In the largest study to date (246 patients), Richter and colleagues showed that pregabalin 600 mg per day over 6 weeks significantly reduced the mean pain score, sleep interference, past week and present pain intensity, and sensory and affective pain scores. At the dose of 150 mg per day, pregabalin was no different from placebo, although this is the recommended starting dose.[162] In the experience of these authors, many patients with painful DPN respond to this dose, but there is a clear minority that requires 300 mg or even 600 mg per day for the best response. The advantage of this drug over gabapentin is the rapid improvement in pain in only 1 to 2 days, which is a result of the greater than 90% bioavailability of the pregabalin compared to only about 33% bioavailability of gabapentin at doses of 2400 mg or more.[163] Figure 3-22 illustrates the

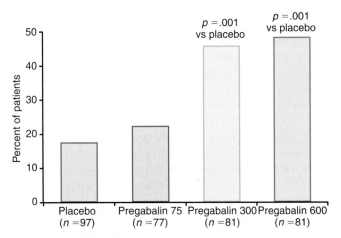

*Last observation carried forward (LOCF) analysis.
All pregabalin doses in mg/d.

Figure 3–22 Pregabalin 50% reduction. In this clinical trial, the 50% responder rates (i.e., the percentage of patients who achieved at least 50% reduction in mean pain score from baseline to end point) in the 300 mg/d and 600 mg/d pregabalin groups were significantly higher than in the placebo group (*p* = .001) in last observation carried forward (LOCF) analysis. The 50% responder rate in the 75 mg/d pregabalin group was not significantly different from that in the placebo group. A response of 30% from baseline has been shown to be clinically meaningful. In Study 029, 33% of placebo patients, 38% of 75 mg/d pregabalin patients, 62% of 300 mg/d pregabalin patients, and 65% of 600 mg/d pregabalin patients had a response of 30% or greater in the LOCF analysis. *(Redrawn with permission from Lesser H, Sharma U, LaMoreaux L, Poole RM: Pregabalin relieves symptoms of painful diabetic neuropathy: A randomized controlled trial. Neurology 63:2104–2110, 2004.)*

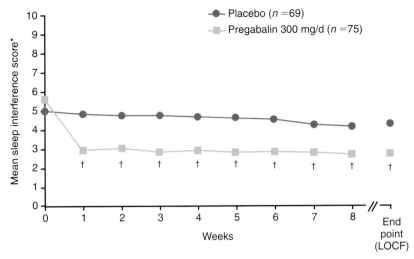

Figure 3-23 **Pregabalin and sleep.** Pregabalin effects on mean weekly sleep interference scores in DPN are noted. After only 1 week of 300 mg pregabalin, the mean sleep interference index fell from approximately 6 to 3, a 50% improvement. The effect continued at this improved level throughout the duration of the trial. *(Redrawn with permission from Rosenstock J et al: Pain 110:628–638, 2004.)*

*Least squares means claculated from the model. †$p \leq .001$.

50% responder rates (i.e., the percentage of patients who achieved at least 50% reduction in mean pain score from baseline to end point) in the 300 mg/d and 600 mg/d pregabalin groups.[164] These rates were significantly higher than that in the placebo group ($p = .001$) in last observation carried forward analysis. The 50% responder rate in the 75 mg/d pregabalin group was not significantly different from that in the placebo group. In general, a 50% reduction of pain score from baseline by 30% or more of the subjects in a study is considered clinically meaningful. Figure 3-23 demonstrates the effect of 300 mg pregabalin on the mean weekly sleep interference scores of subjects with DPN.[160]

Finally in using pregabalin, it is important to note that the drug is cleared by the kidney. Patients with a pretreatment creatinine clearance of less than 60 mL/min need to have a reduced dose of the drug (as is noted in the package insert from the manufacturer). One of the authors has achieved successful pain reduction for DPN with only 25 mg per day in patients on chronic hemodialysis.

Lamotrigine

Only a few studies have been conducted using lamotrigine to treat neuropathic pain. In a small placebo-controlled crossover trial of 14 patients, lamotrigine was added to either phenytoin or carbamazepine to manage patients with intractable postherpetic neuralgia. Eleven of the 13 patients experienced greater pain relief when lamotrigine (added to phenytoin or carbamazepine) was compared to placebo.

In the first open study of lamotrigine as the sole analgesic in painful diabetic neuropathy, Eisenberg and colleagues studied 15 patients and showed a reduction in the visual analogue and numeric pain scales compared to pretreatment measurements. In the study, patients were titrated from 25 mg to 400 mg per day, and pain profiles and sensory testing were performed on seven subsequent office visits. Two patients withdrew from the

study because of adverse effects (rash, dizziness, and ataxia). Most patients continued to use lamotrigine 6 months after the open study was completed.[165] In a randomized, controlled study in 59 patients, the same authors showed statistically significant improvement in several pain profiles in the group receiving lamotrigine at dosages of 200, 300, and 400 mg per day. More adverse effects were reported in the placebo group than in the lamotrigine group.[166]

Side effects reported from lamotrigine use are headache, somnolence, diplopia, ataxia, asthenia, and a rash. Most feared is a Stevens-Johnson syndrome. The drug should be started at 25 mg per day and slowly increased by 25 mg weekly to 200 to 400 mg total dose taken on a twice per day schedule.

Valproic Acid

Kochar and associates reported the first study of valproic acid in the treatment of painful DPN. They assessed valproic acid (1200 mg per day) in 60 patients with type 2 diabetes in a randomized clinical trial, assessing the benefit using the short form of the McGill Pain Questionnaire and nerve conduction studies. At the end of 1 month, significant improvement was observed in the group receiving valproic acid in the short form of the McGill Pain Questionnaire, and no changes were detected in the electrophysiologic testing. The drug was well tolerated except for one patient whose liver function studies rose to abnormal levels.[167] In a contrasting study from Denmark in 31 patients, no difference in total pain was recorded in patients taking 1500 mg of valproic acid per day compared to the placebo group.[168]

Topiramate

Edwards and colleagues reported the results of their study investigating the efficacy of topiramate in treating painful diabetic neuropathy. In this single-center, randomized, controlled trial of 27 subjects, patients were prescribed either topiramate or placebo and were titrated up to their maximum tolerated dose or 200 mg twice daily. Patients were maintained on a stable dosage for 4 weeks. At the conclusion of the study, patients taking topiramate had significantly less pain than did the placebo group and significantly lower scores on the short form of the McGill Pain Questionnaire. Although topiramate was generally well tolerated, more than 25% of the patients in the topiramate group discontinued the study because of adverse effects.[169]

In a large 12-week randomized clinical trial of topiramate compared to placebo in 323 patients, Raskin and colleagues showed that the group receiving topiramate experienced statistically significant reductions of visual analog scale scores. Patients were titrated up to 400 mg per day or maximum tolerated dose. Fifty percent of patients receiving topiramate and 34% of patients receiving placebo responded to treatment defined as a greater than 30% reduction of the pain visual analogue (PVA) scale. Topiramate also reduced worst pain intensity and sleep disruption. The most commonly reported adverse effects were diarrhea, loss of appetite, and somnolence.[170]

Topiramate has the attractive benefit of causing weight loss without disrupting glucose control.[170] In an extension of this trial, 205 patients participated in a 26-week open-label study in which patients initially given placebo were started on topiramate and those taking the active drug continued it. Approximately 60% of patients completed the study. At the final visit, PVA scales, current pain, and sleep disruption scores did not differ significantly between the former topiramate and former placebo groups, implying that pain relief from topiramate is effective and long lasting. Mean weight loss was over 5 kilograms in both groups taking topiramate. Approximately 40% of the subjects discontinued the study, primarily because of side effects.[171]

Collins and colleagues studied the relative efficacy and adverse effect of antidepressants and anticonvulsants in diabetic neuropathy using published reports from several electronic databases. The NNT to achieve at least 50% pain relief with antidepressants was 3.4, and that with anticonvulsants was 2.7. Antidepressants and anticonvulsants showed the same efficacy and only minor side effects in the treatment of diabetic neuropathy.[172]

Topical Agents

Capsaicin

Capsaicin is the active agent in hot peppers. When applied to skin over a prolonged period of time, it depletes substance P, an endogenous neuropeptide necessary for the propagation of pain. This depletion occurs subcutaneously and in the dorsal root ganglia and dorsal horn. The discovery of this phenomenon led to several studies using capsaicin to treat diabetic neuropathy, post-mastectomy pain syndrome, and postherpetic neuralgia. One study showed statistically greater improvement at the final visit in patients with painful diabetic neuropathy who used capsaicin cream four times per day compared to patients who applied an inactive cream.[173] Those results were not replicated in a much smaller study of patients with various types of neuropathies. The major adverse effect of capsaicin cream is its tendency to produce burning, stinging, erythema, and warmth at the site of application. Even though this reaction tends to wane after 1 to 2 weeks, the intensity of the reaction frequently leads to premature discontinuation of the agent and poor patient compliance. At best, if tolerated, capsaicin cream produces only mild to moderate pain relief and often serves best as adjunctive therapy with other agents.

Lidocaine

White and colleagues studied the effectiveness and safety of a 5% lidocaine patch in patients with postherpetic neuralgia, patients with low back pain, and 49 patients with painful diabetic neuropathy. The patch was applied on up to four areas of maximum peripheral pain for 2 weeks. Significant improvements in the Brief Pain Inventory were measured in general activity, mood, walking ability, normal work, relationships with others, and sleep and enjoyment of life in patients with painful diabetic neuropathy. The patch was well tolerated and considered safe.[174] In a similar study of the 5% lidocaine patch, 41 patients with painful diabetic neuropathy improved in four composite measures of neuropathic pain.[175]

Clonidine

Zeigler and colleagues studied the efficacy of transdermal clonidine in patients with painful diabetic neuropathy.[176] Twenty-four patients received either transdermal clonidine (0.3 mg per day) or placebo patches in a two-period crossover study in which each patch was applied for 6 weeks. The mean pain score diminished by only 13% in the clonidine group compared to placebo, a result that was not statistically significant ($p = .11$). Nine patients requested to continue the clonidine patch treatment and were subjected to single or multiple challenges and withdrawals. Seven of the nine patients reported return of pain on withdrawal of the clonidine patch and relief of pain when the patch was reapplied, suggesting that a subset of patients with diabetic neuropathy experience pain relief from topical clonidine patches.[157] In a similar study design, Byas-Smith and colleagues showed little difference in pain relief between the active drug (titrated from 0.1 to 0.3 mg per day) and placebo group in 41 patients with painful diabetic neuropathy. As in the previous study, several patients (12 patients) requested continuation of the clonidine patches. Analysis of this subgroup showed 20% less pain after treatment with clonidine patches than after treatment with placebo.[177] On the basis of these two studies, clonidine patches may be beneficial in a subset of patients with painful diabetic neuropathy.

Tramadol Hydrochloride

Tramadol hydrochloride is a unique pharmacologic agent that acts in two ways: as an opioid agonist and as an activator of monoaminergic spinal inhibition of pain. Although approved only for oral use in the United States, tramadol can be administered intravenously, intramuscularly, and rectally. Its potency is equivalent to that of meperidine. Respiratory depression and addiction are rare complications of tramadol. Adverse effects include dizziness, nausea, sedation, dry mouth, and sweating.

In a multicenter, randomized, double-blind placebo-controlled study comparing tramadol hydrochloride to placebo, tramadol was shown to be statistically better at reducing pain intensity and producing greater pain relief within the study population. The average daily dose tolerated was 210 mg.[178] Patients receiving tramadol scored significantly better on physical and social functioning scales. Treatment with tramadol should begin at 50 mg per day and be slowly advanced to the maximum dose of 100 mg four times a day. In an extension of the previous study, the authors demonstrated duration of pain relief over 6 months.[179]

Antiarrhythmics

Mexiletine

Mexiletine is an antiarrhythmic agent and an orally active local anesthetic agent that is structurally related to lidocaine. Dejgard and colleagues studied 16 patients with painful diabetic neuropathy. Mexiletine was compared to placebo at a dosage of 10 mg/kg/d. Patients receiving mexiletine reported statistically better control of pain, dysesthesia, paresthesia, and nightly exacerbation of pain and better sleep than when taking placebo.[180] Two other studies showed no benefit when mexiletine therapy was used to treat neuropathic pain arising from diabetic neuropathy.[181,182] In a fourth study, only patients who were able to take a high dose of mexiletine (675 mg) achieved significant relief from nocturnal pain and improved sleep. Many patients (13% to 50%) develop side effects when prescribed mexiletine, including nausea, vomiting, headache, chest pain, and palpitations.[183]

Antispasticity Medications

In an animal model of pain, baclofen has shown some analgesic properties. Terrence and colleagues tested baclofen in 15 patients with postherpetic neuralgia and 10 patients with painful diabetic neuropathy. Few patients improved, and the authors concluded that baclofen has little utility as a conventional analgesic for neuropathic pain.[184]

Narcotics

Controversy exists over the place of narcotics in the treatment of chronic pain, especially long-term neuropathic pain. Many physicians avoid their use on the basis of the belief that they are not effective or that their addictive potential is too great. Conversely, other pain experts believe that the potential for addiction is low and that opioid analgesics can be used safely if the amount and frequency of use are carefully monitored.[185] In a randomized, double-blind, crossover trial of controlled-release oxycodone, patients with postherpetic neuralgia who were treated with 30 mg twice per day experienced improvement in their pain.[186] Watson stated that chronic opioid use is acceptable in chronic refractory cases of neuropathic pain if proper guidelines are followed.[187]

Antioxidants

α-Lipoic Acid

Many studies have shown that α-lipoic acid given parenterally at a dose of 600 mg per day reduces neuropathic symptoms and deficits.[188] Conversely, the results from oral use of α-lipoic acid have not been convincing. In the ALADIN II study of α-lipoic acid, using 600 and 1200 mg per day in 65 patients, no improvement was observed in the Neuropathy Disability Score even though statistically significant changes were recorded in the nerve conduction velocity compared to placebo.[189] In ALADIN III, neuropathic deficits were significantly reduced in patients during the parenteral 3-week phase of the study, yet statistically significant reductions of the neuropathic impairment scores were not noted after 6 months of the subsequent oral phase.[190]

The opposite results occurred in the ORPIL study of oral α-lipoic acid. Patients taking 1800 mg per day experienced a reduction of neurologic symptoms and deficits over 3 weeks of treatment. This study has been criticized for the small number of patients who completed the study (22 patients).[191] α-Lipoic acid is well tolerated by most patients. The most common side effects are headache, rash, and gastrointestinal upset.

Experimental Agents

In addition to the above agents, many new compounds are currently undergoing phase 2 and 3 clinical trials. Unfortunately, there are many other compounds that were promising but have been withdrawn from testing because of ineffectiveness or serious adverse events. Table 3-6 summarizes some of the current and potential

TABLE 3-6   Treatment of DPN: Putative Pathogenic Mechanisms*

Abnormality	Compound	Aim of Treatment	Status of RCTs
Polyol pathway ↑	Aldose reductase inhibitors	Nerve sorbitol ↓	
	Sorbinil		Withdrawn (AE)
	Tolrestat		Withdrawn (AE)
	Ponalrestat		Ineffective
	Zopolrestat		Withdrawn (marginal effects)
	Zenarestat		Withdrawn (AE)
	Lidorestat		Withdrawn (AE)
	Fidarestat		Effective in RCTs, trials ongoing
	AS-3201		Effective in RCTs, trials ongoing
	Epalrestat		Marketed in Japan
Myo-inositol ↓	*Myo*-inositol	Nerve *myo*-inositol ↑	Equivocal
Oxidative stress ↑	Alpha-lipoic acid	Oxygen free radicals ↓	Effective in RCTs, trials ongoing
Nerve hypoxia ↑	Vasodilators	NBF ↑	
	ACE inhibitors		Effective in one RCT
	Prostaglandin analogues		Effective in one RCT
	phVEGF165 gene transfer	Angiogenesis ↑	RCTs ongoing
Protein kinase C ↑	Protein kinase C-β inhibitor (ruboxistaurin)	NBF ↑	RCTs ongoing
C-peptide ↓	C-peptide	NBF ↑	Studies ongoing
Neurotrophism ↓	Nerve growth factor (NGF)	Nerve regeneration, growth ↑	Ineffective
	BDNF	Nerve regeneration, growth ↑	Ineffective
LCFA metabolism ↓	Acetyl-L-carnitine	LCFA accumulation ↓	Ineffective
GLA synthesis ↓	Gamma-linolenic acid (GLA)	EFA metabolism ↑	Withdrawn
NEG ↑	Aminoguanidine	AGE accumulation ↓	Withdrawn

*List of compounds and compound status of randomized clinical trials was current only as of April 2005.
AE, adverse event; AGE, advanced glycation end product; BDNF, brain-derived neurotrophic factor; EFA, essential fatty acid; GLA, gamma-linolenic acid; LCFA, long-chain fatty acid; NBF, nerve blood flow; NEG, nonenzymatic glycation; RCT, randomized clinical trial; VEGF, vascular endothelial growth factor.
From Boulton AJM, Vinik AI, Arezzo J, et al: Diabetic neuropathies: A statement by the American Diabetes Association. *Diabetes Care: 28*:956–962, 2005.

treatments for diabetic neuropathy based on "putative pathogenic mechanisms."[6]

Spinal Cord Stimulation

In extremely refractory patients, neurosurgical procedures can be performed to relieve pain. Tesfaye and his group reported their results using spinal cord stimulation of the thoracic or lumbar epidural space in patients with painful DPN. They studied 10 patients, all of whom had experienced a poor response to previous pharmacologic therapies. The investigators reported better pain control in 8 of 10 patients. There was improvement of both background and peak pain at 3, 6, and 14 months and better exercise tolerance at 3 and 6 months. In six patients, spinal cord stimulation alone controlled the pain. In those six patients, their neuropathic pain increased dramatically when the stimulator was turned off, and pain relief returned when the stimulator was reactivated. One patient died 2 months after the start of the study from unrelated causes, and another patient ceased to experience pain relief after 4 months of treatment.[192]

The same investigators restudied the six benefiting patients a mean of 3.3 years post-implantation and once again found dramatic improvement of pain when the stimulator was turned on compared to when it was turned off. Four of the patients were reassessed at 7.5 years with similar impressive results. Two patients had died in the interim from cardiovascular causes. Two complications ensued between the 3.3- and 7.5-year periods:

skin peeling under the transmitter site and electrode damage from trauma.[193]

Surgery

Recently, surgical decompression of nerves in the foot has been promoted as a treatment of pain in patients with diabetic neuropathy. Impressive results have been published, the percentage amelioration of pain being as high as 85% and 92% and improvement of two-point discrimination of 72%.[194-196] Since the presence of a positive percussion sign (Tinel's) at the level of the tarsal tunnel is used to determine candidacy for the operation, it appears that the surgery is performed in most cases to correct a decompressed nerve rather than to treat a diffuse symmetrical polyneuropathy. The American Academy of Neurology recently published a practice advisory stating that only class IV studies (uncontrolled studies, case series, case reports, or expert opinions) exist for the utility of surgical decompression for the treatment of diabetic neuropathy.[197] This review concluded that the data are insufficient to support or refute the procedure. The organization recommended the performance of randomized controlled clinical trials and emphasized the need to distinguish between entrapment neuropathy and peripheral sensorimotor neuropathy.

Cost and Treatment Summary

The cost of medications to manage neuropathic pain must be considered, particularly for patients on fixed

---

BOX 3-4 Summary of Treatment Scheme for Neuropathic Pain

- Discuss the frequent refractoriness of pain to various agents
- Explain trial and error method of using drugs
- Simple to complex medications
- Cheap to expensive medications
- Explain side effects
- Single daily dosing preferred to multiple doses
- Begin with a small dose; titrate judiciously
- Titrate one drug at a time
- Careful dosing in the elderly

---

budgets taking large numbers of expensive drugs. The least expensive drugs used to treat neuropathic pain are ibuprofen, doxepin, phenytoin, carbamazepine, amitriptyline, and imipramine.

In summary, treatment of neuropathic pain is a challenge for both the physician and patient. Many aspects of care should be considered in choosing an appropriate medication, including the severity of pain, age of the patient, potential drug interactions, coexistent medical and surgical disorders, allergies, medication intolerances, and ability to pay for the treatment. Box 3-4 lists a time-proven and effective scheme that this author has found to be helpful to treat neuropathic pain.

Routine Assessment by the Health Care Professional

Early identification and appropriate therapy of the patient who is at increased risk of ulceration and amputation require routine assessment and examination by the health care professional. The health care provider is responsible for lifelong surveillance, examination of the feet at each office visit, risk stratification, and referral for therapeutic footwear and orthoses when needed. The patient's responsibilities include daily foot inspection and obtaining patient education on self-care practices. The ADA has estimated that 50% of the limbs with foot ulcers can be saved if both the health care provider and the patient fulfill their respective responsibilities.

Routine Office Visit Exam

At each office visit the health care provider should examine the patient's feet. To help expedite the exam in the office of nonpodiatric providers, our diabetes clinic has a poster on the wall of each exam room that states: "if you have diabetes, please remove your socks and shoes before the doctor comes in" (Fig. 3-24). We have found this "happy foot" poster to be very effective in ensuring that patients have their feet examined every time they are seen by the provider. In addition to improving patient care, the poster saves the provider time, since many elderly and disabled patients need extra time or

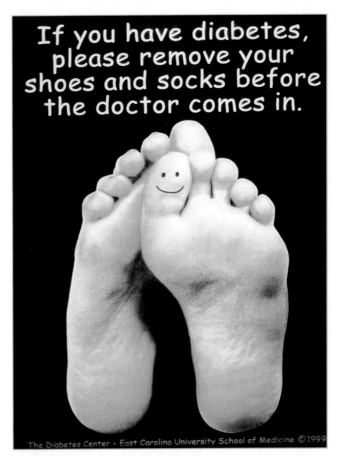

Figure 3-24   **"Happy Foot" poster.** This poster is prominently displayed on the walls of all the exam rooms of the Diabetes Clinic of the Brody School of Medicine at the East Carolina University in Greenville, North Carolina. The endocrinologists in this clinic have found that patients are much more likely to already have their shoes and socks off when the physician enters the exam room. This poster definitely facilitates the foot examination and speeds up the visit. Patients with disabilities are assisted in this effort by the clinic's able and friendly medical assistants.

assistance in removing their socks and shoes. We have found that when patients expect to have their feet examined at every visit, their personal foot hygiene, nail care, and overall concern with their feet improves.

An important part of the office exam in the neuropathic patient is to check for foot deformities. Motor neuropathy can lead to foot deformities from muscle atrophy and imbalance of the muscles. A common deformity is the claw toe deformity (see Figs 3-3 and 3-4). The loss of foot flexor strength allows the foot extensors to contract relatively unopposed. Even at rest, the toes are pulled into a claw position. As this occurs the fat pad is pulled off the metatarsal heads. This may lead to high pressure points under the metatarsal heads, the tips of the toes, and the knuckle of the toe. These are common areas for ulceration. Metatarsal bar orthoses help to pull the fat pad back into place and straighten the toes. Thus, the metatarsal bar can help to prevent ulceration in patients with claw toe deformity.

Other deformities that the health care provider should evaluate include hammer toes, hallux limitus, bunions, Charcot arthropathy, limited joint mobility, abnormal toe position, calluses, and partial foot amputations. Bunions do not allow for proper shoe fitting. Callus formation is secondary to repeated insult from increased pressure. Thus, shoes that fit poorly, shoes that have poor cushioning, going barefoot, and foot deformities can result in heavy callus formation. Although calluses form to better protect the foot, calluses are unyielding, fixed tissue that is more prone to injury from shearing and can actually increase the pressure under the callus even more. It is not uncommon to find an ulcer under a callus.[198]

Charcot foot (see Chapter 12) is a progressive destruction of the bones in the foot. The arch of the foot is usually lost. The misshapen foot and bony protrusions lead to increased pressure points in unusual places on the foot.[199] Any foot deformity contributes to increased pressure and shear stress over the bony prominence, putting the foot at increased risk of ulceration. Foot deformities should be sought, noted, and evaluated at each office visit. These and other foot deformities are discussed in detail elsewhere in this book.

Sensory neuropathy can easily be evaluated via monofilament testing (see Sense of Touch: Monofilament Testing earlier in this chapter).

Figure 3-25 details the importance of monofilament testing. Individuals who were unable to feel the 5.07

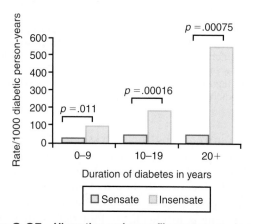

Figure 3–25   Ulceration and monofilament score. In a study of the incidence of plantar ulceration by duration of diabetes and sensitivity to 5.07 monofilament, 358 American Indians were screened with the Semmes-Weinstein 5.07 monofilament. The patients were followed prospectively for lower-limb events and changes in sensation. Insensitivity to the 5.07 monofilament occurred in 19% of the patients screened. Among the insensate group, the odds ratio of subsequent ulceration was 9.9 (95% CI, 4.8 to 21.0) and amputation was 17.0 (95% CI, 4.5 to 95.0) compared to those individuals who were able to feel the 5.07 monofilament. These relationships were maintained when controlling for the duration of diabetes and vascular indices. *(Redrawn with permission from Rith-Najarian SJ, Stolusky T, Gohdes DM: Identifying diabetic patients at high risk for lower-extremity amputation in a primary health care setting: A prospective evaluation of simple screening criteria. Diabetes Care 15:1386–1389, 1992.)*

monofilament (insensate) were at greater risk of ulceration at any duration of diabetes.[200] For this reason, diabetic individuals with insensate feet should obtain custom footwear. Lack of vibration sense over the great toenail carries a similar risk. Monofilaments and tuning fork evaluation should be determined on an annual basis.

In addition to sensory and motor neuropathy, patients with diabetes typically have autonomic neuropathy. Two common consequences of autonomic neuropathy in the diabetic foot are sudomotor dysfunction and changes in vascular flow within the skin of the sole of the foot. Both of these abnormalities lead to dry feet. Dry, cracked, or fissured skin in the feet is a common problem in people with diabetes. The reason is twofold: lack of skin lubrication and redirection of blood flow in the microscopic blood vessels in the skin (Fig. 3-26).

Skin lubrication is maintained by oil and sweat secretion by the sebaceous glands. These sweat glands atrophy in the presence of autonomic neuropathy. This natural lubrication is important for maintaining the health of the skin. The other reason for dry feet is because the AV shunts, which are located in the soles (but not the dorsum) of the feet, are inappropriately dilated. Normally, the sympathetic nerves to these channels keep them tightly shut, and the blood flows to the skin surface through the nutrient capillaries. These channels (AV shunts) are normally used by the body to help protect an individual from very cold weather.

During extreme cold, the body allows these channels to open up and redirects the blood away from the surface of the skin back toward the central (core) part of the body. These channels are located in the earlobes, the fingers, the tip of the nose, and the soles of the feet. Therefore, frostbite occurs in these places first. When the nerves to these channels are damaged from autonomic neuropathy, the channels are not kept consistently shut (i.e., the AV shunts dilate). This allows the blood to bypass the surface of the skin. Bypassing of the surface of the skin causes a lack of integrity to the skin and aids in its becoming dry.

This is also a common reason for cold feet. The combination of poor natural lubrication and reduction in blood flow in the soles of the feet allows the skin to become dry, crack, form fissures, and become hard. The skin serves to protect the feet from injury. If the skin is dry and has lost its integrity for any reason, the foot is at increased risk for damage, sores, lesions, ulcers, infections, and even amputation. Therefore, keeping the feet well lubricated (not wet) is an essential part of prophylactic foot care.

In choosing an agent to help maintain or replace skin moisture, the health care provider must read the label of the product. Sometimes agents added to creams, ointment, and lotions are not the best for feet. Many of the fragrances that are used in these products are alcohol based. As alcohols evaporate, they can dry the skin further. The patient should be instructed that words ending

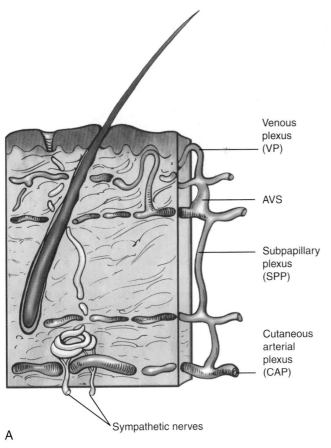

A

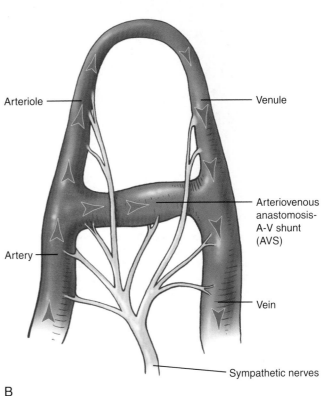

B

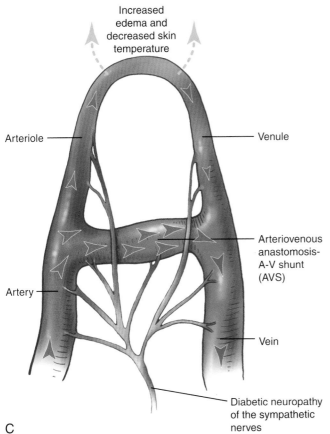

C

Figure 3–26 **AV shunts.** Plantar AV shunts in normal and neuropathic diabetic individuals. **A,** The microvasculature of the sole of the foot. Small subcutaneous arteries penetrate the dermis and anastomoses in the cutaneous arterial plexus (CAP). Arterioles arise from this plexus and ascend to form the subpapillary plexus (SPP). Arteriovenous anastomosis (AV shunts [AVS]) are richly innervated, are under rigid sympathetic control, and connect small arteries and arterioles to small veins and venules, which form a venous plexus (VP). **B,** A schematic model of the normal artery, arteriole, venule, vein, and sympathetically innervated AV shunt. Under normal circumstances, the AV shunt is closed, and blood flow is through the nutrient capillaries. **C,** Proposed mechanism of AV shunting in diabetic neuropathy. A decrease in sympathetic innervation of the richly innervated AV shunts and less innervated arterioles results in relatively greater dilatation of the AV shunt and only a modest dilatation of the arteriole. This leads to a shunting of blood away from the capillary dermal papillae loops (nutrient capillary), a decrease in transcutaneous oxygen tension at the skin, an increase in foot venous oxygen tension, and low skin temperature. *(References: DCCT Research Group: The effect of intensive diabetes therapy on the development and progression of neuropathy. Ann Intern Med 122:561–568, 1995. Harris M, Eastman R, Cowie C: Symptoms of sensory neuropathy in adults with NIDDM in the U.S. population. Diabetes Care 16:1446–1452, 1993. Ohkubo Y, Kishikawa H, Araki E, et al: Intensive insulin therapy prevents the progression of diabetic microvascular complications in Japanese patients with non-insulin-dependent diabetes mellitus: A randomized prospective 6-year study. Diabetes Res Clin Pract 28(2):103–117, 1995. Hassan K, Simri W, Rubenchik I, et al: Effect of erythropoietin therapy on polyneuropathy in predialytic patients. J Nephrol 16(1):121–125, 2003.)*

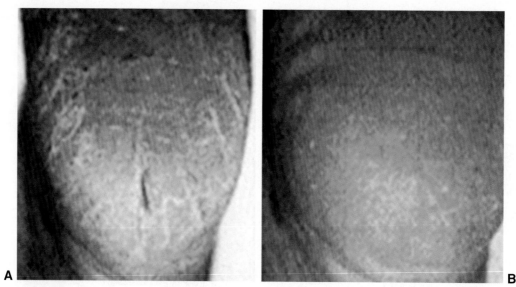

Figure 3–27 Xerosis before and after treatment. **A,** The foot of a subject with grade 7 xerosis prior to treatment with 10% urea and 4% lactic acid in a nongreasy emulsion base (Atrac-Tain cream, available online at http://www.sweenstore.com/atractain.html). Note the presence of fissures. **B,** After 4 weeks of treatment with this product, there was marked improvement. The contralateral foot (not shown), which was treated with only the vehicle (placebo), had no significant change in 4 weeks. *(Data from Pham HT, Exelbert L, Segal-Owens AC, et al: A prospective, randomized, controlled double-blind study of a moisturizer for xerosis of the feet in patients with diabetes. Ostomy Wound Manage 48(5):30–36. 2002.)*

with "-ol" are often alcohols. If any of the first four items on the label ends with the last two letters "-ol," another product should be chosen. Furthermore, words such as "natural," "intensive," "nature's," "diabetic," "diabetes," "pure," "prevention," "dermal," "the best," "formulated," "formula," "secret," "oldest," "doctors," and "physicians" have no bearing on the quality of the product. In addition, petroleum-based products seal the surface of the skin. They keep what little lubrication is made from evaporating too quickly but do not penetrate past the surface of the skin. Thus, petroleum-based products do not replace the moisture in the skin.

Creams or lotions with substances that are known to help replace the moisture to the skin surface and just below the surface of the skin are better than perfumed lotions or petroleum-based products. Most ointments are petroleum based. Animal oils (e.g., lanolin), urea (a substance commonly found in urine), and fats (e.g., stearates) tend to penetrate deep into the skin and moisturize dry skin well. There are many excellent creams and lotions on the market. One lotion that is commonly used is called Lansinoh. This lotion is a form of lanolin and is often used by nursing mothers to avoid cracking of their nipples when breast-feeding.

Other commonly used lanolin-based products include Bag Balm and Udder Butter, which were first used to keep cows' udders soft and pliable. These lanolin-based products appear to be safe and work reasonably well. However, Bag Balm and Udder Butter contain an antibiotic that some health care professionals find less than desirable. Urea is found in many over-the-counter lotions

and creams. Urea appears to be fairly efficacious and safe as a moisturizer. In the opinion of this author, a 20-40 cream or gel of urea available by prescription (Carmol) is one of the better pure lubricants on the market.

Patients with severe dryness from diabetic autonomic neuropathy will often have xerosis. This term, derived from the Greek *xeros*, meaning "dry," is often associated with flaking of the skin and is often recalcitrant to the usual lubricant therapies. A recent prospective randomized, double-blind clinical trial compared the efficacy of a test moisturizer containing 10% urea and 4% lactic acid to that of a placebo emulsion base vehicle in 40 patients with severe xerosis.[201] Subjects had one foot treated with the test product and the other with the placebo for 4 weeks, and the xerosis was documented by photographs and graded on a seven-point scale. The test product, marketed as Atrac-Tain Cream (available online at www.sweenstore.com/atractain), led to a statistically greater improvement in the treated foot. In some patients, deep heel fissures were healed with this product within 4 weeks (Fig 3-27). The authors noted that unfortunately, 25% of their subjects did not apply the cream daily and failed to complete the study. Nonetheless, this study represents the only randomized trial to demonstrate a significant improvement in xerosis by a moisturizing product in a diabetic population.

Risk Stratification

Several classification schemes for foot risk stratification have been proposed and are discussed elsewhere in this

TABLE 3-7 Treatment-Based Diabetic Foot Index

Category	Presentation
0	Minimal or no pathology present
1	Insensate foot
2	Insensate foot with deformity
3	Neuropathy with deformity plus history of prior foot ulcer
4	Insensate injury
5	Infected diabetic foot
6	Dysvascular foot

book. Table 3-7 is a convenient, evidence-based classification.[202] In this system, patients are stratified according to the presence or absence of sensation, deformity, neuropathic ulceration, infection, and vascular disease. Each category corresponds to a recommended treatment regimen and is discussed in Chapters 9, 15, and 28. Evidence exists that the odds ratio of developing a foot ulcer increases as patients exhibit more of the following characteristics: severe peripheral neuropathy (inability to feel a monofilament of 5.07), advanced peripheral vascular disease (absence of pedal pulses, dependent rubor, pallor on elevation, or history of intermittent claudication or rest pain), foot deformity, history of previous foot ulcer or amputation, presence of plantar callus, and/or limited joint mobility syndrome.[59] Health care professionals need to identify feet that are at risk for ulceration and seek methods (see below) to prevent the same.

Proper Footwear

Chapter 13 describes appropriate footwear for people with diabetes in detail. Because of the presence of neuropathy, special protective shoes are often necessary.[203] Custom or modified footwear is important for healing (e.g., total contact casting, removable walker, half-shoe) and for prevention (e.g., extra-depth shoe, custom-molded shoes, custom insoles). Metatarsal bars are commonly used in custom insoles and help to correct the claw toe deformity (see above). Rocker-bottom shoes are also commonly used. The rocker-bottom shoe enables the individual to rock or roll the foot from heel to toe without bending the shoe or creating undue pressures on the foot.

Custom shoes can decrease the reulceration rate from 60% over 3 years to 20% over 3 years.[204] The benefit of special shoes and insoles has been recognized and supported by Medicare. The Medicare-supported Therapeutic Shoe Bill allows for payment for special footwear and insoles made for people with diabetes. The ADA states that the objectives of prescription footwear include (1) to relieve areas of excessive plantar pressure, (2) to reduce shock, (3) to reduce shear stress, (4) to accommodate deformities, (5) to stabilize and support deformities, and (6) to limit motion of joints.

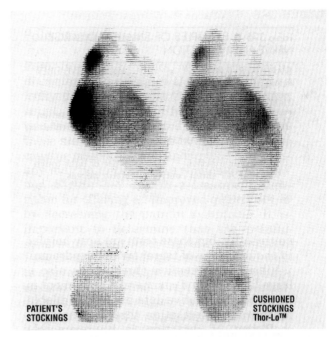

Figure 3–28 Harris Foot Mat. Harris Foot Mat results before and after wearing a cushioned stocking. The Harris Foot Mat is an inexpensive method to document the presence of increased pressure points in an individual. This person had increased pressure points over the first metatarsal head and great toe on the right foot. Use of a cushioned sock (Thor-Lo) greatly decreased the presence of these pressure points. Harris mat determinations are recommended for all diabetic patients on a routine basis. This serves as both information for the health care provider and education and motivation for patients.

In addition to special shoes, socks are very important in protecting insensate feet.

Figure 3-28 illustrates impressions generated utilizing Harris mats. The figure clearly demonstrates the advantage of a cushioned sock (Thor-Lo) over a standard sock. Even in people without neuropathy or foot deformity, well-fitting shoes, especially jogging, tennis, or other cushioned shoes, are essential for avoiding blisters and other foot lesions. Simple habits such as changing the shoes every 4 to 6 hours, breaking in new shoes slowly, and inspecting shoes before wearing each time are also effective preventive measures.

Patient Education

Chapter 30 details the importance and techniques for proper patient education. Table 3-8 summarizes the general principles. Foot soaks; "bathroom surgery"; going barefoot; heating pads; astringents; plastic shoes; and over-the-counter preparations for corns, calluses, and nails should be avoided. It is important for the patient to be actively involved in his or her own care. Proper foot care should be demonstrated by the health care educator and in turn by the patient.

TABLE 3-8 Education for Diabetic Patients with Neuropathy

Appropriate type of exercise	Good communication with health care provider
Wash feet carefully	Dry feet carefully (especially between toes)
Inspect feet every day (especially between toes)	Look for changes in skin color
Feel for increased skin temperature	Avoid extremes in temperature
Trim toenails straight across	Wear proper footwear
Stop smoking	Avoid minor trauma (i.e., no bare feet)
Good nutrition	Learn (read pamphlet or watch video) about proper foot care

The use of a nonbreakable mirror enables the patient to inspect the soles of his or her feet with ease. Specific instructions (such as "Don't go barefoot") are often more practical than are generalities (such as "Avoid hurting your feet"). Liberal use of films, booklets, pamphlets, videos, and handouts is important. The importance of patient education was well illustrated in one study, which showed that simple interventions (patient foot care education provided with written information about proper foot care) reduced serious foot problems by 60% in 1 year.[205]

Although patient education is important in all people with diabetes, it is especially important to provide patient education to individuals with diabetic neuropathy. Devices for activities of daily living, including buttoners, zipper assist devices, mirrors, and bathwater thermometers, can be helpful to a patient when diabetic neuropathy is advanced.

Prognosis and Avoidance of Future Complications

Prognosis

Most of the information about the prognosis of diabetic neuropathy can be found from the results of the DCCT trial, which compared the prognosis of patients with diabetic neuropathy treated with routine insulin to that of patients treated with an aggressive course of four insulin injections per day. Patients who received aggressive treatment achieved stabilization of the neuropathy and fewer progressed to autonomic neuropathy. Several studies have shown that patients with autonomic neuropathy, especially cardiac autonomic neuropathy, have excessive mortality. Cardiac autonomic neuropathy is the most frequent autonomic complication of diabetic neuropathy.[206] It leads to orthostatic hypotension, exercise intolerance, and enhanced intraoperative instability, and it has been hypothesized to cause an increased incidence of silent myocardial infarction, ischemia, and sudden death.[207]

Autonomic neuropathy also contributes to many complications that increase morbidity in patients with diabetic neuropathy. These include poor papillary dark adaptation, gastroparesis, enteropathy, colonic hypomotility, constipation, urinary incontinence, erectile dysfunction, retrograde ejaculation, cold hands and feet, and hypoglycemic unawareness.

Avoidance of Future Complications of Diabetic Neuropathy

The ultimate consequences of diabetic neuropathy can be pain or foot ulcers and amputation. The management of neuropathic pain was discussed above. The greatest challenge to practitioners who care for patients with diabetes is management of the patient with an insensate foot. The avoidance of ulceration and possible amputation in the care of the neuropathic patient includes three essential components: regular assessment of the foot, use of properly prescribed footwear, and patient education. In addition, offering these methods and tools to improve the quality of life for patients with diabetic neuropathy should be considered part of good clinical care.

Summary

In summary, diabetic neuropathy is a major public health problem that is often overlooked by physicians and patients. In the previous edition of this text and in an article that was published in *Diabetes Forecast*, we labeled neuropathy the "forgotten complication" of diabetes.[208] As was previously stated in this chapter, the current situation regarding appreciation for the true prevalence and clinical significance of DPN has not changed significantly since the sixth edition was published. Fortunately, our understanding of the pathogenesis, clinical manifestations, and treatment of DPN is far advanced over that of clinicians in 2001. However, further research is needed to expand our knowledge of the etiologies and pathogenesis of DPN and to discover better methods to prevent the onset and progression of this disorder, independent of glucose control.

Even if diabetes could miraculously be cured or prevented, neuropathy would continue to exist as an important clinical problem for millions of people in the United States and throughout the world. This is one complication of diabetes that should never be forgotten.

ACKNOWLEDGMENTS

The authors wish to thank Kenneth Stone and Amy Long for their assistance with the footnotes, tables, and figures. Also thanks to Mary P. Schumer and to Drs. Michael Pfeifer and Douglas Green for their contributions to the sixth edition of this text.

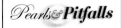

Pearls

- Suspect an alternative (or additional) diagnosis to diffuse diabetic polyneuropathy (DPN) when the patient's symptoms or signs are
  - More unilateral than bilateral
  - More proximal than distal
  - More motor than sensory
  - More localized than diffuse
  - More pronounced with walking than at rest
  - More common in the morning than the evening
  - When there is associated edema
- Weight loss and depression are important manifestations of DPN.
- DPN symptoms and signs may precede the onset of diabetes.
- When treating neuropathic pain, remember that you are managing a patient. Begin medication carefully and in low doses, advancing as tolerated. Try inexpensive medications before prescribing the newest and, most likely, the most expensive therapy. Explain potential side effects at the time of the first visit. Emphasize that complete relief of pain is rare and pain relief of 50% to 75% is considered substantial improvement.
- Pearls regarding reflexes:
  - When the sensory deficit is present proximal to the knees (including loss of knee jerks) the hands are usually involved with DPN.
  - Normal people over age 60 years often lose their Achilles reflexes (ankle jerks).
  - Patients with pain from small fiber DPN may still have normal deep tendon reflexes.
  - Diminished knee and ankle jerks may be reinforced by using the Jendrassik's maneuver (the patient hooks the hands together by the flexed fingers and tries to pull them apart).
- Claw feet are a significant problem because the metatarsal heads bear much of the weight, resulting in a biomechanical instability with a predisposition for callus and ulcers to occur on the metatarsal heads.
- Neuropathic ulcers are typically painless, are generally round in shape with a "punched out" appearance, and almost always form at pressure points.
- Be sure to spread the toes to look for "kissing ulcers" in patients with insensate feet.
- When the patient's pain persists for more than 6 months after therapy is begun:
  - Check to be sure the patient is not smoking.
  - Check to be sure the patient's glucose, blood pressure, and lipids are at target levels.
  - Increase medication to maximal dose and add a second or third medication to the regimen if needed.
- The five indications for custom diabetic shoes are:
  1. Inability to feel the 5.07 monofilament
  2. Deformities
  3. Prior foot ulcer
  4. Any history of amputation
  5. Arterial insufficiency

Pitfalls

- Not all pain in the hands and feet of a diabetic patient is neuropathic pain. Patients with diabetes may have other disorders producing pain in the hands and feet.
- Remember that a patient who feels the 5.07 monofilament might still have DPN but protective sensation is intact.
- The unilateral swollen foot that is painless in the presence of good pulses should not be dismissed without an evaluation for an early Charcot foot.
- Do not assume that focal tenderness is related to DPN. Patients who have an area of focal tenderness should be referred to a podiatrist to rule out another pathologic process (e.g., Morton's neuroma, stress fracture(s), tarsal tunnel syndrome, or plantar fasciitis).
- It is important to note the paradox of severe neuropathic pain in patients who have insensate feet.
- Patients with classic nonhealing neuropathic ulcers may also have an ischemic component, and one should not forget to order an evaluation of their peripheral circulation.
- Gait abnormalities may be from large fiber DPN, but central nervous system disorders need to be ruled out with a complete neurologic evaluation.

References

1. American Diabetes Association: Clinical Practice Recommendations 1995. Diabetes Care 18:8–15,1995.
2. Diabetic Neuropathies: A Statement by the American Diabetes Association. Diabetes Care 28:936–962, 2005.
3. Espinet LM, Osmick MJ, Ahmmed T, Villagra VG: A cohort study of the impact of a national disease management program on HEDIS diabetes outcomes. Dis Manage 8(2):86–92, 2005.
4. Herman WH, Kennedy L, for the Goal A1C Study Group: Underdiagnosis of Peripheral Neuropathy in Type 2 Diabetes. Diabetes Care 28:1480–1481, 2005.
5. www.diabete.org/for-media/2005-press-releases/diabeticneuropathy.jip, accessed 5-10-05.
6. Boulton AJM, Vinik, AI, Arezzo, J, et al: Diabetic neuropathies: A statement by the American Diabetes Association. Diabetes Care 28:956–962, 2005.
7. Boulton AJM, Gries, FA and Jervell, JA: Guidelines for the diagnosis and outpatient management of diabetic peripheral neuropathy. Diabet Med 15:508–514, 1998.
8. DCCT Research Group: The effect of intensive diabetes therapy on the development and progression of neuropathy. Ann Intern Med 122:561–568, 1995.
9. Mayo, CH. Aphorisms of Dr Charles Horace Mayo, 1865–1939 and William James Mayo, 1861–1939. Rochester, Mayo Foundation for Medical Education and Research, 1988.
10. Accessed March 2007 at http://www.painfoundation.org/page.asp?file-QandA/FifthVitalSign.htm.
11. Dyck PJ, Kratz KM, Karnes JL, et al: The prevalence by staged severity of various types of diabetic neuropathy, retinopathy, and nephropathy in a population-based cohort: The Rochester Diabetic Neuropathy Study. Neurology 43:817–824, 1993.
12. Accessed April 2006 at http://www.cdc.gov/diabetes/pubs/estimates05.htm#prev 2005.
13. www.iasp-pain.org/terms, accessed 2005.
14. Serra J: Overview of neuropathic pain syndromes. Acta Neurol Scand 173(suppl):7–11, 1999.
15. Fields HL, Price DD: Toward a neurobiology of placebo analgesia. In Harrington A (ed): The Placebo Effect: An Interdisciplinary Exploration. Cambridge, MA: Harvard University Press, 1997, pp 93–115.
16. Fields HL: Depression and pain: A neurobiological model. Neuropsychiatr Neuropsychol Behav Neurol 4:83–92, 1991.
17. Dyck PJ: Detection, characterization, and staging of polyneuropathy: Assessed in diabetics. Muscle Nerve 11:21–32, 1988.
18. Thomas PK: Metabolic neuropathy. J R Coll Physicians Lond 7:154–160, 1973.
19. Dyck PJ, Karnes J, O'Brien PC: Diagnosis, staging, and classification of diabetic neuropathy and associations with other complications. In Dyck PJ, Thomas PK, Asbury AK, et al (eds): Diabetic Neuropathy. Philadelphia: WB Saunders, 1987, pp 36–44.
20. Feldman EL: Classification of diabetic neuropathy. UpToDate: Classification of diabetic neuropathy. http://www.utdol.com, accessed April 2006.
21. Dyck PJ, Karnes JL, O'Brien PC, et al: The Rochester Diabetic Neuropathy Study: Reassessment of tests and criteria for diagnosis and staged severity. Neurology 42:1164–1170, 1992.
22. Harris M, Eastman R, Cowie C: Symptoms of sensory neuropathy in adults with NIDDM in the U.S. population. Diabetes Care 16:1446–1452, 1993.
23. Pirart J: Diabetes mellitus and its degenerative complications: A prospective study of 4,400 patients observed between 1947 and 1973 Diabetes Care 1:168–188, 1978.
24. Partanen J, Niskanen L, Lehtinen J, et al: Natural history of peripheral neuropathy in patients with non-insulin dependent diabetes mellitus. N Engl J Med 333:89–94, 1995.
25. Börü UT, Recep A, Haluk S, et al: Prevalence of peripheral neuropathy in type 2 diabetic patients attending a diabetes center in Turkey. Endocr J 51:561–567, 2004.
26. Mohan, V, Vijayaprabha R, Rema M: Vascular complications in long-term Southern Indian NIDDM of over 25 years duration. Diabetes Res Clin Pract 31:133–140, 1996.
27. Amos A, McCarty D, Zimmet P: The rising global burden of diabetes and its complications: Estimates and projections to the year 2010. Diabet Med 14:S1–S85, 1997.
28. www.idf.org/home/index.cfm, accessed 12-01-05.
29. Robinson LR, Stolov WC, Rubner DE, et al: Height is an independent risk factor for neuropathy in diabetic men. Diabetes Res Clin Pract 16:97–102, 1992.
30. Sosenko JM, Gadia MT, Fournier AM, et al: Body stature as a risk factor for diabetic sensory neuropathy. Am J Med 80:1031–1034, 1986.
31. Demaine AG: Polymorphism of the aldose reductase gene and susceptibility to diabetic microvacular complications. Curr Med Chem 10:1389–1398, 2003.
32. UK Prospective Diabetes Study Group: Effect of intensive blood glucose control with metformin on complications in patients with type 2 diabetes: UKPDS 34. Lancet 352:854–865, 1998.
33. UK Prospective Diabetes Study Group: Intensive blood glucose control with sulfonylureas or insulin compared with conventional therapy and risk of complications inpatients with type 2 diabetes mellitus: UKDPS 33. Lancet 352:837–853, 1996.
34. Writing Team for the Diabetes Control and Complications Trial/Epidemiology of Diabetes Interventions and Complications Research Group: Effect of intensive therapy on the microvascular complications of type 1 diabetes mellitus. JAMA 287:2563–2569, 2002.
35. Martin C, Cleary P, Green DL, et al: Persistent effects of intensive therapy eight years after The Diabetes Control and Complications Trial (DCCT). Diabetes 53:S2 A57:244, 2004.
36. Martin CL, Albers J, Herman W, et al: Neuropathy among the Diabetes Control and Complications Trial cohort 8 years after trial completion. Diabetes Care 29:340–344, 2006.
37. The Diabetes Control and Complications Trial/Epidemiology of Diabetes Interventions and Complications Research Group: Retinopathy and nephropathy in patients with type 1 diabetes four years after a trial of intensive therapy. N Engl J Med 342:381–389, 2000.
38. Ohkubo Y, Kishikawa H, Araki E, et al: Intensive insulin therapy prevents the progression of diabetic microvascular complications in Japanese patients with non-insulin-dependent diabetes mellitus: A randomized prospective 6-year study. Diabetes Res Clin Pract 28(2):103–117, 1995.
39. Nakayasu W, Akinori H, Takafumi K, et al: Cost-effectiveness of intensive insulin therapy for type 2 diabetes: A 10-year follow-up of the Kumamoto study. Diabetes Res Clin Pract 48:201–210, 2000.
40. Tasfaye, S, Chaturvedi, N, Eaton, S et al: Vascular risk factors and diabetic neuropathy N Engl J Med 352:341–350, 2005.
41. Koike H, Mori K, Misu K, et al: Painful alcoholic polyneuropathy with predominant small-fiber loss and normal thiamine status. Neurology. 56:1717–1732, 2001.
42. Koike H, Iijima M, Sugiura M, et al: Alcoholic neuropathy is clinicopathologically distinct from thiamine deficiency neuropathy. Ann Neurol 54:19–29, 2003.
43. Adler AI, Boyko EJ, Ahroni JH, et al: Risk factors for diabetic peripheral sensory neuropathy: Results of the Seattle Prospective Diabetic Foot Study. Diabetes Care 20:1162–1167, 1997.
44. Young RJ, Zhou YQ, Rodriquez E, et al: Variable relationship between peripheral somatic and autonomic neuropathy in patients with different syndromes of diabetic polyneuropathy. Diabetes 35:192–197, 1986.
45. Gane E, Bergman R, Hutchinson D: Resolution of alcoholic neuropathy following liver transplantation. Liver Transp 10:1545–1548, 2004.
46. Pirzada NA, Morgenlander JC: Peripheral neuropathy in patients with chronic renal failure: A treatable source of discomfort and disability. Postgrad Med 102(4):249–250, 255–257, 26, 1997.
47. Hassan K, Simri W, Rubenchik I, et al: Effect of erythropoietin therapy on polyneuropathy in predialytic patients. J Nephrol 16(1):121–125, 2003.
48. Locatelli F, Pozzoni P, Del Vecchio L: Renal replacement therapy in patients with diabetes and end-stage renal disease. J Am Soc Nephrol 15(suppl 1):S25–S29, 2004.
49. Muller-Felber W, Landgraf R, Scheuer R, et al: Diabetic neuropathy 3 years after successful pancreas and kidney transplantation. Diabetes 42(10):1482–1486, 1993.
50. Navarro X, Sutherland DE, Kennedy WR: Long-term effects of pancreatic transplantation on diabetic neuropathy. Ann Neurol 42:727–736, 1997.
51. DCCT Research Group: The effect of intensive treatment of diabetes on the development and progression of long-term compli-

cations in insulin-dependent diabetes mellitus. N Engl J Med 329:977–986, 1993.

52. Report of the Expert Committee on the Diagnosis and Classification of Diabetes Mellitus. Diabetes Care 20:1183.2, 1997.

53. Genuth S, Alberti KG, Bennett P, et al: Follow-up report on the diagnosis of diabetes mellitus. Diabetes Care 26:3160–3167, 2003.

54. Borch-Johnsen K: The new classification of diabetes mellitus and IGT: A critical approach. Exp Clin Endocrinol Diabetes 109(suppl 2):S86–S93, 2001.

55. Zhang P, Engelgau M, Valdez R, et al: Costs of screening for prediabetes among U.S. adults: A comparison of different screening strategies. Diabetes Care 26:2536–2542, 2003.

56. Singleton JR, Smith AG, Russell J, Feldman EL: Polyneuropathy with impaired glucose tolerance: Implications for diagnosis and therapy. Curr Treat Options Neurol 7(1):33–42, 2005.

57. Singleton JR, Smith AG, Bromberg MB: Painful sensory polyneuropathy associated with impaired glucose tolerance. Muscle Nerve 24(9):1225–1228, 2001.

58. Polydefkis M, Griffin JW, McArthur J: New insights into diabetic polyneuropathy. JAMA 290(10):1371–1376, 2003.

59. Alexander CM, Landsman PB, Teutsch SM, Haffner SM, Third National Health and Nutrition Examination Survey (NHANES III), National Cholesterol Education Program (NCEP): NCEP-defined metabolic syndrome, diabetes, and prevalence of coronary heart disease among NHANES III participants age 50 years and older. Diabetes 52(5):1210–1214, 2003.

60. Haslbeck KM, Schleicher E, Bierhaus A, et al: The AGE/RAGE/NF-(kappa)B pathway may contribute to the pathogenesis of polyneuropathy in impaired glucose tolerance (IGT). Exp Clin Endocrinol Diabetes 113(5):288–291, 2005.

61. Beggs J, Johnson PC, Olafsen A, Watkins CJ: Innervation of the vasa nervorum: Changes in human diabetics. J Neuropathol Exp Neurol 51:612–629, 1992.

62. Cameron NE, Cotter MA: Metabolic and vascular factors in the pathogenesis of diabetic neuropathy. Diabetes 46(suppl 2):S31–S37, 1997.

63. Johnson PC, Beggs JL: Pathology of the autonomic nerve innervating the vasa nervorum in diabetic neuropathy. Diabet Med 10(suppl 2):S56–S61, 1993.

64. Hotta N, Koh N, Sakakibara F, et al: Prevention of abnormalities in motor nerve conduction and nerve blood-flow by a prostacyclin analog, beraprost sodium, in streptozotocin-induced diabetic rats. Prostaglandins 49:339–349, 1995.

65. Cameron NE, Cotter MA, Robertson S: Angiotensin converting enzyme inhibition prevents development of muscle and nerve dysfunction and stimulates angiogenesis in streptozotocin-diabetic rats. Diabetologia 35:12–19, 1992.

66. Cameron NE, Cotter MA, Robertson S: Rapid reversal of a motor nerve conduction deficit in streptozotocin-diabetic rats by the angiotensin converting enzyme inhibitor lisinopril. Acta Diabetol 30:46–48, 1993.

67. Reja A, Tesfaye S, Harris ND, Ward JD: Is ACE inhibition with lisinopril helpful in diabetic neuropathy? Diabet Med 12:307–309, 1995.

68. Tomlinson DR, Dewhurst M, Stevens EJ, et al: Reduced nerve blood flow in diabetic rats: Relationship to nitric oxide production and inhibition of aldose reductase. Diabet Med 15:579–585, 1998.

69. Yoshida M, Sugiyama Y, Akaike N, et al: Amelioration of neurovascular deficits in diabetic rats by a novel aldose reductase inhibitor, GP-1447: Minor contribution of nitric oxide. Diabetes Res Clin Pract 40:101–112, 1998.

70. Tesfaye S: Epidemiology and etiology of diabetic peripheral neuropathies: Adv Stud Med 4(10G):S1014–S1021, 2004.

71. Tesfaye S, Harris N, Jakubowski JJ, et al: Impaired blood flow and arterio-venous shunting in human diabetic neuropathy: A novel technique of nerve photography and flouroscien angiography. Diabetologia 36:1266–1274, 1993.

72. Tesfaye S, Malik R, Harris N, et al: Arteio-venous shunting and proliferating new vessels in acute painful neuropathy of rapid glycemic control (insulin neuritis). Diabetologia 39:329–335, 1996.

73. Xia P, Inoguci T, Kern TS, et al: Characterization of the mechanism for the chronic activation of diacylglycerol-protein kinase C pathway in diabetes and hypergalactosemia. Diabetes 43:1122–1129, 1994.

74. Greene, DA, Lattimer SA: The polyol pathway in dysfunction of diabetic peripheral nerve. Diabet Med 2:206–210, 1985.

75. Cole JA, Walker RE, Yordy MR: Hyperglycemia-induced changes in Na+/myo-inositol transport, Na(+)-K(+)-ATPase, and protein kinase C activity in proximal tubule cells. Diabetes 44:446–452, 1995.

76. Ishii H, Koya D, King GL: Protein kinase C activation and its role in the development of vascular complications in diabetes mellitus. J Mol Med 76:21–31, 1998.

77. Koya D, King GL: Protein kinase C activation and the development of diabetic complications. Diabetes 47:859–866, 1998.

78. Pirart J: Diabetes mellitus and its degenerative complications: A prospective study of 4,400 patients observed between 1947 and 1973. Diabetes Care 1:168–188, 1978.

79. Williams B, Gallacher B, Patel H, Orme C: Glucose-induced protein kinase C activation regulates vascular permeability factor mRNA expression and peptide production by human vascular smooth muscle cells in vitro. Diabetes 46:1497–1503, 1997.

80. Danis RP, Bingaman DP, Jirousek M, Yang Y: Inhibition of intraocular neovascularization caused by retina ischemia in pigs by PKC beta inhibition with LY333531. Ophthalmol Vis Sci 39:171–179, 1998.

81. Hata Y, Rook SL, Aiello LP: Basic fibroblast growth factor induces expression of VEGF receptor KDR through a protein kinase C and p44/p42 mitogen-activated protein kinase-dependent pathway. Diabetes 48:1145–1155, 1999.

82. Bursell SE, Takagi C, Clermont AC, et al: Specific retinal diacylglycerol and protein kinase C beta isoform modulation mimics abnormal retinal hemodynamics in diabetic rats. Invest Ophthalmol Vis Sci 38:2711–2720, 1997.

83. Koya D, Jirousek MR, Lin YW, et al: Characterization of protein kinase C beta is form activation on the gene expression of transforming growth factor-beta, extra cellular matrix components, and prostanoids in the glomeruli of diabetic rats. J Clin Invest 100:115–126, 1997.

84. Joy SV, Scates AC, Bearelly S, et al: Ruboxistaurin, a protein kinase C beta inhibitor, as an emerging treatment for diabetes microvascular complications. Ann Pharmacother 39(10):1693–1699, 2005.

85. Cameron NE, Cotter MA: Comparison of the effects of ascorbyl μ-linolenic acid and μ-linolenic acid in the correction of neurovascular deficits in diabetic rats. Diabetologia 39:1047–1054, 1996.

86. Cameron NE, Cotter MA, Hohman TC: Interactions between essential fatty acid, prostanoid polyol pathway and nitric oxide mechanisms in the neurovascular deficit of diabetic rats. Diabetologia 39:172–182, 1996.

87. The γ-Linolenic Acid Multicenter Trial Group: Treatment of diabetic neuropathy with γ-linolenic acid. Diabetes Care 16:8–15, 1993.

88. Cameron NE, Cotter MA, Basso M, Hohman TC: Comparison of the effects of inhibitors of aldose reductase and sorbitol dehydrogenase on neurovascular function, nerve conduction and tissue polyol pathway metabolites in streptozotocin-diabetic rats. Diabetolgia 40:271–281, 1997.

89. Goldfarb S, Zihadeh FN, Kern EFO, Simmons DA: Effects of polyol-pathway inhibition and dietary myo-inositol on glomerular hemodynamic function in experimental diabetes mellitus in rats. Diabetes 40:465–471, 1991.

90. Obrosova I, Faller A, Burgan J, et al: Glycolytic pathway, redox state of NAD (P)-couples and energy metabolism in lens in galactose-fed rats: Effect on an aldose reductase inhibitor. Curr Eye Res 16:34–43, 1997.

91. Sima AA, Greene DA, Brown MB, et al: The Tolerestat Study Group: Effect of hyperglycemia and the aldose reductase inhibitor Tolerestat on sural nerve biochemistry and morphometry in advanced diabetic peripheral polyneuropathy. J Diabetes Complications 7:157–169, 1993.

92. Hansen, SH: The role of taurine in diabetes and the development of diabetic complications. Diabetes Metab Res Rev 17:330–346, 2001.

93. Pfeifer MA, Schumer MP, Gelber DA: Aldose reductase inhibitors: The end of an era or the need for different trial designs? Diabetes 46(suppl)2:S82–S89, 1997.

94. Judzewitsch RG, Jaspan JB, Polonsky KS, et al: Aldose reductase inhibition improves conduction velocity in diabetic patients. N Engl J Med 308:119–125, 1983.

95. Pfeifer MA, Peterson H, Snider H, et al: Long-term open-label sorbinil therapy prevents the progression of diabetic neuropathy. Diabetes 37:45, 1988.

96. Chung SS, Chung SK: Aldose reductase in diabetic microvascular complications. Curr Drug Targets 6(4):475–486, 2005.
97. Yorek MA, Wiese TJ, Davidson EP, et al: Reduced motor nerve conduction velocity and Na(+)-K(+)-ATPase activity in rats maintained on L-fructose diet: Reversal by myo-inositol supplementation. Diabetes 42:1401–1406, 1993.
98. Greene DA, Lattimer SA, Carroll PB, et al: A defect in sodium-dependent amino acid uptake in diabetic rabbit peripheral nerve: Correction by aldose reductase inhibitor or myo-inositol administration. J Clin Invest 85:1657–1665, 1990.
99. Kim J, Kyriazi H, Greene DA: Normalization of Na(+)-K(+)-ATPase activity in isolated membrane fraction from sciatic nerves of streptozocin-induced diabetic rats by dietary myo-inositol supplementation in vivo or protein kinase C agonists in vitro. Diabetes 40:558–567, 1991.
100. Kim J, Rushovich EH, Thomas TP, et al: Diminished specific activity of cytosolic protein kinase C in sciatic nerve streptozocin-induced diabetic rats and its correction by dietary myo-inositol. Diabetes 40:1545–1554, 1991.
101. Cameron NE, Leonard MB, Ross IS, Whiting PH: The effects of sorbinil on peripheral nerve conduction velocity, polyol concentrations and morphology in the streptozotocin-diabetic rat. Diabetologia 29:168–174, 1986.
102. Clements, RS Jr, Bell DS: Diabetic neuropathy: Peripheral and autonomic syndromes. Postgrad Med 71:50–52, 60–67, 1982.
103. Sima AA, Lattimer SA, Yagihashi S, Greene DA: Axo-glial dysfunction: A novel structural lesion that accounts for poorly reversible slowing of nerve conduction in the spontaneously diabetic bio-breeding rat. J Clin Invest 77:474–484, 1986.
104. Yagihashi S, Kamijo M, Ido Y, Mirrleese DJ: Effects of long-term aldose reductase inhibition on development of experimental diabetic neuropathy: Ultra-structural and morphometric studies of sural nerve in streptozocin-induced diabetic rats. Diabetes 39:690–696, 1990.
105. Friedman EA: Advanced glycosylated end products and hyperglycemia in the pathogenesis of diabetic complications. Diabetes Care 22(suppl 2):B65–B71, 1999.
106. Honing ML, Morrison PJ, Banga JD, et al: Nitric oxide availability in diabetes mellitus. Diabetes Metab Rev 14:241–249, 1998.
107. Canal N, Nemni R: Autoimmunity and diabetic neuropathy. Clin Neurosci 4:371–373, 1997.
108. Jaeger C, Allendorfer J, Hatziagelaki E, et al: Persistent GAD 65 antibodies in longstanding IDDM are not associated with residual beta-cell function, neuropathy or HLA-DR status. Horm Metab Res 29:510–515, 1997.
109. Zanone MM, Burchio S, Quadri R, et al: Autonomic function and autoantibodies to autonomic nervous structures, glutamic acid decarboxylase and islet tyrosine phosphatase in adolescent patients with IDDM. J Neuroimmunol 87:1–10, 1998.
110. Vinik AI, Anandacoomaraswamy D, Ullal J: Antibodies to neuronal structures: innocent bystanders or neurotoxins? Diabetes Care 28(8):2067–2072, 2005.
111. Apfel SC: Neurotrophic factors and diabetic peripheral neuropathy. Eur Neurol 419(suppl 1):27–34, 1999.
112. Freeman R: Human studies of recombinant human nerve growth factor and diabetic peripheral neuropathy. Eur Neurol 41(suppl 1):20–26, 1999.
113. Pittenger G, Vinik A: Nerve growth factor and diabetic neuropathy. Exp Diabesity Res 4:271–281, 2003.
114. Cameron NE, Eaton SE, Cotter MA, Tesfaye S: Vascular factors and metabolic interactions in the pathogenesis of diabetic neuropathy. Diabetologia 44:1973–1988, 2001.
115. Kato N, Makino M, Mizuno K, et al: Serial changes of sensory nerve conduction velocity and minimal F-wave latency in streptozotocin-induced diabetic-rats. Neuorsci Lett 244:169–172, 1998.
116. Singhal A, Cheng C, Sun H, Zochodme DW: Near nerve local insulin prevents conduction slowing in experimental diabetes. Brain Res 763:209–214, 1997.
117. Obrosova I, Faller A, Ostrow E, et al: Glycolytic pathway, redox state of NAD (P)-couples and energy metabolism in lens in galactose-fed rats: Effect of an aldose reductase inhibitor. Curr Eye Res 16:34–43, 1997.
118. Cardiac Arrhythmia Suppression Trial (CAST) Investigators: Preliminary report: Effect of encainide and flecainide on mortality in a randomized trial of arrhythmia suppression after myocardial infarction. N Engl J Med 321:406–412, 1989.
119. Clemens R: Dietary myo-inositol intake and peripheral nerve function in diabetic neuropathy. Metabolism 28(suppl 1):477–483, 1979.
120. Graf J, Halter JB, Pfeifer MA, et al: Glycemic control and nerve conduction abnormalities in non insulin dependent diabetic subjects. Ann Intern Med 94:307–311, 1981.
121. Lang AH, Forsstrom J, Bjorkqvist SE, Kuusela V: Statistical variation of nerve conduction velocity: An analysis in normal subjects and uremic patients. J Neurol Sci 33:229–241, 1977.
122. Brownlee M: The pathobiology of diabetic complications: A unifying mechanism. Diabetes 54(6):1615–1625, 2005.
123. Hayden MR, Tyagi SC: Neural redox stress and remodeling in metabolic syndrome, type 2 diabetes mellitus, and diabetic neuropathy. Med Sci Monit 10(12):RA291–RA307, 2004.
124. Uemura S, Matsushita H, Li W, et al: Diabetes mellitus enhances vascular matrix metalloproteinase activity: Role of oxidative stress. Circ Res 88:1291–1989, 2001.
125. Pfeifer MA, Ross D, Schrange J, et al: A highly successful and novel model for the treatment of chronic painful peripheral neuropathy. Diabetes Care 16:1103–1115, 1993.
126. Feldman EL, Stevens MJ, Greene DA: Pathogenesis of diabetic neuropathy. Clin Neurosci 4:365–370, 1997.
127. Livingston WK: Pain Mechanisms: A Physiological Interpretation of Causalgia and Its Related States. New York: MacMillan, 1943, pp 1–253.
128. Dyck PJ, Lais AC, Ohta M, et al: Chronic inflammatory polyradiculoneuropathy. Mayo Clin Proc 150(11):621–637, 1975.
129. Sharma KR, Cross J, Farronay O, et al: Demyelinating neuropathy in diabetes mellitus. Arch Neurol 59:758–765, 2002.
130. Hendriksen PH, Oey PL, Wieneke GH, et al: Subclinical diabetic neuropathy: Similarities between electrophysiological results of patients with type 1 (insulin-dependent) and type 2 (non-insulin-dependent) diabetes mellitus. Diabetologia 35:690–695, 1992.
131. Diabetes Control and Complications Trial Research Group: The effect of intensive diabetes therapy on the development and progression of neuropathy. Ann Intern Med 22:561–568, 1995.
132. Asbury AK, Porte D: Report and recommendations of the San Antonio Conference on Diabetic Neuropathy. Diabetes Care 11(7):592–597, 1988.
133. Reeves ML, Seigler DE, Ayyar DR, Skyler JS: Medial plantar sensory response: Sensitive indicator of peripheral nerve dysfunction in patients with diabetes mellitus. Am J Med 76:842–846, 1984.
134. Galer, BS: Neuropathic pain of peripheral origin: Advances in pharmacologic treatment. Neurology 45(suppl 9):S17–S25, 1995.
135. Gilron I, Bailey J, Weaver DF, Houlden RL: Patients' attitudes and prior treatments in neuropathic pain: A pilot study. Pain Res Manage 7(4):199–203, 2002.
136. Vinik A: Clinical review: Use of antiepileptic drugs in the treatment of chronic painful diabetic neuropathy. J Clin Endocrinol Metab 90:4936–4945, 2005.
137. inflammatory drugs in the therapy of diabetic neuropathy. Arch Intern Med 147:1442–1444, 1987.
138. Egbunike IG, Chaffee BJ: Antidepressants in the management of chronic pain syndromes. Pharmacotherapy 10:262–270, 1990.
139. Max MB, Culnane M, Schafer SC, et al: Amitriptyline relieves diabetic neuropathy pain in patients with normal or depressed mood. Neurology 37(4):589–596, 1987.
140. Max MB, Lynch SA, Muir J, et al: Effects of desipramine, amitriptyline, and fluoxetine on pain in diabetic neuropathy. N Engl J Med 326:1250–1256, 1992.
141. Spiegel K, Kalb R, Pasternak G: Analgesic activity of tricyclic antidepressants. Ann Neurol 13:462–465, 1983.
142. Rowbotham MC, Goli V, Kunz NR, Lei D: Venlafaxine extended release in the treatment of painful diabetic neuropathy: A double-blind, placebo-controlled study. Pain 110(3):697–706, 2004.
143. Westanmo AD, Gayken J, Haight R: Duloxetine: A balanced and selective norepinephrine- and serotonin-reuptake inhibitor. Am J Health Syst Pharm 62:2481–2490, 2005.
144. Goldstein DJ, Lu Y, Detke MJ, et al: Duloxetine vs. placebo in patients with painful diabetic neuropathy. Pain 116:109–118, 2005.
145. Wernicke J, Rosen A, Lu Y, et al: The safety of duloxetine in the long-term treatment of diabetic neuropathic pain [abstract]. J Pain 5(suppl 1):48, 2004.
146. Ellenberg, M: Treatment of diabetic neuropathy with diphenylhydantoin. N Y State J Med 68(20):2653–2655, 1968.

147. Chadda VS, Mathur MS: Double blind study of the effects of diphenylhydantoin sodium on diabetic neuropathy. J Assoc Physicians India 26:403–406, 1978.

148. Saudek CD, Werns S, Reidenberg MM: Phenytoin in the treatment of diabetic symmetrical polyneuropathy. Clin Pharmacol Ther 22:196–199, 1977.

149. Rull JA, Quibrera R, Gonzalex-Millan H, Castaneda OL: Symptomatic treatment of peripheral diabetic neuropathy with carbamazepine (Tegretol®): Double blind crossover trial. Diabetologia 5:215–218, 1969.

150. Wilton TD: Tegretol in the treatment of diabetic neuropathy. S Afr Med J 48:869–872, 1974.

151. Beydoun A, Kobetz SA, Carrazana EJ: Efficacy of oxcarbazepine in the treatment of painful diabetic neuropathy. Clin J Pain 20(3):174–178, 2004.

152. Dogra S, Beydoun S, Mazzola J, et al: Oxcarbazepine in painful diabetic neuropathy: A randomized, placebo-controlled study. Eur J Pain 9(5):543–554, 2005.

153. Gu Y, Huang LY: Gabapentin actions on N-methyl-D-aspartate receptor channels are protein kinase C-dependent. Pain 93(1):85–92, 2001.

154. Backonja M, Beydoun A, Edwards KR, et al: Gabapentin for the symptomatic treatment of painful neuropathy in patients with diabetes mellitus: A randomized controlled trial. JAMA 280(21): 1831–1836, 1998.

155. Gorson KC, Schott C, Herman R, et al: Gabapentin in the treatment of painful diabetic neuropathy: A placebo controlled, double blind, crossover trial. J Neurol Neurosurg Psychiatry 166:251–252, 1999.

156. Backonja M, Glanzman RL: Gabapentin dosing for neuropathic pain: Evidence from randomized, placebo-controlled clinical trials. Clin Ther 25(1):81–104, 2003.

157. Dallocchio C, Buffa C, Mazzarello P, Chiroli S: Gabapentin vs. amitriptyline in painful diabetic neuropathy: An open-label pilot study. J Pain Symptom Manage 20: 280–285, 2000.

158. Morello CM, Leckband SG, Stoner CP, et al: Randomized double-blind study comparing the efficacy of gabapentin with amitriptyline on diabetic peripheral neuropathy pain. Arch Intern Med 159(16):1931–1937, 1999.

159. Zareba G: Pregabalin: A new agent for the treatment of neuropathic pain. Drugs Today (Barc) 41(8):509–516, 2005.

160. Rosenstock J, Tuchman M, LaMoreaux L. Sharma U: Pregabalin for the treatment of painful diabetic peripheral neuropathy: A double-blind, placebo-controlled trial. Pain 110:628–638, 2004.

161. Frampton JE, Scott LJ: Pregabalin in the treatment of painful diabetic peripheral neuropathy. Drugs 64(24):2813–2820, 2004.

162. Richter RW, Portenoy R, Sharma U, et al: Relief of painful diabetic peripheral neuropathy with pregabalin: A randomized, placebo-controlled trial. J Pain 6(4):253–260, 2005.

163. Wesche D, Bockbrader H: Linear PK profile and bioavailability of gabapentin vs. pregabalin. Presented at 24th Annual Scientific Meeting of the American Pain Society, Boston, March 30–April 2, 2005.

164. Lesser H, Sharma U, LaMoreaux L, Poole RM: Pregabalin relieves symptoms of painful diabetic neuropathy: A randomized controlled trial. Neurology 63:2104–2110, 2004.

165. Eisenberg E, Alon N, Ishay A, et al: Lamotrigine in the treatment of painful diabetic neuropathy. Eur J Neurol 5:167–173, 1998.

166. Eisenberg E, Lurie Y, Braker C, et al: Lamotrigine reduces painful diabetic neuropathy: A randomized, controlled study. Neurology 57:505–509, 2001.

167. Kochar DK, Jain N, Agarwal RP, et al: Sodium valproate in the management of painful neuropathy in type 2 diabetes: A randomized placebo controlled study. Acta Neurol Scand 106:248–252, 2002.

168. Otto M, Bach FW, Jensen TS, Sindrup SH: Valproic acid has no effect on pain in polyneuropathy: A randomized, controlled trial. Neurology 62:285–288, 2004.

169. Edwards KR, Glantz MJ, Button J, et al: Efficacy and safety of topiramate in the treatment of painful diabetic neuropathy: A double-blind, placebo-controlled study. Neurology 54(suppl 3): A81, 2000.

170. Raskin P, Donofrio PD, Rosenthal NR, et al: Topiramate vs placebo in painful diabetic neuropathy: Analgesic and metabolic effects. Neurology 63:865–873, 2004.

171. Donofrio PD, Raskin P, Rosenthal NR, et al: Safety and effectiveness of topiramate for the management of painful diabetic peripheral neuropathy in an open-label extension study. Clin Ther 27:1420–1431, 2005.

172. Collins SL, Moore RA, McQuay HJ, Wiffen P: Antidepressants and anticonvulsants for diabetic neuropathy and postherpetic neuralgia: A quantitative systematic review. J Pain Symptom Manage 20(6):449–458, 2000.

173. Capsaicin Study Group: Treatment of painful diabetic neuropathy with topical capsaicin: A multicenter, double-blind, vehicle-controlled study. Arch Intern Med 151:2225–2228, 1991.

174. White WT, Patel N, Drass M, Nalamachu S: Lidocaine patch 5% with systemic analgesics such as gabapentin: A rational polypharmacy approach for the treatment of chronic pain. Pain Med 4(4):321–330, 2003.

175. Argoff CE, Galer BS, Jensen MP, et al: Effectiveness of the lidocaine patch 5% on pain qualities in three chronic pain states: Assessment with the Neuropathic Pain Scale. Curr Med Res Opin 20(suppl 2):S21–S28, 2004.

176. Zeigler D, Lynch SA, Muir J, et al: Transdermal clonidine versus placebo in painful diabetic neuropathy. Pain 48:403–408, 1992.

177. Byas-Smith MF, Max MB, Muir J, Kingman A: Transdermal clonidine compared to placebo in painful diabetic neuropathy using a two-stage "enriched enrollment" design. Pain 60(3):267–274, 1995.

178. Harati Y, Gooch C, Swenson M, et al: Double-blind randomized trial of tramadol for the treatment of the pain of diabetic neuropathy. Neurology 50:1842–1846, 1998.

179. Harati Y, Gooch C, Swenson M, et al: Maintenance of the long-term effectiveness of tramadol in treatment of the pain of diabetic neuropathy. J Diabetes Complications 18(3):601–613, 2000.

180. Dejgard A, Petersen P, Kastrup J: Mexiletine for treatment of chronic painful diabetic neuropathy. Lancet 1(8575–6):9–11, 1988.

181. Wright JM, Oki JC, Graves L III: Mexiletine in the symptomatic treatment of diabetic peripheral neuropathy. Ann Pharmacother 31(1):29–34, 1997.

182. Stracke H, Meyer UE, Schumacher HE, Federlin K: Mexiletine in the treatment of diabetic neuropathy. Diabetes Care 15(11): 1550–1555, 1992.

183. Jarvis B, Coukell AJ: Mexiletine: A review of its therapeutic use in painful diabetic neuropathy. Drugs 56(4):691–707, 1998.

184. Terrence CF, Fromm GH, Tenicela R: Baclofen as an analgesic in chronic peripheral nerve disease. Eur Neurol 24(6):380–385, 1985.

185. Portenoy RK: Opioid therapy for chronic nonmalignant pain: A review of the critical issues. J Pain Symptom Manage 11:203–217, 1996.

186. Watson CP, Babul N: Efficacy of oxycodone in neuropathic pain: A randomized trial in postherpetic neuralgia. Neurology 50(6):1837–1841, 1998.

187. Watson CP: The treatment of neuropathic pain: Antidepressants and opioids. Clin J Pain 16(2 suppl):S49–S55, 2000.

188. Halat KM, Dennehy CE: Botanicals and dietary supplements in diabetic peripheral neuropathy. J Am Board Fam Pract 16(1):47–57, 2003.

189. Reljanovic M, Reichel G, Rett K, et al: Treatment of diabetic polyneuropathy with the antioxidant thioctic acid (alpha-lipoic acid): A two year multicenter randomized double-blind placebo-controlled trial (ALADIN II). Alpha Lipoic Acid in Diabetic Neuropathy. Free Radic Res 31(3):171–179, 1999.

190. Ziegler D, Hanefeld M, Ruhnau KJ, et al: Treatment of symptomatic diabetic polyneuropathy with the antioxidant alpha-lipoic acid: A 7-month multicenter randomized controlled trial (ALADIN III Study). ALADIN III Study Group. Alpha-Lipoic Acid in Diabetic Neuropathy. Diabetes Care 22(8):1296–1301, 1999.

191. Ruhnau KJ, Meissner HP, Finn JR, et al: Effects of 3-week oral treatment with the antioxidant thioctic acid (alpha-lipoic acid) in symptomatic diabetic polyneuropathy. Diabet Med 16(12): 1040–1043, 1999.

192. Tesfaye S, Watt J, Benbow SJ, et al: Electrical spinal-cord stimulation for painful diabetic peripheral neuropathy. Lancet 348(9043):1698–1701, 1996.

193. Daousi C, Benbow SJ, MacFarlane IA: Electrical spinal cord stimulation in the long-term treatment of chronic painful diabetic neuropathy. Diabet Med 22(4):393–398, 2005.

194. Weiman TJ, Patel VG: Treatment of hyperesthetic neuropathic pain in diabetics. decompression of the tarsal tunnel. Ann Surgery 1995; 221:660–665, 1995.

195. Wood WA, Wood MA: Decompression of peripheral nerves for diabetic neuropathy in the lower extremities. J Foot Ankle Surg 42:268–275, 2003.

196. Dellon AL: Diabetic Neuropathy: Review of a surgical approach to restore sensation, relieve pain, and prevent ulceration and amputation. Foot Ankle Int 25:749–755, 2004.

197. Chaudhry V, Stevens JC, Kincaid J, So YT: Practice advisory: Utility of surgical decompression for the treatment of diabetic neuropathy. Report of the Therapeutics and Technology Assessment Subcommittee of the American Academy of Neurology. Neurology 66:1805–1808, 2006.

198. Grunfeld C: Diabetic foot ulcers: Etiology, treatment, and prevention. Adv Intern Med 37:103–132, 1992.

199. Murray HJ, Boulton AJ: The pathophysiology of diabetic foot ulceration. Clin Podiatr Med Surg 12:1–17, 1995.

200. Rith-Najarian SJ, Stolusky T, Gohdes DM: Identifying diabetic patients at high risk for lower-extremity amputation in a primary health care setting: A prospective evaluation of simple screening criteria. Diabetes Care 15:1386–1389, 1992.

201. Pham HT, Exelbert L, Segal-Owens AC, et al: A prospective, randomized, controlled double-blind study of a moisturizer for xerosis of the feet in patients with diabetes. Ostomy Wound Manage 48(5):30–36, 2002.

202. Armstrong DG, Lavery LA, Harkless LB: Treatment-based classification system for assessment and care of diabetic feet. J Am Podiatr Med Assoc 86:311–316, 1996.

203. Janisse DJ: Prescription insoles and footwear. Clin Podiatr Med Surg 12:41–61, 1995.

204. Levin M: Diabetic foot wounds: Pathogenesis and management. Adv Wound Care 10:24–30, 1997.

205. Litzelman DK, Slemenda CW, Langefeld CD, et al: Reduction of lower extremity clinical abnormalities in patients with non-insulin-dependent diabetes mellitus: A randomized, controlled trial. Ann Intern Med 119:36–41, 1993.

206. Valensi P: Diabetic autonomic neuropathy: What are the risks? Diabetes Metab 24(suppl 3):66–72, 1998.

207. Ziegler D: Diagnosis and treatment of diabetic autonomic neuropathy. Curr Diab Rep 1(3):216–227, 2001.

208. Tanenberg RJ, Pfeifer MA: Neuropathy: The "forgotten complication." Diabetes Forecast. 53:56–60, 2000.

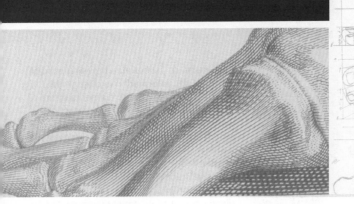

HEMORHEOLOGY: PRINCIPLES AND CONCEPTS

DONALD E. MCMILLAN ■

The foot needs blood in order to function. Blood is a fluid that is distributed through the body by the pumping action of the heart. Fluids are a broad class of materials that behave by flowing when acted on by any driving force. Fluids differ from solids because solids resist continuing movement by generating a force through the magnitude of their internal deformation (Fig. 4-1). Fluids continue to move because their resistance to motion is generated by the motion itself. Even solids will flow (or break) when they are placed under sufficient force.

The systematic examination of flow is the scope of the scientific discipline called rheology, taken from *rheos*, the Greek word for "flow" or "current." The study of blood's flow properties is called hemorheology. Blood has physical flow properties that are unique, and these unique properties are affected by disease states such as diabetes. We will review here the features of blood flow and its control that may help in understanding and managing foot problems in diabetes.

The Concept of Blood Flow

Many fluids, including air and water, behave in a very regular way when acted on by force. They are referred to as newtonian because their response is analyzable by using Newton's laws. In addition to formulating three basic laws for planetary motion (*Book I: The Motion of Bodies*), Newton experimented with movement of fluids, specifically water (*Book II: The Motion of Bodies in Resisting Mediums*). He found a simple and direct relationship between applied force and responsive motion, like that expected from his second law of motion. The ratio of such a fluid's resistive force, σ, to its responsive motion or shear rate, γ (see the section entitled "Blood as a Shear Thinning Fluid," below) is

$$\eta = \frac{\sigma}{\dot{\gamma}}$$

where η is the fluid's viscosity, is normally stable at constant temperature. Blood does not respond so simply and hence is said to be nonnewtonian. Nonnewtonian fluids make up a broad class. We have day-to-day contact with many of them, principally as foods, inks, and cosmetics. None of the other nonnewtonian materials behave exactly like blood.

Blood has unique cellular and plasma components. Its dominant cells are erythrocytes. They typically form 40% of blood's volume. Leukocytes form less than 1% of the volume but become very important in the microcirculation. Electrolytes and glucose are osmotically important, affecting red cell size, but they make only a very small direct contribution to blood's flow properties. Proteins in blood have effects on blood flow linked both to their shape and to their concentration. This happens because they interact with red cells on the basis of their shape. The protein–red blood cell mixture in blood generates

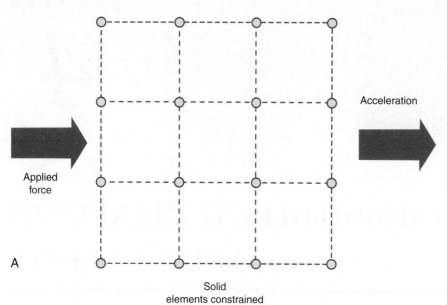

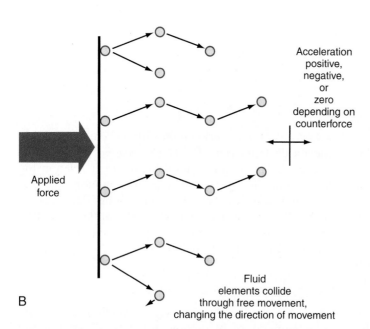

Figure 4–1 Difference between solid (**A**) and fluid (**B**) deformation is diagrammed. In solid deformation, the elements of the material are held in place by interactions with their neighbors and resist movement more and more with greater displacement until the solid is disrupted. If no disruption occurs, the solid returns to its original shape by elastic recovery. A fluid resists deformation in proportion to the rate of displacement of its constituents relative to each other as long as there is time for the random motion of the elements relative to each other to dissipate the original momentum.

different flow responses depending on vessel size and flow rate.

Blood is designed to flow and to deliver oxygen to the tissues. But it must also stop flowing when necessary. This happens regularly following trauma, during menstruation, and after parturition. To do this, blood contains platelets to plug small defects in the vessel walls, such as venipuncture sites and shaving nicks. Larger defects require local blood vessel constriction and the coagulation of the blood. A feature that helps to slow local blood flow is the marked rise in blood flow resistance (viscosity; see Fig. 4-5 later in the chapter) when flow is slowed. This feature of blood is conferred to it by the plasma proteins, especially fibrinogen. Fibrinogen is also responsible for clot formation. In disease states such as diabetes and in

pregnancy, fibrinogen levels rise, and blood viscosity at low flow (shear) rates becomes elevated.[1,2] Fibrinogen and some closely related proteins have been associated cross-sectionally with diabetic complications.[3] Fibrinogen is also now well documented as a risk factor for cardiovascular disease in nondiabetics.[4,5] Reports show it to have a similarly predictive role in diabetes.[6–8]

Inertial Versus Viscous Flow

Different blood flow properties are either more or less important in specific flow situations, particularly those that are seen in blood flow in the leg and foot. A review of both nonnewtonian fluid and circulatory flow concepts can help us to understand which blood flow properties are most affected by diabetes. Fluid flow is commonly influenced by inertia, a property that is linked to mass. Fluids, like all materials in motion, try to continue movement in a straight line.

In the circulation, there are very few straight paths, so blood usually cannot maintain straight-line flow. It changes direction by using its motion energy and its surrounding vessel walls to generate pressure gradients. These pressure gradients cause blood flow to change in direction. Flow-redirecting pressure gradients are seen mainly in large arteries and veins. In capillaries, change in flow direction is controlled by viscous drag generated by using the inner wall of the turn.

The relative importance of inertia and viscous drag to the flow of newtonian fluids was systematized by the 19th century work of Sir Osborne Reynolds, who studied liquid flow in straight tubes.[9] He showed that three factors controlled the relative importance of viscosity to inertia in linear flow: the velocity of the fluid, u; the diameter of the tube, d; and the kinematic viscosity of the fluid, v. Kinematic viscosity is the fluid viscosity divided by the fluid's density. The relationship is usually represented by an equation as the flow's Reynolds number, Re:

$$Re = \frac{u\,d}{v}$$

The ratio of the product of velocity and tube diameter to the kinematic viscosity has no dimension if the units that are used are the same and the fluid is newtonian. The Reynolds number portrays the relative importance of inertia and viscosity to flow in tubes and in structures roughly similar to tubes: the blood vessels (Table 4-1).

A flow at a Reynolds number that is less than 0.01 is characterized by a nearly uniform shearing motion. Direction change is mediated by the resistive force generated by local differences in rate of shearing. In contrast, flows with a Reynolds number of 100 or more change direction through inertia-generated pressure gradients.

Two important patterns are generated by the contrast between the high Reynolds flow (>100) seen in arteries and the low Reynolds flow (<0.01) seen in capillaries and small veins. Flow eddies are limited to larger vessels. Eddying has two effects. It causes the flow at the vessel wall to be uneven, increasing the local pressure drop. It also mixes blood locally, an important need in blood's oxygen delivery and other transport functions. In small veins and venules, this mixing is absent. The flow is layered, as is easily seen in fluorescein studies of the retina. Injected dye returns more rapidly after it passes through shorter and more direct vessel loops. The outer layers of the retinal venules fill with dye first, and almost no mixing occurs.[3]

Nonmixing of blood can also be expected in most microvessels in the foot, but capillary flow is a little more complex. Red blood cells pass through capillaries one at a time. They are greater in diameter (8 μm) than true capillaries (usually 4 to 6 μm). The erythrocytes must deform to pass through a capillary. They tend to fill it completely. Their movement disturbs the layered flow of the local plasma. The result is a flow that acts to mix plasma between red cells, called bolus flow.[10] This mixing effect enhances oxygen's passage into tissues. By this means, blood is uniquely well designed to defeat the lack of fluid mixing at low Reynolds flow by using red cells to force the needed mixing. This helps to explain why blood can be more viscous than hemoglobin solutions made from it by destroying red cell membranes and still supply oxygen more effectively than oxygen-binding macromolecules in plasma.

Blood flow in arterioles and small veins falls between the two extremes discussed above (see Table 4-1). Both inertial and viscous effects are important. Changes in local flow rate affect mixing efficiency, but slowing always reduces mixing and causes the tangential wall force due to viscous drag to decline.

Arteries to the Leg and Foot

Foot blood flow supplies three major tissue components: skin, muscle, and bone. Little is known specifically about blood flow to foot bones; it is often assumed to be modest and stable. On the other hand, muscle flow is closely related to contractile activity, rising strikingly in parallel with oxygen consumption during intrinsic foot muscle contraction. Skin blood flow is determined principally by body core and environmental temperature, rising with the need to dissipate heat. It can change at least as strikingly as the flow associated with intrinsic muscle activity in the foot. A severalfold rise in foot flow is generated by vigorous walking or running.

It is useful to picture the circulation to the foot with both blood flow and blood's flow properties in mind. Blood passes to the foot through the arteries. The aorta gives rise to the common iliac and then the external iliac and femoral arteries. The superficial femoral branch passes medially and posteriorly through the adductor canal to become the popliteal artery. Below the knee, the popliteal artery gives rise to three arteries (Fig. 4-2). All

TABLE 4-1   Blood Vessel Reynolds Numbers

Size of Vessel	Reynolds Number (Range)*
Intracardiac	400–1500
Aorta, large arteries	500–5800
Muscular arteries	100–1000
Primary arterioles	0.05–1.0
Small arterioles	0.07–0.7
Capillaries	~0.001
Small venules	0.05–0.5
Moderate-sized veins	50–500
Large veins	200–900

*Large Reynolds number flows (>100) are subject to much more inertial influence than are lower Reynolds flows, whereas Reynolds number flows < 0.01 are dominated by viscous drag. Reynolds number flows > 2000 are capable of generating turbulent patterns if tube length is long enough. Reynolds number flows around 1 (0.1 to 10) are mixtures of viscous and inertial behavior.

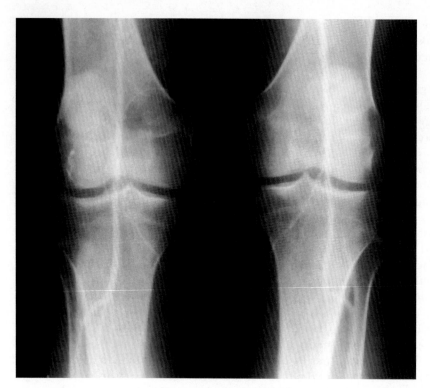

Figure 4–2   Arteriogram of both knee areas shows how the popliteal artery gives rise to three branches after it passes behind the knee. A fork-like configuration on the left deserves the name trifurcation, while on the right, the early takeoff of the anterior tibial and size disparity between the smaller posterior tibial and larger peroneal artery destroy the appropriateness of the name, also illustrating the variability of the arterial anatomy.

three supply the foot, but two normally carry most of the flow. The anterior tibial artery changes direction abruptly as it passes forward and then downward with the antero-lateral muscles of the leg. It then passes to the front of the ankle, where it becomes the dorsalis pedis artery, supplying the dorsal and even plantar foot. The posterior tibial and peroneal arteries arise more directly as medial and lateral branches of the popliteal artery. The posterior tibial artery (medial in Fig. 4-2) is normally considerably larger. It passes behind the ankle's medial malleolus to supply the plantar foot and its muscles. The peroneal artery (lateral in Fig. 4-2) passes behind the lateral malle-olus to supply the less muscular lateral foot. The upper leg's arterial anatomy is responsible for some features of arterial pressure around the ankle. The pressure is highest in the large and direct posterior tibial artery. A slightly lower pressure is usually found in the dorsalis pedis artery. Intraluminal pressure is not infrequently low or ultrasonically undetectable in the peroneal arteries at the ankle.

Two leg artery problems develop in diabetes. The more common is atherosclerotic occlusion. It is dispro-portionately distal in diabetes, affecting the branches of the popliteal more than the iliac and femoral arteries.[11] The development of occlusive disease below the knee enlarges the collateral arteries around the knee. Only infrequently is disease at this low level associated with symptoms of intermittent claudication.[11] Two reasons exist for this absence. First, the low site of occlusion impairs calf flow less than higher blockages do. Second, pain appreciation is reduced by diabetic neuropathy, and this can hide the symptoms. Clinical problems are commonly

associated with ankle artery pressures below 80 mm Hg. At lower arterial perfusion pressure, injury- or infection-mediated gangrene is sometimes the initially recognized event. Several features of diabetic blood flow contribute to the low pressure and to gangrene development. Their detection can justify new treatments effective in reducing obstruction (see Tables 4-3, 4-4, and 4-5 later in the chapter).

The second diabetes-associated problem is arterial wall calcification. This abnormality develops in the middle layer rather than the inner layer of the vessel wall. It interferes with leg blood pressure evaluation. Leg artery calcification also changes the distal arterial flow pattern and limits maximum blood flow to the foot.[12] Expansion of the artery wall during local systole is pre-vented, so larger rises in systolic pressure and greater systolic flow are delivered to the microvessels of the foot. Wall expansion is important in preventing athero-sclerosis, so arterial calcification interacts with gravity-mediated rises in intraluminal pressure to set the stage for plaque development at the branches of the popliteal artery.

The plantar forefoot has a deep arterial arch con-necting the posterior tibial and dorsalis pedis terminal branches like the one in the palm of the hand that con-nects radial and ulnar arteries. This arch may be throm-bosed by local infection. Blood problems generated by diabetes appear to add to this likelihood. Distal throm-bosis can result in digital artery occlusion and toe gan-grene even when proximal foot arteries are completely patent, but leg artery occlusion is a far more common cause of gangrene.

Blood Flow in Leg Veins

Venous return in the leg has some unusual features linked to the dependent position that the lower limbs normally occupy. The saphenous veins have valves, an anatomic feature that is shared with the superficial forearm veins. The anatomic situation of the deep leg veins below the trifurcation is more unusual. They are not only valved but also paired and ensheathed in common with their associated arteries (venae comitantes). This allows the arterial pulse to act to propel deep leg vein blood toward the heart. Arterial stiffening interferes with this mechanism. The result is a rise in intraluminal leg vein pressure. Walking also assists deep vein blood to return to the heart. Loss of muscle due to diabetic neuropathy therefore further reduces blood return. Subcutaneous tissue pressure has been measured and found normally to be less than 3 mm Hg,[13] a value that is well below the oncotic pressure of the plasma. With a higher venous pressure in the ankle and foot, more fluid passes into the tissues, and the efficiency of the lymphatic system is put to the test. This system is also equipped with valves and in health has the ability to contract and pump the lymph.

Effects of Autonomic Neuropathy on Flow

Diabetes is commonly followed by damage to the sympathetic nerves that control blood flow to the feet. The vasoconstrictive response to standing is substantially reduced[14] (Fig. 4-3). When a nondiabetic person stands up, skin blood flow to the feet drops to about 20% of resting supine flow. Reduced autonomic activity in diabetes interferes with this degree of vasoconstriction, so flow to the skin of the feet while standing remains high.[14,15] This means that leg artery flow in the standing position is unusually high in diabetes at the same time that gravity raises intraluminal leg artery pressure by more than 100 mm Hg. The unusually high intraluminal pressure stretches the arterial wall and reduces its degree of expansion with systole. Persistently high flow acts with reduced wall motion to favor atherosclerotic plaque formation[16] that can develop in leg arteries that would otherwise be protected by reduced flow.

Loss of this reflex may explain why atherosclerotic plaques cause more blockage in the leg than thigh arteries in diabetes and why leg artery atherosclerosis, in contrast with coronary disease, is commonly related in diabetes to disease duration as well as to age.[17] The autonomic neuropathy that allows persistently high foot blood flow in the standing posture[14] is probably also responsible for lowering nutritional flow relative to shunt microvessel flow in the foot in long-standing diabetes.[18]

The Role of Leukocytes in Blood Flow

Leukocytes have unusual importance in the microcirculation. White cells are kept in the main stream by the well-mixed flow that is present in large arteries and veins.

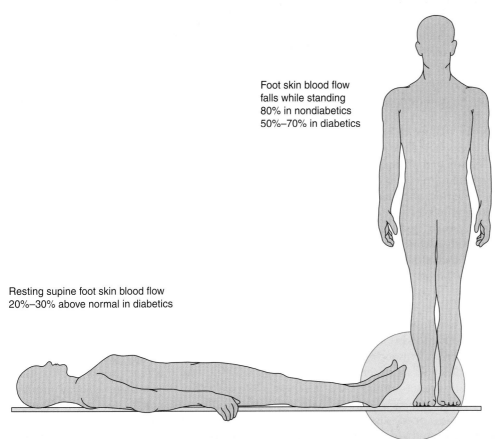

Foot skin blood flow falls while standing
80% in nondiabetics
50%–70% in diabetics

Resting supine foot skin blood flow
20%–30% above normal in diabetics

Figure 4–3 Figures portray two features of leg and foot blood flow in diabetes that may contribute to the development of leg artery disease in diabetes. Resting (not maximal) skin blood flow is usually high in diabetes, but on standing, the normal approximately 80% fall in skin blood flow fails to develop, favoring substantially higher leg artery flow in diabetes when the subject is standing.

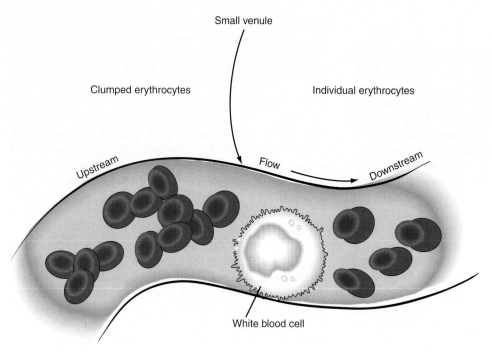

Small venule

Clumped erythrocytes

Individual erythrocytes

Upstream   Flow   Downstream

White blood cell

WBC adherent or rolling slowly

Figure 4–4   Leukocytes tend to stay longest in small venules, where they generate small clusters of erythrocytes by slowing their passage. The erythrocytes are forced to disaggregate to pass the standing or slowly moving white blood cell.

But in smaller vessels, leukocytes tend to make contact with the vessel wall and then roll along if flow is sufficiently rapid. They tend to rest against the wall where flow is slow (in modest-sized venules). The tendency for leukocytes to be near the wall of small vessels is enhanced by high plasma fibrinogen levels,[19] raising the resting leukocyte count in small venules in diabetes.

Adherence of leukocytes to venule walls places them in the path of returning red cells, forcing the small aggregates of erythrocytes that have just passed through capillaries or shunt vessels and are clumped together (Fig. 4-4) to disaggregate again in order to pass the resting leukocytes.[20]

The leukocyte's microcirculatory role as an impeder of movement of red cells as they begin their return to the heart is furthered by fibrinogen. Fibrinogen promotes red cell aggregation. Two other agents that directly influence the leukocyte's role as a microcirculation obstructer are adrenalin and leukocyte-activating peptides. Adrenalin alters microcirculatory flow and pressure. Both injected and endogenous epinephrine dislodge white cells that are resident in venules, reducing local flow resistance and raising the circulating white blood cell count. Leukocyte activation, by peptides such as f-Met*Leu*Phe that signal their increased responsiveness to chemoattractant chemicals and their ability to synthesize strong oxidants, also increases their adherence to vessel walls. Their activation may even result in permanent occlusion of tissue if arterial pressure is insufficient to dislodge them when they become lodged in arterioles and capillaries.[21] This is an attractive mechanism to explain the development of toe gangrene in advanced diabetic occlusive leg artery disease. Both activated monocytes

and granulocytes can contribute to capillary nonperfusion in diabetic retinopathy.[22] Pharmacologic agents that can reverse the leukocyte's activation state and thereby improve microvascular flow have a role in management of advanced diabetic leg artery disease by affecting this phenomenon.

Blood as a Shear Thinning Fluid

We have pointed out physical, physiologic, and anatomic components of the diabetic foot's circulation. We now discuss more specific features of blood flow and the effects of diabetes on them. As has already been mentioned, blood is much more resistant to flow at low than at high shear rates. This property is called shear thinning. *Shear* is a word that is used to describe the component of motion within a material that distorts its planes rather than simply changing the relative positions of two points. The rate of distortion of local surfaces during fluid motion is referred to as *shear rate*. Movement of a small fluid area relative to an adjacent area occurs at one inverse second (the unit of shear rate) if the two areas move relative to each other in both position and rotation the same distance as the distance between them. If a similar amount of motion takes only 10 msec, then the local shear rate is 100 inverse seconds (100 sec^{-1}). For a newtonian fluid, the viscosity or ratio of resistive force generated locally by internal fluid motion is constant. This means that 100 times as much force-resisting flow develops at 100 sec^{-1} as at 1 sec^{-1}. Blood is shear thinning (Fig. 4-5), and the flow resistance ratio is only about 20 because its viscosity falls fivefold from 1 sec^{-1} to 100 sec^{-1}. Overall, blood is typically at least 25 times as thick or vis-

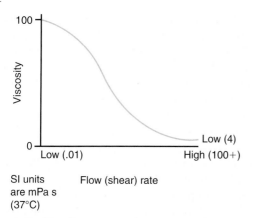

Figure 4–5 Blood's nonnewtonian property of shear thinning is diagrammed. At high flow rates, blood is only five or six times as thick as water, but its flow resistance grows 25-fold as its internal motion slows. This property is useful in blood's need to flow easily and yet stop flowing after injury. A newtonian fluid would produce a horizontal line.

cous at very low shear rate (0.01 sec^{-1}) as it is at high shear rate (500 sec^{-1}).

The basis for blood's shear thinning behavior is the interaction of its red cells during flow. At hematocrits below 10%, blood shows little shear thinning, and a 40% to 55% suspension of erythrocytes in saline is also almost newtonian. But as either the concentration of red cells rises to over 60% or plasma globulins are added, red cell suspensions become progressively more shear thinning, their low shear rate viscosity rising higher and higher. The basis for the rise is increasing contact between erythrocytes during flow. In the absence of globulins, each erythrocyte's negative surface charge actively reduces contact with neighbors unless crowding by a hematocrit above 60% forces contact. Plasma globulins overcome the negative red cell charge, while albumin has little effect other than to stabilize red cell shape. Other large molecules that similarly enhance red cell contact during flow at low shear rate include dextran (a large carbohydrate molecule) and polyvinylpyrrolidinone (a pyrrole polymer). The plasma globulins share large size and substantial flow eccentricity (molecular elongation) with dextran and polyvinylpyrrolidinone. This physical property also causes increased attractiveness of red cell membranes for each other.

Plasma Proteins and Shear Thinning

Molecular size and elongation affect the protein concentration required to produce red cell aggregation. Fibrinogen is the most potent plasma globulin. Polyvinylpyrrolidinone (360,000 daltons) is ten times as potent as the dextran (150,000 daltons) commonly used in laboratory studies. Fibrinogen and other globulins generate blood's shear thinning properties. Haptoglobin is the most important of the globulins that remain in serum after clotting. In diabetes, all three plasma components

favoring increased erythrocyte contact during low shear rate flow—fibrinogen, haptoglobin, and total globulin—are elevated. Total globulin elevation reflects, at least in part, a reduction in plasma albumin. Therefore, diabetic blood typically shows more shear thinning (higher viscosity at low shear rate) than does nondiabetic blood,[2] being 25% more viscous at low shear rate. A recent study compared viscosity at a single shear rate (9 sec^{-1}) of blood from diabetic people with and without foot ulcers and showed higher blood viscosity in the former group.[23]

Increased low shear rate blood viscosity alters blood flow by reducing the shearing motion near the center of steady flow. This effect is very modest. Increased shear thinning burdens flow at low to normal rates less than 2%, the burden decreasing as flow rate rises. The pressure rise that is required to overcome this resistance increase is also less than 2%. This means that variations in plasma protein composition with age, gender, individual genetic predisposition, diabetes, and pregnancy have only this level of direct linkage to blood pressure and do not directly generate measurable changes in cardiac output.

Flow Destabilization

Blood has another continuously present nonnewtonian flow property that is of interest in addition to shear thinning (Table 4-2). Many nonnewtonian fluids lower fluid drag. *Drag* is a word that is used to describe the increased

TABLE 4-2 Types of Nonnewtonian Blood Flow Properties

A. Time independent (always present during flow)
  1. *Shear thinning* (lower viscosity at higher flow rate)
     Red blood cells interact with plasma globulins to try to aggregate at low flow rates, raising the viscosity. Red blood cells stretch progressively as flow rate rises, becoming more streamlined and continuing to lower blood viscosity.
  2. *Flow destabilization* (favors or opposes kinetically mediated change)
     Fluids fail to flow smoothly at high rates of absolute motion, developing irregular patterns with greater pressure drops. Substances that make the fluid nonnewtonian can affect this property, altering the fluid's ability to flow smoothly in curvilinear vessels, a major feature of artery and vein blood flow.

B. Time dependent (present as flow changes and shortly thereafter)
  1. *Viscoelasticity* (elastic strain energy stored as flow increases)
     Elastic erythrocytes (or stretchable molecules in other fluids) are deformed by the initiation or increase of flow rate. Red cell shape change reduces blood's initial resistance to flow but causes a persistence of internal force as a result of cell motion after the fluid's overall motion has ceased.
  2. *Transient resistance* (increased resistance to flow onset or restoration)
     Nonspherical elements in a fluid (erythrocytes in blood) become oriented to the flow as it is initiated or restored. Red blood cell orientation takes less time but more energy as blood's flow rate increases. Rapid red blood cell relaxation from flow orientation in blood causes its resistance to restarting flow to rise much more rapidly than that of other thixotropic fluids, important in arterial flow.

pressure drop generated by newtonian fluids during tube flow at high Reynolds numbers. At Reynolds numbers above 2,000, flow becomes unstable, with local eddies forming and dissipating through the flow. This disturbance causes flow resistance to rise roughly as the 1.4 power of flow velocity.[9] Some substances that make the fluid nonnewtonian also lower this turbulence-related drag when added to the system.[24,25] Red cells might reduce blood's drag in arteries by damping eddies, but the Reynolds number never achieves a value sufficiently high to make drag clearly important. On the other hand, early destabilization in curving flow (as opposed to straight flow) is seen in many nonnewtonian flows. Fortunately, blood is as stable as newtonian fluids during curvilinear flow, and diabetes has no measurable effect on this flow property.[26]

Time-Based Flow Properties of Blood

Blood also has two time-based flow properties: viscoelasticity and transient resistance (Table 4-2). Both are affected by diabetes. Time-based flow properties are seen only for brief periods when flow conditions change. They are not detectable during steady flow but affect blood flow only when it is pulsatile rather than steady. The pulsatility of blood flow in arteries gives these flow properties special importance in these vessels.

Blood Viscoelasticity

Viscoelasticity is responsible for blood's unusually low initial resistance to flow at low shear rate.[27] Because elastic behavior is characteristically reversible, blood's low initial flow resistance is associated with an essentially symmetric dissipation of resistive force when flow stops. While it is clearly visible only at low shear rate, viscoelastic behavior is a feature of flow initiation at all flow rates. To understand what is happening, we return to the concept of fluid deformation as principally the motion of one fluid area relative to another. Blood contains red cells and plasma, but only plasma can continue to move in this manner. Red cells begin to deform, but their solid shape causes them to resist further deformation. They simply achieve a new average shape while flowing. This shape is lost as flow ceases. Erythrocyte shape change is easier to accomplish than is plasma deformation at flow onset, so the flow resistance of blood is initially low, but the saving in early resistance shows up when flow stops as a shear stress tail.

While commonly represented as individual red cell deformation, blood's viscoelastic deformation initially involves red cell rouleaux. Red cells normally form rouleaux when flow has stopped. Red cell suspensions that do not form rouleaux show much less viscoelasticity. At low shear rate (<0.5 sec^{-1}), diabetic blood forms rouleaux more vigorously and is more viscoelastic than is nondiabetic blood. This difference becomes less evident as shear rate rises. The total elastic strain energy that is stored at flow initiation rises continuously up to at least 30 sec^{-1} but less rapidly above 0.5 sec^{-1}.

Blood's Transient Resistance

A number of fluids that have solid components or that gel easily manifest a property called thixotropy,[28] a word coined from Greek to describe fluids and suspensions that fall in flow resistance after they are initially sheared (Fig. 4-6). Good examples are found around the kitchen.

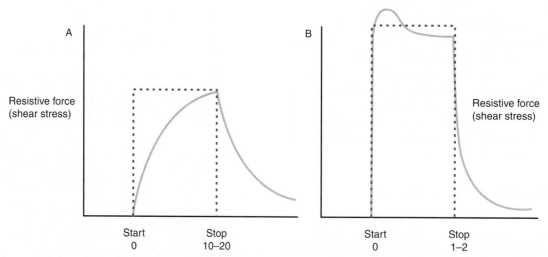

Figure 4–6   Blood's viscoelasticity (**A**) and transient resistance (**B**) are diagrammed. The *thicker lines* show blood's behavior, and the *thinner dashed lines* show a newtonian fluid of similar viscosity to indicate the normal response. At slow onset of flow (shear rate: 0.01 to 0.1 sec^{-1}), red cell bending dominates the fluid's interior motion, reducing its early resistance to deformation. But as flow ceases, the red cells restore their shape and orient more randomly, accounting for the slow decline in internal force that is seen. At faster onset of flow (shear rate 0.2 to 30 sec^{-1}), red cell bending is dominated by the need to orient the cells to rapidly developing flow. This need is directly linked to the rotation of the cells into line and therefore peaks sharply, as shown. The slow red blood cell–based relaxation that is seen at the end of flow is proportionately smaller but still portrays blood's viscoelastic character.

Two such materials are mustard and ketchup. When stirred or shaken, both will thin and pour more easily for a few minutes.

Blood was found to be thixotropic a number of years ago, but it does something that no other thixotropic fluid does as well: It recovers its increased flow resistance very quickly, literally between heartbeats. For that reason, this property has been renamed transient flow resistance.[29] Thixotropy has been shown to be caused by the extra work needed to align red cells into the plane of flow as flow begins or restarts. Transient resistance is recovered rapidly because elastic red cells move out of the plane of flow as flow slows or stops as they relax elastically. A large part of blood's transient resistance is mediated by growing contact between red cells as they lose the orientation they maintained during flow.

Transient resistance is the blood flow property most strikingly affected by diabetes. It is elevated about 30%.[30] Its major direct effects are in the arterial system, where flow is clearly burdened more by increased transient resistance than it is benefited by a higher initial drop in flow resistance from increased elasticity in diabetes.[30] But it also has effects whose magnitude have not yet been assessed in local flow situations in which flow velocity suddenly changes at arterial and arteriolar branch sites. In these flow areas, inertial and transient resistance effects are additive. The hemorheologic effects of diabetes should be largest in large artery areas where flow is suddenly accelerated.

Reduced Erythrocyte Deformability in Diabetes

One of the truly unique features of diabetic blood is the reduced ability of diabetic red blood cells to pass through capillary-sized glass tubes[31] and filters.[32–35] This defect is associated with two other red cell abnormalities. Diabetic red cells also manifest greater flow resistance at low shear rate when resuspended in an artificial medium.[36,37] Most interesting of all is a slowing and reduced ability to form doublets,[38] the first stage of rouleau formation. This kind of motion is most susceptible to thermodynamic analysis. It indicates that diabetic erythrocyte membranes resist rate of bending about twice the normal amount.[38] This means that diabetic red cells are slow to change shape as they enter capillaries, explaining the higher pressure at the arteriolar end of the capillaries that is seen in diabetic limbs even before mural sclerosis has developed.[39]

The basis for the abnormal behavior of diabetic red cells remains unclear. There is evidence that diabetic red cells are more glycated than are normal red cells.[40] But rapid reversibility by insulin administration[33,34,41] and the uniformity of reduced red cell deformability in 4-μm glass tube flow[31] argue that glycation might not be the basis for the observed reduced deformability. The mechanism has importance because most studies have shown that the erythrocyte deformability problem is reduced

when glucose control is better. If a mechanism other than glycation is responsible, then a management strategy other than tight glucose control becomes possible.

Leukocyte Deformability in Diabetes

Diabetic red cell filtration studies were susceptible to leukocyte-plugging artifacts, suggesting initially that increased numbers of leukocytes in diabetes might be responsible for slowing filtration of diabetic blood.[42] But changes in technique to deal with this still allowed reduced red cell filterability to be demonstrated.[43–45] In the meantime, leukocytes were reported to have slowed passage through capillary-sized (5-μm) filters in diabetes.[46] Chemical activation alters leukocyte behavior,[22] further burdening clinical analysis. Further studies have not made the situation clear. The effect of age is of the same magnitude as the diabetes effect in one study[47] and it eliminated the diabetes effect in another.[48] A recent report confirmed the initial observation but could show no difference when the white cells were divided into polymorphonuclear and mononuclear components.[49] A linkage between the age and activation effects has not been shown yet.

In the microcirculation, leukocytes normally pass through small arteriolevenular shunt vessels rather than true capillaries. Both red and white cells tend to be directed into the shunt vessels by the higher flow that these vessels experience while tissues are at rest. With less arterial pressure from leg artery disease in diabetes, leukocyte shunting loses efficiency, raising leukocyte residency frequency and duration in true capillaries,[21] a phenomenon that can lead to permanent tissue damage.[21] This becomes particularly important in the foot. The cutaneous vessels that are responsible for heat loss are mainly shunt vessels, while the nutritional vessels are true capillaries.[18] Foot skin nutrition is disproportionately compromised by diabetic leg artery disease.[18] Activation of leukocytes by infection can turn marginal blood flow into toe gangrene. This result illustrates how problems can add to each other to lead to amputation.

Treatment Considerations

As was described above, many hemorheologic changes in diabetes have been linked in their severity to poor glucose control. But few randomized tests of the effects of improved glucose control on hemorheologic parameters have been carried out. The cross-sectional and prospective data already cited[4,8] argue that close control of blood glucose should reduce or prevent rheologically mediated vascular complications of diabetes. But our large study of Diabetes Control and Complications Trial (DCCT) patients failed to show any plasma protein level benefit of intensive treatment in type 1 diabetes.[50]

Exercise (Table 4-3) is reported to lower blood viscosity through plasma protein changes.[50–54] Both fibrinogen[51–53]

TABLE 4-3 Nonpharmacologic Hemorheologic Management

1. *Exercise*
   Generalized hemoconcentration and intravascular hemolysis in the feet occur during activity, but fibrinolysis increases as physical condition improves with training.[51–54]
2. *Diet*
   Diabetes control accompanied by an appropriately low fat diet decreases VLDL (triglyceride)[82] and its stimulated endothelial PAI-1 synthesis.[56]
3. *Protein intake*
   When adequate and timely, good-quality protein allows a normal albumin synthesis rate when combined with insulin.[57,58]
4. *Garlic/onion oil* (allyl propyl disulfide)
   When consumed in diet, this acts to lower plasma free fatty acids and increase fibrinolysis.[83]
5. *Trans-unsaturated fatty acids*
   Present in margarine and other foods, these have been shown to lower plasma fibrinogen levels in rats.[83]
6. *Fish oil and supplements*
   These act to lower blood viscosity,[17,59,62] fibrinogen,[61] and red cell flow resistance[64] and membrane fluidity.[64]
7. *Smoking cessation*
   Fibrinogen and haptoglobin fall slowly after smoking stops in parallel with declining cardiovascular risk.[84]
8. *Vitamins and nutrients* (often considered food supplements)

TABLE 4-4 Parenteral Agent Hemorheologic Management

1. *Hemodilution*
   A therapy designed to reduce blood viscosity by lowering hematocrit without decreasing blood volume and oxygen delivery. It is normally accomplished by removal of blood and replacement of plasma by an excess of low-molecular-weight dextran (40,000 daltons) or another oncotically active material. This is done to expand the plasma volume without raising blood viscosity. This management has been used in stroke,[85] peripheral arterial disease,[86,87] and retinal vein thrombosis[88] with varying degrees of success. Its ultimate methodology and role in disease management are still being explored.[65]
2. *Plasmapheresis*
   Undesirable plasma components, usually proteins, are removed by phlebotomy. Red blood cells are separated by centrifugation and returned to the patient during the procedure; the plasma is either processed to remove specific substances and returned to the patient or replaced by salt-poor albumin. Treatment effectiveness depends on the half-life of the material being removed and the benefit derived from the feasible amount of lowering. The technique has been used to remove immune proteins,[89] lipoproteins,[90] and acts to lower plasma fibrinogen,[66] but it is both costly and inconvenient for the patient.
3. *Enzyme administration*
   a. Streptokinase, used in treating early acute myocardial infarction,[91] causes fibrinogen to fall to very low levels, altering blood flow properties.[68,92]
   b. Urokinase, also used in acute myocardial infarction, has less antibody interference and less drop in fibrinogen[93] and blood viscosity[92] than streptokinase.
   c. Alteplase (tissue plasminogen activator), also used in acute myocardial infarction, has much less effect on fibrinogen and blood flow properties than streptokinase.[68]
   d. Ancrod (Arvin) has been used in treating peripheral artery disease.[94,95]
   e. Piyavit (enzyme from medicinal leeches) lowers blood viscosity and platelet aggregation.[65]

and haptoglobin[54] are reported to fall. Haptoglobin's fall is thought to involve the feet; red cells are damaged as they pass through plantar capillaries as the feet hit the ground. Hemoglobin released binds to haptoglobin, and both are cleared from the bloodstream by the reticuloendothelial system.

Nutritional choices are also thought to affect blood viscosity. Lowering the traditional U.S. dietary fat intake results in less serum triglyceride.[55] Lowering of very low-density lipoprotein triglyceride levels leads in turn to reduced levels of plasminogen activator inhibitor 1 (PAI-1), the major component of plasmin-mediated clot dissolution and fibrinogenolysis. Very low-density lipoprotein is a direct stimulator, slowing PAI-1 formation by endothelial cells.[56] Adequate protein intake is necessary for normal serum albumin levels.[57,58] Consumption of high levels of fish[59] or its associated ω-3 unsaturated fatty acids[60–62] is reported to lower blood viscosity, but effects of the levels of dietary intake achieved by most Americans have not been studied. The fish oil effect appears to be mediated by triglyceride lowering[25] and erythrocyte membrane lipid changes.[63,64]

A number of parenteral regimens are used to manage serious hemorheologic problems (Table 4-4). Low-molecular-weight dextran, available as 40,000-dalton average Rheomacrodex, has been used in Europe to expand plasma volume as red cells are removed to lower the hematocrit and reduce blood's flow resistance. Alternative plasma expanders based on starch and other large molecules have also been examined.[65]

Plasmapheresis is often used to lower the level of a particular plasma protein. Fibrinogen levels remain subnormal for 2 to 3 days, while plasma complement and other clotting components are restored in 1 day.[66]

The use of plasmin-activating enzymes to dissolve intravascular clots has become commonplace. Most of these agents also lower blood and plasma viscosity in parallel with their clot-dissolving action, an effect that is considered to benefit microcirculatory flow.[67] Streptokinase, acting throughout the plasma volume, produces a more striking change than urokinase and tissue plasminogen activator (t-PA; Alteplase) because the latter has a strong tendency to bind to thrombi.[68]

Information about oral pharmacologic agent effects on blood flow properties and fibrinogen levels is shown in Table 4-5. It has been growing steadily but remains far from complete. I have unpublished data that show that sulfonylurea drugs improve blood viscosity at the same time that they normalize glucose control. Hypoglycemia mediates additional changes in the flow properties of blood that are less desirable. They include increased blood and plasma viscosity, rising von Willebrand factor and t-PA levels, and falling PAI levels without change in fibrinogen level.[69]

Table 4-5 lists aldose reductase inhibitors, which are used in diabetic neuropathy management in some countries, anabolic steroids, benzoic acid derivatives, and a series of agents that are used principally in Europe to treat intermittent claudication. They are also commonly

TABLE 4-5   Oral Medication Hemorheologic Management

Aldose reductase inhibitors
 Sorbinil: lowers fibrinogen, improves red cell filterability[96]
 Ponalrestat (statil): improves red cell suspension viscosity[97]

Anabolic steroids
 Furazabol: activates fibrinolytic system, lowers fibrinogen[98]
 Stanozolol: activates fibrinolytic system, lowers fibrinogen[4]

Anionic amphophiles
 Aspirin: suppresses fibrinogen synthesis,[82] reduces RBC
   aggregation,[99] enhances RBC flow through glass capillaries[100]
 Calcium dobesilate: lowers fibrinogen[101] and blood viscosity,[101,102]
   reduces red cell aggregation[99]

Anticlaudicants
 Buflomedil: lowers fibrinogen, WBV, WBC activation[103,104]
 Defibrotide: produces a fall in fibrinogen in claudication patients[4]
 Dipyridamole: improves filterability of processed red cells in
   vitro[105]
 Pentoxifylline: lowers fibrinogen[75,76] by a mechanism other than
   activating fibrinolysis,[82] opposes WBC activation[74]
 Suloctidil: lowers fibrinogen, mechanism not clear[106]
 Ticlopidine: lowers fibrinogen in claudication, transient ischemia
   (TIA) patients[4,107]

Anticonvulsants
 Valproic acid: acts on liver, probably stops fibrinogen synthesis[108]

Antihypertensives
 β-Blockers
  Celiprolol: lowers fibrinogen in hypertension management[4]
  Propranolol: lowers fibrinogen and increases fibrinolysis
    together[4]
 Calcium inhibitors
  Diltiazem: reported to lower blood viscosity, basis not clear[109]
  Flunarizine: reported to lower blood viscosity, basis not clear[110]
  Nimodipine: WBV falls without fall in plasma viscosity or
    fibrinogen[111]
 Central agents
  Clonidine: lowers fibrinogen modestly, basis not clear[83]

Antioxidants
 Idebenone: improves red cell filterability, aggregability, lowers
   plasma viscosity[112]
 Probucol: lowers fibrinogen and factor VIII in Watanabe rabbits[113]

Biguanides
 Buformin: increases fibrinolysis, decreases fibrinogen[19]
 Metformin: reported to increase fibrinolysis by lowering PAI-1[71]
 Phenformin: reported to increase fibrinolysis, not available in the
   United States[70]

Ergot derivatives
 Dehydroergocryptine: decreases RBC flow resistance in acidosis
   and hyperosmolar states[114]

Fibric acid derived triglyceride-lowering drugs
 Bezafibrate: lowers fibrinogen, more in hypertriglyceridemia[115,116]
 Ciprofibrate: lowers fibrinogen, more in hypertriglyceridemia[4]
 Clofibrate: lowers fibrinogen, more in hypertriglyceridemia[4,80]
 Fenofibrate: lowers fibrinogen, more in hypertriglyceridemia[4,67]
 Gemfibrozil: reported to raise fibrinogen level[81]

HMG-reductase inhibitors
 Lovastatin: raises fibrinogen while improving red cell
   filterability[117]; lowers plasma viscosity and red cell aggregation
   but does change fibrinogen[44]; has its effect influenced by
   lipoprotein(a) level[118]
 Pravastatin: lowers fibrinogen, plasma viscosity[119]; produces no
   change[120]
 Simvastatin: does not change fibrinogen level[16]

Vitamins, nutrients
 Ligustrazine (herb component): lowers whole blood viscosity,
   cause not clear[121]
 Niceritrol (nicotinic acid + PETN): lowers fibrinogen in diabetes[4]
 Nicotinic acid: lowers fibrinogen level in parallel with
   triglyceride[83,122]
 Troxerutin: reduces red cell clumping in diabetic retinopathy,[123]
   reverses WBC wall adhesions in diabetic rats[82]

WBV, whole blood viscosity; *WBC*, leukocytes; *RBC*, erythrocytes.

employed as vasodilators. A number of antihypertensive drugs used in diabetes have been reported to affect blood flow properties. Some of their therapeutic effects may ultimately be explained by this mechanism, but their major hypotensive effects appear to be from their influence on vascular smooth muscle. The biguanide drugs, recently reintroduced in diabetes management in the United States, have all been shown to lower plasma fibrinogen levels by increasing fibrinolysis.[19,70,71] Agents that are used in controlling hyperlipidemias and also commonly used in diabetes management make up a large fraction of the table.

The agent in Table 4-5 that is used most frequently in leg and foot disease in diabetes in the United States is pentoxifylline, a xanthine derivative with adenosine agonist effects. It has been shown to improve intermittent claudication.[72] Its effect was initially thought to be generated by improved red cell deformability,[73] but more recent work has suggested that the agent's adenosine action reverses leukocyte activation.[74] Such an inactivation could also help to explain its reported ability to lower fibrinogen.[75,76]

The major feature of Table 4-5 is the effect of many drugs on plasma fibrinogen levels. The mechanism for

drug action in lowering or raising plasma fibrinogen is of interest. It is hinted at by an analysis of the cited reports. Fibrinogen is synthesized by the liver and after introduction into the plasma volume has a half-life of 2 to 4 days, a short period for plasma proteins. Valproic acid's effect in lowering fibrinogen is likely to be by direct suppression of hepatic protein synthesis, since it has been reported to disrupt liver metabolism and structure in idiosyncratic hepatotoxic reactions through generation of toxic metabolites.[77]

Cytokines, especially interleukin-6 (IL-6), interact with surface receptors on hepatocytes to increase both fibrinogen and haptoglobin synthesis.[78] Pentoxifylline may act by reducing leukocyte-mediated signaling[74] by IL-6 and its resultant fibrinogen and haptoglobin synthesis.

The mechanism of effect of many other drugs listed in Table 4-5 appears to be more complex. The relatively short half-life of fibrinogen and associations between hypertriglyceridemia and the coagulation process[79] argue that plasma fibrinogen is lost early in good part because the coagulation process is initiated and/or the enzyme plasmin has been activated. Either mechanism can lead to a fall in plasma fibrinogen level. Plasmin's activation is usually accomplished by t-PA, an enzyme whose two kringles encourage its attachment to coagulated fibrin. This enzyme is efficiently opposed by PAI-1. Both enzymes are principally products of the endothelium that lines the vascular space. Evidence that PAI-1 is directly stimulated from endothelial cells in culture by very low-density lipoprotein[56] creates a potential explanation for the effect of many of the drugs in Table 4-5. But a past report indicting suppression of hepatic synthesis in clofibrate's fibrinogen-lowering action[80] and the ability of gemfibrozil to lower triglyceride while raising fibrinogen[81] suggest that the situation is more complex.

Fibrinogen is a well-documented risk factor that predicts future cardiovascular disease[4,5] that both alters blood's flow properties and accelerates its coagulability. Drug effects on its blood level should receive at least as much attention as drug effects on serum cholesterol. Hemorheologic treatment is currently a decade or more behind management of hyperlipidemia. The interaction of antihyperlipidemic agents with blood fibrinogen levels should assist us in speeding our assimilation of information that will allow us to understand how to restore the health of the feet and other parts of the body through which blood passes in the diabetic patient.

References

1. McMillan DE: Hemorheological studies in the Diabetes Control and Complications Trial. Clin Hemorheol 13:147–154, 1993.
2. McMillan DE, Utterback NG, Stocki J: Low shear rate blood viscosity in diabetes. Biorheology 17:355–362, 1980.
3. Nielsen NV: The normal fundus fluorescein angiogram and the normal fundus photograph. Acta Ophthalmol 64(suppl 180):1–30, 1986.
4. Cook NS, Ubben D: Fibrinogen as a major risk factor in cardiovascular disease. Trends Pharmacol Sci 11:444–451, 1990.
5. Yarnell JWG, et al: Fibrinogen, viscosity, and white blood cell count are major risk factors for ischemic heart disease. Circulation 83:836–844, 1991.
6. McMillan DE, Malone JI, Rand LI: Progression of diabetic retinopathy is linked to rheologic plasma proteins in the DCCT. Diabetes 44:54A, 1995.
7. McMillan DE, Malone JI, Steffes MW: Plasma fibrinogen and total globulin are elevated in albuminuria in the DCCT. Diabetes 44:23A, 1995.
8. Schmechel VH, Beikufner P, Panzram G: Langsschnittuntersuchungen zur progrenstischen bedeutung des plasmafibrinogens beim diabetes mellitus. Z Ges Inn Med Jahrg 39:453–457, 1984.
9. Schlichting H: Boundary Layer Theory. New York: McGraw-Hill, 1979.
10. Lew HS, Fung YC: The motion of the plasma between the red cells in the bolus flow. Biorheology 6:109–119, 1969.
11. Marinelli MR, et al: Noninvasive testing vs clinical evaluation of arterial disease. JAMA 241:2031–2034, 1979.
12. Christensen NJ: Muscle blood flow, measured by xenon-133 and vascular calcifications in diabetics. Acta Med Scand 183:449–454, 1968.
13. Wiederhielm CA, Weston BV: Microvascular, lymphatic, and tissue pressures in the unanesthetized mammal. Am J Physiol 225:992–996, 1973.
14. Tooke JE, Rayman G, Boolell M: Blood flow abnormalities in the diabetic foot: Diagnostic aid or research tool? In Connor H, Boulton AJ (eds): The Foot in Diabetes. New York: John Wiley, 1987, pp 23–31.
15. Rayman G, Hassan A, Tooke JE: Blood flow in the skin of the foot related to posture in diabetes mellitus. Br Med J 292:87–90, 1986.
16. McDowell IFW, et al: Simvastatin in severe hypercholesterolaemia: A placebo controlled trial. Br J Clin Pharmacol 31:340–343, 1991.
17. Bild DE, et al: Lower-extremity amputation in people with diabetes epidemiology and prevention. Diabetes Care 12:24–31, 1989.
18. Fagrell B, et al: Vital capillary microscopy for assessment of skin viability and microangiopathy in patients with diabetes mellitus. Acta Med Scand Suppl 687:25–28, 1984.
19. Fahraeus R: The suspension-stability of the blood. Acta Med Scand 55:1–228, 1921.
20. Schmid-Schonbein GW, et al: The interaction of leukocytes and erythrocytes in capillary and post-capillary vessels. Microvasc Res 19:45–70, 1980.
21. Schmid-Schonbein GW: Capillary plugging by granulocytes and the no-reflow phenomenon in the microcirculation. Fed Proc 46:2397–2401, 1987.
22. Schroder S, Palinski W, Schmid-Schonbein GW: Activated monocytes and granulocytes, capillary nonperfusion, and neovascularization in diabetic retinopathy. Am J Pathol 139:81–100, 1991.
23. Giansanti R, et al: Haemorheological profile and retinopathy in patients with diabetic foot ulcer. Clin Hemorheol 15:73–80, 1995.
24. Lumley JL, Kubo I: Turbulent drag reduction by polymer additives: A survey. In Gampert B (ed): The Influence of Polymer Additives on Velocity and Temperature Fields. New York: Springer-Verlag, 1984, pp 3–21.
25. Sellin RHJ, Moses RT: Drag Reduction in Fluid Flows. Chichester, UK: Ellis Horwood, 1989.
26. McMillan DE, et al: Taylor-Couette flow stability of diabetic blood. Clin Hemorheol 9:989–998, 1989.
27. McMillan DE, Utterback NG: Maxwell fluid behavior of blood at low shear rate. Biorheology 17:343–354, 1980.
28. Mewis J: Thixotropy: A general review. J Non-Newtonian Fluid Mech 6:1–20, 1979.
29. McMillan DE, Strigberger J, Utterback NG: Rapidly recovered transient flow resistance: A newly discovered property of blood. Am J Physiol 253: H919–H926, 1987.
30. McMillan DE, Utterback NG: Viscoelasticity and thixotropy of diabetic blood measured at low shear rate. Clin Hemorheol 1:361–372, 1981.
31. McMillan DE, Utterback NG, La Puma J: Reduced erythrocyte deformability in diabetes. Diabetes 27:895–901, 1978.
32. Barnes AJ, et al: Is hyperviscosity a treatable component of diabetic microcirculatory disease? Lancet 2:789–791, 1977.
33. Juhan I, et al: Effects of insulin on erythrocyte deformability in diabetics: Relationship between erythrocyte deformability and platelet aggregation. Scand J Clin Lab Invest 41:159–164, 1981.
34. Lipovac V, et al: Influence of lactate on the insulin action on red blood cell filterability. Clin Hemorheol 5:421–428, 1985.
35. Volger E, Schmid-Schonbein H: Mikrorheologisches verhalten des blutes beim diabetes mellitus. Dtsch Gesellshaft Inner Med 80:963–966, 1974.
36. McMillan DE, Utterback NG: Impaired flow properties of diabetic erythrocytes. Clin Hemorheol 1:147–152, 1981.
37. Rillaerts E, et al: Increased low shear rate erythrocyte viscosity in insulin dependent diabetes mellitus. Clin Hemorheol 8:73–80, 1988.
38. McMillan DE, Utterback NG, Mitchell TP: Doublet formation of diabetic erythrocytes as a model of impaired membrane viscous deformation. Microvasc Res 26:205–220, 1983.
39. Tooke JE: Microvascular dynamics in diabetes mellitus. Diabetes Metab 14:530–534, 1988.
40. McMillan DE, Brooks SM: Erythrocyte spectrin glycosylation in diabetes. Diabetes 31:64–69, 1982.
41. Baldini P, et al: Insulin effects on human red blood cells. Mol Cell Endocrinol 46:93–102, 1986.
42. Stuart J, et al: Filtration of washed erythrocytes in atherosclerosis and diabetes mellitus. Clin Hemorheol 3:23–30, 1983.
43. Diamantopoulos EJ, Raptis SA, Moulopoulos SD: Red blood cell deformability index in diabetic retinopathy. Horm Metabol Res 19:569–573, 1987.
44. Koppensteiner R, Minar E, Ehringer H: Effect of lovastatin on hemorheology in type II hyperlipoproteinemia. Atherosclerosis 83:53–58, 1990.
45. Stuart J, Juhan-Vague I: Erythrocyte rheology in diabetes mellitus. Clin Hemorheol 7:239–245, 1987.

46. Ernst E, Matrai A: Altered red and white blood cell rheology in type II diabetes. Diabetes 35:1412–1415, 1986.
47. Missirlis Y, Kaleridis V: Polymorphonuclear leukocyte deformability in type II diabetes mellitus and in ageing. Clin Hemorheol 14:489–496, 1994.
48. MacRury SM, et al: Deformability of leukocyte subpopulations in type 1 (insulin-dependent) and type 2 (non-insulin-dependent) diabetic patients. Clin Hemorheol 14:539–544, 1994.
49. Caimi G, et al: Rheological and metabolic leucocyte determinants in diabetes mellitus. Clin Hemorheol 15:53–60, 1995.
50. McMillan DE, Malone JI: Hemorheological effects of intensive diabetes management in the DCCT. Clin Hemorheol 14:481–488, 1994.
51. Hornsby G, et al: Exercise conditioning reduces plasma fibringen in noninsulin-dependent diabetes mellitus. Diabetes 37(suppl 1): 240a, 1988.
52. Schneider SH, et al: Impaired fibrinolytic response to exercise in type II diabetes: Effects of exercise and physical training. Metabolism 37:924–929, 1988.
53. Volger E, Pfafferott C: Effects of acute physical effort versus endurance training on blood rheology in coronary heart disease patients. Clin Hemorheol 10:423, 1990.
54. Wolf PL, et al: Changes in serum enzymes, lactate, and haptoglobin following acute physical stress in international-class athletes. Clin Biochem 20:73–77, 1987.
55. American Diabetes Association: Nutrition recommendations and principles for people with diabetes mellitus. Diabetes Care 20:S15–S20, 1997.
56. Stiko-Rahm A, et al: Secretion of plasminogen activator inhibitor 1 from cultured human umbilical vein endothelial cells is induced by very low density lipoprotein. Arteriosclerosis 10:1067–1073, 1990.
57. Hutson SM, et al: Regulation of albumin synthesis by hormones and amino acids in primary cultures of rat hepatocytes. Am J Physiol 252:E291–E298, 1987.
58. Jeejeebhoy KN, et al: The comparative effects of nutritional and hormonal factors on the synthesis of albumin, fibrinogen and transferrin. Clin Symp 9:217–247, 1973.
59. Kobayashi S, et al: Epidemiological and clinical studies of the effect of eicosapentaenoic acid (epa c20:5 ω-3) on blood viscosity. Clin Hemorheol 5:493–505, 1985.
60. Cartwright IJ, et al: The effects of dietary O-3 polyunsaturated fatty acids on erythrocyte membrane phospholipids, erythrocyte deformability and blood viscosity in healthy volunteers. Atherosclerosis 55:267–281, 1985.
61. Radack K, Deck C, Huster G: Dietary supplementation with low-dose fish oils lowers fibrinogen levels: A randomized, double-blind controlled study. Ann Intern Med 111:757–758, 1989.
62. Woodcock BE, et al: Beneficial effect of fish oil on blood viscosity in peripheral vascular disease. Br Med J 288:592–594, 1984.
63. Kamada T, et al: Dietary sardine oil increases erythrocyte membrane fluidity in diabetic patients. Diabetes 35:604–611, 1986.
64. Popp-Snijders C, et al: Fatty fish-induced changes in membrane lipid composition and viscosity of human erythrocyte suspensions. Scand J Clin Lab Invest 46:253–258, 1986.
65. Kameneva MV, et al: Piyavit-a complex preparation from the medicinal leech improves blood rheology and decreases platelet aggregation. Clin Hemorheol 15:633–640, 1995.
66. Wood L, Jacobs P: The effect of serial therapeutic plasmapheresis on platelet count, coagulation factors, plasma immunoglobulin, and complement levels. J Clin Apheresis 3:124–128, 1986.
67. Arntz HR, et al: Influence of fenofibrate on blood rheology in type II hyperlipoproteinemia. Clin Hemorheol 10:297–307, 1990.
68. Jan KM, et al: Altered rheological properties of blood following administrations of tissue plasminogen activator and streptokinase in patients with acute myocardial infarction. Circulation 72:417, 1985.
69. Fisher BM, et al: Effects of acute insulin-induced hypoglycemia on haemostasis, fibrinolysis and haemorheology in insulin-dependent diabetic patients and control subjects. Clin Sci 80:525–553, 1990.
70. Fearnley GR, Chakrabarti R: Fibrinolytic treatment of rheumatoid arthritis with phenformin plus ethyloestrenol. Lancet 2:757–761, 1966.
71. Vague P, et al: Metformin decreases the high plasminogen activator inhibition capacity, plasma insulin and triglyceride levels in non-diabetic obese subjects. Thromb Haemost 57:326–328, 1987.
72. Porter JM, et al: Pentoxifylline efficacy in the treatment of intermittent claudication: Multicenter controlled double-blind trial with objective assessment of chronic occlusive arterial disease patients. Am Heart J 104:66–72, 1982.
73. Ehrly AM: The effect of pentoxifylline on the deformability of erythrocytes and on the muscular oxygen pressure in patients with chronic arterial disease. J Med 10:331, 1979.
74. Nash GB, et al: Effects of acute Trental infusion on white blood cell rheology in patients with critical leg ischaemia. Clin Hemorheol 11:309, 1991.
75. Bachet P, Lancrenon S, Chassoux G: Fibrinogen and pentoxifylline. Thromb Res 55:161–163, 1989.
76. Ferrari E, et al: Effects of long-term treatment (4 years) with pentoxifylline on haemorheological changes and vascular complications in diabetic patients. Pharmatherapeutica 5:26–39, 1987.
77. Eadie MJ, Hooper WD, Dickinson RG: Valproate-associated hepatotoxicity and its biochemical mechanisms. Med Toxicol 3:85–106, 1988.
78. Castell JV, et al: Recombinant human interleukin-6 (IL-6/BSF-2/HSF) regulates the synthesis of acute phase proteins in human hepatocytes. FEBS Lett 232:347–350, 1988.
79. Simpson HCR, et al: Hypertriglyceridaemia and hypercoagulability. Lancet 1:786–790, 1983.
80. Pickart L: Suppression of acute-phase synthesis of fibrinogen by a hypolipidemic drug (clofibrate). Int J Tissue React 3:65–72, 1981.
81. Stringer MD, Rampling MW, Kakkar VV: Rheological effects of gemfibrozil in occlusive arterial disease. Clin Hemorheol 10:339, 1990.
82. Berthasult, et al: Hemorheological abnormalities in rats with experimental mild diabetes: Improving effect of troxerutine and α-tocopherol. Clin Hemorheol 14:83–92, 1994.
83. Pickart L: Fat metabolism the fibrinogen/fibrinolytic system and blood flow: New potentials for the pharmacological treatment of coronary heart disease. Pharmacology 23:271–280, 1981.
84. Meade TW, Imeson J, Stirling Y: Effects of changes in smoking and other characteristics on clotting factors and the risk of ischaemic heart disease. Lancet 2:986–988, 1987.
85. Strand T, et al: A randomized controlled trial of hemodilution therapy in acute ischemic stroke. Stroke 15:980–989, 1984.
86. Ernst E: Hemodilution for peripheral arterial occlusive disease. Clin Hemorheol 12:35–40, 1992.
87. Yates CJP, et al: Increase in leg blood-flow by normovolaemic haemodilution in intermittent claudication. Lancet 2:166–168, 1979.
88. Hansen LL, Wiek J, Wiederholt M: A randomized prospective study of treatment of nonischaemic central vein occlusion by isovolaemic haemodilution. Br J Ophthalmol 73:895–899, 1989.
89. Schwab PJ, Okun E, Fahey JL: Reversal of retinopathy in Waldenstrom's macroglobulinemia by plasmapheresis. Arch Ophthalmol 64:515–521, 1960.
90. Seidel D, et al: The HELP-LDL-apheresis multicentre study, an angiographically assessed trial on the role of LDL-apheresis in the secondary prevention of coronary heart disease. Part I. Eur J Clin Invest 21:375–383, 1991.
91. I.S.A.M. Study Group: A prospective trial of intravenous streptokinase in acute myocardial infarction (I.S.A.M.). N Engl J Med 314:1465–1471, 1986.
92. Arntz HR, et al: The effects of different thrombolytic agents on blood rheology in acute myocardial infarction. Clin Hemorheol 11:63–78, 1991.
93. Mathey DG, et al: Intravenous urokinase in acute myocardial infarction. Am J Cardiol 55:878–882, 1985.
94. Lowe GDO: Drugs in cerebral and peripheral arterial disease. BMJ 300:524–528, 1990.
95. Lowe GDO, et al: Subcutaneous Ancrod therapy in peripheral arterial disease: Improvement in blood viscosity and nutritional blood flow. Angiology 30:594–599, 1979.
96. Robey A, et al: Sorbinil partially prevents decreased erythrocyte deformability in experimental diabetes mellitus. Diabetes 36:1010–1013, 1987.
97. Rillaerts EG, Vertommen JJ, De Leeuw IH: Effect of statil (ICI 128436) on erythrocyte viscosity in vitro. Diabetes 37:471–475, 1988.
98. Abiko Y, Kumada T: Enhancement of fibrinolytic and thrombolytic potential in the rat by an anabolic steroid, furazabol. Thromb Res 8:107–114, 1976.

99. McMillan DE, Utterback NG, Wujek JJ: Effect of anionic amphophiles on erythrocyte properties. Ann N Y Acad Sci 416: 633–641, 1983.

100. Rao PR, et al: Aspirin analogues and flow of erythrocytes through narrow capillaries. Clin Hemorheol 15:877–887, 1995.

101. Vinazzer H, Hachen HJ: Influence of calcium dobesilate (Doxium) on blood viscosity and coagulation parameters in diabetic retinopathy. Vasa 16:190–192, 1987.

102. Benarroch IS, et al: Treatment of blood hyperviscosity with calcium dobesilate in patients with diabetic retinopathy. Ophthalmic Res 17:131–138, 1985.

103. Capecchi PL, et al: Buflomedil prevents ischaemia-dependent changes in blood rheology and neutrophil reactivity: A possible adenosine-mediated mechanism. Clin Hemorheol 15:221–333, 1995.

104. Van Acker K, Rillaerts E, De Leeuw I: The influence of buflomedil on blood viscosity parameters in insulin-dependent diabetic patients: A preliminary study. Biomed Pharmacother 43:219–222, 1989.

105. Saniabadi AR, Fisher TC, Rimmer AR, et al: A study of the effect of dipyridamole on erythrocyte deformability using an improved filtration technique. Clin Hemorheol 10:263, 1990.

106. Roncucci R, et al: Effects of long-term treatment with suloctidil on blood viscosity, erythrocyte deformability and total fibrinogen plasma levels in diabetic patients. Arzneim-Forsch Drug Res 29:682–684, 1979.

107. Boisseau MR, et al: Hemorheologically active substances, their profile and clinical impact. Clin Hemorheol 14:171–180, 1994.

108. Sussman NM, McLain LW Jr: A direct hepatotoxic effect of valproic acid. JAMA 242:1173–1177, 1979.

109. Ernst E, Matrai A: Diltiazem alters blood rheology. Pharmatherapeutica 5:213–216, 1988.

110. De Cree J, et al: The rheological effects of cinnarizine and flunarizine in normal and pathologic conditions. Angiology 30:505–515, 1979.

111. Forconi S, et al: Effect of treatment with the calcium-entry blocker nimodipine on cerebral blood flow (spect) and blood viscosity of patients affected by cerebral chronic vascular insufficiency. Clin Hemorheol 11:787, 1991.

112. Nagakawa Y, et al: Effect of idebenone on hemorheologic variables in geriatric patients with cerebral infarction. Clin Hemorheol 11:351, 1991.

113. Mori Y, et al: Hypercoagulable state in the Watanabe heritable hyperlipidemic rabbit, an animal model for the progression of atherosclerosis. Thromb Haemost 61:140–143, 1989.

114. Li A, Sahm U, Artmann GM: Dihydroergocryptine maintains erythrocyte fluidity in acidotic and hyperosmolar buffer solutions modelling hypoxic and ischemic microcirculation. Clin Hemorheol 15:133–146, 1995.

115. Almer LO, Kjellstrom T: The fibrinolytic system and coagulation during bezafibrate treatment of hypertriglyceridemia. Atherosclerosis 61:81–85, 1986.

116. Specht-Leible N, et al: Fibrinogen and bezafibrate: A pilot study in patients following percutaneous transluminal coronary angioplasty (PTCA). Clin Hemorheol 13:679–685, 1993.

117. Beigel Y, et al: Lovastatin therapy in heterozygous familial hypercholesterolaemic patients: Effect on blood rheology and fibrinogen levels. J Intern Med 230:23–27, 1991.

118. Koenig W, et al: The effects of lovastatin on blood rheology. Clin Hemorheol 11:785, 1991.

119. Jay RH, Rampling MW, Betteridge, DJ: Abnormalities of blood rheology in familial hypercholesterolaemia: Effects of treatment. Atherosclerosis 85:249–256, 1990.

120. Arntz HR, et al: Influence of pravastatin on blood rheology in type II hypercholesterolemia. Clin Hemorheol 11:785, 1991.

121. Zhao C, et al: The hemorheological study of ligustrazine treatment in diabetic subjects. Clin Hemorheol 9:615, 1989.

122. Sirs JA, Boroda C: Variations of blood rheology in diabetic patients on nicofuranose. Clin Hemorheol 11:191, 1991.

123. Ledevehat C, Vimeux M, Bondoux G: Hemorheological effects of oral troxerutin treatment versus placebo in venous insufficiency of the lower limbs. Clin Hemorheol 9:543, 1989.

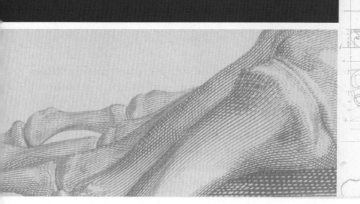

ATHEROSCLEROSIS AND THROMBOSIS IN DIABETES MELLITUS: NEW ASPECTS OF PATHOGENESIS

JOHN A. COLWELL, TIMOTHY J. LYONS, RICHARD L. KLEIN, ■

MARIA F. LOPES-VIRELLA, AND RUDOLF J. JOKL

The development of atherosclerosis is accelerated in diabetes mellitus, leading to increased morbidity and mortality and excessive health care costs. Virtually all of the large vessels are involved in this process, and clinical manifestations may be apparent as a result of atherosclerotic narrowing and/or thrombosis of coronary, cerebral, renal, and leg vessels.

These factors have led to a renewed interest in factors present in the diabetic state that might help to explain the acceleration of this process. Work in diabetes has been facilitated by new concepts about the pathophysiology of the process of atherosclerosis in the nondiabetic state.

Review articles and our chapters in previous editions of this text[1] have considered atherosclerosis in depth and should be consulted for older references.[1–3] This chapter provides updated information about the factors associated with the diabetic state that may underlie accelerated atherosclerosis and thrombosis and suggests a pathogenetic scheme that builds on knowledge of these processes in the nondiabetic state. The emphasis is on changes in the endothelium, on qualitative and quantitative changes in lipids and lipoproteins, on glycation and glyco-oxidation, and on altered platelet function, coagulation, and fibrinolysis in diabetes mellitus.

Historical Perspective

Clinicians have long recognized that peripheral vascular disease is an extremely serious medical complication. Advanced calcification of the aorta was found in a mummy from ancient Egyptian times (approximately 1290 to 1223 B.C.[4]). It is reported that in 400 B.C., Hippocrates "cut away the mortified parts," presumably in patients with gangrene after trauma or vascular occlusion. The first evidence of an amputation was a picture in the *Field Book of Wound Surgery* in 1517, showing the technique of Hans von Gersdortt. It was clear by the 17th century that amputations were indicated not only after traumatic injury, but also for foot ulcers and abscesses. In the mid-1800s, Syme performed his celebrated amputation at the ankle joint, ether anesthesia was introduced, and an association of diabetes with gangrene was described by Marchal. By 1891, Heidenhain had published a thorough review of diabetes and arteriosclerosis of the legs and had recommended levels for amputation if gangrene was found.[5,6]

Autopsy studies prior to 1930 in diabetic patients showed that 29% of them had gangrene at the time of death, and data from the Joslin Clinic between 1923 and

1969 indicated that amputations accounted for 22% to 40% of major surgical operations in their diabetic patients.[7] In Bell's classic autopsy study of 2130 diabetic individuals who had died from 1911 through 1955, gangrene was found in 21% and was 53 to 71 times more common than in nondiabetic individuals.[8]

As time has progressed, diagnostic techniques have improved. Cross-sectional studies have indicated that about 15% to 30% of a heterogeneous group of type 2 diabetes mellitus patients may have evidence of peripheral vascular disease when studied by noninvasive techniques.[2,9–12] The disease appears to progress as a function of age, duration of diabetes, or both when extrapolation from cross-sectional data is done. Longitudinal data are limited but suggest that the rate of progression may be about 2.5% per year in newly diagnosed white, type 2 subjects in the United States, whereas it may reach 5% to 7% per year in type 2 diabetic populations who are followed up after the disease is present.[13] In any case, longitudinal studies agree that macrovascular complications involving both the leg and coronary vessels progress with increasing duration of diabetes.

Risk Factors for Peripheral Vascular Disease in Diabetes

Studies of risk factors provide insight into the pathogenesis of peripheral vascular atherosclerosis in diabetes and are reviewed elsewhere in this volume (see Chapter _). In addition to the influences of age and duration of diabetes, several studies have indicated that hypertension and cigarette smoking, two classic risk factors for cardiovascular disease, are also predictive of peripheral vascular disease.[2] These correlations have been seen in populations as geographically diverse as those of Rochester, Minnesota;[14] Seattle, Washington,[9] Munich, Germany;[11] Kuopio, Finland;[15] and Framingham, Massachusetts.[16] Hyperglycemia does not appear to be an independent risk factor for peripheral vascular disease. Indeed, in some populations, such as that of Japan, peripheral vascular disease is rarely seen in type 2 diabetes, despite long-standing hyperglycemia.[2] Studies in the United States and Germany have not established that either fasting glucose or glycosylated hemoglobin (HbA_{1c}) values are good predictors of progression of peripheral vascular disease in type 2 diabetes.[9,11]

Altered lipid and lipoprotein profiles are frequently seen in type 2 diabetic subjects, with or without peripheral vascular disease. Several large-scale studies indicate that certain lipid-lipoprotein changes might be important risk factors for peripheral vascular disease in diabetes mellitus. In a cross-sectional study of 252 individuals with type 2 diabetes, elevated plasma triglyceride levels and decreased high-density lipoprotein (HDL) cholesterol levels emerged as possible risk factors for peripheral vascular disease.[9] In a 5-year prospective study in Finland,

claudication was associated with increased plasma cholesterol, very low-density lipoprotein (VLDL) cholesterol, decreased HDL cholesterol,[17] and increased VLDL triglyceride and low-density lipoprotein (LDL) triglyceride levels.[15] Multivariate analysis revealed that high LDL triglyceride and VLDL cholesterol levels had independent associations with claudication. On the other hand, negative correlations with lipids and either prevalence or incidence of peripheral vascular disease has been reported in some studies.[14]

Hyperinsulinemia has been implicated as an independent vascular risk factor in many epidemiologic studies.[18–21] Generally, prospective studies have used ischemic heart disease and vascular deaths, rather than peripheral vascular disease, as the vascular end points of interest. In one large cross-sectional study, the greatest risk for coronary heart disease and peripheral vascular disease was seen in diabetic and nondiabetic subjects with the highest plasma C peptide levels.[22] Thus, although data in diabetic subjects with peripheral vascular disease are limited, it is possible that endogenous hyperinsulinemia might interact with other risk factors to accelerate macrovascular disease. There are many reviews of this issue, which should be consulted for details.[23–25]

Thus, there are mixed messages from epidemiologic studies of peripheral vascular disease in diabetes. It is likely that this state of affairs is caused by confounding factors, including (1) end points such as claudication and amputation, which are late-stage events; (2) the likelihood that pathogenesis differs in type 1 diabetes, impaired glucose tolerance, and type 2 diabetes; (3) the probability that multiple risk factors such as hyperglycemia, lipid disturbances, hypertension, and cigarette smoking interact; and (4) the frequent association of diabetic neuropathy with vascular insufficiency in many patients with diabetes. Nevertheless, epidemiologic data suggest that an atherogenic mix of lipids and lipoproteins may, in particular, contribute to peripheral vascular disease and that hypertension, smoking, and perhaps hyperglycemia may interact to accelerate the process. Such leads from epidemiologic studies have stimulated research on precise mechanisms that might be involved in the pathogenesis of atherosclerosis in diabetes mellitus.

Pathogenesis of Atherosclerosis

Research in the last two decades suggests that atherosclerosis is a chronic inflammatory process that can be converted into an acute clinical event by plaque rupture.[26] The earliest atherosclerotic lesion is the fatty streak that, although not clinically significant on its own, plays a significant role in the events that lead to plaque progression and rupture. Formation of fatty streaks is induced by the transport of lipoproteins across the endothelium and their retention in the vessel wall. Schwenke and colleagues[27] have shown that for any given plasma lipoprotein concentration, the degree of lipoprotein retention in the artery wall is more important than the rate of transport of the same lipoprotein into the artery wall. Frank and colleagues[28] demonstrated, using ultrastructural techniques, that LDL can be rapidly transported across an intact endothelium and becomes trapped by the extracellular matrix of the subendothelial space.[29] Once LDL is transported across the artery wall and binds to the extracellular matrix, lipid oxidation is initiated, since microenvironment conditions that exclude plasma-soluble antioxidants are established.[30] With oxidation of LDL, endothelial cells are stimulated to release potent chemoattractants, such as monocyte-chemoattractant protein 1, monocyte-colony stimulating factor,[31] and GRO,[32] and these chemoattractants promote the recruitment of monocytes into the subendothelial space. Recruitment of these cells, owing to their enormous oxidative capacity, leads to further oxidation of LDL. The more heavily modified LDL is cytotoxic to endothelial and smooth muscle cells,[33,34] and it is no longer recognized by the LDL receptor. It is taken up by macrophage scavenger receptors, leading to massive accumulation of cholesterol in macrophages and to their transformation into foam cells, the hallmark of the atherosclerotic process.[35,36] Besides promoting the transformation of macrophages into foam cells, oxidized LDL is a potent inducer of inflammatory molecules and stimulates the immune system, leading to the formation of antibodies and, as a consequence, to the formation of immune complexes. These complexes may play a crucial role not only

in foam cell formation, but also in macrophage activation and thus in the rupture of atheromatous plaques, as described later in this chapter. Figure 5-1 illustrates some of these concepts.

Diabetes accelerates the sequence of events described above in many ways. Both LDL transport through the endothelium and retention in the subendothelial space are enhanced in diabetes. The rate of transport depends not only on the plasma concentration of LDL, but also on its size as well as on the permeability of the endothelium. Small, dense LDL particles permeate more efficiently through the endothelium owing to their size. Dense LDL levels are increased in both type 1 and type 2 diabetes, mostly when the patients are in poor glycemic control.[37,38] Furthermore, increased LDL transport rate due to increased permeability of the endothelium is also observed in diabetes, since increased vascular permeability is one of the earliest abnormalities that occurs in vessels exposed to high glucose concentrations.[39] Besides increased rate of transport, the degree of retention of LDL by the matrix is also markedly increased in diabetes. It has been shown that collagen-linked advanced glycation end-products (AGEs), which are increased in diabetes, can act as reactive "foci" to covalently trap circulating serum proteins, including LDL, leading to its increased retention in the subendothelium.[40,41] AGE products are derived from oxidation of Amadori products, a stable product that results from the nonenzymatic reaction of glucose with primary amino acids. The amount of glycated adducts on amino acids varies directly with the ambient glucose concentration

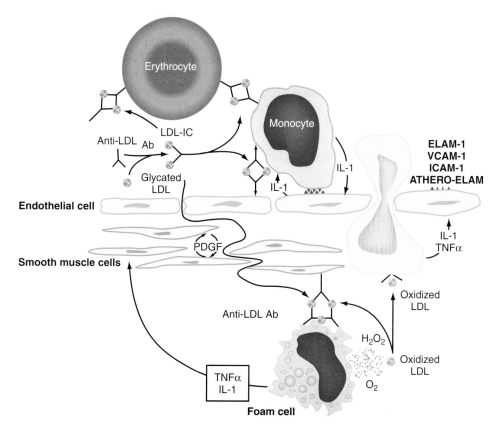

Figure 5–1 New concepts about the pathogenesis of atherosclerosis, with emphasis on the roles of monocyte-derived macrophages, cytokines, immune complexes, glycation and oxidation of LDL, and endothelial adhesion proteins.

and therefore is increased in diabetes mostly in patients with poor glycemic control. Furthermore, AGE-LDL, like heavily oxidized LDL, is cytotoxic, and it is a powerful chemoattractant for monocytes/macrophages, thus inducing monocyte recruitment from the circulation across normal endothelium.[42]

AGE-LDL and oxidized LDL may also induce endothelial dysfunction. On occupancy of macrophage receptors, AGE-LDL induces the release of tumor necrosis factor (TNF), interleukin-1 (IL-1), platelet-derived growth factor (PDGF), and immunoglobulin growth factor 1.[43,44] These mediators, in turn, promote the expression of adhesion molecules and the recruitment of nearby connective tissue cells, inducing their proliferation and activating them to produce extracellular matrix components. AGEs will also lead to the downregulation of the surface anticoagulant thrombomodulin and to the increase of procoagulant tissue factor.[42] AGEs were also found to chemically inactivate nitric oxide (NO) or endothelium-derived relaxing factor.[45]

Infusion of AGE products in rabbits has also been shown to induce a variety of vascular changes. In endothelial cells, these included increased expression of vascular cell adhesion molecule-1 (VCAM-1) and intercellular adhesion molecule-1 (ICAM-1), mainly in areas affected by atheroma.[46] Further supporting the significance of these interactions, it has been shown that blockade of receptor for AGE products (RAGE) can inhibit AGE product–induced impairment of endothelial barrier function and consequent hyperpermeability. Inhibition of AGE product formation by using antioxidants has a similar effect.

Modified lipoproteins may also induce endothelial dysfunction indirectly by triggering an immune response that leads to auto-antibody formation. Immune complexes (ICs) formed by association of the modified lipoproteins with the respective antibodies are able to stimulate macrophages and release large amounts of TNFα and IL1β as well as of oxygen active radicals.[47,48] The release of these cytokines leads to increased expression of adhesion molecules,[49,50] a hallmark of endothelial dysfunction. Levels of TNFα and IL1β released as well as the respiratory burst are considerably higher than those induced by other immune complexes or by free modified lipoproteins. Time course studies of cytokine release and mRNA expression in macrophages exposed to modified LDL immune complexes suggest that the synthesis and release of TNFα and IL1β is under independent control.[48] TNFα was released almost immediately after addition of LDL-IC to the macrophages, coinciding with early expression of TNFα mRNA, detectable 30 minutes after stimulation. In contrast, IL-1β was detected in only macrophage supernatants 8 hours after exposure to LDL-IC, and the onset of expression of IL-1β mRNA was also delayed in comparison to that of TNFα mRNA. Wide variations in the amounts of TNFα released by monocyte-derived macrophages from different donors was observed, sug-

gesting that the genetic background plays an important role in these cell mediated responses.

The release of cytokines by activated macrophages can contribute to atherogenesis and endothelial dysfunction by a variety of mechanisms other than increased expression of adhesion molecules.[49–51] IL-1 has been reported to stimulate the synthesis and cell surface expression of procoagulant activity and platelet activating factor by endothelial cells.[52,53] This can result in enhanced interactions with granulocytes, increased vascular permeability,[54] induction of IL-1 release from endothelial cells by a positive feedback mechanism,[55] and induction of PDGF-AA, which can be indirectly responsible for fibroblast and smooth muscle cell proliferation through an autocrine growth regulating mechanism.[56] TNFα can induce cellular responses similar to those of IL-1, such as cell surface expression of procoagulant activity[57] and production of IL-1 by endothelial cells.[58]

In addition to IL-1 and TNFα, activated monocytes and macrophages have been shown to secrete other products, such as interferon-α (IFN-α), growth factors such as fibroblast growth factor and PDGF-BB,[59–61] transforming growth factor,[62] modulatory substances such as PGE$_2$,[63] proteases,[64] collagenases,[65] and oxygen radicals.[66] Several of these mediators have been shown to have effects that could be directly related to the development of atherosclerosis. PDGF-BB, released by monocytes/macrophages, besides playing a role in stimulating smooth muscle cell proliferation, can also increase endocytosis, cholesterol synthesis, and LDL receptor expression in mononuclear cells. Transforming growth factor-β stimulates matrix production by smooth muscle cells. Besides cytokines and growth factors, activated macrophages overexpress CD40, an important modulator of the inflammatory response in the vessel wall, on interaction with CD40 ligand. It is well known that in acute coronary syndromes, the levels of CD40 ligand are elevated, and recently, increased levels of CD40 ligand were found in a group of 39 patients with diabetes and angiographically documented coronary artery disease.[67] Treatment with rosiglitazone but not with placebo was able to significantly decrease the levels of CD40 ligand in the same patients.[67]

Another consequence of the activation of macrophage by immune complexes containing modified forms of LDL is perturbation of cell cholesterol homeostasis that leads to the transformation of macrophages into foam cells. Foam cell formation is a key event in atherosclerosis. In vitro, both insoluble and soluble (red blood cell adsorbed) LDL-IC prepared with rabbit apoB antibodies induce profound alterations in lipoprotein metabolism and in the cholesterol homeostasis of monocyte-derived macrophages.[68,69] These observations were recently reproduced by using LDL-IC prepared with human copper-oxidized LDL and purified human oxLDL antibodies.[47] The increased accumulation of cholesterol esters (CE) in human macrophages exposed to LDL-IC is secondary to an increased uptake of the LDL complexed with antibody, followed by altered intracellular metabolism of the particle.[70] In the initial stages, the intracellular accumulation of CE reflects the accumulation of intact LDL; in later stages, the cell accumulates cholesteryl esters generated by de novo esterification of the free cholesterol released during lysosomal hydrolysis of LDL, and a foam cell is formed. LDL-IC taken up by macrophages as a consequence of their interaction with the FcγI receptor.[71] Surprisingly, while inducing foam cell formation, the LDL-IC also stimulate a considerable increase (approximately 20-fold) in LDL receptor activity.[69,72] The increase in LDL receptor activity seems to be specifically induced by LDL-IC and not by other types of immune complexes.[69,70]

The role of immune complexes in the development of arteriosclerosis in humans has been studied mainly by measuring antibodies against oxidized LDL. Antibodies to oxidized LDL have been described to occur naturally in humans[73] and to be detectable in a higher proportion of patients with advanced atherosclerosis, mostly in those with inflammatory reaction to the atherosclerotic plaques.

The levels of oxLDL antibodies have been repeatedly reported to correlate with different end points that are considered evidence of atherosclerotic vascular disease, progression of carotid atherosclerosis, or risk for the future development of myocardial infarction.[74–79] According to Maggi and colleagues, a significantly higher level of oxidized LDL antibodies is measured in patients with carotid atherosclerosis compared to normal controls, and the highest levels were found in patients with associated hyperlipidemia and hypertension.[75] Salonen and colleagues[76] reported a direct relationship between the titer of autoantibodies to MDA-LDL and the rate of progression of carotid atherosclerosis. Lehtimaki and colleagues reported higher levels of oxidized LDL antibodies in patients with angiographically verified coronary disease.[77] According to Erkkilä and colleagues, oxLDL antibody levels were significantly elevated in men with myocardial infarction.[78] In type 2 diabetic patients, Bellomo and colleagues found higher levels of oxLDL and MDA-LDL antibodies compared to healthy controls.[79] Antibodies against 2-furoyl-4(5)-(2-furanyl)-1H-imidazole, a specific model compound of AGE, and to AGE-modified proteins have been detected in the sera of diabetic and euglycemic subjects,[80,81] but the levels of AGE-LDL antibodies were lower in diabetics than in controls in one of the studies.[81] It must be noted that several other studies have yielded contradictory data, showing either no correlation between modified LDL antibodies and end points of atherosclerotic disease or even inverse correlations.[82–90]

The inverse correlations between modified LDL antibody levels and atherosclerosis, together with data obtained in laboratory animals suggesting that modified LDL antibodies are predominantly of the noninflammatory IgM isotype[91] and human studies claiming that IgM antibodies to modified LDL might predominate over IgG antibodies[92] and have a protective effect in relation to the development of atherosclerosis,[93] have led to considerable speculation, including the possibility of "vaccination" against atherosclerosis.[94] This seems highly unwarranted, because of several other lines of evidence. First, the proposed protective murine IgM antibodies are predominantly reactive with oxidized phospholipids, while human antibodies reacting with modified lysine groups have been extensively characterized.[95,96] Second, when the isotype distribution of modified LDL antibodies has been studied under stringent conditions, using affinity chromatography-purified antibodies, the predominant isotypes are IgG1 and IgG3, followed by IgM.[95,96] Given the TH2 dependency and proinflammatory characteristics of these two IgG subclasses of antibodies,[97] the postulated protective role of antimodified LDL antibodies becomes untenable. The balance between IgG and IgM LDL antibodies may have some pathogenic relevance, however, as is suggested by recent reports showing that common carotid and femoral intima-media thickness are directly related to the levels of IgG oxLDL antibodies and inversely related to the levels of IgM oxLDL antibodies.[98] Also of interest is the fact that the levels of IgG oxLDL and MDA-LDL antibodies are associated with the metabolic syndrome and smoking.[99]

A clearer perspective about the pathogenic role of modified LDL antibodies seems to emerge when the levels of circulating antigen-antibody complexes (immune complexes, IC) containing modified forms of LDL (LDL-IC) are measured.[89,100–103] LDL-IC levels have been reported to be increased in patients with coronary artery disease[103] and in diabetic patients who have nephropathy[103] or who develop coronary artery disease over an 8-year period.[89] The composition of IC isolated from the sera of diabetic patients by precipitation with polyethlylene-glycol has demonstrated a significant enrichment in carboxymethyl lysine and MDA-lysine,[96] suggesting that oxLDL and AGE-LDL are involved in IC formation. This is supported by the detection in the IC of significantly elevated concentrations of oxLDL and AGE-LDL IgG antibodies of higher affinity than those that remain free in the supernatant.[96,100,103]

The advantages and disadvantages of the measurement of LDL-IC versus the measurement of serum modified LDL antibodies have been recently summarized,[100] but it needs to be stressed that there is ample evidence showing that LDL-IC are proinflammatory, thus supporting the measurement of LDL-IC as more directly related to the pathogenic potential of LDL antibodies than the measurement of free circulating antibodies. The evidence supporting the proinflammatory characteristics of LDL-IC has been obtained in in vitro studies using both rabbit apo B antibodies and purified human oxLDL antibodies to prepare ox-LDL-IC. Using LDL-IC prepared with rabbit antibodies, we demonstrated their ability to induce of foam cell formation.[68,69] The transformation of human monocyte-derived macrophages into foam cells can be induced either by insoluble LDL-IC presented to the macrophages as large aggregates or by LDL-IC adsorbed to red blood cells. Both types of LDL-IC may be formed in vivo. Subendothelial LDL deposits are likely to include LDL-IC formed in situ, and these are probably large insoluble aggregates. Soluble LDL-IC present in the circulation are likely to be adsorbed to red blood cells via C3b receptors and other nonspecific interactions. Once absorbed to red blood cells, LDL-IC are transported to organs that are rich in tissue macrophages where the LDL-IC can be transferred to phagocytic cells expressing Fc receptors.[47,97]

Besides contributing to foam cell formation and progression of atherosclerotic plaques, IC containing modified LDL are very likely involved in plaque rupture. In recent years, angiographic studies on patients with acute myocardial infarction led to the surprising finding that frequently, the atherosclerotic lesion that gave rise to the occlusive thrombus did not have high-grade stenosis.[104–106] These studies led to the concept that the composition of atherosclerotic plaques is more important than their size in triggering plaque rupture and acute vascular events.

The thickness and collagen content of the fibrous cap as well as the size of the lipid core are the most important elements in determining plaque vulnerability. Vulnerable plaques that are prone to rupture have a thin fibrous cap, owing to a marked decrease in collagen content, and their lipid core usually occupies more than 40% of the plaque area. Thus, mechanisms that contribute to decrease the collagen content of plaques have been the focus of considerable attention in recent years.

Collagens are synthesized and assembled by vascular smooth muscle cells and degraded by collagenases. Thus, both decreased production of collagen by smooth muscle cells, as well as enhanced degradation of collagen by collagenases, can contribute to plaque vulnerability.[107] It has been shown that the expression of collagens in smooth muscle cells is regulated by cytokines and growth factors.[108] Transforming growth factor-β and PDGF stimulate the synthesis of collagen types I and III, whereas IFN-γ markedly decreases collagen biosynthesis.[108] Studies examining the pathology of atherosclerotic lesions and studies with cell culture systems indicated that IFN-γ, which is released by activated T cells, inhibits smooth muscle cell proliferation and collagen expression in smooth muscle cells.[109,110] IFN-γ also promotes apoptosis of smooth muscle cells.[111] These findings provided important evidence for understanding the relative paucity of smooth muscle cells in vulnerable regions of atherosclerotic plaques. Decreased synthesis of collagen is not, however, the only mechanism leading to the decreased collagen content in vulnerable atherosclerotic plaques. As was mentioned before, increased degradation of collagen by collagenases is also an important factor. Most of the collagen (50% to 75%) in a normal artery is type I collagen.[112,113] Interstitial collagenase, or metalloproteinase (MMP-1), is an important proteinase specialized in the initial cleavage of collagens, mainly type I. Other metalloproteinases, such as MMP-2 and MMP-9, catalyze further the breakdown of collagen fragments or activate MMP-3 and MMP-10 and other members of the MMP family, promoting the degradation of a broad spectrum of matrix constituents, such as proteoglycans and elastin. MMP activity is also regulated by tissue inhibitors of MMP.[114] MMP-1 has been found in vulnerable regions of atherosclerotic plaques, suggesting that this collagenase plays a role in plaque destabilization.[115] We have recently shown that oxidized LDL and oxLDL-IC stimulate the expression of MMP-1 in human vascular endothelial cells at a transcriptional level. That increased expression is associated with a marked increase in collagenase activity.[116–118]

A few studies have investigated MMP levels and activities in diabetes. Serum levels of MMP-2, MMP-8, and MMP-9 are increased in patients with type 2 diabetes,[119] and MMP-9 levels and activity are increased in aortas from streptozotocin-diabetic rats compared to controls.[120] Another group of proteases, the cathepsins, may also be involved in causing plaque rupture. The cathepsins are cysteine proteinases that degrade elastin and fibrillar collagen. Cathepsins K, L, and S all have potent elastolytic activity. Cathepsin S is the most potent elastase known,[121] whereas cathepsin K cleaves collagen I and III.[122] The cathepsins were originally thought to function only in acidic lysosomes, but recent research shows that they can be released by macrophages.[123] Macrophages in human lesions contain abundant immunoreactive cathepsin K and S,[124] and atherosclerotic lesions from apoE-deficient mice express cathepsins B, D, L, and S.[125] Cathepsin B has even been suggested as a biomarker of vulnerable plaques.[126] Expression levels of cathepsins C and D are upregulated in aneurysms,[127] which also contain lower levels of the endogenous cysteine protease inhibitor cystatin C.[128] Furthermore, human smooth muscle cells (SMCs) in culture can be stimulated to secrete active cathepsin S by IL-1β or IFN-γ.[124] Together, these findings suggest that the cathepsins might be involved in causing plaque rupture or aneurysms. So far, the presence of cathepsins and cystatin C in lesions from patients with diabetes has not been studied.

Another possible mechanism of plaque rupture is increased cell death. Contrary to what was conventionally accepted, it has recently been shown that "apoptotic" cells can release cytokines and that, following apoptosis, an inflammatory response in the arterial wall induced by the overexpression of Fas-associating death domain protein, one of the signaling molecules in the apoptotic pathway may occur.[129] Furthermore, apoptotic cells have a potent procoagulant activity due to the redistribution of phosphatidylserine on the cell surface during apoptosis, which leads to increased tissue factor activity, a key element in the initiation of coagulation. During cell apoptosis, shedding to the lipid core of membrane apoptotic microparticles that are rich in PS, which carry almost all tissue factor activity, is responsible for the procoagulant activity of the plaque.[130] Luminal endothelial cell apoptosis is also likely responsible for thrombus formation on eroded plaques without rupture. The increased expression of tissue factor is not limited to the plaque, however, but it is also found in circulating monocytes in patients with acute coronary syndromes.[131] Whether or not diabetes enhances the expression of tissue factor in circulating monocytes or in plaques is not known.

Endothelium

Vascular endothelial cells participate in a number of important homeostatic and cellular functions such as the coagulation of blood, the activity of leukocytes, platelet reactivity, capillary permeability, and regulation of vascular smooth muscle tone. The tonic regulation of vascular smooth muscle cells might be influenced by the endothelium through the release of potent vasorelaxing agents such as endothelium-derived relaxing factor and prostacyclin (PGI_2) and vasoconstrictors, including thromboxane and endothelin.

Endothelium-Derived Relaxing Factor

The potent vasorelaxation action of endothelium-derived relaxing factor was first demonstrated by Furchgott and Zawadzki[132] and was later determined to be the free radical species NO.[133,134] Nitric oxide is synthesized by endothelial cells from the terminal guanidine nitrogen terminal of the amino acid L-arginine by the endothelium isoform of NO synthase (eNOS).[135,136] The demonstration that NO is the mediator of endothelium-derived relaxing factor has stimulated new investigations into abnormal vascular physiology.

Vascular complications are the leading cause of increased mortality in patients with diabetes mellitus. Endothelial dysfunction, characterized by impaired endothelium-dependent vasoreactivity, is the first sign of blood vessel damage that precedes morphologic changes of the vessel wall.[137,138] Reduced bioavailability of NO contributes to the changes in vascular tone and is considered to be one of the central features common to vascular disease.

There are numerous factors that may influence either the production of NO or the diffusion of NO to its cellular targets. When LDL isolated from healthy subjects, from diabetic subjects, or modified by oxidation were incubated with cultured endothelial cells, NO release into the medium was significantly reduced.[139] Chylomicron remnants have a negative effect on NO,[140] while VLDL[141] and HDL[142,143] enhance NO biosynthesis. These in vitro studies are supported by the observation that HDL restores endothelial function in hypercholesterolemic

men.[144] Lipoprotein effects on NO release in vivo may differ however, as intense LDL-cholesterol-lowering therapy with HMG-CoA reductase inhibitors did not improve NO-dependent endothelial function.[145] NO production might be influenced by the availability of substrate for eNOS. The K_M of eNOS for substrate L-arginine is approximately 2.9 μM, while the cytoplasmic levels of arginine are 600 to 900 μM, suggesting that L-arginine concentration should not be rate limiting for eNOS activity. Regardless, L-arginine ameliorated the LDL-induced downregulation of eNOS activity in endothelial cells.[139] Similarly, infusion of L-arginine in both type 2 diabetic patients and healthy subjects increased NO availability.[146] The supplementation of L-arginine might be effective because analysis of the kinetics of the conversion of arginine to NO in type 2 diabetic patients appears to be altered in comparison to nondiabetic subjects.[147] Folic acid administration might also stimulate NO availability. The active form of folic acid, 5-methyltetrahydrofolate, restores the function of uncoupled eNOS, although the exact mechanism is not known. Acute administration of folate to patients with type 2 diabetes improved NO-dependent vasodilation.[148] The results of these two investigations of effects of dietary supplements on NO function provide a rationale for initiation of studies to determine whether these supplements influence future cardiovascular events in diabetic patients.

There is substantial evidence that acute hyperglycemia attenuates endothelium-dependent vasodilatation,[149,150] and the variable degree of hyperglycemia at the time of measurement in different studies might affect endothelium-dependent vascular responses in patients. Studies of intact coronary arteries that were conducted ex vivo demonstrated that acute elevation of glucose concentration increases NO release by enhancing eNOS activity through increased intracellular sodium concentrations via sodium/glucose cotransporter-1.[151] But hyperglycemia also might influence the transport of NO to its cellular targets and thus affect its bioavailability. The main pathways for NO metabolism to enable its transport from regions of high production downstream to the microcirculation are (1) oxidation of oxyhemoglobin to form methemoglobin and nitrate ion, (2) combination with deoxyhemoglobin to form nitrosyl hemoglobin, and (3) nitrosylation of thiol groups on hemoglobin and other proteins to form S-nitrosothiols.[135] In diabetes, increased levels of superoxide radicals also may be present that quickly combine with NO to produce damaging peroxynitrite. The hyperglycemia of diabetes accelerates the glycation of plasma proteins, including hemoglobin, which might change its affinity toward NO. The binding of NO to hemoglobin was studied across a range of glycation levels in vitro (HbA_{1c} 5.9% to 9.8%) and in type 1 diabetic patients and healthy subjects.[152] Nitrosyl hemoglobin levels were increased in diabetic patients and the increase in nitrosyl hemoglobin was correlated positively with HbA_{1c} level in studies that were conducted both in vitro and in vivo. Subsequent studies by other investigators concluded also that NO is bound by red blood cell hemoglobin but that binding is proportional to S-nitrosohemoglobin content, not nitrosyl hemoglobin content.[153] Fueling the debate, a third mechanism of NO inactivation that invokes the reaction of nitrite with the heme group of deoxyhemoglobin has also been proposed.[154] Thus, while the mechanisms might differ, these studies conclude that the bioavailability of NO in diabetic patients might be influenced by the level of glycemic control through its inactivation by complexing with glycated hemoglobin or other plasma proteins. The disparities in the roles of NO metabolites that have been reported may result primarily from the methods of detection or assay that were employed,[155] and this has elicited a call for reform and unity in methodology to more critically address the important questions surrounding NO metabolism. Clearly, the results of these studies raise questions and debate,[156] and more research is required in this critical area.

Endothelial cell eNOS requires not only arginine as a substrate, but also several cofactors, including NADPH, calcium, and tetrahydrobiopterin [$(6R)$-5,6,7,8-tetrahydro-L-biopterin] (BH_4) for normal activity. BH_4 seems to modulate eNOS activity. In the absence of sufficient BH_4, eNOS changes its functional profile and, instead of oxidizing L-arginine, the enzyme reduces molecular oxygen to superoxide anion. Superoxide radicals quickly combine with NO to produce damaging peroxynitrite.[157] In patients with type 2 diabetes, BH_4 administration improved endothelium-dependent vasodilation by increasing NO activity.[158] Similar effects on endothelium-dependent vasodilation were obtained when the precursor to BH_4, sepiapterin, was utilized.[159] These data suggest collectively that endothelial dysfunction in diabetes might also result from an absolute or relative deficit in the availability of the eNOS cofactor BH_4.[160]

The above review of the literature suggests a strong association between diabetes and NO metabolism. Recently, there has been intensive investigation of the impact of diabetes complications on NO levels.[161,162] Basal NO levels are increased in type 2 diabetes patients and are significantly increased in patients with proliferative retinopathy compared to those with nonproliferative or no retinopathy.[163] This might result in part because elevated glucose levels increase NO production in retinal endothelial cells,[164,165] but the metabolic fate of the NO is unknown. A considerable body of evidence indicates that microalbuminuria is strictly associated with a generalized vascular dysfunction.[161,162] In this regard, serum nitrate and nitrite levels and index of NO production were significantly elevated in type 1 diabetic patients with microalbuminuria compared to patients without or to healthy control subjects.[166] Serum nitrate and nitrite levels also were independently associated with both albumin excretion rate and glomerular filtration rate,

suggesting a link between NO and glomerular filtration. When nitrate and nitrite levels were determined in urine from patients with type 2 diabetes and from healthy controls,[167] levels were higher in both microalbuminuric and normoalbuminuric patients than in controls and were positively associated with glomerular filtration rate. In agreement with observed increases in nitrate and nitrite levels in urine, immunohistochemical stain intensities for eNOS also were significantly increased in glomerular endothelial cells of microalbuminuric patients compared with control subjects.[168]

Obesity is becoming more prevalent in the developed world because of the abundance of food and the decrease in physical activity. Obesity is a risk factor for cardiovascular disease. The precise mechanism by which obesity promotes cardiovascular disease is not known but might result from the insulin resistance syndrome, which frequently accompanies the overweight state. Obesity, and especially the insulin resistance syndrome, may involve impaired endothelial function.[169] There is ample evidence that NO concentrations are increased in spontaneously hypertensive rats;[170] furthermore, these animals are insulin resistant. It was suggested that this NO response might represent an adaptive effort to combat the hypertensive state by stimulating vasodilation. Alternatively, it might also represent one of the myriad responses to insulin resistance. One early study in hypertensive patients determined that the ability of insulin-resistant patients with hypertension to avoid a significant salt-induced increase in blood pressure was dependent on their ability to increase NO secretion.[171] Type 2 diabetes is a well-recognized state of insulin resistance, and there is conflicting data suggesting that NO production is normal and/or increased in patients and/or animal models of the syndrome.[172,173] Plasma concentrations of NO were found to be increased in patients with type 2 diabetes but not in nondiabetic subjects with insulin resistance.[174] These results are in contrast to those found in an earlier investigation of nondiabetic, insulin-resistant subjects.[175] The reason for these contradictory results is not certain but might be related to differences in methodology used to quantitate NO and to determine the extent of insulin resistance. Clearly, more research is necessary to determine the role of NO in the insulin resistance syndrome.

Prostacyclin

PGI_2, another potent vasorelaxant, is produced by the two rate-limiting cyclooxygenases, COX-1 and COX-2, which form the prostaglandin endoperoxide, PGH_2. PGH_2 is transformed enzymatically into PGI_2 by PGI_2 synthase in blood vessels or into thromboxane A_2 by thromboxane A_2 synthase in platelets. In blood vessels, especially in the larger arteries, the predominant prostaglandin is PGI_2. As was extensively reviewed in our chapter in an earlier edition of this text,[1] PGI_2 production by the vasculature of diabetic patients is reduced. We also suggested previously that the decrease in PGI_2 production might result from the lack of a then-unidentified factor that had been described in plasma.[176] The existence, but unfortunately not the identity, of this factor is strongly supported by recent studies of transgenic mice that are devoid of both eNOS and COX-1.[177] This experimental strategy should exclude the enzymatic sources of NO and PGI_2. Nonetheless, these mice maintain a mechanism by which acetylcholine can hyperpolarize, relax, and vasodilate resistance blood vessels, suggesting that a substance other than NO or PGI_2 must be involved. This "third factor" that still provides local control of vascular homeostasis in the absence of NO and PGI_2 might be the controversial substance called endothelium-derived hyperpolarizing factor. The true identity of this factor, however, still remains a mystery. Details of the investigations of endothelium-derived hyperpolarizing factor are beyond the scope of this review but have been reviewed in depth elsewhere.[178–180] Endothelium-derived hyperpolarizing factor might, in fact, not be an enzymatically derived "factor" that can diffuse like NO or PGI_2 from endothelial cells. Rather, it might be a phenomenon that begins as a calcium-activated event that hyperpolarizes the endothelium and a signal that is transferred to the smooth muscle by potassium or via gap junctions. Only future research will resolve this mystery.

Reduced PGI_2 concentrations in diabetes might also result from decreased levels of prostacyclin-stimulating factor (PSF). As we reported in our chapter in the previous edition of this text,[181] PSF levels were significantly reduced in patients with type 2 diabetes and in coronary arteries from patients with ischemic heart disease. The mechanism by which PSF expression was reduced in the vascular wall with atherosclerosis was not evident. In the development of atherosclerosis, however, LDL modified by oxidation (oxLDL) is found in atherosclerotic lesions and is considered to play a major role in atherogenesis. Lysophosphatidylcholine (LysoPC) is a major constituent lipid of oxLDL and is present in atherosclerotic plaques. It has been associated with many of the atherogenic effects of oxLDL. Recent studies determined the effects of LysoPC on PSF expression in cultured vascular smooth muscle cells.[182] LysoPC, but not phosphatidylcholine or native LDL, reduced PSF expression in a dose dependent manner. Calphostin C, a protein kinase C inhibitor, restored the reduction of PSF expression by LysoPC, suggesting that LysoPC-induced reduction of PSF expression is mediated by PKC activation.

PGI_2 is quite active biologically, but it is chemically unstable, and its half-life in vivo is quite short. Recently, beraprost sodium, a stable analogue of PGI_2, was developed, and a flurry of investigations of its action and efficiency ensued, as we reported previously.[181] Recent studies in streptozotocin-induced diabetic rats demonstrated that oral administration of beraprost sodium restored endothelial dysfunction[183] and attenuated glomerular hyperfiltration.[184] The compound also improved blood flow in the limbs of type 2 diabetic patients.[185] A long-term (24-month) administration regimen of the analogue decreased albuminuria in 27 patients with type 2 diabetes.[186] The effects of beraprost on endothelial cell dysfunction, measured as VCAM-1 expression in cultured cells and plasma concentration in type 2 diabetes patients, were determined.[187] Beraprost significantly reduced VCAM-1 expression in cultured endothelial cells and repressed the binding of monocytes to these cells. Type 2 diabetic patients ($n = 11$) who had atherosclerotic change of carotid arteries were enrolled for an open, prospective study of the analogue. Patients receiving beraprost for three years exhibited significantly lower VCAM-1 concentrations than those who did not receive the compound. Most important, the increase in carotid artery intimal medial thickness was significantly less in patients who received the PGI_2 analogue than that in patients who did not, suggesting that beraprost might have beneficial effects on the progression of atherosclerosis in diabetic patients.

Thromboxane A_2

Maintenance of vascular tone and the luminal diameter of a blood vessel are dependent on the net balance of vasoconstrictor and vasodilator forces. The endothelium also contributes to the local regulation of the vasculature by releasing endothelium-derived contracting factors. Two major vasoconstrictor molecules that are released by the endothelium are thromboxane A_2 (TXA2) and endothelin. In our chapter in an earlier edition of this text, we detailed studies that concluded that plasma levels of TXA2 were significantly increased in diabetic patients.[176] In patients with diabetes, TXA2 is routinely considered to be derived both from hyperaggregable platelets and from the arterial wall. However, human monocytes also can synthesize TXA2 as the major cyclooxygenase metabolite of arachidonic acid.[188] Monocytes isolated from type 2 diabetic patients were found to secrete significantly more TXA2 than those isolated from control subjects.[189] Thus, the monocyte may also contribute to the pathogenesis of occlusive vascular disease in diabetes.

The thiazolidinedione class of drugs includes peroxisome-proliferator-activated receptor gamma activators and selective ligands. As a class, they are associated with multiple antidiabetic actions, including enhancing insulin sensitivity and improving hyperglycemia and hyperlipidemia. Prostaglandin J_2, a prostaglandin D_2 metabolite, is an endogenous ligand of peroxisome-proliferator-activated receptor gamma, and studies in diabetic rats concluded that troglitazone, a thiazolidinedione, increased prostaglandin I_2 and prostaglandin E_2 production.[190] Subsequent studies demonstrated that troglitazone also reduced TXA2 release from platelets.[191] The mechanism of the action and its subsequent impact on vascular disease progression remain to be determined.

Endothelin-1

Endothelin (ET) was first described in 1988,[192] and there has been a virtual explosion of research involving this potent vasoconstrictor during the ensuing years. ET and NO function in negative feedback loops for each other, each acting to limit the action of the other.[193] Therefore, ET might contribute to endothelial regulation both directly through its vasoconstrictor effects and indirectly through it inhibitory effects on NO production. Reports of ET levels in diabetic patients are inconsistent; levels that were found were increased, decreased, or similar in comparison to those in healthy subjects.[194] The endothelin system is complex, as three ET isoforms (ET-1, ET-2, and ET-3) are encoded by three distinct genes and are secreted as precursors to be processed subsequently by proteolytic enzymes. The endothelins regulate cellular metabolism via specific cell surface receptors (ET_A, ET_B, ET_C), of which only ET_A and ET_B are expressed by mammals. The ET_A receptors are localized primarily on vascular smooth muscle cells and regulate vasoconstriction, while ET_B receptors are expressed predominantly by vascular endothelial cells and are involved in vasodilation as activation of the receptor leads to NO release. Thus, vasoregulatory action of the endothelins in vivo could be the outcome of a number of factors, including type of receptor involved, number of receptors, and tissue involved.

Recently, a series of studies were conducted to determine whether impaired NO bioavailability in obesity and type 2 diabetes results from effects of ET on NO production.[195] Study participants included nondiabetic lean (body mass index < 26 kg/m^2 for men or < 28 kg/m^2 for women; $n = 20$) or obese ($n = 20$) control subjects and type 2 diabetic patients ($n = 14$). Vascular reactivity was measured as leg blood flow by using a catheter inserted into the femoral vein. The relative contribution of NO to resting vascular tone was determined by measuring leg blood flow before and after administration of L-NMMA (N^G-monomethyl-L-arginine), a competitive inhibitor on NOS. Leg blood flow was similar in the three groups and decreased equally after L-NMMA administration, suggesting that the relative contribution of NO to vascular tone was similar across the three groups. This is not unexpected because, as was stated above, the literature is clearly divided on the question of whether NO production is altered in obesity and type 2 diabetes. Studies were then conducted after blocking ET-1 action with BQ123, a high-affinity competitive inhibitor of ET-1 type A receptors. Maximal doses of BQ123 were used to provide near-maximal and equivalent reduction in blood vessel resistance across the three study groups so that the resulting increase in vein blood flow was similar between the groups. The NOS inhibitor L-NMMA was then added to the BQ123 infusion to study blood flow with both ET_A and NOS antagonism. This significantly reduced leg blood flow in all three groups, but blood flow, and therefore, most important, blood vessel resistance, increased significantly more in obese subjects. This suggests that obese individuals have an increased underlying capacity of the production of NO. In support of this hypothesis, chemically determined total NO flux was also stimulated in the obese group during infusion of BQ123; NO flux in the lean and type 2 diabetes groups was unaffected. A third series of control studies was undertaken with obese subjects by infusing phentolamine, an α-adrenergic receptor antagonist, to determine whether alterations in NO tone seen during infusion of BQ123 were a nonspecific response to vasodilation rather than a specific effect of ET receptor antagonism. Nonspecific vasodilation with phentolamine failed to induce venous resistance to blood flow, as did the ET-blocker, BQ123. Thus, augmentation of NO in obese individuals was confirmed. One possibility for augmented NO availability in obese subjects is increased production through ET-1 action on ET_B receptors, which have been shown to mediate ET-induced vasodilation in healthy individuals. The above-described studies did not block ET_B receptors; therefore, this hypothesis cannot be excluded. However, because this effect was not observed in lean control subjects, it is unlikely that the effect resulted from increased ET_B-mediated NO production. In summary, these studies suggest that in obesity, ET contributes to ET dysfunction through indirect effects on NO availability in addition to the previously demonstrated direct vasoconstrictor effects.

Considerable research has investigated associations between ET and diabetic complications.[194,196] However, the results of these studies are not in total agreement. This might result, in part, from differences in the diabetic populations studied. However, the type of assay, the difference between commercial assay kits used to quantitate endothelin, and variations between individual laboratories all may influence the determination of ET concentration. Until these inconsistencies are resolved, the relationship between diabetes and ET will remain uncertain.

Cell Adhesion Molecules

Endothelial cells elaborate leukocyte-specific adhesion molecules both constitutively and in response to cytokines and other mediators.[197] Cellular adhesion molecules mediate the attachment and transmigration of leukocytes across the endothelial surface and are hypothesized to play an important role in the initiation of atherosclerosis.[198] Binding of leukocytes to the endothelium requires the interaction of integrin on the surface of leukocytes with ICAM, VCAM, and the selectins on the endothelial cells. Soluble forms of these adhesion molecules are present in endothelial cell culture supernatants and human sera, and levels of soluble E-selectin,[199] VCAM,[200] and ICAM[199] correlate to their membrane-bound expression.

As we detailed previously,[181] levels of circulating adhesion molecules are generally increased in patients with type 1 or type 2 diabetes. Atherothrombosis is widely considered a chronic inflammatory disease and diabetes is an important risk factor for atherothrombosis. Levels of inflammatory markers are increased in type 1 diabetes, and this increase might result, in part, from hyperglycemia. However, it is not known what other factors determine the increased inflammatory activity in type 1 diabetes. The EURODIAB Prospective Complications Study, a large cohort of European patients with type 1 diabetes, recently investigated two determinants of inflammatory activity in this type 1 diabetes cohort. The first evaluated conventional risk factors for atherothrombosis, including glycemic control. They also measured endothelial dysfunction by determining plasma concentrations of soluble VCAM and E-selectin.[201] The markers of inflammatory activity (C-reactive protein, IL-6, and TNF-α) were associated with conventional risk factors, including gender, diabetes duration, level of glycemic control, body mass index, HDL cholesterol (inversely), triglycerides, and systolic blood pressure. This study also demonstrated that the plasma levels of the adhesion molecules, considered an index of endothelial dysfunction, were also strongly and independently associated with these inflammatory markers. This suggests that endothelial dysfunction plays an important role in the inflammatory activity associated with type 1 diabetes. One interpretation of these findings is that endothelial dysfunction causes increased inflammatory activity. However, because of the cross-sectional design of the study, the possibility that inflammation causes increased expression of adhesion molecules, and thus endothelial dysfunction, cannot be excluded. A recent longitudinal study in type 2 diabetic patients demonstrated that inflammation and endothelial dysfunction are mutually interrelated and progress with time without one clearly preceding the other.[202] This suggests that in diabetes, inflammation induces endothelial dysfunction and that endothelial dysfunction may increase inflammatory activity, thus creating a vicious circle. Regardless, these results suggest that treatment regimens in type 1 diabetes should not only aim to decrease inflammatory activity through treatment of conventional risk factors, but also strive to improve endothelial function.

Although the clinical consequences of atherothrombosis such as infarct or stroke usually occur in adults, the atherogenic process actually begins during childhood. Risk factors for atherosclerosis appear during childhood, and atherosclerosis is accelerated in children in whom multiple risk factors for the disease are present.[203] The concentrations of soluble forms of ICAM, VCAM, E-selectin, P-selectin, and L-selectin were determined in children and adolescents with attendant atherosclerosis risk factors (obesity, hypertension, and diabetes) and compared with levels in healthy controls.[204] Elevated plasma concentrations of ICAM, VCAM, and E-selectin were found in the group of children with attendant risk factors. Most important, the highest concentrations of these molecules appeared in obese children with coexisting hypertension. Thus, it appears that endothelial activation is associated with risk factors for atherosclerosis even in the early stages of development of the disease.

Plasma concentrations of adhesion molecules are elevated in patients with type 2 diabetes. The influence of glucose tolerance status (insulin resistance) on plasma concentration of adhesion molecules was determined in patients with coronary heart disease confirmed by coronary angiography.[205] Glucose tolerance status was determined after oral glucose tolerance testing. Glucose tolerance testing confirmed the presence of frank type 2 diabetes in 8 subjects and impaired glucose tolerance in 35 others. In agreement with previous studies, the concentrations of soluble adhesion molecules were significantly elevated in patients with type 2 diabetes compared to those with impaired glucose tolerance or normal glucose tolerance ($n = 35$). The concentration of VCAM increased significantly with the progression of altered glucose metabolism and was highest in type 2 diabetes patients, but no association was found with ICAM concentration. The concentration of E-selectin was significantly associated with both fasting and postchallenge glucose concentrations. These studies suggest that impaired glucose tolerance might also be associated with endothelial activation and thus contribute to atherogenesis in these patients.

The above review of the literature suggests that endothelial activation is associated with atherosclerosis development in diabetes and, most important, that this association might be influenced by glucose tolerance status. Numerous studies have investigated the associations between soluble adhesion molecules and hypertension, obesity, and dyslipidemia, all of which are features of insulin resistance syndrome. Discussion of this literature is beyond the scope of this chapter, but the reader is encouraged to consult a recent review for details.[206]

Glycoxidation/Lipoxidation of Vascular Structural Proteins

Glycation, glycoxidation, and lipoxidation of vascular wall structural proteins might also be important in atherogenesis, not only by altering the characteristics of the vessel wall, but also by affecting its interaction with plasma constituents. The combined stresses that lead to these modifications may be described as "carbonyl stress," as has recently been reviewed.[207,208] With age, collagen becomes more insoluble, thermally stable, and resistant to enzymatic attack.[209] Evidence is accumulating that these changes result from glucose-derived cross-links, formed via the browning or glycoxidation process. These changes are apparently irreversible once they have occurred.[210] This is consistent with the exaggeration of aging changes in collagen in the presence of diabetes. Glycoxidation of vascular connective tissues may contribute to accelerated atherosclerosis in various ways.

Abnormal Vascular Rigidity and Tone

Monnier and colleagues found an association between skin collagen fluorescence in type 1 diabetic patients and both arterial stiffness (assessed in vivo) and elevated systolic and diastolic blood pressures.[211] Oxlund and colleagues[212] demonstrated increased aortic stiffness in patients with type 1 diabetes at autopsy but did not measure glycoxidation products. Decreased elasticity and compliance of arteries and arterioles in diabetes might be due in part to enhanced glucose-mediated cross-linking and might contribute to the development of hypertension. Arterial stiffness and hypertension combined might result in abnormal shear stresses and endothelial damage, predisposing to injury and atherogenesis. In smaller vessels, similar stresses might contribute to the development of diabetic retinopathy, nephropathy, and neuropathy and to microvascular disease in the foot. Collagen glycoxidation products appear to quench the activity of NO (endothelium-derived relaxing factor) both in vitro and in vivo,[45] potentially causing impairment of endothelium-mediated vasodilation and abnormalities in vascular tone, flow dynamics, perfusion, and blood pressure, all of which might contribute to arterial and arteriolar damage.

Covalent Binding of Plasma Constituents

Endothelial injury causes permeation of plasma constituents into the vessel wall and covalent binding to connective tissue glycoxidation products. Brownlee and colleagues[40] found increased binding of LDL to glycated versus control collagen; and in diabetic compared to nondiabetic animals, cross-linking of LDL to aortic collagen was increased 2.5-fold. Once trapped in a high-glucose environment in the vessel wall, LDL particles may undergo extensive glycoxidation/lipoxidation. Free radical chain reactions in the trapped LDL might damage its constituent lipids and also neighboring structural proteins and cells. It has been shown, for instance, that products of lipid peroxidation stimulate collagen cross-linking,[213] and recent work from our group suggests that they might directly mediate cross-link formation.[214] Further, modified LDL might induce altered gene expression in vascular cells[215] that might promote atherogenesis. These interwoven mechanisms might lead to various vicious cycles in the diabetic milieu, leading to damage of arteries and small vessels and later to in situ formation of lipoprotein-immune complexes, further accelerating foam cell formation. Figure 5-2 illustrates many of these concepts.

The Receptor for Advanced Glycation End-Products

Monocytes/macrophages are strongly implicated in the development of atherosclerotic lesions. AGE products in vessel walls are chemotactic to monocytes, inducing them to migrate through the vascular endothelium.[216] A specific receptor for AGE products on monocytes/macrophages was identified by Vlassara and colleagues in 1986.[217] Macrophages expressing this receptor might phagocytose proteins and even entire cells expressing glycoxidation products.[218] Consistent with this, AGE products in vessel walls have been localized immunologically to intracellular locations in macrophages, smooth muscle cells, and foam cells derived from these cells. Since the first RAGE on endothelial cells was cloned in 1992, several others have been characterized in detail. Many of the consequences of increased AGE product formation in diabetes might be mediated through interactions with these various AGE receptors,[219] and the different receptors might trigger different changes in gene expression.[220] AGE product/receptor interactions in macrophages might induce release of cytokines, TNF-α, and IL-1[44]; these might mediate growth and remodeling and accelerate the atherosclerotic process. They might also induce production of prothrombotic tissue factor by macrophages, an action that can be inhibited by antioxidants.[221] In T lymphocytes, AGE product/receptor interactions induce synthesis of IFN-γ, which can enhance immune-mediated mechanisms of tissue injury.[222] In rat renal mesangial cells, AGE products stimulate increased collagen production, an effect that is probably mediated by transforming growth factor-α and by PDGF.[223] Receptor-mediated actions of AGE products have also been implicated in the development of diabetic retinopathy.[224–226] Infusion of AGE products in rabbits produced a variety of vascular changes. In endothelial cells, these included increased expression of VCAM-1 and ICAM-1, effects that are seen predominantly in areas affected by atheroma.[46] The induction of VCAM-1 is dependent on AGE product/receptor interactions, and VCAM-1 antigen is elevated in diabetic plasma.[227] Further supporting the significance of these interactions, it has been shown that blockade of RAGE can inhibit AGE product-induced impairment of endothelial barrier function and consequent hyperpermeability, and use of soluble RAGE may hold therapeutic promise.[228] Inhibition of AGE product formation using antioxidants has a similar effect.[229]

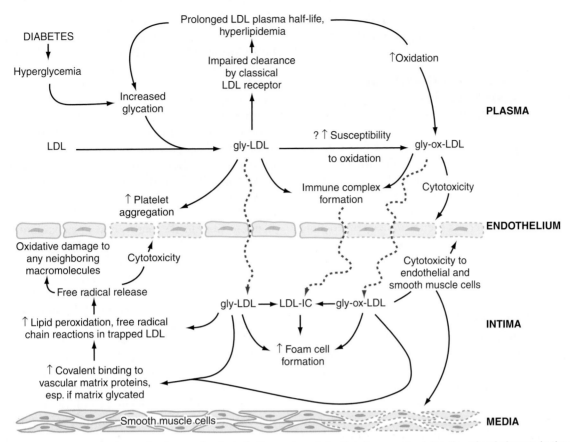

Figure 5–2 A postulated scheme for the mechanism of atherosclerosis in diabetes, emphasizing the role of glucose in the process.

Renal Impairment

Accumulation of glycoxidation products in skin collagen is associated with renal impairment in diabetes,[211,230–232] suggesting a possible causative role for these products in diabetic nephropathy. Supporting this, infusion of AGE product–modified albumin in rodents induces renal changes (glomerular sclerosis, albuminuria) similar to those occurring in diabetic renal disease.[233] It also induces upregulation of glomerular mRNA for laminin and collagen,[234] proteins that accumulate in glomerulosclerosis. Diabetic nephropathy, and other forms of renal disease, are characterized by a considerable increase in the expression of RAGE in various renal cell types, many of which do not normally express this receptor.[235] In addition to the kidney-specific effects, if a generalized collagen or other connective tissue protein abnormality is a common underlying mechanism for both micro-albuminuria and atheroma, this could partly explain the observation that microalbuminuria is a risk factor for macrovascular disease. A recent prospective study employing kidney biopsies supported a role for carbonyl and oxidative stress in promoting diabetic nephropathy.[236] The hypertension and lipid abnormalities that are characteristic of renal impairment may contribute further to the development of atherosclerosis.

Glycoxidation of Collagen and Diabetic Complications: Alternative Hypotheses

Many studies demonstrate associations between the levels of fructose-lysine (FL) and glycoxidation products in collagen and the presence or severity of several diabetic complications. The data are compatible with, but do not prove, the hypothesis that these products might contribute to complications, including accelerated macrovascular disease. FL, often regarded as a relatively harmless precursor of damaging glycoxidation products, might contribute indirectly. Alternatively, increased FL and the presence of complications might be related only insofar as both arise from a common origin: either prolonged hyperglycemia itself or other associated metabolic derangements. In contrast, glycoxidation and lipoxidation products significantly alter the properties of collagen, and so a direct causative role in the development of complications is easier to envisage, yet the case has not been proven. Glycoxidation products might simply reflect long-term glycoxidative/lipoxidative stresses; these stresses might cause disease primarily by cumulative effects on substrates other than collagen. Alternatively, complications might arise in association with hyperglycemia but via mechanisms that are not related to glycoxidation. In this case, glycoxidation products in collagen would represent only a record of past events. A recent paper from the DCCT/EDIC study[237] sheds light on this question.

Is It Possible to Inhibit the Glycation and Browning of Vascular Structural Proteins?

If carbonyl stress is indeed a significant risk factor in the development of macrovascular and microvascular complications of diabetes, then reducing this stress would clearly be desirable; it would mitigate recurrent damage to short-lived species, such as LDL, and cumulative damage to long-lived species, such as collagen. Possible means to inhibit the glucose-mediated, lipid-mediated, and "oxidative" components of carbonyl stress may be considered separately.

Reducing Glucose-Mediated Stress

Most obviously, glycemic control should be optimized, minimizing FL formation and reducing concentrations of glucose vulnerable to autoxidation. As well as decreasing formation of FL, existing FL levels may be reduced; improved glycemic control has been shown to reduce FL content within a few months even in long-lived proteins.[210] Decreased FL should decrease subsequent formation of glycoxidation products. Optimal glycemic control is an established goal in the management of diabetic patients. In relation to changes in connective tissue proteins, this conclusion is further reinforced by the recent studies from the DCCT/EDIC study.[238,237]

Reducing Lipid-Mediated Stress

Lipoxidative modification of proteins and other molecules may be minimized by decreasing substrate available for oxidative damage and making it more resistant to oxidation. Thus, the plasma lipid profile should be optimized by dietary and pharmacologic means and by dietary measures to minimize oxidizability of the fatty acid constituents of lipoproteins and cell membranes. Reaven and colleagues have shown that if monounsaturated fats are substituted for dietary polyunsaturated or saturated fats, LDL is less susceptible to oxidative damage.[239] The recent publication of results from the Collaborative Atorvastatin Diabetes Study (CARDS) trial reinforces the importance of tight control of plasma lipoprotein levels to prevent vascular complications in diabetic patients.[240]

Reducing Oxidative Stress

There is little direct evidence concerning the efficacy of any treatment aimed to reduce oxidative damage to proteins and lipids in diabetes. Vitamin C (ascorbate) is thought to be the most important aqueous antioxidant.[241] Plasma vitamin C and platelet vitamin E, the most important fat-soluble free radical scavenger, tend to be abnormally low in diabetic patients.[242,243] Dietary supplements of these vitamins may represent a cheap, low-risk intervention. However, under some circumstances, vitamin C might act as a pro-oxidant,[244] and there are insufficient grounds to recommend its routine use in diabetic patients. In the case of vitamin E (α-tocopherol), while there is significant circumstantial evidence in favor of its use in diabetic patients to reduce oxidative stress and perhaps to slow atherogenesis and the development of microvascular complications, the results of clinical trials have been disappointing. Under some circumstances, vitamin E might have pro-oxidant effects.[245] Probucol might be effective in reducing lipid peroxidation[246] and might have a protective effect in the vessel wall;[247–249] however, it seems to have few advantages over vitamin E. Butylated hydroxytoluene might also have similar effects;[250,251] coenzyme Q (ubiquinone), which detoxifies the tocopheroxyl radical (the product of vitamin E oxidation), can also inhibit LDL oxidation. While it might have a role to play, this has not been clearly defined.[252] Other agents inhibiting the toxic consequences of lipid peroxidation or inhibiting oxidation itself, might be developed as a result of improved understanding of the chemistry involved.[253]

Scavenging Reactive Carbonyls

Aminoguanidine is a scavenger of reactive carbonyl groups, especially of dicarbonyl compounds (e.g., glyoxal formed by oxidative decomposition of fructose-lysine, Schiff base, or fatty acids or 3-deoxyglucosone formed by decomposition of fructose-lysine), species that might mediate advanced carbonyl reactions. It can prevent the formation of glycoxidation and lipoxidation products and can interrupt vicious cycles of oxidative damage. In vitro, it may inhibit both collagen cross-linking[254] and lipid peroxidation.[255,256] In cell culture, we showed that at concentrations as low as 1 μmol/L, it can significantly inhibit the cytotoxicity that develops in LDL when it is exposed to glycoxidative stress.[257] The same low concentrations can also inhibit the toxicity of simulated hyperglycemia (25 mmol/L glucose) toward retinal vascular cells (unpublished observations). The results suggest that the observed toxicities might be mediated by oxidation products of LDL and glucose, respectively, and that these products are present at very low concentrations. In vivo, aminoguanidine can inhibit the development[258,259] and progression[260] of diabetic retinopathy in streptozotocin-diabetic rats and can also inhibit the development of diabetic nephropathy[261,262] and neuropathy.[263,264] Unfortunately, while aminoguanidine showed some evidence of a beneficial effect on renal function in a clinical trial,[265] it did not prove sufficiently safe for human consumption. Another class of experimental agents, the "leumedins" (N-[fluorenyl-9-methoxycarbonyl] amino

Fibrinolytic System

The fibrinolytic system controls the patency of the vascular tree by plasmin degradation of fibrin deposits and of thrombi. The generation and activities of plasmin are regulated mainly by the production of two critical proteins by the vascular endothelium: t-PA and the main inhibitor of t-PA, PAI-1. t-PA converts inactive plasminogen into plasmin at the site of fibrin formation. One critical regulator of thrombosis is likely to be the capacity for endogenous fibrinolysis. One hypothesis is that small amounts of fibrin are constantly deposited on the endothelium and that these fibrin deposits are continually dissolved, resulting in a dynamic balance between coagulation and fibrinolysis.

Impaired fibrinolytic activity is characterized by low t-PA activity and high PAI-1 antigen and activity. Studies in humans have shown that t-PA antigen concentration (associated with high PAI-1 and low basal or stimulated t-PA activity) might increase as a consequence of preclinical atherosclerosis and might be a marker of future coronary and cerebrovascular events. Impaired fibrinolysis is an independent risk factor for myocardial infarction in both nondiabetic and diabetic subjects. Low fibrinolytic activity is a leading determinant of ischemic heart disease in young men. t-PA antigen has been found to have a higher predictive value of mortality in patients with established coronary disease than do cholesterol, triglycerides, fibrinogen, blood pressure, diabetes, or smoking.

Conditions that favor enhanced thrombus formation have been frequently documented in type 2 diabetic patients, including decreased global plasma fibrinolytic activity, decreased plasma t-PA activity, higher basal t-PA antigen, insufficient t-PA release from endothelium under stress, and excess plasma PAI-1 antigen or activity in plasma, platelets, or arterial wall.[284] It has been suggested that normal t-PA and PAI-1 activity levels might be selective factors that influence the survival of diabetic patients. Most studies have been conducted in patients with type 2 diabetes. Decreased fibrinolytic function in type 2 diabetes correlated with the presence and severity of angiopathies. Lower exercise-induced levels of plasma t-PA have been found in early diabetic nephropathy. In patients with type 1 diabetes, higher t-PA antigen levels were associated with the presence of peripheral vascular disease, and increased PAI-1 activity was seen in the presence of microalbuminuria. There appears to be hormonal regulation of PAI-1 gene expression and protein synthesis. Insulin has been shown to induce PAI-1 mRNA expression in hepatocytes, leading to an increased release of this protein by liver cells. Some evidence for this effect of insulin has been shown in some in vivo studies but not in others. There is a correlation between PAI-1 and plasma insulin levels in obese individuals. Studies have shown a correlation between PAI-1 and plasma triglyceride levels. Longitudinal studies are needed on the relationships of obesity, plasma glucose, insulin, triglycerides, and PAI-1 in the syndrome of centripetal obesity and insulin resistance.

In vitro studies with cultured endothelial cells have provided some insights into regulation of t-PA and PAI-1 release by lipoproteins. VLDLs harvested from normal individuals will cause release of t-PA and PAI-1 from cultured endothelial cells, whereas VLDLs from hypertriglyceridemic individuals will not. Similar studies showed that endothelial production of PAI-1 is increased by incubation in vitro with VLDL obtained from hyperglycemic patients. Stimulation of endothelial release of t-PA and PAI-1 with desmopressin acetate in type 2 diabetic subjects with hypertriglyceridemia causes a decreased plasma t-PA activity and an elevated PA-1 response when compared with normal controls. Other studies implicated glycoxidized LDL, high levels of free fatty acids, increased oxygen species, and several cytokines as factors altering production of tPA or PAI-1 in diabetes.

The source of physiologically active PAI-1 in plasma is probably the endothelium. Elevated levels might reflect endothelial damage. On the other hand, liver cells and abdominal adipose tissue synthesize and release PAI-1, and studies of PAI-1 in plasma, serum, and platelets have shown that the concentration of PAI-1 antigen in platelets is very high and that platelets account for 93% of PAI-1 antigen in whole blood. Platelet PAI-1 exists primarily in an inactive form.

Discussion

What does all of this mean? Is diabetes characterized by a hypercoagulable state? If so, could this underlie the predisposition toward thrombosis that is often seen in diabetes? What is the effect of therapy? Can we prevent macrovascular thrombosis?

Clearly, the final answers to all of these questions are not apparent. There is still a lot of work to do. Generalization is dangerous for a number of reasons. First, in clinical studies, it is important to differentiate data obtained from type 1 and type 2 diabetic subjects in view of the major differences in pathophysiology between these two syndromes. Second, there is great heterogeneity within type 1 diabetic populations. In some cases, studies are done in prepubertal children; other studies involve adults of short duration; others involve type 1 diabetic individuals with nephropathy, retinopathy, neuropathy, or macrovascular disease. Third, there is even greater heterogeneity within type 2 diabetic populations. Thus, individuals may be obese or nonobese; have low, normal, or elevated plasma insulin or lipid levels; be free from microvascular or macrovascular disease; be treated with diet, oral agents, or insulin; or have clinically apparent or unapparent microvascular or macrovascular disease. Furthermore, the majority of studies are cross-sectional, and this may give misleading data because of patient selection. Longitudinal data are limited and extremely difficult and costly to pursue. Duration of type 2 diabetes may be difficult to assess.

Nevertheless, from the studies cited in this review and in other sources,[1-3,23,285,286] some trends are apparent. First, even when an abnormal mean value for platelet function or index of coagulation is found and the subjects are well defined (e.g., type 1 diabetes free from clinical vascular disease), there are many patients with normal activity or levels, no matter what parameter is measured. On the other hand, there is a certain consistency in reported results in uncomplicated type 1 diabetic subjects with hyperglycemia, and there is increasing evidence that in these individuals, insulin therapy might return altered values to or toward normal. By probing results from a number of different studies in different type 1 diabetic populations, some interesting findings emerge. When studied in vivo, insulin administration to hyperglycemic type 1 diabetic subjects has been found to produce changes in platelet function, the intrinsic coagulation system, and fibrinogen dynamics that could reduce the tendency toward intravascular thrombosis. These findings provide a theoretical basis for intensive insulin therapy in type 1 diabetic subjects. On the other hand, studies in type 2 diabetes are limited. It must be recognized that it will require properly designed, multicenter collaborative trials to definitely answer the question as to whether intensive insulin therapy will alter thrombotic events in type 1 or type 2 diabetic individuals.

In light of current knowledge, however, it is generally accepted that one reasonable approach to the prevention of thrombotic events is the use of agents such as aspirin, which irreversibly acetylates platelet cyclo-oxygenase and thereby inhibits platelet thromboxane production. Currently, there are more than 200 studies with antiplatelet agents in nondiabetic and in diabetic individuals, in which major vascular events such as strokes, myocardial infarctions, and vascular death have been monitored before and after antiplatelet therapy. Results have been compared with those obtained in individuals receiving placebo therapy. There is general agreement, as indicated by meta-analyses of published data, that antiplatelet therapy is a safe and effective way to prevent future cardiovascular events in diabetic or nondiabetic individuals who have had one vascular event.[287,288] Thus, pooled data suggest that vascular morbidity can be lowered about 25%, nonfatal myocardial infarctions about 30%, and vascular mortality approximately 15% after antiplatelet therapy when it is used as a secondary prevention strategy.[287,288] It is generally believed that the benefits of antiplatelet therapy outweigh the risks in diabetic subjects who are at high vascular risk.[289] There is no evidence that aspirin therapy will accentuate diabetic retinopathy or vitreous hemorrhage. Although use of aspirin as a primary prevention strategy is still somewhat controversial, studies in nondiabetic individuals suggest that this is safe and worthwhile if coronary event risk is greater than 1.5% per year.[290]

Summary

Is it presumptuous to attempt to define the pathogenesis of atherosclerosis in diabetes mellitus? One could adopt this view because the pathogenesis in nondiabetic individuals is a subject of active research and therefore is open to changing views. Extrapolation from these current postulates to a disease state as complicated and heterogeneous as diabetes mellitus could therefore be dangerous, inaccurate, and misleading. In addition, investigators are limited by a variety of factors in their search to delineate mechanisms involved in the atherosclerotic process in humans. Access to normal arterial tissue for in vitro studies has been limited, and noninvasive techniques for assessing the degree and extent of early lesions of atherosclerosis in vivo are under development. Longitudinal studies are compromised by these limitations in technique and by the slow progression of the atherosclerotic process. These factors have led investigators to rely on correlative relationships and studies using cell systems that might not be directly transferable to the atherosclerotic process in humans. Further, pathogenesis of atherosclerosis may differ in vessels from various sites. The issue is further complicated by the fact that animal models are limited; much of the work has been done in animal species in which atherosclerosis is a difficult lesion to produce. Clinical trials in diabetes that will provide useful information are now under way, but existing studies have usually been secondary prevention trials in patients with very advanced vascular disease. Primary prevention of atherosclerosis is of greatest importance.

Nevertheless, the situation is improving. Advances in surgical technique in humans, with close coordination of investigators from various disciplines, have led to the availability of fresh human tissue from coronary bypass patients and other individuals who have undergone major surgery. Tissue culture techniques allow investigators to directly study the metabolism and function for critical components of the human arterial tree and to objectively manipulate variables involved in the atherosclerotic process. Noninvasive techniques for assessing the vascular system in humans are undergoing refinement and are becoming more available to clinical investigators. Techniques of molecular biology are opening up new approaches to the genetic influences on atherosclerosis. An explosion of biochemical and physiologic information about prostanoids and their derivatives and about lipids, lipoproteins, and apolipoproteins has occurred in recent years. Improved animal models of atherosclerosis and diabetes mellitus exist, and work using animals such as monkeys and pigs is beginning to appear. Clinical trials are moving in the direction of primary rather than secondary prevention and target glucose, lipids, lipoproteins, platelets, and prostanoids. All of these are postulated to be operative in atherosclerosis associated with diabetes mellitus.

An explosion of information on endothelial function, immune complexes, cytokines, adhesion proteins, glycation, and glycoxidation has occurred and has led to newer concepts. Alterations in the coagulation and fibrinolytic systems might predispose diabetic subjects to vascular thrombosis. As work in these very active areas of research continues, it is likely that improved methods of preventing or forestalling the development of accelerated macrovascular disease in diabetes will emerge.

References

1. Colwell JA, et al: New concepts about the pathogenesis of atherosclerosis in diabetes mellitus. In Levin ME, O'Neal LW (eds): The Diabetic Foot, 4th ed. St. Louis: Mosby-Year Book, 1988, pp 51–70.
2. Colwell JA: Peripheral vascular disease in diabetes mellitus. In Davidson J (eds): Clinical Diabetes Mellitus. New York: Thieme Medical Publishers, 1986, pp 357–375.
3. Colwell JA, Winocour PD, Lopes-Virella MF: Platelet function and platelet interactions in atherosclerosis and diabetes mellitus. In Rifkin H, Porte D (eds): Diabetes Mellitus: Theory and Practice. New York: Elsevier, 1989, pp 249–256.
4. Levin ME, Powers MA: Hypertension and diabetes: Then and now. Diabetes Spectrum 3:274, 1990.
5. Davis NS Jr: Diabetic gangrene. JAMA 31:103–105, 1898.
6. Lawson RA: Amputations through the ages. Aust N Z J Med 42:221–230, 1973.
7. Wheelock FC, Marble A: Surgery and diabetes. In Marble A, White P, Bradley RF, et al (eds): Joslin's Diabetes Mellitus, 11th ed. Philadelphia: Lea & Febiger, 1971, pp 599–620.
8. Bell ET: Incidence of gangrene of the extremities in nondiabetic and diabetic persons. Arch Pathol Lab Med 49:469–473, 1960.
9. Beach KW, et al: The correlation of arteriosclerosis obliterans with lipoproteins in insulin-dependent and noninsulin-dependent diabetes. Diabetes 28:836–840, 1979.
10. Epstein FH, et al: Epidemiological studies of cardiovascular diseases in a total community: Tecumseh, Michigan. Ann Intern Med 62:1170–1187, 1965.
11. Janka HU, Standl E, Mehnert H: Peripheral vascular disease in diabetes mellitus and its relation to cardiovascular risk factors: Screening with the Doppler ultrasonic technique. Diabetes Care 3:207–213, 1980.
12. Melton LJ, et al: Incidence and prevalence of clinical peripheral vascular disease in a population-based cohort of 56 diabetic patients. Diabetes Care 3:650–654, 1980.
13. Osmundson PJ, et al: Course of peripheral occlusive arterial disease in diabetes. Diabetes Care 2:143–152, 1990.
14. Palumbo PJ, et al: Progression of peripheral occlusive arterial disease in diabetes mellitus: What factors are predictive? Arch Intern Med 151:717–721, 1991.
15. Uusitupa MIJ, et al: 5-year incidence of atherosclerotic vascular disease in relation of general risk factors, insulin level, and abnormalities in lipoprotein composition in non-insulin-dependent diabetic and nondiabetic subjects. Circulation 82:27–36, 1990.
16. Garcia ML, et al: Morbidity and mortality in diabetics in Framingham population: Sixteen year follow-up study. Diabetes 23:105–111, 1974.
17. Biesbroeck RC, et al: Specific high affinity binding of HDL to cultured human skin fibroblasts and arterial smooth muscle cells. J Clin Invest 71:525, 1983.
18. Ducimetier P, et al: Relationship of plasma insulin levels to the incidence of myocardial infarction and coronary heart disease mortality in a middle-aged population. Diabetologia 19:205–210, 1980.
19. Fontbonne AM, et al: Insulin and cardiovascular disease: Paris prospective study. Diabetes Care 6:461–469, 1991.
20. Pyorala K: Relationship of glucose tolerance and plasma insulin to the incidence of coronary heart disease: Results from two population studies in Finland. Diabetes Care 2:131–141, 1979.
21. Welborne TA, Wearne K: Coronary heart disease incidence and cardiovascular mortality in Busselton with reference to glucose and insulin concentrations. Diabetes Care 2:154–160, 1979.
22. Standl E, Janka HV: High serum insulin concentrations in relation to other cardiovascular risk factors in macrovascular disease of type 2 diabetes. Horm Metab Res 17(suppl):46–51, 1985.
23. Colwell JA, et al (eds): Workshop on insulin and atherogenesis. Metabolism 12(suppl 1):1–91, 1985.
24. Stolar MW: Atherosclerosis in diabetes: The role of hyperinsulinemia. Metabolism 2(suppl 1):1–9, 1988.
25. Stout RW: Insulin and atheroma: An update. Lancet 1:1077, 1987.
26. Berliner JA, et al: Atherosclerosis: Basic mechanisms: Oxidation, inflammation and genetics. Circulation 91:2488–2496, 1995.
27. Schwenke DC, Carew TE: Initiation of atherosclerotic lesions in cholesterol-fed rabbits: II. Selective retention of LDL vs selective increases in LDL permeability in susceptible sites of arteries. Arteriosclerosis 9:908–918, 1989.
28. Frank FS, Fogelman AM: Ultrastructure of the intima in WHHL and cholesterol-fed rabbit aortas prepared by ultra-rapid freezing and freeze-etching. J Lipid Res 30:967–978, 1989.
29. Nievelstein PFEM, et al: Lipid accumulation in rabbit aortic intima 2 hours after bolus infusion of LDL: A deep-etch and immunolocalization study of rapidly frozen tissue. Arterioscler Thromb 11:1795–1805, 1991.
30. Navab M, et al: Monocyte transmigration induced by modification of low density lipoprotein in co-cultures of human aortic wall cells is due to induction of monocyte chemotactic protein 1 synthesis and is abolished by high density lipoprotein. J Clin Invest 88:2039–2046, 1991.
31. Rajavashisth TB, et al: Induction of endothelial cell expression of granulocyte and macrophage colony-stimulating factors by modified low density lipoproteins. Nature 344:254–257, 1990.
32. Schwartz D, et al: The role of a *gro* homologue in monocyte adhesion to endothelium. J Clin Invest 94:1968–1973, 1994.
33. Henriksen T, Evensen SA, Carlander B: Injury to human endothelial cells in culture induced by LDL. Scand J Clin Lab Invest 39:361–364, 1979.
34. Hessler JR, Robertson AL Jr, Chisolm GM: LDL-induced cytotoxicity and its inhibition by HDL in human vascular smooth muscle and endothelial cells in culture. Atherosclerosis 32:213–218, 1979.
35. Fogelman AM, et al: Malondialdehyde alteration of LDL leads to cholesterol ester accumulation in human monocytes/macrophages. Proc Natl Acad Sci U S A 77:2214–2218, 1980.
36. Hoff HF, et al: Modification of LDL with 4-hydroxynonenal induces uptake by macrophages. Arteriosclerosis 9:538–549, 1989.
37. James RW, Pometta D: Differences in lipoprotein subfraction composition and distribution between type I diabetic men and control subjects. Diabetes 39:1158–1164, 1990.
38. James RW, Pometta D: The distribution profiles of very low and low density lipoproteins in poorly controlled male, type 2 (non-insulin-dependent) diabetic patients. Diabetologia 34:246–252, 1991.
39. Bucala R, Vlassara H: Advanced glycosylation end products in diabetic renal and vascular disease. Am J Kidney Dis 26:875–888, 1995.
40. Brownlee M, Vlassara H, Cerami A: Nonenzymatic glycosylation products on collagen covalently trap low-density lipoprotein. Diabetes 34:938–941, 1985.
41. Brownlee M, Pongor S, Cerami A: Covalent attachment of soluble proteins by non-enzymatically glycosylated collagen: Role in the in situ formation of immune complexes. J Exp Med 158:1739–1744, 1983.
42. Esposito C: Endothelial receptor-mediated binding of glucose-modified albumin is associated with increased monolayer permeability and modulation of cell surface coagulant properties. J Exp Med 170:1387–1407, 1989.
43. Doi T, et al: Receptor-specific increase in extracellular matrix production in mouse mesangial cells by advanced glycosylation end products is mediated via platelet-derived growth factor. Proc Natl Acad Sci U S A 89:2873–2877, 1992.

44. Vlassara H, et al: Cachectin/TNF and IL-1 induced by glucose-modified proteins: Role in normal tissue remodeling. Science 240:1546–1548, 1988.

45. Bucala R, Tracey KJ, Cerami A: Advanced glycosylation products quench nitric oxide and mediate defective endothelium-dependent vasodilatation in experimental diabetes. J Clin Invest 87:432–438, 1991.

46. Vlassara H, et al: Advanced glycation endproducts promote adhesion molecule (VCAM-1, ICAM-1) expression and atheroma formation in normal rabbits. Mol Med 1:447–456, 1995.

47. Virella G, et al: Pro-atherogenic and pro-inflammatory properties of immune complexes prepared with purified human oxLDL antibodies and human oxLDL. Clin Immunol 105:81–92, 2002.

48. Virella G, et al: Activation of human monocyte-derived macrophages by immune complexes containing low density lipoprotein. Clin Immunol Immunopathol 75:179–189, 1995.

49. Beekhuizen H, van Furth R: Monocyte adherence to human vascular endothelium. Leukoc Biol 54:363–378, 1993.

50. Pohlman T, et al: An endothelial cell surface factor(s) induced in vitro by lipopolysaccharide, interleukin-1 and tumor necrosis factor increases neutrophil adherence by a CDw18-dependent mechanism. J Immunol 136:4548–4553, 1986.

51. Davies MJ, et al: The expression of the adhesion molecules ICAM-1, VCAM-1, PECAM, and E-selectin in human atherosclerosis. J Pathol 171:223, 1993.

52. Bevilacqua MP, et al: Interleukin-1 induces biosynthesis and cell surface expression of procoagulant activity in human vascular endothelial cells. J Exp Med 160:618–622, 1984.

53. Breviario F, et al: IL-induced adhesion of polymorphonuclear leukocytes to cultured human endothelial cells: Role of platelet-activating factor. J Immunol 141:3391–3397, 1988.

54. Martin S, et al: IL-1 and INF- increase vascular permeability. Immunology 64:301–305, 1988.

55. Warner SJC, Auger KR, Libby P: Interleukin-1 induces interleukin-1: II. Recombinant human interleukin-1 induces interleukin-1 production by adult human vascular endothelial cells. J Immunol 139:1911–1917, 1987.

56. Raines EW, Dower SK, Ross R: Interleukin-1 mitogenic activity for fibroblasts and smooth muscle cells is due to PDGF-AA. Science 243:393–396, 1989.

57. Hansson GK, et al: Immune mechanisms in atherosclerosis. Arteriosclerosis 9:567–578, 1989.

58. Nawroth PP, et al: Tumor necrosis factor/cachectin interacts with endothelial cell receptors to induce release of interleukin-1. J Exp Med 165:1363–1375, 1986.

59. Stevenson HC, et al: Analysis of human blood monocyte activation at the level of gene expression. J Exp Med 161:503–513, 1985.

60. Nathan CF, Murray HW, Cohn ZA: The macrophage as an effector cell. N Engl J Med 303:622–626, 1980.

61. Ross R, et al: Localization of PDGF-B protein in macrophages in all phases of atherogenesis. Science 248:1009–1012, 1990.

62. Assoian RK, et al: Expression and secretion of type beta transforming growth factor by activated human macrophages. Proc Natl Acad Sci U S A 84:6020–6024, 1987.

63. Ferreri NR, Howland WC, Spiegelberg HL: Release of leukotrienes C4 and B4 and prostaglandin E2 from human monocytes stimulated with aggregated IgG, IgA, and IgE. J Immunol 136:4188–4193, 1986.

64. Musson RA, Shafran H, Henson PM: Intracellular levels and stimulated release of lysosomal enzymes from human peripheral blood monocytes and monocyte-derived macrophages. J Reticuloendothel Soc 28:249–264, 1980.

65. Werb Z, Bonda MJ, Jones PA: Degradation of connective tissue matrices by macrophages: I. Proteolysis of elastin, glycoproteins, and collagens by proteinases isolated from macrophages. J Exp Med 152:1340–1357, 1980.

66. Nakagawara A, Nathan CF, Cohn ZA: Hydrogen peroxide metabolism in human monocytes during differentiation in vitro. J Clin Invest 68:1243–1252, 1981.

67. Marx N, et al: Effect of rosiglitazone treatment on soluble CD40L in patients with type 2 diabetes and coronary heart disease. Circulation 107:1954–1957, 2003.

68. Griffith RL, et al: LDL metabolism by macrophages activated with LDL immune complexes: A possible mechanism of foam cell formation. J Exp Med 168:1041–1059, 1988.

69. Gisinger C, Virella GT, Lopes-Virella MF: Erythrocyte-bound low density lipoprotein (LDL) immune complexes lead to cholesteryl ester accumulation in human monocyte derived macrophages. Clin Immunol Immunopathol 59:37–52, 1991.

70. Lopes-Virella MF, et al: Enhanced uptake and impaired intracellular metabolism of LDL complexed with anti-LDL antibodies. Arterioscler Thromb 11:1356–1367, 1991.

71. Lopes-Virella MF, et al: The uptake of LDL-IC by human macrophages: Predominant involvement of the FcgRI. Atherosclerosis 135:161–170, 1997.

72. Huang Y, Ghosh M, Lopes-Virella MF: Transcriptional and post-transcriptional regulation of LDL receptor gene expression in PMA-treated THP-1 cells by LDL-IC. J Lipid Res 38:110–120, 1997.

73. Salonen JT: Is there a continuing need for longitudinal epidemiologic research: The Kuopio ischaemic heart disease risk factor study. Ann Clin Res 20:46–50, 1988.

74. Palinski W, et al: Antisera and monoclonal antibodies specific for epitopes generated during oxidative modification of low density lipoprotein. Arteriosclerosis 10:325–335, 1990.

75. Maggi E, et al: LDL oxidation in patients with severe carotid atherosclerosis: A study of in vitro and in vivo oxidation markers. Arterioscler Thromb 14:1892–1899, 1994.

76. Salonen JT, et al: Autoantibody against oxidized LDL and progression of carotid atherosclerosis. Lancet 339:883–887, 1992.

77. Lehtimaki T, et al: Autoantibodies against oxidized low density lipoprotein in patients with angiographically verified coronary artery disease. Arterioscl Thromb Vasc Biol 19:23–27, 1999.

78. Erkkilä AT, et al: Autoantibodies against oxidized low-density lipoprotein and cardiolipin in patients with coronary heart disease. Arterioscl Thromb Vasc Biol 20:204–209, 2000.

79. Bellomo G, et al: Autoantibodies against oxidatively modified low-density lipoproteins in NIDDM. Diabetes 44:60–66, 1995.

80. Palinski W, et al: Immunological evidence for the presence of AGE in atherosclerotic lesions of euglycemic rabbits. Arterioscler Thromb Vasc Biol 15:571–582, 1995.

81. Turk Z, et al: Detection of autoantibodies against advanced glycation endproducts and AGE-immune complexes in serum of patients with diabetes mellitus. Clin Chim Acta 303:105–115, 2001.

82. Virella G, et al: Anti-oxidized low-density lipoprotein antibodies in patients with coronary heart disease and normal healthy volunteers. Int J Clin Lab Res 23:95–101, 1993.

83. Boullier A, et al: Detection of autoantibodies against oxidized low-density lipoproteins and of IgG-bound low density lipoproteins in patients with coronary artery disease. Clin Chim Acta 238:1–10, 1995.

84. Uusitupa MIJ, et al: Autoantibodies against oxidized LDL do not predict atherosclerosis vascular disease in non-insulin-dependent diabetes mellitus. Arterioscl Thromb Vasc Biol 16:1236–1242, 1996.

85. van de Vijver LP, et al: Autoantibodies against MDA-LDL in subjects with severe and minor atherosclerosis and healthy population controls. Atherosclerosis 122:245–253, 1996.

86. Leinonen JS, et al: The level of autoantibodies against oxidized LDL is not associated with the presence of coronary heart disease or diabetic kidney disease in patients with non-insulin-dependent diabetes mellitus. Free Radic Res 29:137–141, 1998.

87. Festa A, et al: Autoantibodies to oxidised low density lipoproteins in IDDM are inversely related to metabolic control and microvascular complications. Diabetologia 41:350–356, 1998.

88. Wu R, et al: Autoantibodies to OxLDL are decreased in individuals with borderline hypertension. Hypertension 33:53–59, 1999.

89. Lopes-Virella MF, et al: Antibodies to oxidized LDL and LDL-containing immune complexes as risk factors for coronary artery disease in diabetes mellitus. Clin Immunol 90:165–172, 1999.

90. Hulthe J, et al: Antibodies to oxidized LDL in relation to carotid atherosclerosis, cell adhesion molecules, and phospholipase A(2). Arterioscl Thromb Vasc Biol 21:269–274, 2001.

91. Shaw PX, et al: Natural antibodies with the T15 idiotype may act in atherosclerosis, apoptotic clearance, and protective immunity. J Clin Invest 105:1731–1740, 2000.

92. Wu R, Lefvert AK: Autoantibodies against oxidized low density lipoproteins (oxLDL): Characterization of antibody isotype, subclass, affinity and effect on the macrophage uptake of oxLDL. Clin Exp Immunol 102:174–180, 1995.

93. Palinski W, Witztum JL: Immune responses to oxidative neoepitopes on LDL and phospholipids modulate the development of atherosclerosis. J Intern Med 247:371–380, 2000.
94. Hansson GK: Vaccination against atherosclerosis: science or fiction? Circulation 106:1599–1601, 2002.
95. Virella G, et al: Immunochemical characterization of purified human oxidized low-density lipoprotein antibodies. Clin Immunol 95:135–144, 2000.
96. Virella G, et al: Autoimmune response to advanced glycosylation end-products of human low density lipoprotein. J Lipid Research 443:487–493, 2003.
97. Virella G, Tsokos G: Immune complex diseases. In G. Virella (ed): Medical Immunology, 5th ed. New York: Marcel Dekker, 2002, pp 453–471.
98. Hulthe J, Bokemark L, Fagerberg B: Antibodies to oxidized LDL in relation to intima-media thickness in carotid and femoral arteries in 58-year-old subjectively clinically healthy men. Arterioscler Thromb Vasc Biol 21:101–107, 2001.
99. Fagerberg B, Bokemark L, Hulthe J: The metabolic syndrome, smoking, and antibodies to oxidized LDL in 58-year-old clinically healthy men. Nutr Metab Cardiovasc Dis 11: 227–235, 2001.
100. Virella G, Lopes-Virella MF: Lipoprotein autoantibodies: Measurement and significance. Clin Diag Lab Immunol 10:499–505, 2003.
101. Szondy E, et al: Occurrence of anti-low density lipoprotein antibodies and circulating immune complexes in aged subjects. Mech Ageing Dev 29:117–123, 1985.
102. Tertov VV, et al: Low density lipoprotein-containing circulating immune complexes and coronary atherosclerosis. Exp Mol Pathol 52:300–308, 1990.
103. Atchley D, et al: Oxidized LDL–anti-oxidized LDL immune complexes and diabetic nephropathy. Diabetologia 45:1562–1571, 2002.
104. Falk E: Why do plaques rupture? Circulation 86(suppl III):III-30–III-42, 1992.
105. Giroud D, et al: Relation of the site of acute myocardial infarction to the most severe coronary arterial stenosis at prior angiography. Am J Cardiol 69:729–732, 1992.
106. Little WC, et al: Can coronary angiography predict the site of a subsequent myocardial infarction in patients with mild-moderate coronary artery disease? Circulation 78:1157–1166, 1988.
107. Libby P: Molecular bases of the acute coronary syndromes. Circulation 91:2844–2850, 1995.
108. Amento EP, et al: Cytokine positively and negatively regulate interstitial collagen gene expression in human vascular smooth muscle cells. Arterioscler Thromb 11:1223–1230, 1991.
109. Hansson GK, Holm J, Jonasson L: Detection of activated T lymphocytes in the human atherosclerotic plaques. Am J Pathol 135:169–175, 1989.
110. van der Wal AC, et al: Site of intimal rupture or erosion of thrombosed coronary atherosclerotic plaques is characterized by an inflammatory process irrespective of the dominant plaque morphology. Circulation 89:36–44, 1994.
111. Fuster V, Lewis A: Conner Memorial Lecture. Mechanisms leading to myocardial infarction: Insights from studies of vascular biology. Circulation 90:2126–2146, 1994.
112. Morton LF, Barnes M:. Collagen polymorphism in the normal and diseased blood vessel wall. Investigation of collagens types I, III and V. Atherosclerosis 42:41–51, 1982.
113. Hanson AN, Bentley JP: Quantitation of type I to type III collagen ratios in small samples of human tendon, blood vessels, and atherosclerotic plaques. Anal Biochem 130:32–40, 1983.
114. Matrisian LM: The matrix-degrading metalloproteinases. BioEssays 14:455–463, 1992.
115. Sukhova G, et al: Colocalization of the interstitial collagenase MMP-1 and MMP-13 with sites of cleaved collagen indicates their role in plaque destabilization. Circulation 98(suppl):1–48, 1998.
116. Huang Y, Mironova M, Lopes-Virella MF: Oxidized LDL stimulates matrix metalloproteinase-1 expression in human vascular endothelial cells. Arterioscler Thromb Vasc Biol 19:2640–2647, 1999.
117. Huang Y, et al: Fc-gamma receptor cross-linking by immune complexes induces matrix metalloproteinase-1 in U937 cells via mitogen-activated protein kinase. Arterioscler Thromb Vasc Biol 20:2533–2538, 2000.
118. Huang Y, et al: Oxidized LDL differentially regulates MMP-1 and TIMP-1 expression in vascular endothelial cells. Atherosclerosis 156:119–125, 2001.
119. Marx N, et al: Antidiabetic PPAR-activator rosiglitazone reduces MMP-9 serum levels in type 2 diabetic patients with coronary artery disease. Arterioscler Thromb Vasc Biol 23:283–288, 2003.
120. Uemura S, et al: Diabetes mellitus enhances vascular matrix metalloproteinase activity: Role of oxidative stress. Circ Res 88:1291–1298, 2001.
121. Shi GP, et al: Molecular cloning and expression of human alveolar macrophage cathepsin S, an elastinolytic cysteine protease. J Biol Chem 267:7258–7262, 1992.
122. Kafienah W, et al: Human Cathepsin K cleaves native type I and II collagens at the N-terminal end of the triple helix. Biochem J 331:727–732, 1998.
123. Reddy VY, Zhang QY, Weiss SJ: Pericellular mobilization of the tissue-destructive cysteine proteinases, cathepins B, L, and S, by human monocyte-derived macrophages. Proc Natl Acad Sci U S A 92:3849–3853, 1995.
124. Sukhova GK, et al: Expression of the elastolytic cathepsins S and K in human atheroma and regulation of their production in smooth muscle cells. J Clin Invest 102:576–583, 1998.
125. Jormsjo S, et al: Differential expression of cysteine and aspartic proteases during progression of atherosclerosis in apolipoprotein E-deficient mice. Am J Pathol 161:939–945, 2002.
126. Chen J, et al: In vivo imaging of proteolytic activity in atherosclerosis. Circulation 105:2766–2771, 2002.
127. Gacko M, Glowinski S: Cathepsin D and cathepsin L activities in aortic aneurysm wall and parietal thrombus. Clin Chem Lab Med 36:449–452, 1998.
128. Shi GP, et al: Cystatin C deficiency in human atherosclerosis and aortic aneurysms. J Clin Invest 104:1191–1197, 1999.
129. Schaub FJ, et al: Fas/FADD-mediated activation of a specific program of inflammatory gene expression in vascular smooth muscle cells. Nature Med 6:790–796, 2000.
130. Tedgui A, Mallat Z: Apoptosis as a determinant of atherothrombosis. Thromb Haemost 86:420–426, 2001.
131. Moons AH, Levi M, Peters RJ: Tissue factor and coronary heart disease. Cardiovasc Res 53:313–325, 2002.
132. Furchgott RF, Zawadzki JV: The obligatory role of endothelial cells in the relaxation of arterial smooth muscle by acetylcholine. Nature 299:373–376, 1980.
133. Ignarro LJ, et al: Endothelium-derived relaxing factor produced and released from artery and vein is nitric oxide. Proc Natl Acad Sci U S A 84:9265–9269, 1987.
134. Palmer RMJ, Ferrige AF, Moncada S: Nitric oxide release accounts for the biological activity of endothelium-derived relaxing factor. Nature 327:524–526, 1987.
135. Moncada S, Palmer RMJ, Higgs EA: Nitric oxide: Physiology, pathophysiology, and pharmacology. Pharmacol Rev 43:109–142, 1991.
136. Palmer RMJ, Ashton DS, Moncada S: Vascular endothelial cells synthesize nitric oxide from L-arginine. Nature 333:664–666, 1988.
137. Naseem KM: The role of nitric oxide in cardiovascular diseases. Mol Aspects Med 26:33–65, 2005.
138. Llorens S, Nava E: Cardiovascular diseases and the nitric oxide pathway. Curr Vasc Pharmacol 1:335–346, 2003.
139. Ji Y, et al: Inhibition of endothelial nitric oxide generation by low-density lipoprotein is partially prevented by L-arginine and L-ascorbate. Atherosclerosis 176:345–353, 2004.
140. Goulter AB, et al: Chylomicron-remnant-like particles inhibit the basal nitric oxide pathway in porcine coronary artery and aortic endothelial cells. Clin Sci (Lond) 105:363–371, 2003.
141. Takahashi M, et al: Very low density lipoprotein enhances inducible nitric oxide synthase expression in cytokine-stimulated vascular smooth muscle cells. Atherosclerosis 162:307–313, 2002.
142. Mineo C, et al: High density lipoprotein-induced endothelial nitric-oxide synthase activation is mediated by Akt and MAPkinases. J Biol Chem 278:9142–9149, 2003.
143. Yuhanna IS, et al: High-density lipoprotein binding to scavenger receptor-BI activates endothelial nitric oxide synthase. Nat Med 7:853–857, 2001.
144. Spieker LE, et al: High-density lipoprotein restores endothelial function in hypercholesterolemic men. Circulation 105:1399–1402, 2002.
145. Balletshofer BM, et al: Intense cholesterol lowering therapy with HMG-CoA reductase inhibitor does not improve nitric oxide dependent endothelial function in type 2 diabetes: A multicenter, randomized, double-blind, three-arm, placebo-controlled clinical trial. Exp Clin Endocr Diab 113:324–330, 2005.

146. Cassone Faldetta M, et al: L-arginine infusion decreases plasma total homocysteine concentrations through increased nitric oxide production and decreased oxidative status in Type 2 diabetic patients. Diabetologia 45:1120–1127, 2002.

147. Avogaro A, et al: L-arginine-nitric oxide kinetics in normal and type 2 diabetic subjects: A stable-labeled 15N arginine approach. Diabetes 52:795–802, 2003.

148. van Etten RW, et al: Impaired NO-dependent vasodilation in patients with Type II (non-insulin-dependent) diabetes mellitus is restored by acute administration of folate. Diabetologia 45:1004–1010, 2002.

149. Akbari CM, et al: Endothelium-dependent vasodilatation is impaired in both microcirculation and macrocirculation during acute hyperglycemia. J Vasc Surg 28:687–694, 1998.

150. Williams SB, et al: Acute hyperglycemia attenuates endothelium-dependent vasodilatation in humans in vivo. Circulation 97:1695–1701, 1998.

151. Taubert D, et al: Acute effects of glucose and insulin on vascular endothelium. Diabetologia 47:2059–2071, 2004.

152. Milsom AB, et al: Abnormal metabolic fate of nitric oxide in type 1 diabetes mellitus. Diabetologia 45:1515–1522, 2002.

153. James PE, et al: Vasorelaxation by red blood cells and impairment in diabetes: Reduced nitric oxide and oxygen delivery by glycated hemoglobin. Circ Res 94:976–983, 2004.

154. Cosby K, et al: Nitrite reduction to nitric oxide by deoxyhemoglobin vasodilates the human circulation. Nat Med 9:1498–1505, 2003.

155. Rogers SC, et al: Detection of human red blood cell-bound nitric oxide. J Biol Chem 29:26720–26728, 2005.

156. Gladwin MT, Schechter AN: NO contest: Nitrite versus S-nitrosohemoglobin. Circ Res 94:851–855, 2004.

157. Rodriguez-Manas L, et al: Effect of glycaemic control on the vascular nitric oxide system in patients with type 1 diabetes. J Hypertens 21:1137–1143, 2003.

158. Heitzer T, et al: Tetrahydrobiopterin improves endothelium-dependent vasodilation by increasing nitric oxide activity in patients with type II diabetes mellitus. Diabetologia 43:1435–1438, 2000.

159. Bagi Z, Koller A: Lack of nitric oxide mediation of flow-dependent arteriolar dilation in type 1 diabetes is restored by sepiapterin. J Vasc Res 40:47–57, 2003.

160. Werner ER, et al: Tetrahydrobiopterin and nitric oxide: Mechanistic and pharmacological aspects. Exp Biol Med 228:1291–1302, 2003.

161. Farkas K, et al: Endothelial nitric oxide in diabetes mellitus: Too much or not enough? Diabetes Nutr Metab Clin Exper 13:287–297, 2000.

162. Maejima K, et al: Increased basal levels of plasma nitric oxide in type 2 diabetic subjects: Relationship to microvascular complications. J Diabetes Complications 15:135–143, 2001.

163. Ozden S, et al: Basal serum nitric oxide levels in patients with type 2 diabetes mellitus and different states of retinopathy. Can J Ophthalmol 38:393–396, 2003.

164. Pricci F, et al: Oxidative stress in diabetes-induced endothelial dysfunction involvement of nitric oxide and protein kinase C. Free Radic Biol Med 35:683–694, 2003.

165. Du Y, et al: Diabetes-induced nitrative stress in the retina, and correction by aminoguanidine. J Neurochem 80:771–779, 2002.

166. Chiarelli F, et al: Increased circulating nitric oxide in young patients with type 1 diabetes and persistent microalbuminuria: Relation to glomerular hyperfiltration. Diabetes 49:1258–1263, 2000.

167. Apakkan Aksun S, et al: Serum and urinary nitric oxide in type 2 diabetes with or without microalbuminuria: Relation to glomerular hyperfiltration. J Diabetes Complications 17:343–348, 2003.

168. Hiragushi K, et al: Nitric oxide system is involved in glomerular hyperfiltration in Japanese normo- and micro-albuminuric patients with type 2 diabetes. Diabetes Res Clin Prac 53:149–159, 2001.

169. Shankar SS, Steinberg HO: Obesity and endothelial dysfunction. Semin Vasc Med 5:56–64, 2005.

170. Potenza MA, et al: Insulin resistance in spontaneously hypertensive rats is associated with endothelial dysfunction characterized by imbalance between NO and ET-1 production. Am J Physiol Heart C 289:H813–H822, 2005.

171. Facchini FS, et al: Blood pressure, sodium intake, insulin resistance, and urinary nitrate excretion. Hypertension 33:1088–1012, 1999.

172. Williams IL, et al: Obesity, atherosclerosis and the vascular endothelium: Mechanisms of reduced nitric oxide bioavailability in obese humans. Int J Obesity 26:754–764, 2002.

173. Vincent MA, Montagnani M, Quon MJ: Molecular and physiologic actions of insulin related to production of nitric oxide in vascular endothelium. Cur Diab Rep 3:279–288, 2003.

174. Chien WY, et al: Increased plasma concentration of nitric oxide in type 2 diabetes but not in nondiabetic individuals with insulin resistance. Diabetes Metab 31:63–68, 2005.

175. Zavaroni I, et al: Plasma nitric oxide concentrations are elevated in insulin-resistant healthy subjects. Metabolism 49:959–961, 2000.

176. Colwell JA, et al: New concepts about the pathogenesis of atherosclerosis in diabetes mellitus. In Levin ME, O'Neal LW, Bowker JH (eds): The Diabetic Foot, 5th ed. St. Louis: Mosby Year Book, 1993, pp 79–114.

177. Scotland RS, et al: Investigation of vascular responses in endothelial nitric oxide synthase/cyclooxygenase-1 double-knockout mice: Key role for endothelium-derived hyperpolarizing factor in the regulation of blood pressure in vivo. Circulation 111:796–803, 2005.

178. Triggle CR, Ding H: Endothelium-derived hyperpolarizing factor: Is there a novel chemical mediator? Clin Experim Pharm Physiol 29:153–160, 2002.

179. Busse R, et al: EDHF: Bringing the concepts together. Trends Pharm Sci 23:374–380, 2002.

180. Cohen RA: The endothelium-derived hyperpolarizing factor puzzle: A mechanism without a mediator? Circulation 111:724–727, 2005.

181. Colwell JA, et al: Atherosclerosis and thrombosis in diabetes mellitus: New aspects of pathogenesis. In Bowker JH, Pfeifer MA (eds): The Diabetic Foot, 6th ed. St. Louis: Elsevier Health Sciences, 2000, pp 65–106.

182. Hashimoto T, et al: Lysophosphatidylcholine inhibits the expression of prostacyclin stimulating factor in cultured vascular smooth muscle cells. J Diab Complications 16:81–86, 2002.

183. Matsumoto K, et al: Impaired endothelial dysfunction in diabetes mellitus rats was restored by oral administration of prostaglandin I2 analogue. J Endocrinol 175:217–223, 2002.

184. Yamashita T, et al: Beraprost sodium, prostacyclin analogue, attenuates glomerular hyperfiltration and glomerular macrophage infiltration by modulating ecNOS expression in diabetic rats. Diabetes Res Clin Pract 57:149–161, 2002.

185. Aso Y, et al: Changes in skin blood flow in type 2 diabetes induced by prostacyclin: Association with ankle brachial index and plasma thrombomodulin levels. Metabolism 50:568–572, 2001.

186. Owada A, Suda S, Hata T: Effect of long-term administration of prostaglandin I(2) in incipient diabetic nephropathy. Nephron 92:788–796, 2002.

187. Goya K, et al: Effects of the prostaglandin I2 analogue, beraprost sodium, on vascular cell adhesion molecule-1 expression in human vascular endothelial cells and circulating vascular cell adhesion molecule-1 level in patients with type 2 diabetes mellitus. Metabolism 52:192–198, 2003.

188. Fu JY, et al: The induction and suppression of prostaglandin H2 synthase (cyclooxygenase) in human monocytes. J Biol Chem 265:16737–16740, 1990.

189. Konieczkowski M, Skrinska VA: Increased synthesis of thromboxane A2 and expression of procoagulant activity by monocytes in response to arachidonic acid in diabetes mellitus. Prostag Leukotr Essent Fatty Acids 65:133–138, 2001.

190. Fujiwara T, Ohsawa T, Takahashi S: Troglitazone, a new antidiabetic agent possessing radical scavenging ability, improved decreased skin blood flow in diabetic rats. Life Sci 63:2039–2047, 1998.

191. Hishinuma T, Yamazaki Y, Mizugaki M: Troglitazone has a reducing effect on thromboxane production. Prostag Lipid Mediat 62:135–143, 2000.

192. Yanagisawa M, et al: A novel potent vasoconstrictor peptide produced by vascular endothelial cells. Nature 332:411–415, 1988.

193. Markewitz BA, Michael JR, Kohan DE: Endothelin-1 inhibits the expression of inducible nitric oxide synthase. Am J Physiol 272:L1078–L1083, 1997.

194. Khan AS, Chakrabarti S: Endothelins in chronic diabetic complications. Can J Physiol Pharmacol 81:622–634, 2003.

195. Mather KJ, et al: Interactions between endothelin and nitric oxide in the regulation of vascular tone in obesity and diabetes. Diabetes 53:2060–2066, 2004.

196. Lam H-C, et al: Role of endothelin in diabetic retinopathy. Curr Vasc Pharm 1:243–250, 2003.

197. Schram MT, Stehouwer CDA: Endothelial dysfunction, cellular adhesion molecules and the metabolic syndrome. Horm Metab Res 37(suppl 1):49–55, 2005.

198. Blankenberg S, Barbaux S, Tiret L: Adhesion molecules and atherosclerosis. Atherosclerosis 170:191–203, 2003.

199. Leeuwenberg JF, et al: E-selectin and intracellular adhesion molecule-1 are released by activated human endothelial cells in vitro. Immunology 77:543–549, 1992.

200. Schmidt AM, et al: Advanced glycation endproducts interacting with their endothelial receptor induce expression of vascular cell adhesion molecule-1 (VACM-1) in cultured human endothelial cells and in mice: A potential mechanism of the accelerated vasculopathy of diabetes. J Clin Invest 96:1395–1403, 1995.

201. Schram MT, et al: The EURODIAB Prospective Complications Study Group: Vascular risk factors and markers of endothelial function as determinants of inflammatory markers in type 1 diabetes. Diab Care 26:2165–2173, 2003.

202. Stehouwer DC, et al: Increased urinary albumin excretion, endothelial dysfunction, and chronic low-grade inflammation in type 2 diabetes: Progressive, interrelated, and independently associated with risk of death. Diabetes 51:1157–1165, 2002.

203. Berenson GS, et al: Association between multiple cardiovascular risk factors and atherosclerosis in children and young adults: The Bogalusa Heart Study. N Engl J Med 338:1650–1656, 1998.

204. Glowinska B, et al: Soluble adhesion molecules (sICAM-1, sVCAM-1) and selectins (sE selectin, sP selectin, sL selectin) levels in children and adolescents with obesity, hypertension, and diabetes. Metab Clin Exper 54:1020–1026, 2005.

205. Kowalska I, et al: Circulating E-selectin, vascular cell adhesion molecule-1, and intercellular adhesion molecule-1 in men with coronary artery disease assessed by angiography and disturbances of carbohydrate metabolism. Metabolism 51:733–736, 2002.

206. Schram MT, Stehouwer CDA: Endothelial dysfunction, cellular adhesion molecules and the metabolic syndrome. Horm Metab Res 37(suppl 1):49–55, 205.

207. Lyons TJ, Jenkins AJ: Glycation, oxidation and lipoxidation in the development of the complications of diabetes mellitus: A "carbonyl stress" hypothesis. Diabetes Rev 5:365–391, 1997.

208. Lyons TJ: Glycation, carbonyl stress, EAGLEs, and the vascular complications of diabetes. Sem Vasc Med 2:175–189, 2002.

209. Hamlin CR, Kohn RR: Evidence for progressive, age-related structural changes in post-mature human collagen. Biochim Biophys Acta 236:458–467, 1971.

210. Lyons TJ, et al: Decrease in skin collagen glycosylation with improved glycemic control in patients with insulin-dependent diabetes mellitus. J Clin Invest 87:1910–1915, 1991.

211. Monnier VM, et al: Relations between complications to type I diabetes mellitus and collagen-linked fluorescence. N Engl J Med 314:403–408, 1986.

212. Oxlund H, et al: Increased aortic stiffness in patients with type 1 (insulin-dependent) diabetes mellitus. Diabetologia 32:748–752, 1989.

213. Hicks M, et al: Increase in crosslinking of nonenzymatically glycosylated collagen induced by products of lipid peroxidation. Arch Biochem Biophys 268:249–254, 1989.

214. Requena JR, et al: Lipoxidation products as biomarkers of oxidative damage to proteins during lipid peroxidation reactions. Nephrol Dial Transplant 11(suppl 5):48–53, 1996.

215. Song W, et al: Effect of native LDL and modified LDL on mRNA expression of genes in human retinal pericytes. Invest Ophthalmol Vis Sci 46:2974–82, 2005.

216. Kirstein M, et al: Advanced protein glycosylation induces transendothelial human monocyte chemotaxis and secretion of platelet-derived growth factor: Role in vascular disease of diabetes and aging. Proc Natl Acad Sci U S A 87:9010–9014, 1990.

217. Vlassara H, Brownlee M, Cerami A: Novel macrophage receptor for glucose-modified proteins is distinct from previously described scavenger receptors. J Exp Med 164:1301–1309, 1986.

218. Vlassara H, et al: Advanced glycosylation end products on erythrocyte cell surface induce receptor-mediated phagocytosis by macrophages: A model for turnover of aging cells. J Exp Med 166:539–549, 1987.

219. Hudson BI, et al: Diabetic vascular disease: It's all the RAGE. Antioxid Redox Signal 7:1588–600, 2005.

220. Valencia JV, et al: Divergent pathways of gene expression are activated by the RAGE ligands S100b and AGE-BSA. Diabetes 53:743–751, 2004.

221. Ichikawa K, et al: Advanced glycosylation end products induced tissue factor expression in human monocytes. Diabetes 45(suppl 2):128A, 1996.

222. Imani F, et al: Advanced glycosylation endproduct-specific receptors on human and rat T-lymphocytes mediate synthesis of interferon gamma: Role in tissue remodeling. J Exp Med 178:2165–2172, 1993.

223. Throckmorton DC, et al: PDGF and TGF-beta mediate collagen production by mesangial cells exposed to advanced glycosylation end products. Kidney Int 48:111–117, 1995.

224. Chibber R, Molinatti PA, Kohner EM: Potential role of glucose-mediated proteins in the pathogenesis of diabetic retinopathy. Diabetes 45(suppl 2):15A, 1996.

225. Stitt AW, et al: Intracellular advanced glycation endproducts (AGEs) co-localize with AGE-receptors in the retinal vasculature of diabetic and AGE-infused rats. Diabetes 45(suppl 2):15A, 1996.

226. Yamagishi S, et al: Receptor-mediated toxicity to pericytes of advanced glycosylation end products: A possible mechanism of pericyte loss in diabetic microangiopathy. Biochem Biophys Res Commun 213:681–687, 1995.

227. Hori O, et al: Advanced glycation endproducts interacting with their endothelial receptor induce expression of vascular cell adhesion molecule-1 (VCAM-1) in cultured human endothelial cells and in mice: A potential mechanism for the accelerated vasculopathy of diabetes. J Clin Invest 96:1395–1403, 1995.

228. Hudson BI, Schmidt AM: RAGE: A novel target for drug intervention in diabetic vascular disease. Pharm Res 7:1079–86, 2004.

229. Wautier JL, et al: Receptor-mediated endothelial cell dysfunction in diabetic vasculopathy: Soluble receptor for advanced glycation end products blocks hyperpermeability in diabetic rats. J Clin Invest 97:238–243, 1996.

230. Makita Z, et al: Advanced glycosylation end products in patients with diabetic nephropathy. N Engl J Med 325:836–842, 1991.

231. McCance DR, et al: Maillard reaction products and their relation to complications in insulin dependent diabetes mellitus. J Clin Invest 91:2470–2478, 1993.

232. Sell DR, et al: Pentosidine formation in skin correlates with severity of complications in individuals with long-standing IDDM. Diabetes 41:1286–1292, 1992.

233. Vlassara H, et al: Advanced glycation end products induce glomerular sclerosis and albuminuria in normal rats. Proc Natl Acad Sci U S A 91:11704–11708, 1994.

234. Yang CW, et al: Administration of AGEs in vivo induces genes implicated in diabetic glomerulosclerosis. Kidney Int 49:S55–S58, 1995.

235. Abel M, et al: Expression of receptors for advanced glycosylated end-products in renal disease. Nephrol Dial Transplant 10:1662–1667, 1995.

236. Beisswenger PJ, et al: Susceptibility to diabetic nephropathy is related to dicarbonyl and oxidative stress. Diabetes 54:3274–3281, 2005.

237. Genuth S, et al: Glycation and carboxymethyllysine levels in skin collagen predict the risk of future 10-year progression of diabetic retinopathy and nephropathy in the diabetes control and complications trial and epidemiology of diabetes interventions and complications participants with Type 1 diabetes. Diabetes 54:3103–3111, 2005.

238. Writing Team for the Diabetes Control and Complications Trial/Epidemiology of Diabetes Interventions and Complications Research Group: Effect of intensive therapy on the microvascular complications of type 1 diabetes nellitus. JAMA 287:2563–2569, 2002.

239. Reaven P, et al: Effects of oleate-rich and linoleate-rich diets on the susceptibility of low density lipoprotein to oxidative modification in mildly hypercholesterolemic subjects. J Clin Invest 91:668–676, 1993.

240. Colhoun HM, et al: On behalf of the CARDS investigators. Rapid emergence of effect of atorvastatin on cardiovascular outcomes in the Collaborative Atorvastatin Diabetes Study (CARDS). Diabetologia 48:2482–2485, 2005.

241. Frei B, England L, Ames BN: Ascorbate is an outstanding antioxidant in human plasma. Proc Natl Acad Sci U S A 86:6377–6381, 1989.

242. Jennings PE, et al: Vitamin C metabolites and microangiopathy in diabetes mellitus. Diabetes Res 6:151–154, 1987.

243. Karpen CW, et al: Production of 12 HETE and vitamin E status in platelets from type 1 human diabetic subjects. Diabetes 34:526–531, 1985.

244. Young IS, Torney JJ, Trimble ER: The effect of ascorbate supplementation on oxidative stress in the streptozotocin diabetic rat. Free Radic Biol Med 13:41–46, 1992.

245. Bowry VW, Stocker R: Vitamin E in human low-density lipoprotein: When and how this antioxidant becomes a pro-oxidant. Biochem J 288:341–344, 1992.

246. Parthasarathy S, et al: Probucol inhibits oxidative modification of low density lipoprotein. J Clin Invest 77:641–644, 1986.

247. Carew TE, Schwenke DC, Steinberg D: Antiatherogenic effect of probucol unrelated to its hypocholesterolemic effect: Evidence that antioxidants in vivo can selectively inhibit low density lipoprotein degradation in macrophage-rich fatty streaks and slow the progression of atherosclerosis in the Watanabe heritable hyperlipidemic rabbit. Proc Natl Acad Sci U S A 84:7725–7729, 1987.

248. Kita T, et al: Probucol prevents the progression of atherosclerosis in Watanabe heritable hyperlipidemic rabbit, an animal model for familial hypercholesterolemia. Proc Natl Acad Sci U S A 84:5928–5931, 1987.

249. Kuzuya M, et al: Probucol prevents oxidative injury to endothelial cells. J Lipid Res 32:197–204, 1991.

250. Björkhem I, et al: The antioxidant butylated hydroxytoluene protects against atherosclerosis. Arterioscler Thromb 11:15–22, 1991.

251. Freyschuss A, et al: Antioxidant treatment inhibits the development of intimal thickening after balloon injury of the aorta in hypercholesterolemic rabbits. J Clin Invest 91:1282–1288, 1993.

252. Thomas SR, Neuzil J, Stocker R: Cosupplementation with coenzyme Q prevents the prooxidant effect of α-tocopherol and increases the resistance of LDL to transition metal-dependent oxidation initiation. Arterioscler Thromb Vasc Biol 16:687–696, 1996.

253. Coffey MD, et al: In vitro cell injury by oxidized low density lipoprotein involves lipid hydroperoxide-induced formation of alkoxyl, lipid, and peroxyl radicals. J Clin Invest 96:1866–1873, 1995.

254. Brownlee M, et al: Aminoguanidine prevents diabetes-induced arterial wall protein cross-linking. Science 232:1629–1632, 1986.

255. Bucala R, Cerami A: Phospholipids react with glucose to initiate advanced glycosylation and fatty acid oxidation: Inhibition of lipid advanced glycosylation and oxidation by aminoguanidine. Diabetes 41(suppl 1):23A, 1992.

256. Bucala R, et al: Inhibition of advanced glycosylation by aminoguanidine reduces plasma LDL levels in diabetes. Clin Res 41:183A, 1993.

257. Lyons TJ, Li W: Aminoguanidine and the cytotoxicity of modified LDL to retinal capillary endothelial cells. Diabetes 43(suppl 1):112A, 1994.

258. Hammes HP, et al: Aminoguanidine inhibits the development of accelerated diabetic retinopathy in the spontaneous hypertensive rat. Diabetologia 37:32–35, 1994.

259. Hammes HP, et al: Aminoguanidine treatment inhibits the development of experimental diabetic retinopathy. Proc Natl Acad Sci U S A 88:11555–11558, 1991.

260. Hammes HP, et al: Secondary intervention with aminoguanidine retards the progression of diabetic retinopathy in the rat model. Diabetologia 38:656–660, 1995.

261. Edelstein D, Brownlee M: Rapid communication: Aminoguanidine ameliorates albuminuria in diabetic hypertensive rats. Diabetologia 35:96–97, 1992.

262. Soulis-Liparota T, et al: Retardation by aminoguanidine of development of albuminuria, mesangial expansion, and tissue fluorescence in streptozotocin-induced diabetic rat. Diabetes 40:1328–1334, 1991.

263. Cameron NE, et al: Effects of aminoguanidine on peripheral nerve function and polyol pathway metabolites in streptozotocin diabetic rats. Diabetologia 35:946–950, 1992.

264. Kihara M, et al: Aminoguanidine effects on nerve blood flow, vascular permeability, electrophysiology, and oxygen free radicals. Proc Natl Acad Sci U S A 88:6107–6111, 1991.

265. Bolton WK, et al: Randomized trial of an inhibitor of formation of advance glycation end products in diabetic Nephropathy. Am J Nephrol 24:32–40, 2004.

266. Burch RM, et al: N-(fluorenyl-9-methoxycarbonyl) amino acids, a class of anti-inflammatory agents with a different mechanism of action. Proc Natl Acad Sci U S A 88:355–359, 1991.

267. Navab M, et al: A new anti-inflammatory compound, Leumedin, inhibits modification of low density lipoprotein and the resulting monocyte transmigration into the subendothelial space of cocultures of human aortic wall cells. J Clin Invest 91:1225–1230, 1993.

268. Stitt A, Gardiner TA, et al: The AGE inhibitor pyridoxamine inhibits development of retinopathy in experimental diabetes. Diabetes 51:2826–2832, 2002.

269. Degenhardt TO, et al: Pyridoxamine inhibits early renal disease and dyslipidemia in the streptozotocin-diabetic rat. Kidney Int 61:939–950, 2002.

270. Thallas-Bonke V, et al: Attenuation of extracellular matrix accumulation in diabetic nephropathy by the advanced glycation end product cross-link breaker ALT-711 via a protein kinase C-dependent pathway. Diabetes 53:2921–2930, 2004.

271. Li YM, et al: Opsonization and removal of serum AGEs by coupling to lysozyme. Diabetes 45(suppl 2):239A, 1996.

272. Mitsuhashi T, et al: Depletion of reactive advanced glycation end-products (AGEs) from diabetic uremic sera by a lysozyme-linked matrix. Diabetes 45(suppl 2): 47A, 1996.

273. Vasan S, et al: Design, synthesis, and pharmacological activity of a novel class of thiazolium-based compounds that cleave established AGE-derived protein crosslinks. Diabetes 45(suppl 2):28A, 1996.

274. Steinberg D: Antioxidants and atherosclerosis: A current assessment. Circulation 84:1420–1425, 1991.

275. Smith MA, et al: Advanced Maillard reaction end products, free radicals, and protein oxidation in Alzheimer's disease. Ann N Y Acad Sci 738:447–454, 1994.

276. Calzada C, et al: 12(S)-hydroperoxyeicosatetraenoic acid increases arachidonic acid availability in collagen-primed platelets. J Lipid Res 42:1467–1473, 2001.

277. Fibrinogen Studies Collaboration: Plasma fibrinogen level and the risk of major cardiovascular diseases and nonvascular mortality: An individual participant meta-analysis. JAMA 294:1799–1809, 2005.

278. Klein RL, et al: Fibrinogen is a marker for nephropathy and peripheral vascular disease in type 1 diabetes: Studies of plasma fibrinogen and fibrinogen gene polymorphism in the DCCT/EDIC cohort. Diabetes Care 26:1439–1448, 2003.

279. Jones RL: Fibrinopeptide-A in diabetes mellitus. Diabetes 34:836–843, 1985.

280. Paramo JA, et al: Prothrombin fragment 1+2 is associated with carotid intima-media thickness in subjects free of clinical cardiovascular disease. Stroke 35:1085–1089, 2004.

281. Ceriello A, et al: Hyperglycemia-induced thrombin formation in diabetes: The possible role of oxidative stress. Diabetes 44:924–928, 1995.

282. Ceriello A, et al: Fibrinogen plasma levels as a marker of thrombin activation in diabetes. Diabetes 43:430–432, 1994.

283. Villanueva GB, Allen N: Demonstration of altered antithrombin III activity due to nonenzymatic glycosylation at glucose concentration expected to be encountered in severely diabetic patients. Diabetes 37:1103–1107, 1988.

284. Pandolfi A, et al: Plasminogen activator inhibitor type 1 is increased in the arterial wall of type II diabetic subjects. Arterioscler Thromb Vasc Biol 21:1378–1382, 2001.

285. Colwell JA, Halushka PV: Platelet function in diabetes mellitus. Br J Haematol 44:521–526, 1980.

286. Ostermann H, van de Loo J: Factors of the haemostatic system in diabetic patients: A survey of controlled studies. Haemostasis 16:386–416, 1986.

287. Antiplatelet Trialists' Collaboration: Collaborative overview of randomized trials of antiplatelet therapy: I. Prevention of death,

myocardial infarction, and stroke by prolonged antiplatelet therapy in various categories of patients. BMJ 308:81–106, 1994.

288. Antiplatelet Trialists' Collaboration: Collaborative meta-analysis of randomized trials of antiplatelet therapy for prevention of death, myocardial infarction, and stroke in high risk patients. BMJ 324:71–86, 2002.

289. Colwell JA: Aspirin therapy in diabetes. Diabetes 20:1767–71, 1997.

290. Sanmuganathan PS, et al: Aspirin for primary prevention of coronary heart disease: Safety and absolute benefit related to coronary risk derived from meta-analysis of randomized trials. Heart 85:265–71, 2001.

THE BIOMECHANICS OF THE FOOT IN DIABETES MELLITUS

PETER R. CAVANAGH AND JAN S. ULBRECHT ■

Introduction

The aim of this chapter is to provide a biomechanical framework on which an understanding of the causes, treatment, and prevention of foot injury in patients with diabetes can be built. Although peripheral vascular disease has long been implicated in lower-limb problems in the diabetic patient, it is now well recognized that the majority of injuries to the foot, principally ulcers, are a consequence of mechanical trauma that the patient does not recognize because of neuropathy. Diabetes-related distal symmetric polyneuropathy results in a loss of protective sensation, and subsequently, a number of biomechanical risk factors conspire to cause injury. Thus, biomechanics has great relevance to neuropathic injury.[1-4]

Most skin injuries that are seen on the feet of patients with diabetic neuropathy occur in the forefoot, with approximately equal distribution on the dorsal and plantar surfaces.[5] Those on the plantar surface are frequently at sites of high pressure under the foot.[6-12] Many of the ulcers on the dorsum are at sites of high pressure at which the patient's footwear creates a lesion,[13] meaning that the majority of foot ulcers have, in large part, a biomechanical etiology. This has been known for some time, owing mainly to the writing of Brand and his colleagues,[14,15] who emphasized the role of repetitive stress in foot injury. Subsequent developments have shown that biomechanics can make a significant contribution to managing the foot in diabetes. Tools are available to make measurements of pressure under the bare foot during walking and, more important, to make measurements inside the shoes of patients who have been prescribed footwear to prevent

ulceration or reulceration. There has been rapid growth in the understanding of why people with diabetes have higher pressures under their feet than do those without diabetes. The topic of shear stress as a possible mechanism of skin injury is being revisited, and the biomechanical consequences of peripheral neuropathy for posture and gait are being explored. Experimental determinations of tissue properties are expanding our knowledge of the effects of diabetes on the mechanical behavior of skin, collagen, and adipose tissue, and objective assessment of footwear designs is providing an understanding of how best to intervene to prevent or treat injury. Evidence dealing with all of these issues (Table 6-1) will be presented in this chapter. It is also extremely important that biomechanical issues be considered when new treatments for wounds on diabetic feet are being evaluated.[16]

In this chapter, and on the DVD that accompanies the book, we describe how the forces that injure the foot are generated, how they may cause injury, and how they might be measured and modified to achieve healing and, better still, to prevent injury. Our concentration is on the topics on which evidence is available to support our assertions. However, by necessity, we also mention a number of areas that are in need of further biomechanical study, and we will attempt to provide some hypotheses to guide such study. We intend to keep this chapter firmly directed at clinical reality, because a frequent (and usually valid) criticism of biomechanical and bioengineering texts is their inaccessibility to clinicians. After a brief discussion of the mechanics of gait and a review of plantar pressure measurement, we discuss the mechanical factors that are

TABLE 6-1   A Summary of the Evidence for Biomechanical Factors Involved in the Processes of Ulceration, Healing, and Prevention

Factor	References
Ulceration	
Elevated peak plantar pressure: a major risk factor	6, 7, 11, 12, 88
Factors affecting peak barefoot plantar pressure	
Thickness of plantar tissue	130, 131, 153
Foot deformity	112, 114
Callus	106, 161
Limited joint mobility	151, 152
Body weight (low correlation)	27, 114
Gait parameters (speed, stride length, etc.)	112
Tissue changes from prior ulceration	161
Threshold normal pressure for injury (estimated at 750 kPa)	83
Pressure-induced dorsal injury is caused by footwear	13
Hallux pressure during turning may be significantly higher than during straight walking	95
Elevated pressure causes tissue ischemia	Studies in progress
Shear stress contributes to neuropathic injury	Studies in progress
Ulcer Healing	
Pressure relief is required	228
The total-contact cast is effective at pressure relief and healing	59, 229, 244
Other pressure relief devices	264
Ideal healing rates can be predicted	230
Ulcer Prevention	
Appropriate footwear reduces plantar pressure	43, 68, 75, 292, 301, 320, 328, 344
Socks reduce plantar pressure	337
Removal of callus reduces plantar pressure	106
In-shoe pressure facilitates footwear modification	72, 73
Shear stress can be modified by proper footwear fit	Studies in progress
Prophylactic metatarsal head resection is associated with acute Charcot foot	408

kPa, kilopascal.

responsible for the development of foot injuries in diabetes. Following a consideration of the role of unloading in ulcer healing, we turn to the mechanics of footwear. Finally, we discuss some issues in clinical biomechanics, including what to look for in a foot examination. We conclude with a discussion of the role of surgery in altering the biomechanics of the foot.

Gait: Internal and External Mechanics

Why Study Gait Mechanics?

Most foot injuries occur while the patient is walking and are caused by the forces that are generated during gait. Thus, a natural place to begin the discussion of injury is with an overview of the mechanics of gait. When we watch a patient ambulate in the clinic, we are attempting to assess certain aspects of the external mechanics of the patient's gait. What we actually see are the limb movements in space, which bear little relationship to the most important quantities in the current context, that is, the injurious stresses in the tissue, which could be labeled the internal mechanics. Yet it is worth dwelling briefly on the external mechanics of gait, because observation and, preferably, measurement can sometimes provide insight into the reasons for high forces and pressures during gait.

Kinematics

A number of techniques are available to track the spatial position of targets attached to segments of the lower limb during gait.[17–19] Most commonly, reflective markers are used and tracked by high-speed videography (Fig. 6-1A). This method, called motion capture, allows joint motion in the foot to be measured quantitatively during normal function rather than depending on inferences from a static examination. For example, the pattern of dorsiflexion and plantarflexion of the first metatarsophalangeal (MTP) joint in a diabetic patient during gait is shown in Figure 6-1B. Very few such measurements of foot movement in diabetes have actually been performed to date, although the techniques are widely used in orthopedic biomechanics for the study of conditions such as cerebral palsy[20,21] and joint replacement.[22,23]

The example just chosen is quite relevant to the current context, because plantar ulceration of the hallux is a common occurrence in patients with diabetic neuropathy.[24,25] Dorsiflexion at the first MTP joint is essential during the toe-off phase of gait. When the ability of that joint to dorsiflex is mechanically limited, very high pressure must be expected under the hallux during toe off, a common finding in patients who ulcerate in this region (Fig. 6-1C). An understanding of the necessary range of dorsiflexion of the first MTP joint during gait, taken together with a static measurement of dorsiflexion at that joint, can provide insight into why high plantar pressure may occur at that particular site.

Forces at the Foot

Although the likelihood of high pressure between a region of the foot and the ground can be inferred from an analysis of movement, as described earlier, neither the eye nor the most sophisticated video analysis system can measure these forces and pressures, because it is only the consequences of force that can actually be "seen." The area of mechanics in which the forces that cause movement are studied is called *kinetics*, whereas the label *kinematics* is applied to studies (e.g., those described earlier) in which the movement per se is measured. The most frequently measured and studied forces are the external forces between the foot and either the ground or the footwear. Less frequently, internal forces in tissues or

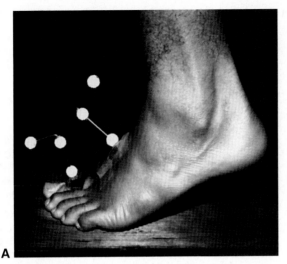

A

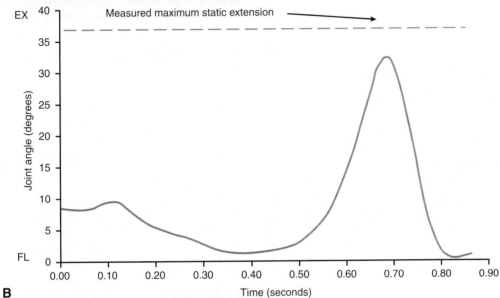

B

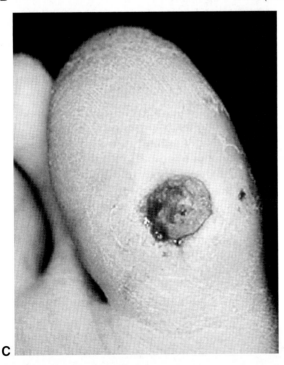

C

Figure 6–1 **A,** Foot with targets attached for automated video analysis of motion of the first metatarsophalangeal joint (MTPJ1). At least three targets must be placed on each segment of interest (or on a base firmly attached to it). If the targets are visible in two or more video cameras, the three-dimensional locations of the targets can be obtained automatically by computer analysis of the resulting images and the unique position of the segment in space can be determined. **B,** Dynamic flexion-extension pattern of MTPJ1 during slow barefoot walking in a patient with diabetic neuropathy and limited joint mobility. Measurements were made by using automated analysis of video, as described above. The *dashed line* represents the maximum extension (37 degrees) measured statically during physical examination. Note that the maximum dynamic value is approximately 90% of the static value. EX, extension; FL, flexion. **C,** An ulcer under the hallux in a patient with limited joint mobility of MTPJ1.

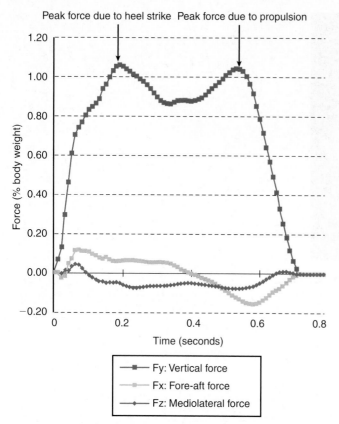

Figure 6-2 shows:
Peak force due to heel strike   Peak force due to propulsion

Legend:
- Fy: Vertical force
- Fx: Fore-aft force
- Fz: Mediolateral force

Figure 6-2 Three components of ground reaction force underneath one foot during a single step. The step begins with heel strike at time 0 and ends with toe off. The three components of the force are fore-aft shear component (Fx), vertical component (Fy), and mediolateral shear component (Fz). Note that the vertical component is six times larger than the anteroposterior shear and 15 times larger than the mediolateral shear. The *left arrow* marks the peak vertical force after heel strike; the *right arrow* marks the peak vertical force during the late part of the step cycle and is used for calculation of pressure as shown in Figure 6-3.

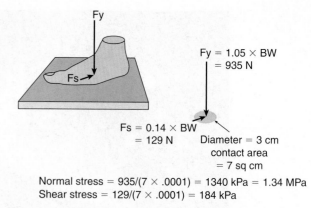

$Fy = 1.05 \times BW = 935$ N

$Fs = 0.14 \times BW = 129$ N

Diameter = 3 cm
contact area = 7 sq cm

Normal stress = $935/(7 \times .0001) = 1340$ kPa = 1.34 MPa
Shear stress = $129/(7 \times .0001) = 184$ kPa

Figure 6-3 Schematic of a rocker-bottom Charcot foot in contact with the ground during the late-support phase of gait at the instant shown by the *right arrow* in Figure 6-2. If the contact area is assumed to be circular with a diameter of 3 cm, the normal stress will be 1.34 MPa, and the shear stress will be 184 kPa. BW, body weight; Fs, net shear force; Fy, vertical force.

forces between the articulating surfaces of joints can be measured, estimated, or modeled.

When the foot strikes the ground in gait, Newton's third law tells us that equal forces will be experienced by both the foot and the ground. Because it is more convenient to measure the force with an instrument mounted on the ground than on the foot, a device called a "force platform" is frequently found in gait laboratories. As is demonstrated in Figure 6-2, the force measured by a force platform during a single foot contact is usually expressed in three components: vertical (or normal, to use the engineering term), anteroposterior shear, and mediolateral.

Pressure: The Harm Done by Force

The forces shown in Figure 6-2 can be thought of as the mechanical input to the foot, yet their magnitude does not necessarily reflect the risk of injury. As the late Paul Brand so aptly said, "Pressure is the critical quantity that determines the harm done by the force."[26] The link between force and pressure is, of course, the area of

force application. Much more damage can be done by a force transmitted through a few plantar prominences than by the same force distributed over a larger area of the plantar surface. Consequently, plantar pressure measurement is a topic of critical interest in the field of diabetes-related foot injury, and we examine below the way in which such measurement can be achieved.

Average pressure is calculated by dividing the applied force by the area over which it acts. What is widely called *plantar pressure* in the diabetes literature is known in mechanical terms as *normal stress:* "stress" because it is the result of force applied to a defined area and "normal" because it is measured at right angles to the supporting surface. Shear stress is calculated in the same manner but using the magnitude of the shear force and its area of application, which may be the same as that for the normal stress. For example, consider the effects of the peak ground reaction forces shown in Figure 6-2 on a rocker-bottom foot with concentrated force application to a midfoot prominence. As is shown in Figure 6-3, the calculation leads directly to estimates of large "normal" and "shear" stresses. In practice, however, the areas of application are rarely known, and as we have previously shown,[27] similar calculations of pressures based on body weight or ground reaction forces and total foot area are not valid because "effective foot area" is much smaller than the area of the footprint. Plantar pressure must therefore be measured directly rather than being estimated. Although plantar pressure is routinely measured in all patients in the senior author's diabetic foot clinic, we are still frequently surprised by the discrepancies between our preconceptions of how a particular foot functions and the evidence from direct plantar pressure measurement. Identifying a clinically apparent plantar bony prominence does not guarantee that a high pressure exists in that region; conversely, and more important, the absence of any obvious bony deformity is no guarantee that low pressures are exerted on the region.

Plantar Pressure Measurement

Devices Used

Methods for the measurement of plantar pressure have been discussed in detail by ourselves and others.[28–33] Many devices for barefoot and in-shoe plantar pressure measurement are commercially available,[30,34,35] and all of them require the use of a computer and usually proprietary software. Although several different principles of measurement of pressure are used in the manufacture of the sensors that make up the devices,[30] in the majority, a matrix of transducers is used. For barefoot measurement, the patient walks onto the platform and continues walking. In this situation, information from a single foot contact is collected. For in-shoe measurement, the matrix of transducers is manufactured into a thin, pliable "insole," which is placed in the shoe in direct contact with the foot. In this case, information from multiple steps can be obtained.[30]

Two other devices for measuring plantar pressure have been proposed; both are simple and do not require a computer. The first has a single discrete sensor and a voltage meter.[36] No validation of this approach has yet appeared. The second, called the Podotrack®, is in the tradition of the Harris mat[37] and gives a "semiquantitative" estimate of pressure distribution.[38] It consists of a three-layer sandwich on which the patient's foot leaves an impression in different shades of gray. The device was found to be highly specific (>92% for three independent observers) but not very sensitive (32%, 36%, and 69% for three observers). Thus, the probability of underestimating pressure was high. In a later study,[39] the same authors found that training the observers could increase sensitivity to greater than 90%. Vijay and colleagues[40] have reported on the use of this device in a clinical setting.

When any of these instruments is used, attention must be given to many technical considerations: dynamic range, sampling rate, spatial resolution, frequency response, linearity, hysteresis, temperature sensitivity, reliability, and reproducibility. All these factors have been reviewed elsewhere.[31,32] Of particular importance is an understanding of the relevance of effective sensor size on the pressure measured. Generally speaking, the smaller the sensor, the larger is the apparent pressure recorded in the same region of the same foot.[31–34] Thus, normative data must be developed specifically for each instrument that is used and such data cannot be interchanged.

This important point has been investigated theoretically by Lord.[41] Starting with data from an optical pedobarograph with a spatial resolution of approximately 400 pixels per square centimeter, she then created virtual sensors of progressively increasing dimensions to model the effect of transducer size and demonstrated that a sensor with dimensions of 10×10 mm is likely to underestimate the actual plantar pressure (as measured by the optical pedobarograph) by 30% to 40%. In a similar study, Davis and colleagues[42] found that sensors with an effective size of greater than approximately 6×6 mm would result in significant error in the estimate of pressure compared to a device with 5- $\times$ 5-mm sensors.

This unfortunate situation, in which different results are obtained from the same foot under the same conditions, is analogous to that in which falsely high blood pressures are obtained with inappropriately small blood pressure cuffs. This state of affairs is unlikely to be resolved in the near future unless manufacturers agree on standard platform characteristics. Unfortunately, a single correction factor to convert estimates from two different systems to a common base will not be appropriate for all regions of the foot. This is because in systems with large area sensors, a pressure that is applied to a small area (such as a prominent metatarsal head [MTH] will be effectively averaged over a whole large element and will be irreversibly represented as a lower pressure. However, for a region in which pressure is more evenly distributed (such as the heel), two devices with different element sizes will provide approximately the same estimates, and no correction factor will be required. Perry and colleagues[43] made region-by-region corrections to compare pressures measured during barefoot and shod walking using different devices. Only a few comparisons of different devices have been performed.[44,45]

Several devices have been proposed to measure the distribution of shear stress under the foot,[46–49] and the role of shear stresses has also been modeled.[50] However, no single device has yet been demonstrated to have the resolution and durability that are required to understand the presumably complex pattern of plantar shear stresses.

Footwear that offers the possibility of measuring a number of different modalities has been proposed by Mueller and his colleagues,[51,52] who developed an in-shoe device to measure temperature, pressure, humidity, and step count.

Data Collection Issues

Also to be considered for accurate plantar pressure measurement are several aspects of the data collection process that will affect the results. These include stride length (natural or mandated), speed of walking (natural or mandated), and whether first step or midgait have been used.[53,54] In our daily clinical use, we prefer to make the step as "normal" as possible for the subject at that point in time. We recognize that step length and speed will affect plantar pressure; however, we believe that in a clinical setting, measuring the consequences of a "normal" step for that patient at a given point in time is more meaningful than attempting to make the subjects conform to a set of conditions that might be unnatural for them. However, speed can be critically important in making comparisons between different types of footwear, since peak pressure is a function of speed.[55] If the patient chooses to walk more slowly during trials with one particular type of shoes, this can lead to the incorrect impression that the footwear is responsible for the observed reduction in plantar pressure.

Bus and de Lange[53] have studied different methods of collecting plantar pressure and have shown that allowing neuropathic patients to take one or two steps prior to contacting the platform can produce acceptable results. These patients needed the fewest repeat trials with the two-step protocol. Similar experiments have been conducted by Peters and colleagues,[56] who reported comparable peak pressures using the one- and three-step approaches. There were, however, differences in other measures (contact time, pressure-time integral). In general, the one-step protocol was more repeatable.

In their studies of the total-contact cast (TCC), Shaw and colleagues[57] made sure that speed and step length were maintained between conditions, whereas Fleischli and colleagues,[58] Lavery and colleagues,[59] and Baumhauer and colleagues[60] allowed the subjects in their studies of different healing devices to choose their own speed for each of the conditions. Both methods are legitimate, but the results of the studies must be interpreted with these conditions in mind. Shaw and colleagues[57] wanted to understand how a TCC functions and to separate the effects of speed and stride length from those of the cast itself; the other authors were interested in observing the full clinical effect of the intervention being studied.

In our barefoot studies, we have chosen to look at the average of five "first steps,"[32] whereas for in-shoe testing, we average many (approximately 30) steps during normal gait. The reliability of in-shoe pressure measurements was investigated in symptom-free subjects by Kernozek and colleagues.[61] Subjects walked on a treadmill at three speeds. Reliabilities greater than 0.9 in the estimates of peak pressure and force-time integral were achieved by the analysis of data from only eight steps. Putti and colleagues[34] made repeated in-shoe pressure measurements on 50 subjects wearing running shoes, with a 12-day interval between testing sessions. They found a maximum of 15.3% variability (as measured by a coefficient of repeatability) in more than 100 separate variables.

Young and colleagues[62] have shown that plantar callus can significantly increase plantar pressure during walking. It is therefore important that any testing of plantar pressure be preceded by the patient's normal callus care—usually removal by sharp debridement.

Data Analysis

We will now illustrate the collection and analysis of plantar pressure by an example of a patient who has experienced recurrent ulceration under the left first MTP joint. The results of barefoot plantar pressure measurement are shown in Figure 6-4. Note that forefoot pressures are relatively moderate (<400 kilopascals [kPa])

at all sites except MTH1, where a sustained load is applied from before heel off until the end of stance. At approximately 76% of contact time this peak reaches a magnitude greater than 1130 kPa, which is the limit of measurement of the device. The results should be compared to the normal values of 299 kPa (± 137 kPa) for MTH1 reported by Rosenbaum and colleagues[55] for the same device during normal-speed walking (see the discussion of normal values below).

Peak Pressure Plot

It is not yet customary to include digitized movie images of movements in patient charts (although it is entirely feasible to do so on a Web-based client, and it could become routine once all medical records are computerized). Thus, some distillation must be made from the 60 or more images of pressure that are available every second. The peak pressure plot shown in Figure 6-5 is often chosen for this purpose. This plot was created by simply retaining the largest pressure that every sensor on the platform experienced during the entire contact phase. It can be an extremely useful plot, since the peak loading of each region can be seen in a single picture.

Regional Analysis Using Masks

A further derivation from Figure 6-5 is to divide the foot into a number of anatomic regions or masks for a so-called regional analysis. This requires the construction of the masks shown in Figure 6-6. A mask can be as simple as a single square or rectangle that encloses a region of interest on the foot—for example, a hallux, all the metatarsal heads, or the midfoot—where the patient might be experiencing a recurrent ulceration. These masks are created by using commercial software supplied by the device manufacturers (in the diagrams in this chapter, the software that was used is NovelWin from Novel Electronics, Inc., St. Paul, MN). Once the mask has been created, it can be applied to data from one or many foot contacts to generate statistically based estimates of quantities such as peak regional pressures, regional pressure versus time graphs, and force-time impulses (see below).

We suspect that regional analysis might be important because some areas of the foot that are normally involved in weight bearing might be better adapted for this function and might therefore tolerate higher pressure before breakdown. Conversely, the pressure threshold for tissue breakdown might be lower in regions of the foot that are not normally involved in weight bearing. An example would be the tip of a very clawed toe or the midfoot that is exposed to weight bearing because of an underlying Charcot fracture deformity (see Fig. 6-3).

A regional analysis of the data presented in Figures 6-4 and 6-5 is shown in Figure 6-7. In this analysis, the 10 masks shown in Figure 6-6D were applied to five consecutive

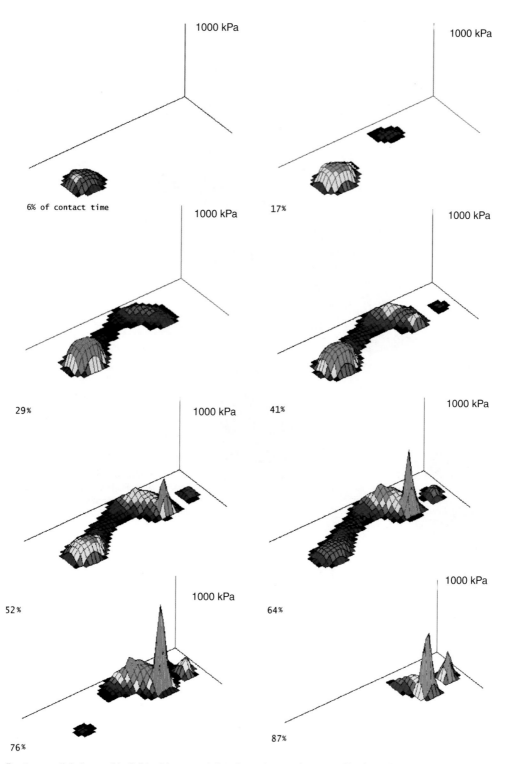

Figure 6–4 Posteromedial views of individual frames of data from the continuous collection of plantar pressure during barefoot walking in a patient who had experienced recurrent ulcers underneath a prominent first metatarsal head on the left foot. (See text for details.)

steps of the left foot. The resulting peak regional pressure analysis (see Fig. 6-7) shows both the mean peak pressures from the five trials and the standard deviations between the five trials. Note that the heel, midfoot, and lesser toe pressures are very consistent in this patient but that the MTH1, lateral MTH, and hallux pressures exhibit high variability. These results suggest that the patient does not have a stereotyped loading pattern on successive steps (see the discussion of variability below).

Analysis of In-Shoe Plantar Pressure

Because most patients wear shoes and often sustain injury while wearing them, the ability to measure pressures

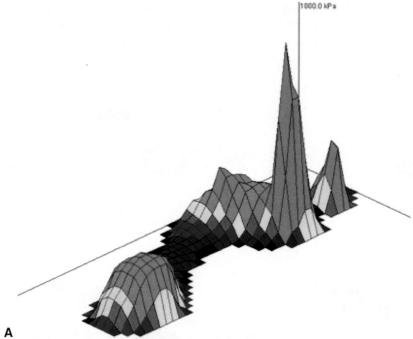

A

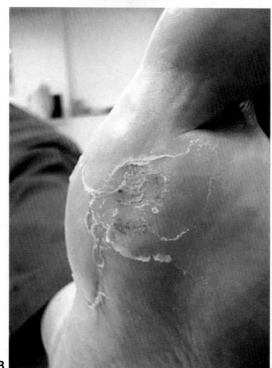

B

Figure 6–5   Peak pressure plot, which summarizes the data shown in Figure 6-4. **A,** In this summary plot, the greatest pressure at each location under the foot from any time in the ground contact is shown in the diagram with the same scale and color key used in Figure 6-4. This display is a useful addition to the patient's chart. **B,** The recently healed ulcer under this patient's left first metatarsal head.

inside the shoe is an important extension of investigative techniques beyond just barefoot measurement. Bauman and Brand[63] and Brand and Ebner[64] used single in-shoe transducers almost 30 years ago; more recently, similar studies have been performed to investigate principles of footwear management.[43,51,65–74] Although these have been principally research studies, devices suitable for clinical use are now available,[1,75] and it is likely that this approach will revolutionize footwear prescription in the future.

In-shoe peak pressures for the patient whose barefoot data are presented in Figures 6-5 through 6-7 are shown in Figure 6-8. The patient was wearing a pair of custom-molded shoes with rigid rocker outsoles and dual-density professional protective technology (PPT) and Plastazote #2 insoles (see the section below on footwear for more discussion of this type of footwear). Note that the peak pressures are still highest at MTH1 but that they have been reduced from greater than 1,000 kPa in barefoot walking to approximately 150 kPa in the

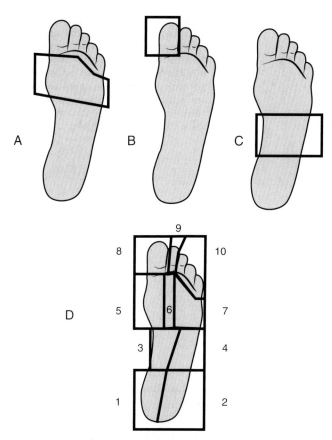

Figure 6-6 Typical masks for regional analysis. **A, B,** and **C** are single masks that examine one anatomic region (metatarsal heads, hallux, and midfoot, respectively). **D,** Ten masks used for regional analysis of plantar pressure (see Fig. 6-7).

shoes. The patient remained healed for many months in these shoes.

Loading Analysis Using Impulse

When we change some component of the patient's foot or footwear, an examination of the peak pressure response tells us "what" has happened rather than "why" it has happened. Analysis of the distribution of loading throughout the period of foot contact using impulse analysis can often provide insight into why a change in peak pressure has occurred. Terminology can be confusing here, because in mechanics, an impulse refers to the product of force and time, not pressure and time. But in a system of pressure transducers with the same area (which is always the case for platforms but not for all in-shoe sensors), pressure and force are directly proportional and can be considered interchangeably with the use of only a single multiplicative constant.

More important, software manufacturers use the terms *pressure-time integral* and *force-time integral* to mean quite different approaches to analysis, each of which gives totally different results. In the EMED analysis programs (Novel Electronics, Inc., St. Paul, MN), use of the pressure-time integral gives information from the single sensor in the foot or region on which peak pressure is exerted. However, use of the force-time integral gives values that represent the summed impulse from every sensor in the entire foot contact area or region (Fig. 6-9).

In either case, the starting point for analysis is the area under the pressure-time curve of a single sensor during the time when the pressure in that sensor registers above a predefined threshold value. This threshold is usually

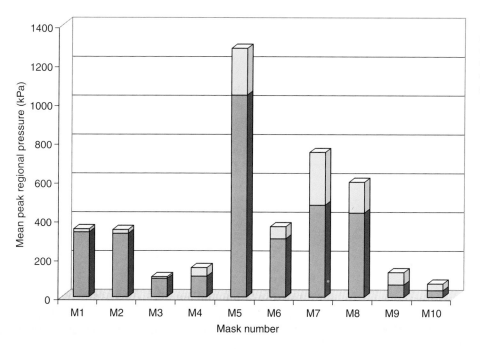

Figure 6-7 A regional peak pressure analysis of the data shown in Figures 6-4 and 6-5 using the masks shown in Figure 6-6D. (Standard deviations from the means of five trials shown in *lighter shading*.)

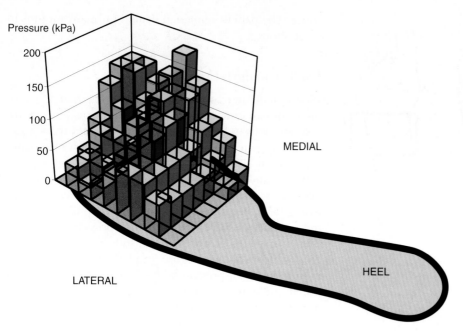

Figure 6–8 In-shoe plantar pressures at a time in the late support phase for the subject whose barefoot data are shown in Figures 6-5 through 6-7. The highest pressures in the foot are still under MTH1, but the peak pressures are reduced by the footwear to only 180 kPa compared to the mean barefoot value of more than 1000 kPa.

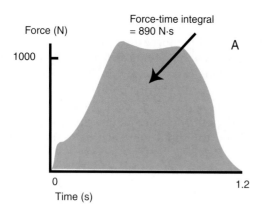

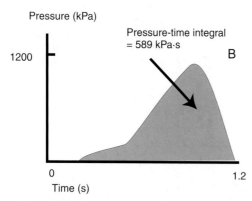

Figure 6–9 **A,** The force-time integral, which describes the total impulse transmitted to the foot by the ground. **B,** The pressure-time integral is simply a summation of the pressure-time curve for the single sensor that recorded the peak pressure during contact. In this case, the sensor is in the forefoot and thus begins to experience loading some time only after initial foot contact. Both of these data sets are for barefoot walking by the subject whose data are shown in Figures 6-4, 6-5, 6-7, and 6-8.

the value that distinguishes signal from noise, but some authors have moved the baseline for integration upward to a value that is considered to represent a boundary between normal and abnormal values[76] (see below). In the case of the pressure-time integral, only the sensor on which peak pressure is exerted is reported in units of kilopascal seconds (kPa · s). For the force-time integral, the pressure-time integrals for all sensors in the defined region (entire foot or region) are summed and multiplied by a constant to express the result in units of Newton seconds (N · s).

Care needs to be taken not only with the selection of the appropriate impulse variables but also with their interpretation. For example, peak pressure and the pressure-time integral can be readily compared between different regions of the foot and different footwear conditions because both refer to the analysis of a single sensor, but the force-time integral for areas that have the same applied pressure may be quite different, depending on the size of the region under consideration. A larger region with the same pressure as a smaller region will yield a larger impulse (e.g., consider the heel and hallux). When comparisons between footwear conditions are being made, the force-time integral can be used only if the two regions for which a comparison is being made are identical in area under the two conditions. An example of impulse analysis in which in-shoe pressure measurement is used to compare different footwear conditions is given in the section below on the biomechanics of footwear.

Duckworth and colleagues[77] measured the time during which plantar pressure was above 981 kPa and showed greater times in patients with a plantar ulcer. Schaff and Cavanagh[78] showed that changes in force-time integral were proportionally much greater than changes in peak pressures in rocker shoes compared to flexible shoes (see the section below on footwear). Shaw and Boulton[76] examined the integral of pressure above a threshold value of 490 kPa in patients with and without prior ulceration. They found much greater percentage increases for impulse variables than for peak pressure variables in the ulcer patients. Thus, although peak pressure data have received by far the most attention to date in studies of the foot in diabetes, analyses that include a time variable might yet prove to be more useful.

Plantar Pressure Gradient

Several investigators have proposed that the difference between plantar pressures in adjacent regions of the foot—sometimes called the pressure gradient—could be an important factor in the etiology of tissue injury. Thomas and colleagues[79] used finite-element analysis (see below) to show normal and shear stress gradients that were 6.25 and 3.3 times greater, respectively, than control, whereas peak normal and shear pressure values were only 0.56 and 0.53 times greater, respectively.

This concept was later explored experimentally by Mueller and his colleagues,[80,81] who reported peak pressure gradients in a group of 20 neuropathic diabetic subjects to be 143% times greater in the forefoot than in the rearfoot, whereas a similar comparison of peak normal pressures was only 36%. Because the correlation between peak pressure and peak pressure gradient was only 0.59, these authors believe that gradient measure might be an independent predictor of plantar tissue risk, reflecting high stress concentrations within the soft tissue. In their 2007 study,[81] the magnitude and depth of the plantar shear stress calculated from peak pressure

measurements were found to be correlated with the pressure gradient ($r = -0.77$ and 0.61, respectively) and the peak pressure ($r = -0.61$ and 0.91, respectively).

Expected Values for Peak Pressure

The results of a regional analysis of peak pressure for a group of asymptomatic subjects walking barefoot at normal speed are shown in Figure 6-10 from the work of Rosenbaum and colleagues.[55] The mean and the mean plus 2 standard deviations (S.D.) are shown on the graph. These data (and all the barefoot peak pressure diagrams in this chapter) were collected with an EMED SF platform (Novel Electronics, Inc., St. Paul, MN) with a sensor area of 0.5 cm². Note that there is considerable between-subject variation in most regions; the coefficients of variation (S.D./mean) in the forefoot are approximately 40%.

A number of other workers have reported pressures in various groups of patients with the EMED SF platform. Armstrong and colleagues[82] reported peak pressures (regardless of their site of occurrence in the foot) of 627 kPa (± 244 kPa) for diabetic patients with no history of ulceration and values of 831 kPa (± 247 kPa) for patients who had ulcerated. Both these mean values are outside the range of mean plus 2 S.D. reported by Rosenbaum and colleagues.[55] Stess and colleagues[12] reported values of peak pressures in the forefoot of 480 kPa (± 18 kPa SEE) in patients with a history of ulcers, and these values are within the range defined by Rosenbaum and colleagues.[55] Armstrong and Lavery[83] found peak pressures of 1000 kPA (± 85 kPa) in Charcot patients, 900 kPa (± 188 kPa) in neuropathic patients with a history of ulceration, 650 kPa (± 256 kPa) in patients with neuropathy but no ulceration, and 450 (± 80 kPa)

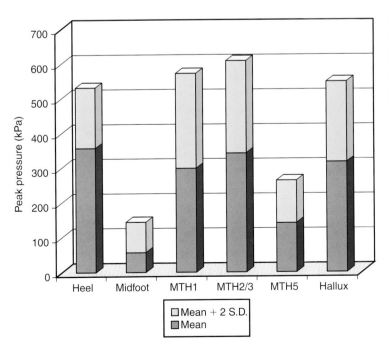

Figure 6–10 Regional analysis of peak pressure (mean and 2 standard deviations) for a group of asymptomatic subjects walking at normal speed from the work of Rosenbaum et al. *(Redrawn with permission from Rosenbaum D, Hautman S, Gold M, et al: Effects of walking speed on plantar pressure patterns and hindfoot angular motion. Gait Posture 2:191–197, 1994, with permission.)*

in diabetic patients with no neuropathy or history of ulceration. Wolfe and colleagues[84] reported the results of plantar pressure analysis on nine patients with Charcot feet and found that peak pressure under many of the feet exceeded the 1270 kPa measurement limit of the EMED-SF platform used.

All four studies described in the previous paragraph used precisely the same measuring device (an EMED-SF platform with a sensor size of 0.5 cm²); therefore, the lower values for peak pressure in patients with ulcers found by Stess and colleagues[12] must have been due to either a difference in measuring protocol or a real difference in patient populations. It is quite likely to be the latter, since we have also found pressures of approximately 500 kPa in neuropathic patients who have ulcerated.[85]

Investigators who have used an optical pedobarograph have generally reported higher values, as would be expected from the higher spatial resolution of the sensors in the optical pedobarograph. Boulton and colleagues[86] suggested that a value of 1080 kPa was a threshold for differentiating between normal and abnormal pressures. This group found that 51% of neuropathic feet in their sample had pressures above this value, and all of those with a history of ulceration exceeded this value. In a clinical study[87] and a later prospective study,[88] Veves and his colleagues used a value of 1207 kPa to distinguish normal from abnormal. They found mean values for peak pressures (regardless of site) of 1108 kPa in neuropathic patients compared to 795 kPa in non-neuropathic diabetic controls; 39% of the neuropathic patients had values above the threshold, compared to 15% of controls. In the prospective study, all patients who had ulcerated showed pressures at baseline greater than 1108 kPa.

Frykberg and colleagues[89] used an F-scan mat system to record peak pressures from various groups of diabetic patients. They used a value of 600 kPa as their threshold for the definition of "abnormal pressures" and found an association between ulceration and high pressure using this approach. Using a similar device, Pham and colleagues[90] found a mean peak pressure of 570 kPa (± 30 kPa) in a prospective study of a large sample of diabetic patients. This group found pressure measurement to be helpful but not robust in predicting ulceration.

Is There a Threshold Pressure for Injury?

Factors That Affect the Threshold

As was discussed above, different investigators have used various threshold values to distinguish normal from abnormal pressures. However, this is not the same as defining a threshold for ulceration. Plantar ulceration has been linked to high plantar pressure in several retrospective studies and in one prospective study.[7,82,83,86,88-92] However, there is no clear agreement yet on the pressure

threshold for ulceration. This lack of accord may be a consequence of several factors. First, as we have noted, results that are obtained by using one pressure platform cannot be extrapolated to other platforms because of the effect of element size. Second, different regions of the foot may have different pressure thresholds for breakdown. Third, the pressure threshold for tissue breakdown may vary, depending on the health of the tissue related to vascular supply, tissue perfusion,[93] amount of glycosylation of the tissues, and scarring. Fourth, shear, although not measured by any of the currently available platforms (see below), may interact with normal forces in ways that are not yet understood. Fifth, the integral or time-pressure product, currently not often calculated, could be more relevant than simple peak pressure.[31,32,76] Sixth, and perhaps most important, barefoot pressures that are measured during a few steps across a pressure platform do not predict the load experienced by the foot. Actual cumulative load during normal daily living depends on each patient's activity level and footwear.

Conventional Approach to Defining Abnormal Values

It is not possible to take the foot pressure distribution of a healthy population and assume that similar values are safe for patients with insensitive feet. Healthy individuals remain ulcer free not necessarily because they have lower plantar pressures but because they can feel pain. As was mentioned earlier, the range of "normal" regional peak pressure values, defined as mean ± 2 S.D., is very wide (see Fig. 6-10), with peak values approaching 600 kPa at several regions. Yet plantar ulcerations can and do occur in the feet of neuropathic patients at sites where peak pressure is as low as 500 kPa, as measured on the EMED SF platform.[84,85]

Evidence for a Threshold Pressure

Although the studies described above that have included patients with a history of ulceration provide some perspective on the issue of a threshold pressure,[12,76,77,83,84,86,88-90] these studies were not specifically designed to explore the issue of ulceration threshold. Armstrong and colleagues[82] analyzed plantar pressures in patients with a history of ulceration and matched each of them with two control diabetic patients without a history of ulceration. Plantar pressure was measured in cases and controls using an EMED SF pressure platform. Peak pressures were significantly higher in cases compared to controls (831 ± 247 kPa versus 627 ± 244 kPa), and measures of skewness indicated an opposite pattern of negative skew for cases (more high pressures) and positive skew for controls (more low pressures). The optimal cutoff point, which balanced sensitivity and specificity in the data, was 700 kPa. However, this value was only 70% sensitive and 65% specific, leaving the authors to conclude that there was no clear value that could be used in screening to predict ulceration. Rather, the higher the pressure, the greater the risk.

These results make great intuitive sense in terms of the skewness described. There will always be patients who ulcerate even at relatively low pressures because of either a traumatic injury or significant walking (either barefoot or in very poor footwear) on a hard surface. Conversely, there will be patients who, because of low activity and/or very protective footwear, will not ulcerate even though experiencing very high barefoot pressures. Thus, barefoot pressure can only predict the degree of risk, which is then modified by level of activity and type and fit of footwear. Therefore, it would be unreasonable to expect to find a clear division between ulcer patients and nonulcer patients based on barefoot level gait measurement.

In a large prospective study of 1666 consecutive patients with diabetes, Lavery and colleagues[94] examined the predictive value of plantar pressure measurement for the identification of patients who will eventually ulcerate. They found that although those who ulcerated did have higher plantar pressure than those who did not (950 versus 850 kPa), peak pressure was not sufficient by itself to identify risk of ulceration. Again, it must be pointed out that this study used barefoot plantar pressure, which, depending on the success and heterogeneity of the footwear used, might not correlate with the in-shoe pressures that patients experience most during a typical day's activity.

Another related point is that barefoot measurements of pressure do not always predict the highest possible pressure. In general, the faster the gait, the higher is the pressure under the foot. At most sites, pressure during barefoot walking predicts pressure for more demanding activities. However, Rozema and colleagues[95] have shown that during turning, for instance, hallux pressure can be very high, even in subjects with low hallux pressure during straight, level gait. This is consistent with the clinical observation that many hallux ulcers occur despite relatively low pressure measured during straight level gait, and this observation will certainly confound any attempt to define hallux ulcer risk on the basis of level gait pressure measurement.

The work of Shaw and Boulton[76] suggests that a consideration of impulse could also be important in trying to define the ulceration threshold.

Caselli and colleagues[96] have shown the ratio of forefoot to rearfoot peak pressures to be a useful index. In the analysis of data from a 30-month prospective study, both peak pressure and the forefoot-to-rearfoot peak pressure ratio were found to be independent predictors of ulceration.

Threshold for Injury: The Future

The actual amount of mechanical trauma needed for tissue breakdown can be assessed only by documenting the trauma to which tissue is exposed at the time of ulceration. The only practical way to do this is to measure cumulative loading to an ulcer site over a prolonged period while the patient is using footwear that is known from clinical experience to be insufficient to prevent ulceration in that patient. The measurement would then need to be repeated in footwear that is known to prevent ulceration. The threshold for tissue breakdown would then be found somewhere between the two conditions. Such data would need to be analyzed in many different ways and include variables for peak pressure, pressure-time integral, time spent over different pressure values, time spent resting, and so on. As was discussed above, barefoot pressure measurement can only ever contribute to estimation of risk, but knowing the true load for tissue breakdown would then, for the first time, allow for more rational footwear prescription. Only footwear that is found by in-shoe load measurement to be safe would be dispensed.

This approach to the determination of ulcer pressure threshold is demonstrated in the case study from the Pennsylvania State University Diabetes Foot Clinics shown in Figure 6-11. The patient's left foot had a classic midfoot Charcot collapse (Fig. 6-11C) with a peak midfoot pressure during barefoot walking (Fig. 6-11D) of 1019 kPa (± 295 kPa). He ulcerated despite wearing a custom-molded shoe (Fig. 6-11A). After healing in a TCC, he was provided with a new custom-molded shoe with a redesigned insole and a patellar-tendon–bearing brace (Fig. 6-11B). He was able to continue his activities of daily life without ulcerating in this shoe-brace combination. Analysis of in-shoe pressure data in these two shoe conditions using a single midfoot mask indicated that peak midfoot pressures in shoe A and shoe B were 190 kPa and ~150 kPa, respectively (Fig. 6-11E). Thus, it appears possible to identify the threshold for ulceration in this patient to be somewhere in the 40-kPa range between ~150 and 190 kPa when measured inside the shoe using a pressure-measuring insole with an average sensor area of approximately 1.5 cm^2.

One additional caveat should be considered. These data were collected during relatively slow level gait, and it is likely that during activities of daily living, the plantar surface would actually be exposed to somewhat higher loads than those measured here, even with the patient wearing the same shoes. Thus, the range of pressure given here as including the ulceration threshold still represents only a window on what is happening. As has already been discussed, injury must in fact depend not just on some measure of loading, but also on the activity and rest pattern.

Is Temperature a Surrogate for Tissue Injury?

It has been suggested that the measurement of foot temperature might be a useful prognostic tool for the indication of impending risk of injury, perhaps reflecting the

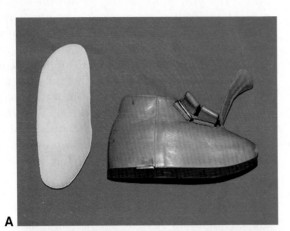

A

Figure 6–11   An approach to the determination of ulcer pressure threshold in a patient with a classic midfoot Charcot collapse of the left foot. **A,** Shoe A, in which the patient ulcerated. **B,** Shoe B, which did not result in an ulcer when used with the patellar tendon–bearing brace. **C,** The plantar surface of the foot showing the midfoot prominence. **D,** A barefoot peak pressure plot using EMED SF showing the elevated pressure under the midfoot prominence. It can be seen that the midfoot is the only region of the foot that experiences significant load during the entire contact. (Panel E on next page.)

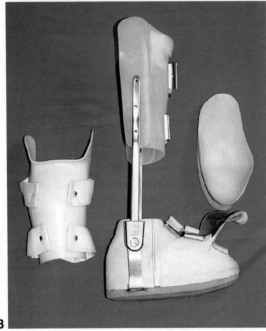

B

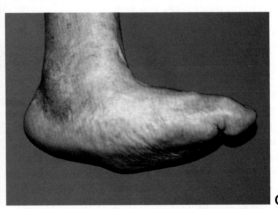

C

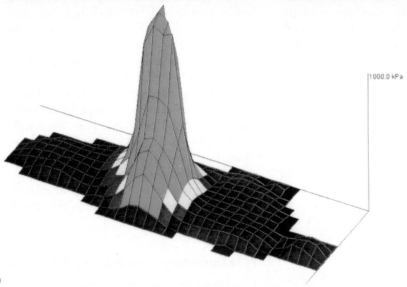

1000.0 kPa

D

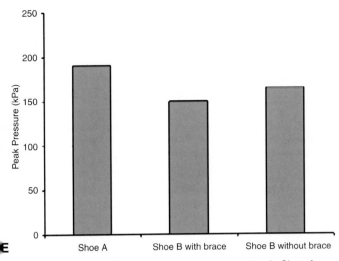

Figure 6–11, cont'd   E, In-shoe peak pressures in Shoe A and in Shoe B with and without the brace. These tests show that this patient's threshold for ulceration was between 150 and 190 kPa as measured inside the shoe. It is uncertain whether it would be safe to allow the patient to ambulate without the brace, since pressure is marginally reduced by the brace.

Summary of Plantar Pressure Measurement

In summary, the use of plantar pressure measurement is vital from the investigational and clinical standpoints. Potential drawbacks in interpreting the results in the literature are interinstrument variability and gait characteristics, such as speed and stride length. From the clinical standpoint, plantar pressure analysis can help to refine the assessment of patient risk and give important information for footwear prescription. In daily practice, plantar pressure measurement can identify areas of high pressure that are unsuspected on clinical examination and that will need to be considered in the footwear prescription. Finally, in-shoe pressure measurement represents a major advance and can refine the process of footwear prescription by defining the exact degree of pressure relief at high-risk areas.

Regarding threshold pressure for injury, it is clear that ulceration has been consistently linked to elevated barefoot peak plantar pressure, but there is no agreement regarding the threshold pressure for injury. The studies to date that addressed risk of ulceration due to plantar pressure were not designed specifically to address this question. Although a consistent ulcer threshold has not been confirmed, the literature suggests that foci of barefoot pressure measurements above 500 to 700 kPa begin to put the patient at increased risk for ulceration. It is certain, however, that peak plantar pressure as a risk factor does not exist in isolation. Patients whose feet are exposed even to low pressures may ulcerate if they engage in risky behaviors such as barefoot walking; conversely, patients with high barefoot pressures who are nonambulatory or who consistently use excellent footwear lower their overall risk of ulceration.

vascular and/or inflammatory reactions to prolonged application of mechanical stress.[97] However, a number of studies have shown that such measurements must be made carefully. Armstrong and colleagues[98] found no difference in skin temperature based on neuropathy, foot laterality, or foot risk category or between people with and without foot deformity and elevated plantar pressure. Sun and colleagues[99] suggested that normalized temperature of the entire plantar surface might be a more reliable indicator than absolute focal temperatures. They also found that the wait time prior to measurement influences the outcome; they suggested that to obtain a truly reliable plantar temperature ("normalized temperature value"), 15 minutes was the minimum acceptable time to allow for the overall mean plantar temperature to stabilize.

Lavery and colleagues[97] provided handheld infrared thermometers to a group of 44 patients, who were then asked to measure plantar temperatures both morning and evening for a period of 6 months. There was only one new ulcer in this group of patients compared to seven ulcers and two Charcot fractures among patients who were given standard therapy. The extent to which simply directing attention to the foot twice daily, rather than to the results of temperature monitoring, was a factor in this improved outcome needs to be further elucidated.

The hypothesis that temperature might be important in the etiology of plantar ulceration has led to the suggestion that forced (intentional) cooling of the feet in a cold water bath might be an effective approach to reducing the risk for tissue damage after a patient engages in activities such as brisk walking.

Where Does Ulceration Occur?

Data on the location of ulcers on the feet of patients with diabetes are available from a series of studies by Ctercteko and colleagues,[92] Birke and Sims[100] (in both Hansen's disease and neuropathic diabetic patients), Calhoun and colleagues,[101] Edmonds and colleagues,[5] Apelqvist and colleagues,[102] and Armstrong and colleagues.[82] Although midfoot ulcers are notably absent from the data presented by Edmonds and colleagues,[5] their series allows comparisons of neuropathic with ischemic ulcers and also presents a comprehensive breakdown of ulcers by location on the foot (Fig. 6-12). Of particular interest from a biomechanical perspective is the fact that ulcers on the dorsal and plantar surfaces are approximately evenly distributed. Since dorsal ulcers are invariably footwear related, this distribution indicates that approximately half of all neuropathic foot ulcers could be avoided very simply by the use of footwear that is appropriately sized. Preventing plantar ulcers also involves appropriate footwear, and in this case, the

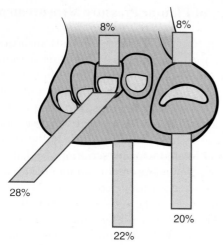

Figure 6–12 The distribution of ulcers in the forefoot from Edmonds and colleagues.[5] The forefoot accounted for 93% of all ulcers in this series. In addition to the locations shown in the figure (plantar and dorsal hallux, plantar and dorsal surfaces, and tips of all toes combined), other forefoot ulcers occurred in the following locations: 2% each on the plantar aspect (other than the tip), sides, and between the toes; on the tip and side of the hallux (4% and 1%, respectively); and on the dorsum of the metatarsal head region (1%).

biomechanical issues are more complex than those affecting dorsal injury prevention (see below).

How Does Foot Injury Occur?

Tissue Ischemia

Although elevated plantar pressure is now accepted as a major factor in the etiopathogenesis of plantar ulcers in diabetic patients, exactly how tissue damage occurs is not well known. Various mechanisms have been discussed by Brand and Coleman,[103] Delbridge and colleagues,[104] Pecoraro and colleagues,[105] and others.[106] It is certain that some regions of the plantar tissue become ischemic when the foot is loaded. A systolic blood pressure of 120 mm Hg is only 15 kPa, and capillary pressure is less than half this value. Reference to Figure 6-10 shows that typical peak plantar pressures in the forefoot during gait are at least 30 times higher, implying that blood flow will be occluded during at least part of the gait cycle. Recovery from this ischemia might be affected by such factors as glycosylation or the state of the microcirculation, which has been shown to be abnormal even in early diabetes.[93]

Factors leading to tissue breakdown have been studied much more systematically by those who are interested in pressure ulcers of the buttocks than by scientists with an interest in the foot. It is believed that pressures as low as 6 to 8 kPa can, when applied for periods of 15 minutes or more, affect the microcirculation, lymph flow, and interstitial transport in the tissues over the ischial tuberosities.

Although the loading pattern in this region is fundamentally different from that which occurs in the foot, the protocols used by Bader[107] to examine recovery of tissue transcutaneous oxygen pressure after repetitive loading would seem to have merit for application to the foot. Delayed recovery of normal tissue oxygenation was found in elderly and neuropathic patients, and this might have been because of the delayed elastic recovery of the aging tissue.

Newton and colleagues[108] have shown that areas of elevated pressure on the plantar surface of the foot experience increased basal skin blood flow, but they were equivocal as to whether this response is protective or maladaptive. These high-pressure areas also had reduced responsiveness to an endothelium-dependent vasodilator.

Other Theories of Tissue Damage

It is also likely that unperceived stresses in the plantar soft tissues can be high enough to actually rupture the microanatomic and macroanatomic structures that are usually protected from damage by the exquisite sensitivity of the plantar aspect of a normal foot. Stepping on a sharp object and actually puncturing the skin would be the most severe and most obvious example. In any case, there can be no doubt that the acute and chronic phases of foot injury deserve more study experimentally than they have received to date.

The classical model of ulceration has been postulated by Delbridge and colleagues.[104] Their theory assumes that the initial event in the formation of a typical neuropathic plantar ulcer is the development of plaque (callus) on the surface of the skin. They believe that tissue breakdown then occurs under the callus and that a cavity filled with plasma and blood develops. In their theory, this cavity enlarges until it causes a rupture of the skin surface, forming an ulcer with a small opening but a larger cavity beneath. This view is certainly congruent with the many preulcers that are seen as hemorrhage into callus.

Davis[109] has hypothesized that the irregular interaction of shear and compressive stresses at the skin surface causes tissue damage by a mechanism that he has likened to one region of a carpet slipping under the action of shear while another region remains stationary because of greater frictional forces.

Landsman and Sage[110] have explored a cellular mechanism for tissue damage. This group presented data from in vitro studies to show that high rates of tissue deformation cause changes in intracellular concentrations of calcium that do not result if the same magnitude of deformation is applied more slowly. The authors hypothesize that the altered intracellular environment may lead to cellular death. For this hypothesis to be verified as a causation of foot ulcers, it would be necessary to show that the tissue of patients with foot ulcers is deformed more rapidly than is nondiabetic tissue during typical activities of daily life.

Mueller and colleagues[80,81] have advanced the notion of "pressure gradient" as an important factor in tissue breakdown. They have shown in a group of neuropathic patients that the ratio of the peak pressure gradient between the forefoot and hindfoot was twice that of the peak pressure ratio.[80] This indicates that the peak pressure gradient might be a more sensitive indicator of tissue exposure to damaging mechanical conditions than peak pressure alone. The effects of peak pressure gradients on shear stresses were examined by Zou and colleagues,[81] using a model of subsurface tissue stress. Such approaches are currently limited by the absence of accurate data on the mechanical properties of the complex plantar tissue layers.

It is interesting to speculate what the different theories might predict about the most appropriate foot-ground interface parameters to measure. For instance, the intermittent ischemia hypothesis would predict that the most important attribute to measure would be time spent above the threshold pressure for vascular occlusion, whereas the direct tissue tearing hypothesis might predict that a small number of very high pressure events would be sufficient to cause the initial damage.

Causes of High Plantar Pressure and Other Contributors to Ulceration Risk

As was noted earlier, pressures generated under apparently healthy feet (see Fig. 6-10) can be high enough to cause ulceration in the presence of neuropathy. It is also true that diabetes, particularly diabetes that is complicated by neuropathy, is associated with higher than normal plantar pressure.[86,111] It is generally believed that diabetes mellitus may alter both the musculoskeletal and soft tissue mechanics in a manner that elevates plantar pressure and makes tissue damage more likely. Few of these effects have been observed in prospective studies; therefore, evidence rests on retrospective analysis and cross-sectional studies.

Structure and Function Relationships

Cavanagh and colleagues[112] examined the relationship between the bony structure of the foot and elevated plantar pressure during controlled-speed barefoot walking in 50 symptom-free adults. A variety of angular and linear measurements were taken from standardized anteroposterior and lateral weight-bearing radiographs. A multivariate statistical technique (stepwise multiple regression) was used to identify the structural variables that are associated with high pressure. Among the strongest predictors of high pressure under the first MTH were soft tissue thickness between the sesamoids and ground, inclination of the metatarsal shaft in a sagittal plane, and frontal plane splay of the first and fifth metatarsals. It is encouraging to find that static

structural measurements of the foot are statistically related to dynamic functional characteristics. This suggests that it might be possible in the future to add such measurements as a component of a larger risk factor profile to predict risk of injury. However, because this approach was able to predict only 38% of the variance in peak plantar pressure at the first MTH, we decided in a second study[113] to add dynamic "functional" variables such as stride parameters, foot motion measures, and electromyographic data as possible predictors. With all of these variables in the regression, 50% of the variation in plantar pressure could be predicted, and structural variables were still dominant in predicting the MTH pressure, whereas both structural and functional variables were important at the hallux and heel.

Ahroni and colleagues[114] have reported a similar study in neuropathic diabetic patients. These investigators measured in-shoe pressure as the patients walked in their own footwear at a freely chosen speed; foot deformity was assessed subjectively by a nurse-practitioner. A wide variety of variables was offered to the subsequent regression models. The inclusion of foot deformity resulted in a significant improvement in the prediction capacity of the model at the MTHs and hallux. However, the maximum amount of explained variance in peak pressure from all variables in the models was only 5.3% to 11.7%. Song and colleagues[115] used the traditional classification of feet as pes planus and pes rectus to show that such groups could be distinguished on the basis of functional measurements. They extended this analysis to neuropathic patients and were again able to distinguish between groups on the basis of functional measurements.

Robertson and colleagues[116] found that plantar soft tissue density as measured from computerized tomographic (CT) scans was lower in individuals with diabetes, but they found no difference in the soft tissue thickness beneath the MTHs between the neuropathic and control groups. Various features of the MTP joints were different between groups.

Mueller and his colleagues[117–121] have used the simultaneous combination of spiral CT and plantar pressure measurements to examine structure-function relationships in neuropathic feet. Smith and colleagues[120] introduced the technique and, in two subjects, were able to generate plantar pressures under the MTHs in the CT scanner that were very similar to those measured in the same subjects during walking. They also measured soft tissue thickness during loading. The required scan times of approximately 20 to 45 seconds are clearly an advantage over magnetic resonance imaging (MRI) scans, which are at least an order of magnitude greater. The approach was subsequently explored with the use of a larger number of subjects,[118] and several structural variables were reliably obtained from the CT scans. Applications of the technique to footwear design have also been explored[74] (see below).

The reliability of MRI to determine the static structure of the foot was assessed by Bus and colleagues,[122] who found relatively good interobserver agreement for a number of variables except interphalangeal angles. Although MRI is traditionally regarded as the primary imaging mode for visualization of soft tissues, the use of CT as a method of measuring the thickness and extent of plantar soft tissues was explored by Bolton and colleagues.[121] They found the approach reliable and reported that the thicknesses of the plantar aponeurosis and flexor hallucis longus tendon were 14% and 10% greater, respectively, in a group of diabetic patients than in controls.

Mueller and colleagues[123] found that MTP joint angle accounted for 19% to 45% of the variance in forefoot peak plantar pressure during barefoot walking in a group of neuropathic diabetic subjects. In the nondiabetic control group, soft tissue thickness, hallux valgus, and forefoot arthropathy were the most useful predictors. The investigators were able to account for 47% to 71% of the variance in peak plantar pressure in the neuropathic subjects and 52% to 83% of the variance in the control group.

Structural Alterations

We discussed earlier that foot structure is a major determinant of plantar pressure. Although some structural factors are independent of diabetes, a number of others that predispose toward elevated pressure appear to be a result of the disease. Obviously, the major collapse of the foot that is seen in Charcot fractures will lead to elevated pressure. However, a number of more subtle changes also appear to contribute. Clawed toes are a frequent clinical finding, and this phenomenon has been ascribed to atrophy of the intrinsic muscles that control the position of the proximal phalanges on the metatarsal bones.[124] In addition to the fact that clawed toes increase the likelihood of dorsal ulceration from footwear, it is hypothesized that the soft tissue "metatarsal cushions"[125] are displaced distally, leaving the condyles of the MTHs exposed. Gooding and colleagues[126,127] have investigated tissue thickness under the MTHs using ultrasound, but the results have been inconclusive. Young and colleagues[128] describe significantly reduced plantar tissue thickness in both neuropathic diabetic patients and those with rheumatoid arthritis and metatarsalgia. The authors were able to account for almost 70% of the variation in plantar pressure at MTH1 on the basis of soft tissue thickness. Kawchuk and Elliott[129] have provided insight into the accuracy and validation of displacements measured by using ultrasonic probes.

The relationship between clawing of the toes and the anterior displacement of the submetatarsal fat pads was finally elucidated in an MRI study by Bus and colleagues[130] (Fig. 6-13), in which an R^2 of 0.63 was found between tissue thickness and MTP joint angle in a group of 42 neuropathic patients. A subsequent study[131] demonstrated that clawed toes and hammertoes were

also associated with a distal-to-proximal load transfer and elevated plantar pressures at the MTHs in neuropathic patients.

Masson and colleagues[132] compared plantar pressure distribution in patients with diabetes and with rheumatoid arthritis. The two groups had a similar prevalence of foot deformity and exhibited similar numbers of patients with plantar pressure above 980 kPa. Thus, this study again links deformity and high plantar pressures. Only the diabetic patients experienced plantar ulceration, of course, because of the coexistence of neuropathy.

In an as yet unconfirmed observation, Taylor and colleagues[133] reported rupture of the plantar fascia in 12 consecutive diabetic patients with clawing of the toes. No such rupture was found in 12 matched control patients with diabetes but without clawing of the toes. If confirmed in a larger study, these observations could reshape our view of the pathogenesis of clawed toes and perhaps cause us to question the role of intrinsic muscle atrophy as the primary determinant of clawed toes and hammertoes. It should also be noted that Kastenbauer and colleagues[134] found no differences in peroneal motor nerve conduction velocity between groups with and without clawing of the toes. If intrinsic muscle atrophy were the cause of the clawing, then a decrease in nerve conduction velocity in the clawed toe group would have been expected. Also, the theory of Taylor and colleagues,[133] that the plantar fascia is a critical element in the transmission of force through the toes, is supported by observations of Hamel and Sharkey.[135]

In a large group of people with diabetes, Ledoux and colleagues[136] found differences in the type and frequency of foot deformities in pes cavus, neutrally aligned, and pes planus feet. Specifically, subjects with pes cavus feet had significantly more prominent MTHs, bony prominences, and clawed toes and hammertoes, and they exhibited great hallux dorsiflexion but decreased hallux plantarflexion. Neutrally aligned feet had, in general, less deformity. In a subsequent study,[137] this same group showed that although foot type was not related to ulcer risk, toe deformity (clawed toes and hammertoes, hallux limitus) significantly increased the risk of ulceration. In contrast, Nube and colleagues[24] found pronated feet to be related to a history of hallux ulceration.

Using ultrasound to measure plantar tissue thickness under the MTHs, Abouaesha and colleagues[138] found that peak plantar pressure can be predicted from tissue thickness with high sensitivity and specificity.

Mueller and associates[117–121,123] have conducted a number of imaging studies, some including simultaneous or supplementary plantar pressure measurement.

Tissue Properties

More direct metabolic consequences of diabetes may also affect plantar soft tissue structure and function. Nonenzymatic glycosylation of many proteins in the body

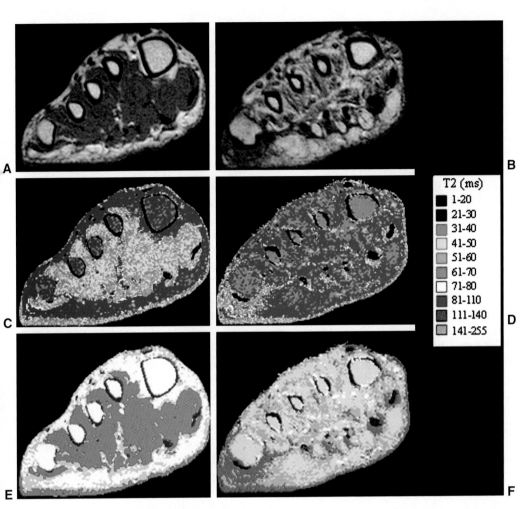

Figure 6–13 Images from the analysis of a nondiabetic control subject (**A, C,** and **E**) and an age- and sex-matched neuropathic subject (**B, D,** and **F**). **A** and **B,** Single-echo anatomic T2 images of a metatarsal cross-section. **C** and **D,** T2 maps generated from 11 spin-echo images with color-coding according to the adjacent legend. In these maps, tendon and cortical bone appear as black (T2 ≤ 30 ms); muscle and skin appear as green, yellow, orange, and red (31 ms < T2 < 70 ms); and fat and trabecular bone appear as white, blue, and dark gray (71 ms < T2 ≤ 140 ms). **E** and **F,** Segmented images from the multicomponent analysis of the T2 maps, with muscle and skin tissue outlined in blue and shaded dark gray. Skin tissue was excluded in the quantification of muscle tissue. *(Reproduced from Bus SA, Yang QX, Wang JH, et al: Intrinsic muscle atrophy and toe deformity in the diabetic neuropathic foot: A magnetic resonance imaging study. Diabetes Care 25(8): 1444–1450, 2002.)*

T2 (ms)

- 1-20
- 21-30
- 31-40
- 41-50
- 51-60
- 61-70
- 71-80
- 81-110
- 111-140
- 141-255

has been demonstrated in patients with diabetes,[139] and this process has been shown to affect the mechanical properties of tissue, usually reducing elasticity. The foot is no exception, and Delbridge and colleagues[140] have shown that keratin in the stratum corneum of the diabetic foot is glycosylated in comparison with nondiabetic skin. Zilberberg[141] found a higher content of the nonenzymatic cross-link pentosidine in plantar skin samples from the amputated feet of diabetic patients compared to those from nondiabetic controls. She also found a trend for skin from diabetic feet to be stiffer, as determined by conventional mechanical testing. This may result in a reduced capacity of the skin for the distribution of pressure.

These results were confirmed by Hashmi and colleagues[142] in a large group of patients with type 2 diabetes. The authors reported increased concentrations of pentosidine in skin samples that were not well correlated with plasma protein glycosylation. Direct measurement of epidermal plasticity indicated lower values in the diabetic patients than in controls. Measures of skin hardness were proposed by Thomas and colleagues,[143] who found relationships between these measures and elevated plantar pressure.

Cheung and colleagues[144] used magnetic resonance elastography to study the mechanical properties of the plantar fat pads. The investigators found a trend towards stiffer values in the tissues of diabetic patients. Changes in the properties in the deep plantar tissues have been implicated in altered foot function in diabetic patients.[145-147] The thickness of the plantar fascia and Achilles tendon was measured by D'Ambrogi and colleagues[147] using ultrasound and compared with measurements of plantar pressure. These authors reported that diabetic patients (including people with and without neuropathy and plantar ulceration) exhibited a significant increase in plantar tissue thickness and a reduction in mobility of the first MTP joint compared to control subjects. Moderate correlations between tissue thickness and joint mobility (r = –0.53) and between tissue thickness and the vertical component of force in the MTHs were reported. Data from what is apparently the same patient group[146] were later reported to show higher correlations between the same parameters. The role of an altered "windlass mechanism" in higher plantar pressures was also illustrated with the same data.[145]

Klaesner and colleagues[148] developed a portable "indentor" that they found to be "reliable, accurate, and sensitive enough" for the determination of the mechanical properties of plantar tissues. This device was then used in combination with a three-element viscoelastic model to quantify plantar stiffness in neuropathic diabetic subjects with a history of plantar ulcers and matched controls.[149] The authors reported that the tissues of diabetic patients were stiffer than those of controls.

Limited Joint Mobility

A further presumed by-product of nonenzymatic glycosylation is the observed limitation of range of movement in many joints of the body in persons with diabetes. Although first demonstrated in the hand,[150] this condition has now been found in the joints of the foot and ankle.[25,151] Anecdotally, limitation of motion in the first MTP joint is frequently associated with ulceration of the hallux in neuropathic patients (see earlier discussion and Fig. 6-1C). Birke and colleagues[152] found that patients with a history of MTH1 ulceration had significantly diminished dorsiflexion range of motion at the first MTP joint. Limited first-ray mobility explained almost 50% of the variance in peak MTH1 plantar pressure.

Decreased subtalar joint mobility has been associated with elevated plantar pressure,[151] although there are indications that protective sensation might allow compensation to occur such that pressure might not necessarily be elevated in the setting of subtalar limited joint mobility without neuropathy.[153]

Chantelau and colleagues[154] reported higher interdigital pressures between the fourth and fifth toes (a common site of ulceration) in patients with limited joint mobility compared to controls and also noted that pressure was higher in shoes with constrained toe caps.

Veves and colleagues[155] have proposed that diabetic Caucasians might be at greater risk of limited joint mobility compared to diabetic African Americans. The increased range of motion at the subtalar and first MTP joints in African American diabetic patients compared to Caucasian patients was accompanied in their relatively small sample (24 African American, 31 Caucasian) by lower plantar pressures.

Although Sabato and colleagues[156] found an association between high pressure and ulceration in patients with Hansen's disease (leprosy), the authors reported that a reduced range of motion at the ankle joint was not associated with ulceration. However, others[151,154] have found that a limited range of motion at several foot and ankle joints in diabetic patients is associated not just with elevated pressure but also with ulceration.

There are some initial indications that pharmacologic interventions might have some impact on limited joint mobility. Nargi and colleagues[157] showed that the use of N-phenacylthiazolium bromide (a substance that cleaves collagen cross-links) in diabetic rats resulted in increased joint mobility.

Curran and colleagues[158] were the first to show that a program of physical therapy might be effective in improving joint movement in diabetic patients with limited joint mobility. Armstrong and colleagues[159] per-formed an uncontrolled study of 10 patients with a history of ulceration and limited joint mobility. After a supervised program of passive range-of-motion exercise performed three times per week for one month and once-daily exercises at home, range of motion at the first MTP joint increased significantly. There was also a reduction in peak forefoot plantar pressures.

Plantar Callus

It has been suggested that neuropathy predisposes patients to the production of excessive plantar keratoses.[160] Alternatively, the formation of callus has been ascribed to elevated shear stress,[125] although experimental evidence for this view is lacking. It is also possible that callus is simply a consequence of elevated vertical pressure, though callus is not found at all sites of high plantar pressure. Whatever the cause of callus may prove to be, evidence has shown that the removal of callus from bony prominences in the forefoot reduces plantar pressure by an average of 29%.[106] It therefore appears that excessive callus acts to elevate pressure, which may result in positive feedback for the production of further callus. This observation confirms the critical importance of callus care in the patient at risk for neuropathic ulceration.

In a prospective study of 63 neuropathic diabetic patients, Murray and colleagues[161] found that on the basis of six patients who ulcerated (seven ulcers), relative risk ratios for developing an ulcer were 4.7 for patients with an area of high pressure, 11.0 for patients with areas of plantar callus, and 56.8 for those with a prior ulcer. This points to the importance of callus in the pathogenesis of ulcers and also suggests that the tissue might become altered after ulceration to make it more susceptible to injury.

Foot Fractures

Several authors have noted a large number of radiographic abnormalities in the feet of neuropathic patients.[162-165] Cavanagh and colleagues[166] found a 12% prevalence of fractures (mostly metatarsal shaft) in neuropathic patients, most of which had not been previously diagnosed. In addition, an 8% prevalence of Charcot joint fractures was found. Fractures can result in alteration of weight bearing and load sharing by regions of the foot that are not specialized for this purpose. Thus, unperceived injury to bone can be a risk factor for elevated plantar pressure and ulceration.

Lower-Limb Weakness

Strength loss in the leg as a result of peripheral neuropathy has been well documented by Andersen and colleagues.[167] These authors studied 58 patients with insulin-dependent diabetes mellitus younger than 65 years old, all with a diabetes duration of greater than 20 years. Patients with neuropathy showed a 21% reduction in ankle dorsiflexor and plantar flexor strength, a 16% reduction in knee extensor strength, and a 17% reduction in knee flexor strength as measured with a Lido isokinetic dynamometer. The most severe strength losses that were noted in individual patients compared to controls were a more than 50% reduction in the plantar flexors. In a subsequent study using MRI, Andersen and colleagues[168] found a 32% reduction in the volume of the dorsal and plantar flexors, with more atrophy apparent distally.

Andreassen and colleagues[169] studied the decline in strength in a group of 30 diabetic patients together with 30 age-matched controls over a 6- to 8-year period. They found progressive declines in plantarflexion and dorsiflexion strength that was related to the severity of neuropathy. The mean annual loss in symptomatic neuropathic patients was 3.3% (± 2.3%) compared to 0.7% (± 1.7%) in controls. Correlations between lower-limb weakness and reduced conduction velocity in the peroneal and tibial nerves were reported by van Schie and colleagues.[170] Foot deformity was also moderately associated with decrements in conduction velocity. In neuropathic patients and those who had experienced foot ulcers, there was greater loss of strength in the tibial rather than peroneal nerve distribution. Interestingly, Cetinus and colleagues[171] found that hand-grip strength, an indicator of upper-limb function, was significantly reduced in the right hands of patients with type 2 diabetes compared to an age-matched control group. Differences on the left side were not significant.

While atrophy of the intrinsic muscles of the foot had long been suspected, our own MRI studies[172] using T_2 mapping have shown that the loss is much more profound than had previously been anticipated. As is shown in Figure 6-13, densely neuropathic patients may lose most of their intrinsic muscles to fatty infiltration. This must have significant consequences for foot function and is likely to contribute to foot deformity.

Prior Ulceration

Previous ulceration is a leading risk factor for future ulceration. The initial ulceration represents tangible proof that the patient has the combination of other risk factors that together produce ulceration. In addition, altered mechanical properties of the new tissue generated during the wound repair process may further increase the risk.[173] Although little is known about the mechanical properties of tissue generated during wound repair,[174] clinically one can feel the adhesion between different tissue layers and the lack of mobility of the skin overlying bony prominences. The exact role of adhesion and scar tissue in causing further tissue breakdown is not well known, but stress concentration is certainly a possible explanation. Thus, scar tissue might act in much the same way that callus appears to act: by transferring large,

concentrated loads to the immediately underlying softer tissue. Thus, the 56.8 risk ratio that is conferred by prior ulceration[161] might reflect scar-tissue–induced abnormalities as well as other risk factors present at the time of initial ulceration. Prior ulceration was also found to be a predictive factor for future ulceration in the risk model developed by Boyko and colleagues[175] (see below).

Shear Stress

Most of the previous discussion concerning the interaction of the foot with the shoe or ground has centered on the normal (vertical) pressures. But as is shown in Figure 6-2, there are also forces during gait, so-called shear forces, that tend to make the foot slip from its relatively fixed position on the ground. These forces generate shear stress separately in the tissues and the shoe materials, which are considered on a theoretical basis in the following discussion. Little is known at present about the magnitude and direction of shear stress during everyday activities or its role in causing plantar injury. This is because until recently, there were only isolated examples in the literature of instrumentation to measure shear stress.[67,176] Many authorities believe that shear stress is an important pathogenic factor in foot injury,[9,125,177] and it should not be ignored simply because there is no satisfactory measurement device at present. As we shall discuss below, shear stress can probably be modulated by the fit of a shoe, and it could emerge that the minimization of shear stress is an important criterion in defining appropriate fit.

Four new devices to measure plantar shear stress have been described during the last decade. Lord and colleagues[178] enhanced the magnetoresistive device (originally proposed by Tappin and colleagues[179]) by allowing measurement to be made in two orthogonal directions. The authors reported values for shear stress of 20 to 60 kPa, which are approximately 10% of the vertical stress values that are commonly encountered. Davis and associates[180,181] have designed and tested a device that is composed of 16 sensors, each 2.54 cm × 2.54 cm, capable of measuring three components of the applied load. They have derived estimates of 15 to 45 kPa for shear stress under the foot in various conditions. Akhlaghi and Pepper[182] describe preliminary results using thin polyvinylidene fluoride piezoelectric film, which has charge outputs proportional to shear stress in two independent directions. Christ and colleagues[183] reported on a device with 64 elements based on the same capacitance approach as platforms for the measurement of normal stress. All four of these devices are currently being used only in research environments, and all have different geometrical and physical characteristics. If any or all of them can be shown to be linear and independent of temperature changes, they might offer a new approach to the measurement of foot-ground interaction and the understanding of the etiology of foot injury.

Body Weight: Is It a Factor?

Cavanagh and colleagues[27] reported a small but statistically significant association between body mass and peak pressure in diabetic patients. Body weight accounted for only 14% of the variance in peak plantar pressure. Similar results were reported by Ahroni and colleagues,[114] who were able to explain only 6% of the variance. This somewhat counterintuitive finding indicates that foot structure is the dominant factor in determining plantar pressure and that the area over which load is distributed is subject to much more dramatic variations than is the load itself. Consider, for example, how a prominent MTH concentrates the forefoot load.

Vela and colleagues[184] asked young, symptom-free subjects to walk with added weight carried in the pockets of a vest while in-shoe plantar pressure was measured. Not surprisingly, they found that plantar pressure increased as a function of added load. This experiment addresses a different issue from that described above. Loads that are artificially added to a constant load distribution system (i.e., the individual subject's foot structure) will always increase peak plantar pressure. However, gain in body weight by an individual patient might or might not increase plantar pressure, depending on whether the plantar architecture is altered (e.g., by the deposition of more adipose tissue in the foot). Thus, in any given patient, body weight alone will be a poor predictor of plantar pressure. A small female weighing 100 pounds can easily exhibit higher plantar pressure than a large male weighing 300 pounds.

Abnormal Posture and Gait

The standing posture of patients with neuropathy is markedly less stable than the posture of control patients with diabetes of the same duration but with minimal neuropathy.[185–187] Simoneau and colleagues[185] have shown that neuropathic patients sway as much with their eyes open and head forward as do nonneuropathic patients in the challenging condition of "eyes closed/head back." This tendency might be a factor in the increased number of falls reported by neuropathic patients[188] and could contribute to the increased number of fractures that have been reported in this group.[165,189,190]

A number of investigators have explored the effects of diabetic neuropathy on gait, and there is considerable speculation that the gait patterns of neuropathic patients could predispose them to injury. Peripheral neuropathy has been shown to be a risk factor for injuries and falls during gait.[191,192] Courtemanche and colleagues[187] reported that neuropathic patients exhibited conservative gait patterns with increased time spent in double support and lower walking speeds. Increased reaction times to secondary tasks during gait were also found, suggesting that the neuropathic patients had to exert more cognitive control over normal gait compared to controls.

Katoulis and colleagues[193] also found smaller knee-joint excursions and lower peaks of vertical and anteroposterior ground reaction forces in neuropathic patients with a history of ulceration compared to nonneuropathic subjects. However, these may have been effects of speed, since the neuropathic patients walked significantly more slowly than did those in the control groups. Shaw and colleagues[194] used matching gait speeds between groups and found slightly higher first peaks in the vertical ground reaction forces of neuropathic patients with a history of ulceration compared to control subjects. Van Schie and colleagues[195] showed that the peak ground reaction forces in the residual limb of unilateral amputees were lower than those on the unaffected side, but the force-time integral was higher, reflecting the altered gait mechanics necessary for ambulation with only one power-input limb.

Various authors have hypothesized that peripheral neuropathy might lead to more variable[1] or less variable[9,103] gait patterns. It has also been hypothesized that less variable gait might contribute to risk of plantar ulceration. Cavanagh and colleagues[196] found that neuropathic patients did not exhibit abnormal variability of in-shoe plantar pressure patterns during shod walking, but by studying 10-minute epochs of continuous gait, Dingwell[197] found increased kinematic variability at the ankle joint in neuropathic patients.

Taken together, these studies show that neuropathic gait might be somewhat different from nonneuropathic gait and does exhibit, if anything, slightly more variability compared to normal, thus refuting the hypothesis that less variable plantar loading due to neuropathy at a subconscious level contributes to ulceration. Of course, patients with loss of protective sensation do not vary their gait at a conscious level in response to pain. Neuropathy does cause unstable posture. However, despite the widely agreed-upon role of sensory feedback in gait,[198] patients with diabetic neuropathy are able to ambulate in a nonchallenging situation in a manner remarkably similar to that of their nonneuropathic counterparts. The frequent anecdotal reports from patients that they "do not know where their feet are" and that they "bump their feet into things" must mean that gait studies to date have failed to successfully characterize the result of proprioceptive deficits. It is likely that the increased number of fractures in neuropathic patients is at least partly the result of these mechanisms.

Impaired balance and gait were found to be related in a small study of people with diabetes.[199] Diabetes was among the combination of diseases that were shown to be predictive of poor recovery of gait and balance after rehabilitative treatment.[200]

A number of studies have shown that neuropathic patients choose to walk more slowly than age-matched controls;[201,202] therefore, certain findings showing alterations in gait kinematics and kinetics might actually be speed-related effects. Rao and colleagues[203] found that diabetic subjects walking at the same speed as controls exhibited a similar range of ankle motion, despite the finding of reduced range of motion on static examination. The investigators believe that diabetic subjects used strategies such as shortening their stride length and reducing their push-off power to modulate plantar loading.

Kwon and colleagues[202] reported earlier onset of calf muscle activity and greater co-contraction in muscles spanning the knee and ankle joints in neuropathic patients compared to controls and suggested that this might be a "safety" strategy to compensate for loss of sensory input. Richardson and colleagues[204–207] have conducted a number of studies on neuropathic gait. They found that neuropathic diabetic patients exhibited increased variability in step width and other gait parameters in poorly illuminated settings.[205] The authors have also demonstrated that challenging environments (irregular surfaces and low lighting) magnify gait differences between older women with and without peripheral neuropathy in a manner that is correlated with the severity of peripheral neuropathy.[206]

There are indications that even when the increased risk of falls is controlled for, the risk of fracture at multiple sites in women with type 2 diabetes is increased.[208] Kanade and colleagues[209] have discussed the risks and benefits of walking as an exercise program for people with diabetes. In a group of older disabled women, Volpato and colleagues[210] found that diabetes was an independent risk factor that increased the risk of falling. The neuropathic status of these individuals was not reported. In another study,[211] older men with a longer duration of diabetes were found to have an enhanced risk of frequent falls.

Footwear

Uccioli and colleagues[212] conducted a prospective study of patients with previous ulceration. Patients were randomly assigned to wear either their own shoes or extra-depth shoes with custom-molded insoles. After 1 year, reulceration in the two groups was 58.3% for the group wearing their own shoes and 27.7% in the extra-depth shoe group. Since reimbursement for special footwear was extremely limited in Italy prior to this study, the authors justified their protocol of assigning patients to wear shoes in which they had already ulcerated by the need to influence public health policy. Such a protocol would probably not, and should not, be approved by Institutional Review Boards in the United States, since it is now clear from this and a number of other studies[13] that poorly-fitting footwear can play a key role in causing ulceration.

Ill-fitting footwear has been identified as the root cause of 21% to 76% of ulcers and/or amputations.[213–217] McGill and colleagues[218] followed a group of 472 patients (250 with neuropathy and 222 without) for 2 years and identified trauma from footwear as the major cause in 54% of the 34 ulcers that occurred (6.3% and 0.5%

annual incidence in the neuropathic and nonneuropathic groups, respectively).

Activity

It seems logical that increased activity would increase the risk of ulceration, since the accumulated mechanical stress during a given time period would be greater. However, studies to date have indicated that the picture is somewhat more complex. Lemaster and colleagues[219] collected self-report activity data on a cohort of patients enrolled in a footwear study[220] and reported that activity appeared to be inversely related to ulcer risk. A number of limitations of this study, discussed elsewhere,[221] together with the questionable accuracy of self-report activity data, suggest that these results should be viewed with caution.

However, some of these findings were confirmed by Armstrong and colleagues,[222] who studied 100 patients who were judged to be at risk for neuropathic ulceration. The patients wore an activity monitor for at least 25 weeks, during which time the eight patients who experienced ulceration took approximately 40% fewer steps per day than those who did not experience ulceration. The authors found that the variability in the number of steps per day increased in the 2 weeks prior to ulceration and suggested that "peaks and valleys" of activity might lead to tissue damage. Similarly, a case study by Lott and colleagues[223] showed a dramatic increase in weight-bearing activity on the day of ulcer recurrence.

The somewhat controversial hypothesis that a certain threshold level of tissue stress is protective for ulceration has been advanced by Maluf and Mueller.[224] In a study comparing the activity levels of 10 neuropathic patients with ulcer history and 10 patients without ulcer history, these authors found that the patients with prior ulcers were significantly less active than were those without a history of ulceration. Other factors could be responsible for this difference, and the hypothesis that plantar soft tissues respond to increased stress with hypertrophy in a similar manner to muscle and bone should be directly testable.

The potential importance of level of activity in foot pathology has led to the suggestion that one might need to prescribe the "dose" of activity, just as one would the dose of a prescription drug.[225,226]

Predictive Models

In a prospective study with a mean duration of follow-up of 3.28 years, Boyko and colleagues[175] reported 216 foot ulcers in 1285 diabetic (mostly male) veterans. The significant predictors of ulcer were high HbA1C levels, impaired vision, prior foot ulcer, prior amputation, monofilament insensitivity, tinea pedis, and onychomycosis.

Ledoux and colleagues[137] reported toe deformities (fixed hammertoes or clawed toes and hallux limitus) to be associated with increased risk of ulcer occurrence. Similarly, Nube and colleagues[24] found pronated feet to be related to a history of hallux ulceration, whereas a restricted range of motion at the first MTP joint was not.

Summary of Causes of High Pressure and Ulceration

In summary, a variety of structural and functional factors in the foot and leg interact to result in elevated plantar pressure, or they can cause skin injury directly. Among the most important variables is soft-tissue thickness. Other important anatomic and functional factors include the degree of foot deformity and gait parameters such as speed and instability.

Underlying tissue properties that are thought to have an effect include inelasticity due to nonenzymatic glyco-sylation, resulting in limited joint mobility, particularly at the first MTP joint and subtalar joints. Plantar callus is a visible marker for high plantar pressure, perhaps owing its existence to elevated pressure and itself causing an estimated 30% increase in pressure. Scar formation from prior ulceration could result in a focus of elevated pressure. Finally, body weight has not been found to contribute significantly to elevated peak plantar pressure.

Although vertical pressure has been measured in almost every study to date, it is believed that future evaluation of shear forces will further illuminate the pathogenesis of ulceration.

Ulcer Healing: Biomechanical Considerations

The Need for Load Relief

Ulcers develop on neuropathic feet because of trauma that the patient does not feel, and it makes sense that ulcers cannot heal if mechanical trauma is ongoing. It is now generally agreed that the terms *chronic ulcer* and *non-healing ulcer* are misnomers when applied to feet with adequate vascular supply.[227] The evidence for this statement comes from the many studies of total-contact casting (TCC) (see the section on the total-contact cast below), which is probably the most effective and certainly the best studied method of mechanically protecting plantar neuropathic ulcers. De Block and colleagues[228] found that only 3% of a large group of ulcer patients that they studied actually had "chronic" foot ulcers that were resistant to appropriate treatment. If a typical neuro-pathic plantar ulcer fails to heal by approximately 8 weeks, either it is being ineffectively treated or the patient is not being compliant with the treatment regimen. In a review, Sinacore[229] summarized 13 studies that described the efficacy of the TCC in the treatment of 389 neuropathic ulcers. Even though many ulcers had been present for months and even years prior to instituting TCC treat-

ment, the reported healing rates were 77% to 100% in 5 to 7 weeks.

By studying uncomplicated ulcers in patients who have remained in a TCC to complete wound closure, we have been able to define "ideal healing curves" for plantar wounds of different initial sizes.[230] (Uncomplicated ulcers were those without infection, with good vascular supply, and with continuous healing all the way to closure.) These curves, shown in Figure 6-14, are derived from the following equation:

$$r = b_0 + b_1 \times r_0 + b_2 \times t + b_3 \times r_0 \times t$$

This equation expresses the equivalent radius (r) of the ulcer at the time (t) in days after presentation. Equivalent radius is the radius of a circle whose area is the same as the (usually noncircular) ulcer. Where r_0 is the equivalent radius at day 0, the constants b_0, b_1, b_2, and b_3 were determined to be:

$b_0 = -0.74$
$b_1 = 1.04$
$b_2 = -0.10$
$b_3 = -0.012$

Ideal healing curves such as those shown in Figure 6-14 allow healing data for a given patient to be plotted against the ideal. In the clinic, the equivalent radius of a wound can be estimated by measuring the widest (D_w) and narrowest (D_n) diameter and dividing the sum of these measurements by 4.

If the patient's data deviate significantly into the area 1, 2, and 3 standard errors away from the mean (shown as dotted lines on the graph), then the treatment and the patient's compliance and behavior need to be reevaluated. That is not to say that all wounds must or can heal "ideally." Compromises might have to be made in patient care, possibly leading to a healing rate that is less than ideal, and such an approach may be acceptable to both the patient and the care provider. Nevertheless, having an ideal standard is useful even in such a case, since it allows judgments to be made as to how much of a compromise is actually involved. An example of actual healing data for a large midfoot ulcer is shown in Figure 6-14C.

The above equation can be rewritten to predict the time to healing (t_h):

$$t_h = -(b_0 + b_1 \times r_0)/(b_2 + b_3 \times r_0)$$

A table of days to healing for ulcers of different initial sizes is presented in Table 6-2, and the corresponding graph is shown in Figure 6-15. Such an approach to wound measurement has also been recommended as part of a comprehensive wound management protocol.[231]

The most common reason for failure to heal a neuro-pathic ulcer is lack of effective pressure relief at the ulcer site, owing either to the failure of the clinician to prescribe the correct measures or to patient nonadherence. The following section will examine ways in which load can be relieved from an active ulcer.

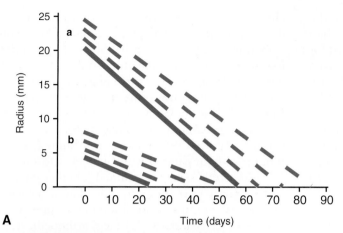

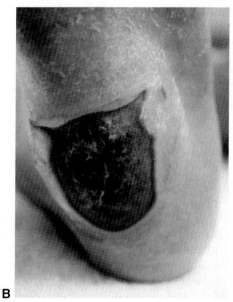

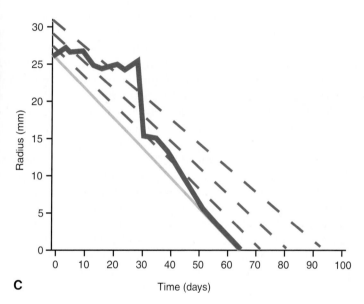

Figure 6–14   **A,** Ideal healing curves for plantar wounds with initial sizes of 5-mm and 20-mm equivalent radii, from Hsi and colleagues. [230] The *dashed lines* associated with each curve are 1, 2, and 3 standard errors from the mean. **B,** A large midfoot ulcer at the initial visit. **C,** The ulcer shown in Figure 6-14B was healed in a TCC with the healing curve shown. Note that progress was not along the ideal curve until drainage was controlled at approximately day 30.

TABLE 6-2   **Ideal Healing Times for Ulcers of Different Initial Sizes**

Initial Size (Equivalent Radius) (mm)	Initial Area (cm²)	Time to 50% Reduction in Radius (days)	Time to Complete Healing (days)
2.5	0.2	4.7	14.3
5	0.8	12.3	27.9
10	3.1	21.2	43.9
15	7.1	26.3	53.1
20	12.6	29.6	59.0
25	19.6	31.9	63.2
30	28.3	33.6	66.2

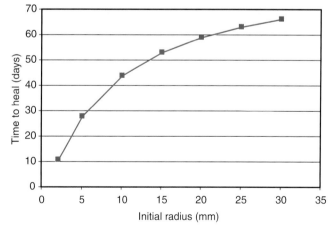

Figure 6–15   Days to healing for ulcers of different initial sizes.

The Total-Contact Cast

The TCC was originally believed to equalize loading of the plantar surface by ensuring total contact of the plantar skin with the cast material,[232] thereby minimizing pressure at an ulcer site. The device was not developed by Paul Brand, but he and his associates popularized its use, first in India in the treatment of patients with Hansen's disease and later in the United States in the treatment of the ulcerated diabetic neuropathic foot.[232] In early publications on the TCC, emphasis was placed on the "total contact," and it was recommended that the cast be made of plaster because it is more malleable than fiberglass. Later, outer layers of fiberglass were added for strength. Most centers now make the whole cast from fiberglass,[57,233–235] without apparent detriment in clinical outcomes. For further information on the use of TCC, see Chapter 13.

The precise mechanism of unloading in the TCC has now been studied by measuring plantar pressure inside the cast. A common design feature of the TCC is to pad the ulcer area with a soft foam before putting the cast on.[236,237] This, in essence, creates a void under the ulcer. In a group of healthy subjects, Shaw and colleagues[57] demonstrated pressure alteration in the forefoot at an MTH "ulcer site" in a TCC from approximately 350 kPa barefoot to approximately 50 kPa (a reduction of 86%). Neither peak pressure nor impulse (total force transmitted during a step) was equalized across the plantar surface in the TCC. Although some of the unloading that was seen in the forefoot was due to transfer of load to other parts of the foot (particularly the heel), approximately 30% of the unloading was actually due to the transferring of load from the leg directly to the cast walls, and much of the effect was due to the "void" created by the foam under the "ulcer." Midfoot peak pressure was reduced by 28% (from 92 kPa to 66 kPa, NS), but this result cannot be reasonably extrapolated to what might happen in patients with high midfoot pressure due to a Charcot fracture or a similar prominence. Heel pressure was reduced markedly (by 49%, from 354 kPa to 181 kPa), but the overall heel impulse was markedly increased (52%) because of increased time of loading. The authors did not report any peak pressure-time integrals.

In a comprehensive study of 25 patients with recently healed forefoot ulcers, depending on the site, Lavery and colleagues[59] found average pressure reductions of 81% to 92% in a TCC compared to a thin rubber-soled canvas oxford shoe at the previous ulcer sites. The average pressures in the canvas shoe were 271 kPa at the hallux, 438 kPa at MTH1, and 506 kPa at MTH2-5, whereas the corresponding average pressures at these sites in the TCC with a plastic walking heel were 49, 59, and 39 kPa, respectively. There was a small benefit in terms of pressure relief to the use of a TCC with a plastic walking heel compared to a TCC with a canvas cast shoe over it. Armstrong and Stacpoole-Shea[238] reported on the heel pressures in this cohort. Mean peak pressures of the group were reduced by 33% (from approximately 275 kPa to 185 kPa), but the pressure-time integral was not changed (meaning that loading at the point of peak pressure in the TCC was much longer than that in the canvas shoe).

Cogley and colleagues[239] noted a 91% reduction in forefoot plantar pressure in five subjects in a TCC compared to barefoot walking, and they actually reported an increase in heel pressure, but it was not statistically significant. Baumhauer and colleagues[60] noted forefoot pressures in a TCC of approximately 85 to 155 kPa.

However, their protocol called for casting in 5 to 10 degrees of dorsiflexion at the ankle, which could be responsible for these somewhat higher forefoot pressures than those reported in the other studies. Almost all other descriptions of the TCC procedure call for casting with the ankle in a neutral position (e.g., Coleman et al.,[232] Burnett[240]). In the Baumhauer study, no data were given for baseline barefoot or similar pressures. Martin and Conti[241] reported that a TCC significantly lowered midfoot pressure in patients with Charcot deformity.

Three studies have examined whether or not truly "total contact" is required to unload an ulcer. Conti and colleagues[242] reported no difference in pressure reduction between standard short-leg orthopedic casts and TCCs both in asymptomatic subjects and in patients with midfoot collapse due to Charcot fracture.[241] Making the same comparison, Cogley and colleagues[239] also found no difference in forefoot pressure relief in five subjects (TCC: 91% reduction, short-leg cast: 88% reduction), and similar results had been reported much earlier by Birke and colleagues.[243]

In all of the biomechanical studies just summarized, the emphasis has been on pressure relief, and there can be no doubt that removing injurious forces from the wound is central to healing. However, in all these studies, only peak pressure was measured. Impulse and shear could also be important factors and might also be reduced in a TCC. Shortened stride length and less walking in general because of the weight and clumsiness of the cast might also be of benefit. Another potential benefit of the TCC that has not been confirmed by clinical studies is reduction of edema. Finally, an important advantage of the TCC over other means of pressure relief is ensured patient adherence.

Many studies have highlighted the clinical efficacy of the TCC approach, and their summary in 1996 by Sinacore[229] is discussed above. The work of Mueller and colleagues[244] deserves special mention, since, to date, theirs has been the only randomized controlled trial of TCC therapy published. Forty patients with plantar neuropathic ulcers were randomized to receive either good wound care plus a TCC or good wound care alone. The patients who were not casted were instructed to avoid putting any weight on the ulcerated foot and were given crutches or walkers to that end. They were also given protective footwear in case they should step on the affected foot. The average duration of the ulcers before entry into the study was 155 days in the TCC group and 175 days in the standard-care group. Despite the effort to encourage the control group not to put weight on the foot with the ulcer, in the TCC group 19 of 21 ulcers healed in 42 ± 29 days, whereas in the control group, only 6 of 19 ulcers healed in 65 ± 29 days.

Since 1996, several other studies have been published that further demonstrate the benefits of the TCC and provide some insights into other factors that affect ulcer healing time. Lavery and colleagues[245] reported on a series that included 25 neuropathic plantar ulcers with a mean surface area of 7.7 ± 4.0 cm^2 and a duration of 88.5 ± 98.3 days and 22 patients with Charcot fractures and ulcers with a mean surface area of 10.3 ± 4.6 cm^2 and duration of 17.7 ± 12.9 days. All of the ulcers that were enclosed in a TCC healed in 38.8 ± 21.3 days, and all of the Charcot-related ulcers healed in a TCC in 28.4 ± 13.0 days. Short duration, small size, and association with a Charcot fracture all predicted a shorter healing time. A related study[246] reported that among the 25 noninfected ulcers, higher plantar pressures at the ulcer site predicted a longer duration of casting until healing. Sinacore[247] reported on a series of patients with various fixed deformities of the foot. He found a gradient of healing times for ulcers: 35 ± 12 days in the forefoot, 73 ± 23 days in the midfoot, and 90 ± 12 days in the rearfoot, with an overall average of 67 ± 29 days. The extent of the fixed deformity was also correlated with healing time. Caravaggi and colleagues[234] followed 50 patients with neuropathic foot ulcers to healing in a fiberglass TCC. All the ulcers healed in 58.5 ± 38.0 days, and size predicted time to healing. Patients preferred fiberglass casts to plaster casts. Finally, Lin and colleagues[248] reported that a group of 21 patients with neuropathic foot ulcers who were randomly selected from those that healed using a TCC in their clinic did so, on average, in 43.5 days. The authors found that the sole cause of nonhealing of a forefoot plantar ulcer in their series was inability to dorsiflex at the ankle (dorsiflexion range of motion in nonhealers was –20 degrees to –5 degrees; in those who healed, it was –5 degrees to +10 degrees). Fourteen of the 15 ulcers that had failed to heal initially did so in an average of 39.3 days after a tendo-Achilles lengthening (TAL) procedure (and ongoing TCC). It is perhaps relevant that Lin and colleagues[248] applied the TCC with 5 degrees of dorsiflexion at the ankle, whereas others describe TCCs applied with the ankle in a neutral position.[232,240]

Exact and consistent data on the complications of the TCC are hard to come by. Reported rates of complications vary from 6% to 43%,[229] and this variability depends on what is reported as a complication. Minor abrasions are common and heal in the next TCC. Major abrasions are rare, and the devastating complication of a major unrecognized infection is very rare, as are falls that lead to new fractures.

To summarize the pressure and clinical data on the TCC, it is reasonable to conclude that the TCC is very effective at reducing forefoot and probably midfoot plantar pressure and at healing plantar ulcers. The data are less clear with respect to heel ulcers. It might be that to accomplish efficient healing of a heel ulcer in a TCC, a significant foam cover creating a void under the ulcer (as is done routinely in many but not all centers) might be particularly useful, since, although heel pressure was reported to be decreased in a TCC in at least two studies, one study found increased impulse and the other found no improvement in the pressure-time integral in a TCC that was intimately molded at the heel. Many centers report that their results are as good with all-fiberglass TCCs as with plaster TCCs. Both the clinical data of Lin and colleagues[248] and the pressure data of Baumhauer and colleagues[60] suggest that the efficacy of the TCC in healing forefoot ulcers may depend critically on the angle at which the ankle is fixed with respect to the available range of dorsiflexion. In those two studies, the TCC was applied with dorsiflexion at the ankle. Lin and colleagues[248] found unusually poor healing compared to other studies, and Baumhauer and colleagues[60] found relatively high forefoot pressures in a TCC compared to other studies. On the basis of the available data, there seems to be no reason to cast with the ankle in dorsiflexion, and the possibility that a few degrees of plantarflexion could be additionally helpful should be explored. The pressure studies of Birke and colleagues,[243] Conti and colleagues,[241,242] and Cogley and colleagues[239] with standard short-leg casts, as well as the study of Shaw and colleagues,[57] suggest that the "total contact" concept might not be as critical to healing casts as had previously been thought.

The TCC can be bivalved by making a saw cut on the medial and lateral midlines, in effect making a "clamshell" type of front section that is held in place by Velcro™ straps. This approach has both advantages (ease of removal for bathing or sleeping) and disadvantages (perhaps too easy for noncompliant patients to remove at inappropriate times). A loosely applied bivalved cast probably does not unload the plantar surface as well as does a full TCC (see above discussion of Shaw and colleagues[57]). To date, no quantitative comparison of pressure relief in the two devices has been performed. Another version of a bivalved cast, in which the front shell is not replaced, is called a walking or "Carville" splint.[249,250] In a small study, Foster and colleagues[251] found that five of seven ulcers with a duration of 32 ± 31 weeks healed in a splint in 11 ± 8 weeks, whereas four of seven ulcers with a duration of 29 ± 16 weeks healed in a TCC in 7 ± 16 weeks.

Other forms of casts are also used, particularly a cast boot that does not extend above the ankle.[249,252-254] The mechanism of action of the cast boot is different from that of the TCC because no load can be shared by the leg. Usually, a large cutout around the ulcer site is made in the thick foam padding lining the boot, and this technique probably serves to mechanically isolate the wound. Plantar pressure was measured in a small study of five volunteers in a cast boot, and pressure reduction in the forefoot compared to a bare foot was only approximately 50% of the barefoot value, which is unlikely to be enough to promote good healing.[239] However, in one clinical study of a cast boot,[252] 35 of 40 patients healed in a mean of 3 months (range 1 to 8 months), and in another study,[255] ulcers that healed did so by 130 days, despite a mean ulcer duration prior to entry into the study of 912 days.

Another unloading method that uses casting is the MABAL shoe proposed by Hissink and colleagues.[256] The authors describe a removable fiberglass "combicast" that is applied to the ulcerated foot over a thick felted foam dressing. A rocker outsole is attached, and the cast ends below the level of the malleoli. Velcro™ straps are used to stabilize the shoe to the foot. A better than 90% healing rate, with a mean healing time of 34 days (range 7 to 75 days), was reported for a group of 23 ulcers with a mean area of 2 cm².

Armstrong and colleagues[257] reported significantly better healing in neuropathic plantar ulcers in patients using a TCC compared to a removable cast walker or a half-shoe (89.5%, 65%, and 58.3% complete healing in 12 weeks). The authors also reported markedly less activity of patients using the TCC compared to the half-shoe but not the removable cast walker.

The lack of adoption of total contact casting into the broader scope of practice has often been attributed to the provider's unwillingness to risk the occurrence of iatrogenic ulcers. However, a study of 70 consecutive neuropathic patients who received an average of 5.7 sequential casts[258] has shown that in skilled hands, the procedure is safe for the patient. Twenty-two complications were noted, for an overall initial complication rate of 5.5% per cast. These included seven new ulcers on bony prominences (pretibial and malleolar), six new midfoot ulcers, four forefoot/toe ulcers, and five hindfoot ulcers. In no case was a preexisting ulcer made worse, and all but one of the iatrogenic ulcers healed within 3 weeks, often during continued casting. Application of the TCC using a pressure-relieving foam disk in the area of high plantar pressure results in less pressure at these sites and might improve healing times.[259]

The TCC was shown to be superior to removable cast walkers or half-shoes in a study of the number of ulcers healing in a 12-week period.[260] The number of steps per day was less in patients who wore a cast, and this could be a significant factor in accelerated healing. In a retrospective study of nonischemic, noninfected ulcer healing in 180 patients with the Scotchcast boot, Knowles and colleagues[261] found a mean time to healing of 130 days (± 107 days). As was expected, superficial wounds healed faster than deep wounds, although 36 wounds (20%) did not heal.

All the removable devices can be used in the setting of infected wounds, since they allow for frequent dressing changes and wound inspection. Once infection is under control and the patient is clearly improving on antibiotics, it is a matter of clinical judgment as to whether a full TCC with frequent changes should be employed for optimal wound protection.

Other Approaches to Unloading

The absence of information on pressure thresholds for healing complicates the interpretation of studies of the various unloading devices. Strictly avoiding putting any weight on the affected limbs (i.e., non-weight-bearing) should be completely efficacious, but in a clinical setting, it is never as good as a TCC.[244] This might be because the TCC has other benefits over non-weight-bearing, but more likely, it is a function of some steps taken by the insensate patient despite his or her best efforts. Clinical experience suggests that when non-weight-bearing is to be part of the protocol, very specific and explicit instructions need to be given to the patient about how to accomplish non-weight-bearing in each situation they may encounter at home, at work, at night, and so on. It is a matter of clinical experience that patients who put weight of even a few steps per day on the ulcerated foot do not heal particularly well. Balance is also compromised in neuropathic patients; therefore, any intervention that requires the patient to balance on one leg could be dangerous.

Knowles and colleagues[261,262] and Armstrong and Lavery and associates[263,264] discuss a number of approaches to unloading the foot. Many footwear interventions for healing can benefit by the added use of a mobility aid, such as crutches or a wheelchair. A novel approach to unloading has been suggested by Roberts and Carnes,[265] who designed an "orthopaedic scooter." This device consists of a metal frame attached to a trolley with four small wheels and an adjustable-height padded channel on which patients can rest their lower leg and foot while propelling themselves with the contralateral foot. A similar device has been used by others,[266] and the design has also been refined with the addition of a brake (Roll-A-Bout Corp., Boca Raton, FL).

Chantelau and colleagues[267] describe the use of half-shoes in the healing of forefoot plantar ulcers. These shoes offer support only under the hindfoot and midfoot, leaving the forefoot suspended. Despite the risk of blunt trauma to the forefoot and of the additional load added to the midfoot, these shoes appear to be successful in healing forefoot ulcers. In the study by Chantelau and colleagues,[267] 96% of patients healed, with a mean time to ulcer closure of 70 days. Because of the inherent instability of this approach, the investigators insisted that patients also use crutches. Needleman[268] presented a retrospective case series of 33 patients who had been treated with a "half-shoe" (called an Integrated Prosthetic and Orthotic System; IPOS, Niagara Falls, NY). In that study, 77% of patients healed in an average of 8 weeks. Among the complications from wearing the IPOS shoe were balance problems or falls (eight of the 33 patients reviewed), new ulcers or preulcers (four of 33 patients), and bone pain (two patients). Needleman also presented a comparison of charges for a course of treatment. The figures he proposed (as of 1997) were $82 plus the cost of daily wound care for the IPOS shoe, $800 to $1400 plus four to seven episodes of wound care for the TCC, and approximately $1000 plus daily wound care for the bivalved cast. He also estimated the cost of hospital bed rest at $390 per day plus daily wound care and a one-time charge for crutches plus daily wound care. This figure is already a significant underestimate of actual costs in many hospitals. A full cost-benefit analysis is not possible because of the lack of comparative data for wound healing by these different methods.

An important point to make about half-shoes is that they are not all created equal. In the studies of Chantelau and colleagues[267] and Needleman,[268] the shoes used had no support surface for the forefoot (true half-shoes). Fleischli and colleagues[269] studied unloading in terms of plantar pressure in the Darco half-shoe. This version of the half-shoe has a forefoot support, but in reality, it is a negative-heel shoe with a large rocker (see the section of this chapter on footwear). Pressure reduction in this type of shoe as reported by Fleischli and colleagues[269] was only 64% to 66% compared to a canvas shoe. The published healing data mentioned above were on true half-shoes.[267,268]

A number of braces and orthosis-like devices have also been explored as alternatives to TCCs. Most of these have a rigid rocker or roller sole, some method of attachment of vertical members up the sides or back of the leg, and a soft insole. Among the devices that have been most studied are the Aircast brace,[58,60,270] the CAM walker,[270] the DH walker,[58,270] and the Easy Step walker.[271]

The Aircast brace has four inflatable chambers that are designed to provide an enhanced fit to the leg, but there are no published data to support this feature as being additionally helpful in plantar pressure relief or commenting on its clinical efficacy. However, Lavery and colleagues[270] noted a 60% to 73% reduction of plantar pressure at forefoot ulcer sites among 25 subjects with recently healed ulcers and an approximately 26% reduction in the heel peak pressure without a change in the pressure-time integral[238] compared to a canvas oxford with a thin rubber sole. The absolute forefoot peak pressures in the device were 111 to 150 kPa, significantly higher than TCC pressures in the same subjects (53 to 83 kPa). The heel peak pressures were approximately 200 kPa in the Aircast brace, 275 kPa in the canvas shoe, and 185 kPa in the TCC. In a similar study, Baumhauer and colleagues[60] found similar forefoot pressures (approximately 65 to 155 kPa) in the brace in 10 healthy volunteers, and these values were not significantly different from TCC pressures (but see the earlier discussion of the TCC technique used in this study).

The insole of the DH walker consists of small hexagonal foam columns that can be removed to provide pressure relief for an ulcer. Although this has been shown to be effective when brand new in normal subjects in terms of pressure relief, care is needed when the device is used clinically to ensure that columns surrounding the ulcer site do not collapse into the void, resulting in a significant loading of the ulcer site. Again, no published clinical data are available. However, forefoot pressure relief in the DH walker, as demonstrated by Lavery and colleagues,[270] was in the range of 77% to 84%, with absolute pressures

of 64 to 83 kPa. Similarly, Fleischli and colleagues[58] noted pressure reductions of 76% to 85% in 26 patients with recently healed ulcers, with absolute peak pressures of 49 to 77 kPa at the ulcer sites in the device. Both studies used a simple canvas shoe for comparison. Armstrong and Stacpoole-Shea[238] reported that heel pressures in the DH walker were 195 kPa compared to a shoe baseline of 275 kPa.

Saltzman and colleagues[272] reported reduced pressures under a Charcot midfoot prominence when using a patellar tendon–bearing brace, and Guse and Alvine[273] have also recommended such a brace to unload plantar ulcers. Further studies need to be conducted to determine the optimal design characteristics of such devices for unloading the foot, since a poorly designed or fitted device may result in little unloading. In fact, Saltzman and colleagues[272] noted that the longer a device had been used, the looser the cuff and the less well the brace functioned to unload the foot. Landsman and Sage[274] have presented some successful case studies in which an ankle-foot orthosis was used during the healing of plantar ulcers in patients with Charcot fractures. Their pressure measurements showed that the brace offered considerable relief at the ulcer site compared to a shoe alone.

Morgan and colleagues[275] described a device called the Charcot Restraint Orthotic Walker (CROW), which has some similarity to a bivalved TCC. It is constructed from a bivalved polypropylene shell, but in contrast to the TCC or Carville splint, there is a layer of deep padding under the footbed, and the outsole is rockered. These authors and others[276] described the successful use of the CROW as a follow-up to TCCs in patients with Charcot fractures. It has been speculated that the CROW could be used to treat ulcers, but such use is not supported by any published data. A similar device was used by Boninger and Leonard[277] to treat Charcot fractures and ulcers. Healing of 12 ulcers was very slow in this small study (eight ulcers healed in an average of 10 months).

Various types of felt and foam dressings are used at a number of centers for healing plantar ulcers.[278,279] This approach consists of adhering a bilayer of felt and foam to the patient's foot (foam layer next to the skin). A region of pressure relief is created by removing the foam and felt material from the area of the ulcer, thus transferring load to the surrounding tissue. A surgical shoe is then worn to accommodate the bulk of the dressing. No large controlled study of this method exists, but a number of anecdotal reports suggest that it can be effective for patients who insist on remaining ambulatory during ulcer healing. Without providing specific data, Ritz and colleagues[280] state that more than 90% of neuropathic plantar ulcers can be healed in an average of 8 weeks by using the felted-foam approach. In a study comparing 10 patients with plantar ulcers due to Hansen's disease treated with traditional care plus felt dressings to seven patients treated without felt, Kiewied[281] noted that at 4 weeks, five of the 10 patients had healed with felt dressings, whereas none of the other seven patients had healed given traditional care only. Fleischli and colleagues[58] noted off-loading of between 34% to 48% in terms of forefoot peak pressure at previous ulcer sites when felt dressings were compared to walking in simple canvas shoes. This therapy is also said to be helpful for healing nonplantar wounds. However, some experts have expressed concern about the possible edge effects of such dressings, particularly when used on the plantar surface of the foot.[282,283]

Connelley[36] has suggested from anecdotal observations that a pressure of 55 kPa (8 psi) measured inside footwear during walking will allow plantar ulcers to heal. This value is similar to those presented above for unloading in the TCC, Aircast brace, and DH walker (although different devices were used by these investigators to measure the pressure; see the earlier discussion on this issue). For a discussion of the implementation of alternatives to the TCC, see Chapter 13.

The recognition that many patients will not use removable devices that are designed to off-load during ulcer healing,[284] together with the lack of adoption of the TCC, have led Armstrong and his colleagues to propose what they have called an Instant Total Contact Cast[285] or an Irremovable Cast Walker.[286,287] This modification entails using a conventional off-loading technique at the plantar surface together with a boot or walker. The walker is then wrapped with several turns of cast tape so that the patient is discouraged from removing the walker until the next office visit. Such a device was shown in one study to heal 80% of plantar ulcers in 12 weeks[286] and to result in significantly faster healing than occurs with a removable cast walker.[287]

Most of the methods for off-loading the plantar ulcer described in this section have the advantage over the TCC that they can be easily removed and can therefore be used in the setting of infected ulcers, where frequent wound inspection and dressing changes are essential.

Unloading the Plantar Ulcer: A Summary

Uncomplicated neuropathic ulcers should heal easily if given proper mechanical protection. The best-studied and best-established method for protecting the plantar neuropathic wound is the TCC.[288] Extensive data on normal healing in a TCC have been presented here, and some of the design features of the TCC have also been discussed. Interestingly, equalization of pressure across the plantar surface is probably not an important feature of the cast, and "total contact" might not be key. The TCC is labor intensive and therefore expensive, and it can lead to serious complications, such as unrecognized infection and iatrogenic lesions.

Only a few of the other methods discussed above for protecting the plantar surface are supported by clinical

data; even then, only small numbers of patients have been studied. The half-shoe for healing plantar forefoot ulcers has been evaluated the most, but as was discussed above, not all brands or types of half-shoes are likely to be equally efficacious. Several other commercial devices—in particular, the Aircast brace and DH walker—appear promising in terms of peak pressure relief, but that is not the same as clinical efficacy (particularly if peak pressure turns out not to be the key variable that determines tissue breakdown). Many experts support the use of felt and foam dressings.

As was discussed earlier, patients with neuropathy fall more often, have more injuries, and sway more during standing than do people without neuropathy. All the devices that are intended to unload a neuropathic ulcer would seem intuitively to be likely to increase the risk of falling just because of their ungainliness, and this hypothesis is supported for the TCC with a plastic heel by Lavery and colleagues,[289] who demonstrated approximately 20% more sway in patients during standing in a TCC with a plastic heel compared to standing in a simple canvas sports shoe. Interestingly, use of a TCC with a cast shoe, a "CAM" type cast walker, and a Darco half-shoe had little effect on postural sway. It still seems prudent to pay attention to the risk of falling and injury in all patients who are being treated for neuropathic plantar ulcers. However, casting with a cast shoe may be preferable in patients at very high risk for falling compared to casting with a plastic heel (but it should be recalled that a TCC with a cast shoe does not reduce pressure as well as does a TCC with a plastic heel).[59]

Patients who have ulcerated often continue to wear footwear that had been prescribed to prevent ulceration. It is the common clinical experience that patients who are using their own shoes do not heal, even though the shoes might be good enough to prevent recurrence. It is worthwhile to consider this point in terms of what is known about pressure relief that can be achieved in a TCC compared to "therapeutic" shoes. The data that we just reviewed for pressure relief in a TCC show that 80% to 90% of the peak plantar pressure can be removed in a cast, whereas in sport shoes, that figure is around 30% and might be no more than 50% in therapeutic shoes.

Footwear: Theoretical Background

That footwear is thought to be so central to injury prevention in diabetes is emphasized by the fact that another chapter in this book deals with the various aspects of footwear design and prescription (see Chapter 28). Footwear can cushion the plantar surface from the injurious high pressures that we discussed above and, through proper or improper fit, can prevent or cause dorsal injury. Footwear can thus be critical in preventing the first injury in patients with newly diagnosed neuropathy and becomes an issue of lifetime concern for a patient who has experienced a neuropathic ulcer. Given the emphasis on the practical aspects of footwear in other chapters, in this section, we describe some of the principles behind the action of footwear and explore ways in which some science may be applied to this area, which has been widely described as an art.

Cushioning: Static and Dynamic

If asked to choose a single word to describe the objective of footwear for the neuropathic foot, many workers in the field would probably choose the term *cushioning*. Yet the definition of cushioning in a footwear context is elusive; it has no units, it is not easily measured, and it is often misinterpreted. Webster's dictionary[290] offers the definition "to protect against force or shock" and goes on to define a cushion as "an elastic body for reducing shock." This definition might be paraphrased in more mechanical terms as "controlling the energy of a collision." To understand the inadequacy of this definition and to seek a better one, it is helpful to divide the contact of the shoe and the ground into two distinct phases: a dynamic phase, which starts at heel strike and ends at foot flat, and a quasi-static phase, which includes the remainder of ground contact. It might come as a surprise that late stance and toe off are considered quasi-static, but compared with the high-impact forces of heel contact,[291] the rather slowly changing forces of the second part of stance have minimal dynamic components.

The major difference between these two phases is that the net force acting on the foot through the shoe can be reduced by the cushioning effect of footwear during the dynamic phase, but the net force during the quasi-static phase cannot be changed. However, during both phases, the net force can be distributed so that local pressures on the foot are reduced. By *net force*, we mean the total, at any instant in time, of all the forces acting on each part of the foot. For example, if there were forces of 300 N and 200 N on the forefoot and hindfoot, respectively, at 0.3 second after foot strike, a net force of 500 N would be acting, and this could be recorded by a force platform, as shown in Figure 6-2.

To appreciate the difference between the dynamic and static phases, consider the two situations shown in Figure 6-16. In Figure 6-16A, an egg is dropped from the same height onto surfaces of successively softer characteristics. On the hard surface, it breaks, but on the foams, the impact is cushioned, and breakage does not occur. The appropriate models are of a mass with velocity v and acceleration g, contacting first a rigid link and then springs of stiffness k_1 and k_2 (where $k_1 > k_2$). Hypothetical force-time curves show that the peak force at impact would be reduced and the time to peak force would be increased. Both effects are forms of cushioning that can occur in a dynamic situation.

In the static situation, a flat plate is shown placed atop the same materials (Fig. 6-16B). Despite the fact that the plate sinks more deeply into the softer foams, the net (or total) force acting on the plate is the same in each case and is equal to its weight.

In the case of a collision, as occurs at heel strike, Webster's definition of cushioning is appropriate, because we are concerned with managing the energy of the collision to reduce the force exerted on the foot. Certainly, therapeutic shoes can be cushioned in this way, but we know that neuropathic ulceration rarely occurs in the heel regions, except for ulcers caused by continuous application of pressure (similar to decubitus ulcers in the bedridden patient), which have a different etiology. Thus, collision energy is not really what causes ulcers. Because the static example (see Fig. 6-16B) shows that net force cannot be reduced during the midstance phase when forefoot plantar pressures are largest (see Fig. 6-5), we must search elsewhere to find a definition of cushioning that is relevant to the prevention of neuropathic foot injury.

Footwear as a Distributor of Force

This search leads to a definition of cushioning that is based on distribution of force (and accompanying reduction of pressure) rather than attenuation of net force. As was mentioned earlier, the term *net* is key to understanding the action of footwear because, although the net force acting on the forefoot at any instant in time may remain the same, the local forces acting on individual anatomic structures, which, when totaled, must equal the net force, can be altered dramatically by footwear.

A further model of cushioning in the context of forefoot deformity is proposed in Figure 6-17. If a bony prominence such as the head of a plantarflexed metatarsal bone contacts a rigid surface, most of the ground reaction force will be applied to the small area of the bony prominence, with resultant large local pressures (Fig. 6-17A). Patients are always encouraged to avoid walking barefoot for precisely this reason. The model of this foot in a conventional (nontherapeutic) shoe is shown in Figure 6-17B. The uniform stiffness of the midsole material (i.e., its spring constant k) is so large that even though the shoe deforms slightly, the amount of deformation is not enough to engage the adjacent spring elements with the foot so that the load can be shared. Thus, no pressure reduction occurs.

When a compliant material is placed in the shoe, the situation becomes much more favorable for the soft tissue of the foot. The appropriate model now consists of a series of springs with lower spring constants than before, arranged in parallel with each other (Fig. 6-17C). Because the spring constant is smaller, more deformation will occur, allowing adjacent spring elements to begin to share the load as the material under the bony prominence is compressed. This action results in the so-called accommodative behavior of shoes for the neuropathic

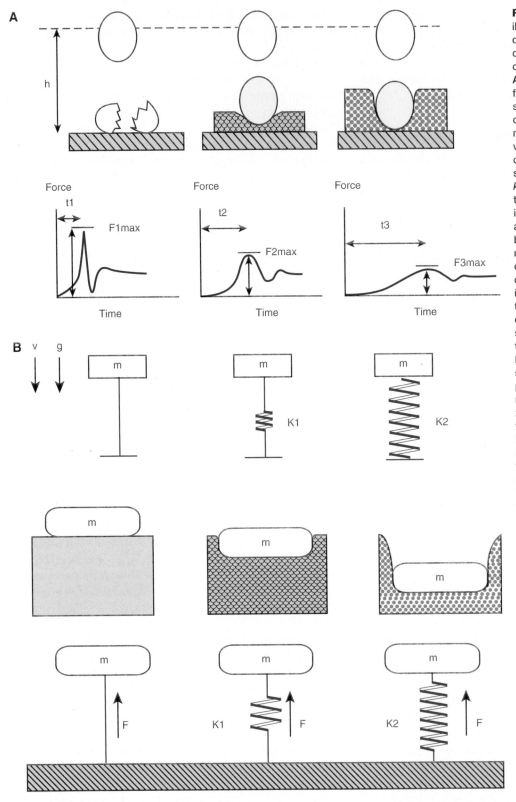

Figure 6–16 Schematic illustrations on the effects of different types of cushioning during the dynamic phase and quasi-static phase of contact. *A,* Dynamic phase. Egg falling from the same height onto surfaces of successively softer characteristics. The appropriate models are of a mass with velocity *v* and acceleration *g,* contacting first a rigid link, then springs of stiffness k_1 and k_2 ($k_1 > k_2$). Hypothetical force-time curves show that the peak impact force would be reduced and the time to peak force would be increased by the softer material; however, the area under each curve (which represents the change in momentum of the egg) is the same in each case. Thus, in the dynamic phase (as occurs during gait primarily only at foot strike), soft materials can change the peak force acting on the foot. *B,* Static phase. Flat plate standing on materials of progressively increasing softness: rigid; stiffness, k_1; stiffness k_2 ($k_1 > k_2$). Note that despite the fact that the plate sinks more deeply into the softer material, the net (total) force acting on the plate is the same in each case and is equal to its weight. Therefore, in the static phase of foot contact with the ground (as occurs in the later phases of support), soft materials cannot change the total force acting on the foot but can affect the distribution of the force (see also Fig. 6-17).

foot. The total force from all the spring elements at any instant will be the same as the force in Figure 6-17A, but the local pressure (force in each spring element divided by its area of application) will be reduced.

This situation in Figure 6-17C clearly is not perfect, because the greater compression of the spring element under the prominence will still result in greater local pressure. The available options are to increase the length of the adjacent springs (Fig. 6-17D) or to reduce both the stiffness and the length of the spring under the prominence (Fig. 6-17E). In practice, the first of these options is easier to achieve, because the deformation

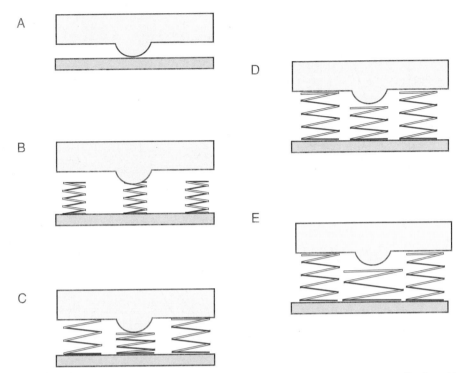

Figure 6–17   Role of footwear during the quasi-static phase of ground contact in cushioning by distribution of load. **A,** Schematic cross section of a foot with a plantar prominence resting on a flat, rigid surface. **B,** Conceptual model of the foot in contact with a rigid shoe. Spring elements are all the same and extremely stiff. Even though slight deformation occurs under the prominence, this does not cause enough deflection to bring other regions of the foot-shoe interface into the load-bearing process. Thus, the pressure under the prominence is as high as in **A,** because the total force still is transmitted through this region. **C,** When a more compliant material is placed in the shoe, the appropriate model now consists of springs with lower spring stiffness than before in parallel with each other. Because the spring stiffness is smaller, more deformation will occur, and as the material under the bony prominence is compressed, adjacent spring elements begin to share the load. This action results in the "accommodative" behavior of shoes for the neuropathic foot. The force that is transmitted through the prominence now will be less. **D,** An alternative solution (shown for the almost unloaded foot) is to reduce the length of the spring under the prominence and/or increase the length of the springs away from this region so that all springs will engage immediately on loading. This occurs with a molded insole, with which load sharing begins as soon as the foot is loaded and peak pressures are reduced. **E,** A better solution still is to make the spring under the prominence both shorter and less stiff. This reduces the loading on the prominence and increases loading on other structures. This occurs with a composite insole that incorporates different material under the bony prominence.

range over which a less stiff spring could work is limited by the room in the shoe. Molding of the insole to the shape of the foot is the practical embodiment of this theory. This process brings the insole up to meet the parts of the plantar aspect that would otherwise not share in the load-bearing process. A firm molded insole should in theory equalize loading. However, relative movement between foot and footbed would bring prominent parts of the foot into contact with raised parts of the rigid insole, leading to tissue damage. Thus, we depend on soft materials that modify their contour and keep the load shared between adjacent regions even when shearing movements occur. The "softness" of various insole materials is compared in Figure 6-18D.[292]

It has been shown that socks must be considered in this equation,[293,294] because use of special thick socks alone can reduce barefoot peak pressures by approximately 30%. One can conceptualize the way in which socks achieve this as being similar to how insoles have their effect: by providing a large number of short springs that can bring new, albeit small, regions of the foot sur-

rounding bony prominences into a weight-bearing role.

Even with a well-molded insole (e.g., Plastazote backed with PPT), there will still be elevated pressures under bony prominences compared with the adjacent regions. This occurs because the molding results in a thin, compressed layer of material under the prominence, which probably acts as a stiffer spring and will give greater force for a given compression than the uncompressed material in surrounding areas. There are currently no data in the literature on the mechanical characteristics of moldable materials after they have been reduced in thickness.

From the point of view of equalizing the pressure in different areas of the foot, the ideal foot-shoe interface would be a hydrostatic cushion (a fluid-filled bag) that could adapt to local curvatures and apply equal loads to all regions of the foot. This principle has been implemented in the area of pressure ulcers of the buttocks,[295] and there are reports of investigations into fluid-filled insoles.[296] However, fluid has no ability to resist movement of the foot in the anteroposterior or mediolateral

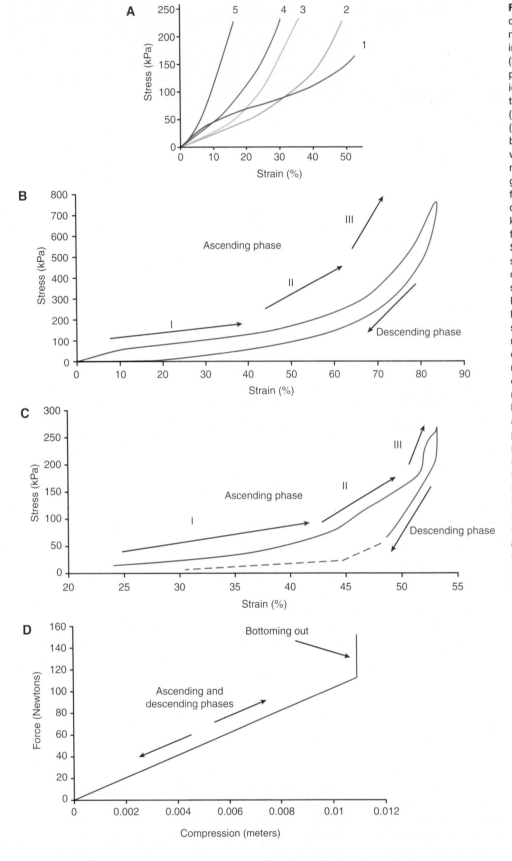

Figure 6–18   Results of compression tests for several insole materials (**A**), a material used in insole construction (Plastazote #1) (**B**), the human heel pad (**C**), and a perfect spring (**D**). Note that the idealized spring is linear and follows the same path during the ascending (loading) and descending (unloading) phases but that a bottoming-out point is reached at which force increases sharply with minor change in compression. The gradient of the spring (change in force divided by change in deformation) in its linear portion is known as spring stiffness. Graphs for materials have a standard form: Stress is plotted on the Y axis and strain on the X axis. No single value can be used to characterize the slopes of the curves for the Plastazote material and the human heel pad, because these curves get steeper in three phases (i.e., the materials become stiffer) as more compression occurs. Stiffness (or modulus) can be calculated for each of these phases. Both insole material and the heel show hysteresis, meaning that loading and unloading follow different paths. The variations in mechanical properties of typically used insole materials are apparent from **A**. The materials shown are (1) Poron (PPT), (2) Spenco, (3) Plastazote #1, (4) Plastazote #2, and (5) Soft Pelite. *(Adapted from Sanders JE, Greve JM, Mitchell SB, Zachariah SG: Material properties of commonly-used interface materials and their static coefficients of friction with skin and socks. J Rehabil Res Dev 35(2):161–176, 1998.)*

directions, providing a very unstable platform for the foot. The insole's depth would also have to be great enough to prevent bottoming out. These problems do not appear to be insurmountable, however, with an appropriate restraint applied through the upper and with the kind of depth that is already incorporated into a rocker shoe. The problem of excessive weight of the fluid-filled insoles could prove more difficult to resolve.

Properties in the Plane of the Ground

The example of lack of control in the "fluid bag" brings us to the last additions to the conceptual model of the shoe-foot interface: damping and spring stiffness in the anteroposterior and mediolateral directions. We note from the stress-strain experiments on both a shoe material and the heel (see Fig. 6-18) that these structures exhibit hysteresis, showing that energy-absorbing (damping) elements are present. Hysteresis is said to occur when the behavior of a material is different during loading and unloading. Perfect springs store all of the available energy when they deform and return that energy during the rebound phase. If no damping were present in the earlier example of the falling egg (see Fig. 6-16), the egg would rebound from the foam cushions up to its initial height.

Whereas springs store energy, dampers redirect it. The first law of thermodynamics tells us that energy cannot be created or destroyed; it can only be transformed. Energy that is used to deform a damper is converted to heat and therefore cannot be usefully recovered as mechanical energy. When a viscous element is cyclically loaded, stress and strain are not in phase, and a characteristic loop is developed (see Fig. 6-18B). The area that is enclosed by the loop is a measure of how much energy has been lost. Practically speaking, the damping elements control the rate of compression of the spring and its tendency to oscillate or bounce. They are usually represented as dashpots (Fig. 6-19), which in our model would be in parallel with the spring. Thus, each spring element in our cushioning models of Figures 6-16 and 6-17 should be replaced by the combined element shown in Figure 6-19A.

Finally, we turn to the issue of stiffness and damping in shear directions. The potential role of shear stress in causing foot injury was discussed earlier, and we consider here how footwear may affect shear stress. As long as there is sufficient friction between the insole and the foot or sock, points on the foot will tend to remain in contact with the same points on the surface of the insole when shear forces are applied, causing the insole material to experience shear strain. When there is not enough friction, the foot will, of course, slip. Exactly how much strain occurs for a given shear stress will be determined by the stiffness of the material in shear, and this can be added conceptually to our unit element by a spring in the horizontal plane, as shown in Figure 6-19B. In the examples that were discussed previously, the spring con-

stant of the horizontal components would be extremely small in the hydrostatic cushion, extremely large on a rigid surface, and intermediate in value in traditional insole materials. Providing a material that allows an appropriate amount of shear strain to occur is a critically important factor in the specification of an insole. There will also be a damping action in the horizontal plane, as shown by the added horizontal dashpot in Figure 6-19C, which represents the final configuration of a conceptual model that is appropriate for the consideration of cushioning in the shoe. The complete conceptual model, which incorporates different spring constants under the bony prominence, as well as compliance and damping in both vertical and horizontal directions, is shown in Figure 6-19D.

Although the concepts of individual springs and dampers are useful for discrete conceptual models, when the materials are continuous, the compression modulus and shear modulus are better quantities for the characterization of the vertical and horizontal spring stiffness. Values for these quantities are not common knowledge at the present time, although, as will be discussed in the next subsection, information on the material properties of insoles is now available,[292,297,298] and it is expected that compression and shear moduli will become the basis for a more quantitative approach to footwear design and manufacture in the near future.

Tissue and Material Properties

Many of the presumed reasons for elevated plantar pressure in diabetes have to do with changes in the plantar soft tissues, whereas footwear is prescribed to redistribute plantar forces and thereby lower plantar pressures. Thus, a deeper understanding of the properties of footwear materials and the plantar tissues—in particular, how they respond to force—is key in providing further insight into why high pressure may occur and how it can be dealt with. The excellent chapter by Thompson[299] in the fourth edition of this book is recommended as a good primer on tissue mechanics, as is the more mathematical treatment presented by Sharkey.[300]

When a force is applied to an object, some deformation always occurs. If the material is very hard (e.g., bone), the deformation might not be visible to the naked eye, but if the material is soft (e.g., the heel pad), deformation is obvious. Because both the area over which the force is applied and the initial length of the material will affect the outcome of a given interaction, engineers have chosen to standardize the approach to these kinds of problems using the quantities stress and strain. As was discussed earlier, stress is synonymous with pressure and is calculated by dividing force by the area over which it acts. Strain is simply fractional deformation, calculated by dividing the change in length by the original length. Thus, stress causes strain; it is important that these terms not be used interchangeably.

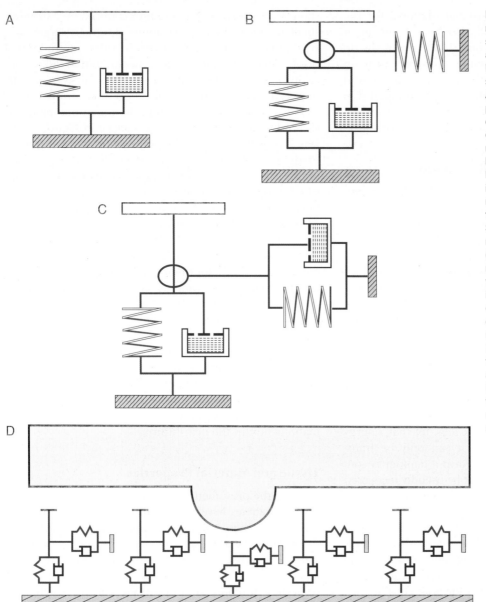

Figure 6-19 Single-spring models cannot describe shear stress or the hysteresis noted in actual materials (see Fig. 6-18). However, refinements to such simple models are possible. **A,** Damping element is added in parallel with the spring. This controls the rate at which the spring compresses and controls the rebound. It also can model hysteresis in the materials. **B,** Stiffness of the material in shear is modeled by a spring that is rounded at one end and attached to the vertical element at the other. Stiffness of the spring can be measured as the shear stiffness (or modulus) in actual shoe materials. **C,** Final model element with both compliance and damping in both vertical and horizontal directions. (See text for further details.) **D,** Refined large conceptual model of the foot in cross section. Load sharing will begin as soon as the foot is loaded in both horizontal and vertical directions. Damping is incorporated into each element, and the spring constants of the materials under the prominence are smaller than those elsewhere.

The field of solid mechanics examines the relationship between stress and strain in materials. In a biologic context, it is most developed in the area of tensile (elongation) testing of hard tissues; for example, both experimental and theoretical determinations of the effects of stress on bone are well documented.[300] In contrast, soft tissues have received less attention, particularly in compression, and little is known about the mechanical properties of the tissues of the plantar surface of the foot. The same is true for the mechanical properties of the materials that are typically put in contact with the foot, such as polyethylene foam (e.g., Plastazote) and urethane foam (e.g., PPT). Both soft tissues and these materials are complex because they exhibit large deformation, nonlinearity, and viscoelastic behavior—all properties that make theoretical approaches difficult.

Figure 6-20 shows theoretical examples of deformation (strain) under the action of stress. A normal (vertical) stress causes both compression in the direction of the stress and expansion at right angles to the stress. When a shear stress is applied (Fig. 6-20C), the entire material "rotates"; that is, it experiences the most absolute deflection at the free surface and possibly zero deflection at the opposite surface. In general, tissues in the foot will experience both shear and normal stress (Fig. 6-20D), with resultant compression along the line of normal stress, expansion at right angles to the stress, and "rotation" simultaneously. The same will be true of insole materials.

The mechanical properties of materials can be characterized by performing controlled tests on uniformly shaped samples such that the strain resulting from a

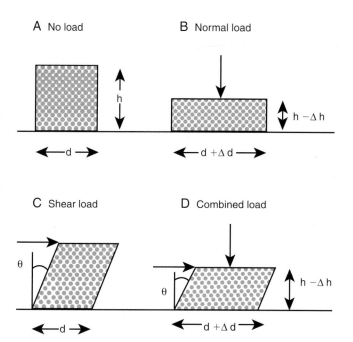

Figure 6-20   Tissue deformation (strain) under the action of stress. From the unloaded position (**A**), normal stress applied to the top of the cube (**B**), causes compression in the direction of the stress by an amount Δd. When a shear stress is applied (**C**), the entire material "rotates," and the deflection is measured by the angular change θ. In the general case (**D**), tissue in the foot will express all consequences of stress; compression along the line of normal stress, expansion at right angles to the stress, and rotation will occur simultaneously.

known stress can be measured. In the present application, compression and shear tests are most relevant, although these are less frequently conducted than are tension tests. Tests can be done either in vitro or, in some cases, in vivo.

Examples of the results of compression tests for a perfect spring, an insole material (Plastazote I closed-cell polyethylene foam), and the human heel pad are shown in Figure 6-18. Note that the graphs for materials have a standard form. Stress is plotted on the Y axis in units of force divided by area (kilopascals in the SI system), and strain is plotted on the X axis in dimensionless form (change in thickness divided by initial thickness).

The relationship between stress and strain in the working range of a perfect spring is linear (see Fig. 6-18A), and this curve can therefore be described by a single constant equal to the gradient of the curve, the so-called spring constant. Notice, however, that in this idealized spring, a point is reached when further application of force causes no further change in thickness, and the spring is said to be "bottomed out."

In almost all biologic tissues and in most insole applications, the materials are nonlinear in compression. The particular form of nonlinearity that is most often seen is the stiffening of materials as strain increases (see Figs. 6-18B and 6-18C). When stress is high enough to cause materials to reach the part of their range at which they become extremely stiff (see Fig. 6-18C), this is the equiv-

alent of the spring's bottoming out. Although an objective in insole design is to avoid bottoming out, prolonged use causes degradation of material, which may bring it closer to the bottoming-out regions.[297,298,301]

The curve for Plastazote #1 shown in Figure 6-18B is clearly nonlinear and therefore cannot be described by a single "spring constant." As this figure shows, a variety of slopes (equivalent to spring constants) can be used to characterize these curves, and their values describe the stiffness of the materials over different regions of their operating ranges. If we compare Plastazote #1 with Pelite, another insole material, we find that Pelite is three times stiffer than Plastazote #1 in the middle part of the range. Similar tests can be performed with the materials being subjected to shear stress.

There are several points of interest about the heel pad data (see Fig. 6-18C). Note that the early part of the curve (phase I) is quite flat. This indicates that very little stress is required to produce significant strain. The tissue then seems to stiffen, first along one line (phase II) and then along another, steeper line (phase III). The anatomic correlates of this behavior remain to be identified. A comparison of the heel pad data with the insole material is also of interest. Note that the initial stiffness of the heel pad is less than that of the insole material, the phase II slope is about equal, and the phase III slope is stiffer.

Another major departure from perfect spring behavior is that both the insole material and the heel pad follow different paths during loading and unloading. This feature, which is discussed above, is known as hysteresis and results in energy loss during repeated loading and unloading.

Although some data describing the mechanical properties of commonly used shoe materials are available,[297,298,301] most prescribers and fabricators follow an empirical approach to insole and shoe manufacture at the present time. However, reference to such data will become vital as more quantitative methods of footwear design become possible. Similarly, investigation of the mechanical properties of the plantar soft tissues will be helpful in ascertaining the presumed role of soft tissue change in the increase in plantar pressure associated with diabetes. With better understanding of the relationship between these relatively simple material characteristics and cushioning, it should be possible to pick the correct material for a given situation.

A method for the estimation of the stiffness of plantar tissues during MRI measurements has been proposed by Gefen and colleagues.[302] This approach involves estimating the force applied by a spherical indenter using a photoelastic technique while deformation is simultaneously measured from MRI. Gefen has also examined the deformation of the plantar fascia in vivo using a pressure-sensitive optical gait platform in combination with a radiographic fluoroscopy system.[303] He estimated a maximum strain of approximately 12% in the region of toe off and reported values for stiffness of 170 ± 45 N/mm. Using similar techniques, strain in the heel pad was estimated to be approximately 40% during walking.[304] Direct measurement of the force transmitted by the plantar fascia were made in cadaver feet during gait simulation by Erdemir and colleagues,[305] who estimated the loads to be 96% ± 36% of body weight.

Ledoux and colleagues[306] have used quasi-linear viscoelastic theory to characterize the properties of plantar tissue and reported significant differences between the heel and all other areas. Subject-specific finite-element models of the heel pad were developed by Erdemir and colleagues[307] and were used to estimate nonlinear material properties describing the hyperelastic behavior of each heel. Diabetic and control values were not significantly different.

Computer Models of Foot and Shoe Biomechanics

The models that were presented earlier are useful to help understand the concepts behind therapeutic footwear interventions in the diabetic patient. They do not, however, allow direct predictions of the efficacy of different approaches to be made, because they lack the quantitative detail and sufficient complexity to approximate the real situation. The two most accessible methods currently available to assess different types of footwear are (1) to use different materials in experiments with patients and measure plantar pressure at the interface of the foot with the inside of the shoe and (2) to try to predict plantar pressure from known forces, material properties, and tissue architecture by computerized modeling. Most previous models have attempted to explore the effects of major structural or surgical changes. Little has been done on the modeling of events leading to tissue breakdown in the normal foot with relatively normal gross structure but with important changes in the plantar adipose tissue, for example.

Although calculations of the effects of stress on uniform rigid solids (e.g., beams and plates) are routinely performed in engineering, the effects of stress on multiple layers of soft, irregular, nonlinear, viscoelastic tissues are more problematic. We have explored a technique known

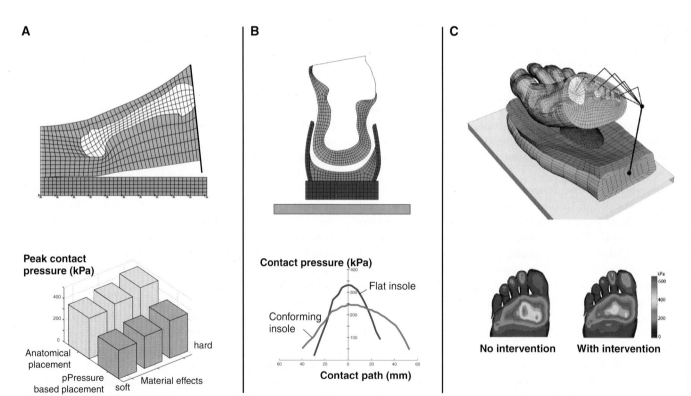

Figure 6–21   **A,** A two-dimensional finite-element model of the metatarsal head region provided design guidelines for pressure-relieving midsole plugs. Placement of the plugs was found to be more critical than was material selection; pressure-based placement resulted in superior performance compared to anatomically based placement. **B,** A two-dimensional finite-element model of the hindfoot region was used to examine the influence of insole conformity, thickness, and material properties on contact pressures. Conformity was found to be the most important design variable. **C,** Three-dimensional finite-element models are necessary to test the efficacy of interventions that provide sophisticated load transfer mechanisms. This example shows the evaluation of a metatarsal pad design and placement illustrating the pressure reduction achieved by this intervention. *(A, Adapted from Erdemir A, Saucerman JJ, Lemmon D, et al: Local plantar pressure relief in therapeutic footwear: Design guidelines from finite element models. J Biomech 38(9):1798–1806, 2005. B, Adapted from Goske S, Erdemir A, Petre M, et al: Reduction of plantar heel pressures: Insole design using finite element analysis. J Biomech 39(13):2363–2370, 2006. C, Adapted from Budhabhatti S, Erdemir A, Cavanagh PR: Computational prediction of in-shoe pressures with and without a metatarsal pad. [Abstract]. XXI Meeting of the International Society of Biomechanics, Taipei, Taiwan, July 1–5, 2007.)*

as finite-element analysis,[308] and some of the preliminary results from this technique are shown in Figure 6-21. The basic approach is to divide the problem into small geometric elements (in either two or three dimensions) that can be mathematically characterized one at a time by a sophisticated computer program. First, the geometry and mechanical properties of each element are defined; the boundary conditions and external loads are then added, and the program is set in motion. The model allows the combined effects of all these factors to be used in the prediction of the resulting deformations and stresses at any point in the model.

The particular benefit of this approach is that any of the input parameters can be varied at will and a set of new predictions can thus be obtained. In the example shown in Figure 6-21A, a two-dimensional model of the second ray has been formulated. All of the plantar soft tissues have been given a combined "bulk" property, and friction between the outer layer and the footwear has been incorporated into the model. A "plug" with material properties that can be modified has been placed under the MTH as a cushioning device. The plug is centered either directly under the MTH prominence or at the center of the focal pressure distribution (which is more posterior because of the shear forces in the late stage of the stance phase). The results show that a "pressure-based" placement is superior to an "anatomically based" placement and also that plug placement is more critical than the material used.

Thompson and colleagues[309] also used finite-element modeling to explore the effects of changes in the mechanical properties of skin and other soft tissues as a result of diabetes. They predicted an approximately 25% increase in stresses at the skin–adipose tissue interface in the subcalcaneal tissue for diabetic patients with stiffer skin and more compliant adipose tissue. Finite-element analysis was also employed by Patil and colleagues,[310] who chose to concentrate on stresses in the tarsal bones with various simulated muscle actions. This approach has some potential for understanding damage to the bones of neuropathic feet.

Finite-element models of the second and third rays were developed by Actis and colleagues.[311] They used an approach that allowed the complexity of the element shape functions to be varied in different regions of the mesh and used models with different levels of complexity. Some of the soft tissues were represented with nonlinear materials; footwear was also included in their models. The authors found a good fit between measured and predicted plantar pressures. Finite-element foot models have also been developed by Gefen and colleagues.[312,313] Five plane-strain models, one through each ray of the foot, were constructed with the use of assumptions of homogeneous, isotropic, elastic materials with nonlinear properties for the plantar tissues. The authors used this model to estimate tissue stresses during standing and to demonstrate the elevated plantar pressure that results from increased tissue stiffness. Estimates of internal stresses from such models need to be interpreted cautiously because of the complexity of the internal structure, which cannot yet be adequately modeled. In a more recent model, Yarnitzky and colleagues[312] have developed a hierarchal modeling system that initially uses a macromodel of the entire foot to estimate forces in the plantar fascia at various points in the stance phase. These forces become the boundary conditions in the micromodel, which is a finite-element simulation to determine tissue deformation and stresses.

Cheung and colleagues[314,315] developed a three-dimensional finite-element model of the human ankle-foot complex and interfaced it with simulated footwear. The model was unique in that it included a simulation of almost all the foot bones and many of the ligaments, together with soft tissues. The investigators used the model to examine the effects of different mechanical properties on plantar pressure[316] and found an approximately 34% increase in plantar pressure with an approximate fivefold increase in tissue stiffness. The pressure-relieving effects of a customized insole were also simulated, and a reduction of approximately 40% in peak plantar pressure under the MTHs was predicted using an insole constructed from a material with a Young modulus of 0.3 MPa compared to a rigid surface of 1000 MPa.

Dai and colleagues[50] varied the frictional characteristics of the foot-shoe interface in their three-dimensional finite-element model to simulate the effect of wearing socks. They demonstrated that the shear force on the forefoot could be reduced by a factor of 10 by using low-friction socks with a coefficient of friction of 0.04 compared to socks with a value of 0.54.

The benefits of finite-element models for simulation of multiple conditions were demonstrated by Erdemir and colleagues,[317] who developed guidelines for local plantar pressure relief using soft "plugs" placed underneath regions of plantar prominence. These authors investigated 36 plug designs, a combination of three materials, six geometries, and two placements using a two-dimensional finite-element model. Such an experiment would have been very difficult to perform on human subjects. The results indicated that plugs placed on the basis of plantar pressure measurements were more likely to be effective than those positioned according to the anatomic landmarks. The benefits of tapering and material section were also demonstrated.

Goske and colleagues[318] used a similar approach to the design of footwear to reduce heel pressure. Plantar pressures under the heel were predicted by using two-dimensional plane-strain finite-element modeling for 27 insole designs. Among the variables that were examined were conformity, insole thickness, and insole material. Conformity of the insole on the medial and lateral borders of the heel was found to be the most important design variable. Peak pressures were relatively insensitive to insole material selection.

Biomechanical Studies of Footwear

The previous section reviewed, in mostly theoretical terms, the principles that might be employed in the design of the foot-shoe interface. We will now review what is known about the biomechanical effects of frequently employed footwear modifications. The foot-shoe interface, outsole modifications, and modifications of the shoe's upper portion will be discussed. Chapter 28 emphasizes the clinical perspective of footwear prescription.

Insoles

Several authors have studied the mechanical properties of commonly used insole materials. The classical approach to mechanical testing of materials is to subject them to progressively increasing stress and to measure the amount of strain that results. When this is done for typical insole materials, a characteristic sigmoid curve is generated (see Fig. 6-18). The material is initially relatively stiff to small stresses; it then has a period of being less stiff in response to midrange stresses; finally, as compaction of the material occurs, it becomes very stiff (showing little strain) in response to further increases in stress. Thus, insole materials have a nonlinear response to loading, and this is perhaps why the responses have not been used by insole designers—because a single number cannot characterize the entire stress-strain behavior. The "operating range" of different insole materials is not yet clear in terms of compression, but it is almost certain that many soft materials (particularly those in thin insoles) are used beyond 50% compression, which will move them to the stiff region of the curves (see Fig. 6-18).

Campbell and colleagues[297] were the first to attempt to define insole materials in a rigorous engineering manner. They subjected 31 foamed rubber and plastic materials to accelerated aging (including heat, sustained compression, and cyclic loading), using both novel tests and formal protocols such as ASTM D395.[319] Materials were placed into four groups based on the magnitude of changes that occurred with the various duty cycle tests. Reduction in thickness following sustained compression ranged from barely measurable change (Poron 20125, also known as PPT) to approximately 50% (Aliplast, Cetite, Ethafoam, Evasote, Neoprene, and Pelite). The reduction in thickness following cyclic compression tests varied from almost zero (Poron 20125) to more than 80% (Pelite, Evasote, Ensolite, and Aliplast).

Leber and Evanski[320] examined the pressure reduction properties of seven commonly used insole materials using a Harris-Beath mat in patients with metatarsalgia. They attempted to quantify the results using the calibration procedures proposed by Silvino and colleagues.[37] The range of pressure reduction that was measured was between 28% and 53%. The most effective materials identified were PPT, Spenco, and Plastazote.

Another significant effort to characterize a number of materials used for insoles was conducted by Sanders and colleagues.[292] These authors examined 11-mm-diameter by 4-mm-thick specimens of eight commonly used materials in a 1-Hz cyclic loading protocol up to pressures of 220 kPa for 60-minute periods. Coefficients of friction between the material and skin, material and sock, and skin-sock interface were also determined. Recovery from the compression set was assessed 1 hour and 168 hours after the 60-minute compression test. The results of the compression tests are shown in Figure 6-22.[292] The shapes and stiffness of the curves varied considerably. There was appreciable deformation in some of the materials after the 60-minute tests, but most materials recovered well in 168 hours (although several recovered poorly in 1 hour). Sanders and colleagues[292] include in their article a comprehensive description of the chemical composition of the various materials.

Brodsky and colleagues[301] examined the response of five commonly used insole materials to repeated compression and repeated shear and compression combined. They proposed that the ideal material would exhibit a combination of durability and moldability. After 10,000 cycles, loss of thickness ranged from zero (for PPT) to 55% (Plastazote #1). These results have important implications for the replacement of insoles at regular intervals, since it is clear that many regularly used insole materials lose their effectiveness rapidly with use.

Foto and Birke[321] conducted a survey of health professionals who treat diabetic patients to determine the most commonly used multidensity materials (such as a layered

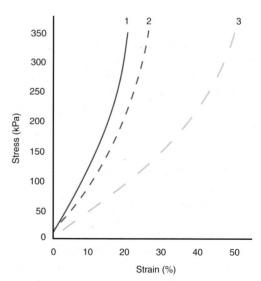

Figure 6–22 The results of simulated wear tests on insole materials. Stress-strain curves for a sample of dual-density material (Poron and Plastazote #2) after cycling under a 350-kPa stress for 40 cycles (1), 10,000 cycles (2), and 100,000 cycles (3). Note the increase in stiffness of the material as cycling increases shown by the steeper curves. *(Adapted from Foto JG, Birke JA: Evaluation of multidensity orthotic materials used in footwear for patients with diabetes. Foot Ankle Int 19:836–841, 1998.)*

TABLE 6-3 Percent Loss in Performance During Dynamic Compression of Dual-Density Insole Materials on Repeated Cycles

Number of Cycles	Materials				
	a	b	c	d	e
1000	7%	13%	8%	4%	22%
10,000	12%	22%	27%	36%	50%
100,000	26%	25%	36%	49%	61%

Source: From Foto and Birke.[298]
a is Poron + Plastazote #2.
b is Spenco + Microcel Puff Lite.
c is Plastazote #1 + Poron.
d is Plastazote #1 + Poron + Microcel Puff.
e is Plastazote #1 and Plastazote #2.

combination of Plastazote #2 and Poron). They then devised a testing method[298] to measure how the materials behaved when new compared to how they behaved when aged in terms of their mechanical properties. The authors presented stress-strain curves for the various materials after 40 cycles, 10,000 cycles, and 100,000 cycles and examined each material against their criterion that the material should be capable of maintaining a dynamic strain of 50% or less at a stress of 350 kPa. The key findings of the study are summarized in Table 6-3 and Figure 6-22. The authors concluded that the Poron/Plastazote #2 and Spenco/Microcel Puff Lite combinations exhibited the best dynamic material deformation and compression set properties of all the materials tested, and from those examined, these materials were the preferred choice to be used in insoles for diabetic patients. Lavery and colleagues[59] have also described a methodology for the evaluation of the change in material properties over time.

The practitioner will often choose materials on the basis of whether or not they can be molded to match a positive cast of the foot. These thermoplastic properties are fundamental to the formulation of the polymers that are used, but few data are readily available regarding ease of molding and temperature requirements, and so on; nor has the efficacy of molded insoles been well studied. Hewitt[322] examined the peak pressures under the feet of neuropathic patients as they walked in insoles molded in the heel and arch areas versus flat insoles of approximately the same thickness. He found mixed results, with MTH pressures being relieved in some patients by the molded insole, whereas other patients showed increases in peak pressure. Pitei and colleagues[68] found that peak pressure was decreased by ethylene vinyl acetate insoles compared to the patients' conventional street shoes by 31% when new and by 50% as they became molded to the foot during breaking-in.

The basic philosophy of most molded-insole approaches is to increase the load in "safe regions" to decrease the load over "at-risk" regions. A simply molded insole offers, at least in theory, the same support to all points under the foot (although the compression of each region of the

insole will differ, depending on the load immediately above it and the thickness). However, molding can also be "exaggerated" or customized; in other words, areas of the foot that are considered safe can be loaded preferentially. This modification can be accomplished with extra support in a safe area (e.g., metatarsal pads, bars, or more individualized insole buildup) or with an extra relief under the at-risk area (i.e., plugs of a softer material or simply thinning of the material to provide less contact between the foot and insole).

The most popular class of "extra loading" devices is the metatarsal pad that is placed under the metatarsal shafts to unload the MTHs. The traditional metatarsal pad can be quite effective in relieving MTH pressure if it is correctly placed and the patient can tolerate it. Edington[323] examined MTH peak pressures as patients walked barefoot across a pressure platform with metatarsal pads of various dimensions directly attached to their feet. For pads that were placed 3/16 to 1/4 inch behind the palpated third MTH, he found significant and substantial reductions in peak pressure at the MTHs (53 kPA for 3/16-inch pads and 80 kPa for 5/16-inch pads). Holmes and Timmerman[324] found reductions between 12% and 60% in MTH peak pressures using a protocol similar to that of Edington.[323] They also reported that three of their 10 subjects showed either no change or an increase in MTH pressure and speculated that this was because of incorrect positioning of the pad. Chang and colleagues,[325] using an in-shoe protocol, found only minor reductions in plantar pressures with metatarsal pads. This result might have been due to positioning of either the pad or the small discrete sensors that were used, which had a metal disc backing. The importance of placement of the pad was further emphasized by the experiments of Hsi and colleagues,[326] who found that placement of the pad approximately 8 mm proximal to the region of elevated MTH pressure resulted in no significant reduction of plantar pressure. When the pad was moved to be "just proximal" to the region of peak pressure, a significant pressure relief was obtained. Jackson and colleagues[327] examined the pressure-relieving effects in the central MTHs of both metatarsal pads and bars in patients with rheumatoid arthritis. The investigators placed the pad or bar 5 mm proximal to the MTH of interest and found significant reduction in plantar pressure, use of the bar providing the greatest relief.

Frykberg[328] has presented preliminary data to suggest that a rockered insole could be effective in reducing plantar pressure under the forefoot, and this device could be considered to be a prefabricated metatarsal bar. Lord and Hosein[71] have provided insight into the redistribution of plantar pressure that can occur with customized insoles.

As was discussed above, the effective thickness of an insole can be increased under an area of particular concern by using a firmer, less compressible material under areas of the foot that are judged to be able to take greater loads and using softer materials under the area of concern. For instance, a two-layer composite insole could have a firm material as its base, a thin layer of soft material over the whole surface, and a soft material all the way through to the base layer at the area of concern. Such a relief or plug can be extended into the midsole of the shoe and can take any shape needed. A small circular plug might be used under an MTH, whereas a large plug involving a third of the insole could be used for a foot that is badly deformed by a Charcot fracture (Fig. 6-23). Little is known about the ideal geometry and material properties required for such plugs, and there is concern that a ring of high stress can be created at the edges of the plug.[329]

The thickness of insoles is usually limited by the space available in the shoe, but this can be substantial (up to half an inch) in a super-extra-depth shoe. No study has systematically examined the effects of insole thickness on pressure relief in a large group of patients with different characteristics. Our own data, which were used to validate the finite-element models described earlier, suggest that the effect will be different depending on the foot deformity and baseline pressure of the patient. Lemmon and colleagues[308] used PPT insoles of various thicknesses in two individuals with markedly different MTH2 plantar pressures. The results indicated a steeper gradient of pressure versus insole thickness in a patient with reduced submetatarsal tissue and higher baseline plantar pressure compared to an individual with more plantar tissue. A reduction of approximately 6 kPa/mm versus 2 kPa/mm was obtained in the two individuals.

As was expected on a theoretical basis, the thicker the insole, the less was the incremental improvement in pressure reduction per millimeter of added thickness. For the subject with lower barefoot peak pressure, adding thickness beyond 12.5 mm (0.5 inch) led to little incremental improvement in pressure. However, for the indi-vidual with higher barefoot peak pressure, the curve was still reasonably steep, even around 12.5 mm (0.5 inch), indicating continuing benefit from increasing insole thickness. Although this work is preliminary, it under-scores the importance of insole thickness, which was pre-dicted theoretically (see Computer Models, previously). In our own clinics, we do not use insoles that are less than 6.25 mm (0.25 inch) thick for any at-risk patient, and we try to approach the 12.5-mm (0.5-inch) thickness for all high-risk patients. In the individual with higher baseline pressure in the study by Lemmon and col-leagues,[308] the overall pressure reduction (from the mod-erate value of only 279 kPa) from the 12.5-mm insole was 25%. This could be expected to be even higher for an individual with still higher baseline pressures, since the pattern of greater plantar pressure relief by the same intervention for feet with higher baseline pressure has been found in other studies.[330]

Conti[331] has pointed out that there are many unan-swered questions regarding appropriate insole prescrip-tion, and Janisse[332] has described a number of practical implementations of the theories discussed above. He also provides recommendations for the manufacture of a variety of therapeutic footwear devices. Some of these approaches (including metatarsal pads) were used by Ashry and colleagues,[333] who examined four different insole designs in a group of 11 patients with great-toe amputation. Surprisingly, the authors found no significant differences in peak plantar pressures with their various interventions. This could be due to the poor perform-ance characteristics of the device they used for in-shoe pressure measurement,[334] but their conclusion that insole modification is unwarranted would seem to be premature.

It is noteworthy that the use of even simple athletic shoes has been observed to reduce the incidence of callus[335] and in three studies has been found to reduce pressures by 25% to 30% on average compared to use of leather-soled shoes or the subjects' own over-the-counter shoes.[68,69,330] In addition, Perry and colleagues[330] found that the peak pressure reduction in the forefoot as a result of cushioned running shoes compared to leather oxfords (expressed as percent reduction) was much greater in individuals with high initial peak pressure. For example, those with peak MTH1 pressures of 200 kPa in oxfords typically experienced little change in running shoes, but those with peak pressures of 600 kPa in oxfords experienced pressure reduction of approximately 50% in running shoes. Thus, the combination of insole and midsole in these shoes can often be effective, particularly in patients with higher baseline pressure, in reducing pressure below the level of injury threshold.

Fluid-filled insoles have been described,[296] but no data are available on their performance in diabetic patients. There is also a complete class of commercial over-the-counter devices that purport to combine molding, relief, load transfer, and support; but the efficacy of these

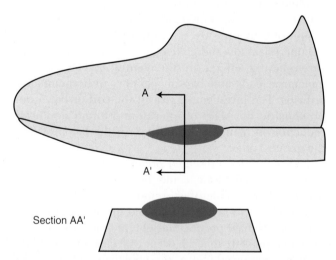

Figure 6–23 A compliant insole plug under a prominent area in the midfoot of the patient whose plantar pressures were shown in Figure 6-11. A schematic cross section of the shoe is also shown.

devices has not been tested in published studies of either pressure reduction or clinical efficacy.

Our own studies[75] suggest that customized insoles of appropriate design can play a significant role in pressure and impulse reduction at the MTHs if load can be transferred to the arch and other regions of the foot. Loading at the heel also seems particularly amenable to reduction by insoles that provide a "cupping" of the heel. A case study demonstrating redistribution of load away from the first MTH in a patient with recurrent ulceration and elevated pressure at this location is presented in Figure 6-24. The customized insole in this case incorporated molding, a metatarsal pad, pressure relief under the MTHs, and a substantial buildup in the medial arch area. A Novel PEDAR system was used to measure in-shoe pressure.

During barefoot walking, this patient's MTH1 plantar pressure was 1058 kPa. Even with a 1/4-inch PPT insole, the peak pressure at this location was 552 kPa, much higher than in-shoe pressures that are usually observed in this region. Figure 6-24C shows a comparison between the regional plantar pressures in the 1/4-inch PPT flat

insole and in the customized insole during normal walking in the same shoe. The largest changes that occurred were in the medial midfoot, where increased load was being taken by the built-up arch in the customized insole. The peak pressure in this region increased by 61.2% (from 72 to 115 kPa). Although this change is substantial, it is small in comparison to the change in force-time integral, which increased by 1041% (from 3.9 to 44.5 N · s). This and other features in the insole resulted in a decrease of peak pressure in the patient's region of concern, MTH1, by 37% (from 552 to 348 kPa). The MTH1 force-time integral showed a somewhat lower (24%) percentage reduction (from 100.2 to 76.6 N · s). A useful insight is gained by expressing the regional force-time integrals in the MTH1 and medial arch as a percentage of the total force-time integrals in all regions. For the flat insole, this approach indicates that the MTH1 and midfoot were responsible for 17% and 4%, respectively, of the force-time integrals in the flat insole. In the molded insole, these values change to 13% and 12%, respectively, reflecting the unloading of MTH1 and the transfer of load to the medial arch. In

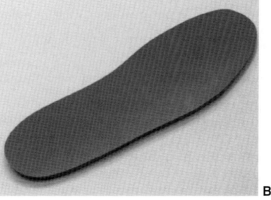
A

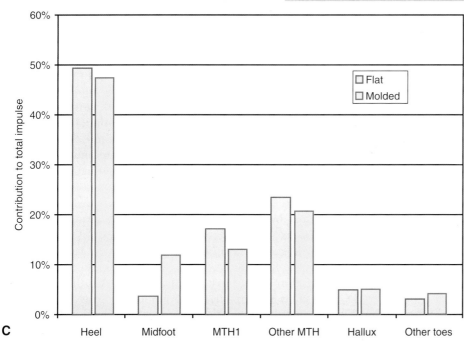

B

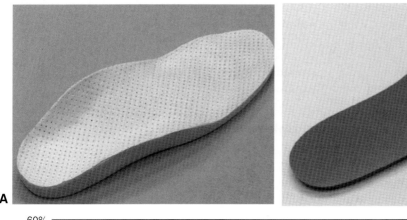
C

Figure 6–24   A case study showing redistribution of load away from a high-risk region. The graphs show a comparison of plantar pressure in the same shoe with a molded insole (**A**) and a flat insole (**B**) in a patient who had previously ulcerated at the first metatarsal head. **C,** Peak pressure at MTH1 was markedly reduced in the molded insole but increased at other sites. The contribution of each region to the total force-time integral or impulse shows that the midfoot increased its load-sharing role in the molded insole while other regions were reduced or unchanged. (See text for further details.)

many respects, the prescription of insoles can be characterized as a process of experimental load transfer until enough load relief to prevent injury has occurred. As was discussed earlier, we can now document changes caused by footwear in peak pressure, pressure-time integral, force-time integrals, time over a certain pressure, and so on. However, the relative importance of each quantity and the absolute relief required to prevent injury are not yet clear. Custom insoles significantly reduced the peak pressures and force-time integrals at the first MTH in this study,[75] yet there was considerable variability in the success of the intervention, only seven of 21 feet experiencing reductions in both pressure and integral.

Although shear stress is difficult to measure, approaches to reducing shear stress have been proposed. Lavery and colleagues[336] have described the use of multilayer viscoelastic insoles, in which the middle layers had low-friction characteristics to enable the foot to move relative to the shoe.

In summary, when prescribing an insole for an individual at risk for neuropathic ulceration, one must consider the material or combination of materials, thickness, molding, supports (e.g., metatarsal pads), and reliefs (e.g., plugs). This is a useful and important checklist to consider when a prescription is being written. Even though we know something about the individual effects of these various insole attributes, as was just reviewed, there are very few data on how they should be most efficaciously combined. In the absence of such data, it is reasonable to take cost into consideration. Flat insoles are relatively inexpensive, even when thick, whereas the more customized an insole is, the more expensive it generally is.

Another point that is worthy of emphasis is that in the entire discussion of insoles, only reduction of the loading forces to areas of the plantar surface at risk was considered. Insoles or in-shoe orthoses are often made in settings other than the neuropathic foot to correct or control the motions of the foot. Such "corrections" load one part of the foot more than another and thereby increase pressure in areas that, in a neuropathic foot, might not necessarily be able to tolerate higher pressures. Thus, in the neuropathic foot, any such correction or control must be performed with extreme caution and only with very good reason.

Socks

Socks should be considered as part of the cushioning system. Veves and colleagues[294,337,338] have shown in patients with either diabetes or rheumatoid arthritis that special padded socks can significantly reduce plantar pressures. In their initial studies, 10 neuropathic subjects with plantar pressures greater than 980 kPa wore specially padded socks for 6 months. Reductions of 31.3% in peak forefoot plantar pressure were found when the socks were new. After 3 and 6 months of wear, the socks had lost some of their efficacy and offered reductions in peak pressure of only 15.5% and 17.6%, respectively. Patient acceptance of the socks was good, and no patient developed an ulcer during the study. The authors also experimented with the use of over-the-counter padded sport socks designed for tennis and running and found that if the socks had high-density padding, a reduction of 17% could be achieved when the socks were new. In studies of patients with rheumatoid arthritis,[338] peak forefoot pressures and perceived pain were both significantly reduced in padded socks. In all of these studies, the patients' own socks (usually thin) had no significant effect on plantar pressure.

A study of multilayered "protective foot care socks" found that there was a 10% reduction in peak plantar pressure in a group of high-risk diabetic patients.[339] As was noted earlier, socks can also markedly reduce friction between the foot and the shoe,[50] indicating an additional reason why they may exert a beneficial action.

Stacpoole-Shea and colleagues[340] measured pressure distribution during a benchtop simulation of compression of seamless and seamed sock material between two flat plates. They reported a 10-fold concentration of pressure at the seams and recommended that neuropathic patients should use seamless socks. It is obviously important that shoes with enough room in the toebox should be used by patients for whom padded socks are prescribed. Otherwise, significant injury to the dorsum of the toes can result.

Outsole Modifications

The discussion of footwear so far has concentrated principally on the interface between the foot and the shoe, and there is no doubt that this is the most important aspect of footwear for the neuropathic foot. However, a number of investigators have shown either clinically or through direct measurement of plantar pressure that outsole modifications can also have an important effect in preventing injury.[65,66,78,341–343] The most common of these is the rigid rocker-bottom shoe or a variant thereof called a roller, which was advocated by Dr. Paul Brand[103] for many years. The rocker has a break in the contour of the outsole, whereas the roller has a smooth curve (Fig. 6-25). The general principle behind these designs is that they allow the patient to walk with minimum motion of the joints of the foot. In particular, no extension of the MTP joints is required during the phase of forefoot weight bearing, and this appears to reduce forefoot pressures by up to 50% compared to walking in flexible shoes.[66,78,342,343]

It is not known, however, whether the lack of motion in the foot joints is important or whether other factors predominate. It is frequently said that the rigid sole, usually accompanied by a molded insole, loads the entire foot throughout the stance phase. This is certainly not true, but pressure measurements have confirmed that

A

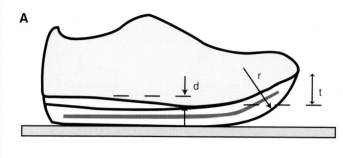

B

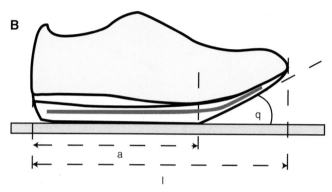

Figure 6-25 Design parameters for rigid shoes. **A,** A roller shoe with a constant curvature outsole, radius *r*, in the forefoot region. The heel-forefoot height differential is *d*, and the toe spring, *t*, is defined as the height of the anterior tip of the shoe sole above the plane of the ball of the foot. **B,** A rocker shoe with a rocker angle beginning at a ratio of (*a/l*) of shoe length. The rigid roller or rocker effect should be achieved by minimizing toe spring, since this high toe spring probably increases toe pressures.

the duration of loading in all areas except the forefoot is increased in a rocker shoe.[78] These increases in loading time are marked in the hindfoot and midfoot but only small in the toes. The hindfoot and midfoot force-time integrals are also dramatically increased, indicating the change in load sharing that is taking place; in contrast, the force-time integral at the forefoot is markedly decreased. Thus, the actual changes in loading that occur with rocker shoes have been determined.

However, functional effects of several important design variables remain to be fully explored. These

include the location of the rocker or roller axis along the anteroposterior axis of the shoe, the angle of the rocker or roller axis with respect to the anteroposterior axis, the amount of toe spring (see below), the height of the outsole at the rocker or roller axis (and thereby the angle of the rocker or the anteroposterior curvature of the roller), and the height differential of the sole between heel and the rocker/roller axis. In addition, it has been shown that a given shoe can actually increase the load under some parts of the foot while reducing it elsewhere.[78] Another extremely important issue is that individual variability in response to rigid shoes is significant. Thus, the process of prescribing shoes for a given individual is complex.[343]

The characteristics of roller placement and geometry have been addressed systematically by Coleman[65] and by Nawoczenski and colleagues[66] (Table 6-4). Both studies examined the effects of these shoe design variables in young, healthy male volunteers using the same brand of footwear. Coleman controlled for cadence (80 steps per minute) but not speed or stride length, whereas Nawoczenski and colleagues did not mention gait parameters. Plantar pressures were measured in both studies by using discrete transducers. Coleman placed the roller axis "just behind the fifth MTH" (probably at approximately 60% of shoe length); Nawoczenski and colleagues explored take-off points of 50% and 60%.

As is apparent from Table 6-4, there were remarkable differences between the results of Nawoczenski and colleagues[66] and those of Coleman[65] for the same type of footwear modifications. The effect demonstrated by Nawoczenski and colleagues was always much less than that shown by Coleman. Although there may have been differences in speed, cadence, and stride length between the two studies, the most striking difference might have been design of the toe spring, defined as the height of the anterior tip of the shoe sole above the plane of the ball of the foot (see Fig. 6-25). It appears that Coleman maintained the "normal" toe spring of the shoes used in his study but that Nawoczenski and colleagues manufactured their shoes with 20 degrees of toe spring. On the

TABLE 6-4 Effects of Roller Shoes on Plantar Pressure Reduction

			Pressure Reduction Expressed as % from Control					
Author	Take-Off (% of shoe length from heel)	Radius (% of shoe length)	Hallux	MTH1	MTH2	MTH3	MTH4	MTH5
C	60%**	60%***	−21%		−31%		−34%	
N*	60%	75%	−5%	−7%		−12%		−10%
C	60%**	77%***	−15%		−24%	−25%		
N*	60%	125%	−3%	−2%		−8%		−6%
N*	50%	75%	−11%	−9%		−26%		−13%
N*	50%	60%	−8%	−4%		−28%		−12%

* % Effects estimated from a figure in Nawoczenski et al.[66]
** Estimated on the basis of data from van Schie et al.[343]
*** Estimated on the basis of assumed shoe size #10 measuring 30 cm.
C, Coleman.[65]
N, Nawoczenski et al.[66]

basis of the photograph in the article by Nawoczenski and colleagues,[66] this was probably more toe spring than that initially built into the shoes. Since Coleman's results showed more pressure relief, it would appear that rigid shoes should be built with minimal toe spring. (This conclusion is supported by the observations of Bauman and Brand,[63] who found only a 6% to 14% reduction in forefoot pressure by a wooden rigid rollered sandal with significant toe spring, whereas they found pressure reductions of 29% to 41% in wooden flat shoes with a roller.) Concerning take-off and radius parameters, it appears from these two studies that with the 60% take-off, the shortest radius tested was best (60%) but that the 50% take-off might be better than 60% in terms of maximizing pressure reduction.

Another important parameter of rocker and roller shoe design that is somewhat related to toe spring is the differential in height between the heel and the forefoot of the insole/midsole/outsole combination (see Fig. 6-25). In most commercially manufactured shoes, the rear part of the foot is at least 1/4 to 3/8 inch above the forefoot, and the upper is made to fit this design. Patients do not like shoes that appear high, and one way to make rollered and rockered shoes appear less high is to even out this difference by making the heel no higher than the forefoot. The efficacy of this alteration has never been addressed experimentally.

In the studies mentioned above, Coleman[65] examined three rocker shoe designs, and Nawoczenski and colleagues[66] examined one. A modular shoe has been proposed for the investigation of the effects of different outsole configurations without altering the foot-shoe interface.[344] Using this device, van Schie and colleagues[343] systematically explored the pressure distributions inside nine different rigid rocker shoe designs and compared them with the control condition of a flexible, nonrockered extra-depth shoe with the same flat insole. Speed of walking between trials in this study was kept constant. Peak pressure was reduced by rocker shoes compared to control at most forefoot locations but was increased in the midfoot and heel. Axis location was found to have an important effect, particularly on hallux pressures. There was a mean trend toward optimal reduction of pressure in one of the rocker shoe conditions at each anatomic location, but the axis position for this optimal placement was variable across subjects and anatomic locations. Most configurations of the rocker shoe were superior to the control shoe, but no single configuration was optimal for all subjects at all sites or even at the same site. These results suggested that some form of in-shoe plantar pressure measurement would be ideal to ensure a rigid rocker-bottom shoe design that is optimized. On average, the best axis location for reducing MTH pressure was in the region of 55% to 60% of shoe length, whereas for the toes, it was 65%. Van Schie and colleagues[343] proposed a conceptual model linking the various rocker design parameters and their effects (Fig. 6-26).

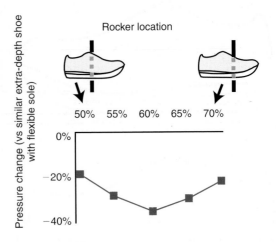

Figure 6-26 Experimental results of a study to examine the effects of variation in the placement of a rocker shoe axis. Peak pressure at the first metatarsal head is shown as a function of rocker axis location. Note that all peak pressures in this region were reduced by at least 20%, but there was an optimal location for the axis where pressure relief was maximized.

The results of the studies that have explored effects of rocker shoe design on pressure relief are presented in Table 6-5. For reasons that have not been fully explained, hallux pressure reduction in the study of van Schie and colleagues[343] was much less than in the other studies. The summary data as presented in the table neither add to nor detract from the conclusion of van Schie and colleagues that hallux pressure is best relieved by the 65% take-off rocker. Although none of the other studies systematically explored the effect of the take-off position on plantar pressure, the results of all the studies are similar with respect to pressure reduction at the MTHs, and in general, these summary data confirm that the best pressure reduction at the MTHs occurs with the 55% to 60% take-off point. The 65% take-off rocker may be acceptable at MTH1 through 4 but perhaps not at MTH5. Whether MTH5 would be better relieved by a more proximal rocker has not been extensively addressed, though Sims and Birke[342] noted, in apparent agreement with van Schie and colleagues,[343] that "progressive decrease in pressure was noted as the rocker apex was moved posteriorly ... the 3[d] MTH showed a decrease at all positions, but ... rocker placement had minimal effect on ... pressure at 5th MTH." The expected result—that the higher the rocker (and therefore the greater the rocker angle) the better the pressure relief—is a clear trend.

As van Schie and colleagues[343] also observed, pressure reduction depends on gait style. The preferred use of the rocker shoe is to dwell on the flat portion of the sole until the last stages of stance. This should then be followed by a rapid rocking forward on the "knife edge" of the rocker and then toe off of the support foot. However, some patients appear to rock forward and spend considerable time applying load on the anterior

TABLE 6-5   Effects of Roller Shoes on Plantar Pressure Reduction

Author	Take-Off (% of shoe length from heel)	Rocker Angle (deg)	Hallux*	MTH1	MTH2	MTH3	MTH4	MTH5
				Pressure Reduction Expressed as % from Control				
v	70%	20	−4%	−19%	−38%	−38%		
v	70%	30	−12%	−23%	−40%	−41%		
Average				−21%	−39%	−40%		
v	65%	20	−1%	−26%	−43%	−44%		
S	67%	24	−32%	−29%		−33%		12%
v	65%	26	−19%	−31%	−48%	−49%		
N	**65%	30	−32%	−16%		−25%		−6%
Average				−25%	−45%	−38%		3%
C	**60%	15	−16%		−36%	−35%		
C	**60%	20	−23%		−45%	−45%		
v	60%	20	4%	−29%	−46%	−48%		
v	60%	22	−2%	−35%	−52%	−56%		
C	**60%	30	−37%		−51%	−49%		
Average				−32%	−46%	−46%		
v	55%	20	8%	−28%	−47%	−50%		
v	55%	21	6%	−30%	−51%	−56%		
Average				−29%	−49%	−53%		
v	50%	20	23%	−19%	−39%	−45%		

* Averages are not calculated for the hallux data because of the unexplained differences among the studies.
** Estimated based on data from van Schie et al.[343]
C, Coleman.[65]
N, Nawoczenski et al.[66]
S, Schaff and Cavanagh.[78] Reported results for medial, middle, and lateral forefoot.
v, van Schie et al.[343] Reported results for lateral MTHs rather than 3, 4, and 5 individually.

TABLE 6-6   Comparison of Rocker and Roller Shoes of the Same Height

Author		Hallux	MTH1	MTH2	MTH3	MTH4	MTH5
		Pressure Reduction Expressed as % from Control					
C (0.75" height)	15° Rocker	−16%		−36%	−35%		
**60% take-off	77% R ***Roller	−15%		−24%	−25%		
Difference		−1%		−12%	−10%		
C (1.25" height)	20° Rocker	−23%		−45%	−45%		
**60% take-off	60% R ***Roller	−21%		−31%	−34%		
Difference		−2%		−14%	−11%		
N* (0.75")	30° Rocker 65% take-off	−32%	−16%		−25%		−6%
	60% R Roller 50% take-off	−8%	−4%		−28%		−12%
Difference		−24%	−12%		3%		6%

* % Effects estimated from a figure in Nawoczenski, et al.[66]
** Estimated based on data from van Schie et al.[343]
*** Estimated based on assumed shoe size #10 measuring 30 cm.
C, Coleman[65], lower and higher shoes.
N, Nawoczenski et al.[66]
R, Radius.

flattened portion of the outsole. This tendency is believed to be associated with an increase in pressure under the forefoot and highlights the importance of training the patient to use a rocker shoe correctly. Taking short strides is probably the key to successful use of a rocker shoe, since it is more likely that the patient will use the rocker appropriately (without maintaining the flat area of the front part of the shoe in contact with the ground). These same observations and comments were made much earlier by Bauman and colleagues.[15]

We have observed a patient with remarkable "out-toeing" and an MTH1 ulcer. A standard rocker was not successful at keeping this patient's ulcer healed, and observation revealed that design modifications to the shoe were required. With the standard rocker axis orientation (with respect to the anteroposterior axis), this patient rolled right over MTH1. We changed the axis of the rocker to be perpendicular to the foot position at toe off (approximately 25 degrees to the anteroposterior axis). In-shoe plantar pressure at that site was markedly reduced, and the patient has remained healed in the modified shoe while continuing his out-toed gait.

Only in the studies of Coleman[65] and Nawoczenski and colleagues[66] were the effects of rockers and rollers compared by using the same methodology. In the three comparisons shown in Table 6-6, rockers generally, but not always, yielded somewhat better results than rollers at reducing pressure. The mean difference in pressure reduction was –9% at the hallux and –7% at the MTHs, or about –8% overall, favoring rockers.

The alterations in kinetics and kinematics of gait while walking in rocker shoes has been studied by Van Bogart and colleagues.[345] These authors found increased cadence, decreased stride length, and alterations in knee and ankle joint kinematics with accompanying changes in power characteristics at all joints in the late stance phase.

A careful reader will notice that many footwear modifications can reduce plantar pressure significantly and might speculate that simply adding these reductions can lead to pressures below zero. Obviously, that is not reasonable. In the absence of data on combinations of modifications, it might be reasonable to assume that each added modification reduces pressure further by its own percent effect from the baseline of the previous modification. The basis for this hypothesis is the study by Perry and colleagues,[43] in which the lower the initial pressure, the lower were both the absolute and the percent pressure reductions.

Fit of Footwear

Proper fit in shoes and other footwear is a critical issue in the prevention of both dorsal and plantar ulcers. Despite its importance, fit is usually left to the subjective opinion of the fitter and the wearer. When the fitter is inexperienced and the wearer has limited sensation, it is clear that this approach can lead to a less than perfect outcome. A shoe with ideal fit would control the motion of the foot relative to the weight-bearing surface without applying any pressure whatsoever to the dorsum of the foot. This is not possible in practice, however; therefore, a working definition of shoe fit might be "a covering for the dorsum of the foot that minimizes the application of pressures to the dorsum while controlling mediolateral and anteroposterior foot movement." The only study that has examined nonplantar pressure in diabetic patients is that mentioned above by Chantelau and colleagues.[154] Jordan[346] has measured dorsal pressure in relation to comfort in nondiabetic subjects, and her methodology could be readily applied to the issue of dorsal ulceration. It is desirable and expected that such measurements will become routine in footwear prescriptions for high-risk patients in the near future.

In the absence of experimental data on shoe fit, the following represents a working hypothesis of the role of fit of the upper in providing a safe shoe. Although relief of pressure over bony prominences is an obvious need, a less frequently expressed role of the upper might be to limit the amount of shear strain that the tissue on the plantar aspect of the foot experiences. As is shown in Figure 6-27, in the presence of shear forces, the upper acts on the dorsum of the foot to generate opposing

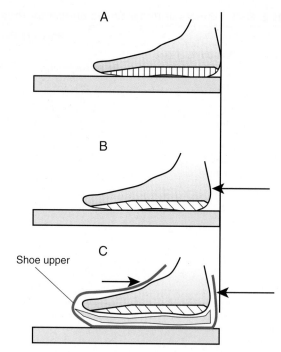

Figure 6–27 Hypothesis for the role of the shoe upper and a soft insole in reducing the shear strain of the plantar tissues. Soft tissues on the plantar surface of the foot are shown with schematic shading to indicate the amount of shear stress experienced. From the resting position on a flat surface with minimum shear stress in the tissues (**A**), an anteriorly directed shear force applied to a foot with no upper (**B**) causes forward movement of the foot about the fixed plantar surface, which will lead to high shear stress in the tissues. If the same force is applied to a foot in a shoe with an upper and a compliant insole (**C**), the resulting shear stress is reduced because the upper applies a restraining force to the foot once the insole has allowed forward movement. Note that there would be no reduction in the shear of the plantar tissue without the restraint of the shoe upper. Thus, the shoe and the insole together reduce the amount of shear stress in the plantar tissues and possibly the risk of injury. This hypothesis can be investigated experimentally.

forces. This has the effect of reducing the forward movement of the foot against the shoe compared with what would occur with the shoe platform alone, consequently reducing the amount of shear strain in the plantar tissues. An insole that allows shear strain will facilitate this forward movement of the foot relative to the shoe and allow the upper to "engage" the dorsum at a lower value of shear strain. Because excessive shear strain in the tissue is likely to be damaging, the combination of an appropriate insole and a well-fitting upper has the potential to reduce plantar injury on the basis of the principles described here rather than from a simple cushioning approach. If the upper does not fit correctly or the insole does not permit shear strain, this role can be lost; if the upper fits too tightly, direct injury to the dorsum of the foot can result.

In practice, the shoe fitter attempts by palpation to establish that any bony prominences will be given adequate pressure relief and to locate the position of the most distal toe. Once this latter position has been determined, there must be some attempt to determine how much relative movement between foot and shoe will occur with the given combination of insole materials, upper, gait, and physical characteristics of the patient. At present, almost no quantitative tools are available to assist with this extremely complex process.

Modifications to the upper that are intended to accommodate dorsal deformities include extra-depth shoes, stretching of the upper, soft leather "windows," and custom molding; these are discussed elsewhere in this book.

Plantar Pressure Measurement in Footwear Prescription

In-shoe plantar pressure measurement, as reported in the scientific literature, has been applied most frequently to the evaluation of off-loading devices that are designed to heal ulcers (see the section of this chapter on ulcer healing) and to the elucidation of the general effects of various footwear design features (see the earlier part of this section). Such efforts to evaluate prescription footwear quantitatively date back more than 40 years to the work of Bauman and colleagues.[15] However, there have been only a few reports[70,72] of the use of this methodology in the prescription of shoes for individual patients, perhaps because this method does not fit the randomized controlled trial approach that dominates many scientific journals. This dearth of data is unfortunate because, although the definition of general principles from experimental studies is important, we believe that the care of individual patients could be greatly enhanced by in-shoe pressure measurement. In our foot clinics, we use in-shoe pressure measurement for patients who have proven extremely difficult to keep from reulcerating. Although we rarely know the threshold for ulceration (but see the case study in the earlier section on ulcer threshold), we invariably have a shoe in which the patient has already ulcerated. Therefore, the goal for the design of new footwear is to provide substantial pressure relief compared to that shoe. An example of this approach is shown in Figure 6-11.

We have recently explored approaches that go beyond the conventional shape-based design of therapeutic insoles toward a method that uses both plantar pressure and shape.[73] In particular, we have devised algorithms to design metatarsal supports based on the contours of the pressure distribution under the metatarsal heads (Fig. 6-28). Initial results (Botek et al 2007, in press) suggest that this approach is highly effective in relieving pressure.

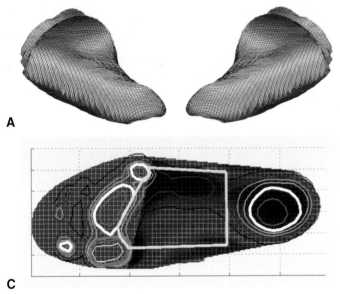

A

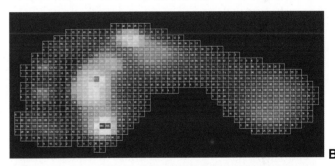

B

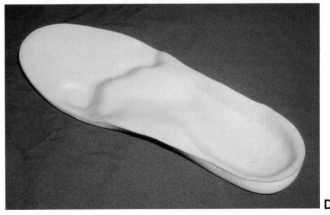

D

C

Figure 6–28   A new approach to the prescription and manufacture of custom insoles. **A,** Results of a digital scan of both feet. **B,** Plantar pressure profile from a right foot contact during walking, showing elevated pressure under the first, second, and fifth metatarsal heads (MTHs). **C,** Shape (continuous color surface) and plantar pressure (contours) combined and trimmed to a shoe outline. The yellow leading edge is the basis for a metatarsal support designed to unload the high MTH pressures based on the measured plantar pressure contours. The "tail" of the intervention is smoothly and automatically merged into the foot shape. **D,** The finished insole manufactured on a computer-controlled milling machine. *(Reproduced from Cavanagh PR, Owings TM: Nonsurgical strategies for healing and preventing recurrence of diabetic foot ulcers. Foot Ankle Clin 11(4):735–743, 2006, with permission.)*

Acceptance of Therapeutic Footwear

Compliance with the wearing of prescription footwear is obviously a key to successful treatment. Chantelau and Haage[347] reported that patients who were compliant in the use of prescribed therapeutic footwear (reported use for more than 60% of the day) experienced significantly fewer ulcer recurrences than did noncompliant patients.

Very few studies of psychological factors involved in the acceptance of prescription footwear are available, but obviously, even the most sophisticated biomechanical approach to footwear design will fail if the shoes are not worn. It is true that many styles of footwear that are currently prescribed to diabetic patients in the United States are not aesthetically pleasing. Several European manufacturers of extra-depth shoes are providing much more attractive styles, which could promote better patient compliance. Williams and Nester[348] have reported that style is a very important factor in shoe choice among diabetic patients. McLoughlin and colleagues[349] reported a remarkable gender difference in compliance with therapeutic footwear in the United Kingdom. In an audit performed 2 years after an initial footwear prescription, records indicated that whereas 71% of men received new shoes, only 35% of women obtained a repeat prescription. Again, 65% of women failed to attend a foot review clinic, whereas male attendance was described as "much better." Johnson and colleagues[350] have pointed out that patients and health care professionals often have differing perspectives in terms of the expectations and realities of preventive behavior.

Summary of Footwear Biomechanics

In summary, from the biomechanical perspective, the primary goal of footwear is to redistribute force over a large area (i.e., reduce pressure), thereby cushioning foci of elevated pressure. Ideally, this would involve redistributing the pressure throughout the surface of the foot by using an insole that conformed to all curvatures of the foot. Such a hydrostatic insole model has the drawback of not resisting shear stress, however. The spring and damper concepts help in the understanding of foot-shoe interface material design, but progress is also rapidly being made in the area of computerized modeling for footwear design.

Many basic principles of footwear design for the neuropathic foot remain to be elucidated. The uncertainty over the positioning of the rocker axis is a good example of why more objective research is needed in this field before footwear can be designed according to established principles rather than simply being based on designs from clinical experience. Many of the ideas outlined in this section on footwear need to be confirmed by further experimental investigations. The entire field of therapeutic footwear biomechanics is still in a primitive stage, in which trial and error is the principal modus operandi. This is not a satisfactory situation for either patient or provider, and it frequently results in a long and frustrating search for a solution that will keep the patient healed. One can only hope that the continued application of technologies such as biomechanical modeling, pressure measurement, materials testing, and foot shape measurement will result in a more complete understanding of the principles of different approaches and faster convergence toward appropriate interventions.

Clinical Biomechanics: What to Look for and What to Do About It

So far, we have discussed the biomechanics of gait, of the soft tissues of the foot, of various devices for healing neuropathic plantar ulcers, and of footwear, all in the context of understanding the cause and options for treatment and prevention of diabetic foot injury. At each point, we have tried to describe potential clinical implications. The goal of the next section of this chapter is to pull together the information that has been provided so far into a coherent, usable clinical strategy. The reader might also wish to consult a monograph by Warren and Nade,[351] which offers much practical advice on the treatment of neuropathic limbs.

The key permissive factor in diabetic foot injury is loss of protective sensation because of the distal symmetric peripheral neuropathy that can result from diabetes. The degree of nerve damage can be assessed in many ways, and it has been proposed that to fully define the degree of neuropathy, an objective assessment of symptoms, function, and electrophysiologic tests should be performed.[352] However, in the context of defining the level of sensory loss that allows an injury to go unperceived, simple functional sensory tests appear to provide the best discrimination.[32,86,100,353,354] Loss of protective sensation has been defined in terms of touch-pressure sensation using the Semmes-Weinstein monofilaments[100,353] and in terms of vibration perception threshold using the Biosthesiometer (Biomedical Instruments, Newbury, OH)[86,355] and the Vibratron (Physitemp Instruments, Clifton, NJ).[353]

We use primarily the Semmes-Weinstein monofilaments and believe that in clinical practice, this simple tool provides the quickest and best method of confirming and measuring loss of protective sensation. In several studies using a method-of-limits protocol rather than a "forced-choice" protocol,[32,100] the 10-g monofilament was found to be discriminatory. We believe that this extremely simple and inexpensive tool should be in the office of all physicians who care for patients with diabetes. Just as an annual examination of the retina is viewed as essential to good care, an annual assessment of sensory level in the feet should be seen as critical.[356] If the patient can perceive the 10-g monofilament at multiple sites in the feet, he or she can be considered to require little or no additional special foot care. An exception to this would be a patient with good sensation but very ischemic feet, for whom even a simple cut or blister, even though it would be painful, might lead to gangrene and amputation. Regardless of an ability to feel pain and recognize injury, that patient needs to be educated about sensible foot care. Likewise, a patient with good sensation who wears shoes that are inappropriate even for a healthy person, such as those with high heels and a cramped toebox, should also receive education about healthy foot care habits and reasonable footwear styles as an investment for the future.

A number of clinical recommendations for the patient with loss of protective sensation, which are based on biomechanical principles, are contained in two important documents that have emerged from the activities of the American Diabetes Association's Council on Foot Care.[357,358] The first of these[357] is concerned with preventive foot care and identifies several biomechanical risk factors of which the clinician should be aware. The components of an adequate foot examination are also discussed. The second[358] is the result of a Consensus

Development Conference on Diabetic Foot Wound Care, and many of the recommendations on off-loading the ulcerated foot parallel the remarks made in the section of this chapter on ulcer healing. In a 2006 publication, we described what the practicing physician should know about foot biomechanics[359] and how an examination should be conducted. Once the loss of protective sensation has been identified, a detailed evaluation of foot structure and function and of gait and footwear is essential. From sources described at the start of this paragraph and on the evidence described in this chapter, the following sections have been compiled to help the clinician determine what to look for. Many of these clinical recommendations are components of a brief examination that we have called "the Two-Minute Foot Exam" (Table 6-7).

Plantar Pressure

On the basis of the many studies linking high barefoot pressure to ulceration, it makes sense to measure barefoot plantar pressure in all patients with loss of protective sensation if equipment is available. The best study that defines risk is that of Armstrong and colleagues.[82] They suggest that a pressure of 750 kPa provides the best level of discrimination between low-risk and high-risk patients

TABLE 6-7   A "Two-Minute Foot Exam" to Check for Biomechanical and Other Risk Factors Once a Patient Has Been Judged to Be at Risk Because of Significant Neuropathy or Vascular Disease

Evaluation Component	Details	Action
1. Examine all surfaces	Look for: Ulcer Callus Hemorrhage into callus Blister Maceration between toes Other breaks in the skin Skin infection Edema, erythema, elevated temperature	Prescribe unweighting device to heal ulcer (see Figs. 6-8 and 6-9) Remove callus (sharp debridement and/or dremmel or emery board) Treat skin infection or injury Refer if Charcot fracture suspected
2. Examine the nails	Look for: Fungal infections Ingrown toenails Evidence of injury from self nail care	Consider treating fungal infections Advise against self-care of nails Suggest chiropody care
3. Identify foot deformity	Look for: Prominent metatarsal heads Clawed toes or hammertoes Rocker-bottom foot deformity Hallux valgus and bunions Prior amputation	The presence of foot deformity will dictate footwear specifications (see text and Table 6-8)
4. Examine the shoes Have the patient put shoes and socks on as the last component of the examination. This will show the patient's ability to examine his or her own feet.	Look for: Drainage into socks Worn-out (flattened) insoles Shoes that are leaning badly to one side Poorly fitting shoes (too tight, too loose, too short, not enough room for the toes) Gait pattern	Prescribe appropriate footwear if necessary (see text and Table 6-8) Suggest replacement shoes if necessary
5. Establish need for education	Ask: Why do you think I am concerned about your feet? Do you walk without shoes at home? Who takes care of your nails?	Schedule patient for education visit with diabetes educator or nurse if understanding is lacking or if behaviors are unacceptable

Adapted from Cavanagh PR, Ulbrecht JS, Caputo GM: What the practising physician should know about diabetic foot mechanics. In Boulton AJM, Connor H, Cavanagh PR (eds): The Foot in Diabetes, 3rd ed. Chichester, UK, John Wiley & Sons, 2000, p. 46.

(as measured by using an EMED SF system). They do point out, however, that the higher the pressure, the higher the risk, and that there is no clearly "safe" pressure. We have used barefoot pressure assessment routinely in patients with loss of protective sensation for several years, and we tend to think of pressure greater than 500 kPa as conferring some risk at forefoot or midfoot sites. At the hallux, clearly, high pressures confer risk, but low pressures there do not exclude risk, since the hallux behaves differently during activities of daily living than during level walking.[95] The recommendation to perform barefoot plantar pressure measurement on all patients with loss of protective sensation must be tempered somewhat by the fact that there has been no prospective study showing better patient outcomes due to plantar pressure testing.

Recent surveys of approaches to unloading have been given by Lavery and Murdoch,[360] van Schie,[361] van Deursen,[362] Cavanagh and colleagues,[4,73,363] Elftman,[364] and McGuire.[365,366] The need for better evidence in this area was highlighted in a Cochrane review by Spencer,[367] who found limited evidence for a variety of pressure-relieving interventions intended for the prevention and treatment of diabetic foot ulcers.

However, the lack of attention to off-loading has been widely blamed for equivocal or poor results in a number of healing trials, and this has led to the suggestion that there should be a standard off-loading protocol in all clinical trials of advanced wound-healing products.[16] Beuker and colleagues[368] compared off-loading in four devices designed for plantar ulcer healing: a custom-molded insole shoe, a cast MABAL shoe, a prefabricated pneumatic walking brace, and a bivalved total-contact cast. The control device was a standard orthotic shoe with a 10-mm-thick hard, flat insole made from ethylene vinyl acetate. Although all devices significantly unloaded the region of interest compared to control, there were significant differences in the magnitude of unloading between the devices, the bivalved cast showing the most unloading.

Particular attention should be given to elevated plantar pressure in the intact foot of a patient with unilateral amputation. Kanade and colleagues[369] have shown that even though a group of 21 patients with transtibial amputations walked more slowly than did a control group, they exhibited higher peak plantar pressures. Van Deursen[362] has pointed out that in addition to conventional orthotic approaches, plantar pressure can also be reduced by reduction in walking speed, alteration of the foot rollover process during gait, and transfer of load from the foot to the leg or to assistive devices.

The current popularity of vacuum-assisted (negative-pressure) wound closure has led to an examination of techniques that can provide both vacuum and off-loading of plantar pressure.[370,371] Although the primary purpose of dressings has heretofore been in direct treatment of the wound (through either delivery of healing agents or the enhancement of the wound environment), there has recently been interest in dressings that also unload the wound.[372,373]

If plantar pressure measurement is not available, a clinical assessment of all the factors that contribute to high pressure and therefore to ulceration (as reviewed above in the section on causes of high pressure) is needed. This includes clinical assessment of foot or toe deformity, the soft tissue plantar cushion, the range of motion of key joints, callus and preulcers, and, of course, ulcers and scar tissue. Even when plantar pressure measurement is available, assessment is needed of strength, balance, and the patient's intended activity level, including special activities such as golfing, horse riding, and similar pursuits. In each of the following subsections, we first offer what the clinician needs to assess, followed by some intervention options. Therapeutic footwear is, of course, an option that can be used to deal with all of the abnormalities that cause high pressure; footwear is dealt with separately in its own subsection. Many of the deformities can also be treated by surgery (see the section below on surgery).

Foot Deformity

High pressure on both the dorsal and plantar surfaces is the immediate cause of most skin injury. The key foot deformities that must be identified as potential risk factors for foot injury are shown in Table 6-7. On the dorsal aspect of the foot, skin breakdown is usually the result of deformity, the most common of which is clawing of toes. On occasion, the toes will actually become dorsally dislocated, and standard off-the-shelf shoe fit is usually not possible in that situation. At the very least, extra-depth shoes must be prescribed and worn. Although uncommon, bony prominences on the dorsal aspect of the midfoot are very troublesome because this region of the foot is likely to be particularly involved in the transfer of propulsive forces from the foot through footwear to the ground during gait. Such dorsal prominences are sometimes seen in patients with Charcot fractures. Bunions, secondary to hallux valgus, are important deformities, particularly when associated with a wide forefoot. They are usually covered by very little soft tissue, making shoe fitting difficult.

Another important deformity is that of forefoot supination or pronation (rotation of the plane of the MTHs so that they are no longer in the same plane as the hindfoot).[374] When the forefoot is in supination, MTH5 tends to hit the ground first during gait, so higher plantar pressure in this region would be predicted. Similarly, when the forefoot is in pronation, one could predict higher plantar pressure under MTH1. However, this is a good example of how very difficult it is to predict plantar pressure from just an examination of the foot. The pressures just implied will, in fact, depend on whether the supination or pronation is fixed or flexible—in other words, on how difficult it is to bring all the MTHs onto the ground during stance and gait. Plantarflexed metatarsal bones (particularly the first) can also result in focal areas of pressure if the deformity is relatively rigid.

Unusual deformities or prominences frequently imply underlying fractures that are often not noted by the patient,[166] and radiographs of a patient with a major deformity are mandatory. Unusual prominences of the midfoot are of particular relevance because they are usually an indication of an underlying Charcot fracture. In the acute stages of a Charcot process, the foot is also erythematous, hot, and swollen, but in the "healed" stage of a Charcot fracture, these findings are absent.

Soft Tissue Changes

Bones can appear to be prominent either because of deformity or because of changes in the soft tissues overlying the bones. The plantar surface is normally well padded with soft tissue, so some attempt at an examination of the soft tissues there is important. Because most ulcers occur under the hallux and MTHs, these are the regions that should be inspected most carefully.

Because there is an association between soft tissue thickness under an MTH and peak plantar pressure in that region,[112,113,128] an assessment of the quantity of the soft tissues under the MTHs is relevant. In a healthy young foot, the MTHs are not visible through the plantar skin or palpable to a light stroking movement by the examiner's finger across them. As the toes become clawed as a consequence of intrinsic muscle atrophy and/or tearing of the plantar fascia, the plantar fat pad slides forward away from the MTHs, so the tissue between the skin and the MTHs becomes thinner. In an extreme case, the MTHs will be directly palpable, seeming to be covered by skin only. On average, pressure under an MTH that is covered only by skin will be much greater than when there is a good amount of healthy plantar tissue between the MTH and the contact surface. As was discussed earlier, the quantity and quality of the plantar soft tissues may also be affected by glycosylation. Tissue "quality" may be an important factor, but there are no ways to measure this parameter at present. Scarring and adhesions of the soft tissues of the plantar surface can also be detected clinically; because of the possible consequences to plantar soft tissue function and thus to ulceration, we teach our patients to try to mobilize scar tissue by massage. Scarring implies, of course, that an ulcer had been present, identifying that patient as almost certainly still having all the characteristics necessary for further ulceration.

An intriguing anecdotal approach to the alleviation of soft-tissue deficits using injected liquid silicone has been reported for a number of years by Balkin and colleagues.[375–377] Recently, a controlled study of this approach reported that patients who had been injected with sili-

cone had lower MTH pressures up to 12 months after the treatment.[378] If this procedure can be shown to be medically safe, it would appear to offer a useful way to reduce plantar pressure at MTH prominences. The same group[379] conducted a 24-month follow-up study of 14 patients who had received six injections of 0.2 mL of liquid silicone under sites of plantar MTH callus and compared them with a placebo group of patients who had been injected with saline. The authors found that although peak plantar pressures were reduced in comparison to baseline in the silicone group at 12 months, there was no difference at 24 months.

Callus

Even though the etiology of callus is not clear, the fact that callus contributes to high plantar pressure has been demonstrated.[161] Furthermore, in the study of Murray and colleagues,[161] the presence of callus in a patient with loss of protective sensation conferred a very high risk ratio for ulceration. It is therefore strongly recommended that callus be looked for and that appropriate measures be taken to prevent, limit, and remove it. Appropriate footwear prevents callus,[335] and one measure of how efficacious footwear is, short of preventing ulceration, is prevention of callus. One can feel very confident that a patient is doing well if callus is being prevented. Patients can contribute to limiting callus by daily self-care: filing the callus with an emery board or pumice stone. Removal of callus is also a very important part of professional foot care.

An extremely important sign in the evaluation of the neuropathic foot is hemorrhage into a callus, also called a preulcer. Although this condition can be quite subtle at times, its existence implies that enough trauma has occurred to cause tissue damage. Therefore, hematoma in a callus must be taken as seriously as an ulcer; it is an ulcer "but for a few more steps." Health care providers must share their concern about such a lesion with their patients as part of patient education, teaching patients how to recognize this lesion and report it immediately.

Limited Joint Mobility

Limited joint mobility is statistically associated with higher plantar pressure.[25,151,152] The possible mechanisms for this association have been discussed. Although direct prediction of plantar pressure from measurement of the range of motion of a joint is not possible, there is nevertheless one measurement that is probably worthwhile: the measurement of hallux dorsiflexion. The normal range of hallux dorsiflexion is approximately 50 degrees in relation to the ground when measured with a simple goniometer.[380] Marked reductions of hallux dorsiflexion are associated with high hallux pressure.[25] One would similarly predict that a reduction in ankle dorsiflexion would tend to increase forefoot plantar pressure.

In general, however, this is not convincing on a patient-by-patient basis, probably because many other factors contribute to forefoot pressure. On the other hand, if a patient is having ongoing problems with recurrent forefoot ulceration, the discovery of a very limited range of dorsiflexion at the ankle might lead to a recommendation for TAL (see the section below on surgery). For completeness, both range of ankle dorsiflexion, with the knee flexed and extended, and subtalar range of motion should be assessed. Since accuracy and interrater reliability are controversial topics in such measurements,[381] those made by a single examiner are preferable. Certain measurements (e.g., subtalar neutral position) may be almost worthless because of lack of appropriate landmarks.

There is now preliminary evidence that passive range of motion and other exercises could be effective in increasing the range of motion of the joints of the foot and perhaps also in reducing plantar pressure during walking.[158,159]

Weakness and Balance

Although much emphasis in the evaluation and treatment of the diabetic patient is placed on sensory neuropathy, patients with a significant motor component to their neuropathy can also display major functional problems with the feet. A quick evaluation of the patient's ability to rise repeatedly on the toes from a neutral standing position is a worthwhile component of the clinical examination to reveal triceps surae weakness. Loss of strength of the ankle dorsiflexors will be apparent in gait, during which foot drop, a steppage gait, or both will be seen. Patients with foot drop can injure their toes by dragging them on the ground; this can be prevented if good shoes are always worn. Falling because of the toes catching on the ground can be prevented by using an ankle-foot orthosis.

Sensory neuropathy also affects the afferent nerves relevant to balance, as was reviewed earlier, and neuropathic patients fall more often than do those without neuropathy. Patients should therefore be asked whether or not they have fallen recently. The traditional Romberg test with the eyes open and closed can also be revealing. A detailed monofilament test using multiple monofilaments of different thicknesses that can establish the threshold for touch sensation (rather than just the presence or absence of protective sensation) can be reasonably predictive of postural stability.[185] However, in the clinic, it is worth remembering that a patient who cannot feel the 10-g monofilament can be expected to sway while trying to stand still as much as a nonneuropathic patient would sway with his or her eyes closed and head back.[185] If there does appear to be a risk for falling, the provision of an assistive device such as a cane or a walker would seem intuitively reasonable. Patients often report that they feel more stable when their shoes are rockered rather than rolled, but we have no quantitative data to support this observation. Patients with short amputations, such as a transmetatarsal amputation (TMA), also report less of a balance problem with an ankle-foot orthosis of some type. Mueller and colleagues.[382] found that an ankle-foot orthosis led to the best biomechanical function in such patients. Although there are no articles in the literature on strength or balance training in patients with diabetes, there are many studies showing the benefits of both these interventions in elderly individuals.[383] It is reasonable to assume that diabetic patients with strength and balance problems would benefit from such a program.

In an intervention study, Richardson and colleagues[207] found that older patients with peripheral neuropathy demonstrate improved gait characteristics with the use of a cane, ankle orthoses, or touch of a vertical surface while walking under challenging conditions. There are some initial indications that the addition of "noise" to the somatosensory system can have positive effects on function.[384,385] This observation has led to a demonstration in diabetic patients that conventional measures of balance control can be improved by the addition of noise transmitted in the form of vibration to the plantar aspect of the feet.[386] It remains to be seen whether this novel finding can be translated into a successful intervention to reduce falls.

Activity and Gait

An important question to ask patients is how much they use their feet and in what activities. It is important to ask about both the amount and type of use because, for example, much greater forces are transmitted through the plantar tissues from running than from walking.[95] A patient who is bed- or chair-bound might not need sophisticated footwear to protect the feet, whereas a very athletic patient who has significant foot problems might have to consider altering his or her behavior as well as footwear. We have, at times, made rigid roller-bottom modified golf shoes with molded insoles as well as English-style riding boots to allow patients to continue as normal a lifestyle as possible while minimizing the risk to their feet. Chair- or bed-bound patients have their own particular problems, however. Heel decubitus ulcers are well known, but decubitus ulcers can also develop over the malleoli in patients who have a preference for lying on one side or the other. These ulcers will not heal until pressure from lying in bed or on a recliner chair is relieved.

Watching the patient walk before prescribing footwear or any other intervention is obviously highly relevant and useful, since most foot injuries occur during gait. Even though much can be inferred about foot function from the static examination described so far, weakness, balance problems, and any unusual gait due to hip or knee problems become apparent only during walking.

There is a single report[387] that aerobic exercise over an extended period of time might retard the development of peripheral neuropathy, but more studies are clearly warranted.

Shoes and Footwear Prescription

The topic of footwear prescription is dealt with more comprehensively in Chapter 28. Recent reviews of therapeutic footwear options for people with diabetes have been provided by Boulton and Jude[388] and by Cavanagh and colleagues.[363,389,390] There are indications that at least in the United States in the late 20th century, Medicare footwear benefits were underused[391] and that informing patients of the availability of the benefits can increase usage.[392]

The role of therapeutic footwear in the prevention of ulceration was questioned in a study by Reiber and colleagues.[220] However, a number of aspects of this study have themselves been questioned.[221,393] In particular, the definition of an ulcer, the neuropathic status of the patients in the study, and the nature and efficacy of the footwear intervention were significant limitations to the study. Subsequently, Maciejewski and colleagues[394] reviewed the literature on the benefits of therapeutic footwear and pointed to the lack of definitive, well-designed studies. This confirms the earlier observations of Spencer.[367]

An interesting set of observations regarding shoe sizing was made by Nixon and colleagues,[395] who found in a study of 440 consecutive podiatry patients (the majority being male military veterans, 58% of whom had diabetes) that only 25% of patients wore appropriately sized shoes. People with current diabetic foot ulceration were five times more likely to have poorly fitting shoes than were those without a wound. The most appropriate approach to casting the feet for the prescription of custom insoles was explored by Tsung and colleagues.[396,397] These authors found that foot-shape-based insoles were superior to flat insoles in pressure reduction and that semi-weight-bearing casts resulted in a superior product compared to non-weight-bearing and full-weight-bearing casts.

We will now discuss some recommendations that flow from the various biomechanical studies that were mentioned in earlier parts of the chapter. It is through shoes that the forces of gait that can potentially damage the foot are transmitted from the ground, and it is therefore in shoes that most injuries occur. Shoes can protect from injury, but they can also cause injury directly. A thorough examination of footwear must be considered an essential component of the clinical biomechanical examination of the patient who is at risk for neuropathic injury.

Concepts of fit must be applied to the clinical situation, with particular attention to dorsal deformities, clawed toes, and forefoot width. Construction of the insole will depend on what the clinical situation demands, but an insole that is already being used must be examined for excessive wear (bottoming out). This can provide insight into the location of high plantar pressure and will also suggest that a particular type of insole is not sufficient (e.g., if it bottoms out very quickly) or is simply too old.

Evaluation of the wear of both the outsoles and uppers of the shoes worn by a patient can also be helpful. Excessive wear of the outsole is probably a consequence of relative movement ("scuffing") during the early and late phases of foot contact and is probably not helpful in predicting where high plantar pressure occurs. Deformations of the upper, however, are often extremely useful because they are evidence of shear forces tending to move the foot off the platform of the shoe. Significant uncompensated supination and pronation deformities of the forefoot can usually be inferred from deformations in the shoe upper.

The approach to footwear prescription should be graded. The simplest intervention for a patient who is at risk for ulceration would be a good-fitting, well-cushioned pair of athletic shoes. A number of studies have shown that wearing athletic shoes can reduce plantar pressure[43,68,69] and lead to fewer calluses.[335] Thus, athletic shoes can be the first line of defense if the patient's foot fits well in the upper. The next step is to provide extra-depth shoes, which typically add from 1/4 to 1/2 inch of space to the toebox, thus allowing for accommodation of significant dorsal deformity or thicker insoles. It is generally advisable to replace the insoles that are supplied with these shoes with a thick foam insole. The next level of complexity in footwear is to make a custom-molded and/or customized insole (see the section on footwear above). Patients who are still not adequately protected will need the outsoles of their depth shoes made rigid and either rockered or rollered (see below). Finally, feet with significant deformity or feet that need a very thick insole will need custom-molded shoes. As is apparent from the foregoing discussion, a large majority of patients can be accommodated by using footwear that is available over the counter from a therapeutic shoe supplier. The manufacture of molded and customized insoles, however, requires specialist care. This fact is implied in the footwear pyramid presented in Figure 6-29.

We believe that the factors that drive a decision regarding which of the above types of footwear to prescribe are a combination of the patient's activity level and plantar pressures (Table 6-8). If barefoot plantar pressure measurement is not available, then deformity can be used as a surrogate measure for elevated pressure. The more active the patient and the higher the plantar pressure (or the greater the deformity), the more sophistication is needed in the footwear. As is apparent from Table 6-8, the process of footwear prescription is not an exact science. The table represents the consensus of several clinicians, but there are few data to support it, so the table allows much latitude. Only when the ulceration threshold has been defined in terms of some measure of loading in a shoe (see the section on threshold) will it

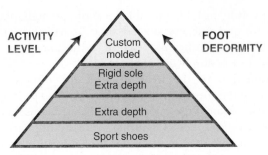

Figure 6-29   The footwear pyramid. The width of the base of each segment is proportional to the number of patients who can be accommodated in the type of footwear indicated. Thus, custom-molded shoes are reserved for a small group of patients who cannot be accommodated by any of the other designs, which increase in complexity from the base upward. Activity level and foot deformity (which is a surrogate measure for plantar pressure) are used to define the appropriate footwear for a given patient.

be possible to prescribe footwear with precision. In the meantime, the proof of the shoe is in its wearing. In other words, whether a shoe is efficacious or not can be judged only by whether an ulcer or, preferably, callus, blister, redness, or preulcer can be prevented.

The literature regarding rocker and roller outsole shoes was presented earlier. There is conclusive evidence that shoes with rigid soles and a curved or rockered outsole are effective in relieving plantar pressure, and clinical experience suggests that such footwear can help to keep patients from experiencing recurrent ulceration.[65,66,78,341–343]

In summary, taking all of the studies of rocker and roller shoes together, we currently recommend the following in the design of rigid footwear:

1. *Minimize toe spring.* Pending definitive investigation of this variable, this recommendation is suggested by comparing the studies of Coleman[65] and Nawoczenski and colleagues.[66]

TABLE 6-8   The Interaction of Plantar Pressure (or Deformity) and Activity Level in the Selection of Appropriate Footwear

	Footwear and Footbed Options		
Deformity	**Low Activity** (Household/Minimal Ambulator)	**Moderate Activity** (Community Ambulator)	**High Activity** (Active Ambulator)
None No deformity	• Standard shoe w/soft insole (usually an athletic shoe)	• Standard shoe w/soft insole (usually an athletic shoe) • Standard shoe w/added flat insole • Standard shoe w/added molded insole	• Standard shoe w/added flat insole • Standard shoe w/added molded insole • Extra-depth shoe w/flat insole • Extra-depth shoe w/molded insole
Moderate Limited hallux motion Prominent metatarsal heads Severe clawed toes or hammertoes Callus Single lesser ray amputation Plantar bony prominences Hallux valgus Dystrophic nails Dorsal exotoses	• Standard shoe w/soft insole (usually an athletic shoe) • Standard shoe w/added flat insole • Standard shoe w/added molded insole • Extra-depth shoe w/flat insole	• Standard shoe w/added flat insole • Standard shoe w/added molded insole • Extra-depth shoe w/flat insole • Extra-depth shoe w/molded insole • Custom-molded shoe w/custom-molded insole Additional features (+/–) • Compliant plugs • Roller soles	• Standard shoe w/added molded insole • Extra-depth shoe w/flat insole • Extra-depth shoe w/molded insole • Custom-molded shoe w/custom-molded insole Additional features (+/–) • Compliant plugs • Differential insoles • Roller soles *Lifestyle modifications*
Severe Charcot ≥ Ray amputation ≥ First ray/multiple	• Extra-depth shoe w/flat insole • Extra-depth shoe w/molded insole • Custom-molded shoe w/custom-molded insole • Unweighting orthosis (e.g., a PTB)	• Extra-depth shoe w/molded insole • Custom-molded shoe w/custom-molded insole • Unweighting orthosis (e.g., a PTB) Additional features (+/–) • Compliant plugs • Differential insoles • Roller soles • Rocker soles	• Custom-molded shoe/w custom-molded insole • Unweighting orthosis (e.g., a PTB) Additional features (+/–) • Compliant plugs • Differential insoles • Roller soles • Rocker soles *Refer to specialist for management* *Requires lifestyle and/or job modification*

Note: Patient history of previous plantar ulcers may require a more aggressive approach to protection than the prescription footwear options suggested in this table.
PTB, patellar tendon–bearing brace.
Source: Reproduced from Brill LR, Cavanagh PR, Doucette MM, Ulbrecht JS: Treatment of Chronic Wounds. Number 5 in a series of monographs. Prevention, Protection and Recurrence Reduction of Diabetic Neuropathic Foot Ulcers. East Setauket, NY, Curative Technologies, Inc., 1994, p 9.

2. *Maintain the heel/forefoot height difference of the original shoe, but pick a shoe with minimal initial difference to avoid ending up with very high shoes.* This recommendation is made empirically, since no published evidence is available. There is concern that altering the heel/forefoot height difference might cause problems with the upper, since this difference was inherent in the original shoe design.

3. *Consider adjusting the axis of the rocker/roller with respect to the long axis of the shoe to accommodate for significant toe-out.* This particularly makes sense if the area of concern is MTH1, but again, no published evidence is available to support this recommendation at present.

4. *Teach patients who use rocker shoes not to dwell on the forward flat part of the rocker for support.* This recommendation has been suggested by van Schie and colleagues[343] and much earlier by Bauman and Brand.[63] Shortening the stride will promote this goal.

5. *Rockers are preferred over rollers.* Rocker shoes of the same height probably reduce pressure more than rollers do (perhaps by an additional 8% from baseline; see Table 6-6), and rockers are less labor-intensive to make.

6. *Consider flaring out the outsole of rollers and rockers.* This is done for added stability.

7. *Consider in-shoe pressure measurement in difficult cases and certainly if a shoe "failed."* This recommendation is suggested because of the individual variability in response to rocker and roller shoes as demonstrated, for instance, by van Schie and colleagues.[343]

8. *Try the suggested rocker and roller designs in* Table 6-9. Most patients will not recognize Shoe 1 as "abnormal." Whereas the take-off point in Shoe 2 favors the toes and hallux, relief at the MTHs should be reasonable (Table 6-5), and using the take-off point of 65% allows the shoe to have a very reasonable height. Shoes 3 to 5 all have the same height, but the different shoes are biased toward different clinical situations. Finally, Shoe 6 is very high and cosmetically troublesome for many patients but can be considered in extreme cases, perhaps with a brace and/or an assistive device that will prevent ankle sprains and falls.

Patients with partial amputations of the foot need special footwear attention, but little quantitative work has been done to explore optimal design characteristics for this group of patients. Mueller and colleagues[382] examined a number of functional measures in patients with TMA wearing six different types of shoes (short- and full-length shoes with different inserts to take up the residual space in the shoe). The investigators reported that appropriate footwear could significantly improve the function of patients with TMA. The best overall performance and patient acceptance was with a full-length shoe with a total-contact insert and a rigid rocker-bottom sole. Footwear with an ankle-foot orthosis proved to be most effective in reducing pressures on the residual foot, but patients did not like the reduced range of ankle motion. Similarly, although a short shoe was biomechanically effective, patients complained of the cosmetics of short shoes; they preferred a full-length shoe with toe filler. The very high complication rate after foot-shortening surgery[398] suggests that pressure measurement could be extremely useful in the management of such patients. Some of the more unusual amputations (e.g., the Chopart [midtarsal] and Syme [ankle] disarticulations) present special biomechanical challenges in footwear management, and it is often because of the difficulties faced in providing adequate footwear that these procedures are not performed more frequently. Based principally on the work of Mueller and colleagues,[382] our clinical recommendations for patients with short feet secondary to TMA are shown in Table 6-10. Unfortunately, these suggestions still contain many principles that are untested by rigorous study.

As was discussed and illustrated in the section above on plantar pressure measurement, in-shoe pressure measurement can be invaluable to guide footwear prescription in patients who reulcerate in newly provided footwear.

It is extremely important to realize that insoles degrade, sometimes rapidly, with normal use. An insole that is protective when prescribed can become dangerous after a few months or sometimes even weeks. The clinician should be vigilant for signs of bottoming out of the insole to the point at which it appears to provide little cushioning and distribution of load. At present, Medicare provisions allow each patient one pair of extra-depth shoes and three pairs of insoles per calendar year. It is not known whether this is sufficient for a typical patient.

It is worth noting in closing that just because shoes are "special," that does not make them right. Unfortunately,

TABLE 6-9   Recommendations for the Design of Rigid Shoes with Rocker and Roller Outsoles

Shoe #	Shoe Description	Height* at Fulcrum (approx. cm)	Clinical Indications
1	Roller, 60% take-off, 75% radius	2.25	Low level of concern; cosmetically almost not noticeable
2	Rocker, 65% take-off, 20°	2.75	"Standard" rocker
3	Roller, 60% take-off, 60% radius	3.25	High risk but will not accept rocker over roller
4	Rocker, 60% take-off, 20°	3.25	High risk; MTHs greater concern than hallux
5	Rocker, 65% take-off, 22.5°	3.25	High risk; hallux and toes greater concern than MTHs
6	Rocker, 65% take-off, 25°	3.75	Extremely high risk; use boot or ankle-foot orthosis for stability

* Height at fulcrum is for a size 10 male shoe 30 cm in length; it will be less for smaller shoes.
Degree indications are for rockers, % radii for rollers.

TABLE 6-1O   Footwear Recommendations for Patients with Short Feet Secondary to Transmetatarsal Amputation

	Shoe Description	Clinical Indications
1	Flexible full-length depth sports shoe, simple insole*	Reasonably long TMA; patient not very active; dorsal fit not a concern; stability not a concern
2	Full-length shoe, upper based on fit needs, appropriate insole,* rigid rocker with outsole height at rocker fulcrum such that a 20° rocker would result if take-off was at 60%. Place rocker axis just proximal to TMA line.	"Standard" shoe; however, this shoe should be strongly discouraged if rocker axis would be at less than 50% of shoe
3	Same as 2 but with AFO built into shoe	Offer to patient for better stability
4	Less than full-length custom-molded shoe; upper based on fit needs; appropriate insole*; 20° rigid rocker with take-off just proximal to TMA line, such that this is 65% of shoe length**	A compromise between a full-length shoe and a short shoe for patients with short TMA
5	Same as 4 but with AFO built into shoe	Offer to patient for better stability
6	Short custom-molded shoe; upper based on fit needs; appropriate insole; 20° rigid rocker with take-off at 75%	For use with short TMAs
7	Same as 6 but with AFO built into shoe	Offer to patient for better stability

* Based on needs to reduce plantar pressure.
** Example: TMA foot 16 cm long, axis of rocker at 15 cm, 15 cm = 65%; therefore, full length of shoe is 15*100/65 = 23 cm.
AFO, ankle-foot orthosis; TMA, transmetatarsal amputation.

many specialist clinics still see patients with recurrent ulceration wearing special (and often expensive) shoes that are simply inappropriate for their condition.

Adherence and Education

It has become increasingly clear that the success of biomechanical interventions to reduce the morbidity of foot complications is heavily dependent on patient behavior and adherence as well as provider behavior.[399] An important study by Armstrong and colleagues[284] showed that patients with plantar ulcers may take more than 70% of their daily steps unprotected during ulcer healing. Out of a mean total of 1219 ± 821.1 steps, the patients wore a removable cast walker that had been provided for only 345 ± 219 of these steps. Adherence to the use of therapeutic footwear also appears to be dismal. Patients studied by Knowles and Boulton[400] self-reported that they wore their shoes for only 25% of their total active time. Both studies indicate that the very best intervention might fail because of patients' poor adherence to treatment recommendations.

Wrobel and colleagues[401] have provided some very important organizational characteristics that appear to have played a role in the success of the Department of Veterans Affairs' effort to reduce foot complications, and a comprehensive approach to ulcer care is described by Singh and colleagues.[402] Vileikyte and her colleagues[403–405] stress the need for the patient to understand the disease process that is causing loss of sensation in order to maximize their compliance with advice regarding prevention. Elftman[364] has also remarked that patients are often "unaware of the neuropathic pathway until it causes a complication," and this should not be the case.

Surgery to Alter Biomechanics

Recent discussion of surgical treatment of biomechanical problems has been presented by Salamon and

Saltzman,[406] Brodsky,[407] and Cavanagh and colleagues.[4] Since both dorsal and plantar ulceration often occurs over bony prominences, it is not surprising that "prophylactic" bone surgery in patients with neuropathy and deformity has been proposed. It is difficult to quantify the absolute risk of a first ulcer occurring, and the surgical benefit (of a bunion procedure, for instance) in terms of ulcer prevention as well as the risk of bone-altering procedures has not been clearly established. There are concerns, however, about surgery in the neuropathic foot causing Charcot fractures (see below). It seems prudent to advise against truly prophylactic surgery, although this recommendation might change as more data become available. However, at some point after an ulcer develops, it might be appropriate to consider surgery to alter the biomechanics of the foot to cure an ulcer and/or prevent recurrence. Obviously, the higher the odds that an ulcer will recur and the more safe and beneficial the procedure is, the more likely it is that surgery will lead to a good outcome. Unfortunately, just as is the case for footwear prescription, this type of decision is a matter of experience and judgment rather than a matter of precise rules.

What do we know about the risks and benefits of various surgical procedures? Of considerable concern is a report by Fleischli and colleagues[408] describing a case series of 22 dorsiflexion metatarsal osteotomies for treatment of chronic persistent or recurrent forefoot ulcers. The authors reported a 68% complication rate, the most prevalent complication being a Charcot fracture "with rapid destruction of the midfoot." Presumably, many of these Charcot fractures were induced by the surgical and/or rehabilitation procedure. Since the majority of the ulcers were Wagner Grade 1 or 2 (i.e., superficial or deep to tendon, capsule, or bone without osteomyelitis or deep abscess), the evidence cited elsewhere in this chapter would suggest that at least 90% of these ulcers should have healed in 6 to 8 weeks with a standard TCC regimen unless complicated by noncompliance, significant vascular disease, or significant infection. The probability that the ulcers would have remained healed cannot be estimated, but healing should certainly have been possible. This report further confirms the position against truly prophylactic surgery on the neuropathic patient.

Actual removal of some or all MTHs has been recommended by some for patients with recurrent forefoot ulcers. Patel and Weiman[409] used an EMED SF platform to show that peak pressures at the site of single MTH resections were significantly reduced without any significant increase in pressure at adjacent sites. Giurini and colleagues[410] have also reported a successful series of patients on whom this procedure was performed. In contrast, we have presented case studies of patients with panmetatarsal head resection in whom the peak pressures were markedly elevated at several sites under the MTH remnants (Fig. 6-30), with subsequent almost intractable recurrent ulceration.[411] Our suspicion is that this procedure is very technique dependent, but further study is required to confirm this.

A surgical approach to the treatment of midfoot Charcot fractures has become much more commonplace in the last decade. Using a cadaver model, Marks and colleagues[412] have shown that a plantar third tubular midfoot plate provides better stabilization for midfoot instability than does screw fixation, and they have applied this approach to Charcot patients. Myerson and colleagues[413] describe a series of 68 patients who were treated by open reduction and arthrodesis, TCC, or amputation. These authors state that surgical salvage of feet with Charcot fractures, once bony coalescence has begun, is reasonable and appropriate. Sammarco and Conti[414] also reported a series of 27 feet in which surgical repair was performed; a complication rate of approximately 30% was described. Early and Hansen[415] reported on an average 28-month follow up (range 6 to 84 months) of 21 feet with midfoot collapse on which reconstruction with reduction, fusion, and internal fixation was performed. Seventy percent of the patients with midfoot ulcers healed without incident, and there were no recurrent midfoot ulcers in the follow-up period. There is, as yet, no published study in which presurgical and postsurgical biomechanical assessment has been performed in a group of Charcot patients who have been surgically reconstructed. Such a study is certainly needed to provide information on the kind of plantar pressure reduction that is required to create a plantar surface that is viable for weight bearing. So far, the clinical results are very encouraging. For further discussion of this issue, see Chapter 23.

TAL has long been mentioned anecdotally as a means of relieving forefoot pressure in patients with a history of chronic forefoot ulceration. In cadaveric feet, simulated contracture of the posterior calf musculature has been shown to create increases in the loading of the forefoot.[416] Lin and colleagues[248] performed percutaneous TAL and follow-up TCC on 15 patients with forefoot ulcers who initially failed to heal in a TCC. All but one of the ulcers progressed to healing in a mean of 39 days. There was no ulcer recurrence in this group of patients at a mean follow-up time of 17.3 months. Armstrong and colleagues[417] reported on 10 similar patients with recurrent forefoot ulceration. Forefoot plantar pressure was reduced by 230 kPa following percutaneous TAL, and mean range of dorsiflexion was increased by approximately 9 degrees. "Calcaneal gait" has been mentioned as a complication of TAL.[418]

In a randomized clinical trial, Mueller and colleagues[419] reported changes in functional limitations after TAL, but patients receiving TAL with a TCC reported lower physical functioning at 8 months after ulcer healing than subjects receiving TCC alone. The authors suggested that TAL patients may therefore require additional physical therapy. Temporary reductions of 27% forefoot pressure at 3 weeks after TAL surgery but 34% increases in heel pressure were reported by Maluf and colleagues.[420] Hindfoot pressure increases persisted over an 8-month follow-up, but the forefoot pressure, the plantar flexor moment, and power increased significantly. The authors hypothesized that

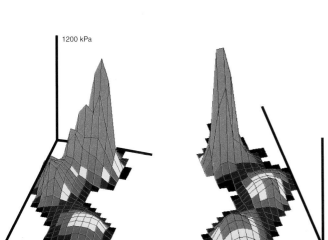

1200 kPa

1200 kPa

Figure 6–30 Peak pressures during walking from the feet of a patient who had undergone bilateral panmetatarsal amputation. Note the regions of extremely high pressure under the distal metatarsal shafts, indicating that pressure relief does not necessarily accompany this procedure.[41]

"the initial decrease in forefoot pressure, followed by progressive reloading of forefoot tissues as plantar flexor muscles regain strength after TAL, may help to reduce the risk of ulcer recurrence in patients with diabetes."[420] Salsich and colleagues[421] found that TAL resulted in a temporary increase in ankle dorsiflexion range of motion and a temporary reduction in concentric plantar-flexor peak torque and passive torque at 0 degree of dorsiflexion. Both of these values returned to preoperative baselines after 8 months. In a study by Holstein and colleagues,[422] TAL surgery was performed in 63 diabetic patients who had 69 ulcerated feet with a mean duration of 48 months. At 12-month median follow-up, there was a healing rate of 80%. Acute transfer ulcers to the heel occurred in 47% of patients with complete anesthesia of the heel pad. The authors concluded that even though lengthening the Achilles tendon is effective in healing plantar neuropathic ulceration, patients with complete anesthesia of the heel pad should not undergo that procedure.

Orendurff and colleagues[423] found from studies on a group of 27 diabetic patients that only 14% of the variance in forefoot plantar pressure could be accounted for by equinus deformity. Therefore, they recommended caution in using TAL procedures to relieve forefoot pressure. These findings contradict those of Lavery and colleagues,[424] who reported that patients with equinus deformity (defined as less than 0 degree of dorsiflexion) had significantly higher plantar pressures than did those without the deformity. TAL has also been recommended for patients with Charcot neuroarthropathy,[425] but this approach remains to be explored quantitatively.

All the procedures mentioned above fit more or less into the category of attempting to reconstruct anatomy. Not mentioned so far are procedures to straighten clawed toes or hammertoes to prevent recurrent ulcers of the toe tips. We find these procedures very helpful, but there are no supporting data for them. Ablative procedures, usually due to infection, ischemia, or both, are often necessary. What is known about the biomechanical consequences of amputation procedures and what are the principles that should govern amputation site selection and method? More often than not, the choice of a site for amputation is governed by a bias for preserving tissue at all costs, without regard to subsequent function. This often leaves the patient and the orthotist with the impossible task of living with and dealing with a foot that cannot be maintained in a healed condition. A good example would be a foot with amputation of multiple medial rays. Ideally, only defined amputations with well-described surgical methods, defined biomechanical consequences, and well-established footwear approaches should be used, but too little is currently known about the consequences of amputation (other than extreme examples such as that just described) to make clear recommendations.

Even minor amputation surgery of the forefoot is associated with significant secondary deformity. Quebedeaux

and colleagues[426] and Lavery and colleagues[427] reported more deformities of the second and third toes and the lesser MTP joints, and more elevated pressures under the MTHs and toes in feet with hallux amputations, compared to the intact contralateral sides. They also found that ulcers were much more common on the amputated side. Similarly, Armstrong and Lavery[428] reported that a history of surgical procedures within the foot (digital or ray amputation distal to the tarsometatarsal joint) was associated with an odds ratio of 9.8 for limited joint mobility or rigid deformity compared to controls who had never had a foot amputation. Peak pressures were also higher in the feet with amputation. However, this study was not designed to establish a cause-and-effect relationship. Similarly, Lavery and colleagues[427] reported elevated pressure under the MTHs and toes in feet with a hallux amputation compared to the contralateral side.

It is not surprising that the mechanics of feet that have undergone partial midfoot amputation are also altered. Garbalosa and colleagues[429] reported elevated forefoot pressure in patients with unilateral TMA compared to their intact side. These investigators also found reduced functional dorsiflexion during gait in the TMA feet. Both these findings suggested that careful footwear management after TMA is essential, but it is also possible that better surgical technique (e.g., incorporation of TAL or tendon transfers, as has been suggested), might improve outcomes. Mueller and colleagues[430] reported that patients with TMA showed reduced ranges of motion and reduced joint moments and power during gait compared to control patients, although, again, speeds were not controlled. Mueller and Sinacore[431] presented a biomechanical rationale for problems during rehabilitation and shoe prescription of patients with TMA. Kelly and colleagues[432] found no difference in the timing of peak pressure between subjects with intact feet and those with TMA (80% ± 5% of stance phase). Transmetatarsal amputation was associated with an 87% complication rate in a retrospective review of 101 cases (in 90 patients) by Pollard and colleagues.[433] Predictors of healing included a palpable pedal pulse and restriction of amputation to the transmetatarsal site, whereas end-stage renal disease was a predictor of failure to heal.

First MTP joint arthroplasty as a curative procedure for plantar ulceration of the hallux interphalangeal joint has been shown by Armstrong and colleagues[434] to result in faster healing than standard nonsurgical care, which consisted of moisture-retentive dressings and an unloading device. Armstrong and colleagues[435] conducted a comparative chart review of 40 patients with uninfected, nonischemic ulcers under MTH5 who had been treated conservatively or by resection of the MTH. The authors reported faster healing (5.8 ± 2.9 versus 8.7 ± 4.3 weeks) and a lower risk of ulceration (4.5% versus 27.8%) in the surgical group.

As was implied above, it is logical to assume that surgical correction of deformity should be useful in

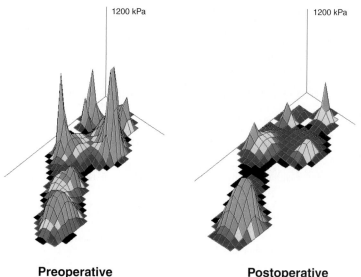

1200 kPa

1200 kPa

Preoperative

Postoperative

Figure 6–31   Preoperative and postoperative peak pressures during walking from a patient who underwent a dorsal wedge osteotomy of the first metatarsal, an arthroplasty of MTH2, and a tendo-Achilles lengthening. Note the marked reduction in forefoot peak pressures but the increased heel pressure.

prevention of neuropathic ulceration and reulceration. However, much remains to be learned before specific recommendations can be made. An example from our own clinical practice of plantar pressure measurements in a patient who has undergone surgery is presented in Figure 6-31.

Concluding Remarks

It is our hope that the techniques and principles presented here will make the biomechanical aspects of etiology and prevention of foot injury in the setting of diabetic neuropathy more understandable and hence more accessible to those who are involved in the treatment of diabetic foot problems. Much remains to be learned. Some of the immediate challenges for the future include the quantification of tissue properties, the definition of objective algorithms for footwear prescription, the reduction of high ulcer recurrence rates, and the introduction of simple in-shoe pressure measurement into a clinical environment. Present economic forces that require clinicians to spend less time with patients will also mean that careful justification will need to be made for additional measurements performed in the clinic. However, it is anticipated that the acceptance of quantitative approaches in what was formerly seen frequently as a subjective field will eventually benefit patients.

ACKNOWLEDGMENTS

Our research on the diabetic foot has been supported by the American Diabetes Association, the National Institutes of Health, and Convatec, Inc (Skillman, NJ).

Declaration of Potential Conflict of Interest: The authors both have an equity interest in DIApedia LLC (State College, PA).

References

1. Cavanagh PR, Simoneau GG, Ulbrecht JS: Ulceration, unsteadiness, and uncertainty: The biomechanical consequences of diabetes mellitus. J Biomech 26(suppl 1):23–40, 1993.
2. Frykberg RG: Biomechanical considerations of the diabetic foot. Lower Extremity 2:207–214, 1995.
3. Payne CB: Biomechanics of the foot in diabetes mellitus: Some theoretical considerations. J Am Podiatr Med Assoc 88(6): 285–289, 1998.
4. Cavanagh PR, Lipsky BA, Bradbury AW, Botek G: Treatment for diabetic foot ulcers. Lancet 366(9498):1725–1735, 2005.
5. Edmonds ME, Blundell MP, Morris ME, et al: Improved survival of the diabetic foot: The role of a specialised foot clinic. Q J Med 60(232):763–771, 1986.
6. Barrett JP, Mooney V: Neuropathy and diabetic pressure lesions. Orthop Clin North Am 4:43–47, 1973.
7. Stokes IAF, Faris IB, Hutton WC: The neuropathic ulcer and loads on the foot in diabetic patients. Acta Orthop Scand 46(5):839–847, 1975.
8. Veves A, Murray H, Young MJ, Boulton AJM: Do high foot pressures lead to foot ulcerations?: A prospective study [abstract]. Diabetologia 34(suppl 2):A40, 1991.
9. Brand PW: Repetitive stress in the development of diabetic foot ulcers. In Levin ME, O'Neal LW (eds): The Diabetic Foot, 4th ed. St. Louis, Mosby, 1988, pp 83–90.
10. Boulton AJM: The pathogenesis of diabetic foot problems: An overview. Diabet Med 13(suppl 1):S12–S16, 1996.
11. Smith L, Plehwe W, McGill M, et al: Foot bearing pressure in patients with unilateral diabetic foot ulcers. Diabet Med 6:573–575, 1989.
12. Stess RM, Jensen SR, Mirmiran R: The role of dynamic plantar pressures in diabetic foot ulcers. Diabetes Care 20(5):855–858, 1997.
13. Apelqvist J, Larsson J, Agardh C-D: The influence of external precipitating factors and peripheral neuropathy on the development and outcome of diabetic foot ulcers. J Diabetes Complications 4(1):21–25, 1990.
14. Brand PW: Insensitive Feet: A Practical Handbook on Foot Problems in Leprosy. London, Leprosy Mission, 1981.
15. Bauman J, Girling E, Brand PW: Plantar pressures and trophic ulceration: An evaluation of footwear. J Bone Joint Surg Am 45-B(4):652–673, 1963.
16. Armstrong DG, Boulton AJ: Pressure offloading and "advanced" wound healing: Isn't it finally time for an arranged marriage? Int J Low Extrem Wounds 3(4):184–187, 2004.

17. Chester VL, Biden EN, Tingley M: Gait analysis. Biomed Instrum Technol 39(1):64–74, 2005.

18. Krag MH: Quantitative techniques for analysis of gait. Automedica 1985;6:85–97.

19. McBride ID, Wyss UP, Cooke TDV, et al: First metatarsophalangeal joint reaction forces during high-heel gait. Foot Ankle 1991;11(5):282–288.

20. Rose SA, DeLuca PA, Davis RB, et al: Kinematic and kinetic evaluation of the ankle after lengthening of the gastrocnemius fascia in children with cerebral palsy. J Pediatr Orthop 13:727–732, 1993.

21. Chambers HG, Sutherland DH: A practical guide to gait analysis. J Am Acad Orthop Surg 10(3):222–231, 2002.

22. Simon SR: Quantification of human motion: gait analysis: Benefits and limitations to its application to clinical problems. J Biomech 37(12):1869–1880, 2004.

23. Andriacchi TP, Yoder D, Conley A, et al: Patellofemoral design influences function following total knee arthroplasty. J Anthroplasty 12(3):243–249, 1997.

24. Nube VL, Molyneaux L, Yue DK: Biomechanical risk factors associated with neuropathic ulceration of the hallux in people with diabetes mellitus. J Am Podiatr Med Assoc 96(3):189–197, 2006.

25. Birke JA, Cornwall MA, Jackson M: Relationship between hallux limitus and ulceration of the great toe. J Orthop Sports Phys Ther 10(5):172–176, 1988.

26. Brand PW: The diabetic foot. In Davidson JK (ed): Clinical Diabetes Mellitus: A Problem Oriented Approach. New York, Thieme Medical Publishers, 1986, pp 376–382.

27. Cavanagh PR, Sims DS, Sanders LJ: Body mass is a poor predictor of peak plantar pressure in diabetic men. Diabetes Care 14(8):750–755, 1991.

28. Alexander IJ, Chao EYS, Johnson KA: The assessment of dynamic foot-to-ground contact forces and plantar pressure distribution: A review of the evolution of current techniques and clinical applications. Foot Ankle 11(3):152–167, 1990.

29. Betts RP, Franks CI, Duckworth T: Foot pressure studies: Normal and pathologic gait analyses. In Jahss MH (ed): Disorders of the Foot and Ankle, 2nd ed, vol 1. Philadelphia, WB Saunders, 1991, pp 484–519.

30. Cavanagh PR, Hewitt FG J, Perry JE: In-shoe plantar pressure measurement: A review. The Foot 2:185–194, 1992.

31. Cavanagh PR, Ulbrecht JS: Plantar pressure in the diabetic foot. In Sammarco GJ (ed): The Diabetic Foot. Philadelphia, Lea and Febiger, 1991, pp 54–70.

32. Cavanagh PR, Ulbrecht JS: Biomechanics of the diabetic foot: A quantitative approach to the assessment of neuropathy, deformity, and plantar pressure. In Jahss MH (ed): Disorders of the Foot and Ankle, 2nd ed. Philadelphia, WB Saunders, 1991, pp 1864–1907.

33. Cavanagh PR, Ulbrecht JS: Clinical plantar pressure measurement in diabetes: Rationale and methodology. The Foot 4:123–135, 1994.

34. Putti AB, Arnold GP, Cochrane L, Abboud RJ: The Pedar((R)) in-shoe system: Repeatability and normal pressure values. Gait Posture 25(3):401–405, 2007.

35. Blackwell B, Aldridge R, Jacob S: A comparison of plantar pressure in patients with diabetic foot ulcers using different hosiery. Int J Low Extrem Wounds 1(3):174–178, 2002.

36. Connelley LK Jr: Verifying successful off-loading of neuropathic pressure ulcers [letter]. J Am Podiatr Med Assoc 89(3):147–149, 1999.

37. Silvino N, Evanski PM, Waugh TR: The Harris and Beath footprinting mat: Diagnostic validity and clinical use. Clin Orthop 151:265–269, 1980.

38. van Schie CHM, Vileikyte L, Abbott CA, et al: Comparing a new simple plantar pressure measuring device with pedobarographically measured pressures [abstract 1005]. Diabetologia 39(suppl 1): A264, 1996.

39. van Schie CHM, Abbott CA, Vileikyte L, et al: A comparative study of the Podotrack, a simple semiquantitative plantar pressure measuring device, and the optical pedobarograph in the assessment of pressures under the diabetic foot. Diabet Med 16:154–159, 1999.

40. Vijay V, Seena R, Lalitha S, et al: A simple device for foot pressure measurement: Evaluation in South Indian NIDDM subjects [letter]. Diabetes Care 21:1205–1206, 1998.

41. Lord M: Spatial resolution in plantar pressure measurement. Med Eng Phys 19:140–144, 1997.

42. Davis BL, Cothren RM, Quesada P, et al: Frequency content of normal and diabetic plantar pressure profiles: Implications for the selection of transducer sizes. J Biomech 29(7):979–983, 1996.

43. Perry JE, Ulbrecht JS, Derr JA, Cavanagh PR: The use of running shoes to reduce plantar pressures in patients who have diabetes. J Bone Joint Surg Am 77-A:1819–1828, 1995.

44. Young MJ, Murray HJ, Veves A, Boulton AJM: A comparison of the Musgrave and optical pedobarograph systems for measuring foot pressures in diabetic patients. The Foot 3:62–64, 1993.

45. McPoil TG, Cornwall MW, Yamada W: A comparison of two in-shoe plantar pressure measurement systems. Lower Extremity 2:95–103, 1995.

46. Wang WC, Ledoux WR, Sangeorzan BJ, Reinhall PG: A shear and plantar pressure sensor based on fiber-optic bend loss. J Rehabil Res Dev 42(3):315–325, 2005.

47. Perry JE, Hall JO, Davis BL: Simultaneous measurement of plantar pressure and shear forces in diabetic individuals. Gait Posture 15(1):101–107, 2002.

48. Razian MA, Pepper MG: Design, development, and characteristics of an in-shoe triaxial pressure measurement transducer utilizing a single element of piezoelectric copolymer film. IEEE Trans Neural Syst Rehabil Eng 11(3):288–293, 2003.

49. Mackey JR, Davis BL: Simultaneous shear and pressure sensor array for assessing pressure and shear at foot/ground interface. J Biomech 39(15):2893–2897, 2006.

50. Dai XQ, Li Y, Zhang M, Cheung JT: Effect of sock on biomechanical responses of foot during walking. Clin Biomech 21(3):314–321, 2006.

51. Maluf KS, Morley RE Jr, Richter EJ, et al: Monitoring in-shoe plantar pressures, temperature, and humidity: Reliability and validity of measures from a portable device. Arch Phys Med Rehabil 82(8):1119–1127, 2001.

52. Morley RE Jr, Richter EJ, Klaesner JW, et al: In-shoe multisensory data acquisition system. IEEE Trans Biomed Eng 48(7):815–820, 2001.

53. Bus SA, de Lange A: A comparison of the 1-step, 2-step, and 3-step protocols for obtaining barefoot plantar pressure data in the diabetic neuropathic foot. Clin Biomech 20(9):892–899, 2005.

54. Stehr M, Dietz HG, Morlock MM: Clinical application of pressure distribution measurements during full gait [abstract]. Program of the 2nd EMED User Meeting, 1991.

55. Rosenbaum D, Hautmann S, Gold M, Claes L: Effects of walking speed on plantar pressure patterns and hindfoot angular motion. Gait Posture 2(3):191–197, 1994.

56. Peters EJ, Urukalo A, Fleischli JG, Lavery LA: Reproducibility of gait analysis variables: One-step versus three-step method of data acquisition. J Foot Ankle Surg 41(4):206–212, 2002.

57. Shaw JE, Hsi WL, Ulbrecht JS, et al: The mechanism of plantar unloading in total contact casts: Implications for design and clinical use. Foot Ankle Int 18:809–817, 1997.

58. Fleischli JG, Lavery LA, Vela SA, et al: Comparison of strategies for reducing pressure at the site of neuropathic ulcers. J Am Podiatr Med Assoc 87(10):466–472, 1997.

59. Lavery LA, Vela SA, Fleischli JG, et al: Reducing plantar pressure in the neuropathic foot: A comparison of footwear. Diabetes Care 20(11):1706–1710, 1997.

60. Baumhauer JF, Wervey R, McWilliams J, et al: A comparison study of plantar foot pressure in a standardized shoe, total contact cast, and prefabricated pneumatic walking brace. Foot Ankle Int 18(1):26–33, 1997.

61. Kernozek TW, LaMott EE, Dancisak MJ: Reliability of an in-shoe pressure measurement system during treadmill walking. Foot Ankle Int 17:204–209, 1996.

62. Young MJ, Cavanagh PR, Thomas G, et al: Callus and elevated dynamic plantar pressures: Does chiropody help? [abstract]. Diabet Med 8(suppl 1):45A, 1991.

63. Bauman JH, Brand PW: Measurement of pressure between foot and shoe. Lancet 1:629–632, 1963.

64. Brand PW, Ebner JD: Pressure sensitive devices for denervated hands and feet. J Bone Joint Surg Am 51-A(1):109–116, 1969.

65. Coleman WC: The relief of forefoot pressures using outer shoe sole modifications. I: Patil KM, Srinivasa (eds): Proceedings of the International Conference on Biomechanics and Clinical Kinesiology of Hand and Foot. Madras, India, Indian Institute of Technology, 1985, pp 29–31.

66. Nawoczenski DA, Birke JA, Coleman WC: Effect of rocker sole designs on plantar forefoot pressures. J Am Podiatr Med Assoc 78:455–460, 1988.

67. Pollard JP, Le Quesne LP, Tappin JW: Forces under the foot. J Biomed Eng 5:37–40, 1983.

68. Pitei DL, Watkins PJ, Foster AVM, Edmonds ME: Do new EVA moulded insoles or trainers efficiently reduce the high foot pressures in the diabetic foot? [abstract 87]. Diabetes 45(suppl 2):25A, 1996.

69. Kastenbauer T, Sokol G, Auinger M, Irsigler K: Running shoes for relief of plantar pressure in diabetic patients. Diabet Med 5:518–522, 1998.

70. Sarnow MR, Veves A, Giurini JM, et al: In-shoe foot pressure measurements in diabetic patients with at-risk feet and in healthy subjects. Diabetes Care 7(9):1002–1006, 1994.

71. Lord M, Hosein R: Pressure redistribution by molded inserts in diabetic footwear: A pilot study. J Rehabil Res Dev 31(3):214–221.

72. Mueller MJ: Therapeutic footwear helps protect the diabetic foot. J Am Podiatr Med Assoc 87(8):360–364, 1997.

73. Cavanagh PR, Owings TM: Nonsurgical strategies for healing and preventing recurrence of diabetic foot ulcers. Foot Ankle Clin North Am 11(4):735–743, 2006.

74. Mueller MJ, Lott DJ, Hastings MK, et al: Efficacy and mechanism of orthotic devices to unload metatarsal heads in people with diabetes and a history of plantar ulcers. Phys Ther 86(6):833–842, 2006.

75. Bus SA, Ulbrecht JS, Cavanagh PR: Pressure relief and load redistribution by custom-made insoles in diabetic patients with neuropathy and foot deformity. Clin Biomech 19(6):629–638, 2004.

76. Shaw JE, Boulton AJM: Pressure time integrals may be more important than peak pressures in diabetic foot ulceration [abstract A21]. Diabet Med 13(suppl 7):S22, 1996.

77. Duckworth T, Boulton AJM, Betts RP, et al: Plantar pressure measurements and the prevention of ulceration in the diabetic foot. J Bone Joint Surg Am 67-B(1):79–85, 1985.

78. Schaff PS, Cavanagh PR: Shoes for the insensitive foot: The effect of a "rocker bottom" shoe modification on plantar pressure distribution. Foot Ankle 11(3):129–140, 1990.

79. Thomas VJ, Patil KM, Radhakrishnan S: Three-dimensional stress analysis for the mechanics of plantar ulcers in diabetic neuropathy. Med Biol Eng Comput 42(2):230–235, 2004.

80. Mueller MJ, Zou D, Lott DJ: "Pressure gradient" as an indicator of plantar skin injury. Diabetes Care 28(12):2908–2912, 2005.

81. Zou D, Mueller MJ, Lott DJ: Effect of peak pressure and pressure gradient on subsurface shear stresses in the neuropathic foot. J Biomech 40(4):883–890, 2007.

82. Armstrong DG, Peters EJG, Athanasiou KA, Lavery LA: Is there a critical level of plantar foot pressure to identify patients at risk for neuropathic foot ulceration? J Foot Ankle Surg 37(4):303–307, 1998.

83. Armstrong DG, Lavery LA: Elevated peak plantar pressures in patients who have Charcot arthropathy. J Bone Joint Surg Am 80-A:365–369, 1998.

84. Wolfe L, Stess RM, Graf PM: Dynamic pressure analysis of the diabetic Charcot foot. J Am Podiatr Med Assoc 81:281–287, 1991.

85. Hsi WL, Ulbrecht JS, Perry JE, et al: Plantar pressure threshold for ulceration risk using the EMED SF platform [abstract 324]. Diabetes 42(suppl 1):103A, 1993.

86. Boulton AJM, Hardisty CA, Betts RP, et al: Dynamic foot pressure and other studies as diagnostic and management aids in diabetic neuropathy. Diabetes Care 1983;6(1):26–33, 1983.

87. Veves A, Fernando DJS, Walewski P, Boulton AJM: A study of plantar pressures in a diabetic clinic population. The Foot 2:89–92, 1991.

88. Veves A, Murray HJ, Young MJ, Boulton AJM: The risk of foot ulceration in diabetic patients with high foot pressure: A prospective study. Diabetologia 35:660–663, 1992.

89. Frykberg RG, Lavery LA, Pham H, et al: Role of neuropathy and high foot pressures in diabetic foot ulceration. Diabetes Care 1998;21:1714–1719, 1998.

90. Pham H, Lavery LA, Harvey C, et al: Risk factors of foot ulceration in a large diabetic population: two year prospective follow-up [abstract 284]. Diabetologia 41(suppl 1):A73, 1998.

91. Boulton AJM, Betts RP, Franks CI, et al: The natural history of foot pressure abnormalities in neuropathic diabetic subjects. Diabetes Res 5:73–77, 1987.

92. Ctercteko GC, Dhanendran M, Hutton WC, Le Quesne LP: Vertical forces acting on the feet of diabetic patients with neuropathic ulceration. Br J Surg 68:608–614, 1981.

93. Tooke JE, Brash PD: Microvascular aspects of diabetic foot disease [review]. Diabet Med 13(suppl 1):S26–S29, 1996.

94. Lavery LA, Armstrong DG, Wunderlich RP, et al: Predictive value of foot pressure assessment as part of a population-based diabetes disease management program. Diabetes Care 26(4):1069–1073, 2003.

95. Rozema A, Ulbrecht JS, Pammer SE, Cavanagh PR: In-shoe plantar pressures during activities of daily living: Implications for therapeutic footwear design. Foot Ankle Int 17(6):325–359, 1996.

96. Caselli A, Pham H, Giurini JM, et al: The forefoot-to-rearfoot plantar pressure ratio is increased in severe diabetic neuropathy and can predict foot ulceration. Diabetes Care 25(6):1066–1071, 2002.

97. Lavery LA, Higgins KR, Lanctot DR, et al: Home monitoring of foot skin temperatures to prevent ulceration. Diabetes Care 27(11):2642–2647, 2004.

98. Armstrong DG, Lavery LA, Wunderlich RP, Boulton AJ: 2003 William J. Stickel Silver Award: Skin temperatures as a one-time screening tool do not predict future diabetic foot complications. J Am Podiatr Med Assoc 93(6):443–447, 2003.

99. Sun PC, Jao SH, Cheng CK: Assessing foot temperature using infrared thermography. Foot Ankle Int 26(10):847–853, 2005.

100. Birke JA, Sims DS: Plantar sensory threshold in the ulcerative foot. Lepr Rev 57:261–267, 1986.

101. Calhoun JH, Cantrell J, Cobos J, et al: Treatment of diabetic foot infections: Wagner classification, therapy, and outcome. Foot Ankle 9(3):101–106, 1988.

102. Apelqvist J, Castenfors J, Larsson J, et al: Wound classification is more important than site of ulceration in the outcome of diabetic foot ulcers. Diabet Med 6:526–530, 1989.

103. Brand PW, Coleman WC: The diabetic foot. In Rifkin H, Porte D Jr (eds): Ellenberg and Rifkin's Diabetes Mellitus: Theory and Practice, 4th ed. New York, Elsevier Science, 1990, pp 792–811.

104. Delbridge L, Ctercteko G, Fowler C, et al: The aetiology of diabetic neuropathic ulceration of the foot. Br J Surg 72:1–6, 1985.

105. Pecoraro RE, Reiber GE, Burgess EM: Pathways to diabetic limb amputation: Basis for prevention. Diabetes Care 13(5):513–521, 1990.

106. Young MJ, Cavanagh PR, Thomas G, et al: The effect of callus removal on dynamic plantar foot pressures in diabetic patients. Diabet Med 9:55–57, 1992.

107. Bader DL. The recovery characteristics of soft tissues following repeated loading. J Rehabil Res Dev 27(2):141–150, 1990.

108. Newton DJ, Bennett SP, Fraser J, et al: Pilot study of the effects of local pressure on microvascular function in the diabetic foot. Diabet Med 22(11):1487–1491, 2005.

109. Davis BL: Foot ulceration: Hypotheses concerning shear and vertical forces acting on adjacent regions of skin. Med Hypotheses 40:44–47, 1993.

110. Landsman A, Sage R: High strain rate tissue deformation and its role in formation and treatment of foot ulcerations in patients with diabetes [abstract 255]. Diabetes 45(suppl 2):71A, 1996.

111. Boulton AJM, Betts RP, Franks CI, et al: Abnormalities of foot pressure in early diabetic neuropathy. Diabet Med 4:225–228, 1987.

112. Cavanagh PR, Morag E, Boulton AJM, et al: The relationship of static foot structure to dynamic foot function. J Biomech 30(3):243–250, 1997.

113. Morag E, Cavanagh PR: Structural and functional predictors of regional peak pressures under the foot during walking (ISB Keynote Paper 1997). J Biomech 32(4):359–370, 1999.

114. Ahroni JH, Boyko EJ, Forsberg RC: Clinical correlates of plantar pressure among diabetic veterans. Diabetes Care 22(6):965–792, 1999.

115. Song J, Hillstrom HJ, Secord D, Levitt J: Foot type biomechanics: Comparison of planus and rectus foot types. J Am Podiatr Med Assoc 86(1):16–23, 1996.

116. Robertson DD, Mueller MJ, Smith KE, et al: Structural changes in the forefoot of individuals with diabetes and a prior plantar ulcer. J Bone Joint Surg Am 84-A(8):1395–404, 2002.

117. Hastings MK, Commean PK, Smith KE, et al: Aligning anatomical structure from spiral X-ray computed tomography with plantar pressure data. Clin Biomech 18(9):877–82, 2003.

118. Commean PK, Mueller MJ, Smith KE, et al: Reliability and validity of combined imaging and pressures assessment methods for diabetic feet. Arch Phys Med Rehabil 83(4):497–505, 2002.

119. Smith KE, Commean PK, Robertson DD, et al: Precision and accuracy of computed tomography foot measurements. Arch Phys Med Rehabil 82(7):925–929, 2001.

120. Smith KE, Commean PK, Mueller MJ, et al: Assessment of the diabetic foot using spiral computed tomography imaging and plantar pressure measurements: A technical report. J Rehabil Res Dev 37(1):31–40, 2000.

121. Bolton NR, Smith KE, Pilgram TK, et al: Computed tomography to visualize and quantify the plantar aponeurosis and flexor hallucis longus tendon in the diabetic foot. Clin Biomech 20(5):540–6, 2005.

122. Bus SA, Maas M, Lindeboom R: Reproducibility of foot structure measurements in neuropathic diabetic patients using magnetic resonance imaging. J Magn Reson Imaging 24(1):25–32, 2006.

123. Mueller MJ, Hastings M, Commean PK, et al: Forefoot structural predictors of plantar pressures during walking in people with diabetes and peripheral neuropathy. J Biomech 36(7):1009–1017, 2003.

124. Myerson MS, Shereff MJ: The pathological anatomy of claw and hammer toes. J Bone Joint Surg Am 71-A(1):45–49, 1989.

125. Habershaw G, Donovan JC: Biomechanical considerations of the diabetic foot. In Kozak GP, Hoar CS J, Rowbotham JL, et al (eds): Management of Diabetic Foot Problems. Philadelphia, WB Saunders, 1984, pp 32–44.

126. Gooding GAW, Stess RM, Graf PM: Sonography of the sole of the foot: Evidence for loss of foot pad thickness in diabetes and its relationship to ulceration of the foot. Invest Radiol 21:45–48, 1986.

127. Gooding GAW, Stess RM, Graf PM, Grunfeld C: Heel pad thickness: Determination by high-resolution ultrasonography. J Ultrasound Med 4:173–174, 1985.

128. Young MJ, Coffey J, Taylor PM, Boulton AJM: Weight bearing ultrasound in diabetic and rheumatoid arthritis patients. The Foot 5:76–79, 1995.

129. Kawchuk GN, Elliott PD: Validation of displacement measurements obtained from ultrasonic images during indentation testing. Ultrasound Med Biol 24(1):105–111, 1998.

130. Bus SA, Maas M, Cavanagh PR, et al: Plantar fat-pad displacement in neuropathic diabetic patients with toe deformity: A magnetic resonance imaging study. Diabetes Care 27(10):2376–2381, 2004.

131. Bus SA, Maas M, de Lange A, et al: Elevated plantar pressures in neuropathic diabetic patients with claw/hammer toe deformity. J Biomech 38(9):1918–1925, 2005.

132. Masson EA, Hay EM, Stockley I, et al: Abnormal foot pressure alone may not cause foot ulceration. Diabet Med 6:426–428, 1989.

133. Taylor R, Stainsby GD, Richardson DL: Rupture of the plantar fascia in the diabetic foot leads to toe dorsiflexion deformity [abstract 1071]. Diabetologia 41(suppl 1):A277, 1998.

134. Kastenbauer T, Sokol G, Stary S, Irsigler K: Motor neuropathy does not increase plantar pressure in NIDDM patients [abstract]. Program of the 5th EMED User Meeting, 1996.

135. Hamel AJ, Sharkey NA: Proper force transmission through the toes and forefoot is dependent on the plantar fascia. Proceedings of the American Society of Biomechanics, 1999.

136. Ledoux WR, Shofer JB, Ahroni JH, et al: Biomechanical differences among pes cavus, neutrally aligned, and pes planus feet in subjects with diabetes. Foot Ankle Int 24(11):845–850, 2003.

137. Ledoux WR, Shofer JB, Smith DG, et al: Relationship between foot type, foot deformity, and ulcer occurrence in the high-risk diabetic foot. J Rehabil Res Dev 42(5):665–672, 2005.

138. Abouaesha F, van Schie CH, Armstrong DG, Boulton AJ: Plantar soft-tissue thickness predicts high peak plantar pressure in the diabetic foot. J Am Podiatr Med Assoc 94(1):39–42, 2004.

139. Brownlee M: Lilly Lecture: Glycation and diabetic complications. Diabetes Care 43(6):836–841, 1994.

140. Delbridge L, Ellis CS, Robertson K: Nonenzymatic glycosylation of keratin from the stratum corneum of the diabetic foot. Br J Dermatol 112:547–554, 1985.

141. Zilberberg J: Fluorescence and pentosidine content of diabetic foot skin. M.S. Thesis. University Park, Pennsylvania State University, 1998.

142. Hashmi F, Malone-Lee J, Hounsell E: Plantar skin in type II diabetes: An investigation of protein glycation and biomechanical properties of plantar epidermis. Eur J Dermatol 16(1):23–32, 2006.

143. Thomas VJ, Patil KM, Radhakrishnan S, et al: The role of skin hardness, thickness, and sensory loss on standing foot power in the development of plantar ulcers in patients with diabetes mellitus: A preliminary study. Int J Low Extrem Wounds 2(3):132–139, 2003.

144. Cheung YY, Doyley M, Miller TB, et al: Magnetic resonance elastography of the plantar fat pads: Preliminary study in diabetic patients and asymptomatic volunteers. J Comput Assist Tomogr 30(2):321–326, 2006.

145. D'Ambrogi E, Giacomozzi C, Macellari V, Uccioli L: Abnormal foot function in diabetic patients: The altered onset of Windlass mechanism. Diabet Med 22(12):1713–1719, 2005.

146. Giacomozzi C, D'Ambrogi E, Uccioli L, Macellari V:. Does the thickening of Achilles tendon and plantar fascia contribute to the alteration of diabetic foot loading? Clin Biomech 20(5):532–539, 2005.

147. D'Ambrogi E, Giurato L, D'Agostino MA, et al: Contribution of plantar fascia to the increased forefoot pressures in diabetic patients. Diabetes Care 26(5):1525–1529, 2003.

148. Klaesner JW, Hastings MK, Zou D, et al: Plantar tissue stiffness in patients with diabetes mellitus and peripheral neuropathy. Arch Phys Med Rehabil 83(12):1796–801, 2002.

149. Klaesner JW, Commean PK, Hastings MK, et al: Accuracy and reliability testing of a portable soft tissue indentor. IEEE Trans Neural Syst Rehabil Eng 9(2):232–40, 2001.

150. Rosenbloom AL, Silverstein JH, Lezotte DC, et al: Limited joint mobility in childhood diabetes mellitus indicates increased risk for microvascular disease. N Engl J Med 305(4):191–194, 1981.

151. Fernando DJS, Masson EA, Veves A, Boulton AJM: Relationship of limited joint mobility to abnormal foot pressures and diabetic foot ulceration. Diabetes Care 14(1):8–11, 1991.

152. Birke JA, Franks BD, Foto JG: First ray joint limitations, pressure, and ulceration of the first metatarsal head in diabetes mellitus. Foot Ankle Int 16(5):277–284, 1995.

153. Cavanagh PR, Fernando DJS, Masson EA, et al: Limited joint mobility (LJM) and loss of vibration sensation are predictors of elevated plantar pressure in diabetes [abstract 2119]. Diabetes 40(suppl 1):531A, 1991.

154. Chantelau E, Schroer O, Tanudjaja T: Between-toe pressure in patients with limited joint mobility (LJM): The effect of footwear [abstract 1003]. Diabetologia 39(suppl 1):A264, 1996.

155. Veves A, Sarnow MR, Giurini JM, et al: Differences in joint mobility and foot pressures between black and white diabetic patients. Diabet Med 12(7):585–589, 1995.

156. Sabato S, Yosipovitch Z, Simkin A, Sheskin J: Plantar trophic ulcers in patients with leprosy: A correlative study of sensation, pressure and mobility. Int Orthop 6(3):203–208, 1982.

157. Nargi SE, Colen LB, Liuzzi FJ, et al: PTB treatment restores joint mobility in a new model of diabetic cheiroarthropathy [abstract 0072]. Diabetes 48(suppl 1):A17, 1999.

158. Curran F, Nikookam K, Garrett M, et al: Physiotherapy: A novel intervention in diabetic pre-ulceration. In Proceedings of the 2nd International Symposium on the Diabetic Foot, 1995.

159. Armstrong DG, Steinberg JS, Stacpoole-Shea S, et al: The potential benefit of passive range of motion exercises to reduce peak plantar foot pressure in the diabetic foot. In Proceedings of the 3rd International Symposium on the Diabetic Foot, 1999, p 76.

160. Sage RA: Diabetic ulcers: evaluation and management. In Harkless LB, Dennis KJ (eds): Clinics in Podiatric Medicine and Surgery: The Diabetic Foot, vol 4. Philadelphia, WB Saunders, 1987, pp 383–393.

161. Murray HJ, Young MJ, Hollis S, Boulton AJM: The association between callus formation, high pressures and neuropathy in diabetic foot ulceration. Diabet Med 13(11):979–982, 1996.

162. Heath H 3rd, Melton LJ 3, Chu C-P: Diabetes mellitus and risk of skeletal fracture. N Engl J Med 303(10):567–570, 1980.

163. Geoffroy J, Hoeffel JC, Pointel JP, et al: The feet in diabetes: Roentgenologic observations in 1501 cases. Diagn Imaging 48:286–293, 1979.

164. Lithner F, Hietala S-O: Skeletal lesions of the feet in diabetics and their relationship to cutaneous erythema with or without necrosis on the feet. Acta Med Scand 200:155–161, 1976.

165. Cundy TF, Edmonds ME, Watkins PJ: Osteopenia and metatarsal fractures in diabetic neuropathy. Diabet Med 1985;2:461–464.

166. Cavanagh PR, Young MJ, Adams JE, et al: Bony abnormalities in the feet of neuropathic diabetic patients [abstract 5]. In: Bakker K, Nieuwenhuijzen Krusemann AC (eds). The Diabetic Foot. Proceedings of the 1st International Symposium on the Diabetic Foot 1991. Excerpta Medica, Amsterdam, The Netherlands, 1991.

167. Andersen H, Poulsen PL, Mogensen CE, Jakobsen J: Isokinetic muscle strength in long-term IDDM patients in relation to diabetic complications. Diabetes 45:440–445, 1996.
168. Andersen H, Gadeberg PC, Brock B, Jakobsen J: Muscular atrophy in diabetic neuropathy: A stereological magnetic resonance imaging study. Diabetologia 40:1062–109, 1997.
169. Andreassen CS, Jakobsen J, Andersen H: Muscle weakness: A progressive late complication in diabetic distal symmetric polyneuropathy. Diabetes 55(3):806–812, 2006.
170. van Schie CH, Vermigli C, Carrington AL, Boulton A: Muscle weakness and foot deformities in diabetes: Relationship to neuropathy and foot ulceration in caucasian diabetic men. Diabetes Care 27(7):1668–1673, 2004.
171. Cetinus E, Buyukbese MA, Uzel M, et al: Hand grip strength in patients with type 2 diabetes mellitus. Diabetes Res Clin Pract 70(3):278–286, 2005.
172. Bus SA, Yang QX, Wang JH, et al: Intrinsic muscle atrophy and toe deformity in the diabetic neuropathic foot: A magnetic resonance imaging study. Diabetes Care 25(8):1444–1450, 2002.
173. Brown GL, Curtsinger LJ, White M, et al: Acceleration of tensile strength of incisions treated with EGF and TGF-B. Ann Surg 208(6):788–794, 1988.
174. Holm-Pederson P, Viidik A: Tensile properties of and morphology of healing wounds in young and old rats. Scand J Plast Reconstr Surg 6:24–35, 1972.
175. Boyko EJ, Ahroni JH, Cohen V, et al: Prediction of diabetic foot ulcer occurrence using commonly available clinical information: The Seattle Diabetic Foot Study. Diabetes Care 29(6):1202–1207, 2006.
176. Laing P, Cogley D, Crerand S, Klenerman L: The Liverpool shear transducer [abstract]. In Bakker K, Nieuwenhuijken Kruseman AC (eds): The Diabetic Foot: Proceedings of the 1st International Symposium on the Diabetic Foot, May 1991, Noordwijkerhout, The Netherlands Program of the First International Symposium and Workshop, May 3–4, 1991, Noordwijkerhout, The Netherlands. Amsterdam, Excerpta Medica, 1991.
177. Jenkin WM, Palladino SJ: Environmental stress and tissue breakdown. In Frykberg RG (ed): The High Risk Foot in Diabetes Mellitus. New York, Churchill Livingstone, 1991, pp 103–123.
178. Lord M, Hosein R, Williams RB: Method for in-shoe shear stress measurement. J Biomed Eng 14(3):181–186, 1992.
179. Tappin JW, Pollard J, Beckett EA: Method of measuring "shearing" forces on the sole of the foot. Clin Phys Physiol Meas 1(1):83–85, 1980.
180. Davis BL, Perry JE: Development of a device to measure plantar pressure and shear [abstract]. In Häkkinen K, Keskinen KL, Komi PV, Mero A (eds): Book of Abstracts, 15th Congress of the ISB. Jyväskylä, Finland, 1995.
181. Perry JE, Davis BL, Hall JO: Profiles of shear loading in the diabetic foot [abstract]. In Hakkinen K, Keskinen KL, Komi PV, Mero A (eds): Book of Abstracts, 15th Congress of the ISB, Jyvaskyla, Finland.1995, pp 722–723.
182. Akhlaghi F, Pepper MG: In-shoe biaxial shear force measurement: The Kent shear system. Med Biol Eng Comput 34:315–317, 1996.
183. Christ P, Gender M, Seitz P: A 3-D pressure distribution measuring platform with 8x8 sensors for simultaneous measurement of vertical and horizontal forces. In Proceedings of the VI EMED Scientific Meeting, 1998.
184. Vela SA, Lavery LA, Armstrong DG, Anaim AA: The effect of increased weight on peak pressures: Implications for obesity and diabetic foot pathology. J Foot Ankle Surg 37(5):416–420, 1998.
185. Simoneau GG, Ulbrecht JS, Derr JA, et al: Postural instability in patients with diabetic sensory neuropathy. Diabetes Care 17(12):1411–1421, 1994.
186. Uccioli L, Giacomini P, Monticone G, et al: Body sway in diabetic neuropathy. Diabetes Care 18:339–344, 1995.
187. Courtemanche R, Teasdale N, Boucher P, et al: Gait problems in diabetic neuropathic patients. Arch Phys Med Rehabil 77:849–655, 1996.
188. Cavanagh PR, Derr JA, Ulbrecht JS, et al: Problems with gait and posture in neuropathic patients with insulin-dependent diabetes mellitus. Diabet Med 9:469–474, 1992.
189. Cavanagh PR, Young MJ, Adams JE, et al: Radiographic abnormalities in the feet of patients with diabetic neuropathy. Diabetes Care 17(3):201–209, 1994.
190. Schaff P, Wetter O, Haslbeck M: Changes in foot loading and pressure patterns during standing of patients with diabetic neuropathy. In Hotta N, Greene DA, Ward JD, et al (eds): Diabetic Neuropathy: New Concepts and Insights. Amsterdam, Elsevier Science, 1995, pp 279–284.
191. Cavanagh PR, Derr JA, Ulbrecht JS, Orchard TJ: Problems during gait and posture in patients with insulin dependent diabetes mellitus [abstract]. Paper presented at the Fall Meeting (September 6–7) of the British Diabetic Association, Newcastle Upon Tyne, UK, 1990.
192. Richardson JK, Hurvitz EA: Peripheral neuropathy: A true risk factor for falls. J Gerontol A Biol Sci Med Sci 50A(4):M211–M215, 1995.
193. Katoulis EC, Ebdon-Parry M, Lanshammar H, et al: Gait abnormalities in diabetic neuropathy. Diabetes Care 20(12):1904–1907, 1997.
194. Shaw JE, van Schie CHM, Carrington AL, et al: An analysis of dynamic forces transmitted through the foot in diabetic neuropathy. Diabetes Care 21(11):1955–1959, 1998.
195. van Schie CHM, Abbott CA, Vileikyte L, et al: Gait analysis in diabetic unilateral lower limb amputees [abstract 1886]. Diabetologia 40(suppl 1):A-480, 1997.
196. Cavanagh PR, Perry JE, Ulbrecht JS, et al: Neuropathic diabetic patients do not have reduced variability of plantar loading during gait. Gait Posture 7:191–199, 1998.
197. Dingwell JB: Variability and nonlinear dynamics of continuous locomotion: Applications to treadmill walking and diabetic peripheral neuropathy. Ph. D. Dissertation. University Park, Pennsylvania State University, 1998.
198. Rothwell JC, Traub MM, Day BL, et al: Manual motor performance in a deafferented man. Brain 105:515–542, 1982.
199. Petrofsky JS, Cuneo M, Lee S, et al: Correlation between gait and balance in people with and without type 2 diabetes in normal and subdued light. Med Sci Monit 12(7):CR273–CR281, 2006.
200. Di Fazio I, Franzoni S, Frisoni GB, et al: Predictive role of single diseases and their combination on recovery of balance and gait in disabled elderly patients. J Am Med Dir Assoc 7(4):208–211, 2006.
201. Yavuzer G, Yetkin I, Toruner FB, et al: Gait deviations of patients with diabetes mellitus: Looking beyond peripheral neuropathy. Eur Medicophys 42(2):127–133, 2006.
202. Kwon OY, Minor SD, Maluf KS, Mueller MJ: Comparison of muscle activity during walking in subjects with and without diabetic neuropathy. Gait Posture 18(1):105–113, 2003.
203. Rao S, Saltzman C, Yack HJ: Ankle ROM and stiffness measured at rest and during gait in individuals with and without diabetic sensory neuropathy. Gait Posture 24(3):295–301, 2006.
204. Thies SB, Richardson JK, Demott T, Ashton-Miller JA: Influence of an irregular surface and low light on the step variability of patients with peripheral neuropathy during level gait. Gait Posture 22(1):40–45, 2005.
205. Thies SB, Richardson JK, Ashton-Miller JA: Effects of surface irregularity and lighting on step variability during gait: A study in healthy young and older women. Gait Posture 22(1):26–31, 2005.
206. Richardson JK, Thies SB, DeMott TK, Ashton-Miller JA: A comparison of gait characteristics between older women with and without peripheral neuropathy in standard and challenging environments. J Am Geriatr Soc 52(9):1532–157, 2004.
207. Richardson JK, Thies SB, DeMott TK, Ashton-Miller JA: Interventions improve gait regularity in patients with peripheral neuropathy while walking on an irregular surface under low light. J Am Geriatr Soc 52(4):510–515, 2004.
208. Bonds DE, Larson JC, Schwartz AV, et al: Risk of fracture in women with type 2 diabetes: The Women's Health Initiative Observational Study. J Clin Endocrinol Metab 91(9):3404–3410, 2006.
209. Kanade RV, van Deursen RW, Harding K, Price P: Walking performance in people with diabetic neuropathy: Benefits and threats. Diabetologia 49(8):1747–1754, 2006.
210. Volpato S, Leveille SG, Blaum C, et al: Risk factors for falls in older disabled women with diabetes: The women's health and aging study. J Gerontol A Biol Sci Med Sci 60(12):1539–1545, 2005.
211. Quandt SA, Stafford JM, Bell RA, et al: Predictors of falls in a multiethnic population of older rural adults with diabetes. J Gerontol A Biol Sci Med Sci 61(4):394–398, 2006.
212. Uccioli L, Faglia E, Monticone G, et al: Manufactured shoes in the prevention of diabetic foot ulcers. Diabetes Care 18:1376–1377, 1995.

213. Benotmane A, Mohammedi F, Ayad F, et al: Diabetic foot lesions: Etiologic and prognostic factors. Diabetes Metab 26(2):113–117, 2000.

214. Reiber GE: Who is at risk of limb loss and what to do about it? J Rehabil Res Dev 31(4):357–362, 1994.

215. Macfarlane RM, Jeffcoate WJ: Factors contributing to the presentation of diabetic foot ulcers. Diabet Med 14(10):867–870, 1997.

216. Edmonds ME, Blundell MP, Morris ME, et al: Improved survival of the diabetic foot: The role of a specialized foot clinic. Q J Med 60(232):763–771, 1986.

217. Apelqvist J, Larsson J, Agardh CD: The influence of external precipitating factors and peripheral neuropathy on the development and outcome of diabetic foot ulcers. J Diabetes Complications 4(1):21–25, 1990.

218. McGill M, Molyneaux L, Yue DK: Which diabetic patients should receive podiatry care?: An objective analysis. Intern Med J 35(8): 451–456, 2005.

219. Lemaster JW, Reiber GE, Smith DG, et al: Daily weight-bearing activity does not increase the risk of diabetic foot ulcers. Med Sci Sports Exerc 35(7):1093–1099, 2003.

220. Reiber GE, Smith DG, Wallace C, et al: Effect of therapeutic footwear on foot reulceration in patients with diabetes: A randomized controlled trial. JAMA 287(19):2552–2558, 2002.

221. Cavanagh PR, Boulton AJ, Sheehan P, et al: Therapeutic footwear in patients with diabetes. JAMA 288(10):1231, 2002; author reply 1232–1233, 2002.

222. Armstrong DG, Lavery LA, Holtz-Neiderer K, et al: Variability in activity may precede diabetic foot ulceration. Diabetes Care 27(8):1980–1984, 2004.

223. Lott DJ, Maluf KS, Sinacore DR, Mueller MJ: Relationship between changes in activity and plantar ulcer recurrence in a patient with diabetes mellitus. Phys Ther 85(6):579–588, 2005.

224. Maluf KS, Mueller MJ: Novel Award 2002. Comparison of physical activity and cumulative plantar tissue stress among subjects with and without diabetes mellitus and a history of recurrent plantar ulcers. Clin Biomech 18(7):567–575, 2003.

225. Armstrong DG, Boulton AJ: Activity monitors: Should we begin dosing activity as we dose a drug? J Am Podiatr Med Assoc 91(3): 152–153, 2001.

226. Armstrong DG, Gildenhuys A, Holtz-Neiderer K: Computerized activity monitoring preoperatively and postoperatively. J Foot Ankle Surg 43(2):131–133, 2004.

227. Cavanagh PR, Ulbrecht JS, Caputo GM: The non-healing diabetic foot wound: Fact or fiction? Ostomy Wound Manage 1998;44(suppl 3A):S6–S13, 1998.

228. de Block C, van Acker K, de Leeuw I: Chronic diabetic foot ulcers: What is in a name? [abstract 0651]. Diabetes 47(suppl 1):A168, 1998.

229. Sinacore DR: Total contact casting for diabetic neuropathic ulcers. Phys Ther 76(3):296–301, 1996.

230. Hsi WL, Ulbrecht J, Caputo G, et al: Normal healing rates for diabetic neuropathic foot ulcers [abstract 0639]. Diabetes 47(suppl 1):A165, 1998.

231. Brem H, Sheehan P, Rosenberg HJ, et al: Evidence-based protocol for diabetic foot ulcers. Plast Reconstr Surg 117(7 suppl): 193S–209S, 2006; discussion 210S–211S, 2006.

232. Coleman WC, Brand PW, Birke JA: The total contact cast: A therapy for plantar ulceration on insensitive feet. J Am Podiatry Assoc 74:548–552, 1984.

233. Huband MS, Carr JB: A simplified method of total contact casting for diabetic foot ulcers. Contemp Orthop 26(2):143–147, 1993.

234. Caravaggi C, Faglia E, Sacchi G, et al: Effectiveness and tolerability of fiberglass total contact cast in the treatment of neuropathic foot ulcer. Diabetes 47(suppl 1):A169, 1998.

235. Borssen B, Lithner F: Plaster casts in the management of advanced ischaemic and neuropathic diabetic foot lesions. Diabet Med 6:720–723, 1989.

236. Birke JA, Novick A, Hawkins ES, Patout CJ: A review of causes of foot ulceration in patients with diabetes mellitus. J Prosthet Orthot 3:13–22, 1991.

237. Myerson M, Wilson K: Management of neuropathic ulceration with total contact cast. In Sammarco GJ (ed): The Foot in Diabetes. Philadelphia, Lea & Febiger, 1991, pp 145–152.

238. Armstrong DG, Stacpoole-Shea S: Total contact casts and removable cast walkers: Mitigation of plantar heel pressure. J Am Podiatr Med Assoc 89(1):50–53, 1999.

239. Cogley D, Laing P, Crerand S, Klenerman L: Foot-cast interface vertical force measurements in casts used for healing neuropathic ulcers [abstract 58]. In: Bakker K, Nieuwenhuijzen Krusemann AC (eds). The Diabetic Foot. Proceedings of the 1st International Symposium on the Diabetic Foot 1991. Excerpta Medica, Amsterdam, The Netherlands, 1991.

240. Burnett O: Total contact cast. In Harkless LB, Dennis KJ (eds): Clinics in Podiatric Medicine and Surgery: The Diabetic Foot, vol 4. Philadelphia, WB Saunders, 1987, pp 471–479.

241. Martin RL, Conti SF: Plantar pressure analysis of diabetic rocker-bottom deformity total contact casts. Foot Ankle Int 17(8): 470–472, 1996.

242. Conti SF, Martin RL, Chaytor ER, et al: Plantar pressure measurements during ambulation in weightbearing conventional short leg casts and total contact casts. Foot Ankle Int 17(8):464–469, 1996.

243. Birke JA, Sims DS J, Buford WL: Walking casts: Effect on plantar foot pressures. J Rehabil Res Dev 22:18–22, 1985.

244. Mueller MJ, Diamond JE, Sinacore DR, et al: Total contact casting in treatment of diabetic plantar ulcers: Controlled clinical trial. Diabetes Care 12(6):384–388, 1989.

245. Lavery LA, Armstrong DG, Walker SC: Healing rates of diabetic foot ulcers associated with midfoot fracture due to Charcot's arthropathy. Diabet Med 14:46–49, 1997.

246. Armstrong DG, Lavery LA, Bushman TR: Peak foot pressures influence the healing time of diabetic foot ulcers treated with total contact casts. J Rehabil Res Dev 35(1):1–5, 1998.

247. Sinacore DR: Healing times of diabetic ulcers in the presence of fixed deformities of the foot using total contact casting. Foot Ankle Int 19:613–618, 1998.

248. Lin SS, Lee TH, Wapner KL: Plantar forefoot ulceration with equinus deformity of the ankle in diabetic patients: The effect of tendo-Achilles lengthening and total contact casting. Orthopedics 1996;19:465–475, 1996.

249. Sinacore DR, Mueller MJ: Total-contact casting in the treatment of neuropathic ulcers. In Levin ME, O'Neal LW, Bowker JH (eds): The Diabetic Foot, 5th ed. St. Louis, Mosby Year Book, 1993, pp 283–304.

250. Birke JA, Novick A, Graham SL, et al: Methods of treating plantar ulcers. Phys Ther 71:116–122, 1991.

251. Foster A, Eaton C, Gibby D, Edmonds ME: The posterior splinted cast: A new treatment for long-standing neuropathic ulcers [abstract]. Diabet Med 7(suppl 1):35A, 1990.

252. Burden AC, Jones GR, Jones R, Blandford RL: Use of the "Scotchcast boot" in treating diabetic foot ulcers. Br Med J 286: 1555–1557, 1983.

253. Jones GR: Walking casts: Effective treatment for foot ulcers? Practical Diabetes 8:131–132, 1991.

254. Jones R, Beshyah SA, Curryer GJ, Burden AC: Modification of the "Leicester (Scotch Cast) boot." Practical Diabetes 16:118–119, 1989.

255. McGill M, Collins P, Bolton T, Yue DK: Management of neuropathic ulceration. J Wound Care 5:252–254, 1996.

256. Hissink RJ, Manning HA, van Baal JG: The MABAL shoe, an alternative method in contact casting for the treatment of neuropathic diabetic foot ulcers. Foot Ankle Int 21(4):320–323, 2000.

257. Armstrong DG, Nguyen HC, Lavery LA, et al: Off-loading the diabetic foot wound: A randomized clinical trial. Diabetes Care 24(6):1019–1022, 2001.

258. Guyton GP: An analysis of iatrogenic complications from the total contact cast. Foot Ankle Int 26(11):903–907, 2005.

259. Petre M, Tokar P, Kostar D, Cavanagh PR: Revisiting the total contact cast: Maximizing off-loading by wound isolation. Diabetes Care 28(4):929–9230, 2005.

260. Watkinson M: Total contact casts were better than removable cast walkers or half shoes for healing diabetic neuropathic foot ulcers [commentary]. Evid Based Nurs 5(1):15, 2002.

261. Knowles EA, Armstrong DG, Hayat SA, et al: Offloading diabetic foot wounds using the scotchcast boot: A retrospective study. Ostomy Wound Manage 48(9):50–53, 2002.

262. Knowles A: The role of pressure relief in diabetic foot problems. Diabetic Foot 1(2):55–56, 58–60, 62–63, 1998.

263. Armstrong DG, Lavery LA, Harkless LB: Healing the diabetic wound with pressure off-loading. Biomechanics 4:67–74, 1997.

264. Armstrong DG, Lavery LA: Evidence-based options for off-loading diabetic wounds. Clin Podiatr Med Surg 15(1):95–104, 1998.

265. Roberts P, Carnes S: The orthopaedic scooter: An energy-saving aid for assisted ambulation. J Bone Joint Surg Am 72-B(4): 620–621, 1990.

266. Fisher A: Neuropathic plantar ulcers: Relief of weight bearing using an orthopaedic knee scooter [abstract 59]. In: Bakker K, Nieuwenhuijzen Krusemann AC (eds). The Diabetic Foot. Proceedings of the 1st International Symposium on the Diabetic Foot 1991. Excerpta Medica, Amsterdam, The Netherlands, 1991.

267. Chantelau E, Breuer U, Leisch AC, et al: Outpatient treatment of unilateral diabetic foot ulcers with "half shoes." Diabet Med 10:267–270, 1993.

268. Needleman RL: Successes and pitfalls in the healing of neuropathic forefoot ulcerations with the IPOS postoperative shoe. Foot Ankle Int 18(7):412–417, 1997.

269. Fleischli JG, Lavery LA, Vela SA: Biomechanical comparison of treatment strategies to reduce pressures at the site of neuropathic ulcers [abstract 1896]. Diabetologia 40(suppl 1):A-482, 1997.

270. Lavery LA, Vela SA, Lavery DC, Quebedeaux TL: Reducing dynamic foot pressures in high-risk diabetic subjects with foot ulcerations. Diabetes Care 19(8):818–821, 1996.

271. Armstrong DG, Lavery LA: Shoes and the diabetic foot. Practical Diabetol 17(1):23–26, 1998.

272. Saltzman CL, Johnson KA, Goldstein RH, Donnelly RE: The patellar tendon-bearing brace as treatment for neurotrophic arthropathy: A dynamic force monitoring study. Foot Ankle 1992; 13(1):14–21, 1992.

273. Guse ST, Alvine FG: Treatment of diabetic foot ulcers and Charcot neuroarthropathy using the patellar tendon-bearing brace. Foot Ankle Int 18(10):675–677, 1997.

274. Landsman A, Sage R: Off-loading neuropathic wounds associated with diabetes using an ankle-foot orthosis. J Am Podiatr Med Assoc 87(8):349–57, 1997.

275. Morgan JM, Biehl WC 3, Wagner FW Jr: Management of neuropathic arthropathy with the Charcot restraint orthotic walker. Clin Orthop 296:58–63, 1993.

276. Mehta JA, Brown C, Sargeant N: Charcot restraint orthotic walker. Foot Ankle Int 19(9):619–623, 1998.

277. Boninger ML, Leonard JA Jr: Use of bivalved ankle-foot orthosis in neuropathic foot and ankle lesions. J Rehabil Res Dev 33(1):16–22, 1996.

278. Myerly SM, Stavosky JW: An alternative method for reducing plantar pressures in neuropathic ulcers. Adv Wound Care 10(1):26–9, 1997.

279. Guzman B, Fisher G, Palladino SJ, Stavosky JW: Pressure-removing strategies in neuropathic ulcer therapy: An alternative to total contact casting. Clin Podiatr Med Surg 11:339–253, 1994.

280. Ritz G, Kushner D, Friedman S: A successful technique for the treatment of diabetic neurotrophic ulcers. J Am Podiatr Med Assoc 82:479–81, 1992.

281. Kiewied J: Felt therapy for leprosy patients with an ulcer in a pressure area [letter]. Lepr Rev 68:378–381, 1997.

282. Armstrong DG, Athanasiou KA: The edge effect: How and why wounds grow in size and depth. Clin Podiatr Med Surg 15(1):105–108, 1998.

283. Armstrong DG, Liswood PJ, Todd WF: Potential risks of accommodative padding in the treatment of neuropathic ulcerations. Ostomy Wound Manage 41:44–48, 1995.

284. Armstrong DG, Lavery LA, Kimbriel HR, et al: Activity patterns of patients with diabetic foot ulceration: Patients with active ulceration may not adhere to a standard pressure off-loading regimen. Diabetes Care 26(9):2595–2597, 2003.

285. Armstrong DA, Wu SC, Crews RC: New casting techniques: Introduction to the "instant total contact cast." In Boulton AJM, Cavanagh PR, Rayman G (eds): The Foot in Diabetes, 4th ed. Chichester, UK: John Wiley and Sons, 2006, pp 350–354.

286. Katz IA, Harlan A, Miranda-Palma B, et al: A randomized trial of two irremovable off-loading devices in the management of plantar neuropathic diabetic foot ulcers. Diabetes Care 28(3):555–559, 2005.

287. Armstrong DG, Lavery LA, Wu S, Boulton AJ: Evaluation of removable and irremovable cast walkers in the healing of diabetic foot wounds: A randomized controlled trial. Diabetes Care 28(3):551–554, 2005.

288. Caputo GM, Ulbrecht JS, Cavanagh PR: The total contact cast: A method for treating neuropathic diabetic ulcers. Am Fam Physician 55(2):605–611, 1997.

289. Lavery LA, Fleishli JG, Laughlin TJ, et al: Is postural instability exacerbated by off-loading devices in high risk diabetics with foot ulcers? Ostomy Wound Manage 44(1):26–34, 1998.

290. Webster's Collegiate Dictionary, 9th ed. Springfield, MA, Merriam-Webster, 1986.

291. Radin EL, Yang KH, Riegger C, et al: Relationship between lower limb dynamics and knee joint pain. J Orthop Res 9(3):398–405, 1991.

292. Sanders JE, Greve JM, Mitchell SB, Zachariah SG: Material properties of commonly-used interface materials and their static coefficients of friction with skin and socks. J Rehabil Res Dev 35(2):161–76, 1998.

293. Veves A, Masson EA, Fernando DJS, Boulton AJM: Sustained pressure relief under the diabetic foot with experimental hosiery, and comparison of different padding densities [abstract]. Diabet Med 6(suppl 2):3A, 1989.

294. Veves A, Masson EA, Fernando DJS, Boulton AJM: Use of experimental padded hosiery to reduce abnormal foot pressures in diabetic neuropathy. Diabetes Care 12(9):653–655, 1989.

295. Bader DL: Effects of compressive loading regimens on tissue viability. In Bader DL (ed): Pressure Sores: Clinical Practice and Scientific Approach. New York, MacMillan, 1990.

296. Simon SR, Berme N, Sawyer F: Measurement of plantar foot soft tissue properties of patients with diabetic neuropathy for prediction of plantar foot pressures and assessment of plantar ulceration risk. Rehabil Res Dev Prog Rep 34:318–319, 1996.

297. Campbell GJ, McLure M, Newell EN: Compressive behavior after simulated service conditions of some foamed materials intended as orthotic shoe insoles. J Rehabil Res Dev 21(2):57–65, 1984.

298. Foto JG, Birke JA: Evaluation of multidensity orthotic materials used in footwear for patients with diabetes. Foot Ankle Int 19(12):836–841, 1998.

299. Thompson DE: The effects of mechanical stress on soft tissue. In Levin ME, O'Neal LW (eds): The Diabetic Foot, 4th ed. St. Louis, Mosby-Year Book, 1988, pp 91–103.

300. Sharkey NA: Skeletal Tissue Mechanics. New York, Springer-Verlag, 1998.

301. Brodsky JW, Kourosh S, Stills M, Mooney V: Objective evaluation of insert material for diabetic and athletic footwear. Foot Ankle 9(3):111–116, 1988.

302. Gefen A, Megido-Ravid M, Azariah M, et al: Integration of plantar soft tissue stiffness measurements in routine MRI of the diabetic foot. Clin Biomech 16(10):921–925, 2001.

303. Gefen A: The in vivo elastic properties of the plantar fascia during the contact phase of walking. Foot Ankle Int 24(3):238–244, 2003.

304. Gefen A, Megido-Ravid M, Itzchak Y: In vivo biomechanical behavior of the human heel pad during the stance phase of gait. J Biomech 34(12):1661–1665, 2001.

305. Erdemir A, Hamel AJ, Fauth AR, et al: Dynamic loading of the plantar aponeurosis in walking. J Bone Joint Surg Am 86-A(3):546–552, 2004.

306. Ledoux WR, Meaney DF, Hillstrom HJ: A quasi-linear, viscoelastic, structural model of the plantar soft tissue with frequency-sensitive damping properties. J Biomech Eng 126(6):831–783, 2004.

307. Erdemir A, Viveiros ML, Ulbrecht JS, Cavanagh PR: An inverse finite-element model of heel-pad indentation. J Biomech 39(7):1279–1286, 2006.

308. Lemmon D, Shiang TY, Hashmi A, et al: The effect of insoles in therapeutic footwear: A finite element approach. J Biomech 30:615–620, 1997.

309. Thompson DL, Cao D, Davis BL: Effects of diabetic-induced soft tissue changes on stress distribution in the calcaneal soft tissue. In Proceedings of XVII International Society of Biomechanics Congress, 1999, p 12.

310. Patil KM, Braak LH, Huson A: Analysis of stresses in two-dimensional models of normal and neuropathic feet. Med Biol Eng Comput 34:280–284, 1996.

311. Actis RL, Ventura LB, Smith KE, et al: Numerical simulation of the plantar pressure distribution in the diabetic foot during the push-off stance. Med Biol Eng Comput 44(8):653–663, 2006.

312. Yarnitzky G, Yizhar Z, Gefen A: Real-time subject-specific monitoring of internal deformations and stresses in the soft tissues of the foot: A new approach in gait analysis. J Biomech 39(14):2673–2689, 2006.

313. Gefen A: Plantar soft tissue loading under the medial metatarsals in the standing diabetic foot. Med Eng Phys 25(6):491–499, 2003.

314. Cheung JT, Zhang M: A 3-dimensional finite element model of the human foot and ankle for insole design. Arch Phys Med Rehabil 86(2):353–358, 2005.

315. Cheung JT, Zhang M, Leung AK, Fan YB: Three-dimensional finite element analysis of the foot during standing: A material sensitivity study. J Biomech 38(5):1045–1054, 2005.

316. Cheung JT, Zhang M, An KN: Effects of plantar fascia stiffness on the biomechanical responses of the ankle-foot complex. Clin Biomech 19(8):839–846, 2004.

317. Erdemir A, Saucerman JJ, Lemmon D, et al: Local plantar pressure relief in therapeutic footwear: Design guidelines from finite element models. J Biomech 38(9):1798–1806, 2005.

318. Goske S, Erdemir A, Petre M, et al: Reduction of plantar heel pressures: Insole design using finite element analysis. J Biomech 39(13):2363–2370, 2006.

319. Standard Methods of Test for Compression Set of Vulcanized Rubber. ASTM Designation: D-395-68. Washington, DC, American National Standards Compliance, 1971, pp 195–201.

320. Leber C, Evanski PM: A comparison of shoe insole materials in plantar pressure relief. Prosthet Orthot Int 10:135–138, 1986.

321. Foto JG, Birke JA: Who's using what?: An orthotic materials survey. BioMechanics 3:63–68, 1996.

322. Hewitt FG Jr: The effect of molded insoles on in-shoe plantar pressures in rockered footwear. M.S. Thesis. University Park, Pennsylvania State University, 1993.

323. Edington CJ: The effect of metatarsal pads on the plantar pressure distribution of the foot. M.S. Thesis. University Park, Pennsylvania State University, 1990.

324. Holmes GB, Timmerman L: A quantitative assessment of the effect of metatarsal pads on plantar pressures. Foot Ankle 11(3): 141–145, 1990.

325. Chang AH, Abu-Faraj ZU, Harris GF, et al: Multistep measurement of plantar pressure alterations using metatarsal pads. Foot Ankle Int 15:654–660, 1994.

326. Hsi WL, Kang JH, Lee XX: Optimum position of metatarsal pad in metatarsalgia for pressure relief. Am J Phys Med Rehabil 84(7):514–520, 2005.

327. Jackson L, Binning J, Potter J: Plantar pressures in rheumatoid arthritis using prefabricated metatarsal padding. J Am Podiatr Med Assoc 94(3):239–245, 2004.

328. Frykberg RG: Offloading properties of a new rocker insole [abstract 0650]. Diabetes 47(suppl 1):A168, 1998.

329. Loppnow BW: The effect of plugs on reducing pressure under the second metatarsal head. M.S. Thesis. University Park, Pennsylvania State University, 1998.

330. Perry JE, Cavanagh PR, Ulbrecht JS: The use of conventional footwear to relieve plantar pressures in the diabetic foot [abstract]. In Proceedings of the 8th Annual East Coast Clinical Gait Laboratories Conference, Rochester, MN, 1993, pp 121–122.

331. Conti SF: In-shoe plantar pressure measurement and diabetic inlays: A series of questions and a few answers. Biomechanics 3(7):47–48, 74–75, 1996.

332. Janisse DJ: Prescription insoles and footwear. Clin Podiatr Med Surg 12:41–61, 1995.

333. Ashry HR, Lavery LA, Murdoch DP, et al: Effectiveness of diabetic insoles to reduce foot pressures. J Foot Ankle Surg 36(4):268–271, 1997.

334. Xia B, Garbalosa JC, Cavanagh PR: Error analysis of two systems to measure in-shoe pressures [abstract]. In Proceedings of the American Society of Biomechanics,1994, pp 219–220.

335. Soulier SM: The use of running shoes in the prevention of plantar diabetic ulcers. J Am Podiatr Med Assoc 76:395–400, 1986.

336. Lavery LA, Lanctot DR, Constantinides G, et al: Wear and biomechanical characteristics of a novel shear-reducing insole with implications for high-risk persons with diabetes. Diabetes Technol Ther 7(4):638–646, 2005.

337. Veves A, Masson EA, Fernando DJ, Boulton AJM: Studies of experimental hosiery in diabetic neuropathic patients with high foot pressures. Diabet Med 7:324–326, 1990.

338. Veves A, Hay EM, Boulton AJM: The use of specially padded hosiery in the painful rheumatoid foot. The Foot 1:1–3, 1991.

339. Garrow AP, van Schie CH, Boulton AJ: Efficacy of multilayered hosiery in reducing in-shoe plantar foot pressure in high-risk patients with diabetes. Diabetes Care 28(8):2001–2006, 2005.

340. Stacpoole-Shea SJ, Walden JG, Gitter A, et al: Could seamed socks impart unduly high pressure to the diabetic foot? [abstract 0776]. Diabetes 48(suppl 1):A179, 1999.

341. Chantelau E, Kushner T, Spraul M: How effective is cushioned therapeutic footwear in protecting diabetic feet?: A clinical study. Diabet Med 7:355–359, 1990.

342. Sims DS, Birke JA: Effect of rocker sole placement on plantar pressures [abstract]. In Proceedings of the 20th Annual Meeting of the USPHS Professional Association. Atlanta, GA, 1985, p 53.

343. van Schie CHM, Becker MB, Ulbrecht JS, et al: Optimal axis location in rocker bottom shoes [abstract]. Presented to The Diabetic Foot: Second International Symposium, May 1995, Amsterdam 1995.

344. Cavanagh PR, Ulbrecht JS, Zanine W, et al: A method for the investigation of the effects of outsole modifications in therapeutic footwear. Foot Ankle Int 17(11):706–708, 1996.

345. Van Bogart JJ, Long JT, Klein JP, et al: Effects of the toe-only rocker on gait kinematics and kinetics in able-bodied persons. IEEE Trans Neural Syst Rehabil Eng 13(4):542–550, 2005.

346. Jordan C, Bartlett R: The relationship between plantar and dorsal pressure distribution and perception of comfort in casual footwear. Gait Posture 2(4):251, 1994.

346a. Botek G, Owings T, Woerner J, et al. Diabetes 2007, in press.

347. Chantelau E, Haage P: An audit of cushioned diabetic footwear: Relation to patient compliance. Diabet Med 11:114–116, 1994.

348. Williams AE, Nester CJ: Patient perceptions of stock footwear design features. Prosthet Orthot Int 30(1):61–71, 2006.

349. McLoughlin C, Southern S, Lomax G, Jones GR: These shoes are made for walking [abstract 10]. In 6th Malvern Diabetic Foot Conference, 1996.

350. Johnson M, Newton P, Goyder E: Patient and professional perspectives on prescribed therapeutic footwear for people with diabetes: A vignette study. Patient Educ Couns 64(1–3):167–172, 2006.

351. Warren G, Nade S: The Care of Neuropathic Limbs. Pearl River, NY, Parthenon, 1999.

352. American Diabetes Association, American Academy of Neurology: Consensus Statement. Report and recommendations of the 1988 San Antonio Conference on Diabetic Neuropathy (AK Asbury and D Porte, Jr, Co-chairmen). Diabetes Care 11(7):592–597, 1998.

353. Sosenko JM, Kato M, Soto R, Bild DE: Comparison of quantitative sensory-threshold measures for their association with foot ulceration in diabetic patients. Diabetes Care 13(10):1057–1061, 1990.

354. Smieja M, Hunt DL, Edelman D, et al: Clinical examination for the detection of protective sensation in the feet of diabetic patients. J Gen Intern Med 14:418–424, 1999.

355. Bloom S, Till S, Sonksen P, Smith S: Use of a biothesiometer to measure individual vibration perception thresholds and their variation in 519 non-diabetic subjects. Br Med J 288:1793–1795, 1984.

356. American Diabetes Association: Standards of Medical Care in Diabetes: 2006. Diabetes Care 29:S4–S42, 2006.

357. Mayfield JA, Reiber GE, Sanders LJ, et al: Preventive foot care in people with diabetes [technical review]. Diabetes Care 21(12):2161–2177, 1998.

358. American Diabetes Association: Consensus development conference on diabetic foot wound care. Diabetes Care 22(8): 1354–1360, 1999.

359. Cavanagh PR, Ulbrecht JS: What the practising clinican should know about biomechanics. In Boulton AJM, Cavanagh PR, Rayman G (eds): The Foot in Diabetes, 4th ed. Chichester, UK, John Wiley and Sons, 2006, pp 68–91.

360. Lavery LA, Murdoch DP: Conventional offloading and activity monitoring. In Boulton AJM, Cavanagh PR, Rayman G (eds): The Foot in Diabetes, 4th ed. Chichester, UK, John Wiley and Sons, 2006, pp 293–307.

361. van Schie CH: A review of the biomechanics of the diabetic foot. Int J Low Extrem Wounds 4(3):160–170, 2005.

362. van Deursen R: Mechanical loading and off-loading of the plantar surface of the diabetic foot. Clin Infect Dis 39(suppl 2):S87–S91, 2004.

363. Cavanagh P.R., Ulbrecht J.S. Footwear for people with diabetes. In Boulton AJM, Cavanagh PR, Rayman G (eds): The Foot in Diabetes, 4th ed. Chichester, UK, John Wiley and Sons, 2006, pp 336–349.

364. Elftman NW: Orthotic management of the neuropathic limb. Phys Med Rehabil Clin N Am 17(1):115–157, 2006.

365. McGuire JB: Pressure redistribution strategies for the diabetic or at-risk foot: II. Adv Skin Wound Care 19(5):270–277; quiz 277–279, 2006.

366. McGuire JB: Pressure redistribution strategies for the diabetic or at-risk foot: I. Adv Skin Wound Care 19(4):213–221; quiz 222–223, 2006.

367. Spencer S: Pressure relieving interventions for preventing and treating diabetic foot ulcers. Cochrane Database Syst Rev 2000(3):CD002302, 2000.

368. Beuker BJ, van Deursen RW, Price P, et al: Plantar pressure in off-loading devices used in diabetic ulcer treatment. Wound Repair Regen 13(6):537–542, 2005.

369. Kanade RV, van Deursen RW, Price P, Harding K: Risk of plantar ulceration in diabetic patients with single-leg amputation. Clin Biomech 21(3):306–313, 2006.

370. Armstrong DG, Kunze K, Martin BR, et al: Plantar pressure changes using a novel negative pressure wound therapy technique. J Am Podiatr Med Assoc 94(5):456–60, 2004.

371. Armstrong DG, Lavery LA: Decreasing foot pressures while implementing topical negative pressure (vacuum-assisted closure) therapy. Int J Low Extrem Wounds 3(1):12–5, 2004.

372. Van Schie C, Ulbrecht JS: New technologies in wound healing: Pressure relieving dressings. In Boulton AJM, Cavanagh PR, Rayman G (eds): The Foot in Diabetes, 4th ed. Chichester, UK, John Wiley and Sons, 2006, pp 355–359.

373. van Schie CH, Rawat F, Boulton AJ: Reduction of plantar pressure using a prototype pressure-relieving dressing. Diabetes Care 28(9):2236–2237, 2005.

373a. Brill LR, Cavanagh PR, Doucette MM, Ulbrecht JS. Treatment of Chronic Wounds. No. 5 in a series of monographs. Prevention, Protection and Recurrence Reduction of Diabetic Neuropathic Foot Ulcers. East Setauket, NY: Curative Technologies, Inc., 1994.

374. Rose GK: Pes planus. In Jahss MH (ed): Disorders of the Foot & Ankle, Medical and Surgical Management, 2nd ed. Vol. 1. Philadelphia, WB Saunders, 1991, pp 892–890.

375. Balkin SW: Plantar keratoses: Treatment by injectable liquid silicone: Report of an 8-year experience. Clin Orthop 87:235–247, 1972.

376. Balkin SW: Injectable silicone and the foot: A 41-year clinical and histologic history. Dermatol Surg 31(11 Part 2):1555–1560, 2005.

377. Balkin SW, Kaplan L: Injectable silicone and the diabetic foot: A 25-year report. The Foot 1:83–88, 1991.

378. van Schie CHM, Whalley A, Vileikyte L, et al: The efficacy of injected liquid silicone in the reduction of foot pressures and callus formation in the diabetic foot [abstract 1074]. Diabetologia 41(suppl 1):A278, 1998.

379. van Schie CH, Whalley A, Armstrong DG, et al: The effect of silicone injections in the diabetic foot on peak plantar pressure and plantar tissue thickness: A 2-year follow-up. Arch Phys Med Rehabil 83(7):919–923, 2002.

380. Fromherz WA: Examination: Physical therapy of the foot and ankle. In Hunt GC (ed): Clinics in Physical Therapy series, vol. 15. New York, Churchill Livingstone, 1988, pp 75–79.

381. Rothstein JM, Miller PJ, Roettger RF: Goniometric reliability in a clinical setting: Elbow and knee measurements. Phys Ther 63:1611, 1983.

382. Mueller MJ, Strube MJ, Allen BT: Therapeutic footwear can reduce plantar pressures in patients with diabetes and transmetatarsal amputation. Diabetes Care 20(4):637–641, 1997.

383. Mazzeo RS, Cavanagh PR, Evans WJ, et al: Exercise and physical activity for older adults [position stand]. Med Sci Sports Exerc 30(6):992–1008, 1998.

384. Liu W, Lipsitz LA, Montero-Odasso M, et al: Noise-enhanced vibrotactile sensitivity in older adults, patients with stroke, and patients with diabetic neuropathy. Arch Phys Med Rehabil 83(2):171–176, 2002.

385. Collins JJ, Priplata AA, Gravelle DC, et al: Noise-enhanced human sensorimotor function. IEEE Eng Med Biol Mag 22(2):76–83, 2003.

386. Priplata AA, Patritti BL, Niemi JB, et al: Noise-enhanced balance control in patients with diabetes and patients with stroke. Ann Neurol 59(1):4–12, 2006.

387. Balducci S, Iacobellis G, Parisi L, et al: Exercise training can modify the natural history of diabetic peripheral neuropathy. J Diabetes Complications 20(4):216–223, 2006.

388. Boulton AJ, Jude EB: Therapeutic footwear in diabetes: The good, the bad, and the ugly? Diabetes Care 27(7):1832–1833, 2004.

389. Cavanagh PR: Therapeutic footwear for people with diabetes. Diabetes Metab Res Rev 20(suppl 1):S51–S55, 2004.

390. Ulbrecht JS, Cavanagh PR: Shoes and insoles for at-risk people with diabetes. In Armstrong DG, Lavery LA (eds): Clinical Care of the Diabetic Foot. Alexandria, VA, American Diabetes Association, 2005, pp 36–44.

391. Sugarman JR, Reiber GE, Baumgardner G, et al: Use of the therapeutic footwear benefit among diabetic medicare beneficiaries in three states, 1995. Diabetes Care 21(5):777–781, 1998.

392. LeMaster JW, Sugarman JR, Baumgardner G, Reiber GE: Motivational brochures increase the number of Medicare-eligible persons with diabetes making therapeutic footwear claims. Diabetes Care 26(6):1679–1684, 2003.

393. Chantelau E: Therapeutic footwear in patients with diabetes. JAMA 288(10):1231–1232; author reply 1323, 2002.

394. Maciejewski ML, Reiber GE, Smith DG, et al: Effectiveness of diabetic therapeutic footwear in preventing reulceration. Diabetes Care 27(7):1774–1782, 2004.

395. Nixon BP, Armstrong DG, Wendell C, et al: Do US veterans wear appropriately sized shoes?: The Veterans Affairs shoe size selection study. J Am Podiatr Med Assoc 96(4):290–292, 2006.

396. Tsung BY, Zhang M, Mak AF, Wong MW: Effectiveness of insoles on plantar pressure redistribution. J Rehabil Res Dev 41(6):767–774, 2004.

397. Tsung BY, Zhang M, Fan YB, Boone DA: Quantitative comparison of plantar foot shapes under different weight-bearing conditions. J Rehabil Res Dev 40(6):517–526, 2003.

398. Mueller MJ, Allen BT, Sinacore DR: Incidence of skin breakdown and higher amputation after transmetatarsal amputation: Implications for rehabilitation. Arch Phys Med Rehabil 76:50–54, 1995.

399. Wu SC, Armstrong DG: The role of activity, adherence, and off-loading on the healing of diabetic foot wounds. Plast Reconstr Surg 117(7 suppl):248S–53S, 2006.

400. Knowles EA, Boulton AJM: Do people with diabetes wear their prescribed footwear? Diabet Med 13(12):1064–1068, 1996.

401. Wrobel JS, Robbins JM, Charns MP, et al: Diabetes-related foot care at 10 Veterans Affairs medical centers: Must do's associated with successful microsystems. Jt Comm J Qual Patient Saf 32(4):206–213, 2006.

402. Singh N, Armstrong DG, Lipsky BA: Preventing foot ulcers in patients with diabetes. JAMA 293(2):217–228, 2005.

403. Vileikyte L, Leventhal H, Gonzalez JS, et al: Diabetic peripheral neuropathy and depressive symptoms: The association revisited. Diabetes Care 28(10):2378–2383, 2005.

404. Vileikyte L: Psychological and behavioral issues in diabetic foot ulceration. In Boulton AJM, Cavanagh PR, Rayman G (eds): The Foot in Diabetes, 4th ed. Chichester, UK, John Wiley and Sons, 2006, pp 132–142.

405. Vileikyte L, Rubin RR, Leventhal H: Psychological aspects of diabetic neuropathic foot complications: An overview. Diabetes Metab Res Rev 20(suppl 1):S13–S18, 2004.

406. Salamon ML, Salzman CL: The operative treatment of Charcot neuroarthropathy. In Boulton AJM, Cavanagh PR, Rayman G (eds): The Foot in Diabetes, 4th ed. Chichester, UK, John Wiley and Sons, 2006, pp 274–284.

407. Brodsky JW: Surgery for ulceration and infection in the diabetic foot. In Boulton AJM, Cavanagh PR , Rayman G (eds): The Foot in Diabetes, 4th ed. Chichester, UK, John Wiley and Sons, 2006, pp 285–292.

408. Fleischli JE, Anderson RB, Davis WH: Dorsiflexion metatarsal osteotomy for treatment of recalcitrant diabetic neuropathic ulcers. Foot Ankle Int 20(2):80–85, 1999.

409. Patel VG, Weiman TJ: Effect of metatarsal head resection for diabetic foot ulcers on the dynamic plantar pressure distribution. Am J Surg 167:297–301, 1994.

410. Giurini JM, Basile P, Chrzan JS, et al: Panmetatarsal head resection: A viable alternative to the transmetatarsal amputation. J Am Podiatr Med Assoc 83(2):101–107, 1993.

411. Cavanagh PR, Ulbrecht JS, Caputo GM: Elevated plantar pressure and ulceration in diabetic patients after pan-metatarsal head resection: Two case reports. Foot Ankle Int 20(8):521–526, 1999.

412. Marks RM, Parks BG, Schon LC: Midfoot fusion technique for neuroarthropathic feet: Biomechanical analysis and rationale. Foot Ankle Int 19(8):507–510, 1998.

413. Myerson MS, Henderson MR, Saxby T, Short KW: Management of midfoot diabetic neuroarthropathy. Foot Ankle Int 15:233–241, 1994.

414. Sammarco GJ, Conti SF: Surgical treatment of neuroarthropathic foot deformity. Foot Ankle Int 19:102–109, 1998.

415. Early KJS, Hansen ST: Surgical reconstruction of the diabetic foot: A salvage approach for midfoot collapse. Foot Ankle Int 17(6):325–330, 1996.

416. Aronow MS, Diaz-Doran V, Sullivan RJ, Adams DJ: The effect of triceps surae contracture force on plantar foot pressure distribution. Foot Ankle Int 27(1):43–52, 2006.

417. Armstrong DG, Stacpoole-Shea S, Nguyen H, Harkless LB: Lengthening of the Achilles tendon in diabetic patients who are at high risk for ulceration of the foot. J Bone Joint Surg 81-A(4):535–538, 1999.

418. Sobel E, Glockenberg A: Calcaneal gait: Etiology and clinical presentation. J Am Podiatr Med Assoc 89(1):39–49, 1999.

419. Mueller MJ, Sinacore DR, Hastings MK, et al: Effect of Achilles tendon lengthening on neuropathic plantar ulcers: A randomized clinical trial. J Bone Joint Surg Am 85-A(8):1436–1445, 2003.

420. Maluf KS, Mueller MJ, Strube MJ, et al: Tendon Achilles lengthening for the treatment of neuropathic ulcers causes a temporary reduction in forefoot pressure associated with changes in plantar flexor power rather than ankle motion during gait. J Biomech 37(6):897–906, 2004.

421. Salsich GB, Mueller MJ, Hastings MK, et al: Effect of Achilles tendon lengthening on ankle muscle performance in people with diabetes mellitus and a neuropathic plantar ulcer. Phys Ther 85(1):34–43, 2005.

422. Holstein P, Lohmann M, Bitsch M, Jorgensen B: Achilles tendon lengthening, the panacea for plantar forefoot ulceration? Diabetes Metab Res Rev 20(suppl 1):S37–S40, 2004.

423. Orendurff MS, Rohr ES, Sangeorzan BJ, et al: An equinus deformity of the ankle accounts for only a small amount of the increased forefoot plantar pressure in patients with diabetes. J Bone Joint Surg Br 88(1):65–68, 2006.

424. Lavery LA, Armstrong DG, Boulton AJ: Ankle equinus deformity and its relationship to high plantar pressure in a large population with diabetes mellitus. J Am Podiatr Med Assoc 92(9):479–482, 2002.

425. Grant WP, Sullivan R, Sonenshine DE, et al: Treatment of Charcot neuroarthropathy with Achilles tendon lengthening [abstract 1772]. Diabetes 48(suppl 1):A401, 1999.

426. Quebedeaux TL, Lavery LA, Lavery DC: The development of foot deformities and ulcers after great toe amputation in diabetes. Diabetes Care 19(2):165–167, 1996.

427. Lavery LA, Lavery DC, Quebedeax-Farnham TL: Increased foot pressures after great toe amputation in diabetes. Diabetes Care 18:1460–1462, 1995.

428. Armstrong DG, Lavery LA: Plantar pressures are higher in diabetic patients following partial foot amputation. Ostomy Wound Manage 44:30–39, 1998.

429. Garbalosa JC, Cavanagh PR, Wu G, et al: Foot function in diabetic patients after partial amputation. Foot Ankle Int 17:43–48, 1996.

430. Mueller MJ, Salsich GB, Bastian AJ: Differences in the gait characteristics of people with diabetes and transmetatarsal amputation compared with age-matched controls. Gait Posture 7(3):200–206, 1998.

431. Mueller MJ, Sinacore DR: Rehabilitation factors following transmetatarsal amputation. Phys Ther 74(11):1027–1033, 1994.

432. Kelly VE, Mueller MJ, Sinacore DR: Timing of peak plantar pressure during the stance phase of walking: A study of patients with diabetes mellitus and transmetatarsal amputation. J Am Podiatr Med Assoc 90(1):18–23, 2000.

433. Pollard J, Hamilton GA, Rush SM, Ford LA: Mortality and morbidity after transmetatarsal amputation: Retrospective review of 101 cases. J Foot Ankle Surg 45(2):91–97, 2006.

434. Armstrong DG, Lavery LA, Vazquez JR, et al: Clinical efficacy of the first metatarsophalangeal joint arthroplasty as a curative procedure for hallux interphalangeal joint wounds in patients with diabetes. Diabetes Care 26(12):3284–3287, 2003.

435. Armstrong DG, Sangalang MB, Jolley D, et al: Cooling the foot to prevent diabetic foot wounds: A proof-of-concept trial. J Am Podiatr Med Assoc 95(2):103–107, 2005.

436. Budhabhatti S, Erdemir A, Cavanagh PR: Computational prediction of in-shoe pressures with and without a metatarsal pad. [Abstract]. Meeting of the International Society of Biomechanics, Taipei, Taiwan, July 1–5, 2007.

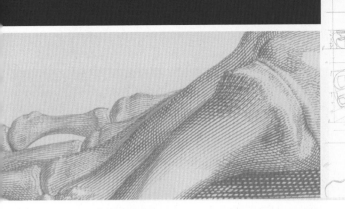

CUTANEOUS MANIFESTATIONS OF DIABETES MELLITUS

MICHELLE DRAZNIN, ROBERT EISON, EMANUAL MAVERAKIS, ∎

AND ARTHUR HUNTLEY

The pathogenesis of diabetic complications remains incompletely understood, with multiple metabolic impairments playing complementary roles. Nonenzymatic glycosylation of various proteins, particularly collagen and elastin, impairs their structure and function in skin, vessels, and nerves. As glucose utilization along insulin-sensitive oxidative and nonoxidative pathways declines (a sine qua non of diabetes), more glucose molecules contribute to the nonenzymatic glycosylation process of numerous proteins. In fact, levels of advanced glycosylation end products in skin and serum have consistently correlated with the severity of microvascular disease in people with type 1 and type 2 diabetes, the strongest association for the risk of progression of diabetic complications being determined by glycated lysine and carboxymethyl-lysine in skin collagen.[1,2] Disruption of the cross-linking of advanced glycosylation end-products is currently under investigation as a means for delaying the cardiovascular and dermatologic complications associated with diabetes.[3]

Conversion of poorly utilized glucose into fructose and subsequently into sorbitol contributes to the osmotic impairment of the intracellular milieu and thus to the pathogenesis of diabetic complications. Inhibition of aldose reductase, an enzyme that is responsible for the conversion of fructose into the sugar-alcohol sorbitol, has long been an approach in preventing diabetic complications. Because excess glucose can also be converted into diacylglycerol, which in turn activates protein kinase C

(with subsequent deleterious serine phosphorylation steps), inhibition of protein kinase C offers another potential therapeutic target in order to prevent and treat diabetic complications. Hyperglycemia also generates significant oxidative stress, impairing endothelial and smooth muscle cell function, compromising the immune system, and enhancing lipid oxidation. This combined influence of oxidative stress, protein kinase C, the sorbitol pathway, and formation of advanced glycosylation end-products leads to the development of diabetic complications.

Finally, functional impairments in microcirculation (diabetic microvascular disease), nerve function (diabetic polyneuropathy), and immune system (reduced host defense) further compromise the structure and function of skin and its elements, leading to many cutaneous manifestations of diabetes.

Cutaneous Infections in Diabetes Mellitus

Before the advent of insulin, the incidence of common pyodermas such as furunculosis, carbunculosis, and erysipelas was much higher for diabetic people than for their nondiabetic counterparts.[4] Today, there is debate as to whether or not diabetic people have an increased rate of cutaneous infections. It is more difficult to eradicate infections in diabetic hosts, however, so their resultant prevalence of infection seems to be higher.

There are several infections that characteristically occur in people with diabetes mellitus, and some threaten life and limb.

Mucocutaneous *Candida* Infections

Yeast infections are common in male and female diabetic patients, often with involvement of the glans penis (balanitis) and the vulva. Vaginal candidiasis is almost universal among women with long-term diabetes, and yeast infections may even be the presenting manifestation of diabetes.[5]

Vulvovaginal *Candida* infection is an especially common problem for the diabetic woman.[6] It is a common cause of pruritus vulvae and almost invariably occurs during glycosuria. Presenting signs include vulvar erythema, which may be accompanied by fissuring with or without satellite pustules. Vaginitis is usually accompanied by a white discharge. Traditional treatment involves normalizing blood sugar as well as treating both the vagina and vulva with topical medication. Since these patients often have a reservoir of *Candida* in the colon, oral nystatin may also be administered. Another option for vaginal candidiasis is oral administration of one dose of 150 mg of fluconazole.

Angular stomatitis due to *Candida* is a classic complication in diabetic children and an occasional complication in diabetic adults. Increased concentrations of salivary glucose reportedly account for its occurrence[7] but not for the predilection for younger patients. Clinically, it is appreciated as white, curd-like material that adheres to erythematous, fissured areas at the angle of the mouth or as white patches on the buccal mucosa and palate. Diagnosis is readily confirmed by examination of a potassium hydroxide preparation. Success in treatment may depend on normalization of blood sugar and the supplemental use of anticandidal lozenges.

The prevalence of *Candida* infection of the hands and feet does not appear to be significantly different for the diabetic population as compared to controls.[8] When it does occur, it usually has one of three presentations. *Candida* paronychia usually involves the hands, but it may occur on the feet. It often begins at the lateral nailfolds as erythema, swelling, and separation of the fold from the lateral margin of the nail. Further infection may result in involvement of the proximal nailfold and separation of the cuticle from the nail. Moisture trapped in the resultant space favors further growth of the yeast and repeated episodes of inflammation. At times, there may be a purulent discharge from the involved nailfold, a clinical finding that suggests bacterial paronychia. The diagnosis of yeast infection can usually be established by performing a KOH preparation on extruded serous material from this space.

Candida infection of the web spaces usually involves the web spaces between the third and fourth digits of the

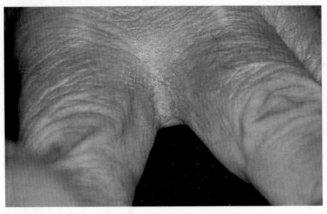

Figure 7–1   *Candida*. This patient has *Candida* infection of the web spaces, involving the web spaces between the third and fourth digits of the hands. This area has a tendency to retain moisture, owing to occlusion from apposing surfaces of skin.

hands or the feet (Fig. 7-1). These areas have a tendency to retain moisture due to occlusion from apposing surfaces of skin. Presumably, the increased glucose content of the skin encourages the establishment of this infection. The clinical appearance is a white patch of skin, often with central peeling. Toe web space involvement is often mistaken for a dermatophyte infection, but the diagnosis can be confirmed on potassium hydroxide preparation.

The third presentation of *Candida* infection of the limbs is involvement in the toenail plates. Although dystrophic toenails are often assumed to be the result of dermatophyte infection, nail plate cultures demonstrate the pathogen to be *Candida* species about 5% of the time. One needs to be careful about making the diagnosis of primary *Candida* infection, however, because cultures might only reflect contaminants or secondary involvement. Clinically, nail plate infections with either dermatophyte or *Candida* species present with distal yellowing or whitening along with thickening of the toenail. Living tissue does not appear to be involved.

Dermatophytosis

Although dermatophyte infections are probably not more common in the diabetic population,[9] they are of special concern. Toe web space infections can lead to inflammation and fissuring that can serve as a portal of entry for bacterial infection in a compromised diabetic foot. The oxygen demand of the subsequent inflammation might exceed the ability of the diabetic microcirculation, leading to gangrene. It is for this reason that tinea pedis should be aggressively managed in patients with neurovascular compromise. This infection should be treated with topical antifungal agents such as terbinafine or imidazoles.

Involvement of the toenails by dermatophytes (onychomycosis) is common among elderly people with diabetes just as it is in the population at large. The infection itself is of little consequence, but the nail dystrophy that results can make proper nail care more difficult for the patient. Currently, the most promising treatment is terbinafine at 250 mg/day for 3 months with monthly liver function test evaluation. Itraconazole at 400 mg/day for 1 week a month for 4 to 6 months can also be used.

Phycomycetes Infections

Hyperglycemia can allow usually nonpathogenic organisms to establish an infection in traumatized skin, occasionally eventuating in gangrene and loss of limb. Diabetic patients with leg ulcers, or nonhealing surgical wounds, especially those of the lower limbs, may have a complicating Phycomycetes infection. Such an infection should be suspected when lower-limb ulcers or posttraumatic lesions are not responding to therapy. Diagnosis can be confirmed by culture and by histologic demonstration of fungal elements invading vascular channels.

Patients with uncontrolled diabetes with ketosis may be predisposed to deep mycotic infections that are opportunistic. Of these, mucormycosis is most often described in association with diabetes. The characteristic presentation is black crusting or pus on the turbinates, septum, or palate. Without treatment, the infection may invade vascular lumens and extend to the maxillary and ethmoid sinuses, the palate, and the orbit. Cerebral involvement occurs in about two thirds of these patients.[10] Treatment consists of correction of acid-base imbalance, aggressive debridement of necrotic tissue, and intravenous amphotericin.

Pseudomonas Infections

Malignant external otitis, an uncommon but serious infection of the external ear canal by *Pseudomonas*, characteristically presents as severe external ear canal pain and purulent discharge in an elderly diabetic patient.[11,12] The infection is thought to begin as a cellulitis of the ear canal, but natural cleavage planes allow progression through the osseous cartilaginous junction. With further extension, the cranial nerves may be involved, especially the facial nerve. About half the affected individuals die of this infection. The treatment of choice consists of surgical debridement and administration of antipseudomonas antibiotics.

Much more common than malignant external otitis, however, is *Pseudomonas* infection of the toe web spaces or colonization under the toenails. Often, people who have onychomycosis develop a lifting of the nail plate from the bed (onycholysis). The resulting space between plate and bed may become colonized with *Pseudomonas*, resulting in a green discoloration of this area. Wood's lamp examination often yields a green fluorescence.

Soaks with dilute vinegar may eradicate superficial infection. In the event of a more advanced cellulitis, oral ciprofloxacin appears to be the treatment of choice.

Corynebacterium Infections

Corynebacterium minutissimum is the etiologic agent of erythrasma, a superficial and often chronic infection. The most common sites are intertriginous areas such as the groin, axillae, and intergluteal and inframammary folds. Diabetes predisposes to this infection, and obese people with diabetes are exceptionally susceptible. Clinically, erythrasma appears as finely scaled, well-defined, erythematous patches. These lesions demonstrate coral red fluorescence on Wood's lamp evaluation. Treatment includes topical clindamycin or erythromycin. Prevention of recurrence is benefited by weight loss and glycemic control.

Dermal and Epidermal Manifestations of Diabetes Mellitus

Pruritus

Generalized pruritus may be the presenting symptom in diabetes mellitus, but it is not considered significantly more common in people with diabetes than in those who do not have the disease.[13] More commonly, diabetes is associated with localized pruritus, such as vulvar pruritus as described above. At times, diabetic neuropathy may be associated with the sensation of pruritus.

Diabetic Thick Skin

People with diabetes tend to have thicker skin than do their nondiabetic counterparts. This observation has three aspects. First, diabetic patients in general have a clinically inapparent but measurable increase in skin thickness. This is not associated with symptoms and goes unnoticed by patients and physicians. Second, a clinically apparent thickening of skin involving the fingers and hands may range from pebbled skin to scleroderma-like skin changes. Third, diabetic scleredema may occur. In this condition, the patient develops a markedly thickened dermis on the upper back region.

The presence of diabetes mellitus is generally associated with measurably thickened skin. By using pulsed ultrasound, it can be demonstrated that diabetic patients have thicker forearm skin than do their age- and sex-matched nondiabetic counterparts.[14] Contrary to the pattern in people who do not have diabetes, skin thickness in diabetes may increase with age (apparently associated with increased duration of diabetes). Of note, most studies have used the upper-limb skin in evaluating skin thickness, and it might not be a valid conclusion that diabetic skin is thickened at other sites.

Hand Skin Thickening

Thickening of skin of the hand is a common occurrence, with a range of manifestations from simple pebbling of the knuckles to the diabetic hand syndrome. The diabetic hand syndrome consists of thickened skin over the dorsum of the digits and limited joint mobility, especially of the interphalangeal joints.[15,16] The earliest description of this phenomenon was apparently the observation that insulin-dependent diabetes was occasionally complicated by painful, stiff hands.[17] Subsequently, Rosenbloom and Frais described three adolescent patients with the syndrome of long-standing diabetes mellitus; restricted joint mobility; thick, tight, waxy skin; growth impairment; and maturational delay.[18] Rosenbloom and colleagues later reported, in a study of 309 people with diabetes (predominantly those with juvenile type 1 diabetes), that 3% had joint limitations and one third of these had thick, tight, waxy skin that the examiner could not tent, mostly involving the dorsum of the hands.[19] This work has been confirmed by other authors, and these observations have been extended to patients with type 2 diabetes mellitus.[20]

Most common is simple thickening of the skin on the dorsum of the hands. At least 30% of diabetic patients have hand skin thickening, and some have demonstrable involvement of the dorsum of the feet. Clinical clues that suggest such a thickening include difficulty in tenting the skin, pebbled or rough skin on the knuckles (Fig. 7-2) or periungual region,[21] and decreased skin wrinkling following immersion in water.[22]

There is significance to the observation of thick skin on the hands and feet in diabetes mellitus. The literature suggests that digital sclerosis (very thick skin) is a marker for retinal microvascular disease. There is, however, a spectrum of thickening of the skin, ranging from that which is only detectable by ultrasound to the more obvious. For less than digital sclerosis, the significance of thick skin in diabetes is uncertain at this time.

Scleredema of Diabetes

Scleredema diabeticorum is a syndrome characterized by a marked increase in dermal thickness on the posterior back and upper neck in middle-aged, overweight, poorly controlled type 2 diabetic subjects (Fig. 7-3). It is not recognized as being related to digital sclerosis, and we found no correlation by ultrasound measurements between back skin and hand skin thickness. Scleredema diabeticorum has a reported prevalence of 2.5% in patients with type 2 diabetes.[23] Histologically, one finds a thickened dermis with large collagen bundles that are separated by wide, clear spaces. There may be increased numbers of mast cells.[24] There are reports of increased, normal, and decreased glycosaminoglycans in affected dermis.[25] It is thought that collagen is irreversibly glycosylated and rendered resistant to degradation by collagenase, leading to excess accumulation.[26]

Lieberman and colleagues suggest that tight glycemic control might decrease skin thickness. They reported that four diabetic patients with thick skin had a decrease

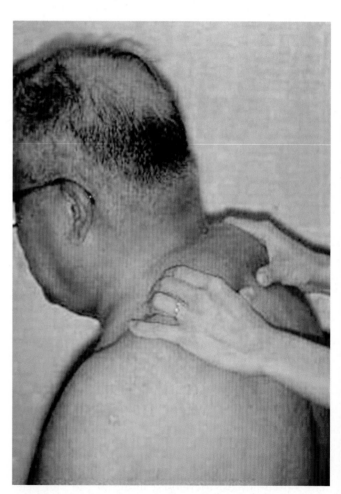

Figure 7–3 Scleredema of diabetes. This patient with type 2 diabetes gave an incidental complaint of limitation of motion of his upper limbs. On examination, this appeared to be due to the shield-like involvement of the upper back, neck, and shoulders with marked dermal thickening. The examiner is demonstrating the inability to tent the skin on the dorsum of the neck.

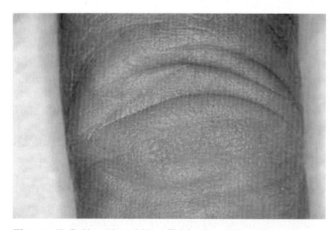

Figure 7–2 Knuckle pebbles. Thickening of the skin on the dorsum of the hand due to many causes, diabetes among them, is often manifested by a pebbling of the skin on the knuckle area. This patient with insulin-dependent diabetes mellitus also has palpably thick skin when tenting is attempted.

of skin thickness following pump administration of insulin with achievement of tighter control.[27] There is no other known treatment for diabetic scleredema. There is no evidence for spontaneous remission.

Yellow Skin

Diabetic skin often has a yellow hue. This is thought to be due to impaired hepatic metabolism of carotene due to elevated blood glucose levels. A diet that is low in carotene should ameliorate this condition. An alternative possible cause of yellow skin might be glycosylation end-products. It is known that proteins that have a long turnover time, such as dermal collagen, undergo glycosylation and become yellow.

Yellow skin is a common finding among patients with diabetes, probably best appreciated on the palms and soles because of sparse competition with melanocytic pigment in these areas. Currently, no significance is associated with this finding other than that of a time proven observation.

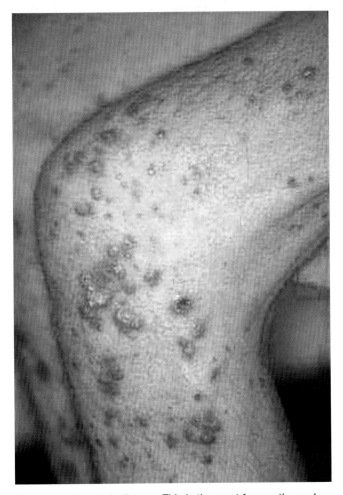

Figure 7–4 Kyrle's disease. This is the most frequently used eponym for perforating dermatitis associated with diabetes. Clinically, this appears as erythematous papules, most frequently located on the lower limbs.

Acanthosis Nigricans

Acanthosis nigricans can be associated with malignancy, but it is more frequently associated with diabetes. The areas that are most often affected are the neck, axillae, intertriginous areas, and extensor surfaces, but the lower lip and chin may also be involved. Clinically, it appears as velvety hyperpigmentation with epidermal thickening.

Acquired Perforating Dermatosis

Acquired perforating dermatosis encompasses all perforating diseases in adults. It is quite frequently associated with diabetes mellitus. This condition is most often encountered in diabetic patients with renal failure. Clinically, this appears as erythematous papules, most frequently located on the lower limbs. Histologically, these papules represent the transepidermal elimination of collagen fibers. Kyrle's disease is the eponym that is frequently used (Fig. 7-4).

Vascular Manifestations of Diabetes Mellitus

People with diabetes have a higher incidence and prevalence of large vessel disease[28] and develop myocardial infarctions and strokes at a much younger age than do their nondiabetic counterparts. Large vessel disease (atherosclerosis) may also be present in the lower limbs, resulting in skin atrophy, hair loss, coldness of the toes, nail dystrophy, pallor on elevation, and mottling on dependence.[29]

Microangiopathy

Microangiopathy is one of the major complications of diabetes mellitus. The small blood vessel changes affecting the retinal and renal vasculature are responsible for blindness and kidney failure. Microvascular pathology has also been assumed to play a role in diabetic neuropathy and in the so-called diabetic foot. Microangiopathy is clinically detected by an eye ground examination that demonstrates the presence of microaneurysms. More severe involvement may demonstrate hemorrhages, exudates, and even some devascularized areas.

The histology of affected diabetic tissue reveals a PAS-positive, thickened capillary basement membrane. Electron microscopy of skeletal muscle capillaries reveals reduplication of the basal lamina. The skin has not been thought to be a good sample source in evaluation of microangiopathy because small blood vessels of the dermis develop less basal lamina thickening than is found in skeletal muscle (which is also easily accessed by using a needle biopsy).

The structural changes that occur in the microcirculation do not seem to account for the full extent of the disease, leading to the concept of functional microangiopathy. Some patients with severe microcirculatory problems such as gangrene of the foot have normal capillaries on skin or skeletal muscle biopsy. Sluggish microcirculation resulting in microvenular dilatation is considered "functional" in that it may be reversed with improved control of diabetes. The clinical manifestations associated with this include retinal venous dilatation, red face, and periungual telangiectasia, all of which may be very early manifestations of the disease and may improve with control of diabetes.

Functional microangiopathy may result from nonenzymatic glycosylation, which affects many blood components, including hemoglobin, red blood cell membrane, fibronectin, fibrinogen, and platelets. Glycosylation of the red blood cell has been shown to inhibit the cell pliability and to decrease the ability of this cell to pass through pores smaller than 7 microns. The lumens of some capillaries may be as narrow as 3 microns, and ordinarily, red blood cells will elongate into a more sausage-like configuration to traverse this loop. Stiffened cell membranes will certainly inhibit or limit this passage.

In addition to stiffened red blood cells, diabetic patients also have increased plasma concentration of fibrinogen as well as capillary leakage, which leads to loss of albumin and water. There is an increased tendency for diabetic platelets to aggregate. The end result is increased whole blood or plasma viscosity and sluggish microcirculation.

In summary, it appears that microangiopathy can be attributed to both structural and functional abnormalities in these vessels. The following discussion will review some of the cutaneous manifestations that may be linked to this microangiopathy.

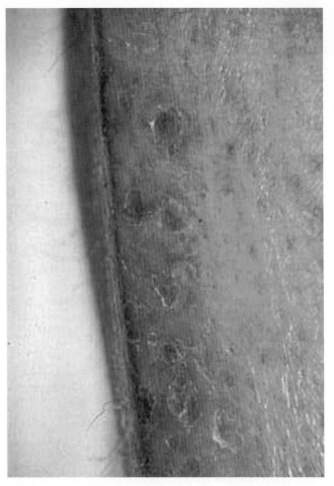

Figure 7-5 Diabetic dermopathy. The presence of many hyperpigmented atrophic macules on the shins is said to be a relatively common finding in patients with diabetes. Antecedent trauma might or might not be recalled by the patient.

Diabetic Dermopathy

Atrophic hyperpigmented macules on the shins, so-called diabetic dermopathy, has been termed the most common cutaneous finding in diabetes.[30] It is usually noted as irregularly round or oval, circumscribed, shallow lesions varying in number from few to many, which are usually bilateral but not symmetrically distributed (Fig. 7-5). They are asymptomatic and often overlooked.

The genesis of these lesions is unclear. Some authors describe a preceding, distinct, red papular eruption that is independent of trauma to the skin.[31] However, Lithner has been able to duplicate these lesions by local thermal trauma.[32] We observe that many patients who develop these depressed hyperpigmented lesions relate antecedent trauma or mild pyoderma such as folliculitis. "Diabetic dermopathy" probably represents posttraumatic atrophy and postinflammatory hyperpigmentation in poorly vascularized skin.

Histologic characteristics of acute lesions include edema of the epidermis and papillary dermis, extravasated erythrocytes, and a mild lymphohistiocytic infiltrate.[33] Older lesions have thick-walled capillaries in the upper dermis, occasional extravasated erythrocytes, and a positive Perl stain for iron.

The significance and prevalence of diabetic dermopathy depend on the operational definition of this entity. Defined as one or more spots, the original description reported their presence in 55% of 293 diabetic patients (65% of males and 29% of females).[34] On the basis of this definition, it has also been shown to occur in 20% of control patients with normal glucose tolerance tests.[35] Thus, defining diabetic dermopathy as one or more spots results in high sensitivity but low specificity for diabetes. In a study that defined dermopathy as the presence of four or more lesions, they were absent in people who did not have diabetes and present in about 14% of those with diabetes (24% of men and 3% of women).[36] The multilesional definition also found a high correlation with retinovascular disease.

Pigmented Purpura

Pigmented purpuric dermatosis is a condition involving the skin on the lower limbs resulting from red blood cell red coloration in one's "complexion" is a function of the degree of engorgement of the superficial venous plexus. Hyperglycemia predisposes to sluggish microcirculation, and affected individuals develop a functional microangiopathy that is clinically evident by venous dilatation.[38] This venous dilatation can be demonstrated in the eye grounds and skin. It may be evident in newly diagnosed diabetic patients, and more important, the vascular engorgement may return to normal when the blood sugar is controlled. In a prospective study of 150 medical hospital admissions, comparing facial redness (none, slightly red, or markedly red) with diabetic parameters (persistent fasting hyperglycemia or a diabetic glucose tolerance curve), of 61 patients with diabetes, 36 (59%) had markedly red faces.[39] Because of normal variation in complexion, this sign is difficult to use as a marker of functional microangiopathy.

Periungual Telangiectasia

One may directly examine the skin to survey the superficial microcirculation. Any area of skin may be examined, but because nailfold capillary loops are in a horizontal axis relative to the skin surface, this area offers an excellent view of the entire microvascular loop (Fig. 7-7). To see past the stratum corneum, it is helpful to first apply mineral oil to the skin surface and wait a few minutes until this layer becomes translucent. One may use a low-power microscope or simply an ophthalmoscope (+40 lens for 10× magnification). In general, the microcirculation of less pigmented individuals is easier to visualize.

One study found venous capillary dilatation in the nailfolds of 49% of 75 diabetic patients compared to 10% of 65 controls.[40] It is important to note that connective tissue diseases may also result in periungual vessel changes but that these changes are morphologically different. In diabetes, one sees isolated homogeneous

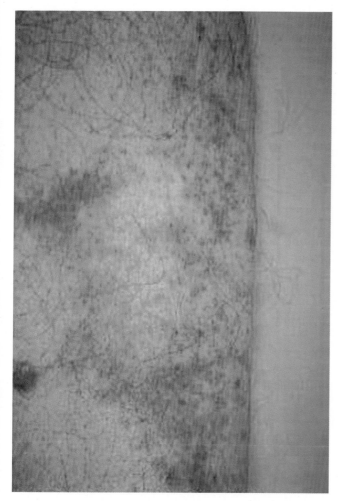

Figure 7–6 Pigmented purpura. Salt and pepper type of yellow-tan hyperpigmentation of the shins in the absence of atrophy is characteristic for pigmented purpura, a common finding, especially in elderly people with diabetes. Patients need not be diabetic to demonstrate this finding. This finding is often seen in conjunction with diabetic dermopathy, so there are some areas of focal atrophy and wide areas of nonatrophic pigmentation.

extravasation from the superficial vascular plexus. It is characterized by multiple tan to reddish small macules (so-called cayenne pepper spots) that coalesce into tan to orange patches. It often extends down to involve the ankles and the dorsum of the feet (Fig. 7-6). It was described as a manifestation in older diabetic patients, about half of whom had diabetic dermopathy.[37] In most of these patients, cardiac decompensation with edema of the legs was determined to be a precipitating factor for the purpura. Except for the frequent association with diabetic dermopathy, this condition appears clinically consistent with Schamberg's disease. This condition also appears to be a marker of structural microangiopathy.

Red Skin and Rubeosis Facei

The prototype functional microangiopathy is facial involvement, the so-called rubeosis facei. The intensity of

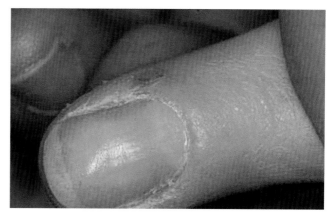

Figure 7–7 Periungual telangiectasia. The nailfold is an excellent site for viewing functional and structural changes in the microvasculature of the skin. This patient illustrates microvascular engorgement and tortuosity involving the proximal nailfold.

engorgement of the venular limbs. In connective tissue diseases, the patterns that are seen are megacapillaries or irregularly enlarged loops.[41]

Venous dilatation of the periungual microcirculation appears to be an excellent indicator of functional microangiopathy. The structural changes of this area are probably represented by venous tortuosity. Thus, a newly diagnosed patient is likely to have simple capillary loops with a dilated venous portion. A long-term diabetic patient who had poor control for a number of years but who now has excellent control may exhibit venous tortuosity without dilatation. More extensive microangiopathy can be heralded by small hemorrhages and by dropout of areas of the microcirculation.

Erysipelas-like Erythema

Another reported phenomenon of microcirculatory compromise in diabetic patients is the development of well-demarcated erythema on the lower leg or dorsum of the foot that correlates with radiologic evidence of underlying bone destruction and incipient gangrene.[42,43] The condition was at first mistaken for erysipelas (hence the name erysipelas-like erythema), but there was no associated pyrexia, elevated erythrocyte sedimentation rate, or leukocytosis. This erythema would seem to be functional microangiopathy localized to an area of macrocirculation compromise.

Other Skin Markers of Diabetes Mellitus

Yellow Nails

As Lithner pointed out, people with diabetes tend to have yellow nails.[43] He noted this phenomenon in half of 36 diabetic patients and in none of 9 controls. Our patients have a similar prevalence of yellow nails, except that we also see it occasionally in elderly controls and in some patients with onychomycosis. Although this phenomenon may occur on all the nails, it is most often evident on the distal aspect of the nail of the hallux (Fig. 7-8).

Clinically, this yellow color is not usually the result of underlying dermatophytosis. Similar to the yellow color observed in diabetic skin, yellowing of the nails probably represents glycosylation end-products. Whereas keratin of the epidermis is present for only 1 month before being shed, that of the nail plate may be present for more than a year. The protein-glucose reaction presumably continues to evolve in the aging nail, resulting in the most yellow pigment at the distal aspect of the slowest-growing nail. The presence of the yellow glycosylation end-products in the nail plate has not been confirmed to date, but one study of fingernails has demonstrated that people with diabetes have high levels of fructose-lysine, another marker of nonenzymatic glycosylation.[44]

Clinically, one appreciates yellow nails of diabetes best on examination of the toenails. Most diabetic patients have some aspect of this yellowing. Minimal involvement consists of distal yellow or yellow-brown discoloration of the hallux nail plate. Marked involvement consists of canary yellow discoloration of all toenails and fingernails. It is not a specific finding in diabetes mellitus, since it can occasionally be observed with normal aging. Like the yellow hue that is appreciated generally in the skin of people with diabetes, the significance of this observation is undetermined.

Diabetic Bullae

Another curious phenomenon in diabetes mellitus is the spontaneous appearance of blisters on the limbs (usually confined to hands or feet). These lesions are not the result of trauma or infection. They tend to heal without treatment (Fig. 7-9).

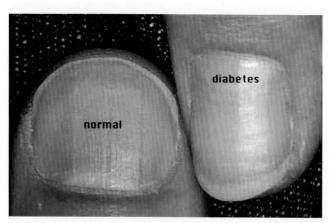

Figure 7-8 Yellow nails of diabetes. For comparison, the examiner's thumbnail is photographed alongside the yellow nail of a person with diabetes.

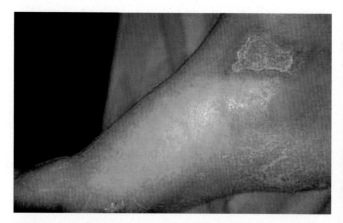

Figure 7-9 Diabetic bullae. This adult-onset diabetic patient had spontaneous onset of multiple bullae on his lower limbs, one of which is illustrated here. These lesions were not secondary to trauma or infection, and they healed without special intervention.

On the basis of epidermal and dermal cleavage levels, there appear to be three types of these blisters. The most common type is spontaneous and nonscarring. They present as clear, sterile blisters on the tips of the toes or fingers and, less frequently, on the dorsal and lateral surfaces of the feet, legs, hands, and forearms. Spontaneous healing occurs within 2 to 5 weeks.[45] These patients were reported to have good circulation to the affected limb and tended to have diabetic peripheral neuropathy. In those patients in whom histopathology has been performed, there is an intraepidermal cleavage without acantholysis.[46,47] The second type of diabetic bullae involves lesions that may be hemorrhagic and heal with scarring and atrophy.[48,49] The reported cleavage plane is below the dermoepidermal junction. A third type described in a case report consists of multiple tender nonscarring blisters on sun-exposed and deeply tanned skin on the feet, legs, and arms. Immunofluorescence and porphyrin studies were negative. Electron microscopy placed the cleavage plane at the lamina lucida.[50]

Necrobiosis Lipoidica

Necrobiosis lipoidica diabeticorum (NLD) is an uncommon manifestation of diabetes mellitus, occurring in about 0.3% of these patients.[51] This skin manifestation is not pathognomonic for diabetes mellitus, since fewer than two thirds of patients with necrobiosis lipoidica are diabetic. Necrobiosis lipoidica has been documented to occur prior to the onset of diabetes mellitus.[52] Certainly, any patient who presents with necrobiosis lipoidica should be evaluated for diabetes.

The initial lesions of NLD begin as well-circumscribed erythematous papules. Evolving radially, the sharply defined lesions have depressed, waxy, yellow-brown, atrophic telangiectatic centers through which the underlying dermal vessels can be visualized. The periphery is slightly raised and erythematous. There may be partial or complete anesthesia of the lesion as well as hypohidrosis and alopecia.[53] Ulceration is reported in about one third of leg lesions, mostly in large lesions following minor trauma. Lesions of NLD sometimes spontaneously resolve, but more often, they do not. They seem to occur and persist independent of degree of glycemic control (Fig. 7-10).

Whereas most lesions of NLD occur on the legs, about 15% of lesions are found elsewhere, including on the hands, forearms, abdomen, face, or scalp. When necrobiosis lipoidica occurs in areas other than the lower limbs, the patient is less likely to have diabetes mellitus.[54]

The histopathology of NLD reveals neutrophilic necrotizing vasculitis in early lesions.[55] With progression, there is collagen degeneration and destruction of adnexal structures. Lesions evolve through granulomatous and sclerotic stages, most of the sclerosis occurring in the lower reticular dermis. The upper dermis contains fatty deposits that give the lesions their yellow color.

Electron microscopy of necrobiosis lipoidica reveals striking changes involving dermal blood vessels consisting of focal degeneration of the endothelial cells lining the microvasculature.[56] These cells have electron lucency and loss of intracellular organelles.

Treatment is used to arrest the progression of the disease. This is most commonly achieved by application of high-potency topical steroids or intralesional injection of steroids into the active margin. Other agents reported include pentoxifylline, high-dose oral nicotinamide,[57] aspirin, and dipyridamole.[58-60] Currently, the most impressive therapeutic option might be oral corticosteroids. Five weeks of oral corticosteroid treatment was described as resulting in complete disease cessation for all of six patients treated.[61] Since the pathophysiology of necrobiosis is not understood, it is difficult to design rational therapy.

Lipodystrophy

Both generalized and partial lipodystrophy, or loss of subcutaneous fat, are associated with diabetes. This is often associated with acanthosis nigricans, hypertrichosis, and hyperhidrosis. Localized lipoatrophy appears as depressed plaques in the skin that may be the result of insulin injections (Fig. 7-11).

Eruptive Xanthomas

Eruptive xanthomas are small yellow papules arising over the extensor surfaces of arms, legs, and buttocks. They occur in the setting of hypertriglyceridemia, a condition that commonly arises in association with uncontrolled diabetes. Treatment of diabetes and resultant normalization of triglyceride levels may lead to disappearance of lesions.

Granuloma Annulare

Granuloma annulare is a granulomatous dermatitis that presents as annular plaques located on the limbs (Fig. 7-12). There is focal degeneration of collagen and elastic fibers associated with this. In a retrospective study of 84 patients, 12% were found to have diabetes, and these patients were more likely to suffer from chronic granuloma annulare than controls.[62]

Diabetic Neuropathy and the Skin

Autonomic Neuropathy

It has been suggested that nonmyelinated nerve fibers, such as those of the autonomic nervous system, may be the first nervous tissue affected in people with diabetes.[63] In clinical practice, evidence of autonomic neuropathy is common as manifested by disturbance of sweating

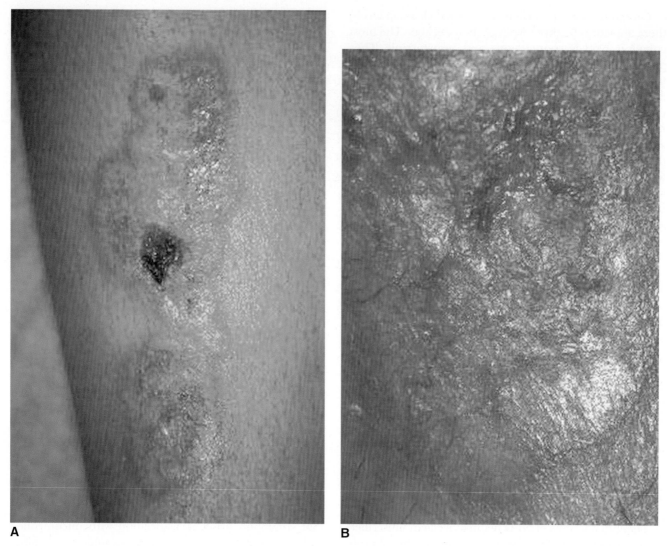

A   B

Figure 7–10 Necrobiosis lipoidica. This patient has waxy tan plaques on both shins. This lesion demonstrates the translucency in the center portion with visibility of underlying blood vessels.

(usually anhidrosis) of the feet. Occasionally, patients complain of oversweating elsewhere, a compensatory mechanism for loss of the ability to temperature regulate in the involved area. It has also been reported that autonomic neuropathy (as measured by quantitation of the sweating deficiency) correlates well with the severity of sensory neuropathy.[64] One can safely assume that patients who have diabetic sensory neuropathy also have accompanying autonomic involvement.

The clinical manifestations of peripheral autonomic neuropathy vary from absence of symptoms to complaints that the feet are abnormally cold, burning, or pruritic. But there is also a problem due to absence of sweating. Perspiration on the feet maintains hydration of the stratum corneum; callosities without hydration tend to become brittle and may fissure, serving as a portal for infection. Thus, symptoms and signs of autonomic peripheral neuropathy in the diabetic patient indicate the need for extra attention to foot care.

Motor Neuropathy

Diabetic motor neuropathy most often affects the foot. The clinical presentation is wasting of the interosseous foot muscles, resulting in two major mechanical problems. The foot tends to splay on weight-bearing, resulting in a wider foot. The toes tend to draw upward, and the plantar fat pads move forward, leaving the metatarsal heads riding on the plantar skin without the benefit of padding.

Motor neuropathy may appear suddenly or occur gradually over several years. Acute and reversible motor neuropathy may follow an episode of ketoacidosis.[65] More commonly, an insidious progression of motor nerve deterioration occurs over many years.

Motor neuropathy in diabetes mellitus is almost always accompanied by sensory involvement. Changes in the shape of the foot follow the imbalance of its internal musculature and result in ill-fitting shoes. If the changes go unnoticed, the patient might continue to wear shoes

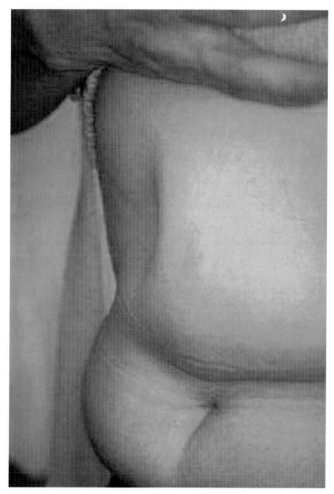

Figure 7–11 Lipoatrophy. This is an example of localized lipoatrophy, which typically appears as depressed plaques in the skin that may be the result of insulin injections.

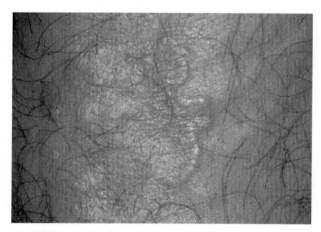

Figure 7–12 Granuloma annulare. This is an example of granuloma annulare presenting on the trunk. This is a granulomatous dermatitis with focal degeneration of collagen and elastic fibers.

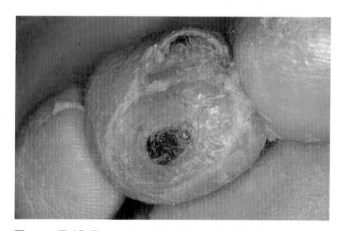

Figure 7–13 The erosion with callus on the tip of the toe is typical of the type of injury resulting from diabetic sensory neuropathy.

that can now traumatize the foot. Because of the accompanying sensory loss, displacement of the plantar fat pads can result in uncushioned weight-bearing at the metatarsal heads. Callosities and eventually ulceration of either the weight-bearing skin or the skin being rubbed by the ill-fitting shoes ensue (neuropathic ulcers). The presence of motor neuropathy of the foot often necessitates the use of special widened shoes with molded inserts to redistribute weight-bearing to accommodate and protect the compromised foot.

Sensory Neuropathy

People with diabetes often develop sensory neuropathy of the feet, especially with long-standing disease. The clinical presentation usually involves tingling and numbness starting in the toes. The level of neuropathy may vary from mild numbness of the distal toes to profound anesthesia and neuropathic ulcers. Thermal sensitivity is also affected.[66]

Although tingling and numbness tend to be the complaint, the lack of sensation may allow trauma to go unnoticed and result in a traumatic ulceration (Fig. 7-13). Depending on the status of the microcirculation, these ulcers may present difficult therapeutic problems. Neuropathic patients who walk barefoot may sustain damage during routine ambulation because they have inadequate sensation and do not withdraw the foot when it encounters noxious stimuli. Occasionally, this unsensed trauma during ambulation results in fracturing the bones of the feet, eventuating into a Charcot foot (Fig. 7-14).

Patients with sensory neuropathy need to be instructed to make sure their shoes are devoid of foreign objects before the shoes are worn. As simple as it sounds, patients who do not follow this rule occasionally sustain severe damage by wearing shoes that, unknown to them, have objects included.

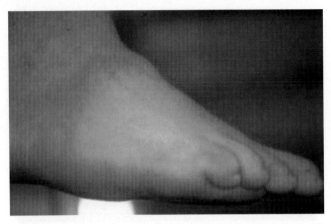

Figure 7-14 Charcot foot. This patient with diabetic motor and sensory neuropathy developed multiple midfoot fractures while running a short distance barefoot. The result is a misshapen foot, as seen here.

Summary

Diabetes mellitus is a common ailment, and virtually all people with diabetes develop skin manifestations of this disease. Many of these manifestations, especially the more common ones, might be explained on the basis of the attachment of glucose to proteins and the subsequent metabolism of this combination, which results in changes in structure, function, and color. It is hoped that the common skin findings described here may eventually be used as indicators of the patient's current and past metabolic status.

References

1. Monnier VM, Sell DR, Genuth S: Glycation products as markers and predictors of the progression of diabetic complications. Ann N Y Acad Sci 1043:567–581, 2005.
2. Brown SM, Smith DM, Alt N, et al: Tissue-specific variation in glycation of proteins in diabetes. Ann N Y Acad Sci 1043:817–823, 2005.
3. Vasan S, Foiles P, Founds H: Therapeutic potential of breakers of advanced glycation end product-protein crosslinks. Arch Biochem Biophys 419(1):89–96, 2003.
4. Greenwood AM: A study of the skin in 500 diabetics. JAMA 89:774–776, 1927.
5. Muller SA, Winkleman RK: Necrobiosis lipoidica diabeticorum: A clinical and pathological investigation of 171 cases. Arch Dermatol 93:272–281, 1966.
6. Sonck CE, Somersalo O: The yeast flora of the anogenital region in diabetic girls. Arch Dermatol 88:846–852, 1963.
7. Knight L, Fletcher J: Growth of Candida albicans in saliva: Stimulation by glucose associated with antibiotics, corticosteroids, and diabetes mellitus. J Infect Dis 123:371–377, 1971.
8. Lugo-Somolinos A, Sanchez JL: Prevalence of dermatophytosis in patients with diabetes. J Am Acad Dermatol 26:408–410, 1992.
9. Alteras I, Saryt E: Prevalence of pathogenic fungi in the toe-webs and toe-nails of diabetic patients. Mycopathologia 67:157–159, 1979.
10. Tomford JW, Whittlesey D, Ellner JJ, Tomashefski JF: Invasive primary cutaneous phycomycosis in diabetic leg ulcers. Arch Surg 115:770–771, 1980.
11. Petrozzi JW, Warthan TL: Malignant external otitis. Arch Dermatol 110:258–260, 1974.
12. Wilson DF, Pulec JL, Linthicum FH: Malignant external otitis. Arch Otolaryngol 93:419–422, 1971.
13. Neilly JB, Martin A, Simpson N, MacCuish AC: Pruritus in diabetes mellitus: Investigation of prevalence and correlation with diabetes control. Diabetes Care 9:273–275, 1986.
14. Collier A, Matthews AM, Kellett HA, et al: Change in skin thickness associated with cheiroarthropathy in insulin dependent diabetes mellitus. Br Med J 292:936, 1986.
15. Huntley AC, Walter RM Jr: Quantitative determination of skin thickness in diabetes mellitus: Relationship to disease parameters. J Med 21(5):257–64, 1990.
16. Brik R, Berant M, Vardi P: The scleroderma-like syndrome of insulin-dependent diabetes mellitus. Diab Metab Rev 7:121–128, 1991.
17. Lundbaek, K: Stiff hands in long term diabetes. Acta Med Scand 158:447–451, 1957.
18. Rosenbloom AL, Frais JL: Diabetes mellitus, short stature and joint stiffness: A new syndrome. Clin Res 22:92A, 1974.
19. Rosenbloom AL, Silverstein JH, et al: Limited joint mobility in childhood diabetes mellitus indicates increased risk for microvascular disease. N Engl J Med 305:191–198. 1981.
20. Fitzcharles MA, Duby S, Wadell RW, et al: Limitation of joint mobility (cheiroarthropathy) in adult noninsulin-dependent diabetic patients. Ann Rheum Dis 43:251–257, 1984.
21. Huntley AC: Finger pebbles: A common finding in diabetes mellitus. J Amer Acad Dermatol 14:612–617, 1986.
22. Clark CV, Pentland B, Ewing DJ, Clark BF: Decreased skin wrinkling in diabetes mellitus. Diabetes Care 7:224–227, 1984.
23. Cole GW, Headley J, Skowsky R: Scleredema diabeticorum: A common and distinct cutaneous manifestation of diabetes mellitus. Diabetes Care 6:189–192, 1983.
24. Cohn BA, Wheeler CE, Briggamon RA: Scleredema adultorum of Buschke and diabetes mellitus. Arch Dermatol 101:27–35, 1970.
25. Konohana A, Kawakubo Y, Tajima S, et al: Glycosaminoglycans and collagen in skin of a patient with diabetic scleredema. Keio J Med 34:221–226, 1985.
26. Venencie PY, Powell FC, Su WP: Scleredema: A review of thirty-three cases. J Am Acad Dermatol 11:128–134, 1984.
27. Lieberman LS, Rosenbloom AL, Riley WJ, Silverstein JH: Reduced skin thickness with pump administration of insulin [letter]. N Eng J Med 303:940–941, 1980.
28. West KM: Epidemiology of Diabetes and Its Vascular Lesions. New York, Elsevier North-Holland, 1978, p 353.
29. Haroon TS: Diabetes and skin: A review. Scott Med J 19:257–267, 1974.
30. Bernstein JE: Cutaneous manifestations of diabetes mellitus. Curr Concepts Skin Disord 1:3, 1980.
31. Bauer M, Levan NE: Diabetic dermangiopathy: A spectrum including pretibial pigmented patches and necrobiosis lipoidica diabeticorum. Br J Dermatol 83:528–535, 1970.
32. Lithner F: Cutaneous reactions of the extremities of diabetics to local thermal trauma. Acta Med Scand 198:319–325, 1975.
33. Binkley GW, Giraldo B, Stoughton RB: Diabetic dermopathy: A clinical study. Cutis 3:955–958, 1967.
34. Melin H: An atrophic circumscribed skin lesion in the lower extremities of diabetics. Acta Med Scand 176(suppl 423):1–75, 1964.
35. Danowski TX, Sabeh G, Sarver ME, et al: Shin spots and diabetes mellitus. Am J Med Sci 251:570–575, 1966.
36. Murphy RA: Skin lesions in diabetic patients: The "spotted leg" syndrome. Lahey Clin Found Bull 14:10–14, 1965.
37. Lithner F: Purpura, pigmentation and yellow nails of the lower extremities in diabetes. Acta Med Scand 199:203–208, 1976.
38. Ditzel J: Functional microangiopathy in diabetes mellitus. Diabetes 17:388–397, 1968.
39. Gitelson S, Wertheimer-Kaplinski N: Color of the face in diabetes mellitus: Observations on a group of patients in Jerusalem. Diabetes 14:201–208, 1965.
40. Landau J, Davis E: The small blood-vessels of the conjunctiva and nailbed in diabetes mellitus. Lancet 2:731–734, 1960.
41. Grassi W, Gasparini M, Cervini C: Nailfold computed videomicroscopy in morpho-functional assessment of diabetic microangiopathy. Acta Diabetol Lat 22:223–228, 1985.
42. Lithner F: Cutaneous erythema, with or without necrosis, localized to the legs and feet: A lesion in elderly diabetics. Acta Med Scand 196:333–342, 1974.

43. Lithner F, Hietala S-O: Skeletal lesions of the feet in diabetics and their relationship to cutaneous erythema with or without necrosis of the feet. Acta Med Scand 200:155–161, 1976.

44. Oimomi M, Maeda Y, Hata F, et al: Glycosylation levels of nail proteins in diabetic patients with retinopathy and neuropathy. Kobe J Med Sci 31:183–188, 1985.

45. Rocca F, Pereyra E: Phlyctenar lesions in the feet of diabetic patients. Diabetes 12:220–222, 1963.

46. Allen GE, Hadden DR: Bullous lesions of the skin in diabetes (bullous diabeticorum). Br J Dermatol 82:216–220, 1970.

47. Cantwell AR, Martz W: Idiopathic bullae in diabetics: Bullosis diabeticorum. Arch Dermatol 96:42–44, 1967.

48. Kurwa A, Roberts P, Whitehead R: Concurrence of bullous and atrophic skin lesions in diabetes mellitus. Arch Dermatol 103:670–675, 1971.

49. James WD, Odom RB, Goette DK: Bullous eruption of diabetes mellitus: A case with positive immunofluorescence microscopy findings. Arch Dermatol 116:1191–1192, 1980.

50. Bernstein JE, Medinica M, Soltani K, Griem SF: Bullous eruption of diabetes mellitus. Arch Dermatol 115:324–325, 1979.

51. Muller SA: Dermatologic disorders associated with diabetes mellitus. Mayo Clin Proc 41:689–703, 1966.

52. Ellenberg M: Diabetic complications without manifest diabetes. JAMA 183:926–930, 1963.

53. Boulton AJ, Cutfield MB, Abouganem D, et al: Necrobiosis lipoidica diabeticorum: A clinicopathologic study. J Am Acad Dermatol 18:530537, 1988.

54. Wilson Jones E: Necrobiosis lipoidica presenting on the face and scalp. Trans St Johns Hosp Dermatol Soc 57:202, 1971.

55. Ackerman AB: Histologic diagnosis of inflammatory skin diseases: A method by pattern analysis. Philadelphia, Lea & Febiger, 1978, pp 424–431.

56. Heng MCY, Allen SG, Song MK, Heng MK: Focal endothelial cell degeneration and proliferative endarteritis in trauma-induced early lesions of necrobiosis lipoidica diabeticorum. Am J Dermatopath 13:108–114, 1991.

57. Handfield-Jones S, Jones S, Peachey R: High dose nicotinamide in the treatment of necrobiosis lipoidica. Br J Dermatol 118:693–696, 1988.

58. Eldor S, Diaz EG, Naparstek E: Treatment of diabetic necrobiosis with aspirin and dipyridamole. N Engl J Med 298:1033, 1978.

59. Fjellner B: Treatment of diabetic necrobiosis with aspirin and dipyridamole. N Engl J Med 299:1366, 1978.

60. Unge G, Tornling G: Treatment of diabetic necrobiosis with dipyridamole. N Engl J Med 299:1366, 1978.

61. Petzelbauer P, Wolff K, Tappeiner G: Necrobiosis lipoidica: Treatment with systemic corticosteroids. Br J Dermatol 126:542–545, 1992.

62. Martin MM: Involvement of autonomic nerve fibers in diabetic neuropathy. Lancet 264:560–565, 1953.

63. Studer EM, Calza AM, Saurat JH: Precipitating factors and associated diseases in 84 patients with granuloma annulare: A retrospective study. Dermatology 193:364–368, 1996.

64. Kennedy WR, Sakuta M, Sutherland D, Goetz FC: Quantitation of the sweating deficiency in diabetes mellitus. Ann Neurol 15:482–488, 1984.

65. Brown MJ, Asbury AK: Diabetic neuropathy. Ann Neurol 15:2–12,1984.

66. Navarro X, Kennedy WR: Evaluation of thermal and pain sensitivity in type I diabetic patients. J Neurol Neurosurg Pshchiatry 54:60–64, 1991.

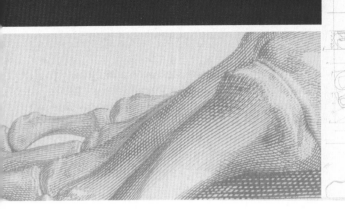

NUTRITIONAL ISSUES IN THE PATIENT WITH DIABETES AND FOOT ULCERS

MARY D. LITCHFORD ■

The signs and symptoms of diabetes with long-term complications, including risk for recurrent infections, foot ulcers with necrosis, and development of gangrene, have been documented by ancient physicians of different cultures. The cause of the diabetes remained a mystery until the late 19th century, when the pancreas was identified as the causative organ. Medical nutrition therapy was the one of the vital intervention strategies for the treatment of diabetes dating back to the second century C.E. The first "diabetic diet" recorded in early medical writings prescribed milk, cereal, starch, autumn fruits, and sweet wines. The diet excluded meats, spring and summer fruits, green vegetables, and concentrated sweets. In 1900, dietary management remained the primary focus of treatment, but the diet changed from a low-protein, high-carbohydrate diet to a calorie-restricted, low-carbohydrate diet consisting of about 850 calories and 10 grams of carbohydrate per day.[1] The discovery of insulin in 1921 dramatically changed the medical nutrition therapy recommendations for management of diabetes. In 1921, the recommended diet was 70% of calories from fat, 10% of calories from protein, and 20% of calories from carbohydrate. The goal for diabetes management in 1921 was glycemic control using a high fat intake rather than reduction of long-term complications from arthrosclerosis.[2]

Medical Nutrition Therapy for Diabetes

Recommendations for optimal management of diabetes remain controversial. Medical nutrition therapy, as a contributor to tight glycemic control, plays a crucial role in the overall management of the acute symptoms of diabetes as well as delaying the long-term complications that contribute to foot ulcers.[3–6] The 2002 American Diabetes Association Clinical Practice Recommendations are the primary standard of care for diabetes management.[3] However, guidelines targeting patients with type 2 diabetes or prediabetes who are overweight or obese have been published by the Joslin Diabetes Center at Harvard Medical School in Boston, Massachusetts.[4] The goals of both sets of recommendations include glycemic control, weight management, blood pressure control, and maintaining a lipid and lipoprotein profile that minimizes the risk of macrovascular complications.[3–6]

Numerous diet systems for diabetes management are available, including the no-concentrated-sweets diet, the carbohydrate-controlled diet, the exchange system, the carbohydrate-counting system, and the glycemic index system. A registered dietitian or other approved medical nutrition therapist must complete a comprehensive nutrition assessment of the patient and determine which system is most appropriate to use. The assessment includes an evaluation of anthropometric data, physical assessment data, biochemical data, and dietary intake of food and fluid. Diabetes education and lifestyle recommendations are individualized for each patient. Follow-up education is required for intervention and reassessment and to ensure compliance with the dietary management plan. The presence of a foot ulcer changes the patient's nutritional needs, but the need for tight glycemic control remains paramount.

Nutrition Basics and Wound Healing

The human body is composed of foods consumed in a lifetime. Adequate macronutrients, micronutrients, and water are required to maintain the body and repair injured tissues. Each component of wound healing must occur in sequence for the wound to progress. The process of wound healing depends on the following:

- Adequate energy for cell proliferation, cell movement, and protein synthesis.
- Adequate protein, amino acids, and peptides for the protein synthesis required for each stage of wound healing.
- Adequate anabolic stimuli, such as growth factors and anabolic hormones.[7]

Research on Nutrition and Wounds

Research on the role of nutrition in wound healing is often inconclusive because malnutrition is not clearly defined. Malnutrition is a complex process that involves more than a decline in dietary intake. Diseases, injuries, medications, and other factors can significantly affect metabolism, creating an internal imbalance that leads to poor nutrient utilization, weight loss, skin breakdown, and poor healing. Unintentional weight loss and protein-energy malnutrition (PEM) are the most frequently observed nutritional deficiencies associated with chronic and non-healing wounds. However, PEM is not always associated with poor healing, and excellent nutrition is not associated with rapid healing.[8–9] Many other factors serve as impediments to healing that are independent of dietary intake and must be considered in evaluating outcomes.

In addition, nutrients play multiple roles in the body rather than being etiology specific, as in the case of medications. Providing dietary supplements to promote wound healing might or might not appear to affect the healing process. However, if the patient has a clinical or subclinical nutrient deficiency or is unable to utilize nutrients efficiently, supplementation may be helpful.[10] Confirmation of most nutrient deficiencies through laboratory analysis is available but can be cost-prohibitive. Despite the controversy, the role of nutrition as an effective intervention strategy to prevent skin breakdown and to promote healing continues to be documented in the literature.[10]

The Agency for Health Research and Quality (AHRQ) *Guidelines for the Treatment of Pressure Ulcers* (1994)[11] identified nutrition assessment and support as one of the three primary components of care in the management of pressure ulcers.

The principles of nutrition assessment and support apply to the patient with a diabetic foot ulcer.

Risk Assessment

Wounds are caused by a combination of factors, including increased pressure on a bony prominence, poor nutrition status and comorbidities including diabetes, vascular disease and neuropathy. Aspects of nutritional status associated with an increased risk for skin breakdown include the following:

- Reduced body mass index (BMI)
- Low body weight
- Low dietary intake of protein
- Low plasma albumin and prealbumin
- Hypocholesterolemia
- Decreased total lymphocyte count
- Nutritional anemias
- Altered ability to self-feed
- Reduced food intake[8–9,12–14]

Venous leg ulcers are commonly seen in individuals with diabetes, congestive heart failure, peripheral vascular disease, and pedal edema. Poor dietary intake and recent weight loss have been reported in more than 20% of patients with venous leg ulcers.[15–16] Even individuals who are overweight may have marginal or poor protein status or nutritional anemias.

Protein-Energy Malnutrition

PEM develops slowly in the patient with inadequate intakes of both protein and energy. It is reasonable to conclude that micronutrient deficiencies also occur with PEM owing to the limited dietary intake. Contributors to PEM may include depression, substance abuse, inability to self-feed, inability to prepare meals, dysphagia, lack of access to food owing to financial hardship, or lack of transportation.[17–18]

PEM alters body composition and the normal way in which the body utilizes protein and fat for fuel. Body composition is divided into fat and fat-free components. Body protein is in the fat-free or lean body mass (LBM) compartment, representing about 75% of total body weight. LBM is 50% to 60% muscle mass by weight, and the rest is bone and tendon. With age, there is natural loss of muscle mass. The majority of LBM is in skeletal muscle mass; however, proteins make up the critical cell structure of muscle, viscera, red blood cells, and connective tissue. Enzymes that direct metabolism and antibodies that maintain immune function are also proteins.[19–21]

Patients with PEM use gluconeogenesis as the primary source of energy. Glucagon, cortisol, and catecholamine levels are increased, and insulin and other anabolic hormones are decreased. Muscle tissue breaks down to release amino acids to drive the gluconeogenesis process. Amino acids enter the citric acid cycle and are converted to acetyl-CoA. Acetyl-CoA is then converted to pyruvate to continue the gluconeogenesis process. Leucine and lysine are converted into ketone bodies and cannot be used for glucose formation. Ketone bodies, acetone, acetoacetate, and β-hydroxybutyrate are used by the brain, heart, and skeletal muscle as an energy source. The catabolism of the body protein is reflected in increased urinary nitrogen loss and decreased plasma albumin, prealbumin, and retinol-binding protein; unintentional weight loss; and skin breakdown.[19–21]

The loss of LBM has deleterious effects on the body. If approximately 10% of LBM is lost, immune function will be impaired, resulting in an increased risk for infection. At this point, free fatty acids are being used for energy, allowing protein to be spared for wound healing. However as LBM decreases to 15%, there is profound weakness, the risk for infection increases, the rate of wound healing decreases, and new wounds appear. With the loss of 20% of total LBM, spontaneous wounds can develop owing to thinning of skin from lost collagen.[19–21]

The most common precipitating cause of PEM in a patient with diabetes is an acute injury or illness leading to the hypermetabolism and increased catabolism of LBM.[22] The body must reabsorb the devitalized tissue and then heal the wound. The wound consumes large quantities of energy during the healing process both by the inflammatory cells and the fibroblasts' production of collagen and matrix. If the body is unable to adapt to preserve LBM, the abnormal hormonal environment will lead to a rapid loss of protein. Calorie and protein needs increase, but energy production is pathologically altered. Substrates such as pyruvate and fatty acids recycle back to glucose and fat instead of being metabolized to CO_2 and H_2O. This results in less adenosine triphosphate and a wasted increase of energy in the form of heat production.[23–25] More calories are needed to prevent weight loss. Protein synthesis is inefficient because 20% to 30% of consumed amino acids are being used for energy production.[26] The progressive loss of LBM and replacement of fat mass is a common problem in patients with diabetes. It is the loss of LBM plus an injury, rather than loss of fat stores, that causes the complications of malnutrition.[20–21,27]

Uncontrolled blood glucose impairs blood flow through the microvascular system at the wound surface by impeding red blood cell permeability and increasing cell wall rigidity. In addition, hemoglobin release of oxygen is impaired, resulting in an oxygen and nutrient deficiency. The underlying disease processes limit nutrient access to the wound site for healing.

Nutritional Management: Macronutrients

Assessment of Calorie Needs

Energy expenditure is measured by indirect calorimetry or calculated using mathematical equations. Indirect calorimetry determines energy expenditure by measuring the body's oxygen consumption and carbon dioxide production using a computerized metabolic cart.[28,29]

Energy expenditure can be calculated by using the Harris-Benedict equation. These regression equations were developed in 1919 by using indirect calorimetry to estimate resting energy expenditure (REE).[30] The accuracy of these equations has been evaluated by numerous researchers.[31–32] The research has demonstrated that the Harris-Benedict equations accurately predict the REE of healthy, adequately nourished persons within +14% of REE measured by indirect calorimetry. In malnourished, ill patients, the Harris-Benedict equations tend to underestimate REE by as much as 22%.[32] The total daily expenditure is based on the REE or BEE. (The terms *BEE* [basal energy expenditure] and *REE* [resting energy expenditure] are used interchangeably.) Factors for injury or activity level are factored into the equation.

Energy needs can be calculated by using empirical formulas. Healthy individuals require approximately 25 calories per kilogram of body weight to meet basal metabolic needs. The AHRQ *Guidelines for the Treatment of Pressure Ulcers* (1994) and the National Pressure Ulcer Advisory Panel guidelines recommend estimating energy needs on the basis of body weight.[11,33]

Recommended Calorie Needs

Recommended calorie levels for wound healing vary from 25 to 30 calories per kilogram of body weight[34] to 30 to 40 calories per kilogram of body weight.[35–36] Tube-fed residents with and without skin breakdown were evaluated for nutritional status by assessing their albumin and hemoglobin levels. Individuals with pressure ulcers had lower albumin and hemoglobin levels despite receiving 32 calories per kilogram of body weight and 1.4 grams of protein per kilogram of body weight.[37] Breslow (1993)[24] reported improved wound healing in nursing home residents receiving 40 calories per kilogram of body weight. The AHRQ *Guidelines for the Treatment of Pressure Ulcers* (1994)[11] recommend 30 to 35 calories per kilogram of body weight for individuals with pressure ulcers who are malnourished.[38]

Calorie needs will vary according to the stage of the wound, the phase of wound healing, comorbidities, age, and current body weight. Severely underweight individuals might require more calories per kilogram than do individuals at or near desirable weight.[39] The elderly patient might require additional calories owing to an inefficient utilization of nutrients or a need for weight gain.

BMI and percentage of desirable body weight are two methods that are used to determine if calorie needs are being met. However, if the body's metabolism is pathologically altered such that nutrient use to make energy is inefficient, the substrates will be recycled to fat and glucose rather than protein. While weight or BMI might be stable, the wound might not be improving.

Assessment of Protein Needs

LBM is metabolically and physiologically active. The body mass is determined by genetics. There are virtually no protein stores in the body. Every protein molecule has a role in maintaining homeostasis. Dietary protein is needed to build new tissue. The healthy adult requires approximately 0.8 grams of protein per kilogram of body weight per day to maintain homeostasis.[40] Stressed and injured patients have greater needs for protein because of the increased needs for protein synthesis and increased losses of amino acids. Urinary nitrogen losses increase after injury.

Elderly people break down more protein daily and have a higher need for protein synthesis to keep up with normal protein losses. The healthy elderly person requires approximately 1.0 grams of protein per kilogram of body weight per day to maintain homeostasis.[41-42] Elderly people experience a decline in the musculoskeletal system as one of the normal physical changes seen with aging. The long-term effect of loss of muscle mass is a decrease in muscle strength and an increased risk for falls.[43] A decline in visceral protein stores is evident after loss of muscle mass due to atrophy.[44-45]

Body proteins that play direct roles in wound healing include albumin, globulin, fibrinogen, and collagen. Albumin and globulin constitute most of the protein within the body and are measured as total protein. Albumin is synthesized in the liver at a rate of 8 to 14 g/day. It makes up approximately 60% of the total protein. Albumin provides approximately 80% of colloidal osmotic pressure of the plasma. Plasma albumin and other high-molecular-weight plasma proteins are typically confined to intravascular space and do not readily cross the capillary membrane. When plasma albumin is low, there is a decrease in oncotic pressure, and water can more easily move into the intravascular space, resulting in edema.[46] The loss of plasma fluid results in hypovolemia, which in turn triggers renal retention of water and sodium. Albumin also serves as a carrier of copper, zinc, calcium, fatty acids, amino acids, metabolites, bilirubin, enzymes, hormones, and medications.

Globulin makes up about 40% of the total protein. Globulin is required for the production of antibodies and is synthesized in the reticuloendothelial system.

Fibrinogen is a plasma protein that is converted by thrombin to fibrin in the presence of calcium ions for clot formation at the wound site. Fibrin is one of the first proteins to arrive at the wound to initiate blood clotting.

The staggered pattern of fibrin at the wound site forms a mesh, allowing red blood cells, platelets, and other factors to congregate at the site and form a blood clot.

Collagen is present in every step of wound healing and is found in the extracellular matrix of tissues and wounds. The amount of collagen synthesized depends on the availability of nutrients and oxygen. Nutrients that are required for protein synthesis include vitamin A, vitamin C, amino acids (especially proline and lysine), iron, copper, and zinc. Adequate perfusion to the wound site is essential for delivery of nutrients for wound healing.[19]

Biochemical Assessment of Protein Status

A patient's protein status is a reflection of the body's ability to synthesize nonessential amino acids and to absorb and utilize essential amino acids. As the protein status declines, the patient is at higher risk for skin breakdown, infection, and delayed wound healing.[47] Changes in plasma albumin, prealbumin, and transferrin are affected by malnutrition and physiologic stress from injury or infection. Stress-induced hypoalbuminemia does not reflect the body's protein status per se; it reflects the body's physiologic response to injury and infection.[48] Plasma levels of albumin, prealbumin, and transferrin decrease in response to infection, injury, or trauma and increase with a decrease in C-reactive protein levels and subsequent recovery of these conditions. The plasma levels do not increase in response to increased intakes of protein or calories when the C-reactive protein level remains elevated.

Albumin

Albumin is the least sensitive measure of protein status, with a half-life of 12 to 21 days. It is affected by hydration status, injury, infection, and inflammatory response. Depressed levels of albumin have been correlated with increased protein needs for individuals who are malnourished.[49] Albumin levels often remain low for extended periods of time after surgery or significant injury in older adults.[50]

Prealbumin

Prealbumin (PAB) is the second most sensitive measure of protein status, with a half-life of 2 to 3 days. However, prealbumin is not a reliable indicator for individuals with chronic renal failure or advanced liver disease. Concurrent corticosteroid treatment or renal insufficiency can falsely elevate prealbumin findings.[45] PAB is a sensitive indicator of protein deficiency and of improvement in protein status with refeeding. When malnutrition is significant, the plasma PAB will usually fall below 10.7 mg/dL. Plasma PAB is not greatly affected by mild renal or liver disease, by fluid compartment shifts, or in patients receiving exogenous albumin. However, as renal disease and liver disease become more significant, the levels do not reflect overall protein status. In addition, iron deficiency does not significantly affect its level. PAB is significantly reduced in hepatobiliary disease, owing to impaired synthesis. It is also reduced with a zinc deficiency, since zinc is required for synthesis of PAB. PAB is a negative acute-phase reactant protein. Plasma levels decrease with surgery, inflammation, malignancy, and protein-wasting diseases of the intestines or kidneys.[51–52]

Retinol-Binding Protein

Retinol-binding protein (RBP) is the most sensitive measure of protein status. It is a low-molecular-weight protein that responds to both protein and calorie restrictions. RBP has a 10-hour half-life and appears to be a better indicator of both short-term and long-term changes in protein status than is albumin, prealbumin, or transferrin. It is typically more affected by energy restriction than by protein deficiency. RBP does not seem to be affected by the acute inflammatory response, like prealbumin or albumin. An elevation in C-reactive protein indicates acute inflammatory response. As long as C-reactive protein is elevated, prealbumin and albumin are significantly depressed.[5] Since RBP is relatively unaffected by the acute inflammatory response, RBP appears to be a more reliable indicator of nutritional status following surgery or injury.[51,54]

RBP is not a reliable indicator of protein status in advanced chronic renal disease. All protein indicators usually show an increase in concentration in advanced kidney disease. These levels do not reflect the patient's protein status. RBP is not a reliable indicator of protein status in advanced liver disorders. The liver has significant stores of RBP and will release the stores as the disease progresses.[52]

Transferrin

Plasma transferrin is an iron-transport protein with a half-life of 8 to 10 days that reflects both protein and iron status. Transferrin increases with iron deficiency and decreases when iron status improves or with protein-energy malnutrition. If a patient has concurrent iron deficiency, it is difficult to determine whether a low transferrin level reflects iron status or protein status. In mild to moderate protein-energy malnutrition, transferrin values may vary, limiting the usefulness of this test. However, markedly low transferrin levels indicate severe protein-energy malnutrition. A value less than 100 mg/dL may be considered a reliable index of severe protein-energy malnutrition.[55]

Total Cholesterol

Other indicators of protein status include total cholesterol, total lymphocyte count, and nitrogen balance. Other laboratory tests that suggest an increased risk for skin breakdown include cholesterol level and total lymphocyte count. The plasma cholesterol level is a reflection of dietary intake, absorption, endogenous synthesis, and excretion. Low levels of total cholesterol or a significant decline in total cholesterol is associated with malnutrition and high mortality. In elderly patients, a total cholesterol level less than 160 mg/dL is a risk factor for skin breakdown when other risk factors are present. Low levels might indicate severe liver disease or a malabsorption syndrome. The low cholesterol level is thought to increase the risk of a variety of nonatherosclerotic diseases because cholesterol or fat-soluble vitamins and detoxifying agents carried in lipoproteins may play a direct role in the immune system.[56–57] However, Hu and colleagues[58] reported that low cholesterol levels were not associated with high mortality among high-functioning community-dwelling older men and women. The population studied by Hu and colleagues[58] was well nourished as indicated by BMI and plasma albumin.

In using total plasma cholesterol as a risk factor for skin breakdown, it is important to consider the lifelong pattern of laboratory test results. Some individuals who are well nourished will have a total plasma cholesterol of less than 160 mg/dL. These individuals would not be at risk for skin breakdown if other factors were not present.[56,59] A significant decline in plasma cholesterol might suggest a change in endogenous synthesis.[45]

Total Lymphocyte Count

Protein-energy malnutrition compromises the immune system and reduces the number of white blood cells, which makes total lymphocyte count of some value. Total lymphocyte count is computed from the results of the complete blood count. The percentage of lymphocytes is multiplied by the total white blood cell count in cubic millimeters.[55] A decline in total lymphocyte count suggests both impaired immune response and worsening protein status.[45]

Nitrogen Balance

For patients with stress-induced hypoalbuminemia, improved nitrogen balance reflects recovery from inflammation, subsequent normalization of inflammatory mediators and a decrease in protein catabolism.[48] For malnourished patients, nitrogen balance may be useful to assess protein status. Under normal conditions, the nitrogen balance value is zero, indicating that the patient is neither losing nor gaining LBM. Negative results indicate that the patient is in negative nitrogen balance, or catabolic. To obtain accurate results, a detailed 24-hour food intake record must be kept. All urine must be collected for the same 24-hour period. Urinary incontinence and other difficulties can render nitrogen balance a relatively impractical test in certain populations.[60]

Recommended Protein Needs

Recommended protein requirements may be based on desirable body weight or actual body weight. If there is a significant difference between actual body weight and desirable body weight, the registered dietitian will use clinical judgment to estimate needs.

The AHRQ *Guidelines for the Treatment of Pressure Ulcers*[11] recommend 1.25 to 1.50 grams of protein per kilogram of body weight for individuals with pressure ulcers who are malnourished.[38] Chernoff and colleagues[35] found that higher intakes of protein, up to 1.8 grams of protein per kilogram of body weight, per day were associated with greater healing rates. Yarkony and Heinemann[61] found that a range of 1.5 to 2.0 grams of protein per kilogram of body weight was needed to heal wounds. Other recommendations are based on a percentage of calories and recommend between 20% to 24% of total calories for wound healing. High-protein enteral formulas with 24% to 25% of calories from protein have demonstrated improved healing of pressure ulcers compared to enteral formulas with 14% to 17% of calories from protein. These findings were especially noted in individuals consuming up to 40 calories per kilogram of body weight.[24,35] However, providing more than 2.0 grams of protein per kilogram of body weight can burden the renal and hepatic systems.[62] Intakes of protein that exceed 2 grams of protein per kilogram of body weight might not be metabolized to increase protein synthesis. Higher intakes of protein without adequate fluid intake might be a risk factor for dehydration in the elderly.[63–65] The optimal level of protein for individuals with pressure ulcers is not known, but the goal should probably lie between 1.2 and 1.8 grams of protein per kilogram of body weight per day.[63] The estimated biologic needs might be unrealistic for the patient to consume via the usual diet or contraindicated because of other medical conditions.

Numerous protein powders and elixirs are available to increase protein intake without significantly increasing the volume of food consumed. Protein supplements vary in biologic quality. The protein supplement products that are selected should meet the Institute of Medicine Recommended Pattern of Essential Amino Acids and have a protein corrected amino acid score (PDCAAS) of 100. The PDCAAS is an indication of the overall quality of a protein because it represents the relative adequacy of its most limiting amino acid. Protein supplements with a PDCAAS of 100 are classified as complete or high biologic value proteins. Protein supplements with PDCAAS of less than 100 are inadequate in one or more essential amino acids.[66–71]

For example, if a particular protein is limiting in methionine/cysteine with an amino acid score of 33, then this protein will provide only 33% of the methionine/cysteine requirement. The practical consequences of this are that in the absence of another source of methionine/cysteine, only 33% of that protein can be used for protein synthesis. The remainder can be used for synthesis of other nitrogen-containing compounds or can be deaminated and used for energy. Giving large quantities of nonessential amino acids can put undue stress on the renal system that is already compromised by diabetes.

Assessment of Fat Needs

The typical American diet tends to be higher in fat content than is recommended by nutrition professionals. However, the patient with skin breakdown might not consume a diet that is adequate in fat or might take supplemental fatty acids such as omega-3 fatty acids for other medical conditions. The role of fat has been examined for its relationship with wound healing. Use of topical oils that contain essential fatty acids as a way to reduce the risk for skin breakdown has also been studied.

Essential fatty acid deficiencies are rare in humans except in patients who are on total parenteral nutrition with inadequate lipid. The research on the role of essential fatty acids in wound healing is based on animal models. Hulsey and colleagues[72] found that essential fatty acid deficiency in rats impaired wound healing of skin, but not colonic anastomoses. However, Porras-Reyes and colleagues[73] concluded that essential fatty acids were not required for wound healing in the rat model. Essential fatty acid deficiencies in humans are not desirable and should be prevented and treated appropriately.

The role of omega-3 fatty acids in wound healing has been examined in animal models as well. Albina and colleagues[74] concluded that rats that were fed a diet rich in omega-3 fatty acids had decreased tensile strength compared to the rats that were fed a diet rich in corn oil. The collagen content was the same for both groups. The omega-3 fatty acids appeared to have a negative effect on wound healing in the animal model.

Omega-3 fatty acids have anti-inflammatory effects and may increase the synthesis of prostaglandins. Decreasing the inflammatory response might result in a weaker response to healing.[75] Supplementation of omega-3 fatty acids can increase the risk of bleeding in patients who take aspirin or other anticoagulant medications.

For the patient with diabetes, supplemental doses of 2 or more grams of omega-3 fatty acids daily may improve the lipid profile. Individuals who were taking daily doses of 2 or more grams of omega-3 fatty acids prior to the development of the wound should consider discontinuing the supplement until cellular proliferation is established.

Nutrient utilization of essential fatty acids through topical applications has been studied in humans.[76] Topical oils containing either linoleic acid or mineral oil were studied for 21 days in 86 intensive care patients who had poor nutritional status and had been identified as being at risk for skin breakdown. The group that received the topical linoleic acid–rich oil was associated with improved skin hydration and elasticity. This group also had a lower incidence of skin breakdown than did the group that received the topical mineral oil.

Recommended Fat Needs

Fat is an essential nutrient to provide essential fatty acids, fat-soluble vitamins, and energy. The role of essential fatty acids and omega-3 fatty acids has not been fully examined in the literature. However, the few animal studies on omega-3 fatty acids suggest that taking supplemental omega-3 fatty acids might negatively affect healing during the inflammatory stage. The *U.S. Dietary Guidelines* recommends diets that contain 30% or fewer calories from fat daily. Low-fat diets might be beneficial to wound healing.[7]

Nutritional Management

Assessment of Hydration Status

Dehydration is a common problem in patients with wounds, owing to the rapid loss of fluid from the wound site. In elderly people, there is a reduced thirst sensation, and commonly ordered medications increased fluid losses. Some patients might have limited access to water, especially if they are unable to communicate their thirst needs. Normal hydration status will optimize wound healing.

Disorders of fluid balance include dehydration and overhydration. Both present challenging physiologic conditions that have medical nutrition therapy interventions. Inappropriate intervention strategies can create additional problems for the adult with a diabetic foot ulcer. Dehydration is the most common fluid electrolyte disorder of frail older adults living in community or institutional settings.[77] Unfortunately, hydration status is often overlooked or misdiagnosed.

Bennett and colleagues[78] conducted a retrospective review of medical records to describe the prevalence, assessment, and risk factors for chronic dehydration in 185 older adults who visited an emergency department over a 30-day period. Results showed that chronic dehydration was present in 48% of the patients. Physicians documented assessment for signs of dehydration in 26% of the dehydrated older adults, but no independent assessments for dehydration were recorded by nurses.

Thomas and colleagues[79] examined the accuracy of the physician's diagnosis of dehydration in older adults. The criterion for dehydration was calculated plasma osmolality greater than 295 mOsm/kg H_2O. Subjects were considered to have intravascular volume depletion if the ratio of blood urea nitrogen (BUN) to plasma creatinine was greater than 20 or the plasma sodium level was greater than 145 mEq/dL.

Thomas and colleagues[79] found that among subjects with a clinical diagnosis of dehydration, only 17% had a plasma osmolarity greater than 295 mOsm, and only 11% had a plasma sodium greater than 145 mEq/dL. A BUN:creatinine ratio greater than 20 was present in 68% of the subjects. Thomas theorized that clinicians appeared to be using the term *dehydration* synonymously with *intravascular volume depletion*. Thomas reported that at least one third of the diagnoses were incorrect.

Accurate assessment of fluid status requires a multidisciplinary approach to ensure that care needs are met. Laboratory test results, physical assessment, anthropometric data, total sodium intake, and total fluid intake and output are essential components of an accurate assessment.

Dehydration is categorized according to the plasma sodium concentration. Variations in plasma sodium reflect the composition of the fluids lost and present different pathophysiologic effects.

The normal concentration of plasma sodium is approximately 135 to 146 mEq/L (135 to 146 mmol/L). The reference range is determined by the laboratory equipment reference standards, calibration methodology, and assays that are used.[45,80–81]

Plasma sodium is categorized as follows:

Isonatremic	130 to 150 mEq/L
Hyponatremic	less than 130 mEq/L
Hypernatremic	greater than 150 mEq/L

Isonatremic dehydration is the most common type of dehydration, representing approximately 80% of reported cases of dehydration. Hypernatremic and hyponatremic dehydration make up between 5% and 10% of reported cases of dehydration.[82]

Isonatremic or Isotonic Dehydration

Isonatremic or isotonic dehydration occurs when sodium and water losses are of the same magnitude in both the intravascular and extravascular fluid compartments. There are no intercellular fluid shifts in isotonic dehydration.[83] This condition is also referred to as combined water and sodium deficit.[84]

Gastrointestinal disturbances causing extreme diarrhea and/or vomiting can trigger isotonic dehydration. This type of dehydration is often seen with food-borne illness, severe bleeding, excessive urine loss, and diuretic therapy. Clinical symptoms include unplanned weight loss, hypotension, orthostatic hypotension, rapid and weak pulse, rapid respirations, oliguria (dark, concentrated, and scanty urine), decreased skin turgor, dry mucous membranes, and altered levels of consciousness. Isotonic dehydration can lead to shock.[46,83]

The plasma sodium levels and plasma osmolality are within normal ranges. Urine specific gravity, plasma

TABLE 8-1 Laboratory Tests Used to Differentiate Different Types of Dehydration

Lab Test	Normal Values	Isotonic	Hypotonic	Hypertonic
Osmolality, serum	285–295 mOsm/kg H_2O; 285–295 mmol/kg H_2O	Normal	< Normal	>295 mOsm/kg H_2O; >295 mmol/kg H_2O
Sodium, serum	136–145 mEq/L; 136–145 mmol/L	Normal	< Normal	> Normal
Hemoglobin	F 12–16 gm/dL; 7.4–9.9 mmol/L M 14–18 gm/dL; 8.7–11.2 mmol/L	> Normal	> Normal	> Normal
Hematocrit	F 37–47%; 0.37–0.47 M 42–52%; 0.42–0.52	> Normal	> Normal	> Normal
Albumin, serum	3.5–5.0 gm/dL; 35–50 gm/L	> Normal	> Normal	> Normal
BUN	10–20 mg/dL; 3.6–7.1 mmol/L	> Normal	> Normal	> Normal
Urine specific gravity	1.005–1.030	> Normal	< 1.005	> 1.031

albumin, BUN, hemoglobin, and hematocrit are all elevated. These patients are not thirsty and do not sense the need for more fluid. Both isotonic fluids and sodium must be given to rehydrate the patient.[46,83] Table 8-1 summarizes the pattern of laboratory test results that is usually seen in isotonic dehydration.[45]

Hyponatremic or Hypotonic Dehydration

Hyponatremic or hypotonic dehydration occurs when the lost fluid contains more sodium than the blood does. Relatively more sodium is lost than fluid. This condition is also referred to as *primary sodium deficit*.[84]

Since the plasma sodium is low, the intravascular water shifts to the extravascular compartment, exaggerating intravascular volume depletion; this can lead to shock. The body's defense against hyponatremia is the renal excretion of sodium-free water. Hyponatremia is more likely to occur in a patient who tends to conserve water.[46,84]

Hypotonic dehydration can occur in the patient who is taking diuretics, is on a sodium-restricted diet, has heat exhaustion or heat stroke, is experiencing diarrhea or vomiting, has excessive sweating, has a renal sodium-wasting syndrome, is on NPO with ice chips for an extended number of days, or has a combination of these contributors. There is typically a reduction in extracellular fluid volume.[83]

Clinical symptoms associated with hyponatremia with decreased extracellular fluid volume include tachycardia, irritability, apprehension, dizziness, personality changes, postural hypotension, dry mucous membranes, cold and clammy skin, tremors, seizures, and coma. The clinical symptoms of hyponatremia typically do not appear until the plasma sodium is less than 120 mEq/L (120 mmol/L). Seizures, coma, and permanent neurologic damage can occur when plasma levels fall below 115 mEq/L (115 mmol/L).[46]

The laboratory tests indicate low plasma sodium, plasma osmolality, and urine specific gravity. Plasma albumin, hemoglobin, hematocrit, and BUN are greater than normal. Urine output is typically greater than normal. Evaluation of urine sodium concentration is helpful because a low level suggests inadequate sodium intake. Giving additional sodium will improve plasma sodium levels. However, if the sodium level in the urine is elevated, the hyponatremia is likely caused by chronic renal failure. Giving additional sodium in the diet will not improve plasma sodium levels and might cause fluid retention.[81]

The treatment for hypotonic dehydration includes giving hypertonic solutions to rehydrate the patient.[83] Table 8-1 summarizes the pattern of laboratory test results that is typically seen in hypotonic dehydration.[45]

Hypernatremic or Hypertonic Dehydration

Hypernatremic or hypertonic dehydration occurs when the lost fluid contains less sodium than the blood. Since the plasma sodium is high, the extravascular water shifts to the intravascular compartment, minimizing intravascular volume depletion. Hypertonic dehydration causes fluid to be drawn out of cells into the bloodstream, causing cellular shrinkage. This condition is also referred to as *volume depletion* or *volume deficit*.[84]

The patient typically has a reduced oral intake of fluids and may have significant losses of fluid from fever or sweating. Symptoms of hypernatremia include intense thirst, fatigue, restlessness, irritability, altered mental status, and coma. Signs of shock are not typically present. The patient may have a low-grade fever, flushed skin, peripheral and pulmonary edema, postural hypotension, tachycardia, increased muscle tone, and muscle twitching.[46]

The laboratory tests that suggest hypertonic dehydration include hypernatremia, hyperosmolality, elevated BUN, elevated BUN:creatinine ratio (assuming that kidney status is normal), elevated plasma albumin, elevated hemoglobin, elevated hematocrit, and increased urine specific gravity.[45] When patients who normally are hyponatremic develop hypertonic dehydration, the plasma sodium level may be within normal ranges. Without historic laboratory data for comparison, the diagnosis of hypertonic dehydration might be missed. Historic laboratory test data are vital to accurately assess the current status of an adult with declining health status. Hypertonic dehydration can also mask nutritional anemias and protein malnutrition because hemoglobin, hematocrit and plasma albumin are affected by the hemodilution. Once hydration status is normalized, these values will fall. It is important to recognize that the changes in hemoglobin, hematocrit, and plasma albumin might be due to a change in hydration status rather than a change in nutritional status. Table 8-1 summarizes the pattern of laboratory test results that is usually seen in hypertonic dehydration.[45]

Recommended Fluid Needs

Fluid needs are calculated on the basis of weight and/or calories consumed. Typically, 25 to 35 cc water per kilogram of body weight or 1 to 1.5 mL of water per calorie consumed are the recommended levels.[85-87] Individuals who consume less than 1000 calories daily will require a minimum of 1500 mL of fluid per day. Additional fluid needs to be added for draining wounds and other losses.

Nutritional Management: Micronutrients

Micronutrients appear to play a significant role in wound healing. Fat-soluble vitamins A, D, E, and K; water-soluble B vitamins; and ascorbic acid are involved in wound healing. Clinicians should observe patients for signs of vitamin or mineral deficiencies. Laboratory tests are available to confirm most vitamin or mineral deficiencies. However, these tests may be cost-prohibitive in the health care setting. Typically, assessment for micronutrient deficiencies is done by observation of physical signs and symptoms of various deficiency states. Dietary history may also be used to document suspected nutrient deficiencies. Individuals with a long history of very poor eating habits or who eat a limited number of foods are at greatest risk for vitamin and mineral deficiencies. The most commonly observed physical signs of malnutrition[17] are outlined in Table 8-2.

Recommendations for Meeting Micronutrient Needs

The AHRQ *Guidelines for the Treatment of Pressure Ulcers*[11] and supportive references recommend a multiple vitamin and mineral supplement as a standard part of the treatment plan if deficiency states are suspected or confirmed. Research published since the AHCRQ *Guidelines for the Treatment of Pressure Ulcers*[11] suggests that the use of selected supplemental micronutrients could enhance wound healing in some individuals.

Water-Soluble Vitamins

Assessment of Needs for Ascorbic Acid

Ascorbic acid (vitamin C) serves a variety of functions critical to wound healing. It stimulates the inflammatory response and improves resistance to infection by

TABLE 8-2 Selected Physical Signs of Malnutrition

Signs and Symptoms	Possible Nutrition-Related Causes
Pale eye membranes	Cyanocobalamin, folacin, iron deficiency
Night blindness, dry eye membranes, dull or soft cornea	Vitamin A, zinc deficiency
Angular fissures, scar at corner of mouth	Niacin, riboflavin, iron, or Vitamin B_6 deficiency
Spongy, swollen, easily bleeding gums	Vitamin C deficiency
Gingivitis	Folacin, cyanocobalamin deficiency
Cheilosis	Riboflavin, folacin, vitamin B_6 deficiency
Changes in tongue including sores, swollen, scarlet or raw	Folacin, niacin deficiency
Smooth tongue with papillae	Riboflavin, cyanocobalamin, vitamin B_6 deficiency
Glossitis of tongue	Iron, zinc, vitamin B_6 deficiency
Pallor of skin	Iron, folacin, cyanocobalamin, vitamin C deficiency
Spoon-shaped nails	Iron deficiency
Poor wound healing	Zinc deficiency
Bilateral edema	Protein deficiency
Limited fat stores, wasted appearance	Protein-energy deficiency
Loss of position, decrease and loss of ankle and knee reflexes, inability to concentrate, defective memory	Thiamin, cyanocobalamin deficiency
Peripheral neuropathy, dementia	Vitamin B_6 deficiency

increasing the white blood cell activity.[88] It plays a role in the hydroxylation of the essential amino acids proline and lysine, which are needed in collagen synthesis.[89] Wound healing involves a dramatic increase in collagen formation to fill the wound. Ascorbic acid deficiency delays wound healing. Ascorbic acid deficiency is rare in the United States, but subclinical states of deficiency are important.[36] Scientific evidence to support the use of ascorbic acid in patients without a deficiency or to accelerate wound healing remains controversial. Ascorbic acid is an antioxidant and appears to protect the wound against inflammatory injury.[19] During the initial inflammatory response, the immune system releases neutrophils to fight potential infection and to clean up the wound site. Neutrophils survive about 6 hours and may cause inflammatory injury as they degrade into free radicals.[19]

Taylor and colleagues[90] reported a positive relationship between supplementation of ascorbic acid and wound healing in 20 surgical patients with pressure ulcers. Patients were randomly assigned to receive either a high dose of ascorbic acid or a placebo. The patients who received the ascorbic acid experienced an 84% reduction in surface area compared to a 43% reduction in the placebo group. Supplementation significantly reduced the size of the pressure ulcer, but complete healing was not included as part of the study. However, Kessels and Knipschild[91] conducted a blind, randomized, controlled trial of 88 patients. They compared outcomes in patients with wounds receiving 10 mg twice per day or 500 mg twice per day of ascorbic acid to enhance healing rates.

After a 12-week trial, improved healing rates were not observed in the group that received ascorbic acid supplements. However, animal studies have supported the role of ascorbic acid in wound healing.[92]

The difference in the outcomes of the studies could be related to ascorbic acid deficiency states in patients with wounds. Selvaag and colleagues[9] evaluated various nutrient deficiencies in geriatric patients with pressure ulcers and found that plasma ascorbic acid levels were significantly lower than those in matched controls. Goode and colleagues[93] assessed baseline status for zinc; vitamins A, C, and E; albumin; and hemoglobin in elderly patients with hip fractures. Of these individuals, 48% developed pressure ulcers. The mean concentration for leukocyte ascorbic acid was significantly lower in those who later developed pressure ulcers. Brocklehurst and colleagues[94] compared mean leukocyte ascorbic acid concentrations and prevalence of pressure ulcers in elderly patients who received ascorbic acid supplements for 12 months compared to a control group. The group that received the supplements had a lower prevalence of pressure ulcers and an increased leukocyte ascorbic acid concentration.

Recommendations for Ascorbic Acid

The Dietary Reference Intakes (DRI) for ascorbic acid has increased for both adult males and females to 90 mg/day and 75 mg/day, respectively. An additional 35 mg/day is recommended for smokers. These levels were increased to provide maximum saturation of ascorbic acid in the body. Ascorbic acid needs can be met with a daily multivitamin supplement that provides 100% of the DRI for most patients.

The Upper Tolerable Intake Levels for ascorbic acid are set at 2000 mg/day.[95] Johnston[96] reported that plasma concentrations for ascorbic acid were higher in individuals who take ascorbic acid supplements than in those who do not: 75 to 80 µmol/L and 45 to 50 µmol/L, respectively. A daily supplement of approximately 1000 mg of ascorbic acid is required to maintain a plasma level of 75 to 80 µmol/L.

Ascorbic acid supplementation is contraindicated in some medical conditions. People who take large doses of ascorbic acid have a greater risk of developing kidney stones. The level of supplementation required to increase the risk for kidney stones is unknown, but even a few hundred milligrams of ascorbic acid per day can result in oxalosis. Oxalosis results in deposits of calcium oxalate in the heart, thyroid, and kidneys. Ascorbic acid provides up to 50% of the oxalic acid the body produces. The other amounts come from dietary intake of oxalates and metabolic pathways that convert glyoxylate to oxalic acid. Renal patients do not excrete oxalic acid. The level of oxalate in the blood is related to the level of ascorbic acid intake. The higher the dietary intake of ascorbic acid, the higher is the level of oxalate in the blood.[97]

Ascorbic acid supplementation is contraindicated for individuals with a history of kidney stones or chronic renal failure.

Assessment for B Vitamin Family

The B vitamin family consists of thiamin (B_1), riboflavin (B_2), niacin, pyridoxine (B_6), folic acid (B_9), cyanocobalamin (B_{12}), pantothenic acid, and biotin. These vitamins serve as cofactors in enzymatic reactions that are critical to the regulation of metabolism. Folic acid and cyanocobalamin are involved in DNA synthesis and, in deficient states, negatively affect red blood cell formation. Deficiencies of folic acid and cyanocobalamin result in macrocytic anemias that significantly decrease the oxygen-carrying capacity of the blood.

The DRI for folic acid is 400 µg/day for adult males and females, and the Upper Tolerable Intake Level is 1000 µg/day. The Food and Drug Administration has required that all enriched food be fortified with 140 µg of folic acid per 100 grams of flour. Decreased plasma folic acid levels are associated with hemolytic anemia, malnutrition, malabsorption syndromes, liver disease, and celiac disease. Megaloblastic anemia will occur after approximately 5 months of folic acid depletion due to increased needs, deficient diet, malabsorption of folic acid, or cyanocobalamin deficiency. Some medications are folic acid antagonists and interfere with nucleic acid synthesis. Box 8-1 lists the most common known folic acid antagonists.[98]

Folic acid needs for most patients with wounds can be met through diet or a daily multiple vitamin with 100% of the DRI for folic acid. Individuals taking medications that are folic acid antagonists will require higher doses of folic acid supplementation. Remember that megadoses of folic acid supplementation can mask a cyanocobalamin deficiency.

The DRI for cyanocobalamin is 2.4 µg/day for adult males and females, and the Upper Tolerable Intake Level is not determinable owing to lack of data on adverse effects. Pernicious anemia may be due to lack of dietary cyanocobalamin or underutilization of cyanocobalamin. Malabsorption of cyanocobalamin is reported in 10%

BOX 8–1 Medications That Are Folic Acid Antagonists

Acetylsalicylic acid
Allopurinol
Colchicine
Hydrocortisone
Phenobarbital
Phenytoin
Sulfamethoxazole
Sulfasalazine
Triamterene
Trimethoprim

BOX 8–2 Medications Associated with Low Serum Cyanocobalamin Levels

Allopurinol
Cimetidine
Phenobarbital
Phenytoin
Primidone

to 30% of adults over age 50 years.[99] The most common etiology is inadequate secretion of intrinsic factor due to a gastric mucosa defect. When cyanocobalamin is ingested, it combines with intrinsic factor and is absorbed in the distal part of the ileum. Without intrinsic factor, cyanocobalamin cannot be absorbed, body stores are depleted, and the body is unable to produce normal red blood cells. However, in about 40% of cases of pernicious anemia, the red blood cells are normocytic.[100–101] The macrocytic red blood cells are produced at a slower rate, have a shorter life span, and carry less hemoglobin. Iron supplementation will not significantly improve hemoglobin levels.

Some medications are associated with low plasma cyanocobalamin levels.[81] Box 8-2 lists the most common medications affecting cyanocobalamin levels.

Cyanocobalamin needs can be met through diet or a daily multiple vitamin with 100% of the DRI for cyanocobalamin. Individuals who take medications that are associated with low plasma levels of cyanocobalamin might require higher doses of supplementation. Oral cyanocobalamin supplements are effective if the body can produce adequate levels of intrinsic factor. If the body is unable to produce adequate levels of intrinsic factor, monthly injections of cyanocobalamin are recommended.

Fat-Soluble Vitamins

Assessment of Needs for Vitamin A

Vitamin A is a stimulant for the onset of the wound-healing process, including epithelialization and fibroblast deposition of collagen. Vitamin A is found in a variety of foods and might not need to be supplemented beyond the DRI except for steroid-retarded wounds, for suspected vitamin A deficiency, and for impaired wound healing following radiotherapy. Suspected vitamin A deficiency states can be confirmed by a low plasma retinol and the results of functional tests such as dark adaptation.

If the patient is taking antimetabolites or corticosteroids, the wound might not heal because of the anti-inflammatory effect of these medications.[102] Glucocorticoids impair most aspects of wound healing, including inflammatory response, fibroblast proliferation, deposition of collagen, capillary regeneration, wound contraction, and epithelial migration.[75,103–105] The detrimental effects of

glucocorticoids vary with the specific type, dosage, and timing.[104] The greater likelihood of impaired healing seems to occur when steroids are given at the time of wounding or between 2 and 4 days after the wound develops.[105–107]

Short-term use of megadoses of vitamin A have been shown to reverse the detrimental effects of corticosteroids but do not decrease the incidence of wound infections or improve delayed wound contraction.[102–103,106–109] It is important to note that systemic vitamin A supplementation can reactivate the inflammatory process and impair the action of the glucocorticoids.

Vitamin A supplementation appears to prevent the impairment of wound healing following local or whole-body radiation therapy in animal models. Taking supplemental vitamin A up to 2 days prior to radiation therapy or following therapy prevented impaired wound healing.[110,111]

Topical application of vitamin A–enriched products has been examined for chronic wounds. Topical vitamin A may be clinically effective for chronic wounds.[102,112,113] It may also play a role in reversing the local steroid effect.[114]

Recommendations for Vitamin A

The DRI for vitamin A appears to meet the needs of most individuals with wounds. However, in patients with a fat malabsorption syndrome, those with suspected or confirmed deficiencies, and those with increased needs, such as patients with burns or chronic infections, may benefit from supplementation of vitamin A at doses of 2300 IU for females and 3000 IU/day for males. The Upper Tolerable Intake Levels for vitamin A have been established at 10,000 IU/day or 3000 RAE.

For high-risk patients, Levenson and Demetriou[103] suggest 25,000 IU/day prior to and after surgery for malnourished patients with gastrointestinal tract dysfunction, all patients with serious injury, patients undergoing surgery that will interfere with alimentation for long periods of time, and patients who develop gut complications after surgery.

For steroid-retarded wounds, megadose supplements of vitamin A are given for a limited period of time. Between 10,000 and 25,000 IU of vitamin A are given orally per day or 10,000 to 15,000 IU intravenously per day for 7 to 21 days. If the wound has not responded, vitamin A should be discontinued.[75,92,102,112]

Assessment of Needs for Vitamin E

There are several alcohol compounds known as tocopherols that possess vitamin E activity. Alpha-tocopherol is the most active of these. The principal function of vitamin E in the body is to act as an antioxidant. Vitamin E maintains cell membrane integrity by preventing peroxidation of polyunsaturated fatty acids contained in the membrane of phospholipids. The role of vitamin E in healing surgical wounds or pressure ulcers is unclear. Deficiency of vitamin E is rare in humans.

Research is limited on the beneficial and detrimental effects of vitamin E supplementation on wound healing. Potential benefits from supplementation are following hyperbaric oxygen therapy. Skin-flap survival improved significantly with a combination of conservative hyperbaric oxygen therapy and moderate vitamin E supplementation in rats compared to groups that did not receive vitamin E.[114] Levy and colleagues[115] demonstrated that vitamin E given prior to hyperbaric oxygen therapy decreased the risk of potential seizures in animal studies.

Supplementation of vitamin E may have detrimental effects on wound healing. Ehrlich and Hunt[116] demonstrated that vitamin E supplementation resulted in decreased rate of collagen synthesis and decreased tensile strength in animal models. The effects of supplementation of vitamin E are similar to those seen with glucocorticoids.[117] Giving megadoses of vitamin A simultaneously seemed to have reversed the negative effects of vitamin E.[116]

Recommendations for Vitamin E

The recommended daily allowance for vitamin E as alpha-tocopherol is 15 mg/day for adult men and women. The Upper Tolerable Intake Level is 1000 mg/day. Intakes of vitamin E greater than 1000 mg/day have been associated with an increased tendency to hemorrhage. Dietary intakes of vitamin E from a variety of foods will most likely meet needs. Individuals with malabsorption syndromes may have increased needs and might benefit from a water-soluble form of vitamin E. A multiple vitamin would most likely meet their needs.

Large doses of vitamin E should not be recommended for individuals with surgical wounds or pressure ulcers unless a deficiency is confirmed. A deficiency state can be confirmed by using laboratory test results as noted in Table 8-3.

Assessment of Needs for Vitamin K

Vitamin K is found in plant-based foods in the form of phylloquinone, or K1. Menaquinone-7, or K2, is synthesized by bacteria in the intestine. Vitamin K is essential for wound healing at the time immediately following wounding for the formation of clot factors II, VII, IX,

and X. Prothrombin (clot factor II) combines with other factors to produce thrombin. Thrombin and fibrinogen form fibrin, resulting in a blood clot.[88]

A deficiency of vitamin K is rare, owing to endogenous synthesis, but it can occur with chronic antibiotic therapy, fat malabsorption, and liver disease. Deficiency symptoms need to be treated aggressively to prevent a potentially lethal hemorrhage. Vitamin K needs for wound healing for most patients can be met with a multivitamin with 100% DRI of 90 µg/day for females and 120 µg/day for males. The Upper Tolerable Intake Level has not been determined.

Micronutrients: Minerals and Trace Elements

Minerals that are involved in wound healing include calcium, magnesium, sodium, potassium, and chloride. Trace elements that are involved in wound healing include zinc, copper, and iron.

Trace Elements

Assessment of Needs for Zinc

Zinc is an essential trace mineral that is involved in cell replication, protein synthesis, collagen synthesis, and immune function. Approximately 20% of the total body zinc stores are found in the skin.[118]

Zinc deficiency has been associated with impaired wound healing.[113,119] The role of zinc in delayed wound healing was first proposed in 1967.[120] Norris and Reynolds[121] evaluated healing rates of pressure ulcers in patients receiving 200 mg of zinc sulfate daily for 12 weeks. In a study using a blind, crossover research design, no significant improvement was demonstrated in the supplemented group.

Haggard and colleagues[122] reported a retrospective study of the effects of zinc supplementation in institutionalized elderly residents with pressure ulcers. Healing rates of residents who were given 440 mg zinc per day were compared to unsupplemented residents. No significant decrease in days required to heal the pressure ulcers was noted.

Hallbook and Lanner[123] reported improvement in healing of chronic venous leg ulcers in patients receiving 220 mg of zinc sulfate daily who had initial plasma zinc levels of less than 100 µg/dL. No benefit was observed in supplemented patients with initial plasma zinc levels greater than 110 µg/dL or the control group. Wilkinson and Hawke[124] reviewed all the randomized controlled trials utilizing zinc supplementation for chronic venous and arterial leg ulcers and concluded that no statistically significant benefit was shown in any of the studies.

Zinc supplementation for patients with wounds remains controversial.[125-126] Although the animal models suggest

TABLE 8-3   Laboratory Test Results for Vitamin E Deficiency

Levels of α-Tocopherol*	Conventional Units	SI Units
Acceptable levels	≥ 7.0 µg/mL	≥ 16.2 µmol/L
Low levels	5.0–7.0 µg/mL	11.6–16.2 µmol/L
Deficient levels	< 5.0 µg/mL	< 11.6 µmol/L

*Use an α-tocopherol to lipid ratio if hyperlipidemia is present.

a link between zinc and wound healing,[126] the same results have not been replicated in human trials.[36,118,121]

Recommendations for Zinc

The DRI[127] for zinc for male and female adults is 11 mg and 8 mg, respectively. Zinc intakes below the recommended daily allowance are commonly reported in elderly people,[11] especially those over the age of 71 years.[128] The median zinc intake from food and the DRI for zinc are approximately 9 mg/day for females and 13 mg/day for males.[99] The Upper Tolerable Intake Level for zinc is 40 mg/day for adult males and females.[99]

Losses of zinc occur with large skin wounds, from diarrhea, and in urine following trauma or closed head injury. Adults who are at greatest risk for a zinc deficiency include elderly people and patients with celiac disease, Crohn's disease, short bowel syndrome, AIDS enteropathy, ileostomy, chronic diarrhea, enteric fistula output, chronic liver disease, cirrhosis, nephrotic syndrome, diabetes, alcoholism, trauma, burns, and sickle-cell anemia. Medications that promote increased losses of zinc include penicillamine, diuretics, diethylenetriamine penta-acetate, and valproate.[98]

Low-dose (25 to 50 mg elemental zinc daily) supplementation or use of a multiple vitamin with the DRI for zinc is warranted when a deficiency state is suspected, when there is an increased need or a significant loss of zinc stores, until epithelialization is well established, or until full closure of the wound. Duration of high-dose supplementation (>100 mg/day) should be limited to 2 to 3 weeks to reduce the risk of adverse effects.[75]

Chronic excessive intakes of zinc can have a negative impact on copper and iron status. Zinc, copper, and iron all compete for the same receptor sites on cells. Too much zinc can cause a copper and iron deficiency because high levels of zinc block the receptor sites, and the cells then do not have access to copper and iron. Copper is required as an enzyme cofactor for collagen cross-linking. A copper deficiency will affect tensile strength and elasticity of skin in the healing wound.

Even low supplemental doses of 25 mg elemental zinc per day over a long time can impair copper absorption.[129] Higher doses of 110 to 165 mg elemental zinc daily for 10 months resulted in copper deficiency in healthy volunteers. However, a copper deficiency was not observed after 6 weeks of 110 to 165 mg elemental zinc daily.[129]

Copper deficiencies are rarely seen except when due to high intakes of supplemental zinc. The high doses of zinc deplete the body of copper. When zinc supplementation is reduced, the body can replace the copper with dietary sources of copper, and wound healing will resume.

Chronic use of megadoses of zinc can result in impaired immune function.[129-132] The immune responses of healthy volunteers were evaluated before and after a 6-week trial of 300 mg elemental zinc. Immune function was impaired following the supplement trial period.[131] However, lower levels of zinc supplementation (100 mg elemental zinc daily for 3 months) did not appear to negatively affect the immune response in an elderly population.[129]

High levels of supplemental zinc also affect lipid profiles. Chandra[131] reported decreased HDL-cholesterol and increased LDL-cholesterol levels in healthy volunteers following a 6-week trial on 300 mg elemental zinc daily. No changes in triglycerides were observed. HDL-cholesterol was also reduced in volunteers taking 160 mg of elemental zinc daily for 6 weeks.[129]

Extremely high doses of elemental zinc are associated with acute symptoms, including nausea, vomiting, epigastric pain, lethargy, and fatigue. Long-term consequences of excessive zinc intake were discussed in the previous section. Short-term use of low-dosage supplements (25 to 50 mg elemental zinc per day) may be helpful in some patients with a suspected zinc deficiency or who have increased needs. Currently, there is no accurate biochemical indicator of zinc status to confirm suspected zinc deficiencies. Plasma zinc levels are affected by acute inflammatory response and hypoalbuminemia owing to redistribution of stores. Homeostatic mechanisms appear to maintain zinc plasma concentrations despite weeks of severe dietary intakes. A decreased plasma alkaline phosphatase is commonly observed with a zinc deficiency, although this test is not specific for zinc status.[45] Needs for wound healing for most patients can be met with a multivitamin with minerals providing 100% of the DRI for zinc.

Assessment of Needs for Copper

The primary function of copper is as a component of enzymes such as cytochrome-C, superoxide dismutase, and lysyl oxide. Lysyl oxide is required for collagen synthesis and formation of collagen cross-linkages, necessary for its tensile strength. Inadequate copper will impair collagen synthesis and delay wound healing. Excess zinc interferes with copper metabolism and the action of lysyl oxidase.

Copper is bound to ceruloplasmin and transported by albumin. A protein deficiency can result in a secondary copper deficiency due to lack of transport. Symptoms of a copper deficiency include hypochromic microcytic anemia, leukopenia, and neutropenia.[88]

Recommendations for Copper

The DRI for copper is 900 mg/day for males and females. Antacids can interfere with copper absorption when used in high dosages.[133] Needs for wound healing for most patients can be met with a multivitamin with minerals providing 100% of the DRI for copper.

Assessment of Needs for Iron

Nutritional anemia is a common problem in patients with wounds. The etiology of anemia may be blood loss, deficient erythropoiesis, or excessive hemolysis.[134] There are four types of nutritional anemias:

- Iron-deficiency anemia
- Anemia of chronic disease
- Pernicious anemia (B_{12} deficiency)
- Megaloblastic anemia (folic acid deficiency)

All four types of anemia have symptoms of low hemoglobin and hematocrit levels. More laboratory tests, such as mean corpuscular volume, plasma iron, total iron-binding capacity, and red cell distribution width, are needed to determine whether the anemia is related to unmet iron needs. If the mean corpuscular volume is elevated or plasma iron is elevated, more tests for plasma levels of folic acid and cyanocobalamin are needed to determine whether the anemia is due to unmet folic acid or cyanocobalamin needs. Once the etiology of the anemia has been determined, proper treatment is essential to meet the needs of the patient.

Iron plays a role in wound healing as a cofactor in hydroxylation of lysine and proline for collagen synthesis. It is also a component of many enzyme systems.[135] However, low hemoglobin levels resulting in impaired oxygen-carrying capacity of cells do not appear to significantly impair wound healing if there is adequate tissue perfusion at the wound site.[104,112,136] Folic acid and cyanocobalamin are involved in DNA and RNA synthesis. Deficient levels are evident in the macrocytic red blood cells, but all cells of the body are potentially affected by megaloblastic and pernicious anemia.

Recommendations for Iron

The recommended daily allowance for iron for adult men and postmenopausal women is 8 mg/day and 18 mg/day for premenopausal women. Individuals who are at risk for iron-deficiency anemia include those with chronic blood loss in the gastrointestinal tract due to cancer, inflammatory bowel disease, peptic ulcers, or parasites; chronic renal failure; poor diet; malabsorption due to celiac disease, Crohn's disease, or short bowel syndrome; and achlorhydria due to atrophic gastritis, gastrectomy, or gastric by-pass. Many medications promote the loss of iron, including chronic aspirin use; proton pump inhibitors, such as omeprazole and lansoprazole; H-2 blockers, such as cimetidine, ranitidine, and famotidine; and high doses of calcium, magnesium, or zinc. Iron is lost in the exudate of large draining wounds.[137]

Iron needs for most patients with wounds can be met through diet or a daily multiple vitamin with minerals providing 100% DRI for iron.

Amino Acids

Assessment of Needs for Amino Acid Supplements

Under physiologic stress, some of the nonessential amino acids become conditionally essential because the body is unable to synthesize enough of these specific amino acids to meet the demands of the body under stress. Arginine and glutamine are two nonessential amino acids that become conditionally essential under physiologic stress. Historically, these amino acids have been used in parenteral and enteral nutrition but not as supplements for individuals eating by mouth. Researchers have examined the role of arginine and glutamine in wound healing.

Assessment of Needs for Arginine

The majority of arginine is produced through a metabolic collaboration between the small intestine and the kidneys. Glutamine, glutamate, and proline can be converted to citrulline by the enterocyte. The intestine-derived citrulline is then released into the general circulation and taken up by the kidney for conversion to arginine, which supplies the body's needs. The synthesis of adequate amounts of arginine requires adequate amounts of its natural precursors, glutamate and proline.[138] Intestinal diseases or provision of nutrition through total parenteral nutrition[138–139] can interfere with arginine synthesis and make it conditionally essential.

In addition, arginine functions as an intermediate in the urea cycle for the detoxification of ammonia. It is the sole substrate for nitric oxide production and is a substrate for the synthesis of the amino acids ornithine and proline. Arginine is a precursor to polyamines and regulator of nucleic acid synthesis. It is the sole substrate for nitric oxide synthase that produces nitric oxide, critical to wound collagen accumulation and acquisition of mechanical strength. Enhanced nitric oxide production activates wound macrophages and neutrophils and leads to improved microvascular hemodynamic changes. The macrophages deliver arginine to the wound via cell lysis. The increased level of arginine activity increases the conversion of arginine to ornithine. Ornithine is a precursor to proline, which is incorporated into collagen.[140–142] Further, it is a secretagogue of hormones such as insulin, growth hormone, and insulin-like growth factor-1.[143]

Arginine has been found to promote healing in healthy adults and elders who are eating sufficient energy and protein. Administering arginine (17 or 24.8 g) to normal middle-aged volunteers for 2 weeks improved collagen synthesis as determined by collagen deposition in a plastic tube implanted in the subcutaneous tissue.[144] In a study of healthy older adults (>65 years of age), administration of 17 g of L-arginine for 2 weeks was shown to improve wound bed protein and hydroxyproline accumulation in subcutaneous catheters and to result in greater lymphocyte responses and elevated levels of insulin-like growth factor-1.[145]

While these studies show the benefit of arginine on artificially induced acute incisional wounds in healthy individuals, it is unknown whether arginine would have the same effect on healing of diabetic ulcers.[143] Also, there are no data that demonstrate that supplemental arginine actually improves healing of wounds sustained following an injury or operation, thus enhancing clinical outcome in patients.[146] Clinical judgment and close follow-up of clinical outcomes are required in recommending arginine for delayed wound healing because of limited evidence-based support. The Food and Nutrition Board found minimal evidence of adverse effects from arginine supplementation at intakes up to 24.8 g/day of free arginine base.[127] Barbul[147] reached a similar conclusion, finding that large doses (e.g., 30 g L-arginine per day) have been used without significant adverse effects but that infrequent gastrointestinal symptoms such as bloating and mild diarrhea have been reported at some of the higher intake levels.

Recommendations for Arginine

Arginine is found in a variety of foods, but the volume of intake required to provide 17 to 24 grams is prohibitive. Arginine is available in pill and powdered forms. The product insert should be consulted to determine the quantity required to provide the recommended level of supplementation.

Standard tube-feeding formulas typically contain 1 to 2 g/L of arginine. Specially formulated enteral formulas contain 12.5 to 18.7 g/L or approximately 2% of calories. Powdered arginine products can be mixed with most liquids and added to commercially prepared enteral formulas.

Assessment of Needs for Glutamine

The body produces approximately 60 to 100 g/day of glutamine daily, especially in muscle and lung.[148–149] Glutamine is catabolized for energy in the intestine, resulting in the production of CO_2, alanine, pyruvate, lactate, and ammonia.[150] Some glutamine will not be utilized for energy by the gut but will be metabolized in the splanchnic tissues to citrulline, arginine, glutamate, or proline,[150] which will be transported via portal blood to the liver.

Glutamine has a number of key functions beyond its incorporation into body proteins. One central function of glutamine is to serve as a nitrogen transport mechanism in the body, carrying both carbon and nitrogen from peripheral tissue to the kidney and liver, which produce NH_3 and urea, respectively. In addition, glutamine is a principal fuel source for enterocytes and immune

tissues (lymph nodes, spleen, thymus, Peyer's patches, and leukocytes). It also is a precursor of the glutamate that is necessary for the production of glutathione in many cell types, including enterocytes, neural cells, liver cells, and lymphocytes.[148]

During catabolic states, the muscle's production of glutamine increases, owing to the activation of muscle protein breakdown and the enzyme glutamine synthetase. There is a dramatic increase in utilization of glutamine, resulting in depletion of muscle glutamine.[151] Since muscle is the source of most body glutamine, the decreased muscle mass found in older individuals might limit the amount of glutamine available during stress conditions. Thus, glutamine supplementation may have a beneficial effect in aged individuals who are injured or under some sort of physiologic stress.[152]

There is considerable evidence that hypercatabolic or hypermetabolic situations are accompanied by a marked depression of muscle intracellular glutamine.[151] It is also clear that glutamine is helpful for patients with a disease state or treatment that threatens the intestinal mucosa, and there is evidence that it might reduce pneumonia, bacteremia, and septic events in patients who are on enteral formula.[153]

Few adverse effects have been reported, despite the substantial number of published investigations in which glutamine has been administered to humans.[154–155] Zeigler and colleagues[156] reported that doses of up to 0.57 g/kg/day (e.g., 40 g/day for a 70-kg man) have been given without any adverse effect being reported. However, the Food and Nutrition Board points out that the published studies of toxicity have not fully taken account of a number of important factors, including the chronic consumption of glutamine.[154] There has been some concern that glutamine supplementation might promote tumor growth by acting as a fuel source, although evidence points to the contrary, and studies have not confirmed this suspicion.[154]

Glutamine supplementation is contraindicated in patients with hepatic failure and chronic renal failure. Blood ammonia levels are of concern if the patient has liver disease. Patients with chronic renal insufficiency might have an altered metabolism of glutamine. Glutamine may also be contraindicated for patients who are taking methotrexate because supplementation might inhibit renal clearance of the drug, resulting in increased plasma levels of the medication.

Recommendations for Glutamine

Fürst and Stehle[151] have suggested a tentative glutamine requirement of ~0.15 to 0.20 g/kg/day after uncomplicated major operations, major injury, or gastrointestinal malfunctions and during cachexia and a requirement of ~0.3 to 0.5 g/kg/day for critical illness. This is somewhat contradictory to the results of Ziegler and colleagues, who concluded that doses lower than 0.285 g/kg/day had no benefit over standard feeding.[156] No studies have examined the role of glutamine supplementation to promote healing of diabetic foot ulcers. Because of limited evidence-based support, clinical judgment and close follow-up of clinical outcomes are required in recommending glutamine for delayed wound healing.

Glutamine is found in a variety of animal products but is destroyed with cooking. Supplemental glutamine is available in powdered form and tablets. The product insert should be consulted for the concentration of glutamine in powders and tablets to determine appropriate daily needs. Glutamine is added to selected commercially prepared tube-feeding formulas. Free glutamine is unstable in solution and is typically available in small amounts in most commercially prepared enteral feedings. Peptide-based products may contain even less glutamine because of the degradation of glutamine during hydrolysis. Powdered glutamine products can be mixed with any liquid and added to commercially prepared enteral formulas.

Combination Amino Acid Therapy

Mixtures of various amino acids have been evaluated in clinical settings for wound healing. A mixture of β-hydroxy-β methylbutyrate (HMB), arginine, and glutamine was shown to be effective in increasing fat-free mass of middle-aged and older patients with advanced-stage cancer[157] and in younger subjects with AIDS-associated wasting.[158] HMB is a metabolite of leucine that has been demonstrated to reduce the rate of proteolysis in animals and humans.[159] Researchers have hypothesized that HMB might increase collagen deposition, inhibit muscle proteolysis, and modulate protein turnover.[160] There did not appear to be any adverse effects of this mixture in the treatment of muscle wasting associated with AIDS or cancer.[161]

Williams and colleagues[160] evaluated the effect on wound healing by giving healthy elderly volunteers a supplement containing 3 g of HMB, 14 g of glutamine, and 14 g of arginine for 14 days. After 2 weeks, there was a significant increase in hydroxyproline content in implanted catheters in the study group, suggesting an increase in collagen deposition in subcutaneous catheters as reflected by hydroxyproline content. However, the total protein deposition in the control group was not significantly different from that in the study group. It is unclear which of the components in the mixture were involved in wound healing or whether the combination created a synergistic effect. It is also important to note that the study was not conducted in individuals with delayed and chronic wounds, that is, pressure ulcers, diabetic ulcers, and the like. More research is needed to determine whether a mixture of arginine, glutamine, and HMB would have the same effect on healing in these patients.

Implications for Practice

Medical nutrition therapy recommendations for patients with diabetic foot ulcers are based on individualized assessment by a registered dietitian or other qualified professional. The AHRQ Guidelines and the recommendations in this chapter serve as a framework from which to begin. However, there is no cookie-cutter approach to healing diabetic foot ulcers. Comorbidities, laboratory test results, and medications must be considered before recommendations are made. All medical nutrition therapy interventions should be reevaluated routinely to determine whether a change needs to be considered.[162]

References

1. King KM, Rubin G: A history of diabetes: From antiquity to discovering insulin. Br J Nurs 12(18):1091–1095, 2003.
2. Burrow GN, Hazlett BE, Phillips MJ: A case of diabetes mellitus. N Engl J Med 306(6):340–343, 1982.
3. American Diabetes Association: Standard of medical care for patients with diabetes mellitus. Diabetes Care 25(10):213–229, 2002.
4. Beaser RS, Ganda OP, Haffner SM: Joslin Diabetes Center Guidelines for Screening and Management of Dyslipidemia Associated with Diabetes. Boston, Josline Diabetes Center, 2005.
5. Diabetes Control and Complications Trial Research Group: The effect of intensive treatment of diabetes complications in insulin-dependent diabetes mellitus. N Engl J Med 329:977–986, 1993.
6. Lawson ML, Gerstein HC, Tsui E, Zinman B: Effect of intensive therapy on early macrovascular disease in young adults with type 1 diabetes. Diabetes Care 22(suppl 1):B35–B39, 1999.
7. Demling RH, DeSanti L: Involuntary weight loss and the non-healing cutaneous wound. Medscape Clinical Update, 1999. Available at http://www.mwdscape.com/viewprogram/714_pnt.
8. Horn SD, Bender SA, Bergstrom N, et al: Description of the national pressure ulcer long-term care study. J Am Geriatr Soc 50:1816–1825, 2002.
9. Selvaag E, Bohmer T, Benkestock K: Reduced serum concentrations of riboflavin and ascorbic acid, and blood thiamine pyrophosphate and pyridoxal-5-phosphate in geriatric patients with and without pressure ulcers. J Nutr Health Aging 6(1):75–77, 2002.
10. Mathus-Vliegen EM: Nutritional status, nutrition and pressure ulcers. Nutr Clin Pract 16:286–291, 2001.
11. AHCPR Clinical Practice Guidelines: Treatment of Pressure Ulcers. Publication 95-0652. Rockville, MD, Agency for Healthcare Research and Quality, 1994.
12. Kalmijn S, Curb JD, Rodriguez K, et al: The association of body weight and anthropometry with mortality in elderly men: The Honolulu heart program. Int J Obes Relat Metab Disord 23:395–402, 1999.
13. Lyder, CH, Preston, J, Grady, JN, et al: Quality of care for hospitalized medicare patients at risk for pressure ulcers. Arch Intern Med 161:1549–1554, 2001.
14. Consortium for Spinal Cord Medicine: Pressure ulcer prevention and treatment following spinal cord injury: A clinical practice guideline for healthcare professionals, 2000. Available at www.pva.org/NEWPVASITE/publications/cpg_pubs/PU.pdf.
15. Wipke-Tevis DD, Rantz CM, Mehr DR, et al: Prevalence, incidence, management and predictors of venous ulcers in the long-term-care population using the MDS. Adv Wound Care 13(5):218, 2000.
16. Wipke-Tevis DD, Stotts NA: Tissue oxygenation, perfusion and position in patients with venous leg ulcers. J Vasc Nurs 16:48–56, 1998.
17. Neidert KC (ed): Nutrition for the Older Adult. Chicago, IL, American Dietetic Association, 2005, pp 8–20.
18. Litchford MD: Common Denominators of Declining Nutritional Status. Greensboro, NC, CASE Software & Books, 2005.

19. Demling RH, DeSanti L: (2001) Protein-energy malnutrition and the nonhealing cutaneous wound. Medscape Clinical Update, 2001. Available at http://www.medscape.com.
20. Wallace JI, Schwartz RS, LaCroix AZ, et al: Involuntary weight loss in older outpatients: Incidence of clinical significance. J Am Geriat Soc 43:329–337, 1995.
21. Kotler D, Tierney AR, Wang J, Pierson RN: Magnitude of cell body mass depletion and timing of death from wasting in AIDS. Am J Clin Nutr 40:444–447, 1989.
22. Kimball MJ, Williams-Burgess C: Failure to thrive: The silent epidemic of the elderly. Arch Psych Nurs 9:99–105, 1995.
23. Cerra F: Hypermetabolism organ failure and metabolic support. Surgery 191:1–28, 1987.
24. Breslow RA, Hallfrisch J, Guy DG, et al: The importance of dietary protein in healing pressure ulcers. J Am Geriatric Soc 41:357–362, 1993.
25. Wolfe R: An integrated analysis of glucose, fat and protein metabolism in severely traumatized patients. Ann Surg 209:63–72, 1989.
26. Wolfe R: Relation of metabolic studies to clinical nutrition: The example of burn injury. Am J Clin Nutr 64:800–808, 1996.
27. Kester P, Caplan R, Souba W, Andrassy R: Metabolic response to trauma. Contemp Orthop 14:53–59, 1987.
28. Lukaski H: Methods for the assessment of human body composition. Am J Clin Nutr 46:163–175, 1987.
29. Lee RD, Nieman DC: Nutritional Assessment, 2nd ed. St. Louis, Mosby, 1996.
30. Harris JS, Benedict, FG: A Biometric Study of Basal Metabolism in Man. Publication 279. Washington, DC, Carnegie Institution of Washington, 1919.
31. Owen OE, Holup JL, D'Alessio DA, et al: A reappraisal of the calorie requirements of men. Am J Clin Nutr 46:875–885, 1987.
32. Roza AM, Shizgal HM: The Harris-Benedict equation reevaluated: Resting energy requirements and the body cell mass. Am J Clin Nutr 40:168–172, 1984.
33. National Pressure Ulcer Advisory Panel: Available at www.naup.org.
34. Evans JM, Andrew KL, Chutka DS, et al: Pressure ulcers: prevention and management. Mayo Clin Proc 70(8):789–799, 1995.
35. Chernoff R, Milton K, Lipschitz D: The effect of a very high-protein liquid formula (Replete) on decubitus ulcer healing in long-term tube-fed institutionalized patients [abstract]. J Am Diet Assoc 90(9):A-130, 1990.
36. Thomas D: The role of nutrition in prevention and healing of pressure ulcers. Clin Geriatr Med 13(3):497–508, 1997.
37. Breslow R: Nutritional status and dietary intake of patients with pressure ulcers: Review of research literature 1943 to 1989. Decubitus 4:16–21, 1991.
38. Breslow RA, Bergstrom N: Nutritional predication of pressure ulcers. J Am Diet Assoc 94(11):1301–1304, 1994.
39. Ahmad A, Duerksen DR, Mounroe S, Bistrian BR: An evaluation of rest energy expenditure in hospitalized, severely underweight patients. Nutrition. 15(5):384–384, 1999.
40. Food and Nutrition Board, National Research Council: Recommended Dietary Allowances, 10th ed. Washington, DC, National Academy Press, 1989.
41. Campbell WW, Ceim CC, Young VR, Evans WJ: Increased protein requirements in elderly people: New data and retrospective reassessments. Am J Clin Nutr 60:501–09, 1994.
42. Castaneda C, Polnikowski GG, Dallal GE, Evans WJ: Elderly women accommodate to a low-protein diet with losses of body cell mass, muscle function and immune response. Am J Clin Nutr 62:30–39, 1995.
43. Evans WJ, Cyr-Campbell D: Nutrition, exercise and healthy aging. J Am Diet Assoc 97(6):623–638, 1997.
44. Cederholm T, Jagren C, Hellstrom K: Outcomes of protein-energy malnutrition in elderly medical patients. Am J Med 98:67–74, 1995.
45. Litchford MD: Practical Applications in Laboratory Assessment of Nutritional Status. Greensboro, NC, CASE Software & Books, 2006.
46. Heitz UE, Horne MM: Fluid, Electrolyte and Acid-Balance. St. Louis, Mosby, 2001.
47. Bergstrom NI: Strategies for preventing pressure ulcers. Clin Geriatr Med 13(3):437–454, 1997.
48. Fuhrman MP, Charney P, Mueller CM: Hepatic proteins and nutrition assessment. J Am Diet Assoc 104:1258–1262, 2004.
49. Niedert KC (ed): Pocket Resource for Nutrition Assessment. Chicago, IL, American Dietetic Association, 2005.
50. Puskarich-May CL, Sullivan DH, Nelson CL, et al: The change in serum protein concentration in response to the stress of total joint surgery: A comparison of older versus younger patients. J Am Geriatr Soc 44:555–558, 1996.
51. Bondestam M, Foucard T, Mehri GM: Serum albumin, retinol-binding protein, thyroxin-binding prealbumin and acute phase reactants as indicators of undernutrition in children with undue susceptibility to acute infections. Acta Paediatr Scand 77:94–98, 1988.
52. Smith FR, Goodman DS, Zaklama JS, et al: Serum vitamin A, retinol-binding protein, and prealbumin concentrations in PCM: I. A functional defect in hepatic retinol release. Am J Clin Nutr 26:973, 1973.
53. Deodhar SD: C-reactive protein: The best laboratory indicator available for monitoring disease activity. Cleve Clin J Med 56:126, 1989.
54. Ingenbleek Y, Van Den Schrieck HG, De Nayer P, DeVisscher M: The role of retinol binding protein in protein calorie malnutrition. Metabolism 24:633–641, 1975.
55. Collins N: Assessment and treatment of involuntary weight loss and protein-energy malnutrition. Adv Skin Wound Care 3(suppl 1):4–10, 2000.
56. Iribarren C, Reed DM, Burchfiel CM, Dwyer JH: Serum total cholesterol and mortality: Confounding factors and risk modification in Japanese-American men. JAMA 273:1926–1932, 1995.
57. Grant MD, Piotrowski ZH, Miles TP: Declining cholesterol and mortality in a sample of older nursing home residents. J Am Geriatr Soc 44:31–36, 1996.
58. Hu P, Seeman TE, Harris TB, Reuben DB: Does inflammation or undernutrition explain the low cholesterol-mortality association in high functioning older person?: MacArthur studies of successful aging. J Am Geriatr Soc 51:80–84, 2003.
59. Verdery RB, Golbderg AP: Hypocholesterolemia as a predictor of death: A prospective study of 224 nursing home residents. J Gerontol Med Sci 46:M84–90, 1991.
60. Rand WM, Pellett PL, Young V: Meta-analysis of nitrogen balance studies for estimating protein requirements in healthy adults. Am J Clin Nutr 77(1):109–127, 2003.
61. Yarkony GM, Heinemann AW: Pressure ulcers. In Stover SL, DeLisa JA, Whiteneck GG (eds): Spinal Cord Injury: Clinical Outcomes from the Model Systems. Gaithersburg, MD, Aspen, 1995, pp 45–52.
62. Kiy AM: Nutrition in wound healing: A biopsychosocial perspective. Nurs Clin North Am 32(4):849–861, 1997.
63. Ayello EA, Thomas, DR, Litchford, MD: Nutritional aspects of wound healing. Home Healthcare Nurse 17(11):719–729, 1999.
64. Lentine K, Wrone EM: New insights into protein intake and progression of renal disease. Curr Opin Nephrol Hypertens 13:333–336, 2004.
65. Long CL, Nelson KM, Akin JM, Geiger JW: A physiological bases for the provision of fuel mixtures in normal and stressed patients. J Trauma 30:1077–1086, 1990.
66. Food and Agriculture Organization of the United Nations: FAO/WHO Expert Consultation: Protein Quality Evaluation. FAO Food and Nutrition Paper 51. Rome, FAO. 1991.
67. Food Policy and Food Science Service, Nutrition Division, FAO: Amino-Acid Content of Foods and Biological Data on Proteins. Food and Agriculture Organization of the United Nations. FAO Nutritional Studies 24. Rome, FAO, 1970.
68. Fürst P, Stehle P: What are the essential elements needed for the determination of amino acid requirements in humans? J Nutr 134:1558S–1565S, 2004.
69. Institute of Medicine, Food and Nutrition Board: Dietary Reference Intakes: Applications in Dietary Assessment. Washington, DC, National Academy Press, 2000.
70. Institute of Medicine, Food and Nutrition Board: Dietary Reference Intakes: Applications in Dietary Planning. Washington, DC, National Academy Press, 2003.
71. Institute of Medicine, Food and Nutrition Board: Dietary Reference Intakes for Energy, Carbohydrate, Fiber, Fat, Fatty Acids, Cholesterol, Protein, and Amino Acids. Washington, DC, National Academy Press, 2002. Available at www.iom.edu/report.asp?id=4340.
72. Hulsey TK, O'Neil JA, Neblett WR, Meng HC: Experimental wound healing in essential fatty acid deficiency. J Pediatr Surg 15(4):505–508, 1980.

73. Porras-Reyes BH, et al (1992). Essential fatty acids are not required for wound healing. Prostaglandins Leukot Essent Fatty Acids 45(4):293–298, 1992.

74. Albina JE, Gladden P, Walsh WR: Detrimental effects of omega-3 fatty acid-enriched diet on wound healing. JPEN J Parenter Enteral Nutr 17(6):519–521, 1993.

75. Lown D: (1998). Wound healing. In Matarese LE, Gottschlich MM (eds): Contemporary Nutrition Support Practice: A Clinical Guide. Philadelphia, WB Saunders, 1998, pp 583–589.

76. Declair V: (1997). Usefulness of topical application of essential fatty acids (EFA) to prevent pressure ulcers. Ostomy Wound Manage 43(5):48–54, 1997.

77. Lavizzo-Mourey R, Johnson J, Stolley P: (1988) Risk factors for dehydration among elderly nursing home residents. J Am Geriatr Soc 36: 213–218, 1988.

78. Bennett JA, Thomas V, Riegel B: Unrecognized chronic dehydration in older adults: Examining prevalence rate and risk factors. J Gerontol Nurs 11:22–28, 2004.

79. Thomas DR, Tariq SH, Makhdomm S, et al: Physician misdiagnosis of dehydration in older adults. J Am Med Dir Assoc 5(2, suppl):S30–S34, 2004.

80. Fischbach F: Manual of Laboratory and Diagnostic Tests, 7th ed. Philadelphia, Lippincott, Williams & Wilkins, 2004.

81. Pagana KD, Pagana TJ: Mosby's Manual of Diagnostic and Laboratory Tests. St Louis, Mosby, 2006.

82. Ellsbury DL, George CS: Dehydration, 2003. Available at eMedicine.com/ped/topic556.htm

83. Maas ML, Tripp-Reimer T, et al: Nursing Care of Older Adults: Diagnoses, Outcomes and Interventions. New York, Elsevier Science Health Science, 2001.

84. American Medical Directors Association: Dehydration and Fluid Maintenance: Clinical Practice Guideline. Columbia, MD, ADMA, 2001.

85. Chernoff R: Nutritional requirements and physiological changes in age: Thirst and fluid requirements. Nutrition Reviews 52(8): 53–55, 1994.

86. Warren JL, Bacon, WE, Harris T: The burden and outcomes associated with dehydration among US elderly. Am J Public Health 84:1265–1269, 1991.

87. Welch, T: Liquid assets: Hydration in the older adult. Consultant Dietitian 22(3):1–8, 1998.

88. Sheffield PJ, Smith AP, Fife CE: Wound Care Practice. Flagstaff, AZ, Best, 2004.

89. Ringsdorf WM, Cheraskin E: Vitamin C and human wound healing. Oral Surg Oral Med Oral Path 53(3):231–236, 1982.

90. Taylor TV, Rimmer S, Day B, et al: Ascorbic acid supplementation in the treatment of pressure sores. Lancet 2(7880):544–546, 1974.

91. ter Riet G, Kessels A, Knipschild P: Randomized clinical trials of ascorbic acid in the treatment of pressure ulcers. J Clin Epidemiol 48(12):1453–1460, 1995.

92. Scholl WM: The effects of moderate and high dose of vitamin C on wound healing in controlled guinea pig model. J Foot Ankle Surg 38(5):33–338, 1999.

93. Goode HF, Burns E, Walker BE: Vitamin C depletion and pressure sores in elderly patients with femoral neck fracture. BMJ 305: 927–31, 1992.

94. Brocklehurst JC, Griffiths LL, Taylor GF, et al: The clinical features of chronic vitamin deficiency: A therapeutic trial in geriatric hospital patients. Gerontologia Clinica 10:309–320, 1968.

95. Monsen E: Dietary reference intakes for the antioxidant nutrients: Vitamin C, vitamin E, selenium and carotenoids. J Am Diet Assoc 100(6):637–640, 2000.

96. Johnston CS: Biomarkers for establishing a tolerable upper intake for vitamin C. Nutr Rev 57(3):71–77, 1999.

97. Pru C, Kjellstrand C: Vitamin C intoxication and hyperoxalemia in chronic hemodialysis patients. Nephron 39:112–116, 1985.

98. Pronsky ZM: Food-Medication Interactions, 13th ed. Birchrunville, PA, Food-Medication Interactions, 2004.

99. Trumbo P, Yates AA, Schlicker S, et al: Dietary reference intakes. J Am Diet Assoc 101(3):294–301, 2001.

100. Carmel R: Prevalence of undiagnosed pernicious anemia in the elderly. Arch Internal Med 156:1097–1100, 1996.

101. Pennypacker LC, Allen RH, Kelly JP, et al: High prevalence of cobalamin deficiency in elderly outpatients. J Am Geriatr Soc 40:1197–1204, 1992.

102. Wicke C, Halliday B, Allen D, et al: Effects of steroids and retinoids on wound healing. Arch Surg 135:1265–1270, 2000.

103. Levenson, SM, Demetriou, AA: Metabolic factors. In Cohen IK, Diegleman RF, Linblad WD, eds: Wound Healing: Biochemical and Clinical Aspects. Philadelphia, WB Saunders, 1992, pp 248–273.

104. Stadelmann WK, Digenis AG, Tobin GR: Impediments to wound healing. Am J Surg 176(suppl 2A):39S, 1998.

105. Ehrlich HP, Hunt TK: Effect of cortisone and vitamin A on wound healing. Ann Surg 167:324–328, 1968.

106. Hunt TK: Vitamin A and wound healing. J Am Acad Dermatol 15(4, pt 2):817–821, 1986.

107. Hunt TK, Ehrlich HP: Effect of vitamin a on reversing inhibitory effect of cortisone on healing of open wounds in animals and man. Ann Surg 170:633–640, 1969.

108. Demetriou AA, Levenson SM, Retura G: Vitamin A and retinoic acid induced fibroblast differentiation in vitro. Surgery 98:931–934, 1985.

109. Ulland AE, Shearer JD, Coulter C, Caldwell MD: Altered wound arginine metabolism by corticosterone and retinoic acid. J Surg Res 70(1):84–88, 1997.

110. Levenson SM, Gruber CA, et al: Supplemental vitamin A prevents the acute radiation-induced defect in wound healing. Ann Surg 200(4):494–511, 1984.

111. Weinzweig J, Levenson SM, Rettura G, et al: (1990). Supplemental vitamin A prevents the tumor-induced defect in wound healing. Ann Surg 211(3):269–276, 1990.

112. Hunt TK, Hopf HW: Wound healing and wound infection: What surgeons and anesthesiologists can do. Surg Clin North Am 77(3):587–606, 1997.

113. Orgill D, Demling RH: Current concepts and approaches to wound healing. Crit Care Med 16(9):899–908, 1988.

114. Stewart RJ, Moore T, Bennett B, et al: Effect of free-radical scavengers and hyperbaric oxygen on random-pattern skin flaps. Arch Surg 129:982–988, 1994.

115. Levy SL, Burnham WM, Bishai A, Hwang PA: The anticonvulsant effects of vitamin E: A further evaluation. Can J Neurol Sci 19(2):201–203, 1992.

116. Ehrlich HP, Hunt T: Inhibitory effects of vitamin E on collagen synthesis and wound repair. Ann Surg 175:235–240, 1972.

117. Havlik RJ: Vitamin E and wound healing. Plastic Surgery Educational Foundation DATA Committee. Plast Reconstr Surg 100(7):1901–1902, 1997.

118. Andrews M, Gallagher-Allred C: The role of zinc in wound healing. Adv Wound Care 12:137–138, 1999.

119. Scholl D, Langkamp-Henken B: Nutrient recommendations for wound healing. J Intraven Nurs 24(2):124–132, 2001.

120. Pories WJ, Henzel JH, Rob CG, Strain WH: Acceleration of wound healing in man with zinc sulfate given by mouth. Lancet 7482:121–124, 1967.

121. Norris JR, Reynolds RE: The effect of oral zinc sulfate therapy of decubitus ulcers. J Am Geriatr Soc 19:793–797, 1971.

122. Haggard J, Houston MS, Williford JH: Retrospective study of the effects of zinc supplementation in an elderly institutionalized population with decubitus ulcer [abstract]. J Am Diet Assoc 99(suppl):A-11, 1999.

123. Hallbook T, Lanner E: Serum-zinc and healing of venous leg ulcers. Lancet 2:780–782, 1972.

124. Wilkinson EA, Hawke CL: Does oral zinc aid in the healing of chronic leg ulcers?: A systemic literature review. Arch Dermatol 134:1556–1560, 1998.

125. Bales C, DiSilvestro RA: Marginal zinc deficiency in older adults: Responsiveness of zinc status indicators. J Am Coll Nutr 13(5): 455–462, 1994.

126. Prasad AS: Zinc: An overview. Nutrition 11:93–99, 1995.

127. Dietary Reference Intakes, 2001. Available at www.nap.edu.

128. Briefel RR, Bialostosky K, Kennedy-Stephenson J, et al: (2000). Zinc intake of the US population: Findings from the third national health and nutrition examination survey, 1988–1994. J Nutr 130(5S, suppl):1367S–73S, 2000.

129. Fosmire GJ: Zinc toxicity. Am J Clin Nutr 51:225–227, 1990.

130. Boukaiba N, Flament AC: A physiological amount of zinc supplementation: Effects on nutritional, lipid and thymic status in an elderly population. Am J Clin Nutr 57:566–572, 1993.

131. Chandra RK: Excessive intake of zinc impairs immune responses. JAMA 252:1443–1446, 1984.

132. Sandstead HH: Requirements and toxicity of essential trace elements, illustrated by zinc and copper. Am J Clin Nutr 61:621–624, 1995.

133. Shils M, Shike M, Ross C, et al: Modern Nutrition in Health and Disease, 10th ed. Philadelphia, Lippincott, 2005.

134. Blackwell S, Hendrix P: Common anemias: What lies beneath. Clin Rev 11(3):53–62, 2001.

135. Lewis B: Nutrition and wound healing. In Kloth LC, McCulloch JM (eds): Wound Healing: Alternatives in Management, 3rd ed. Philadelphia, Davis, 2002, pp 410–425.

136. Marian MJ, Winkler MF: Wound healing. In Gottschlich MM, Matarese LE, Shronts EP (eds): Nutrition Support Dietetics Core Curriculum, 2nd ed. Silver Spring, MD, Aspen, 1993, pp 397–407.

137. Osterweil O: Pressure ulcers and nutrition. In Morley JE, Glick Z, Rubenstein LZ (eds): Geriatric Nutrition: A Comprehensive Review, 2nd ed. New York, Raven Press, 1995. pp 637–650.

138. Reeds PJ: Dispensable and indispensable amino acids for humans. J Nutr 130:1835S–1840S, 2000.

139. Brunton JA, Bertolo RF, Pencharz PB, Ball RO: Proline ameliorates arginine deficiency during enteral but not parenteral feeding in neonatal piglets. Am J Physiol 277:E223–E231, 1999.

140. Albina JE, Mills CD, Barbul A: Arginine metabolism in wounds. Am J Physiol 254:E459–E467, 1988.

141. Kirk SJ, Barbul A: Role of arginine in trauma, sepsis, immunity. JPEN J Parenter Enteral Nutr 14(5):226S–229S, 1990.

142. Schaffer MR, Tantry U, Ahrendt GM: Acute protein-calorie malnutrition impairs wound healing: A possible role of decreased wound nitric oxide synthesis. J Am Coll Surg. 184:37–43, 1997.

143. Stechmiller JK, Childress B, Cowan L: Arginine supplementation and wound healing. Nutr Clin Pract 20:52–61, 2005.

144. Barbul A, Lazarou SA, Efron DT: Arginine enhances wound healing and lymphocyte immune responses in humans. Surgery 108:331–337, 1990.

145. Kirk SJ, Hurson M, Regan M: Arginine stimulates wound healing and immune function in elderly human beings. Surgery 114: 115–60, 1993.

146. Wilmore D: Enteral and parenteral arginine supplementation to improve medical outcomes in hospitalized patients. J Nutr 134:2863S–2867S, 2004.

147. Barbul A: Arginine: Biochemistry, physiology, and therapeutic implications. JPEN J Parenter Enteral Nutr 10:227–238, 1986.

148. Oehler R, Roth E: Glutamine metabolism. In Cynober L (ed): Metabolic and Therapeutic Aspects of Amino Acids in Clinical Nutrition. Boca Raton, FL, CRC Press, 2004, pp 169–182.

149. Van Acker BA, von Meyenfeldt MF, van der Hulst RR, et al: Glutamine: The pivot of our nitrogen economy? JPEN J Parenter Enteral Nutr 23:S45–S48, 1999.

150. Wu G: Intestinal mucosal amino acid catabolism. J Nutr 128:1249–1252, 1998.

151. Fürst P, Stehle P: What are the essential elements needed for the determination of amino acid requirements in humans? J Nutr 134:1558S–1565S, 2004.

152. Walrand S, Boirie Y: Muscle protein and amino acid metabolism with respect to age-related sarcopenia. In Cynober L (ed): Metabolic and Therapeutic Aspects of Amino Acids in Clinical Nutrition. Boca Raton FL, CRC Press, 2004, pp 389–404.

153. Schloerb PR: Immune-enhancing diets: Products, components and their rationales. JPEN J Parenter Enteral Nutr 25:S3–S7, 2001.

154. Institute of Medicine, Food and Nutrition Board: Dietary Reference Intakes for Energy, Carbohydrate, Fiber, Fat, Fatty Acids, Cholesterol, Protein, and Amino Acids. Food and Nutrition Board. Washington, DC, National Academy Press; 2002. Available at www.iom.edu/report.asp?id=4340.

155. Soeters PB, van de Poll MCG, van Gemert WG, Dejong CHC: Amino acid adequacy in pathophysiological states. J Nutr 134:1575S–1582S, 2004.

156. Ziegler TR, Benfell K, Smith RJ, et al: Safety and metabolic effects of L-glutamine Administration in humans. JPEN J Parenter Enteral Nutr 14:137S–146S, 1990.

157. May PE, Barber A, D'Olimpio JT, et al: Reversal of cancer-related wasting using oral supplementation with a combination of β-hydroxy β-methylbutyrate, arginine, and glutamine. Amer J Surg 183:471–479, 2002.

158. Clark RH, Feleke G, Din M, et al: Nutritional treatment for acquired immunodeficiency virus-associated wasting using β-hydroxy β-methylbutyrate, glutamine, and arginine: A randomized, double-blind, placebo-controlled study. JPEN J Parenter Enteral Nutr 24:133–139, 2000.

159. Nissen S, Sharp R, Ray M, et al: Effect of leucine metabolite β-hydroxy-β-methylbutyrate on muscle metabolism during resistance-exercise training. J Appl Physiol 81;2095–2104, 1996.

160. Williams JZ, Abumrad N, Barbul A: Effect of specialized amino acid mixture on human collagen deposition. Ann Surg 236: 369–374, 2002.

161. Rathmacher JA, Nissen S, Panton L, et al: Supplementation with a combination of beta-hydroxy-beta-methylbutyrate (HMB), arginine, and glutamine is safe and could improve hematological parameters. JPEN J Parenter Enteral Nutr 28:65–75, 2004.

162. Litchford MD: The Advanced Practitioner's Guide to Nutrition and Wounds. Greensboro, NC, CASE Software & Books, 2004.

EVALUATION TECHNIQUES

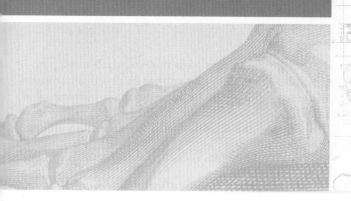

CLASSIFICATION OF FOOT LESIONS IN DIABETIC PATIENTS

JAMES W. BRODSKY ■

Classification of diabetic foot wounds is needed for many purposes. Among the most important is our need to adequately describe the lesions that we treat in order to study patient outcomes as well as to further our understanding of the diabetic foot. Likewise, we need a method to communicate with one another and to compare treatments and their results from one place to another and even from one time to another.

What attributes should the ideal classification system have? First of all, it should be easy to use, practical, and clear. It should be based, as much as possible, on objective criteria and measurements while minimizing subjective assessments in order to enhance its reproducibility in time (intraobserver) and space (interobserver). Last, it should be relevant. Each different class or stage should signify a different diagnostic and/or therapeutic intervention so that it serves as a guide in clinical decision making.

For purposes of tracing factors that might be predictive of outcome, there is a genuine need to consider the many etiologic factors that contribute to the development of diabetic foot wounds. These factors include, but are not limited to, perfusion, presence and extent of gangrene, location and severity of vascular disease, location of the lesion, shape of the wound, wound volume (area × depth), duration, infection, depth of infection, infecting organism(s), nutrition, immunosuppression, effect of other chronic diseases, multisystem involvement, neuropathy, underlying bony deformity, presence of active neuroarthropathy, history of previous lesions, infections and surgeries, gait deviations, abnormalities of pressure under the foot, and joint stiffness. For research purposes, much work remains to be done to determine the relative effect of each of these factors and combinations thereof. In the absence of so much definitive data, we must content ourselves with trying to narrow the scope to areas of a practical nature; factors that we can reliably and reproducibly observe or measure, and factors that have a direct effect on present-day decision making. As our base of knowledge expands, so will our classification systems, reflecting changes in treatment.

Classification Systems

In recent years, numerous authors have grappled with the need for a better classification system for diabetic foot lesions. Each author has contributed significantly to our understanding of the diabetic foot and our methodology for assessment and treatment. Shea described a method of grading pressure ulcers based on their depth and which deeper structures are exposed. This early system gave no consideration to the role of ischemia or vascularity in the healing process but did set a valuable precedent for evaluation of the physical characteristics of a wound.[1]

Forrest and Gambor-Neilssen proposed a wound evaluation system that was clinically sensible but had the same disadvantage of giving no consideration to ischemia.[2] Some authors have also noted that it was not comprehensive in that it did not account for wound severity.[3,4] Knighton and colleagues proposed a complex method of wound evaluation in which several factors are added to create a single wound score for the purpose of evaluating the effectiveness of platelet-derived growth factors in wound healing.[5] While the single wound score makes comparisons easy, other authors noted that it blankets the details, obfuscating rather than illuminating the source of the severity. These same authors noted that many of the factors that are included in the score are cumbersome or subjective, while others are difficult to measure.[3,4]

Pecoraro and Reiber described an elegant wound classification system with 10 classes.[4] This was used as a research tool to track wounds and their contribution to the ultimate outcome of amputation. They identified factors that were associated with more severe final outcomes as well as the characteristics that led to amputation. Other authors have noted that some of the terminology describing the wounds is subjective and difficult to interpret.[3] Many of the 10 classes require the same diagnostic and therapeutic intervention, making the purpose of their distinction unclear. This classification allows some of the same paradoxical combinations as the original Wagner-Meggitt classification, for example, a case with features of both class 1 (intact skin) and class 4 (partial gangrene).

Lavery and colleagues[3] and Armstrong and colleagues[6] described an excellent classification system, in which the wound grades are based on the Wagner-Meggitt system and the stages are separately identified and classified according to the presence of ischemia, infection, or both. This advanced the concept of the depth-ischemia classification, making it slightly more complex but very descriptive. The differences among the stages regarding the presence of infection add an additional indication, in some cases, for surgical intervention, while in cases of grade 2 or 3 lesions, surgery is indicated regardless of the presence or absence of infection. All of these authors and others[1-14] have striven to be more descriptive, more practical, and more comprehensive, and each has contributed significantly to the field of diabetic foot care. Needless to say, further work of many kinds and in many places will continue to refine our understanding.

The greatest challenge to the use of a classification system for diabetic foot wounds is the classic tension between giving it sufficient simplicity to make it practical and incorporating enough detail to make it meaningful. On the one hand, the disadvantage of an overly simplified classification is that it will fail to adequately describe the difference among various kinds of wounds (or patients), so lesions with too much variation among them will be lumped together. On the other hand, an excessively complex system that splits the lesions into too many groups might make the various parts unrecognizable as a part of the whole. Any system that cannot be practically applied can retard rather than advance the main purpose of all our efforts, which is the ability to effectively and efficiently use this knowledge in the daily treatment of actual patients.

Wagner-Meggitt Classification

Wagner and Meggitt developed a classification system in the 1970s at Rancho Los Amigos Hospital in California, which has been known ever since by both names but most commonly in the United States as the "Wagner classification."[10,12,13] It has been the most widely accepted and universally used grading system for lesions of the diabetic foot.[12,13,15] Numerous authors and investigators have since worked to improve our understanding of wounds, particularly diabetic foot wounds, and much progress has been made. Recent work on classification has reflected this intense further thought and research, as was noted above.[1-9,14,16-18]

Owing to its simplicity in use, however, the Wagner classification has become the most widely quoted and utilized system. It has been the foundation on which subsequent work has been built and has functioned for the purpose of communication among investigators and clinicians, allowing comparison among patients in many different locales. The original system has six grades of lesions. The first four grades (grades 0, 1, 2, and 3) are based on the physical depth of the lesion in and through the soft tissues of the foot. The last two grades (grades 4 and 5) are completely distinct because they are based on the extent of lost perfusion in the foot. The vast majority of diabetic foot wounds that are seen in everyday clinical practice are described by the first four grades: 0, 1, 2, and 3. Of these grades, the majority of outpatient treatments are applied to grade 0 and grade 1 lesions, while the deeper and more advanced grade 2 and grade 3 lesions typically require hospitalization and/or surgery. The treatment of grades 4 (partial foot gangrene) and 5 (gangrene of the entire foot) is rather direct: amputation of the gangrenous portion of the foot or limb with concomitant consideration of limb revascularization and treatment of any associated infection.

We owe a debt of gratitude to Wagner and Meggitt for providing the first easily applied classification of diabetic foot lesions. However, there are two concepts in their classification that now deserve revision based on the concept that the extensive experience of the last 20 years. The first is that all grades of diabetic foot lesions from grade 1 ulcers to grade 5 gangrene occur along a progressive continuum. While this might frequently be the case for a grade 1 lesion (superficial ulcer), which advances to a grade 2 lesion (deeper ulcer) and on to a grade 3 lesion (osteomyelitis or abscess), this is not the case with grades 4 and 5. These latter two are ischemic lesions that reflect the diminished vascular status of the foot and are therefore fundamentally unrelated to the nature or progression of the wounds described by the lesser grades. Moreover, these ischemic lesions may exist in the absence of any of the lesser grades. Conversely, grade 4 or 5 may coexist with any of them, so the inclusion of all these grades in a single longitudinal classification not only is illogical, but also obscures our complete understanding of the status of the foot.

For example, a grade 4 lesion (partial gangrene) could be present in a forefoot that is otherwise grade 0 (no break in the skin), grade 1 (a superficial lesion), or even grade 2 or 3. Another example is the problem of classifying the foot that has osteomyelitis but is also partially gangrenous: Is it a grade 3 or grade 4 foot? Even more confusing is the following example: Compare a foot with chronic osteomyelitis of the calcaneus to a foot with gangrene of all the toes. By the Wagner classification, the former is a grade 3 lesion, and the latter is a grade 4. Yet these grades seem inverted when we attempt to understand them as a single progression that mixes wound severity with ischemia. In this example, the grades fail to appropriately depict the relative severity, since the patient with the grade 3 lesion might require a transtibial amputation, while the patient with the grade 4 lesion might need only a transmetatarsal amputation. Vascular pathology absolutely can and must be graded, but again, there is no dependable relationship between the depth of ulcerative lesions (grades 0, 1, 2, and 3) and the ischemia of the foot or lower limb (grades 4 and 5). More important, the grade 5 foot ceases to be a true

foot lesion. Rather, it presents an issue of salvage of the proximal leg.

The second concept that must be corrected, while obvious, needs to be stated: that contrary to the diagrams of the original classification, there are no reliable pathways backward and forward from grade to grade of lesion. For example, a grade 4 lesion (partial gangrene) cannot revert to a grade 2 or 3 lesion, in contrast to a grade 2 lesion, which may revert to a grade 0 as it heals.

Depth-Ischemia Classification

The depth-ischemia classification [8,9] is a modification of the Wagner-Meggitt [10,12,13] classification (Table 9-1). The purposes of this modified classification are (1) to make the classification more rational and easier to use by distinguishing between evaluation of the wound and the vascularity of the foot; (2) to elucidate the distinctions among the grades, especially between grades 2 and 3; and (3) to improve the clinical correlation of appropriate treatments to the grade of lesion. This classification of diabetic foot lesions makes the decision-making path clearer and the information obtained more accessible than is possible with use of the Wagner algorithms.[13] The depth-ischemia classification is utilized in the following manner. Each foot is given both number and letter grades. Their combination describes the physical extent of the wound (number) and the vascularity or ischemia of the foot and limb (letter). First, the soft tissue is inspected, palpated, and graded with a number that

TABLE 9-1   The Depth-Ischemia Classification of Diabetic Foot Lesions

Grade/Definition	Intervention
Depth Classification	
0	
The at-risk foot: previous ulcer or neuropathy with deformity that may cause new ulceration	Patient education, regular examination, appropriate shoe wear and insoles
1	
Superficial ulceration, not infected	External pressure relief: total-contact cast, walking brace, special shoe wear, etc.
2	
Deep ulceration exposing a tendon or joint (with or without superficial infection)	Surgical debridement, wound care, pressure relief if the lesion closes and converts to grade 1 (prn antibiotics)
3	
Extensive ulceration with exposed bone and/or deep infection (i.e., osteomyelitis or abscess)	Surgical debridements; ray or partial foot amputation, IV antibiotics, pressure relief if wound converts to grade 1
Ischemia Classification	
A	
Not ischemic	Observation
B	
Ischemia without gangrene	Vascular evaluation (Doppler, $TcPO_2$ arteriogram, etc.), vascular reconstruction prn
C	
Partial (forefoot) gangrene of the foot	Vascular evaluation, vascular reconstruction (proximal and/or distal bypass or angioplasty), partial foot amputation
D	
Complete foot gangrene	Vascular evaluation, major extremity amputation (TTA, TFA) with possible proximal vascular reconstruction

Each foot is graded both for wound depth (number) and for foot vascularity (letter).
TTA, transtibial amputation (below-knee amputation); TFA, transfemoral amputation (above-knee amputation).
* Modified from Brodsky J: The diabetic foot. In Coughlin MJ, Mann RA (eds): Surgery of the Foot and Ankle, 7th ed. Philadelphia: Mosby, 1999, with permission.

represents the physical extent of the lesion. Second, the limb and foot are evaluated for perfusion.

The first step is based primarily on examination of the foot and its wound or ulcer. The grade 0 foot is a foot that is at risk (Fig. 9-1). This is a foot that either has had a previous ulceration or has the two characteristics that make future ulcerations likely. These are peripheral neuropathy and an area of increased pressure, usually due to a bony prominence. Because neuropathy cannot currently be reversed, the decision making for a grade 0 foot consists of pressure relief to reduce the likelihood of ulceration. A common example is the use of deeper shoes with accommodative, cushioning insoles. A grade 1 lesion is a superficial wound without exposure of any deep structure to sight or to probing (Fig. 9-2). This lesion will usually be treated with some form of pressure relief; classically, this would be a total-contact cast to

redistribute forces over the plantar surface of the foot, thereby partially unweighting the area of high plantar pressure. If the lesion is on the dorsum or border of the foot, that is, a lesion attributable to shoe pressure, then shoe modification might be the intervention. Either way, the decision in a grade 1 lesion is to relieve the underlying pressure that causes the lesion. If there is accompanying infection, even though it is treated appropriately with oral or intravenous antibiotics, the lesion will not heal without relief of the pressure.

Grade 2 lesions are deeper, with exposure of underlying tendon or joint capsule, with or without infection (Fig. 9-3). Determination of infection is secondary at this point, because it does not change the decision-making algorithm. If there are exposed deep structures, then the patient is no longer a candidate for outpatient pressure relief and requires hospitalization for wound debridement and intravenous antibiotics. This decision is the same whether the ulcer is deemed to be infected or not. Grade 3 lesions are the deepest, with exposed bone and/or deep infection, either abscess or osteomyelitis (Figs. 9-4, 9-5). Determination of these three basic wound grades is based on simple physical examination consisting of visualization and gentle probing of the wound with a sterile, blunt instrument. If bone can be palpated in the base of the wound, there is a very high likelihood that osteomyelitis is present.[19]

Once the examiner has described the depth of the wound with the appropriate numeric grade, the second step is to assign a letter grade after evaluating limb perfusion. This "ischemia" portion of the classification is signified by the letter A, B, C, or D. While this might be obvious on the basis of physical examination alone, noninvasive vascular studies such as Doppler ultrasound or transcutaneous oxygen tension might be required. For example, if the patient has bounding dorsalis pedis and

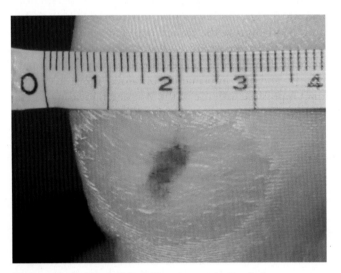

Figure 9–1   Grade 0 foot. The ulcer under the first metatarsophalangeal joint is healed and epithelialized. The patient remains at risk for recurrent or future ulcerations.

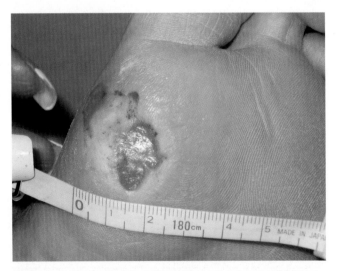

Figure 9–2   Grade 1 foot. The plantar ulcer is superficial and granulating well. There are no deep structures exposed, no infection, and no radiographic evidence of bone erosion.

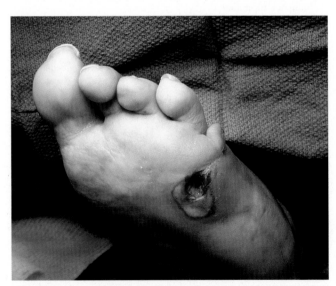

Figure 9–3   Grade 2 foot. The wound is not granulating. The metatarsophalangeal joint capsule is exposed and easily palpated.

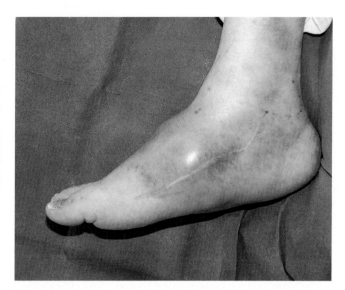

Figure 9-4   Grade 3 foot. The patient has a midfoot Charcot arthropathy and a deep abscess arising from the plantar ulcer.

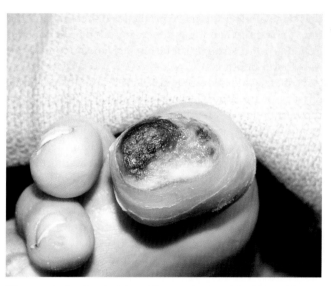

Figure 9-5   Grade 3 foot. Ulcer at the tip of the hallux. The exposed tip of the distal phalanx is brown.

posterior tibial pulses, the foot is almost certainly grade A, that is, without clinically significant ischemia. This is a foot with excellent pulses, color, capillary refill, and hair growth. Grade A lesions do not require vascular evaluation or intervention. If there is obvious gangrene of part (grade C) or all (grade D) of the foot, then these grades are equally easy to assign. The largest number of lesions encountered clinically are grade B, that is, ischemic but not gangrenous. Although this is a wide band within the spectrum, it is not only internally consistent, but also consistent with the ultimate decision-making algorithm that the classification supports. Despite the variation within this grade, it is a rational grouping based on the intervention merited because all of these patients require vascular evaluation using screening tests such as those mentioned above. Thus, it is critical to know both the wound depth and limb vascularity to formulate a proper and successful treatment plan. Depending on the result of these tests, some form of vascular reconstruction might be indicated. We must know whether there is sufficient perfusion for either an external pressure-relieving device or an internal pressure-relieving surgery to be successful. If we are uncertain, we can proceed with neither.

Grade C feet have partial gangrene, and grade D feet are completely gangrenous.. Patients with grade C or D

lesions also require vascular evaluation to determine the distal level of adequate perfusion, that is, the level of potential healing, and to assess the need for revascularization procedures to achieve healing of the most distal amputation possible. The utility of this classification system is that it is straightforward and can be applied to the decision-making process in a sensible fashion. The most immediate necessary decisions are included in this algorithm. The advantage of the depth-ischemia classification is that it is succinct, and once the foot has been graded, the first step in treatment decision making is clear and concise.

The University of Texas classification, discussed above, represents an advance in the treatment of the diabetic foot (Table 9-2). It separates evaluation of ischemia from wound depth and uses the same categories for the latter as does the depth-ischemia classification. As was mentioned earlier in the chapter, it adds consideration of infection to the classification: Stage A has no ischemia or infection, stage B has infection, stage C has ischemia, and stage D has both infection and ischemia. Two studies have been made of this classification system. One showed that outcomes worsened with increasing grade and stage of wounds.[6] The other showed that this classification was more predictive than the original Wagner-Meggitt classification. Most important, the latter study demonstrated

TABLE 9-2   The University of Texas Wound Classification System

	Grade 0	Grade I	Grade II	Grade III
Stage A	Preulcerative or postulcerative lesion completely epithelialized	Superficial wound, not involving tendon, capsule, or bone	Wound penetrating to tendon or capsule	Wound penetrating to bone or joint
Stage B	Infection	Infection	Infection	Infection
Stage C	Ischemia	Ischemia	Ischemia	Ischemia
Stage D	Infection and ischemia	Infection and ischemia	Infection and ischemia	Infection and ischemia

Depth is signified by grade number, horizontally. Infection and ischemia are signified by stage letter, vertically.

that stage of ulcer was more predictive of healing and the time to healing than was grade, that is, that infection and ischemia were stronger determinants of outcome than was wound depth.[3,7]

While classification systems focus on the local characteristics of the wound combined with the perfusion of the foot, much less has been written about the anatomic location of the lesion.[18] Anatomic location has been studied and shown to be less important than the characteristics (classification) of the wounds themselves.[17] However, it is worth noting that diabetic wounds of the forefoot, especially those beyond the distal one third of the metatarsals, commonly have a much higher limb salvage rate and a much lower associated mortality than do more proximal lesions of the foot, even if the actual healing times of the distal and proximal lesions are about the same.[18] Lesions of the hindfoot in particular have a higher rate of transtibial amputation as well as greater difficulty in healing. The treating surgeon or physician should bear in mind the generally increased risk of lesions of both the midfoot and the hindfoot. This risk also points to the multifactorial nature of these wounds and the probability that diabetic foot wounds can never be entirely summarized by a single classification system.

Summary

Classification of diabetic foot lesions is essential to guide clinical decision making. For a classification to be practical, it must be easy to use and provide enough detail to make it applicable to everyday clinical situations. The original system developed by Wagner and Meggitt in the 1970s has been augmented by several authors who have developed systems that are more rational in regard to the relationship of the main factors of wound depth and ischemia. By combining a numerical grade for wound depth with a letter grade denoting the vascular status of the foot, the surgeon can formulate a treatment plan that is likely to be successful.

References

1. Shea J: Pressure sores: Classification and management. Clin Orthop 112:89–100, 1975.
2. Forrest R, Gamborg-Neilssen P: Wound assessment in clinical practice: A critical review of methods and their applications. Acta Med Scand 687:69–74, 1984.
3. Lavery L, Armstrong D, Harkless L: Classification of diabetic foot wounds. J Foot Ankle Surg 356:528–531, 1996.
4. Pecoraro RE, Reiber GE: Classification of wounds in diabetic amputees. Wounds 2:65–73, 1990.
5. Knighton D, et al: Classification and treatment of chronic non-healing wounds: Successful treatment with autologous platelet-derived wound healing factors (PDWHF). Ann Surg 204:322–330, 1986.
6. Armstrong DG, Lavery LA, Harkless LB: Validation of a diabetic wound classification system. Diabetes Care 21(5):855–859, 1998.
7. Armstrong DG, Lavery LA, Harkless LB: Treatment-based classification system for assessment and care of diabetic feet. J Am Podiatr Med Assoc 86:311–316, 1996.
8. Brodsky JW: The diabetic foot. In Mann RA, Coughlin MJ, Saltzman CL (eds): Surgery of the Foot and Ankle. Philadelphia: Elsevier, 2006.
9. Brodsky JW: Outpatient diagnosis and management of the diabetic foot. Instructional Course Lectures. Rosemont, IL: American Academy of Orthopaedic Surgeons 42:43, 1993.
10. Meggitt B: Surgical management of the diabetic foot. Br J Hosp Med 16:227–332, 1976.
11. Oyibo SO, et al: A comparison of two diabetic foot ulcer classification systems. Diabetes Care 24(1):84–88, 2001.
12. Wagner FW Jr: A classification and treatment program for diabetic, neuropathic and dysvascular foot problems. Instructional Course Lectures, vol 28. Rosemont, IL: American Academy of Orthopaedic Surgeons. 1979, pp 143–165.
13. Wagner FW Jr: The diabetic foot and amputations of the foot. In Mann R (ed): Surgery of the Foot. St. Louis: Mosby-Year Book, 1986, pp 421–455.
14. Yarkony G, et al: Classification of pressure ulcers. Arch Dermatol 126:1218–1219, 1990.
15. Calhoun J, et al: Treatment of diabetic foot infections: Wagner classification, therapy and outcome. Foot Ankle 9:101–106, 1988.
16. Alvarez DM, Gilson G, Auletta MJ: Local aspects of diabetic foot ulcer care: Assessment, dressings, and topical agents. In Levin ME, O'Neal, LW, Bowker JH (eds): The Diabetic Foot, 5th ed. St. Louis, Mosby Year Book, 1993.
17. Apelqvist J, Castenfors J, Larsson J, et.al: Wound classification is more important than site of ulceration in the outcome of diabetic foot ulcers. Diabet Med 6:526–530, 1989.
18. Kaufman J, Breeding L, Rosenberg N: Anatomic location of acute diabetic foot infections. Am J Surg 53:109–112, 1987.
19. Grayson ML, Balogh K, Levin E, Karchmer AW: Probing to bone in infected pedal ulcers: A clinical sign of underlying osteomyelitis in diabetic patients. JAMA 273:721–723, 1995.

IMAGING OF THE DIABETIC FOOT

HANNO HOPPE AND JOHN A. KAUFMAN ■

In foot and ankle vascular disease, tendinopathy, neuropathic disease, and infection are common manifestations of diabetes mellitus (Table 10-1).[1] These manifestations often prompt referral for imaging evaluation. Diabetic foot complications, the primary cause of morbidity, mortality, and disability in people who have diabetes, may eventually lead to lower-limb amputation.[2] If amputation becomes necessary, imaging should precisely visualize the extent of infection to reduce amputation to a minimum.[3,4] Over the past decade, magnetic resonance imaging (MRI) has increasingly been used for evaluation of the diabetic foot, including angiography.[5-7] Diabetic foot infection may be especially difficult to distinguish from changes related to neuropathic arthropathy, which is important because management is different.[8] Imaging plays a key role in the distinction of these entities in terms of soft tissue, bony, and articular complications.[9] Radiographs are useful for anatomic information but are neither sensitive nor specific for the detection of early infection.[10] Multidetector row computed tomography (CT) is adequate for the visualization of bony changes and for noninvasive CT angiography (CTA).[11,12] Bone scan provides poor anatomic detail and often vague localization.[13] MRI is relied on primarily as the imaging tool for pedal complications related to diabetes.[6,9]

Magnetic Resonance Imaging

MRI is based on the detection of radiofrequency signals emitted by protons within a powerful static magnetic field. MRI coils and scanning protocols need to be adapted to the patient and the clinical question. For imaging of the ankle, the extremity coil is usually used, with the patient in supine position.[1] A chimney-type coil should be used as the limb coil. A small surface coil is adequate for the forefoot and toes. Instead, a carefully positioned wrist coil can be used if the foot is small and not significantly deformed.

MRI has the ability to create images in any plane with large fields of view. The short-axis view, perpendicular to the toes, is the basis for evaluation of ulcerations and their relationship to bones. T1-weighted imaging is used to evaluate bone marrow changes and subcutaneous fat, and a fat-suppressed T2-weighted image, usually short tau inversion recovery (STIR), is ideally suited to evaluate for edema of bone marrow, soft tissues, and surrounding tendons.[14-17] Sagittal plane and long-axis views parallel to the toes are used to image the metatarsophalangeal and interphalangeal joints in order to visualize septic arthritis. Furthermore, the sagittal plane is adequate to image the midfoot for possible neuropathic involvement, the plantar surface, and the calcaneus.[9] In this plane, T1-weighted and fat-suppressed T2-weighted or STIR imaging should be performed. Axial and coronal planes are recommended for evaluating the malleoli, including the surrounding tendons.[15]

The use of contrast material is recommended with fat-saturated T1-weighted images to visualize the true extent of disease, associated soft tissue, septic arthritis, and tendon involvement and to evaluate for devitalized regions. However, fat-saturated T1-weighted images should be acquired both before and after contrast administration in identical planes to reliably detect areas of abnormal enhancement.[9]

TABLE 10-1   MRI Appearance of Conditions Affecting the Diabetic Foot

Conditions Affecting the Diabetic Foot	Magnetic Resonance Imaging Appearance
Neuropathic osteoarthropathy (acute)	Juxta-articular soft tissue and bone marrow edema on T2 with enhancement (DD: osteomyelitis), joint effusion, erosions
Neuropathic osteoarthropathy (chronic)	Less prominent edema and enhancement, subchondral cysts, bone proliferation, debris and intra-articular bodies, joint deformity with subluxation/dislocation (Lisfranc), neuropathic fractures
Osteomyelitis	Low bone marrow signal on T1 and high signal on T2 with contrast enhancement, cortical disruption, periostitis with circumferential edema and disproportionate contrast enhancement
Septic arthritis	Joint effusion with distention of synovial recesses and intense contrast enhancement, bone marrow edema and enhancement (DD: reactive/osteomyelitis, low signal intensity on T1)
Tendon infection	Circular peritendinous contrast enhancement
Cellulitis	Soft tissue contrast enhancement with fat signal loss on T1 and hyperintense signal on T2
Abscess	Focal isointense or hypointense signal compared with muscle tissue on T1 with fluid equivalent signal on T2 and rim enhancement
Skin callus	Low signal intensity on T1 and low to intermediate signal intensity on T2 focally prominent within subcutaneous fat tissue with enhancement (DD: focal soft tissue infection)
Ulceration	Hyperintense on T2 with peripheral enhancement
Gangrene	Nonenhancement representing devascularization, enhancement of surrounding tissues representing reactive paradoxical hyperemia, small foci of signal void if air within soft tissues
Bone infarction	Well-defined lesion with a serpiginous rim around an area with fat, fluid, or sclerotic bone signal depending on age of infarct
Foreign body granuloma	High signal on T2 and low signal on T1 with marked enhancement, foreign body with signal void
Muscle infarction	Isointense swelling of the involved muscle on T1 and T2, mildly displaced fascial planes, diffuse edema within muscle, perifascial fluid collection, focal mass with peripheral enhancement
Diabetic vascular disease	On MRA, arterial stenosis or occlusion, collateral vessels with slow-forming stenosis

Gadolinium-enhanced magnetic resonance angiography (MRA) is valuable for the evaluation of peripheral diabetic vascular disease.[5,7,18] Advantages of MRA over conventional catheter angiography include the absence of radiation exposure and arterial puncture and the use of nonnephrotoxic contrast material.[19] For MRA of the lower limbs, a peripheral angiographic array coil is used.[20,21] The gadolinium contrast material is injected rapidly through a peripheral vein with a 3D T1-weighted acquisition timed to occur as the contrast enters the arterial circulation.[22] Continuous table movement "chases" the contrast bolus distally and allows for examination of the arteries from the aorta to the foot. However, venous overlay at the level of the calf and foot may occur.[5] Venous contamination can be reduced by using venous compression or so-called hybrid methods.[20,23] By using a hybrid technique, two sets of contrast-enhanced MRA are obtained with separate contrast injections.[19] First, MRA of the calf and foot (Fig. 10-1) is studied, and then two-station MRA of the aortoiliac and thigh regions is performed.[20] The most common method of image analysis is the maximum intensity projection, a postprocessing technique that combines the brightest pixels from each slice in an angiographic image that can be viewed from any angle.[24]

MRA is highly sensitive and specific for the detection of peripheral artery stenosis (Fig. 10-2).[25,26] It has a sensitivity of 100% and a positive predictive value of 92% for arterial lesions requiring intervention.[27] Owing to the limited spatial resolution of MRA, the precise degree of stenosis is typically overestimated, but stenotic lesions that reduce the diameter of the lumen by 50% or more are accurately detected.[28,29] Of interest, MRA visualization of distal runoff vessels in the presence of multilevel inflow occlusions (i.e., aorta to tibial artery) is frequently

superior when compared to conventional angiography.[30] Compared to conventional angiography and CTA, a major limitation of MRA is the inability to visualize intimal calcification, which is an important factor in selecting a distal bypass target.

Computed Tomography

Besides being used for the visualization of bony changes, multidetector row CT is used to perform CTA.[11,12] Lower-limb CTA is the newest technique for peripheral arterial imaging, but it can be obtained with all current multidetector row CT scanners.[31] When patients are mobile, the study can be performed within 15 minutes of room time. The basic principle of CTA is a carefully timed helical acquisition during a rapid peripheral venous infusion of iodinated contrast material. One of the major advantages of CTA is that the source images are simply very thin axial slices with intense vascular opacification. The helical CT data can be visualized as either two-dimensional axial images or by using various two- and three-dimensional postprocessing techniques (Fig. 10-3).[32] Viewing of axial images is mandatory for the assessment of the vessel wall and perivascular structures.[33] This allows a more comprehensive evaluation of the vascular structures than is possible with MRA or conventional angiography.[34] Since CTA of lower-limb arteries has just entered clinical practice, there are only sparse original data on its accuracy in patients. So far, good overall sensitivities and specificities have been reported for hemodynamically relevant steno-occlusive lesions, which were greater than 96%, and there was no evident decrease of performance down to the popliteocrural branches.[35] Results for pedal arteries have not yet been published.

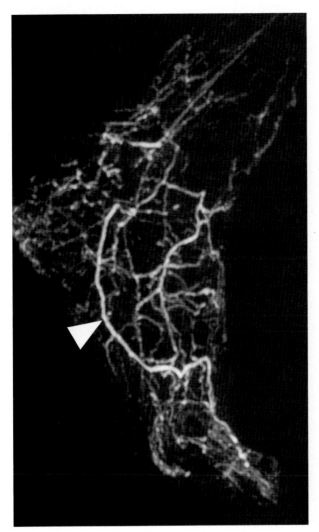

Figure 10–1 Maximum intensity projection of a three-dimensional gadolinium-enhanced MRA of the foot in a patient with severe tibial artery disease shows a patent lateral plantar artery (*arrow*). *(Reprinted with permission from Kaufman JA, Lower-extremity arteries. In Kaufman JA, Lee MJ: The requisites: Vascular and interventional radiology. Philadelphia: Mosby/Elsevier, 2004.)*

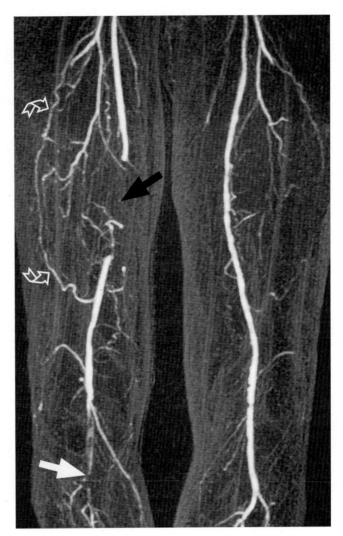

Figure 10–2 Patient with peripheral vascular disease. Gadolinium-enhanced three-dimensional MR angiogram (MRA) of the femoral and popliteal arteries displayed as maximum intensity projection images. MRA demonstrates occlusion of the right superficial femoral artery (*black arrow*) and right popliteal artery (*white arrow*). The occlusion of the right superficial femoral artery is bypassed by collateral vessels originating mainly from the profunda femoral artery (*curved arrows*). *(Reprinted with permission from Kaufman JA: Noninvasive vascular imaging. In Kaufman JA, Lee MJ: The requisites: Vascular and interventional radiology. Philadelphia: Mosby/Elsevier, 2004.)*

One limitation of CTA is a lower spatial resolution than that of conventional angiography. Furthermore, patients with contrast allergy or renal failure may not be candidates for elective studies; this is the case as well for those with contraindications to ionizing radiation, such as patients in the first trimester of pregnancy. Heavily calcified vessels are difficult to evaluate, as bulky intimal calcium can be indistinguishable from the opacified vessel lumen.[35]

Noninvasive Vascular Imaging

For the diagnosis of diabetic vascular disease, conventional angiography, MRA, or CTA can be used.[35–37] Regardless of the modality that is used, arterial stenosis is visualized as focal narrowing of vessel caliber, abrupt

cutoff of flow, or nonvisualization of a branch. Collateral vessels may become apparent in the setting of a slow-forming stenosis.[1]

In diabetic patients, it is common for lower-limb vessels to be diffusely diseased. Surgical revascularization remains the most important therapeutic option for limb salvage in patients with severe arterial occlusive disease.[38] The outcome of distal bypass procedures is greatly affected by the presence or absence of adequate pedal outflow.[39] Therefore, the identification of distal vessels in the foot, including the pedal arch, is crucial for planning advanced distal revascularizations.[24] Failure to properly identify a status that is amenable to recanalization may result in unnecessary amputations. Therefore, preoperative pedal

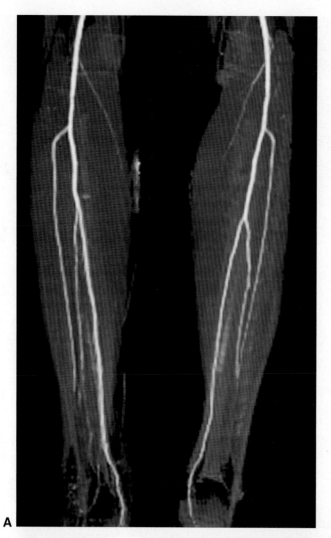

A

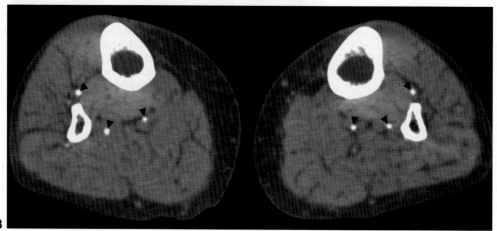

B

Figure 10–3   Coronal maximum intensity projection of a CT angiogram (CTA) of the calves (**A**) showing regular bilateral runoff of the tibial and peroneal arteries. Axial CT image (**B**) acquired during the arterial phase at the level of the calf demonstrating contrast enhancement of the anterior tibial arteries, posterior tibial arteries, and peroneal arteries (*arrowheads*).

imaging should provide a sufficiently detailed depiction of the pedal arteries.[20]

Neuropathic Osteoarthropathy

Diabetes mellitus is the most common cause of neuropathic osteoarthropathy, and the foot and ankle are most commonly affected.[40] Neuropathic osteoarthropathy is an aggressive and deforming arthritis. It is caused by a combination of factors, including repetitive microtrauma and macrotrauma to the articular surfaces and supporting ligaments, peripheral neuropathy with impaired perception of injury, and ischemia with poor healing.[41,42] A sequence of insufficiently healed injuries can cause joint instability and subsequent joint dislocation or subluxation and resultant deformity.[43] Neuropathic osteoarthropathy of the foot usually demonstrates radiographic changes similar to those of osteoarthritis with surrounding bone production, including subchondral sclerosis and osteophytes, intra-articular bodies, and subchondral cysts, which are characteristically more extreme than in typical osteoarthritis.[44] Erosions may form at either the margins or the central portions of the involved joint and may progress to bone destruction or resorption.[44] Neuropathic disease of the foot is likely to present with a mixed pattern of proliferation and erosion, as opposed to primarily erosive or proliferative manifestations seen elsewhere in the body.[10]

In the diabetic foot, neuropathic osteoarthropathy is most common at the Lisfranc joint (tarsometatarsal) in 60% of cases but can also occur in the metatarsophalangeal joints in 30% of cases and in the tibiotalar joints in fewer than 10% of cases.[10,45] Often, neuropathic osteoarthropathy begins in the midfoot, and subluxation usually starts at the second tarsometatarsal joint and proceeds laterally.[42] The ankle, hindfoot, and forefoot may also show neuropathic changes. Frequently, multiple joints are involved, which leads to regional instability.

Neuropathic osteoarthropathy can be classified as either acute or chronic in form, but the two forms may also be superimposed on each other.[45] The acute form presents with a swollen, warm, and tender limb.[42] On MRI, the acute form is characterized by diffuse juxta-articular soft tissue edema.[6] On postcontrast images, the joint capsule and soft tissues are enhanced owing to acute injury or instability, but the subcutaneous tissue typically demonstrates little enhancement.[46] Joint effusion is commonly seen, and erosions may be present. Bone marrow edema and enhancement are typically centered in the subchondral bone, reflecting the articular pattern of disease.[47] In severe cases, prominent edema and enhancement may extend into the periarticular tissue and medullary bone, which can mimic osteomyelitis.[46]

The chronic form of neuropathic osteoarthropathy demonstrated less prominent edema and enhancement on MRI.[46,48] This form is rather characterized by subchondral cysts and bone proliferation with debris or intra-articular bodies.[42] Joint deformity with subluxation or even dislocation is common. Manifestation of neuropathic disease in the Lisfranc joint typically results in superolateral subluxation of the metatarsals, causing a rocker-bottom-type foot deformity, in which the cuboid becomes a weight-bearing structure, eventually leading to callus formation and ulceration beneath the cuboid.[49,50]

In case of simultaneous occurrence of both acute and chronic neuropathic arthropathy, the typical deformity of chronic disease is often present in combination with periarticular soft tissue and bone marrow edema and contrast enhancement, indicating possible acute instability or injury.[1] Neuropathic fractures that are well known to occur in the diabetic foot are avulsion fractures of the posterior calcaneus (Fig. 10-4) and subchondral

fracture of the head of the second metatarsal, similar to Freiberg infraction.[41,51] Furthermore, unusual calcaneal fractures and talocalcaneal joint dissolution as well as talar collapse into the calcaneus, distal fibular fractures, and talar angulation within the ankle mortise are also part of this entity. Another radiographic finding is resorption of the metatarsal heads and phalanges with gradual loss of the ends of the bones and tapering of the shafts, presenting as a "sucked candy" appearance.[52] The extent of osseous changes, including fragment dislocation, angulation, and bone collapse, can be demonstrated by using multidetector row CT with multiplanar reformats. Furthermore, CT, MRI, and bone scintigraphy facilitate an earlier detection of developing neuropathic arthropathy in the foot than is possible with plain radiographs, and immediate off-loading appears to minimize fractures and incapacitating deformities.[53,54] Eventually, massive bony sclerosis, osteophytosis, and osseous debris make it extremely difficult to establish the presence or absence of infection.

Bone scintigraphy of patients with diabetic neuropathic osteoarthropathy of the foot and ankle is characterized by a combination of diffuse and focal increased uptake, similar to that seen with hyperemia and reactive new bone formation.[55] Scintigraphy shows more extensive abnormalities than does radiography, the scan abnormalities sometimes preceding the radiographic changes. While bone scintigraphy is not pathognomonic, it may be useful for follow-up in long-term diabetic patients with peripheral neuropathy.

Osteomyelitis

Pedal ulcers are the most common cause of osteomyelitis of the diabetic foot.[17] Most patients lack clinical symptoms other than ulcer, and the diagnosis of osteomyelitis might be missed.[56] Therefore, imaging is an essential part in the evaluation of osteomyelitis. For patients with clinical suspicion of pedal infection, plain radiographs are usually the initial imaging modality obtained, but radiographic changes of osteomyelitis may be delayed up to 2 weeks, and the sensitivity is poor, because osseous changes become visible on plain radiographs only after 30% to 50% of the bone has been destroyed.[57] On radiographs, demineralization, periosteal reaction, and bony destruction are the classic radiographic triad of osteomyelitis.[1] Periostitis might not be seen in the tarsal bones or the phalanges.[6] Although the accuracy of plain radiography for early diagnosis of pedal osteomyelitis is only about 50% to 60%, radiographs aid in identifying soft tissue calcification, gas, and foreign bodies. Foot deformities can be evaluated by using additional weight-bearing radiographs. Radiographs are readily obtained and relatively inexpensive and, even when not diagnostic, provide important anatomic information that is useful for the interpretation of many of the other studies performed.[58]

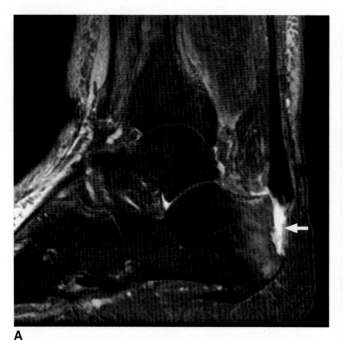

A

Figure 10–4 MRI of the right foot in a patient with posterior calcaneal avulsion fracture at the insertion of the Achilles tendon. The sagittal STIR image demonstrates calcaneal bone marrow edema and a fluid collection posterior to the calcaneus (*arrow*). Diffuse soft tissue edema is present. The coronal gadolinium-enhanced T1-weighted image with fat saturation shows bone marrow enhancement (*arrow*).

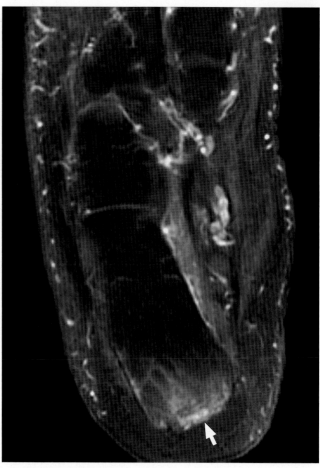

B

For evaluation of osseous changes of the diabetic foot, radiographs should be used in combination with MRI.

Recently, MRI has become the preferred study for evaluation of osteomyelitis of the foot and ankle in patients with diabetes mellitus.[17] Sensitivity ranges from 77% to 100%, and specificity ranges from 79% to 100%.[56,59,60] It has been reported that superimposed factors, such as neuropathic osteoarthropathy, or other inflammatory disease, such as rheumatoid arthritis, may lower the specificity of MRI for osteomyelitis.[10,48,61,62] On MRI, osteomyelitis demonstrates low signal in the bone marrow on T1-weighted images and high signal on T2-weighted images, particularly if fat suppression is used. After administration of contrast material, enhancement becomes visible on fat-suppressed T1-weighted images (Fig. 10-5).[6] Other MRI findings that may be seen with osteomyelitis are cortical disruption and periostitis.[63] Periostitis will be seen as circumferential high signal on T2-weighted images, representing edema with disproportionate contrast enhancement. If periostitis is chronic, edema and enhancement may be thickened.

T2-weighted imaging sequences with fat suppression or STIR sequences are most sensitive for the detection of osteomyelitis. However, T1-weighted images and contrast-enhanced, fat-suppressed, T1-weighted images are more specific and are superior for delineating its extent.[14] In patients with clinically suspected osteomyelitis of the diabetic foot, detection of an abnormal bone marrow signal on MRI usually yields a high sensitivity for the diagnosis of osteomyelitis. On the one hand, many other entities imitate such an alteration of bone marrow signal, such as fracture, tumor, active arthritis or neuropathic disease, infarction, or postoperative change.[10,14,48,56,61,62,64] On the other hand, these entities usually demonstrate a different morphology than osteomyelitis, which enables differentiation in most cases. Correlation with radiographs can be helpful for the identification of a fracture line, a discrete lesion, adjacent arthritis or neuropathic disease, or postoperative metal implants.[63] Clinical inspection of the foot and ankle is indispensable, because in most cases, secondary signs of osteomyelitis such as soft tissue alterations can be found, including skin ulceration, cellulitis, abscess, or sinus tract (Fig. 10-6), which may increase the specificity.[63,65]

In evaluating pedal infection, nuclear medicine examinations are also performed. For the detection of osteomyelitis, three-phase bone scintigraphy is highly sensitive.[66] In the early phases, a regional radiotracer uptake is seen, which is followed by concentration in the underlying bone marrow in delayed phase.[57,59] This test is outstanding for excluding osteomyelitis when there is no increased uptake, except in the setting of severe

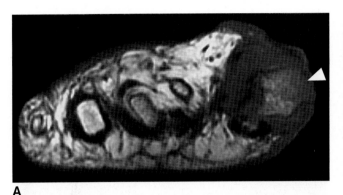 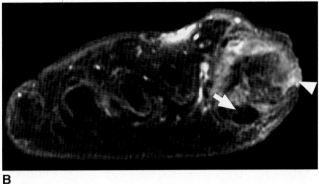

A   **B**

Figure 10–5   Coronal MR images of the right foot. The T1-weighted image (**A**) demonstrates a soft tissue ulcer at the medial aspect of the first metatarsophalangeal joint with lateral dislocation. There is osteomyelitis of the head of the metatarsal with focal cortical disruption of the medial surface with the osseous surface extending through the soft tissue defect (*arrowhead*) and abnormal low signal intensity of the bone marrow. The gadolinium-enhanced T1-weighted image with fat saturation (**B**) shows intense contrast enhancement of the metatarsal head (*arrowhead*), the disrupted joint, and the surrounding tissues. In addition, there is subtle contrast enhancement of the subarticular bone at the base of the proximal phalanx of the great toe (*arrow*).

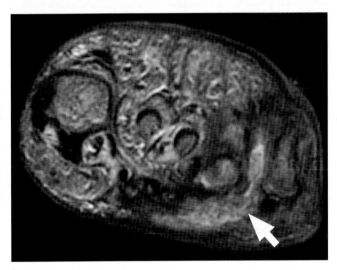

Figure 10–6   T2-weighted MRI with fat saturation (STIR) of the left foot in the coronal plane demonstrating osteomyelitis of the fourth metatarsal with abnormal bone marrow signal intensity and a plantar sinus tract (*arrow*). The soft tissue is swollen, showing diffuse edema.

Septic Arthritis

In the diabetic foot, the majority of cases of septic arthritis are caused by an adjacent soft tissue infection.[56] Septic arthritis is most frequently found in the interphalangeal joints and the metatarsophalangeal joints, predominantly laterally. Septic arthritis of the diabetic foot is most often a consequence of ulceration.[70] On MRI, septic arthritis most commonly becomes apparent as a joint effusion with distention of synovial recesses and intense contrast enhancement.[56] Furthermore, septic arthritis may demonstrate bone marrow edema on T2-weighted images and marrow contrast enhancement, which can be caused by either reactive marrow or osteomyelitis.[6] To differentiate these two entities, a low signal intensity on a T1-weighted image usually indicated the presence of adjacent osteomyelitis.[8,71]

Tendon Infection

MR evidence of tendon infection is present in approximately half the patients who require surgery for pedal infection, and detection of a tendon infection could influence surgical therapy.[15] Of interest, tendons are not a common pathway for the spread of infection, although their sheaths are not uncommonly infected.[9] Septic tenosynovitis occurs mainly in tendons underlying ulcers, especially the peroneal tendons because many ulcers occur at the lateral malleolus.[15] Tendon infection of the Achilles is directly related to posterior ulceration. Septic tenosynovitis can also be seen in patients with septic arthritis of the ankle because of a normal communication between the flexor hallucis longus and ankle joints.[6] MRI imaging of tendon infection typically shows a circular peritendinous contrast enhancement (Fig. 10-7).[15,72] If the contrast enhancement of a tendon is in

vascular disease. Under these circumstances, the addition of a 24-hour image, creating a four-phase bone scan, is recommended.[67] Other processes that result in hyperemia and bone turnover can also cause a positive test, and specificity is comparably low.[13] More encouraging results for the detection of osteomyelitis were reported for labeled blood cell examination in combination with three-phase bone scintigraphy, but both examinations together may be time consuming and costly and lack anatomic information that MRI provides.[10,68] MRI imaging provides a good sensitivity and specificity for diagnosing osteomyelitis in diabetic feet, and it is competitively priced in comparison with other imaging modalities. Furthermore, accurate delineation of extent allows limited surgical resection, making MRI increasingly the preferred diagnostic method.[69]

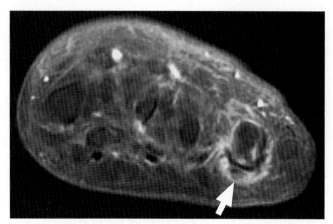

Figure 10–7   Gadolinium-enhanced T1-weighted MRI of the left foot in the coronal plane with fat saturation demonstrating abnormal contrast enhancement of the fourth metatarsal bone and tenosynovitis of the flexor tendon with peritendinous enhancement (*arrow*). There is dislocation of the first metatarsophalangeal joint and lateral subluxation of the second through fourth metatarsophalangeal joints and abnormal contrast enhancement of the soft tissues.

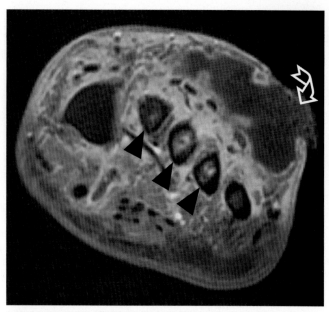

Figure 10–8   Gadolinium-enhanced T1-weighted MRI of the left foot in the coronal plane with fat saturation. A large subcutaneous dorsal abscess with rim enhancement and ulceration (*curved arrow*) is demonstrated adjacent to the extensor tendons. Osteomyelitis is found in the second, third, and fourth proximal metatarsals (*arrowheads*) in addition to diffuse myositis and tenosynovitis in the dorsal and plantar compartments of the foot.

direct contact with adjacent skin ulceration or cellulitis, peritendinous spread of infection is likely.

Abscess

Infected ulcers may cause even more severe soft tissue infections, including cellulitis, sinus tracts, and abscess formation.[9] On MRI, cellulitis becomes apparent as an area of contrast enhancement of the soft tissues with fat signal loss on T1-weighted images and hyperintense signal on T2-weighted images.[15] Focal abscess formation is reported to occur in 10% to 50% of all patients with pedal osteomyelitis.[48,73] MRI characteristics of abscess formation are focal isointense or hypointense signal compared with muscle tissue on T1-weighted images with fluid equivalent signal on T2-weighted images and rim enhancement on gadolinium-enhanced T1-weighted images (Fig. 10-8). Focal abscess formation may be rather small, but there is typically evidence of adjacent soft tissue infection with edema.[16] Abscess formation is significantly more frequent in patients with osteomyelitis and in feet that have been treated surgically.[73]

Skin Callus

In diabetic foot disease, ligamentous and tendon disorders have been shown to cause foot deformities.[9] Subsequently, skin callus may develop in areas of abnormal weight-bearing and friction against footwear. Skin callus is most commonly found underneath the first or second metatarsal heads at the metatarsophalangeal joint and underneath the heel. In case of a midfoot deformity due to

neuropathic arthropathy, callus may develop underneath the cuboid.[6] On MRI, skin callus usually shows low signal intensity on T1-weighted images and low to intermediate signal intensity on T2-weighted images. Callus appears focally prominent within the subcutaneous fat tissue. On postcontrast images, callus may demonstrate enhancement and imitate focal soft tissue infection.

Ulceration

At points of abnormal weight-bearing and friction, callus formation may occur, and the eventual breakdown of callus is accelerated by an alteration in skin turgor and shift of weight and localization of pressure points caused by neuropathy.[74,75] On MRI, signal intensity of ulcers is hyperintense on T2-weighted imaging with peripheral enhancement on fat-suppressed T1-weighted images after contrast. The immunosuppressive setting of diabetes mellitus promotes infection in ulcerations, which may further lead to abscesses, sinus tracts, tendon infections, septic arthritis, and osteomyelitis.[15,56,71,76] While abscess shows the typical MRI signal alterations with fluidlike signal on T2-weighted images and rim enhancement on contrast-enhanced images, the characteristics of a phlegmonous soft tissue infection are a less conspicuous signal on T2-weighted images and rimlike enhancement on contrast-enhanced images.[6]

Gangrene

On contrast-enhanced MRI, gangrene becomes apparent as a region of nonenhancement representing devascularization.[16] Demarcation from normal adjacent tissue is usually abrupt, and the surrounding tissue typically demonstrates reactive paradoxical hyperemia with increased enhancement. Initial MRI findings may look normal in case of ischemia without evident devitalization unless dynamic contrast-enhanced imaging and quantitative image analysis are performed.[6] Soft tissue loss may become apparent with noninfected gangrene, predominantly at the distal digits. In most cases, some induration of the subcutaneous fat with an otherwise normal appearance on T1- and T2-weighted images is seen. Superimposed infection in wet gangrene may demonstrate air within the soft tissues, which becomes apparent as small foci of signal void with blooming on gradient-echo MRI imaging.[77] The classic MRI criteria for osteomyelitis may not apply in patients with devitalized tissue to diagnose infection.

Foreign Body Granuloma

Foreign body granuloma is another type of soft tissue infection in diabetic patients. A foreign body that has entered the superficial or deep soft tissue may be difficult to identify. On MRI, signal characteristics are similar to those of other forms of soft tissue infection, which is high signal intensity on T2-weighted images and low signal intensity on T1-weighted images. In some cases, little to no signal alteration on T2 may be found, although marked enhancement is demonstrated after contrast administration.[9] Occasionally, an area of blooming signal void can be found on MRI representing the foreign body. Since a foreign body can be difficult to detect, radiographic or even CT correlation can help with its identification.

Diabetic Muscle Infarction

Muscle infarction, although uncommon, has been described in the calf and tight muscles of diabetic patients.[78–80] Not infrequently, infarction can recur, involve multiple sites, and be seen bilaterally in up to 30% of affected patients.[81] On MRI, T1- and T2-weighted images demonstrate isointense swelling of the involved muscle, with mildly displaced fascial planes.[82] There is effacement of the fat signal intensity within the muscle. Fat-suppressed T2-weighted images showed diffuse heterogeneous high signal intensity in the muscles, suggestive of edema. Perifascial fluid collection and subcutaneous edema can also be seen in most cases. Following intravenous gadolinium administration, MRI

usually demonstrates a focal area of heterogeneously enhancing mass with peripheral enhancement. Within this focal lesion, linear dark areas can be seen with serpentine enhancing streaks separating them. If the abnormal signal with associated edematous changes is localized to one muscle compartment, compartment syndrome must be considered as a secondary complication.[83]

Bone Infarction

On MRI, bone infarction, which is rather common in the diabetic foot, demonstrates a well-defined lesion with a serpiginous rim around an area (Fig. 10-9), which usually shows a fat signal but may also demonstrate signal characteristics of fluid or sclerotic bone, depending on the age of the bone infarct.[84,85]

Osteomyelitis versus Neuropathic Arthropathy

The differentiation of osteomyelitis from neuropathic arthropathy is difficult. The location of pathologic changes can give direction to further therapeutic management, since neuropathic arthropathy most commonly occurs in the midfoot whereas osteomyelitis is usually found distal to the Lisfranc joint or about the heel.[86] Osteomyelitis of the midfoot is in most cases associated with a foot deformity or with direct spread from ulceration or a sinus tract, which can usually be evaluated on MRI images. Subchondral signal abnormality and joint effusion are found with both osteomyelitis and neuropathic arthropathy, but an abnormality centered at the articulation and involvement of multiple regional joints points the way to neuropathic arthropathy.[6]

The most challenging diagnosis is superimposed infection in patients with neuropathic arthropathy, because neuropathic arthropathy can simulate infection both clinically and radiographically. One possible discriminator is called "ghost sign"; bones that appear vanished on T1-weighted images but are better delineated on T2-weighted and contrast-enhanced imaging and show a diffusely abnormal marrow signal are likely to contain osteomyelitis despite underlying neuropathic arthropathy.[6]

While many MR imaging features coexist in neuropathic arthropathy with and without superimposed osteomyelitis, several findings may serve as useful discriminators in the diabetic foot.[8] The presence of a sinus tract, replacement of soft tissue fat, extensive or diffuse marrow abnormality, thick rim enhancement or diffuse joint fluid enhancement, and joint erosion support superimposed osteomyelitis. On the other hand, an abnormal joint, the preservation of subcutaneous fat, absence of soft tissue fluid collections, presence of subchondral cysts, and presence of intra-articular bodies support neuropathic arthropathy alone, without infection.

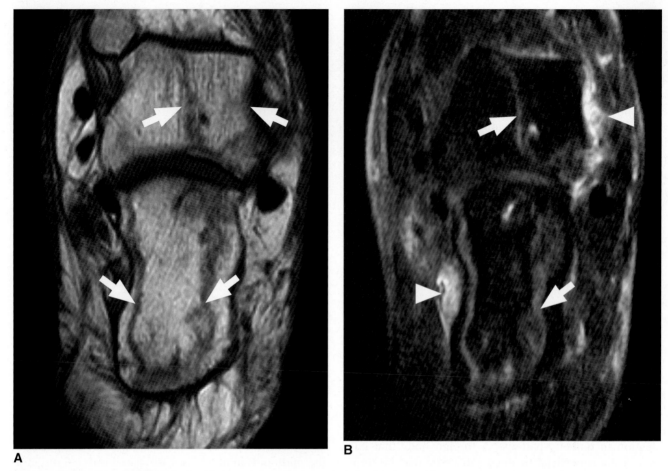

Figure 10–9   Coronal MRI of the left hindfoot demonstrating well-defined lesions with a serpiginous rim (*arrows*) involving the talus and calcaneus on T1-weighted (**A**) and STIR images (**B**) representing bone infarctions. Surrounding edema is present on the STIR image (*arrowheads*).

Summary

Neuropathic osteoarthropathy of the diabetic foot occurs most commonly at the Lisfranc joint. On MRI, the acute form is characterized by diffuse juxta-articular soft tissue edema, joint effusion, and erosion. The chronic form is rather characterized by subchondral cysts and bone proliferation with debris or intra-articular bodies. Joint deformity with subluxation or even dislocation is common. On CT, the extent of osseous changes can be well demonstrated. Bone scintigraphy is not pathognomonic but may be useful for follow-up.

Besides osteomyelitis, diabetic foot infection can manifest as septic arthritis, tendinitis, abscess, callus, ulceration, gangrene, and foreign body granuloma. The classic radiographic triad of osteomyelitis is demineralization, periosteal reaction, and bony destruction. At present, MRI is the preferred study for evaluation of osteomyelitis demonstrating low bone marrow signal on T1-weighted images, high signal on T2-weighted images, and contrast enhancement on fat-suppressed T1-weighted images. MRI provides a good sensitivity and specificity for diagnosing osteomyelitis in the diabetic foot, is competitively priced compared with other imaging modalities, and allows for accurate delineation of extent in order to limit surgical resection to a minimum. Bone scintigraphy has a high sensitivity but low specificity and lacks the anatomic information provided by MRI.

On MRI, the differentiation of osteomyelitis from neuropathic arthropathy can be difficult, particularly when the two occur simultaneously. The presence of a sinus tract, replacement of soft tissue fat, extensive marrow abnormality, thick rim enhancement, diffuse joint fluid enhancement, and joint erosion supports superimposed osteomyelitis. On the other hand, an abnormal joint, the preservation of subcutaneous fat, absence of soft tissue fluid collections, presence of subchondral cysts, and presence of intra-articular bodies support neuropathic arthropathy alone, without infection.

Both MRA and CTA are well suited for noninvasive visualization of peripheral vessels in diabetic foot disease. Arterial stenosis is visualized as focal narrowing of vessel caliber, abrupt cutoff of flow, or nonvisualization of a branch. Collateral vessels may become apparent in the setting of a slow-forming stenosis.

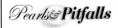

Pearls

- Neuropathic osteoarthropathy occurs most commonly at the Lisfranc joint.
- CT is the preferred study for evaluation of osseous changes.
- The classic radiographic triad of osteomyelitis is demineralization, periosteal reaction, and bony destruction.
- MRI is the preferred study for evaluation of osteomyelitis.
- Both CTA and MRA are well suited for noninvasive visualization of peripheral vessels.

Pitfalls

- Bone scintigraphy has a high sensitivity but low specificity in patients with osteomyelitis.
- On MRI, the differentiation of osteomyelitis from neuropathic osteoarthropathy can be difficult, especially when both occur simultaneously.

References

1. Morrison WB, Ledermann HP: Work-up of the diabetic foot. Radiol Clin North Am 40:1171–1192, 2002.
2. Most RS, Sinnock P: The epidemiology of lower extremity amputations in diabetic individuals. Diabetes Care 6:87–91, 1983.
3. Durham JR, Lukens ML, Campanini DS, et al: Impact of magnetic resonance imaging on the management of diabetic foot infections. Am J Surg 162:150–153, 1991.
4. Horowitz JD, Durham JR, Nease DB, et al: Prospective evaluation of magnetic resonance imaging in the management of acute diabetic foot infections. Ann Vasc Surg 7:44–50, 1993.
5. Tatli S, Lipton MJ, Davison BD, et al: From the RSNA refresher courses: MR imaging of aortic and peripheral vascular disease. Radiographics 23(spec no):S59–78, 2003.
6. Schweitzer ME, Morrison WB: MR imaging of the diabetic foot. Radiol Clin North Am 42:61–71, vi, 2004.
7. Janka R, Fellner C, Wenkel E, et al: Contrast-enhanced MR angiography of peripheral arteries including pedal vessels at 1.0 T: Feasibility study with dedicated peripheral angiography coil. Radiology 235:319–326, 2005.
8. Ahmadi ME, Morrison WB, Carrino JA, et al: Neuropathic arthropathy of the foot with and without superimposed osteomyelitis: MR imaging characteristics. Radiology 238:622–631, 2006.
9. Chatha DS, Cunningham PM, Schweitze, ME: MR imaging of the diabetic foot: Diagnostic challenges. Radiol Clin North Am 43:747–759, ix, 2005.
10. Gold RH, Tong DJ, Crim JR, Seeger LL: Imaging the diabetic foot. Skeletal Radiol 24:563–571, 1995.
11. Catalano C, Fraioli F, Laghi A, et al: Infrarenal aortic and lower-extremity arterial disease: Diagnostic performance of multi-detector row CT angiography. Radiology 231:555–563, 2004.
12. Robertson DD, Mueller MJ, Smith KE, et al: Structural changes in the forefoot of individuals with diabetes and a prior plantar ulcer. J Bone Joint Surg Am 84-A:1395–1404, 2002.
13. Lipman BT, Collier BD, Carrera GF, et al: Detection of osteomyelitis in the neuropathic foot: Nuclear medicine, MRI and conventional radiography. Clin Nucl Med 23:77–82, 1998.
14. Morrison WB, Schweitzer ME, Bock GW, et al: Diagnosis of osteomyelitis: Utility of fat-suppressed contrast-enhanced MR imaging. Radiology 189:251–257, 1993.
15. Ledermann HP, Morrison WB, Schweitzer ME, Raikin SM: Tendon involvement in pedal infection: MR analysis of frequency, distribution, and spread of infection. AJR Am J Roentgenol 179:939–947, 2002.
16. Ledermann HP, Schweitzer ME, Morrison WB: Nonenhancing tissue on MR imaging of pedal infection: Characterization of necrotic tissue and associated limitations for diagnosis of osteomyelitis and abscess. AJR Am J Roentgenol 178:215–222, 2002.
17. Ledermann HP, Morrison WB: Differential diagnosis of pedal osteomyelitis and diabetic neuroarthropathy: MR imaging. Semin Musculoskelet Radiol 9:272–283, 2005.
18. Quinn SF, Sheley RC, Semonsen KG, et al: Aortic and lower-extremity arterial disease: Evaluation with MR angiography versus conventional angiography. Radiology 206:693–701, 1998.
19. Binkert CA, Baker PD, Petersen BD, et al: Peripheral vascular disease: Blinded study of dedicated calf MR angiography versus standard bolus-chase MR angiography and film hard-copy angiography. Radiology 232:860–866, 2004.
20. Meissner OA, Rieger J, Weber C, et al: Critical limb ischemia: Hybrid MR angiography compared with DSA. Radiology 235:308–318, 2005.
21. Fellner FA, Requardt M, Lang W, et al: Peripheral vessels: MR angiography with dedicated phased-array coil with large-field-of-view adapter feasibility study. Radiology 228:284–289, 2003.
22. Rofsky NM, Adelman MA: MR angiography in the evaluation of atherosclerotic peripheral vascular disease. Radiology 214:325–338, 2000.
23. Vogt FM, Ajaj W, Hunold P, Herborn CU, et al: Venous compression at high-spatial-resolution three-dimensional MR angiography of peripheral arteries. Radiology 233:913–920, 2004.
24. Alson MD, Lang EV, Kaufman JA: Pedal arterial imaging. J Vasc Interv Radiol 8:9–18, 1997.
25. Lee HM, Wang Y, Sostman HD, et al: Distal lower extremity arteries: Evaluation with two-dimensional MR digital subtraction angiography. Radiology 207:505–512, 1998.
26. Wyttenbach R, Gianella S, Alerci M, Braghetti A, et al: Prospective blinded evaluation of Gd-DOTA- versus Gd-BOPTA-enhanced peripheral MR angiography, as compared with digital subtraction angiography. Radiology 227:261–269, 2003.
27. Reid SK, Pagan-Marin HR, Menzoian JO, et al: Contrast-enhanced moving-table MR angiography: Prospective comparison to catheter arteriography for treatment planning in peripheral arterial occlusive disease. J Vasc Interv Radiol 12:45–53, 2001.
28. Chiowanich P, Mitchell DG, Ortega HV, Mohamed F: Arterial pseudostenosis on first-pass gadolinium-enhanced three-dimensional MR angiography: New observation of a potential pitfall. AJR Am J Roentgenol 175:523–527, 2000.
29. Wikstrom J, Holmberg A, Johansson L, et al: Gadolinium-enhanced magnetic resonance angiography, digital subtraction angiography and duplex of the iliac arteries compared with intra-arterial pressure gradient measurements. Eur J Vasc Endovasc Surg 19:516–523, 2000.
30. Koelemay MJ, Lijmer JG, Stoker J, et al: Magnetic resonance angiography for the evaluation of lower extremity arterial disease: A meta-analysis. JAMA 285:1338–1345, 2001.
31. Katz DS, Hon M: CT angiography of the lower extremies and aortoiliac system with a multi-detector row helical CT scanner: Promise of new opportunities fulfilled. Radiology 221:7–10, 2001.
32. Hiatt MD, Fleischmann D, Hellinger JC, Rubin GD: Angiographic imaging of the lower extremities with multidetector CT. Radiol Clin North Am 43:1119–1127, ix, 2005.
33. Napoli A, Fleischmann D, Chan FP, et al: Computed tomography angiography: state-of-the-art imaging using multidetector-row technology. J Comput Assist Tomogr 28(suppl 1):S32–45, 2004.
34. Chow LC, Rubin GD: CT angiography of the arterial system. Radiol Clin North Am 40:729–749, 2002.
35. Fleischmann D, Hallett RL, Rubin GD: CT Angiography of peripheral arterial disease. J Vasc Interv Radiol 17:3–26, 2006.
36. Kreitner KF, Kalden P, Neufang A, et al: Diabetes and peripheral arterial occlusive disease: Prospective comparison of contrast-enhanced three-dimensional MR angiography with conventional digital subtraction angiography. AJR Am J Roentgenol 174:171–179, 2000.
37. Kaufman JA, McCarter D, Geller SC, Waltman AC: Two-dimensional time-of-flight MR angiography of the lower extremities: Artifacts and pitfalls. AJR Am J Roentgenol 171:129–135, 1998.
38. Harward TR, Ingegno MD, Carlton L, et al: Limb-threatening ischemia due to multilevel arterial occlusive disease: Simultaneous or staged inflow/outflow revascularization. Ann Surg 221:498–503, 1995.
39. Carpenter JP, Golden MA, Barker CF, et al: The fate of bypass grafts to angiographically occult runoff vessels detected by magnetic resonance angiography. J Vasc Surg 23:483–489, 1996.

40. Jones EA, Manaster BJ, May DA, Disler DG: Neuropathic osteoarthropathy: Diagnostic dilemmas and differential diagnosis. Radiographics 20(spec no):S279–S293, 2000.

41. El-Khoury GY, Kathol MH: Neuropathic fractures in patients with diabetes mellitus. Radiology 134:313–316, 1980.

42. Sella EJ, Barrette C: Staging of Charcot neuroarthropathy along the medial column of the foot in the diabetic patient. J Foot Ankle Surg 38:34–40, 1999.

43. Newman JH: Spontaneous dislocation in diabetic neuropathy: A report of six cases. J Bone Joint Surg Br 61–B:484–488, 1979.

44. Allman RM, Brower AC, Kotlyarov EB: Neuropathic bone and joint disease. Radiol Clin North Am 26:1373–1381, 1988.

45. Armstrong DG, Todd WF, Lavery LA, et al: The natural history of acute Charcot's arthropathy in a diabetic foot specialty clinic. Diabet Med 14:357–363, 1997.

46. Marcus CD, Ladam-Marcus VJ, Leone J, et al: MR imaging of osteomyelitis and neuropathic osteoarthropathy in the feet of diabetics. Radiographics 16:1337–1348, 1996.

47. Yu JS: Diabetic foot and neuroarthropathy: Magnetic resonance imaging evaluation. Top Magn Reson Imaging 9:295–310, 1998.

48. Beltran J, Campanini DS, Knight C, McCalla M: The diabetic foot: Magnetic resonance imaging evaluation. Skeletal Radiol 19:37–41, 1990.

49. Cofield RH, Morrison MJ, Beabout JW: Diabetic neuroarthropathy in the foot: Patient characteristics and patterns of radiographic change. Foot Ankle 4:15–22, 1983.

50. Schon LC, Easley ME, Weinfeld SB: Charcot neuroarthropathy of the foot and ankle. Clin Orthop Relat Res 349:116–131, 1998.

51. Nguyen VD, Keh RA, Daehler RW: Freiberg's disease in diabetes mellitus. Skeletal Radiol 20: 425–428, 1991.

52. Gondos B: The pointed tubular bone, its significance and pathogenesis. Radiology 105:541–545, 1972.

53. Muthukumar T, Butt SH, Cassar-Pullicino VN: Stress fractures and related disorders in foot and ankle: plain films, scintigraphy, CT, and MR imaging. Semin Musculoskelet Radiol 9:210–226, 2005.

54. Chantelau E: The perils of procrastination: Effects of early vs. delayed detection and treatment of incipient Charcot fracture. Diabet Med 22:1707–1712, 2005.

55. Eymontt MJ, Alavi A, Dalinka MK, Kyle GC: Bone scintigraphy in diabetic osteoarthropathy. Radiology 140:475–477, 1981.

56. Ledermann HP, Morrison WB, Schweitzer ME: MR image analysis of pedal osteomyelitis: Distribution, patterns of spread, and frequency of associated ulceration and septic arthritis. Radiology 223:747–755, 2002.

57. Yuh WT, Corson JD, Baraniewski HM, et al: Osteomyelitis of the foot in diabetic patients: Evaluation with plain film, 99mTc-MDP bone scintigraphy, and MR imaging. AJR Am J Roentgenol 152:795–800, 1989.

58. Tomas MB, Patel M, Marwin SE, Palestro CJ: The diabetic foot. Br J Radiol 73:443–450, 2000.

59. Weinstein D, Wang A, Chambers R, et al: Evaluation of magnetic resonance imaging in the diagnosis of osteomyelitis in diabetic foot infections. Foot Ankle 14:18–22, 1993.

60. Levine SE, Neagle CE, Esterhai JL, et al: Magnetic resonance imaging for the diagnosis of osteomyelitis in the diabetic patient with a foot ulcer. Foot Ankle Int 15:151–156, 1994.

61. Daffner RH, Lupetin AR, Dash N, et al: MRI in the detection of malignant infiltration of bone marrow. AJR Am J Roentgenol 146:353–358, 1986.

62. Jelinek J, Pearl AB, Kominsky SJ, Schultz PM: Magnetic resonance imaging of the foot: Rheumatologic disorders mimicking osteomyelitis. J Am Podiatr Med Assoc 86:228–231, 1996.

63. Morrison WB, Schweitzer ME, Batte WG, et al: Osteomyelitis of the foot: Relative importance of primary and secondary MR imaging signs. Radiology 207:625–632, 1998.

64. Seabold JE, Flickinger FW, Kao SC, et al: Indium-111-leukocyte/technetium-99m-MDP bone and magnetic resonance imaging: Difficulty of diagnosing osteomyelitis in patients with neuropathic osteoarthropathy. J Nucl Med 31:549–556, 1990.

65. Craig JG, Amin MB, Wu K, et al: Osteomyelitis of the diabetic foot: MR imaging-pathologic correlation. Radiology 203:849–855, 1997.

66. Newman LG, Waller J, Palestro CJ, G et al: Unsuspected osteomyelitis in diabetic foot ulcers: Diagnosis and monitoring by leukocyte scanning with indium in 111 oxyquinoline. JAMA 266:1246–1251, 1991.

67. Alazraki N, Dries D, Datz F, et al: Value of a 24-hour image (four-phase bone scan) in assessing osteomyelitis in patients with peripheral vascular disease. J Nucl Med 26:711–717, 1985.

68. Jacobson AF, Harley JD, Lipsky BA, et al: Diagnosis of osteomyelitis in the presence of soft-tissue infection and radiologic evidence of osseous abnormalities: Value of leukocyte scintigraphy. AJR Am J Roentgenol 157:807–812, 1991.

69. Morrison WB, Schweitzer ME, Wapner KL, et al: Osteomyelitis in feet of diabetics: Clinical accuracy, surgical utility, and cost-effectiveness of MR imaging. Radiology 196:557–564, 1995.

70. Armstrong DG, Lavery LA: Diabetic foot ulcers: Prevention, diagnosis and classification. Am Fam Physician 57:1325–1328, 1998.

71. Graif M, Schweitzer ME, Deely D, Matteucci T: The septic versus nonseptic inflamed joint: MRI characteristics. Skeletal Radiol 28:616–620, 1999.

72. Wang XT, Rosenberg ZS, Mechlin MB, Schweitzer ME: Normal variants and diseases of the peroneal tendons and superior peroneal retinaculum: MR imaging features. Radiographics 25:587–602, 2005.

73. Ledermann HP, Morrison WB, Schweitzer ME: Pedal abscesses in patients suspected of having pedal osteomyelitis: Analysis with MR imaging. Radiology 224:649–655, 2002.

74. Boulton AJ: The pathogenesis of diabetic foot problems: an overview. Diabet Med 13(suppl 1):S12–S16, 1996.

75. Pitei DL, Foster A, Edmonds M: The effect of regular callus removal on foot pressures. J Foot Ankle Surg 38:251–255, 1999.

76. Grayson ML, Gibbons GW, Balogh K, et al: Probing to bone in infected pedal ulcers: A clinical sign of underlying osteomyelitis in diabetic patients. JAMA 273:721–723, 1995.

77. Morrison WB, Ledermann,HP, Schweitzer ME: MR imaging of the diabetic foot. Magn Reson Imaging Clin N Am 9:603–13, xi, 2001.

78. Lim YW, Thamboo TP: Diabetic muscle infarction of the peroneus brevis: A case report. J Orthop Surg (Hong Kong) 13:14–316, 2005.

79. Kapur S, McKendry RJ: Treatment and outcomes of diabetic muscle infarction. J Clin Rheumatol 11:8–12, 2005.

80. Sahin I, Taskapan C, Taskapan H, et al: Diabetic muscle infarction: An unusual cause of muscle pain in a diabetic patient on hemodialysis. Int Urol Nephrol 37:629–632, 2005.

81. Habib GS, Nashashibi M, Saliba W, Haj S: Diabetic muscular infarction: Emphasis on pathogenesis. Clin Rheumatol 22:450–451, 2003.

82. Kattapuram TM, Suri R, Rosol MS, et al: Idiopathic and diabetic skeletal muscle necrosis: Evaluation by magnetic resonance imaging. Skeletal Radiol 34:203–209, 2005.

83. May DA, Disler DG, Jones EA, et al: Abnormal signal intensity in skeletal muscle at MR imaging: Patterns, pearls, and pitfalls. Radiographics 20(spec no):S295–S315, 2000.

84. Munk PL, Helms CA, Holt RG: Immature bone infarcts: Findings on plain radiographs and MR scans. AJR Am J Roentgenol 152: 547–549, 1989.

85. Abrahim-zadeh R, Klein RM, Leslie D, Norman,A: Characteristics of calcaneal bone infarction: An MR imaging investigation. Skeletal Radiol 27:321–324, 1998.

86. Weishaupt D, Schweitzer ME, Alam F, et al: MR imaging of inflammatory joint diseases of the foot and ankle. Skeletal Radiol 28:663–669, 1999.

Noninvasive Vascular Testing in the Evaluation of Diabetic Peripheral Arterial Disease

Joseph J. Hurley ■

Noninvasive evaluation of lower-limb arterial circulation should provide accurate, reliable answers to three questions regarding diabetic peripheral vascular disease (PAD): (1) the simple presence of PAD of any amount, (2) a prediction of the likelihood of success of wound or minor or major amputation healing with or without concomitant arterial revascularization, and (3) a clear estimation of impending revascularization failure by periodic surveillance. Discernment between diabetic and nondiabetic populations with PAD is important owing to differences in distribution and progression of atherosclerotic PAD in these two distinct groups.[1] Noninvasive vascular testing provides information that can be helpful in initiating wound care management as well as allowing an objective tracking of PAD progression. While many different noninvasive technologies have been suggested to fill this role, pressure measurements and waveforms, transcutaneous oximetry, and duplex ultrasound scanning currently appear to be the most widely accepted and available methods. Each of these tests offers advantages in different aspects of preoperative evaluation and/or postoperative follow-up. Understanding the limitations and pitfalls in interpreting these noninvasive tests (NITs) necessitates a knowledge of the natural history, physical examination findings, and variations in angiographic anatomy with diabetic PDA. The limitations, cost, and availability of these testing methods also are important issues to consider in establishing a noninvasive laboratory.

It is worth emphasizing that NITs do not stand alone but rather supplement information accumulated by methodical history taking coupled with a thorough physical examination.[2] This chapter provides an overview of the current state of the art in utilizing noninvasive testing in the management of diabetic PAD.

Natural History of Diabetic PAD

An estimated 7% of the population (20.8 million people) in this country have diabetes mellitus.[3] These diabetic individuals account for 15% to 17% of patients (including more than 20% of all people aged 60 or older) diagnosed with intermittent claudication, 30% to 50% of patients undergoing lower-limb arterial revascularization,[4,5] (60% to 70% having bypass grafts to arteries below the popliteal artery[6,7]), 15% to 20% of those undergoing carotid arterial intervention, and as many as 50% to 60% of those undergoing major lower-limb amputations;[8] an estimated 82,000 diabetic patients underwent major amputations in 2002. Symptoms of PAD are more likely to appear at an earlier age in diabetic people, as reported by Reunaneu and colleagues,[9] who noted intermittent claudication in 4.3% of diabetic people aged 30 to 59 years compared to only 2.0% of nondiabetic people in the same age group. The prevalence of foot ulceration in the diabetic clinic population is 14% to 15%,[8] with an annual cost of diabetic foot–

associated complications of more than 132 billion dollars yearly.[10]

Beach and colleagues,[11] screening 50- to 70-year-old volunteers, noted that PAD was more prevalent in type 2 diabetic patients (22%) than in controls (3%). Over a 2-year period in these same type 2 patients, the incidence of new PAD in those initially normal (14%) was lower than the incidence of significant progression in those already harboring PAD (87%), as determined by non-invasive testing (ankle-arm index [AAI] less than 0.95, abnormal Doppler derived waveforms, or a decrease of 0.15 in the AAI from previous testing). Finally, type 2 patients with PAD also demonstrated a high incidence of mortality: 22% compared with patients without PAD (4%) during this same study period.

A prospective, minimal 24-month follow-up study conducted by Bendick and colleagues,[12] also employing noninvasive evaluation in diabetic patients, seemingly confirms these results. Using the noninvasive criteria of an AAI less than 0.9, monophasic waveforms, or evidence of progression as indicated by a drop in the AAI of greater than or equal to 0.15, they likewise determined that fewer than 10% of patients who were initially considered to have a normal study developed any evidence of PAD during the study period. In contrast, 76% of those who were identified as having PAD at the start of the trial displayed progression of their arterial disease. The strongest indicator of PAD progression in diabetic individuals is the presence of preexisting PAD. This progression has a high likelihood of continuing over a relatively short time.

The consequences of PAD in diabetic people is also seen in a collected series of 2323 patients undergoing major lower-limb amputation,[13] of whom 54% were diagnosed as having diabetes mellitus.

In this same series, 20% of these individuals had incurred a previous contralateral amputation, while only 37% of the entire series, diabetic and nondiabetic alike, survived for 5 years.

Patients with symptomatic major vessel peripheral vascular disease have a sharply increased risk for coronary and cerebrovascular atherosclerosis. Criqui and colleagues[14] found that the presence of moderately severe to even asymptomatic PAD in the posterior tibial artery increased the risk of coronary artery disease threefold to sixfold. Patients who became symptomatic or harbored severe lower-limb vascular disease had a 10-year risk of death due to coronary heart disease 10 to 15 times greater than that for subjects who were free of large-vessel arterial disease.

McDaniel and Cronenwett[15] noted that even with only the diagnosis of intermittent claudication, mortality was significant after 5 years, revealing a 23% mortality rate in nondiabetic individuals, which jumped to a 49% rate for diabetic individuals.

The implications of diagnosing PAD in a diabetic individual are enormous, including progressive PAD requiring arterial revascularization, minor or major limb amputation, coronary and cerebrovascular disease, and increased mortality.

Clinical Diagnosis of Diabetic Peripheral Arterial Disease

A careful history followed by a thorough physical examination provides the initial suggestions of the possibility of PAD. The location and severity of this occlusive disease can usually be determined at a surprisingly accurate level with the use of history and physical examination alone in experienced hands.[16,17] Historically, the natural progression of arterial insufficiency commences with intermittent claudication. The claudication onset distance decreases until patients start experiencing pain even at rest. The final stage in this progression is the appearance of gangrene or failure of even minor cuts and abrasions to heal while at the same time becoming extremely painful. Unfortunately, since many diabetic individuals have some element of peripheral neuropathy, the stage of rest pain is often lacking, and even lesions at the gangrenous stage can be relatively nonirritating. Commonly, a history of claudication in diabetic patients is later followed by the unheralded appearance of nonhealing wounds or gangrene.

Assessment of claudication demands that the discomfort that is experienced with ambulation is predictable and occurs at virtually the same distance given the identical angle of terrain and gait. Increasing the elevation of terrain (including stairs) or the briskness of gait normally results in a shortened claudication-onset distance. For convenience and the sake of patient communication, we often relate this distance to blocks (i.e., four- to six-blocks claudication, half-block claudication, etc.) It is likewise important to understand that claudication, a word derived from the Latin verb *claudicatio*, meaning "to limp," while usually described as painful, can also be described as weakness, heaviness, or even cramping of the leg muscles. The level of the discomfort often gives a clue to the probable level of arterial narrowing or occlusion. Thigh and buttock claudication suggests an aortoiliac location if bilateral or iliac if unilateral, while calf claudication points to femoral or popliteal involvement. Impotence combined with claudication (Leriche's syndrome) in nondiabetic people is highly suggestive of aortoiliac artery involvement. This syndrome is less reliable in diabetic patients, owing to increased incidence of neurogenic impotence. Rest pain usually implies multilevel disease of a severely stenotic or totally occlusive nature. When present, this pain usually has onset within an hour or two after assuming a supine position. It classically involves the distal forefoot; can be relieved by dangling the foot over the side of the bed, short-distance ambulation, or sleeping in a sitting position; and is repetitive with resuming a supine position.

Rest pain occurs as a result of arterial pressures at the ankle level being inadequate to force blood against gravity to the now upright foot, the toes and distal forefoot being most vulnerable.

Physical findings require observation and palpation. The ischemic foot will display changes in color with elevation and dependency as a result of ischemia-induced deranged autonomic autoregulation. A ruborous foot on dependency blanches rapidly when elevated to 45 degrees above the examination table. The hypoxemia resulting from insufficient blood flow due to PAD is a potent stimulus to vasodilatation, probably the strongest known. Dependent rubor results from the dilated vessels attempting to trap blood for increased oxygen extraction. Two ways of evaluating this in a more objective fashion are capillary refill time and venous refill time. In the supine position, pressure is applied to the skin, and once it is removed, the reappearance of the usual skin color in this area is timed. Capillary refill time is usually considered abnormal when it takes longer than 5 seconds to return to baseline. Venous refill time can be determined by identifying a prominent vein in the foot in a supine patient. The leg is then elevated 45 degrees for 1 minute, following which the patient sits up and hangs the leg over the side of the examination table. The time in seconds between assuming the upright position and the reappearance of the vein bulging above the skin level is recorded. Normal venous refill time is considered to be 20 seconds or less.[18]

Assessment of pulses at the femoral, popliteal, and pedal (dorsalis pedis and posterior tibial) locations should be graded as normal, diminished, or absent. Absent pulses do not necessarily denote hemodynamically significant PAD, since medial layer calcification present in more than 30% of diabetic pedal vessels can prevent palpation of a pulse even in an artery with a normal lumen. Likewise, the presence of pedal pulses does not ensure normal peripheral circulation. Salhi and colleagues,[19] employing noninvasive methods, demonstrated a 10% presence of some PAD in diabetic patients having two detectable pulses and a 20% presence in diabetic patients with one detectable pulse. Only 5% of nondiabetic patients with a single pedal pulse displayed evidence of PAD. Auscultation of the femoral and aortoiliac region for a bruit should be performed. Bruits occur at areas of arterial narrowing, with onset around 50% stenosis and disappearance around 90% stenosis. They provide a clue as to the presence, location, and severity of PAD. Changes in skin, hair, and nails may be a sign of critical ischemia and should be sought. Skin atrophy or rubor, nail thickening, or hair loss all tend to occur with progressive PAD. Boyko and colleagues[2] examined the utility of clinical history taking and physical examination in evaluating PAD in diabetic patients. By using multivariate analysis, the highest probability for finding severe PAD was obtained with the following parameters: patient age (>65 years old), a self-reported history of physician-diagnosed PAD (or more than one-block claudication), peripheral pulse deficit, and abnormal venous filling time. Additionally, they noted that more than 85% of patients with an AAI less than or equal to 0.5 had a history of tobacco abuse.

Diminished peripheral foot pulses and delayed venous filling time were associated with the highest likelihood of having severe (AAI < 0.5) PAD.

Noninvasive Evaluation

Some individuals question any role for noninvasive testing in the clinical assessment and management of diabetic patients with PAD. In 1979, Gibbons and colleagues[20] employing ankle systolic blood pressure measurements evaluated 150 diabetic patients seeking a decisive number to predict the success in selecting an amputation level. Their conclusion, "In the diabetic patient, clinical judgment continues to provide the most accurate and reliable information by which the type of amputation and the likelihood of its success can be judged," was well supported by their clinical material. Mehta and colleagues[21] confirmed the fallibility of ankle pressures in predicting healing of transmetatarsal amputations in diabetes, whereas Barnes and colleagues[22] did likewise for the healing of below-knee amputations. The latter favored the presence of a popliteal pulse. Bone and Pomajzl[23] suggested the value of indexing the potential of healing forefoot amputation using toe pressures derived photoplethysmographically. In their study, eight limbs with digital pressures of less than 45 mm Hg failed to heal. Two of eight (25%) failed to heal in the range of 45 to 55 mm Hg, and all 14 patients who were subjected to forefoot amputation with a pressure greater than 55 mm Hg healed. They also demonstrated the unreliability of ankle systolic blood pressure in predicting amputation success. Hauser and colleagues[24] showed the superiority of transcutaneous oximetry (in clinical decision making over assessment of ankle brachial indices). These and other investigators had a twofold impact: (1) The need for careful clinical evaluation was reemphasized, and (2) the need for better noninvasive testing was suggested. More recently, employment of direct duplex arterial interrogation has aided the growing success with endovascular arterial revascularizations. Its growing role in NIT evaluation of diabetic PAD will be discussed.

Hemodynamic Assessment of Lower-Level Arterial Circulation

Noninvasive hemodynamic assessment of lower-limb circulation involves measuring pressures, recording waveforms, and eliciting the effects of increasing demand on arterial flow (achieved by either exercise or induced reactive hyperemia) and its effect on ankle pressure

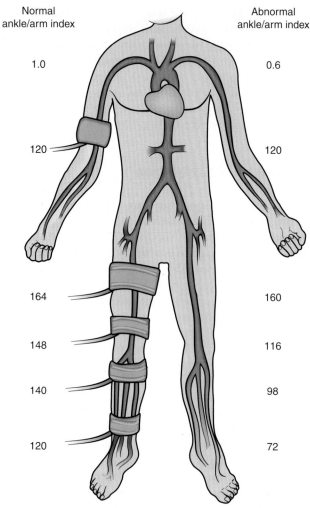

Normal
ankle/arm index

1.0

120

164

148

140

120

Abnormal
ankle/arm index

0.6

120

160

116

98

72

Figure 11–1 Normal condition on the right side of the body with ankle systolic pressure equal to brachial systolic pressure. Ankle pressure divided by arm pressure determines AAI—in this case, 1.0. On the left side, AAI is 0.6, indicating only 60% of expected normal flow at rest. In addition, any gradient greater than 30 mm Hg between two successive cuffs indicates high-grade stenosis or occlusion. Here, 44 mm Hg high-thigh gradient localizes diseased segment to superficial femoral artery. *(From Arizona Heart Institute: Cerebrovascular and peripheral vascular disease: Advanced noninvasive diagnostic techniques, with permission.)*

TABLE 11-1   Determination of Critical Stenosis*

Condition of Measurement	Average Blood Flow (mL/min)	Critical Stenosis Determined by 10% Drop in Flow (%)	Critical Stenosis Determined by 10% Drop in Pressure (%)
Iliac actery	144	85	86
Iliac artery + 1 AV fistula	456	75	74
Aorta + 1 AV fistula	314	86	86
Aorta + 2 AV fistulas	593	79	79
Aorta + 3 AV fistulas	886	73	73

*This table demonstrates the pathophysiology of arterial stenotic disease. Increasing the flow by opening a progressively larger number of arteriovenous (AV) fistulas causes a progressively lesser amount of stenosis necessary to initiate a 10% drop in flow. The validity of using noninvasive pressure measurements to determine flow changes is seen by comparing the last two columns. (Courtesy of Dr. Wesley Moore, Tucson, AZ.)

2. The greater the flow, the less the stenosis necessary to create the same incremental decrease in pressure (Table 11-1).

Thus, more information can be derived when the response to a demand for maximum flow in a limb is elicited. The data of Strandness and Bell[26] as well as others demonstrate that exercise in the presence of arterial occlusive disease proximal to the blood supply of the calf muscles results in a transient decrease in blood pressure at the ankle. It follows that this decrease in ankle pressure provides an objective means for assessing and following the course of PAD in the lower limbs. The magnitude of these changes is a direct function of the work performed coupled with the degree of stenosis or occlusion. In addition, the duration of decreased blood flow after exercise (reactive hyperemia) is a valuable marker of the circulatory system's ability to meet these demands (Fig. 11-2). Normal individuals display little or no postexercise decreased reactive hyperemia. In contrast, patients with critical arteriosclerosis and/or occlusions have markedly prolonged intervals of decreased blood flow response to even minimal exercise demands. The magnitude of the decrease in ankle pressure and its duration are rough guides to the extent of blood flow impairment.[27] Reactive hyperemia can be assessed in individuals who are unable to exercise by inflating a thigh cuff 50 mm Hg greater than systolic pressure for 3 minutes and then reading the serial ankle pressures on release of the pressure. This is known as induced reactive hyperemia.

Further information can be gathered by interpreting waveforms obtained at rest and following exercise (Fig. 11-3). A normal triphasic waveform obtained in conjunction with abnormal pressure results should call the

changes from baseline levels. Segmental pressure measurements (high thigh, above knee, below knee, ankle levels) allow some attempt at accurate identification of the anatomic location of involvement of atherosclerotic disease (Fig. 11-1). Several basic principles are pertinent to understanding the results of noninvasive hemodynamic testing. In a series of canine experiments using multiple in-line arteriovenous fistulas providing a wide range of iliac artery blood flow, Moore and Malone[25] demonstrated the following:

1. The percentage of decrease in blood pressure was the same as the percentage of decrease in blood flow (i.e., blood pressure and blood flow vary directly).

validity of the study into question and require reexamination. Likewise, a deteriorated waveform elicited with normal or elevated systolic pressures suggests the potential for medial calcification (common in diabetic and renal failure patients), suggesting a false elevation of the ankle pressures. Thus, this invalidates this parameter in the assessment of circulatory competency. Waveforms can be obtained and recorded on a strip chart recorder by using photoplethysmography or Doppler velocity flow meters and various-sized pressure cuffs.

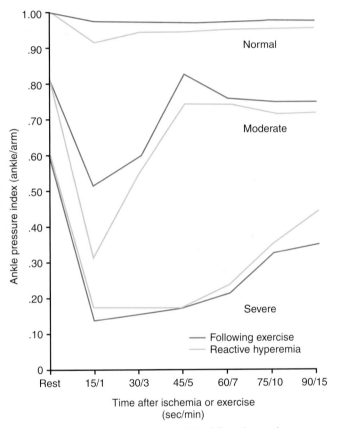

Figure 11–2 Effect of increasing blood flow demands on normal patients and those with moderate and severe peripheral arterial disease. Note the correlation between exercise measured in minutes and reactive hyperemia measured in seconds.

Photoplethysmography

Photoplethysmography employs a transducer that transmits infrared light from an emitting diode into the tissue. Part of the transmitted light is reflected back from the blood within the cutaneous microcirculation and is received by an adjacent phototransistor. The amount of reflected light varies with the blood content of the microcirculation. The output of the phototransistor is A/C, coupled to an amplifier for recording as a pulsatile analogue waveform. This phototransducer is taped to the end of the toe with a double-faced cellophane tape while a small digital blood pressure cuff is placed at the base of the digit (Fig. 11-4). The pressure at which the waveform obliterates corresponds to the digital systolic pressure. The pressure may also be measured by using a digital strain gauge or a peripherally placed Doppler probe.

Doppler Ultrasound

Doppler ultrasound devices consist of two piezoelectric crystals mounted in a probe. By stimulating one of the crystals with an electrical charge, sound waves of various frequencies (all beyond the range of human hearing) are emitted. The second crystal receives the sound waves reflected from moving particles, producing a voltage change. This change can be amplified and converted to analogue waveforms or sound. The higher the frequency emitted by the crystal, the less is the depth of penetration and the narrower is the width investigated. A frequency of 5 MHz or lower gives deep penetration and a comparatively broad beam especially suited for monitoring deep blood vessel flow in the vena cava or iliac veins or for examining peripheral veins. An operating frequency of 10 MHz is less penetrating but permits a sharper focus and is ideal for blood velocity detection in arteries in the lower leg, arms, and digits. The Doppler probe is coupled to the skin with acoustic gel and held at an appropriate angle to the vessel being examined. This angle varies in accordance with the specifications of the individual manufacturers, ranging from 38 to 52 degrees.[28]

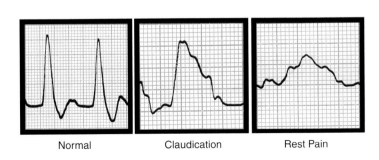

Normal   Claudication   Rest Pain

Figure 11–3 Doppler-derived waveforms from a strip chart recorder. A crisp, rapid systolic upstroke with early reversed flow is depicted in the normal tracing. Broadening of the waveform with a loss of reversed flow, seen with claudicants, deteriorates by further widening and flattening, as seen with the tracing from a patient with rest pain.

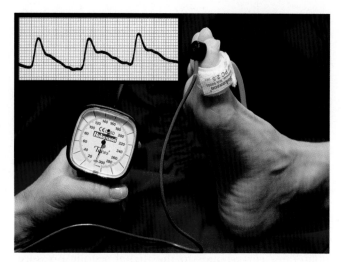

Figure 11–4   Toe pressure recording by using photoplethysmographic technique. The insert reveals a normal tracing at rest. Digital pressure is derived at the point where the waveform disappears with cuff insufflation.

A good seal between the probe and the skin is critical because the sound waves travel poorly through the air. Because there is no ideal probe angle for optimum recording, using a large amount of acoustic coupling gel allows one to vary the angle of insonation to find that point where the audible sound is clearest. A beam of ultrasound travels to the underlying vessel, where it is reflected from red blood cells and shifted in frequency by an amount proportional to the flow velocity of erythrocytes in that vessel. The pitch of the audiofrequency signal produced by the receiving crystal is therefore proportional to the average velocity of the blood flowing within the vessel under study. The Doppler does not record the flow itself but a phase shift. The recorded Doppler signal is used in two ways: (1) to measure segmental systolic pressure and (2) to produce flow velocity waveform patterns for analysis.

Segmental Pressures

Pressure cuffs 12 cm wide are placed at the high thigh level, above the knee, below the knee, and at the ankle level. By listening with the Doppler probe over one of the pedal vessels (dorsalis pedis, posterior tibial, or lateral tarsal arteries), one can obtain the pressure at the level of the inflated cuff. An AAI is obtained by dividing the segmental ankle systolic pressure by the brachial systolic pressure. The usual index recorded should be 1 or just slightly higher. Pressure changes correlate directly with flow, as was previously discussed; thus, an index of 0.5 represents only 50% of the expected blood flow. A gradient of 40 mm Hg or greater between the levels being compared suggests an occlusion or highly stenotic segment. In normal situations, the high thigh pressure is 1.3 times the brachial systolic pressure.

In a paper by Apelquist and colleagues,[29] no upper limit of ankle pressure could be defined in diabetic patients above which value amputation was not necessary or foot ulcers would heal. Toe pressure gave a clearer clue, with primary healing occurring in 85% of patients with toe pressure greater than 45 mm Hg.

Finally, Takolander and Rauwerda,[30] in a review article, surmised probably correctly: "unfortunately in diabetic patients the prognostic value of the ankle pressure may be nil." Medial calcification should always be suspected when an unusually high AAI (>1.15) is found. Decreased ankle pressures have value since there are essentially no falsely decreased pressures. Normal AP and certainly those elevated above brachial systolic pressure need always to be correlated with toe pressure findings.

Toe Pressures

The role of toe pressures with or without pulse waves in predicting the clinical course of rest pain, skin ulcerations, and gangrene in diabetic patients has been extensively examined.[31,32] Holstein and colleagues[33] feel that absolute toe pressures provide a highly accurate method for determining the likelihood of success in the healing of an ulcer or in minor amputation, thus preventing a more proximal, major, potentially disabling amputation. Baker and Barnes[28] seemingly concur with this assessment in diabetic people for the likelihood of minor amputation healing. Bowers and colleagues[34] likewise found a role for toe pressure measurements to confirm the presence of severe clinical deterioration. Defining severe clinical deterioration as rest pain, tissue loss, or gangrene, they found a toe pressure (TSP) of 40 mm Hg or less to have significance. Patients with diabetes in this group had an even significantly higher risk of developing critical ischemia. Meanwhile, Carter and Tate[35] validated the significance of toe systolic pressures and added pulse wave measurements in an attempt to increase accuracy. They decided that toe pressure reflected the overall obstruction in the arterial tree proximal to the digits and was not affected by arterial incompressibility. Adherence to strict study conditions was stressed, with patients resting supine for at least 20 minutes, bodies and limbs covered with a heating blanket in a room with an ambient temperature of approximately 23° C. The presence of diabetes mellitus increased the odds ratio for rest pain, skin lesions, or both after controlling for systolic pressures and wave amplitude. Further, lower toe pulse wave amplitude was significantly related to the occurrence of rest pain, skin breakdown, or both. In summary, rest pain, skin lesions, or both were present in approximately 50% of limbs with toe pressures less than or equal to 30 mm Hg, in 16% of those with pressure of 31 to 40 mm Hg, and in 5% of limbs with arterial disease and toe pressure greater than 40 mm Hg.

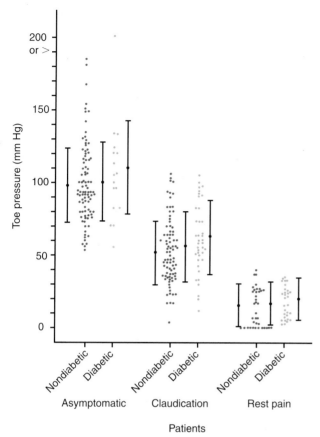

Figure 11-5   Toe blood pressures grouped according to symptoms and presence of diabetes in patients with arterial disease. Mean and standard deviations for the nondiabetic and diabetic subgroups and for the two groups combined are indicated by *vertical bars.* *(From Ramsey DE, Manke DA, Sumner DS: Toe blood pressure: A valuable adjunct to ankle pressure measurement for assessing peripheral arterial disease. J Cardiovasc Surg 24:43, 1983.)*

Ramsey and colleagues[36] discussed the fact that ankle pressure measurements often fail to reflect the severity of peripheral ischemia when the underlying vessels are calcified or with extensive pedal or digital PAD. Using a digital pneumatic cuff and PPG, they concluded that toe pressure measurements obviated this problem. Toe pressure measurements had an average sensitivity of 85% with a specificity of 88% in asymptomatic limbs and 89% and 86% for ischemic limbs. They concluded that a toe pressure greater than 30 mm Hg was indicative of good healing potential and an ankle pressure of less than 80 mm Hg was associated with poor healing. The correlation of toe pressure was essentially the same in both diabetic and nondiabetic limbs (Fig. 11-5). Sahli and colleagues,[19] commenting on ankle pressure measurement in an ongoing screening program for lower-limb PAD in diabetic patients, focused on the value of toe blood pressure assessment. They found that mean AP was higher in both type 1 and 2 diabetic patients than in controls. Toe blood pressure, on the other hand, offers significant advantages compared to ankle blood pressure measure-

ment and is more efficient in detecting diabetic patients with silent PAD.

Personal Experience with Digital Testing of Toe Pressure

We reviewed the predictive value of AAIs and absolute digital systolic pressures in diabetic and nondiabetic patients. In 120 patients undergoing limb salvage procedures, the average AAI preoperatively in diabetic patients was 0.53, increasing to 0.97 postoperatively, with a very wide scatter. This AAI appeared more reliable in nondiabetic individuals; starting at a mean of 0.34 preoperatively (Fig. 11-6), it climbed to 1.03 postoperatively. Photoplethysmographically derived digital pressures were much more predictable and precise in both diabetic and nondiabetic patients.

In the diabetic population, only four patients demonstrated a pressure greater than 40 mm Hg preoperatively (Fig. 11-7), whereas only five remained below this range (only one with less than 30 mm Hg) after successful revascularization.

More recently, McCollum and colleagues[37] confirmed the value of photoplethysmographically derived digital pressures in the assessment of severe ischemia but cautioned that appropriate warming of the foot permitting adequate foot vasodilation was essential to provide accurate gathering of results, so that meaningful conclusions can be drawn. Appropriate testing conditions are critical to every method of noninvasive testing for which reports are available. Vincent and colleagues[38] reported on the use of photoplethysmographically derived digital pressures toe-brachial index, noting that in patients with chronic ulcerations, toe pressures were higher in diabetic patients than in nondiabetic patients. They believed that during pressure measurements, attention must be directed to the patient's state of relaxation, digital skin temperature, and toe position relative to the level of the heart. They emphasized that systolic pressures fluctuated with respiration and activity (e.g., talking). Nielson[39] demonstrated that skin temperature variation from 33° to 24° C caused an average decrease of 10 mm Hg in toe systolic pressures secondary to changes in vasomotor tone. Finally, the same authors revealed diminished toe pressure attributed to hydrostatic forces when measurements were obtained with the patient supine.

Waveform Evaluation

Many approaches to quantitative analysis of waveforms have been suggested, but all have seemingly added little, if any, value over a subjective or qualitative evaluation.[16]

The waveform in the normal state shows a rapid systolic upstroke and usually a peaked appearance. The actual magnitude of the waveform can be affected by the

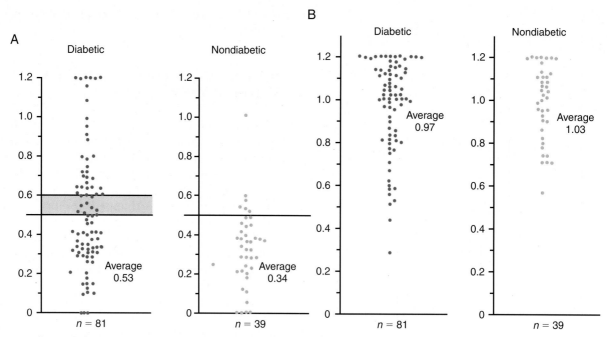

Figure 11–6   A, Preoperative ankle-arm pressure indices (AAIs) display a wide range in diabetic patients as compared with nondiabetic patients, because of medial calcinosis of the vessels causing incompressibility. (Incompressibility >1.2 AAI recorded as 1.2.) **B,** Postoperative indices in nondiabetic patients display a significant change from preoperative levels. The same change to a lesser degree is seen with diabetic individuals.

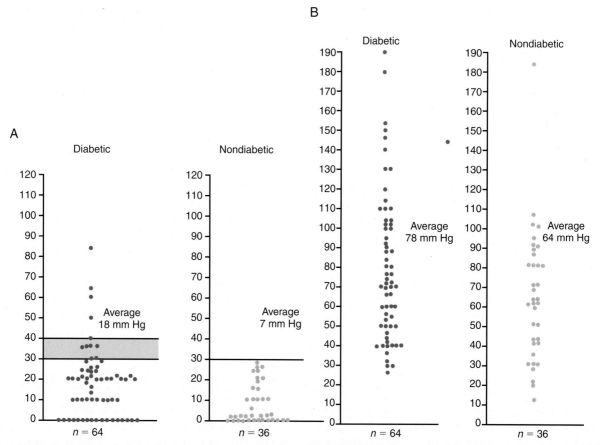

Figure 11–7   A, Absolute toe pressure measurements obtained photoplethysmographically in preoperative diabetic and nondiabetic limb-salvage patients reveal only four patients with a value >40 mm Hg in the diabetic group. **B,** In postoperative patients, there are none with <30 mm Hg and only five patients with <40 mm Hg in the diabetic group. This degree of improvement is not observed in the nondiabetic patient.

depth of the artery (e.g., decreased in obese people), by probe pressure that actually compresses a thin patient's artery, by the probe angle in relation to the artery, or even by the consistency of the vessel being evaluated (e.g., a prosthetic graft will give a distorted picture even when fully patent). Thus, no comparisons of the height of the peak should be attempted. In addition, a normal peripheral waveform will usually show a reversed component as the initial diastolic portion, followed by a small second forward component. The reverse segment is the result of distal resistance, followed by the elastic recoil of the vessel wall. This can sometimes be absent in the normal subject at the ankle level. Deterioration of the waveform can be seen just proximal to an obstructing lesion; distal to the lesion, the waveform is always abnormal, with a loss of the normal rapid systolic upstroke, so the slope is similar to that of the downstroke. In addition, even before these changes, earlier milder stenosis will cause loss of the diastolic components at the popliteal or femoral levels. As the flow deteriorates, waveforms become flattened and then undulating before they totally disappear. Flow and viability may exist despite absent waveforms, because the Doppler probes rarely detect flow at less than 6 mL/minute. Comparing pressures with waveforms helps to avoid errors in interpretations, especially at the high thigh level. Here, a normal waveform coupled with a decreased high thigh pressure suggests good inflow into the common femoral artery with severe stenosis or occlusion of the proximal superficial femoral artery.

Exercise Stress Testing

Exercise can lead to a 10- to 20-fold increase in blood flow through the peripheral arteries. As is apparent in Figure 11-8, increased flows can lower the degree of stenosis necessary to create a given drop in flow or pressure. In addition, limiting factors other than claudication are sometimes demonstrated (decreased pulmonary compliance, arthritic disease, cardiac insufficiency, etc.). A standard treadmill test is done on an incline of 12 degrees at 2 mph.[40] The treadmill test is limited to a maximum of 5 minutes or the onset of chest discomfort, shortness of breath, dizziness, or severe leg pain. The cuffs placed before the stress to determine the resting ankle pressure remain in place during the study. Immediately when the stress is stopped, at 2½ minutes and again at 5 minutes, ankle pressures are determined. The level of exercise necessary to validate claudication is much less than would be routinely encountered in cardiac stress testing. Nevertheless, caution is urged in patients who have coronary artery disease, and it is our policy to have a well-trained nurse or technician in attendance at all times.

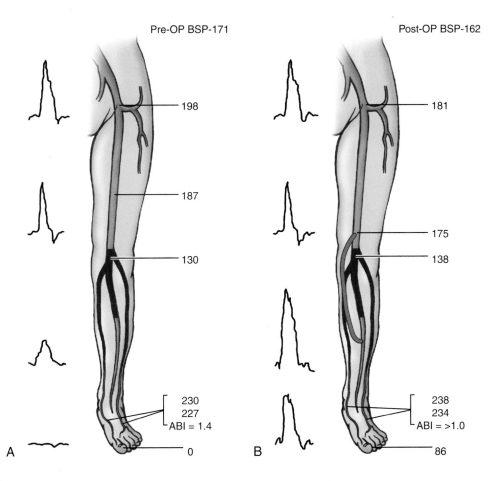

Pre-OP BSP-171   Post-OP BSP-162

Figure 11–8   A, In this example, the classic pattern of distal severe occlusive arterial disease is found with total occlusion of the distal popliteal; the tibial peroneal; and the proximal anterior tibial, posterior tibial, and peroneal arteries. A toe pressure of 0 mm Hg in spite of an ABI of 1.4 makes healing of severe foot ulcers unlikely. **B,** After a popliteal-to-peroneal in situ saphenous vein bypass, the toe pressure is now 86 mm Hg and the ABI remains at 1.4. Total healing of the ulcers occurred within 3 weeks.

In patients with recent contralateral amputations, painful infections, ulcers, digital necrosis, or recent surgery, induced reactive hyperemia can be utilized. The high thigh pressure cuff is inflated to 50 mm Hg over the previously determined resting high thigh pressure. The patient is supine for this study, and the cuff remains inflated for 3 minutes. Ankle pressures are again measured immediately after release of the high thigh pressure cuff and at 15-second intervals for 3 to 5 minutes. Ouriel and colleagues[41] performed a critical evaluation of stress testing in the diagnosis of peripheral vascular disease. They studied 218 patients (372 limbs) and 25 normal subjects (50 limbs) with resting AAI, treadmill exercise, and postocclusive reaction hyperemia to determine reliability and discrimination. They concluded that resting AAI was a simple, accurate, and reproducible test but that routine stress testing was not cost effective, adding little diagnostic information whether one is dealing with claudicants or patients harboring rest pain, ulceration, or gangrene. They suggested that stress testing should be reserved for the small subset of symptomatic patients with normal resting AAI. They also noted that walking distance was not a reproducible measure and that only a weak correlation existed between walking distance and the severity of disease as assessed by resting AAI. A gradual decrease in the use of stress testing has been experienced. It nevertheless can prove useful in situations in which symptoms seemingly contradict physical findings and resting AAI. At times, other etiologies (e.g., pulmonary, cardiac, arthritic) for decreased ambulatory ability are clearly elucidated when the patient reproduces symptoms while undergoing testing.

Regional Tissue Oxygen Perfusion Measurements

Another method to evaluate the state of perfusion of limb tissues and in particular the skin is the measurement of transcutaneous partial oxygen pressure. The transcutaneous partial pressure of oxygen (TCpO2) monitor can instantly read the arterial oxygen value, once it has been set up. The oxygen-sensing part of the TCpO2 electrode is a polarographic electrode consisting of a combined platinum cathode surrounded by a silver ring acting as anode and containing a heating element. A resistor is incorporated for measurement and control of the electrode temperature. An oxygen-permeable but hydrophobic polytetrafluoroethylene membrane separates the skin from the compartment containing both the oxygen-sensing apparatus and a reservoir of potassium chloride solution with a phosphate buffer.[42]

When a polarizing voltage of 630 millivolts is applied to the platinum cathode, a current proportional to the pO2 will be generated by a reduction of oxygen at the cathode, provided that the membrane limits the rate of oxygen diffusion.

The electrode, measuring 9 millimeters in diameter, is affixed to the part of the skin to be studied. The heat input gradually raises the electrode temperature and therefore the local skin temperature to the required 45° C setting. Electrodes can be placed in numerous areas, but at least two must be used. One is placed usually in the anterior upper chest area to serve as a control, while the second electrode is placed at the point of interest to be studied (e.g., the base of a toe with a possible digit amputation, 10 cm below the knee when contemplating potential below-the-knee amputation).

Torneson[43] demonstrated a correlation between digital toe pressures (strain gauge) and TCpO2 measurements in a group of patients harboring critical ischemia. He demonstrated a rough correlation between the two methods for predicting adequate regional perfusion but found that the correlation deteriorated in the more severely ischemic situations. The situation in which the observed TCpO2 was zero yet digital pressures were recorded is explained as a situation in which local oxygen consumption and oxygen delivery are equal. He invoked the concept that gas shunting along with chronic hypoxia removes O_2 totally from the blood before entering the capillary bed, thus allowing the oxygen-empty red cells to tumble uselessly through the capillaries.

Matsen and colleagues[44] felt that the key to understanding and managing the patient with PAD involved the ability to quantify the severity of vascular insufficiency. They noted the effects of limb position changes on the measurement of TCpO2, also noting that at all locations where the TCpO2 was 20 mm Hg or less, a surgical procedure was necessary, either a bypass graft or an amputation.

Hauser and Shoemaker[45] proposed a ratio of study site to chest electrode to arrive at the transcutaneous regional perfusion index. They believed that this would more reliably assess limb oxygenation than direct TCpO2 measurements by obviating the effects of changes in systemic oxygen delivery on the study site TCpO2. They found no overlap, previously a dilemma between responses of normal subjects and patients with claudication. Additionally, they concluded that limb ischemia could be quantified, thus allowing grading of disease severity and surveillance of disease progression.

The TCpO2 levels on the control (anterior chest wall) average about 80% of PaO2 in supine adults. This discrepancy was attributed to the heating electrode causing dermal capillary dilation, oxyhemoglobin dissociation, and enhancement, which increases local oxygen supply and skin oxygen consumption. This magnifies the effect of changes in PaO2 and cardiac output on limb TCpO2.

Mustapha and colleagues[46] used TCpO2 in selecting the most suitable level for major lower-limb amputation.

A TCpO2 reading of 40 mm Hg or greater (at 10 cm below the knee) indicated adequate perfusion of skin that could likely result in a successful below-the-knee amputation. They estimated that a site reading requires an average of 35 minutes.

Byrne and Provan[47] described the use of resting, exercise, and postexercise TCpO2 measurements to distinguish between normal subjects and those with PAD. Abnormal resting TCpO2 levels occurred in 80% of claudicants, all of whom registered a decline in TCpO2 following exercise. A subgroup undergoing contrast angiography (CA) showed that TCpO2 after exercise had a 100% sensitivity and specificity in detecting PVD. If resting values alone are considered, sensitivity falls to 77%. The authors feel that the value of exercise PtcO2 testing was in distinguishing between vascular and other causes of exercise-induced leg pain.

Cino and colleagues[48] studied the use of TCpO2 to diagnose peripheral vascular disease and aid in planning of vascular surgery in both diabetic and nondiabetic patients. They stressed strict protocol, measurements at ambient pressure and temperature, and supine positioning for 15 minutes with readings obtained after the TCpO2 was stable for 5 to 10 minutes. To correct for patient differences in blood oxygen content, blood pressure and cardiac output TCpO2 measurements of the calf and foot were normalized to values measured on the chest, providing a TCpO2 index. They compared the TCpO2 results with those obtained by measurement of absolute ankle pressure and ankle brachial indices and pulse volume recordings but unfortunately did not include the measurement of toe pressures. Predictably, TcpO2 values were superior in identifying the presence of PAD and accurately characterizing different degrees of severity (claudication versus rest pain versus impending gangrene). This held true even in diabetic patients. Healing of amputations was observed where TCpO2 values were greater than 38 mm Hg either preoperatively or after vascular reconstruction. The need for revascularization or predictable failure with ulcer healing was noted with TCpO2 values of less than 30 mm Hg. The authors did comment on the limitation of TCpO2 measurements, which can be influenced by marked edema, hyperkeratosis, cellulitis, and obesity; factors that can reduce thermal conductivity capillary flow and therefore oxygen transmission. They suggest that TCpO2 complements but does not necessarily replace the use of hemodynamic testing.

Hauser and colleagues,[24] studying only a diabetic population, claimed superiority for TCpO2 in NITs in 46 consecutive diabetic patients evaluated. The ability to discriminate severity of disease, likelihood of ulcer healing, or identification of the appropriate amputation level required positional changes of the foot. Employing indexing of values, they found that claudicants could best be discerned from normal patients with leg elevation; but with rest pain and gangrene, the indexed values were quite similar in supine and elevated positions, diverging only with dependent positioning. Comparing TCpO2 to ankle systolic blood pressure measurements and pulse volume recordings yielded a statistically significant ($p < .001$) accuracy level for the former study. Their conclusion was that TCpO2 measurements are the only consistently accurate NIT to evaluate the status of PAD in the diabetic population and "that the foot of a patient with diabetes found to be measurably hypoxic by regional oximetry merits CA irrespective of the pulses or of any other NIT results."

Laser Doppler Velocimetry

Subsequent to attempts to use transcutaneous oximetry, the employment of laser Doppler velocimetry (LDV) alone or in conjunction with TCpO2 was reported. The LDV device emits a monochromic helium-neon laser beam at a frequency of 632.8 nm that is conducted to the skin through a plastic fiberoptic probe. The basis of LDV is that a collimated beam becomes diffusely scattered, absorbed, and broadened when applied to the skin, resulting in Doppler shifts that can be detected by a sensitive photodetector. The Doppler shift is linearly related to the mean velocity of red blood cells within skin capillaries and varies with the angle of the probe to the tissue being monitored. Measurements reflect an average over a semisphere of skin approximately 1 mm in radius. The photo-detected reflected signal is fed into an analogue signal processor, and values are expressed in millivolts. The normal LDV tracing is fairly characteristic, whereas ischemic tissues generate pulse waves of lesser magnitude and amplitude. Karm and colleagues[49] performed LDV measurements in 29 patients (16 diabetic individuals) before they underwent below-knee amputations. Anterior and posterior calf LDV values greater than or equal to 20 mV were associated with successful below-knee amputation wound healing in 25 of 26 patients; all three patients with either anterior or posterior calf LDV values less than 20 mV had below-knee amputations that failed to heal.

Karanfilian and colleagues[32] combined Doppler and LDV measurements in predicting healing of ischemic forefoot ulcerations and amputations in diabetic and nondiabetic patients. Fifty-nine limbs, 63% of which were in nondiabetic patients, were studied. Either transmetatarsal amputation or debridement with or without skin grafting was performed. Criteria for successful healing included a Doppler value of more than 10 mm Hg, a laser Doppler pulse wave amplitude of more than 4 mV, and an ankle systolic pressure of more than 30 mm Hg. With these criteria, the outcome was predicted correctly in 53 of 56 limbs (95%) by Doppler, in 46 of 53 limbs (87%) with LDV, and in 31 of 59 limbs (52.5%) with Doppler ankle pressures.

They concluded that the estimation of skin blood flow by the TCpO2 and LDV is significantly better than Doppler ankle pressure measurements in predicting the healing of forefoot ulcerations and amputations in diabetic and nondiabetic patients.

More recently, Bacharach and colleagues[50] at the Mayo Clinic looked at TCpO2 to predict amputation site healing in lower limbs with arterial occlusive disease. Fifty-eight percent of their patients had diabetes, and testing was obtained with accurate calibration of the equipment in the supine and limb-elevated modes. They found that a TCpO2 value greater than or equal to 40 mm Hg was associated with primary or delayed healing in 50 of 52 limbs (98%) and that a TCpO2 value less than 20 mm Hg was universally associated with failure. Measurement of TCpO2 during limb evaluation improved predictability in limbs with borderline supine TCpO2 values.

Sheffer and Rieger[51] looked at the role of oxygen inhalation and leg dependency in predicting the need for revascularization or the likelihood of successful amputation. While they did not discriminate results on the basis of the presence or absence of diabetes, one third of the patients were diabetic. Satisfactory results were achieved by combining limits for, first, supine (10 mm Hg) and sitting (45 mm Hg) TCpO2 and, second, ankle arterial pressure (60 mm Hg) and supine TCpO2 (10 mm Hg). Oxygen inhalation proved to be of no significant help.

The use of TCpO2 measurements, either absolute, indexed, or with other studies such as laser Doppler velocimetry, has been well studied as a means of evaluating the presence and severity of PAD. While this is intriguing, variables of significant baselines, various adjuncts required, potential impediments, and a lack of a good comparison with digital systolic pressures raise questions about a claimed superiority as a sole noninvasive method to evaluate critical diabetic PAD. Nevertheless, TCpO2 appears to be one valid mechanism that can be employed in the assessment of lower-limb arterial circulatory status in both diabetic and nondiabetic groups.

Duplex Ultrasound Evaluation

Arterial duplex ultrasound scanners provide three types of information: gray-scale-B-mode imaging, color flow imaging, and pulsed and Doppler spectral waveform analysis. The first two types of information are used for localization and characterization of atherosclerotic plaque composition; it is mainly an evaluation of blood flow velocity provided by the latter that is the basis for arterial stenosis algorithms. Pulsed Doppler allows sampling of flow in a small volume of tissue. Duplex-derived velocity measurements require accurate estimation of the Doppler angle, which must be maintained at 60 degrees or less to minimize the angle correction error.

The velocity calculation is a function of the cosine of the angle between the ultrasound beam and the blood flow. At angles greater than 60 degrees, the cosine value changes rapidly, resulting in an increasingly greater potential for error with small additional changes in angle.

When duplex and arteriographic stenosis categories disagree, this might be due to inherent limitations of the arteriogram rather than those of the duplex ultrasound scanner.

Duplex Ultrasound

Color duplex ultrasound (CDUS) scanning of the lower-limb arterial system has evolved not only for diagnosis but also for allowing management decisions and as surveillance of progression of PAD in native arteries and bypass grafts.[52,53] It has assumed a larger role in these situations with increasing utilization of endovascular procedures. Identification of stenosis from occlusion, as well as revealing the location and severity of such lesions, has proven helpful in planning invasive intervention.[54] Additionally, the ability to locate crural arteries for potential bypass sites when even standard angiography has been unsuccessful or, in the face of significant renal insufficiency, where contrast nephropathy is a concern, is becoming more common. Finally, CDUS surveillance of successful lower-limb bypass grafts is the standard for clinical follow-up.

Moneta and colleagues[55] demonstrated CDUS scanning ability to distinguish a 50% or greater stenosis from occlusion in the lower limb. They were able to visualize 99% of arterial segments above the tibial arteries. Overall sensitivities for detecting greater than 50% stenosis ranged from 89% in the iliac vessels to 67% in the popliteal artery. Likewise, stenosis was differentiated from occlusion 98% of the time. Ability to detect occlusion in the tibial vessels was 90% for the anterior and posterior tibial vessels but fell to 82% for the peroneal artery. They noted that the presence of diabetes, kidney failure, or previous vascular disease did not affect the accuracy of this test. Ligush and colleagues[56] pitted CDUS against conventional angiography in planning lower-limb revascularization procedures. With few exceptions, CDUS was able to reliably predict infrainguinal reconstruction strategies. The predictive ability of CA from CDUS in this series was not statistically significant. More recently, Grassbaugh and colleagues,[57] in confirming the findings of Ligush and colleagues, provided CDUS-derived criteria for selections of the most appropriate distal revascularization site, including higher peak systolic velocities, high end diastolic velocities, and greater arterial diameter compared with arteries not selected for bypass grafting and later confirmed as inadequate on subsequent CA. They also noted the failure of CDUS in evaluating the peroneal artery; only five of 10 peroneal arteries ultimately selected as a bypass recipient were correctly identified by CDUS. Additionally, CDUS failed to correctly identify the peroneal artery 20% of the time.

Wilson and colleagues[58] employed CDUS and CA for assessing distal runoff prior to femorocrural bypasses. In a series of 43 consecutive patients undergoing 44 distal revascularizations, CA correctly predicted a suitable runoff vessel in 34 cases but was indeterminate in six and failed to identify runoff in three patients. CDUS correctly predicted a suitable runoff vessel for all 44 grafts. The authors concluded that CDUS imaging is superior to arteriography for preoperative assessment of distal runoff for femorocrural reconstruction. Proia and colleagues,[59] in a series of 23 consecutive patients with critical limb ischemia undergoing infragenicular vein grafts, based these procedures on CDUS as the sole preoperative imaging modality. In only one limb was the target artery abandoned, owing to dense calcifications.

Comparing this group with a group of 50 patients undergoing similar revascularization based on CA findings revealed no statistical difference between 1-year graft patency and limb salvage. They noted that the mean preoperative target artery peak systolic velocity in patent versus failed grafts was 49.18 cm/sec versus 31.9 cm/sec (whereas the mean end diastolic velocity was 22.7 cm/sec versus 14.8 cm/sec, respectively.) Again, these data suggest that target artery velocities might predict successful outcome and improve target selection.

By far the greatest role CDUS scanning plays in management of diabetic PAD involves postoperative surveillance following lower-limb revascularization. Detecting a failing vein bypass graft is critical to allow salvage prior to graft thrombosis. Successful long-term salvage of thrombosed vein grafts is not common, while failing patent grafts consistently display a good long-term assisted primary patency rate. Clinical signs and symptoms appear unreliable in detecting graft failure prior to thrombosis, as do employment of routine ankle and toe pressure measurements. Banddyk and colleagues[60] and then Westerband and colleagues[61] reported that a Doppler-derived low peak systolic velocity (< 40 to 45 cm/sec) and absent diastolic forward flow predicted impending graft failure.

A false decreased peak systolic velocity (PSV) can occur with abnormal widening of the vein graft. B-mode measurements should supply appropriate clues in this circumstance. Mills suggested a postoperative surveillance schedule of every 3 months for the first postoperative year and every 6 months in the second year and beyond with normal functioning grafts. He added high-velocity criteria defined as a peak systolic velocity greater than 300 cm/sec or a velocity ratio of 3.5 (velocity ratio: PSV [at the stenosis]) divided by PSV (at normal vessel preceding stenotic graft segment). He urged concomitant measurement of ankle pressures, AAI, and toe pressures. A decrease in the AAI greater than 0.15 even with normal CDUS mandates CA to identify inflow and outflow lesions or a rare missed graft stenosis.

TABLE 11-2 Vein Graft Surveillance: Duplex Categories of Graft Stenosis*

Stenosis Category	Peak Velocity (cm/sec)	Velocity Ratio (VR)	Interpretation and Management
Normal	<125	1.0–1.4	Normal scan, no action
Low-grade	125–180	1.5–2.4	Abnormal site, rescan in 3 months for progression
Moderate	180–300	2.5–3.4	Consider repair/angiogram, rescan in 6 weeks
Severe	>300	>3.5	Flow-reducing lesion, recommend repair

*Modified duplex ultrasound surveillance categories utilized in our vascular laboratory for detecting possible vein graft stenosis. Additionally, detection of a decreased peak systolic velocity (<40 cm/sec) indicating low flow mandates angiography with possible surgical intervention. (Blood Flow Lab, St. John's Mercy Medical Center, St. Louis, MO.)

Idu and colleagues[62] demonstrated the impact of CDUS on infragenicular vein graft patency in a 5-year experience. One hundred and sixty bypass grafts were monitored with CDUS scanning during the first two postoperative years compared to 41 bypass grafts monitored with clinical assessment alone. The assisted primary patency rate was higher in grafts that underwent CDUS surveillance than in grafts that underwent clinical follow-up (3-year patency rates of 91% and 72%, respectively). Stenosis in bypass grafts greater than 70% in his series resulted in 100% failure without revision and 10% failure with revision.

Duplex ultrasound scanning, usually with color flow, is assuming an even larger role in the diagnosis, selection of distal anastomotic site, and especially postoperative surveillance of lower-limb revascularization. Diabetic individuals make up almost two thirds of those undergoing femorocrural reconstructions. Thus, any improvement in distal bypass grafting has a profound effect on diabetic PAD management. Prevention of graft failure with thrombosis is tantamount to continuing limb salvage in this group, particularly those whose distal anastomosis is sited below the popliteal artery (Table 11-2). CDUS scanning obtains both anatomic and physiologic noninvasive data in a single study.[63] This information, while highly focused, remains critical to the role that noninvasive evaluation plays in the identification of failing distal bypass grafts and following endovascular revascularization procedures. It is safe, reproducible, and exceptionally well tolerated by patients.

Peripheral Noninvasive Investigation

Two questions are raised with regard to noninvasive evaluation in diabetic patients. First, which patients should undergo these studies? Second, which studies should be employed in these investigations? A set of guidelines developed at an international workshop addressed the first question, whereas the second requires understanding of the effectiveness, cost, and effort required of each study.

At an international meeting[18] addressing the assessment of peripheral vascular disease in diabetic patients, the following recommendations for the detection and follow-up of diabetic PAD in a primary care setting were made. The first criterion is claudication.

On an annual basis, diabetic patients should be asked about the presence of exercise-induced calf leg pain that is not present at rest. Patients with lifestyle-limiting, exercise-induced calf pain should be referred to a specialist, a vascular laboratory, or both for special vascular assessment. Second, the presence of any potential signs of critical ischemia (i.e., foot or limb ulceration), the presence of skin changes (nail or skin atrophy or dependent rubor), or the detection of gangrene should lead to a referral for special vascular assessment. Third, palpation of the dorsalis pedis or posterior tibial pulses should be performed on an annual basis for all adult (>18 years old) diabetic patients. An absent or diminished pedal pulse is an indication for performing an ankle-brachial index (ABI) or referral to a vascular laboratory for evaluation if an ABI cannot be determined by the primary care physician.

It is further recommended that, whenever possible, the presence of diminished or absent pulses be confirmed by a second observer or repeat examination before referral. Fourth, auscultation for femoral bruits on an annual basis is recommended for all adult diabetic patients. The detection of femoral bruits is an indication for performing an ABI or, if this is not available, referral to a vascular laboratory. Furthermore, it is recommended that all physician offices that provide routine care to adult diabetic patients should be able to measure ankle-brachial blood pressures to detect PAD. Additional recommendations for obtaining an ABI are any diabetic patient who has newly detected diminished pulses, femoral bruits, or a foot ulcer; any diabetic patient with leg pain of unknown etiology; at baseline examination in all type 1 diabetic patients older than 35 years of age or with more than 20 years' duration of diabetes; and at baseline examination in all type 2 patients over 40 years old. Follow-up for ABI greater than 0.9 is every 2 to 3 years; for 0.5 to 0.9, every 3 to 4 months; and less than 0.5, referral to a vascular specialist, vascular laboratory, or both. If an incompressible artery with an ankle pressure greater than 300 mm Hg or ankle pressure 75 mm Hg above arm pressure is found, repeat in 3 months. If it is still present, these patients should be referred for special vascular assessment (Fig. 11-9).

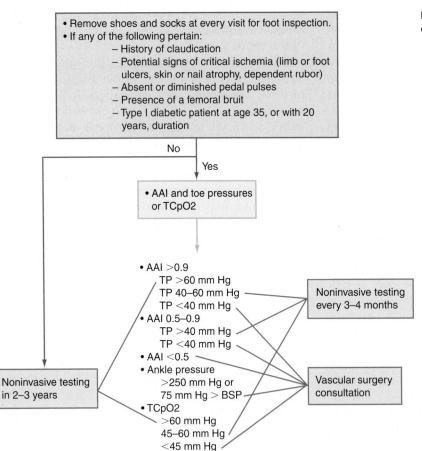

Figure 11–9 Algorithm for office evaluation of diabetic lower-limb arterial disease.

The foregoing has explained which patients should be evaluated and even suggested which initial test should be used. While the ABI is easy and inexpensive to perform, it lacks the ability to allow a more specific assessment of the severity of PAD.[64] This leads to the question of what is the best noninvasive study to employ in investigating PAD in diabetic subjects. The study that is employed depends on the patient's clinical circumstances. Assessing hemodynamically significant iliac artery stenosis and the likelihood of digital amputation success are two vastly different situations requiring different noninvasive procedures. Overall, severity of PAD can be determined with TSP or TCpO2 assessment, which helps to determine the greatest likelihood of healing ulcers or success in digital amputations with or without concomitant limb revascularization.

Both TSP and TCpO2 assessments appear to give approximate as opposed to exact levels for successful management of PAD issues in diabetic individuals. Lack of consensus on an approximate level or the exact determination (absolute level versus indexed findings) to employ in clinical decision making in utilizing these NITs coupled with potentially adverse testing situations calls for a considered approach in their use. Unfortunately, no large study comparing TSP and TCpO2 is available. Both seem to provide information that allows a number below which success without revascularization is unlikely as well as a number indicator above which success is most predictable. We utilize toe pressures and feel that our experience and the literature offered in this article allow the following approach: Below 30 mm Hg, healing is likely in 10% or fewer of our patients, while a toe pressure of 40 mm Hg makes attempts at healing diabetic foot wounds with conservative management or minor digital amputations most likely. We have a "no idea zone" that exists between 30 and 40 mm Hg. Repeat testing has helped to resolve this dilemma in some cases. It might be quite possible that the melding of TCpO2 and TSP studies in this "zone" might deliver a more accurate insight into the appropriate clinical course to take.

Normally, CDUS, segmental pressure measurements, or exercise testing can give reliable information on iliac and femoral popliteal arterial occlusive disease, discerning stenosis from occlusion as well as assessing collateral circulation and location of the lesions. In certain circumstances (contrast dye allergy, renal artery insufficiency), CDUS may supplant CA in preoperative assessment. CDUS may also prove useful in evaluating ambiguous CA results.

Careful attention to testing conditions, including ambient temperature, patient's state of relaxation, and limb positioning, coupled with experienced application of noninvasive techniques, is critical for most of these noninvasive studies. Likewise, physician understanding of the limitations of these noninvasive studies is necessary for applying the results to clinical situations. Unrecognized

ischemia occurs for two reasons: patient error or physician error. Patient error centers on physical findings often in hard-to-examine areas (plantar surface, heel, interdigital spaces) or where significant tissue damage is obscured by severe peripheral neuropathy, as discussed by Pfeifer and Green.[65] Additionally, diabetic retinopathy can frequently deprive patients of their backup sense of vision.

Reliance on the spouse, a family member, or a friend on a regular basis to examine the feet is recommended in this situation.

Physician error can stem from inappropriate interpretation of noninvasive testing as a result of lack of knowledge of their limitations. Most often, this occurs when near-normal or extremely high ankle pressures are equated with no risk of distal ischemia. As you should be aware by now, and to be demonstrated in the examples, extremely high ABIs can be associated with limb-threatening ischemia. Additionally, diabetic individuals deserve a methodical examination of their feet to include the interdigital spaces, plantar surface, and heels of both feet with every visit. The Foot Council of the American Diabetes Association reminds all physicians to remove the shoes and socks of all diabetic patients and inspect the feet whenever these patients are seen in consultation. To this wise admonition should be added that physicians should also understand the applications and limitations of noninvasive testing.

Summary

The enormous cost of diabetic foot problems has been aptly described in preceding chapters. Prevention along with early detection of diabetic PAD should be the cornerstone in managing diabetic foot lesions. Correct application and interpretation of NITs has been described. Examples of common clinical situations and the NIT findings illustrate the vagaries in the evaluation and management of these problems (Figs. 11-8, 11-10).

These examples, while straightforward, illustrate the essence of PAD in diabetic subjects and should be understood. Discussion of the role of magnetic resonance angiography is discussed in the chapter on radiologic intervention (Chapter 16). The greater question involves the implication for progressive PAD and mortality associated with the finding of significant arterial lesions in diabetic subjects. An algorithm for follow-up of diabetic patients depending on their arterial status as well as a table to assess the status of distal revascularization after vein bypass grafting has been supplied (Fig. 11-9). Clearly, this group of patients requires careful, frequent, and methodical follow-up with liberal use and understanding of NITs. It is hoped that, to that end, this chapter will prove beneficial to all who have read it.

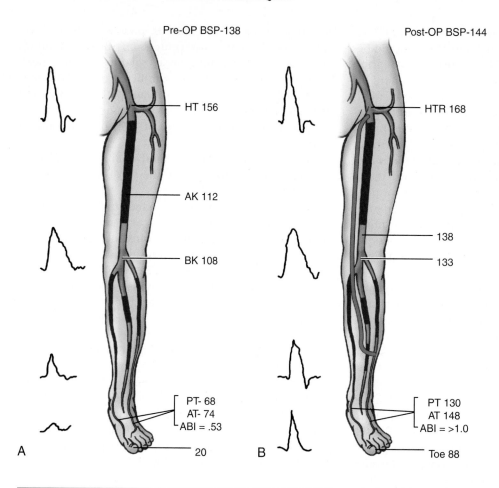

Pre-OP BSP-138

HT 156

AK 112

BK 108

PT- 68
AT- 74
ABI = .53

A

20

Post-OP BSP-144

HTR 168

138

133

PT 130
AT 148
ABI = >1.0

B

Toe 88

Figure 11–10   **A,** This example involves a superficial femoral and three tibial arteries being occluded. A toe pressure of 20 mm Hg makes spontaneous healing of an ulcer of the second toe unlikely. **B,** After a common femoral-to-distal anterior in situ saphenous vein bypass graft, the ABI is now greater than 1.0, and the great toe pressure has risen to 88 mm Hg.

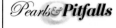 *Pearls&Pitfalls* Achievement of consistently reproducible and accurate interpretations with either toe pressure or transcutaneous oximetry studies is greatly benefited by strict attention to the testing environment. Ideally, patients wait and are examined in a comfortable, soothing room with an ambient temperature of 22° to 24° Celsius. Heightened anxiety or recent exposure to either tobacco products or extreme cold can lead to spuriously lower measurements. Efforts at putting patients at ease, along with a 20- to 30-minute equilibrium in a warm environment (especially on cold days) prior to testing, are advised. Inquiries regarding the recent use of tobacco products should be made and recorded on the chart. A good practice in scheduling a study is to impress on the patient the need to refrain from tobacco use 8 to 12 hours prior to the study. Likewise, dressing warmly on cold days is advised.

References

1. Strandness DE, Priest RE, Gibbons GE: Combined clinical and pathologic study of diabetic and nondiabetic peripheral arterial disease. Diabetes 13:366–372, 1964.
2. Boyko EJ, Ahroni JH, Davignon D, et al: Diagnostic utility of the history and physical examination for peripheral vascular disease among patients with diabetes mellitus. J Clin Epidemiol 50:659–668, 1997.
3. Nathan DMX: Long-term complications of diabetes mellitus. N Engl J Med 328:1676–1685, 1993.
4. Duj JJ, Jimes RA: The role of diabetes in the development of degenerative vascular disease: With special reference to the incidence of retinitis and peripheral vasculitis. Assoc Intern Med 14:1902, 1941.
5. Rosenbloom MS, Flanigan DP, Schuler JJ, et al: Risk factors affecting the natural history of intermittent claudication. Arch Surg 123:867–870, 1988.
6. Logerlo FW, Coffman JD: Current concepts vascular and microvascular disease of the foot in diabetes implications for foot care. N Engl J Med 311:1615–1619, 1984.
7. Hurley JJ, Auer AI, Hershey FB, et al: Distal arterial reconstruction: Patency and limb salvage in diabetics. J Vasc Surg 5:796–802, 1987.
8. Rieber GE, Boyne EJ, Smith DG: Lower extremity foot ulcers and amputations in diabetes. In Harris MI, Cowie CC, Rieber GE, et al (eds): Diabetes in America. Washington, DC: US Government Printing Office, 1995, pp 409–428.
9. Reunanen A, Takkuneu H, Aromaa A: Prevalence of intermittent claudication and its effects on mortality. Acta Med Scand 211:249–257, 1982.
10. National Diabetes Information Clearinghouse: Diabetes. NIH Publ No 06-3892. Bethesda, MD: National Institutes of Health, 2005. E-mail *ndic@info.niddk.nih.gov.*
11. Beach KW, Bedford GR, Bergelin RO, et al: Progression of lower extremity arterial occlusive disease in type II diabetes mellitus. Diabetes Care 11:464–472, 1988.
12. Bendick PJ, Glover JL, Kuebler TW, et al: Progression of atherosclerosis in diabetes. Surgery 93:834–838, 1983.
13. DeFrang RD, Taylor LM, Porter JM: Basic data related to amputations: Basic data underlyng clinical decision-making in vascular surgery. Ann Vasc Surg 2:62–69, 1988.
14. Criqui MH, Langer RD, Fronek A, et al: Mortality over a period of 10 years in patients with peripheral arterial disease. N Engl J Med 326:381–386, 1992.
15. McDaniel MD, Cronenwett JL: Basic data underlying history of intermittent claudication: Basic data underlying clinical decision-making in vascular surgery. Ann Vasc Surg 2:1, 1988.
16. Marinelli MR, Beath KW, Glass MJ, et al: Noninvasive testing vs. clinical evaluation of arterial disease: A prospective study. JAMA 241:2031, 1979.
17. Baker WH, String ST, Hayes AC: Diagnosis of peripheral occlusive disease: Comparison of clinical evaluation and noninvasive laboratory. Arch Surg 113:1308–1311, 1978.

18. Orchard TJ, Strandness DE: Assessment of peripheral vascular disease in diabetes. Diabetes Care 16:1199–1209, 1993.

19. Sahli D, Eliasson B, Svensson M, et al: Assessment of toe blood pressure is an effective screening method to identify diabetic patients with lower extremity arterial disease. Angiography 55:641–651, 2004.

20. Gibbons GW, Wheeloch FC, Siembreda C, et al: Noninvasive predictions of amputation level in diabetic patients. Arch Surg 114:1253, 1979.

21. Mehta K, Hobson RW, Jamil Z, et al: Fallibility of Doppler ankle pressures in predicting healing of transmetatarsal amputations. J Surg Res 28:466–470, 1980.

22. Barnes RW, Thornhill B, Nix L, et al: Prediction of amputation wound healing. Arch Surg 116:80, 1981.

23. Bone GE, Pomajzl MJ: Toe blood pressure by photoplethysmography: An index of healing in forefoot amputations. Surgery 89:569–574, 1981.

24. Hauser CJ, Klein SR, Hehringer CM, et al: Superiority of transcutaneous oximetry in noninvasive vascular diagnosis in patients with diabetes. Arch Surg 119:690–694, 1984.

25. Moore WS, Malone JM: Effect of flow rate and vessel caliber on clinical arterial stenosis. J Surg Res 26:1, 1979.

26. Strandness DE, Bell IW: An evaluation of the hemodynamic response of the claudicating extremity to exercise. Surg Gynecol Obstet 59:325, 1966.

27. Strandness DE: Abnormal exercise response after successful reconstructive arterial surgery. Surgery 59:514–516, 1966.

28. Baker WH, Barnes RW: Minor forefoot amputation in patients with low ankle pressure. Am J Surg 133:331, 1977.

29. Apelquist J, Calentors J, Larson J, Stenstrom A: Prognostic valve of systolic ankle and toe pressures with outcome of diabetic foot ulcers. Diabetes Care 12:373–378, 1989.

30. Takolander R, Rauwerda JA: The use of noninvasive vascular assessment in diabetic patients with foot lesions. Diabet Med 13:539–542, 1996.

31. Jonason T, Ruggvist I: Diabetes mellitus and intermittent claudication: Relation between peripheral vascular cocomplications and location of the occlusive atherosclerosis. Acta Med Scand 281:217, 1985.

32. Karanfilian RG, Lynch TG, Zirul VT, et al: The value of laser Doppler velocimetry and transcutaneous oxygen-tension determination in predicting healing of ischemic forefoot ulcerations and amputations in diabetics. J Vasc Surg 4:511, 1986.

33. Holstein P, Noer I, Tonneses KH, et al: Distal blood pressure in severe arterial insufficiency. In Bergan J, Yao J (eds): Gangrene and severe ischemia of the lower extremities. New York: Grune & Stratton, 1978, pp 95–114.

34. Bowers BL, Valentine RJ, Myers SI, et al: The natural history of patients with claudication with toe pressures of 40 mmHg or less. J Vasc Surg 18:506–511, 1993.

35. Carter SA, Tate RB: Value of toe pulse waves in addition to systolic pressures in the assessment of the severity of peripheral arterial disease and critical limb ischemia. J Vasc Surg 24:258–265, 1996.

36. Ramsey DE, Manke DA, Sumner DS: Toe blood pressure: A valuable adjunct to ankle pressure measurement for assessing peripheral arterial disease. J. Cardiovasc Surg 24:43:200–211, 1983.

37. McCollum PT, Stanley ST, Kent P, et al: Assessment of arterial disease using digital systolic pressure measurements. Ann Vasc Surg 5:349, 1991.

38. Vincent DG, Salles-Cunnha SX, Bernnhard VM, et al: Noninvasive assessment of toe systolic pressures with special reference to diabetes mellitus. J Cardiovasc Surg 24:22, 1983.

39. Nielson PE: Digital blood pressure in normal subjects and patients with peripheral arterial disease. Scand J Clin Lab Invest 36:731, 1976.

40. Ad Hoc Committee on Reporting Standards, Society for Vascular Surgery, North American Chapter. International Society for Cardiovascular Surgery: Suggested standard for reports dealing with lower extremity ischemia. J Vasc Surg 4:80, 1986.

41. Ouriel K, McDonnell AE, Metz CE, et al: A critical evaluation of stress testing in the diagnosis of peripheral vascular disease. Surgery 91:686, 1982.

42. Vesterager, P: Transcutaneous pO2 electrode. Scand J Clin Lab Invest 39:27–30, 1977.

43. Tonneson, K: Transcutaneous oxygen tension in imminent foot gangrene. Acta Anesth Scand 168:107–110, 1978.

44. Matsen FA, Wyss CR, Pedegans LR, et al: Transcutaneous oxygen tension measurement in peripheral vascular disease. Surg Gynecol Obstet 150:525–528, 1980.

45. Hauser C, Shoemaker W: Use of transcutaneous pO2 regional perfusion index to quantify tissue perfusion in peripheral vascular disease. Ann Surg 1197:3, 337–343, 1993.

46. Mustapha NM, Redhead RG, Jansk, Wielogorski JW: Transcutaneous partial oxygen pressure assessment of the ischemic lower limb. Surg Gynecol Obstet 156:582–584, 1983.

47. Byrne P, Provan JL: The use of transcutaneous oxygen tension measurements in the diagnosis of peripheral vascular insufficiency. Ann Surg 200:160–165, 1984.

48. Cino C, Katsamouris A, Megerman J, et al: Utility of transcutaneous oxygen tension measurements in peripheral arterial occlusive disease. J Vasc Surg 1:362–371, 1984.

49. Karm HB, Appel PL, Shoemaker WC: Prediction of below-knee amputation wound healing using noninvasive laser Doppler velocimetry. Am J Surg 158:29–35, 1989.

50. Bacharach JM, Rooke TW, Osmundson PJ, Gloviczki P: Predictive value of transcutaneous oxygen pressure and amputation success by use of supine and elevation measurements. J Vasc Surg 15:558–563, 1992.

51. Shaffer A, Rieger H: A comparative analysis of transcutaneous oximetry (Tcp02) during oxygen inhalation and leg dependency in severe peripheral arterial occlusive disease. J Vasc Surg 16:218–224, 1992.

52. Lui DTM, Glassont R, Grayndler V, et al: Color duplex ultrasonography versus angiography in the diagnosis of lower extremity arterial disease. Cardiov Surg 4:384–388, 1996.

53. Larch E, Minar E, Ahmadi R, et al: Value of color duplex sonography for evaluation of tibioperoneal arteries in patients with femoropopliteal obstruction: A prospective comparison with antegrade intraarterial digital subtraction angiography. J Vasc Surg 25:628–636, 1997.

54. Koelemay MJW, denHarlog D, Prins MH, et al: Diagnosis of arterial disease of the lower extremities with duplex ultrasonography. BR J Surg 83:404–409, 1996.

55. Moneta GL, Yearger RA, Antonovic R, et al: Accuracy of lower extremity arterial duplex mapping. J Vasc Surg 5:275–283, 1991.

56. Liguish J, Scott WR, Preisser JS, Hansen KS: Duplex ultrasound scanning defines operative strategies for patients with limb-threatening ischemia. J Vasc Surg 28:482–491, 1998.

57. Grassbaugh JA, Nelson PR, Rzucidlo EM, et al: Blinded comparison of preoperative duplex ultrasound scanning and contrast arteriography for planning revascularization at the level of the tibia. J Vasc Surg 37:1186–1190, 2003.

58. Wilson YG, George JK, Wilkius DC, Ashley S: Dup0lex assessment of runoff before femorocrural reconstruction. Br J Surg 84:1360–1363, 1997.

59. Proia RR, Walsh DB, Nelson PR, et al: Early results of infragenicular revascularization based soley on duplex arteriography. J Vasc Surg 33:1165–1170, 2001.

60. Bandyk DF, Cato RF, Towne JB, et al: A low flow velocity predicts failure of femoropopliteal and femorotibial bypass grafts. Surgery 98:799–809, 1985.

61. Westerband A, Mills JL, Kistler S, et al: Prospective validation of threshold criteria for intervention in infragenicular vein grafts undergoing duplex surveillance. Ann Vasc Surg 11:44–48, 1997.

62. Idu MM, Blankenstein JD, DeGrer P, et al: Impact of a color-flow duplex surveillance program on infragenicular vein graft patency: A five-year experience. J Vasc Surg 17:42–53, 1993.

63. Moneta GL, Yeager RA, Lee RW, Porter JM: Noninvasive localization of arterial occlusive disease: A comparison of segmental Doppler pressures and arterial duplex mapping. J Vasc Surg 17:578–582, 1993.

64. Mackaay, AJC, Beks PJ, et al: Is toe pressure a better parameter of peripheral vascular integrity than ankle pressure?: Comparison of diabetic with nondiabetic subjects in a Dutch epidemiologic study. J Vasc Technol 19:5–9, 1995.

65. Pfeifer M, Green D: Neuropathy in the diabetic foot: New concepts in etiology and treatment. In Bowker JH, Pfeifer M (eds): The Diabetic Foot, 6th ed. Philadelphia: WB Saunders Company, 2000.

THE CHARCOT FOOT
(PIED DE CHARCOT)

LEE J. SANDERS AND ROBERT G. FRYKBERG ■

A variety of disorders affecting the spinal cord and peripheral nerves have been reported to destroy the protective mechanisms of joints and interfere with the "nutritive" trophic regulation of bone.[1-10] The mechanisms of destruction may be precipitated by a single injury or by repetitive moderate stress applied to the bones and joints of an insensate foot and ankle. The results are fractures, effusions, and ligamentous laxity, followed by erosion of articular cartilage, bony fragmentation, and joint luxation, resulting in collapse of the foot. The presence of peripheral neuropathy and the clinical and laboratory evidence of diabetes mellitus,[11-14] tabes dorsalis,[15,16] leprosy,[7,11,17,18] syringomyelia,[11,15,19] meningomyelocele,[7] congenital insensitivity to pain,[11] chronic alcoholism,[20] spinal cord injury and compression,[1,2-4,11,19] and peripheral nerve injuries[21,22] complete the picture of neuropathic osteoarthropathy, or bona fide Charcot's joint disease. The key characteristic that all these disorders share is the absence or decrease of pain sensation in the presence of uninterrupted physical activity.

As the number of cases of tabes dorsalis has declined, diabetes mellitus has emerged as the leading cause of neuropathic osteoarthropathy today.[11,13,23] The importance of the diabetic form of neuropathic osteoarthropathy was established in 1955 in a report by Miller and Lichtman[13] at the Cook County Hospital and Chicago Medical School. They noted that "whereas tabes of syphilitic origin was formerly the usual cause of these painless deformities of the feet, with complicating soft tissue infections, ulcers and osteomyelitis, the diabetic neuropathic foot is now showing the higher incidence. Perhaps there is greater alertness in recognition."

The Charcot foot remains a poorly understood and frequently overlooked complication of diabetes mellitus that presents a formidable diagnostic and treatment challenge for all members of the health care team. The probability of successful management is greatly increased by a heightened awareness and thorough understanding of the pathogenesis, natural history, and anatomic patterns of neuropathic osteoarthropathy. Identification of high-risk individuals facilitates early implementation of management strategies that are directed toward preventing and minimizing foot deformity, joint instability, ulceration, and disability. Early recognition and timely treatment will often result in a more satisfactory outcome.[24] The key to treatment is prevention of deformity by avoidance of further trauma until the bone and soft tissues heal. The aims of treatment should be to obtain a stable, shoeable foot and to avoid excessive pressure on the skin from a bony prominence. Since William Reily Jordan's linkage of neuropathic osteoarthropathy of the foot and ankle with diabetes mellitus in 1936,[25] the number of case reports has steadily increased. The growing number of cases reflects the prevalence of this disorder as well as increased recognition of Charcot's joint disease.

Historical Perspective

In the early nineteenth century, this disorder was first observed as a rheumatic condition related to a lesion of the spinal cord. Although there might be earlier mention of arthritis associated with venereal or nonvenereal disease, for example, in Sir William Musgrave's Latin dissertation on arthritis (1703),[26] we begin our discussion with early attempts to examine the spinal origin of rheumatism of the foot and ankle. J.K. Mitchell (1798–1858), a physician at the Pennsylvania Hospital in Philadelphia, was the first to experimentally study the spinal origin of rheumatism and to suggest a relationship between caries (tuberculosis) of the spine and arthropathy of the foot and ankle.[27] In 1831, he described his observations of a patient with spinal caries who presented with hot, swollen joints: an ankle on one side and the opposite knee. The usual treatment by leeches, purgatives, and evaporating lotions was disappointing, and Mitchell began to suspect that the cause of the irritation might lie in the affected spine. This led him to investigate the validity of his observations regarding the spinal origin of inflammation. Silas Weir Mitchell (1829–1914), the illustrious son of J.K. Mitchell, provided additional support for his father's observations. Following graduation from the Jefferson Medical College in Philadelphia, S.W. Mitchell continued his education in London and Paris, where he studied with the experimental physiologist Claude Bernard. Mitchell then returned to Philadelphia, where he worked as a contract physician for the Union Army at the Turner's Lane Hospital, the first neurologic research center in the United States. It was here that he observed the effects of gunshot wounds and other injuries of nerves sustained by Union soldiers during the American Civil War. Mitchell, together with his colleagues George Morehouse and W.W. Keen, described alterations in the nutrition of joints related to nerve injuries: "We have ourselves seen cases of spinal injury, in which rheumatic symptoms seemed to have been among the consequences. The indisputable fact (is) that there are rheumatisms depending for existence on neural changes."[21] Silas Weir Mitchell thus helped to establish neurology as a medical specialty and is regarded as one of the most influential physicians in American history. His published observations and those of his father were read with interest by J.-M. Charcot in Paris.

Jean-Martin Charcot (1825–1893) was one of the most celebrated French physicians of the nineteenth century (Fig. 12-1). He transformed the Salpêtrière, a large charitable hospital for women in Paris, into one of the world's greatest teaching centers for clinical neurologic research.[1,28] Charcot's early findings on the tabetic arthropathies were published in 1868 in the *Archives de Physiologie Normale and Pathologique*.[2,3] In this widely cited paper, Professor Charcot presented four case histories and a discussion of the arthopathies associated with pro-gressive locomotor ataxia. Charcot linked the bone and joint changes that are seen in tabetic patients with sclerotic lesions of the spinal cord. He referred to the observations of J.K. Mitchell: "I have observed several facts that seem to confirm Professor Mitchell's observations ... these lesions of the spinal cord which provoke such perturbation, more or less severe, of the nutritional processes in various parts of the body appear however to have a common feature; that is an irritation of the nervous elements of the cord." Charcot's use of the term *nutrition* refers to disturbances of the circulation and vasomotor elements. Charcot also refers to S.W. Mitchell's treatise on gunshot wounds and other injuries of nerves affecting the spinal cord: "one should not forget that the nutritional disturbances caused by a lesion of the spinal cord sometimes involve the joints and will then present in the form of articular changes fairly similar to those produced by acute or subacute articular rheumatism."

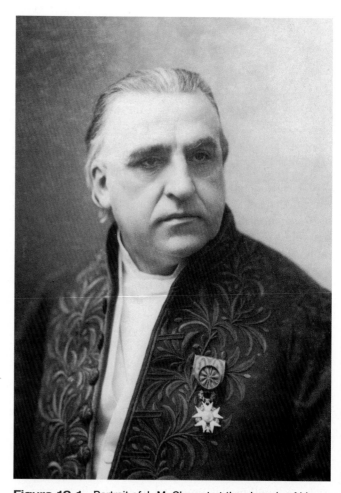

Figure 12–1 Portrait of J.-M. Charcot at the pinnacle of his career. Photograph by Eugène Pirou, Paris. Charcot is wearing a long black coat embroidered in dark green: *l'habit vert*, the academic attire of the French Academy of Sciences. He was elected to membership in l'Académie des sciences (section of medicine and surgery) on November 12, 1883. On his left breast is the French Legion of Honor medal, officer rank. *(From the private collection of Dr. Lee J. Sanders.)*

J.-M. Charcot described his observations of a sudden and unexpected arthropathy, which often began without apparent cause. Lancinating pains in the limbs often preceded the joint affection. He described a sudden onset of generalized tumefaction of the limb with rapid changes in the articular surfaces of a joint. Crepitation in the joint would occur within a few days after onset and would normally precede the development of the characteristic motor incoordination of tabes. Charcot argued that these arthropathies did not result exclusively from the distention of the ligaments and capsules of the joints or from the awkward gait of these patients. "Anatomically, the enormous wear and tear shown by the heads of the bones, the extensive looseness of the ligaments of the joints, and the frequent occurrence of luxations seem to distinguish these arthropathies from the ordinary type of osteoarthritis."[4] Although his 1868 article on tabetic arthropathies is widely referenced in publications on the Charcot foot, there is in fact no mention in this paper of the small bones and joints of the foot and ankle. The first mention of the bone and joint conditions of the tabetic foot, "pied tabetique," was not published by Charcot until 1883.

In August 1881, at the 7th International Medical Congress, in London, J.-M. Charcot received universal acclaim for his research on the tabetic arthropathies. He was given a standing ovation for his demonstration and lecture on multiple joint disease resulting from locomotor ataxia, *Demonstration of Arthropathic Affections of Locomotor Ataxy*.[29,30] Charcot brilliantly illustrated his case presentations with anatomic specimens of bones and joints, clinical photographs, and sections of the spine demonstrating "posterior sclerosis of the cord." He remarked that "fractures of the bones and diseases of the joints appear to belong to the same pathological condition that is to say, when the disease attacks the diaphyses of the bone, the atrophy is shown by fracture; when it attacks the joints we get wasting of the head of the bone with erosion of the surface." What Charcot described was a neuropathic osteoarthropathy, affecting both long bones and their joints. His important contribution to the understanding of spinal arthropathies was recognized in the Transactions of the International Medical Congress, where it was recorded by Sir James Paget that "This disease is, in fact, a distinct pathological entity, and deserves the name, by which it will be known, of 'Charcot's disease.'"[29,30] The terms *Charcot's joint disease* and *Charcot's osteoarthropathy* have since been adopted in reference to all neuropathic arthropathies, regardless of their etiology and anatomic location.

Prior to 1883, virtually all published observations of the bone and joint lesions of ataxic patients were of the long bones of the limbs with their large articulations. However, in November 1883, J.-M. Charcot and Charles Féré published a landmark paper in the *Archives de Neurologie*,[31] in which they described their first observations of the bone and joint conditions of the tabetic foot,

"*pied tabétique.*" The author's (LJS) unpublished translation of the introduction to this paper reads as follows: "Described for the first time, by one of us, the bone and joint conditions of the ataxic are well recognized today, at least their general features, when located on the long bones of the limbs and their large joints. ... Similar changes corresponding to the short bones and small joints of the foot have not yet been the subject of published observations. It is these findings that we wish to call attention to." Charcot and Féré presented four observations of tabetic patients with locomotor ataxia, lancinating pains, and foot deformities. In a fifth observation, they discuss the examination of a skeletal foot in a complex case with extensive bone destruction (Fig. 12-2). This paper marks the first published scientific investigation of the Charcot foot.

Charcot taught that "theories, no matter how pertinent they are, cannot eradicate the existence of facts,"[1] and he believed that "behind the disease of the joint there was a disease far more important in character, and which in reality dominated the situation."[4] This reasoning applies equally well today, with respect to an evidenced-based approach to understanding the pathogenesis, natural history, and treatment of the diabetic Charcot foot.

The association between Charcot's joint disease of the foot and ankle and diabetes mellitus was established in 1936 by William Reily Jordan. In a comprehensive paper entitled "Neuritic Manifestations in Diabetes Mellitus,"[25] Jordan devoted a mere paragraph to Case #10,451, in which he described a 56-year-old woman with diabetes of 14 years' duration and peripheral neuropathy. His patient presented with "a rather typical, painless Charcot joint of the ankle, in addition to chronic osteomyelitis of the foot of an unusual type and without obvious etiology." The similarity of this presentation to that produced by syphilis, in the absence of positive serologic confirmation, led Jordan to believe that this condition was "a diabetic process of a neurologic trophic nature." When Jordan first saw this woman, he noted, "The ankle joint became swollen but not tender. Bits of bone were painlessly extruded from the toes. The lesions would heal but recur, or new ones would develop. The ankle joint became useless and unstable. The process then involved the other ankle and foot." Since this early report by Jordan, the number of case reports of the diabetic Charcot foot has steadily increased.

A National Library of Medicine MEDLINE search for peer-reviewed articles on the Charcot foot, using the MeSH terms "neurogenic arthropathy," "Charcot's joint," and "foot," with publication dates from January 1956 to December 31, 2005, resulted in a total of 328 articles. Careful review of these articles reveals that approximately 23% are not specific to the subject, that is, they mention the Charcot foot but are actually general discussions of diabetic foot disease, wound healing, the adult flatfoot, or surgical management of the foot and ankle. Therefore, approximately 251 peer-reviewed articles on

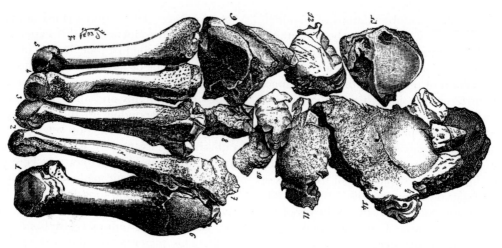

Figure 12-2   Skeleton of an ataxic foot: *1, 2, 3, 4, 5*, metatarsals; *6, 7*, first and second cuneiforms fused to their corresponding metatarsals; *8*, bony fragment, apparently the third cuneiform; *9*, cuboid, represented by an irregular mass; *10, 11*, two fragments of the navicular; *12, 13*, neck and body of the talus. The talar head has disappeared, and the superior surface of the body is completely worn down; *14*, calcaneus. The articular surface of the posterior facet is easily recognizable. There are a number of small osteophytes noted. The anterior facet is completely worn down. *(Charcot J-M, Féré C: Affections osseuses et articulaires du pied chez les tabétiques (pied tabétique): Archives de Neurologie 6(18):305–319, 1883. Courtesy of the New York Academy of Medicine.)*

the Charcot foot were published over this 50-year period. Remarkably, 35% of all indexed articles on the Charcot foot have been published within the last 5 years. Disappointingly, fewer than 10% are research papers, and only two were prospective randomized controlled trials.[32,33] Most of the publications have been review articles, small case reports, discussions of imaging modalities, and discussions of new techniques for surgical management. However, exciting new theories have recently been proposed with respect to the role of proinflammatory cytokines and the RANKL/OPG (receptor activator for nuclear factor kappa B ligand/osteoprotegerin) signaling pathway in the pathogenesis of acute Charcot foot.[34,35]

Unfortunately, there is a lack of consensus on the nomenclature for noninfective bone disease in the neuropathic diabetic foot. Newman described six different names given to conditions of noninfective bone and joint pathology in 67 patients with diabetic neuropathy: "Charcot osteoarthropathy" and "bone loss" were the most common conditions seen.[23] Ali Foster, in the United Kingdom, recently addressed the issue of confusing nomenclature for the Charcot foot and the need for accurate classification.[36] We agree and suggest that uniform terminology be adopted so as to avoid confusion over the diagnosis and treatment of this condition. Although some will not agree with the use of eponyms, their purpose is to honor the great men and women of medicine who first described a disease or pathologic condition. The problem with medical eponyms is that they are usually not descriptive or even necessarily associated with a specific condition. Charcot's name, for example, is linked with at least 15 medical eponyms.[37] Nonetheless, in deference to J.-M. Charcot, our preferences are *Charcot's osteoarthropathy, Charcot's joint disease,* and *the Charcot foot,* with the addition of *diabetic neuropathic osteoarthropathy (DNOAP).* The first term might be the most

appropriate in that it both honors Charcot and accurately refers to a disease of bones ("osteo") and joints ("arthropathy"). Although numerous other names and their variations have been used to describe noninfective neuropathic bone and joint disease of the diabetic foot, in the discussion that follows, the terms *Charcot's osteoarthropathy, Charcot's joint disease, the Charcot foot,* and *diabetic neuropathic osteoarthropathy (DNOAP)* will be used interchangeably.

Burden of the Problem

The prevalence of diagnosed neuropathic bone and joint disease associated with diabetes mellitus has been reported to be 0.08% to 7.5%.[38–41] Pogonowska and colleagues[40] reported on a clinical and radiologic survey of 242 patients in Houston, Texas. They noted that 6.8% of the cases had bone abnormalities classified as "diabetic osteopathy." Forgacs, in a comprehensive literature review of data on 237 patients, estimated that DNOAP occurs in 0.3% to 0.5% of all diabetic patients.[39] Radiographic evidence of lower-limb bone and joint changes was found in 29% of 333 diabetic patients with peripheral neuropathy, reported by Cofield and colleagues.[42] A recent prospective study of 1666 patients from a disease management program in Texas reported that the incidence of Charcot arthropathy was 8.5/1000 per year. This complication was more common in Mexican Americans than in non-Hispanic whites (7.4/1000 versus 4.1/1000; $p = .0001$).[43] It is very likely that there are many more cases of DNOAP that go undetected or misdiagnosed.

The average age reported for the onset of DNOAP is approximately 57 years, the majority of patients being in their sixth and seventh decade.[13,38,39,41,42,44–47] Of greater

TABLE 12-1   Reported Characteristics of Diabetics with Neuropathic Osteoarthropathy

Reference	No. of Cases Reported	Age (years) (Range)	Duration DM (years) (Range)	% Bilateral Involvement
Bailey and Root[38]	17	56 (30–69)	11.5	23.5 4/17
Miller and Lichtman[13]	17	53		5.9 1/17
Sinha et al.[41]	101	2/3s 50s–60s (20–79)	83% > 10 65% > 15	23.8 24/101
Clouse et al.[46]	90	55 (25–78)	18 (1.5–43)	18
Forgács[39]	23	63 (48–79)	14.8 (2–32)	
Cofield et al.[42]	96	56 (27–79)	81% > 10 16 (1–40)	21 20/96
Clohisy and Thompson[45]	18	33.5 (25–52)	20	75 14/18
Sanders and Mrdjenovich[47]	28	79% 50s–60s 57.2 (36–70)	78% > 10 59% > 15 15.1 (1–27)	39.3 11/28

DM, diabetes mellitus.

Modified from Sanders LJ, Frykberg R: Diabetic neuropathic osteoarthropathy: The Charcot foot. In Frykberg RG (ed): The High Risk Foot in Diabetes Mellitus. New York: Churchill Livingstone, 1991, with permission.

significance, the average duration of diabetes at the time of diagnosis of neuropathic bone changes is approximately 15 years, 80% of the patients being diabetic for more than 10 years and 60% for more than 15 years.[38,39,41,42,44–47] Clohisy and Thompson[45] reported on a homogeneous group of 18 adult type 1 (juvenile-onset) diabetic patients with neuropathic osteoarthropathy, an average age of 33.5 years, and a 20-year history of diabetes mellitus. Age therefore does not appear to be as important a factor in the development of DNOAP as does the duration of diabetes mellitus (Table 12-1).

Bilateral involvement has been reported to occur in 5.9% to 39.3% of the heterogeneous cases.[13,41,46,47] Seventy-five percent of the cases reported by Clohisy and Thompson[45] had bilateral involvement, with a very high incidence of serious fractures of the ankle and the tarsal bones. There does not appear to be a significant difference in sex distribution, men and women being affected equally.[48,49]

Natural History (Evolution) of the Charcot Foot

Various descriptions of the development of bone and joint changes associated with neuropathic osteoarthropathies have appeared in the literature over the last century. The terms *atrophic, destructive,* and *hyperemic* have been used to describe acute or early radiographic findings. *Hypertrophic, reparative, proliferative, sclerotic,* and *quiescent* are all terms that are used to describe chronic or late findings.[11,16,49,50] These descriptions are based on clinical, radiologic, and histologic observations as well as the chronicity of disease. Norman and colleagues[14] suggested that neuropathic joints be classified as acute or chronic on the basis of the

suddenness of their onset and speed of development. They stated that "since both reaction to injury and repair occur simultaneously in the joint, two separate phases of development do not take place." What seems to link these opposite states is the process of bony resorption and repair, as determined by the balance of osteoclastic and osteoblastic activity (Fig. 12-3).[51]

The acute phase of neuropathic osteoarthropathy is often precipitated by minor trauma that is unrecognized by the patient.[44,48,49] It is characterized by mild pain, swelling, local heat, erythema, laxity of ligaments, joint effusion, and bone resorption. The clinical picture may be nonspecific and difficult to distinguish from acute gouty arthritis, osteoarthritis, septic arthritis, or cellulitis. Skin temperature elevation of the affected foot has been reported to be approximately 5° C.[44] Nearly all reports confirm the role of trauma in initiating the evolution of neuropathic osteoarthropathy in patients with an underlying neurologic deficit.[11,17,19,49] Patients are usually afebrile with no clinical or laboratory evidence of infection. There may, however, be a mildly elevated erythrocyte sedimentation rate associated with a normal white blood cell count. Sanders and Mrdjenovich[47] reported a mean erythrocyte sedimentation rate of 32 ± 6.7 mm/hour (range: 22 to 41) in a group of 13 neuropathic diabetic patients with bone and joint changes and normal white blood cell counts.

Newman[52] suggested that the earliest changes in the evolution of neuropathic joints involve the soft tissues. He postulated that gross neuropathic changes in the ligaments were responsible for spontaneous dislocation of the foot, which he observed in five cases that occurred without bone destruction. In cases of neuropathic osteoarthropathy that begin with spontaneous dislocations rather than fractures, ligamentous lesions may be

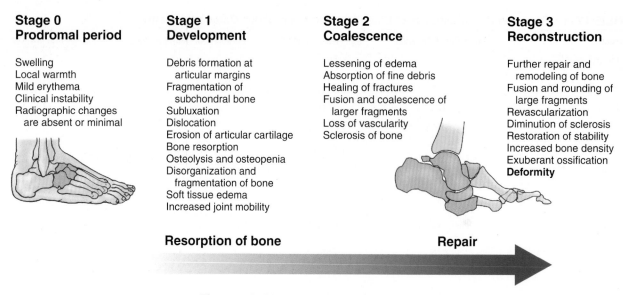

Stage 0
Prodromal period

Swelling
Local warmth
Mild erythema
Clinical instability
Radiographic changes
are absent or minimal

Stage 1
Development

Debris formation at
articular margins
Fragmentation of
subchondral bone
Subluxation
Dislocation
Erosion of articular cartilage
Bone resorption
Osteolysis and osteopenia
Disorganization and
fragmentation of bone
Soft tissue edema
Increased joint mobility

Stage 2
Coalescence

Lessening of edema
Absorption of fine debris
Healing of fractures
Fusion and coalescence of
larger fragments
Loss of vascularity
Sclerosis of bone

Stage 3
Reconstruction

Further repair and
remodeling of bone
Fusion and rounding of
large fragments
Revascularization
Diminution of sclerosis
Restoration of stability
Increased bone density
Exuberant ossification
Deformity

Resorption of bone   **Repair**

Figure 12–3   Evolution of the Charcot foot.

of foremost importance. Ligaments and joint capsule are thought to be stretched by the abnormal stresses applied to the joints, allowing them to go beyond their normal range of motion. They may be further weakened at their attachment to bone by hyperemic resorption, allowing complete dislocation to take place.[19]

Eichenholtz[53] divided the disease process into three radiographically distinct stages: development, coalescence, and reconstruction. The development stage represents the acute, destructive period, which is distinguished by joint effusions, soft tissue edema, subluxation, formation of bone and cartilage debris (detritus), intra-articular fractures, and fragmentation of bone. This phase of bone and joint destruction is induced by minor trauma and aggravated by persistent ambulation on an insensitive foot. The consequence of trauma is a hyperemic inflammatory response, which promotes additional resorption of bone and increases the susceptibility to further injury and progressive deterioration. Nonweightbearing must be initiated during this acute phase of the disease process.

The coalescence stage is characterized by a lessening of edema, absorption of fine debris, and healing of fractures. Clinical and radiographic evidence of coalescence indicates that the reparative phase of healing has begun. The final phase of bone healing is the stage of reconstruction, wherein further repair and remodeling of bone take place in an attempt to restore stability and homeostasis (see Fig. 12-3). Neuropathic osteoarthropathy can be arrested during the development stage. If the disease is diagnosed and treated early, before it has a chance to progress, the result may be minimal joint destruction and deformity.

A stage 0 classification has been proposed, corresponding to the prodromal clinical stage of the Charcot foot, in which the patient presents with a locally swollen, warm, and erythematous foot.[54,55] Radiographic changes are absent, minimal, or very subtle. Technetium 99 bone scan is clearly positive, and indium and gallium scans are negative.[55] This is perhaps the most important stage in the evolution of the Charcot foot for clinicians to recognize, for it is at this point that we can make the greatest difference in secondary prevention, minimizing disability and improving the outcome for the patient.

Late neuropathic bone and joint changes are an exaggeration of those seen in osteoarthritis: cartilage fibrillation, loose body formation, subchondral sclerosis, and marginal osteophytes.[11] These lesions often heal with the formation of hyperplastic dense bone, especially in the midfoot. The early phase of healing is distinguished by the gradual absorption of fine debris and hematoma, with callus formation and the coalescence and reattachment of loose fragments of bone or cartilage. Proliferative changes are characteristic of this phase, the usual findings being intra-articular and extra-articular osteophytes, exostoses, ossification of ligaments and joint cartilage, and marginal lipping at contact points.[8] Proliferation of new bone is often evidenced by exuberant overgrowth (florid ossification) with decreased joint mobility and increased rigidity of the foot. Fusion and rounding of large fragments are late findings.

Pathogenesis of the Charcot Foot

Multiple factors appear to contribute to the development of bone and joint destruction in people with diabetes. Peripheral neuropathy with loss of protective sensation, mechanical stress, autonomic neuropathy with increased blood flow to bone, and trauma have emerged as the most important determinants. Putative factors that may play a role in the development of the diabetic Charcot foot include metabolic abnormalities that weaken bone, renal disease, renal transplantation, corticosteroid-

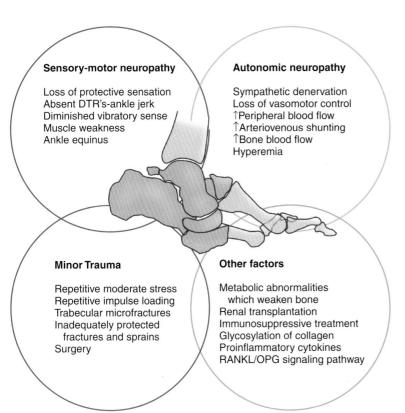

Figure 12–4 Pathogenesis of the Charcot foot.
(Modified from Sanders LJ, Frykberg RG: Diabetic neuropathic osteoarthropathy: The Charcot foot. In Frykberg RG [ed]: The High Risk Foot in Diabetes Mellitus. New York: Churchill Livingstone, 1991, with permission.)

induced osteoporosis, osteoclastogenesis, nonenzymatic glycosylation of bone proteins and extra-articular soft tissues, proinflammatory cytokines, and the RANKL/OPG signaling pathway (Fig. 12-4). Unfortunately, the mechanism for development of neuropathic bone and joint lesions is not entirely understood.

Two mechanisms have been described for the development of bony resorption (osteolysis); one is mediated by increased blood flow to bone, and the other is mediated by unbalanced osteoclastic activity.[34,51,56–59] Infection may cause increased blood flow to bone through granulation tissue, as is often the case with a mal perforans ulcer. The resultant radiographic changes in bone are usually nonspecific. What initially appears to be bone destruction consistent with osteomyelitis might not be caused by direct extension of infection to the bone but might instead represent osteolysis secondary to increased peripheral blood flow, inflammatory hyperemia, granulation tissue, or soft tissue infection.

Bone resorption and joint deformity, especially in the metatarsophalangeal joints, may be associated with trophic ulceration and infection.[8,60] The diagnostic dilemma in these cases is which came first: the osteoarthropathy or the infection. The differentiation of osteoarthropathy from osteomyelitis is often difficult in the presence of overlying soft tissue infection and ulceration; however, newer imaging modalities can assist in making this important distinction.[61–66] Because the presenting symptoms of ulceration and infection often precede radiographic evaluation of the foot, it is often assumed that pathologic bone and joint changes must have occurred secondary to

infection. In their discussion of the role of infection in the pathogenesis of the Charcot foot and ankle, Lippman and colleagues[67] determined that in 4 of their 12 patients, collapse preceded infection. In four other cases, it seemed likely that ulceration and bacterial invasion occurred after the Charcot lesion had been established for some time. Other authors[68,69] have reported similar observations. The role of infection in many of these patients should be viewed as a complication, not as an etiologic factor.[40]

The relationship that exists between certain lesions of the spinal cord and peripheral nerves and the subsequent development of neuropathic joints has been well documented.[1,2–6,15,16,19,22,25,69–71] The presence of peripheral sensorimotor neuropathy characterized by loss of protective sensation, absent deep tendon reflexes, diminished vibratory perception, and muscle weakness sets into motion a series of events that eventually result in the development of Charcot's joint disease. The following discussion is directed at understanding the neurovascular etiology of DNOAP, as well as the possible roles of other important factors that might be less well known.

Increased Peripheral Blood Flow

Autonomic nervous system dysfunction has been noted as an associated finding in patients with neuropathic osteoarthropathy.[2,5,10,13,71–75] Support for the hypothesis that increased blood flow and active bone resorption are responsible for the development of Charcot joint is evidenced by several case reports and experimental data.[23,34–35,39,40,41,76–81] Schwarz and colleagues[50] described the case of a 61-year-old diabetic who developed severe whittling down of the metatarsal bones and proximal phalanges of the left foot after a left lumbar sympathectomy 22 years earlier. Edelman and colleagues[73] reported three cases in which neuropathic osteoarthropathy developed within 2 to 5 years after successful lower limb revascularization. Lippman and colleagues[67] suggested that excess local arterial flow can be a factor contributing to osseous breakdown under stress.

A neurally initiated vascular reflex leading to increased blood flow and active bone resorption has been proposed as an important etiologic factor in the development of bone and joint destruction in neuropathic patients.[5–7,10,49,73] Wartenberg[10] noted a possible role of the sympathetic nervous system in the manifestations of tabes dorsalis, including the production of tabetic joints. He observed local disturbances in sympathetic vessel innervation in unilateral tabetic arthropathies in proximity to the affected joints. "The following pathologic disturbances were found: elevation of the local temperature, rise in the arterial and venous blood pressure, increase in the oscillometric index, anomalies of the sweat secretion and disturbances in the pilomotor reflex."[10]

Normal circulation, with palpable pedal pulses, has consistently been reported in diabetic patients with neuropathic osteoarthropathy.[38,41,44] "Pedal pulses in most of our patients were accentuated. The feet were warm with bounding dorsalis pedis and posterior tibial pulses."[41] The existence of autonomic neuropathy in patients with DNOAP has likewise been reported with regularity.[13,50,69,71]

Evidence exists that autonomic neuropathy with sympathetic denervation resulting in high peripheral blood flow is common in patients with diabetes mellitus.[70–72,74,82–87] Archer and colleagues,[72] at King's College Hospital, London, measured resting foot blood flow in 22 diabetic patients with severe sensory neuropathy using mercury strain gauge plethysmography and Doppler sonogram techniques. They found blood flow to be increased on average five times greater than normal, at 20° to 22° C. They noted that foot skin temperature was also elevated, reflecting the increased circulation.

Edmonds and colleagues,[84] also at King's College Hospital, studied the uptake of methylene diphosphonate labeled with technetium-99m (^{99m}Tc) in 13 neuropathic diabetic individuals and 8 nondiabetic controls. Bone scans were performed, and uptake of radiopharmaceutical was monitored in three phases. Uptake in all three phases (at 2 minutes after injection, at 4 minutes, and at 4 hours) was markedly elevated and confined to the feet in all neuropathic subjects. Increased uptake at 2 and 4 minutes indicated increased blood flow. These investigators concluded that the most likely explanation for their findings was increased bony blood flow secondary to sympathetic denervation. They also noted that severely abnormal autonomic function occurs in association with neuropathic ulceration.[84] High blood flow, vasodilatation, and arteriovenous shunting, which result from sympathetic denervation, could lead to abnormal venous pooling.[87] Boulton and colleagues[82] found mean venous PO$_2$ in the feet of neuropathic subjects with ulcers to be significantly higher than in controls They frequently observed the presence of prominent pedal arteries and distended dorsal foot veins in their diabetic patients who had noninfected neuropathic foot ulcers. These observations led them to believe that arteriovenous shunting with increased venous oxygenation was important in the pathogenesis of ulceration.

Mechanical Stress

Mechanical elements have long been recognized in the etiology of osteoarthritis. Situations that impose chronically increased stress on articular cartilage can act as the inciting primary cause. The repetitive mechanical stress of ambulation with impulsive loading of bone, applied to a foot that has lost protective sensation, results in soft tissue injury (ulcers) and tensile fatigue of cartilage and bone. Trabecular microfractures in the subchondral cancellous bone are the earliest ultrastructural evidence of cartilage damage.[88] The result of healing of these microfractures and remodeling is an increase in the stiffness of the subchondral bone,[89] which reduces bony tissue's normal resilience and ability to absorb shock. Total collapse of the neuropathic foot can occur over a very short period and may be evidenced clinically by depression of the medial longitudinal arch and complaints by the patient that "my arch has fallen."[49]

Any disturbance of the bones and joints of the neuropathic foot that results in bony deformity or alteration of foot mechanics has the potential for causing skeletal and soft tissue lesions.[48] Patients with Charcot's osteoarthropathy will typically have elevated peak plantar pressures.[90] The consequence of increased vertical force and shear stress on the soft tissues overlying prominent bone is ulceration, followed by infection and further collapse of the foot. The degree of injury is determined by the extent of sensory loss, the amount of stress on the joint, the duration of the inflammatory process, and the patient's persistent ambulation in spite of the swelling, redness, and deformity. Cavanagh and colleagues[91] determined that foot deformity rather than body mass is a major determinant for high peak plantar pressures and subsequent ulceration in patients with peripheral neuropathy. A deformed Charcot foot therefore places the limb at significant risk for ulceration and serious complications.[92]

Fractures

Fractures of significant magnitude were responsible for initiating or increasing joint changes in the majority of the 118 cases of neuropathic arthropathy reported

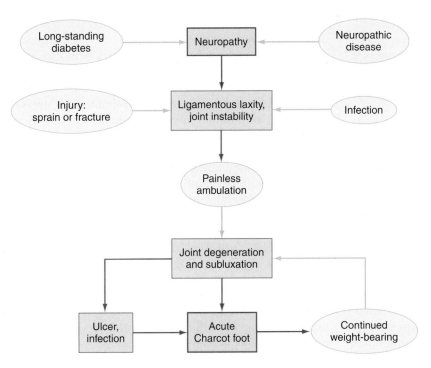

Figure 12–5 Pathogenesis and destructive cycle of the acute Charcot foot. If the trauma of weight-bearing continues, the acute stage is perpetuated, and further deformity will result. Ulcers with subsequent infection complicate this process and contribute to joint disintegration.

by Johnson.[19] He concluded that "the behaviour of the bones and joints in neuroarthropathy can be explained on the basis of the usual responses of these tissues to trauma modified by the presence of decreased protective sensation." Lack of recognition and a cavalier attitude with regard to protection of fractures, sprains, and effusions sustain the atrophic phase and result in bone and joint destruction. As long as the trauma of repetitive stress and weight-bearing continues, resorption outpaces new bone formation, and the destructive cycle continues. Figure 12-5 illustrates a simplified diagram of the pathogenesis and perpetuation of the acute stage by unaltered weight-bearing.

Eleven percent of the cases reported by Newman[23] had spontaneous fractures and dislocations. These cases presented the greatest therapeutic problems compared with other noninfective diseases of bone. Newman stressed the importance of recognizing these conditions and distinguishing them from osteomyelitis. Holmes[93] reported on a series of diabetic patients who had sustained foot and ankle fractures. When there was a delay in diagnosis and treatment, a high incidence of Charcot changes developed. Many such fractures of a minor nature in patients with neuropathy may go undetected and lead to lesser degrees of osteoarthropathy, identified as an incidental finding during routine radiography.[94]

Autonomic neuropathy with loss of vasomotor control and increased peripheral blood flow to bone, coupled with an inflammatory hyperemia of the soft tissues, results in resorption of bone with further weakening. Atrophic bone is easily fractured or fragmented. Frequent spontaneous fractures in neuropathic patients have led some authors[45,51,71,76,86] to believe that intrinsic bone disease may be an etiologic factor.

Equinus Deformity

Grant and colleagues[95] identified fine structural changes in the Achilles tendons of patients with diabetes and peripheral neuropathy, compared to nondiabetic controls. The following ultrastructural changes were observed by electron microscopy: increased packing density of collagen fibrils, decreases in fibrillar diameter, and abnormal fibril morphology. These morphologic abnormalities were thought to be the result of long-term nonenzymatic glycosylation. In addition, the authors suggest that these structural changes could contribute to shortening of the Achilles tendon. Biomechanical test data demonstrate that there is a significant difference in ultimate tensile strength and elasticity between the Achilles tendons of patients with Charcot's osteoarthropathy and non-Charcot controls.[77]

Weakness of the anterior compartment muscles of the leg (ankle dorsiflexors) may have two consequences, one progressing to the other. Initially, a neuropathic foot with weak ankle dorsiflexors exhibits a drop-foot gait with increased force on the forefoot as it slaps to the ground with each step. Simultaneously, myostatic contracture of the gastrocnemius-soleus muscles (triceps surae) occurs unopposed by the ankle dorsiflexors, resulting in increasing ankle equinus.[78,90,96,97] Although there are no data confirming a direct causal relationship between equinus deformity and the development of a Charcot foot, this appears to be a reasonable assumption, especially at the tarsometatarsal and midtarsal joints. Once calf muscle contracture occurs, stress at the tarsometatarsal, naviculocuneiform, and midtarsal joints is increased during rollover in latter stance phase. Conversely, since most investigations measure equinus after the deformity has occurred, we cannot exclude the possibility of a secondary triceps surae contracture occurring after midfoot collapse. Only longitudinal studies of a large diabetes population will be able to determine the true role of equinus in the etiology of Charcot's osteoarthropathy.

Renal Transplantation

Isolated reports have shown an association between renal transplantation with long-term corticosteroid or other immunosuppressive treatment and the subsequent development of neuropathic osteoarthropathy.[45] These reviews show that after renal transplantation, diabetic people have a much higher incidence of Charcot's joint disease than does the nontransplanted diabetic population. Clohisy and Thompson[45] reported on 18 patients with juvenile-onset diabetes and severe neuropathic arthropathy of the ankle and tarsus. Fourteen of these patients had received a renal transplant before the fracture was diagnosed, and none had a history of major trauma. It remains unclear whether corticosteroid-induced osteoporosis or some other metabolic abnormality that tends to weaken bone was the underlying factor responsible for the development of bone and joint destruction in these patients. Further discussion of this subject follows in the section entitled "Pattern V: Calcaneus."

Glycosylation of Collagen

The synthesis of abnormal collagen types that are not usually found in cartilage, bone, ligaments, or other soft tissues might be another possible factor in the development of Charcot's osteoarthropathy. Nonenzymatic glycosylation of proteins associated with chronic hyperglycemia, in particular hemoglobin and dermal collagen, has been reported.[98–102] Digital sclerosis and joint contractures were found to be affecting the hands in 18% of children with type 1 diabetes mellitus.[100] Biopsies of patients with limited joint mobility (LJM) have shown increased crosslinking and glycosylation of collagen.[98] Several authors have studied LJM of the ankle, subtalar, and metatarsophalangeal joints in cross sections of diabetic and nondiabetic patients.[103–105] Characteristically, patients with a history of neuropathic ulceration had significantly less mobility than did those without ulceration or nondiabetic controls, although LJM was not restricted to patients with neuropathy. Fernando and colleagues[104] correlated LJM with higher plantar foot pressures. Sixty-five percent of subjects with both LJM and neuropathy had a history of ulceration. Studies are lacking, however, in patients with Charcot's joint disease, and it is difficult to correlate LJM with the severe hypermobility that is frequently observed in this disorder.

Diminished Bone Mineral Density

Several studies of diabetic patients with neuropathic osteoarthropathy have demonstrated reduced bone mineral density (BMD) associated with excess osteoclastic activity without a concomitant increase in osteoblastic function.[51,71,106] Young and colleagues[71] corroborated the importance of autonomic neuropathy in promoting diminished BMD in patients with peripheral neuropathy. Patients with active Charcot feet had significantly greater deficits in autonomic parameters than did their non-Charcot neuropathic counterparts. Furthermore, BMD in both lower limbs of Charcot patients was less than that found in matched non-Charcot subjects. Since BMD was lower in the affected limb of Charcot patients in contrast to the contralateral side, we must consider that a treatment effect might be responsible rather than a true causative effect.[71] Forst and colleagues[86] observed diminished BMD in the lower limbs of individuals with type 1 diabetes as compared to age- and sex-matched controls. Additionally, a link between decreased BMD in the femoral neck and neuropathy was found. Gough and colleagues,[51] investigating markers of osteoclastic and osteoblastic activity in neuropathic osteoarthropathy, determined that patients with acute Charcot feet had significantly higher levels of osteoclastic activity than did patients with chronic deformities, diabetic controls, and healthy subjects. There were no significant elevations for the osteoblastic marker in any of the groups. Although excess osteoclastic activity alone cannot be considered causative for neuropathic osteoarthropathy, the authors suggest that there is an uncoupling of bone resorption and deposition during the active stage of this process and that such markers of bone metabolism might be used to monitor disease activity.

Petrova and coworkers at King's College Hospital recently measured calcaneal BMD in both feet of patients with unilateral Charcot osteoarthropathy.[107] Calcaneal bone density, temperature, and vibration thresholds were compared between 17 patients with type 1 diabetes and unilateral osteoarthropathy and 47 type 1 controls and between 18 patients with type 2 diabetes and 48 type 2 controls. They found that BMD in the affected Charcot foot was lower, compared with the unaffected foot, in both type 1 and type 2 diabetic patients. In patients with type 1 diabetes, bone density of the unaffected foot was reduced in comparison with that in patients with type 2 diabetes. As expected, the body mass index was lower in type 1 patients than in type 2 patients.

Herbst and coworkers[108] investigated the relationship between BMD and fracture/dislocation patterns of DNOAP of the foot and ankle. They examined the effect of osteopenia on the development of fracture versus dislocation patterns of presentation. Dual-energy X-ray absorptiometry scans were performed on the contralateral femoral neck or distal radius of 55 consecutive patients presenting with a newly diagnosed Charcot foot or ankle. Twenty-three patients presented with a fracture; an equal number presented with dislocation; and nine presented with mixed fracture-dislocation. They found that the fractures were associated with peripheral deficiency of BMD (significantly lower *t*-scores), and a dislocation pattern was associated with normal BMD. Fractures predominated at the ankle and forefoot, whereas dislocations were more common in the midfoot.

These findings raise two important questions: (1) Should routine monitoring of bone density be performed in high-risk diabetic patients? (2) Should antiresorptive pharmacologic agents be used as a preventive measure to stop bone resorption and prevent the development of an acute Charcot foot? Prospective, randomized, controlled multicenter trials are necessary to answer these questions. The potential benefit of bisphosphonates and calcitonin for the treatment of the acute Charcot foot will be discussed later, in the section entitled "Treatment Recommendations."

Patterns of Bone and Joint Destruction

Five characteristic anatomic patterns of bone and joint destruction have been observed to occur in diabetic people with neuropathic osteoarthropathy.[47,49] Sanders and Frykberg[47,49] compiled information on the distribution of bone and joint involvement in neuropathic diabetic people, reported in the English literature, as well as cases from a Department of Veterans Affairs retrospective study, and developed the following anatomic classification: pattern I, forefoot; pattern II, tarsometatarsal joints; pattern III, naviculocuneiform, talonavicular, and calcaneocuboid joints; pattern IV, ankle and/or subtalar joint; and pattern V, calcaneus. Two of these patterns, I and II, are frequently associated with bony deformity and ulceration. The most frequent joint involvement is seen in patterns I, II, and III, and the most severe structural deformity and functional instability are seen in patterns II and IV. Pattern V osteopathy is the least common and may be seen as an isolated fracture of the calcaneus or in association with involvement of other tarsal bones. These anatomic patterns may be seen singly or in combination in any given individual (Fig. 12-6).

Pattern I: Forefoot

This commonly occurring pattern of osteoarthropathy is characterized by involvement of the interphalangeal joints, phalanges, metatarsophalangeal joints, or distal metatarsal bones. Radiographic findings in this location are typically atrophic and destructive in nature, characterized by osteopenia, osteolysis, juxta-articular cortical bone defects, subluxation, and destruction. Pattern I involvement has been reported to occur in 26% to 67% of all affected sites.[13,42,47,62] These studies include those of Miller and Lichtman,[13] with 47.6% (10 of 21); Sanders and Mrdjenovich,[47] with 30% (20 of 66); and Cofield and colleagues,[42] with 67% (73 of 116). Sinha and colleagues[41] reported metatarsophalangeal joint involvement in 26.8% (34 of 127) of all affected sites.

Plantar ulceration is a common finding associated with neuropathic osteoarthropathy of the forefoot. Cofield and colleagues[42] reported that 91% of their patients with radiographic evidence of metatarsophalangeal joint involvement had underlying ulcers. It might not be readily apparent whether the bone and joint changes preceded or developed as a result of the ulceration. This finding might, in fact, be a cutaneous marker for neuropathic osteoarthropathy of the forefoot. Newman and colleagues[109] assessed the prevalence of osteomyelitis in 35 diabetic patients with 41 foot ulcers (38 classic mal perforans ulcers). As determined by bone biopsy and culture, these investigators found that osteomyelitis underlay 68% of the foot ulcers. All patients with exposed bone had osteomyelitis. Digital findings include concentric resorption of bone that may be seen as a characteristic hourglass appearance of the phalangeal diaphyses. The bases of the proximal phalanges broaden to form a cup around the metatarsal head (Fig. 12-7).[50,110]

Resorption of the distal metatarsal bones and phalanges is characteristic of atrophic, destructive DNOAP. This is evidenced on anteroposterior radiographs as a pencil-like tapering of the metatarsal bones with a sucked candy stick appearance (Fig. 12-8). The histopathologic picture reveals erosion of articular cartilage, periarticular fibrosis, increased vascularity, synchronous resorption of bone, and new bone formation. There is disorganization of subchondral bone, with bony resorption and a fatty marrow. Chronic ulceration and infection may be associated with these changes.

Pattern II: Tarsometatarsal Joints

Pattern II osteoarthropathy involves subluxation or fracture-dislocation of the tarsometatarsal (TMT or Lisfranc's) joints[89] and is often associated with plantar ulceration at the apex of the collapsed cuneiforms or cuboid. Tarsometatarsal involvement has been reported to occur in 15% to 48% of cases of DNOAP.[13,41,42,44,89] This pattern of neuropathic osteoarthropathy occurs with greater frequency in diabetic patients than in patients with leprosy (Hansen's disease). Unlike the TMT joint pattern associated with Hansen's disease, this pattern is rarely caused by "definite violence."[17]

The normal anatomic relationships of the TMT joints are illustrated in Figure 12-9. The second metatarsal base is securely recessed in the intercuneiform mortise. This tenon-in-mortise construct creates a very stable keystone for the midfoot. Disturbance of this relationship weakens the foot and allows for dorsolateral displacement of the metatarsal bones on the cuneiforms and cuboid followed by architectural collapse.

Early changes in the TMT joints may be subtle and consistent with incipient osteoarthritis; there may be slight dorsal prominence of the metatarsal bases with local swelling and increased skin temperature. The base

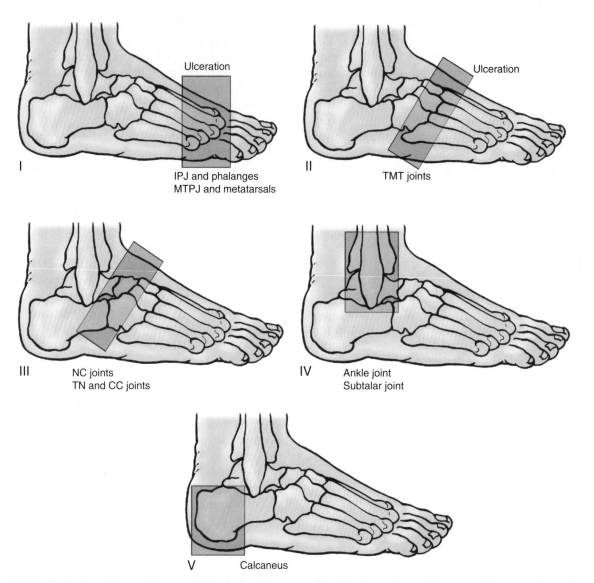

Figure 12–6 Anatomic patterns of bone and joint destruction reported in diabetic patients with neuropathic osteoarthropathy of the foot and ankle. Patterns I and II are frequently associated with bony deformity and ulceration. The most frequent joint involvement is seen in patterns I, II, and III, the most severe structural deformity and functional instability being associated with patterns II and IV. CC, calcaneocuboid; IPJ, interphalangeal joints; MTPJ, metatarsophalangeal joints; NC, naviculocuneiform; TMT, tarsometatarsal; TN, talonavicular. *(Modified from Sanders LJ, Frykberg RG: Diabetic neuropathic osteoarthropathy: The Charcot foot. In Frykberg RG [ed]: The High Risk Foot in Diabetes Mellitus. New York: Churchill Livingstone, 1991, with permission.)*

of the second metatarsal becomes laterally displaced from its normal recessed position in the intercuneiform mortise, and all of the metatarsals are shifted laterally on the lesser tarsus with their bases overriding the cuneiforms. There may be evidence of total disintegration of the cuneiforms, with collapse of the midfoot and a resultant rocker bottom foot deformity. Late changes include degenerative arthritis with fragmentation.

A fracture or minimal subluxation of the base of the second metatarsal, even from ostensibly insignificant trauma, may precede collapse of the TMT joints, as is seen in the following case. A 66-year-old neuropathic diabetic man presented with mild swelling and erythema on the dorsum of his right foot after a fall in his kitchen. Radiographs revealed a laterally displaced fracture of the

second metatarsal base (Fig. 12-10). The patient was placed in a plaster cast, nonweight-bearing, with crutches for 6 weeks. During this time, he was poorly compliant and refused further treatment. Within 8 months, the patient's midfoot collapsed.

The following case represents an acute neuropathic osteoarthropathy affecting the TMT articulations. A 63-year-old neuropathic male with a 15-year history of diabetes mellitus, poorly controlled with insulin, presented to the emergency room with acute erythema, swelling, increased skin temperature, and deformity of his right foot. He reported having mild pain and no history of trauma. The patient, a unilateral transtibial amputee, was afebrile with an elevated blood glucose level of 447 mg/dL. Radiographs revealed a TMT joint dislocation,

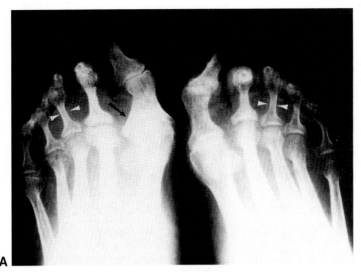

Figure 12-7 **A,** Concentric resorption of bone involving proximal phalangeal shafts of the lesser toes (*arrowheads*). Note the hourglass appearance of the phalanges. Note also the broadening of the phalangeal base of the hallux and cupping of the first metatarsal head (*arrow*). Proliferative changes of the second metatarsal head are also noted. **B,** Graphic illustration of radiographic findings.

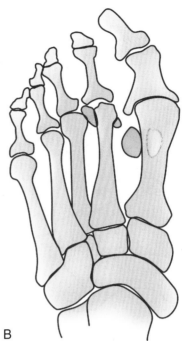

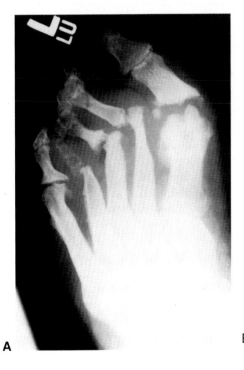

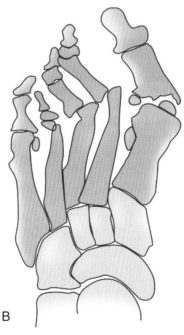

Figure 12-8 **A,** Anteroposterior radiograph reveals osteolytic destruction of all metatarsophalangeal joints, with pencil-like tapering of the metatarsal shafts resembling a sucked candy stick. **B,** Graphic representation of radiographic findings. *(From Sanders LJ, Frykberg RG: Diabetic neuropathic osteoarthropathy: The Charcot foot. In Frykberg RG [ed]: The High Risk Foot in Diabetes Mellitus. New York: Churchill Livingstone, 1991, with permission.)*

with all of the metatarsal bases shifted laterally on the lesser tarsus. The lateral radiograph revealed plantar dislocation of the cuneiforms and navicular, with dorsal displacement of the metatarsal bases. The patient was admitted to the hospital for conservative management of the right foot, an unsuccessful attempt at closed reduction of the dislocation, and control of his diabetes. In spite of efforts to immobilize the limb and to limit weight-bearing, he continued to walk on his right lower limb. Within 6 months, total collapse of the foot

occurred, along with extrusion of the medial cuneiform. Ulceration developed from shear forces over the prominent medial cuneiform (Fig. 12-11).

Pattern III: Naviculocuneiform, Talonavicular, and Calcaneocuboid Joints

Pattern III involves the naviculocuneiform and midtarsal joints and is frequently characterized by dislocation of the navicular bone or by disintegration of the

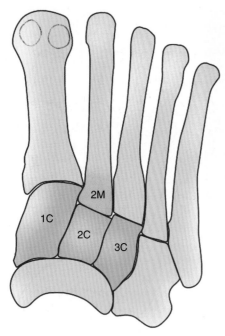

Figure 12–9   Normal anatomy of the tarsometatarsal (Lisfranc's) joints. Note the recessed position of the second metatarsal base in the intercuneiform mortise. C, cuneiform; M, metatarsal.

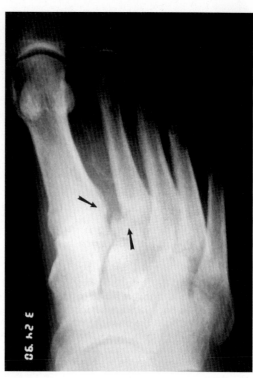

Figure 12–10   Laterally displaced fracture of the second metatarsal base (*arrows*).

naviculocuneiform joints. Sanders and Mrdjenovich[47] reported naviculocuneiform, talonavicular, or calcaneocuboid involvement in approximately 32% of the affected joints (21 of 66 sites) in 28 cases. Very early radiographic changes of impending Charcot's joint destruction may be evidenced by osteolysis of the naviculocuneiform joints. Typical fragmentation, osteolysis, and sharply defined osseous debris are visible on the lateral radiograph (Fig. 12-12). Observation of this finding signals the need for nonweight-bearing cast immobilization of the foot. Ignoring this finding may result in progressive deterioration of the lesser tarsal bones and ultimate collapse of the midfoot.

Isolated midtarsal joint dislocations associated with neuropathic diabetics have been reported by several authors.[19,52,111] Lesko and Maurer[111] reported their experience with eight talonavicular dislocations, in which the displacements of the navicular were variously described as inferomedial, mediodorsal, or medial. Fragmentation of bone frequently accompanies these dislocations. Talonavicular dislocation may be seen alone or in association with involvement of the naviculocuneiform joints, disintegration of the cuneiform bones, or deterioration of the head and neck of the talus (Fig. 12-13).

A combination of patterns II and III is represented in Figure 12-14. Note the dramatic collapse of the midfoot with a rocker bottom appearance. Ulceration of the skin occurred at the apex of the rocker. The tarsometatarsal, naviculocuneiform, talonavicular, and calcaneocuboid joints are all involved.

Pattern IV: Ankle and Subtalar Joints

Pattern IV involves the ankle joint with or without subtalar joint involvement and accounts for only 3% to 10% of the reported cases.[13,16,41,42,47,49,98,112] This pattern invariably results in severe structural deformity and instability of the ankle. Associated medial or lateral malleolar fractures precipitate disintegration of the ankle joint. Charcot's joint disease of the ankle may develop suddenly without any appreciable external cause, with spontaneous swelling and localized redness of the foot and ankle. Patients will initially notice swelling and deformity of the affected ankle, with little pain. They often continue to walk on the affected limb until the collateral ligaments stretch or tear and there is erosion of bone and cartilage with collapse of the joint. Steindler's[16] observations of foot and ankle fractures in patients with tabetic joints caused him to conclude that "the greatest pathological changes correspond to the maximum of mechanical stress ... in the direction of the greatest weight-bearing." He noted two types of destruction: one in the direction of the long axis of the leg, breaking down the talus and calcaneus, and the other evidenced by collapse of the forefoot and tarsus. Free bodies were seen in the ankle joint in 8 of 21 cases.

Harris and Brand[17] noted that if during weight-bearing, "the posture of the foot is disturbed by external forces or paralysis, an abnormal position results, and the new weight stream will cross the trabecular lines so that minor fractures occur more readily and ligaments may

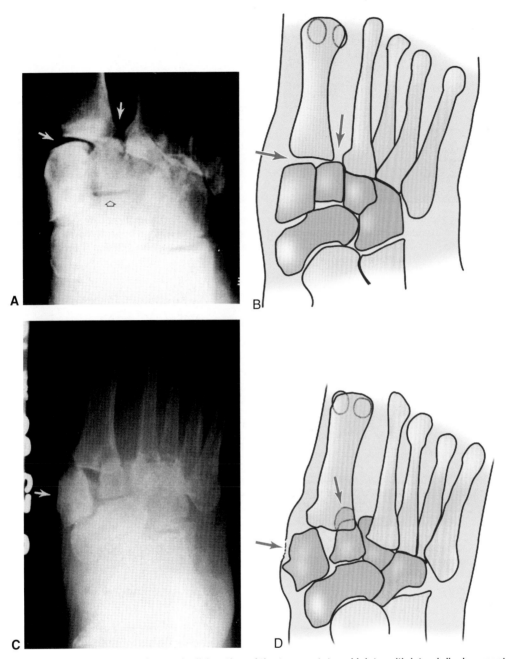

Figure 12–11   A, Anteroposterior radiograph reveals dislocation of the tarsometatarsal joints, with lateral displacement of the metatarsal bases on the cuneiforms and cuboid. The second metatarsal base is completely displaced from the intercuneiform mortise, with the first metatarsal base articulating with the medial half of the second cuneiform (*arrows*). Note distal migration of the second cuneiform (*arrowhead*). **B,** Graphic illustration of radiographic findings in **A. C,** Anteroposterior radiograph taken 6 months after initial presentation. There has been extensive deterioration of the tarsometatarsal, navicular cuneiform, and midtarsal joints. Note extrusion of the medial cuneiform (*arrow*). The second cuneiform has eroded its way into the plantar-lateral aspect of the first metatarsal base. **D,** Graphic illustration of radiographic findings in **C.** *(From Sanders LJ, Frykberg RG: Diabetic neuropathic osteoarthropathy: The Charcot foot. In Frykberg RG [ed]: The High Risk Foot in Diabetes Mellitus. New York: Churchill Livingstone, 1991, with permission.)*

rupture." They described "a relatively rapid and catastrophic disintegration of the proximal tarsal bones allowing the tibia to grind its way through the foot to the ground."

Even trivial trauma associated with an ankle sprain or a relatively minor fracture can result in instability of the ankle joint, with resultant collapse and disintegration.[13,17,19] Miller and Lichtman[13] described a case in which total

destruction of the ankle joint resulted after surgical intervention for a fractured medial malleolus. Johnson[19] reported the case of a 55-year-old woman who, 8 weeks after a sprained left ankle, developed complete displacement of the medial malleolus with grinding away of one half of the talus and part of the distal end of the tibia.

Rapid disintegration of the ankle joint occurred in a 59-year-old neuropathic woman with a 15-year history of

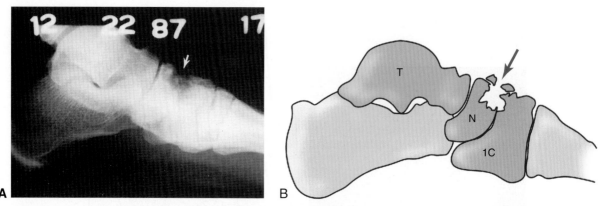

Figure 12–12   **A,** Osteolytic destruction of the naviculocuneiform joints (*arrow*). Fragmentation, osteolysis, and sharply defined osseous debris are noted. **B,** Graphic illustration of radiographic findings. 1C, first cuneiform bone; N, navicular bone; T, talus. *(From Sanders LJ, Frykberg RG: Diabetic neuropathic osteoarthropathy: The Charcot foot. In Frykberg RG [ed]: The High Risk Foot in Diabetes Mellitus. New York: Churchill Livingstone, 1991, with permission.)*

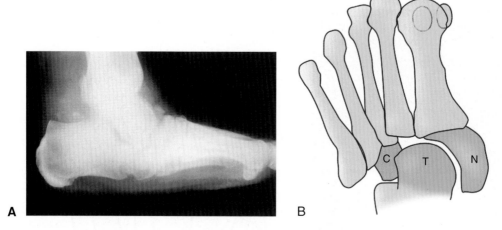

Figure 12–13   **A,** Disorganization of the talonavicular and calcaneocuboid joints. **B,** Graphic illustration of talonavicular dislocation with inferomedial displacement of the navicular bone.

diabetes mellitus. Her chief complaints were pain, redness, and swelling of her left foot and ankle of 1 week's duration. There was no history of trauma; however, she had recently been treated by her family physician for "an infected blister" on her left fifth toe. The infection resolved promptly, but shortly thereafter, pain and swelling developed over the lateral aspect of her foot and ankle. The patient had bounding pedal pulses and a dense peripheral neuropathy. Radiographs revealed osteopenia of the tarsal bones, with evidence of osteoarthritis of the tarsometatarsal joints. A radionucleotide scan with methylene diphosphonate labeled with ^{99m}Tc revealed very high uptake in the left ankle and tarsal bones as well as marked uptake in the asymptomatic right ankle. Blood cultures and an ankle joint aspirate obtained on admission grew *Staphylococcus aureus*. The opinion of an infectious disease consultant was that a septic arthritis was overlying a DNOAP.[113] In spite of appropriate treatment with parenteral antibiotics, bed rest, elevation of the limb, and nonweight-bearing casts, progressive deformity

of the left ankle ensued. The clinical picture was characterized by lateral bulging and instability of the ankle, with medial displacement of the foot and fragmentation of bone. Radiographs and clinical photographs revealed extensive joint destruction with dislocation of the foot to the medial side of the leg (Fig. 12-15).

Pattern V: Calcaneus

Pattern V osteopathy is the least common anatomic presentation (~2%), and is characterized by an extra-articular avulsion fracture of the posterior tubercle of the calcaneus.[45,76,114–116] Although this pattern is not an arthropathy, it is appropriately included in this classification, by definition of the Charcot foot as a neuropathic osteoarthropathy. J.-M. Charcot noted that "fractures of the bones and diseases of the joints appear to belong to the same pathological condition."[30]

Harris and Brand,[17] in their paper on patterns of tarsal disintegration associated with Hansen's disease, used the

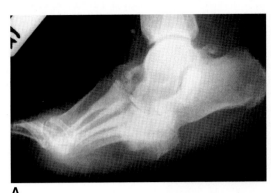

A

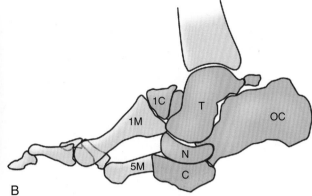

B

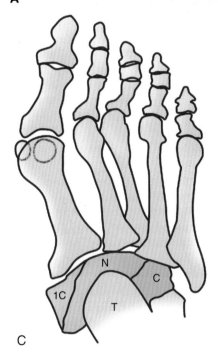

C

Figure 12–14 **A,** Lateral radiograph demonstrates collapse of the tarsometatarsal, naviculocuneiform, talonavicular, and calcaneocuboid joints (combination of patterns II and III). **B** and **C,** Graphic illustrations of radiographic findings, with identification of involved structures. C, cuboid; 1C, medial cuneiform; M, metatarsal; N, navicular; OC, calcaneus; T, talus. *(**A** and **B** from Sanders LJ, Frykberg RG: Diabetic neuropathic osteoarthropathy: The Charcot foot. In Frykberg RG [ed]: The High Risk Foot in Diabetes Mellitus. New York: Churchill Livingstone, 1991, with permission.)*

positional designation "posterior pillar" to describe this fracture pattern. They attributed increased vulnerability of the calcaneus to fracture in an insensitive foot to (1) increased force on the heel caused by the patient's landing more heavily on an insensitive foot, (2) continued walking on a fractured bone, and (3) previous or concurrent ulceration "which may have weakened the bone by hyperemic decalcification or may allow infection and osteomyelitis to complicate the fracture." Kathol and colleagues[114] reported on 21 diabetic patients with calcaneal fractures, of which 18 were nontraumatic and 14 were limited to the posterior third of the calcaneus. This fracture pattern occurs in the same plane as a calcaneal fatigue fracture, with displacement and rotation of the posterior tuberosity. The term *calcaneal insufficiency avulsion fracture* was coined by Kathol's group to describe this unique fracture pattern.[114]

A bilateral calcaneal fracture was reported by Coventry and Rothacker[115] in a 45-year-old neuropathic woman with juvenile-onset diabetes. El-Khoury and Kathol[76] reported on four patients with spontaneous, unusual

avulsion fractures of the posterior tubercle of the calcaneus, "where the avulsed fragment migrated superiorly due to the constant pull of the Achilles tendon." These patients had diminished pain and vibratory perception. Clohisy and Thompson[45] reported 19 calcaneal fractures in 18 neuropathic type 1 (juvenile-onset) diabetic patients who had no history of major trauma to their limbs. Five of these patients had bilateral calcaneal fractures. In 17 limbs, the calcaneal fractures were seen together with fractures of more than one other tarsal bone. Fourteen of the patients in this study had undergone renal transplant surgery before the fracture was diagnosed.

Thompson and colleagues,[112] in a retrospective review of 55 neuropathic kidney transplant patients, found a 20% incidence of skeletal disease among diabetic patients, the highest incidence occurring in the third and fourth years after transplantation. They reported seeing three calcaneal fractures in 11 patients with neurotrophic joint disease. The initial manifestation in all patients was a pathologic fracture, usually in a bony

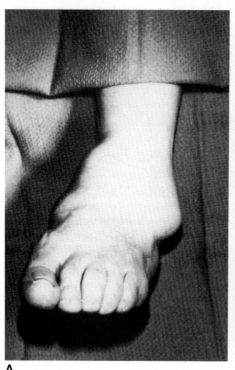

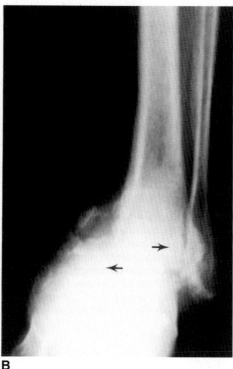

A   **B**

Figure 12–15 **A,** Unstable neuropathic left ankle, with lateral bulging. **B,** Anteroposterior radiograph reveals extensive joint destruction with fragmentation of bone. Note dislocation of the joint (*arrows*), with the foot displaced medially. *(From Sanders LJ, Frykberg RG: Diabetic neuropathic osteoarthropathy: The Charcot foot. In Frykberg RG [ed]: The High Risk Foot in Diabetes Mellitus. New York: Churchill Livingstone, 1991, with permission.)*

metaphysis, that is, adjacent to a joint. Only later did they see actual joint destruction that seemed to result from the subchondral collapse associated with the initial fracture.

A calcaneal insufficiency avulsion fracture of the posterior tubercle of the right calcaneus occurred spontaneously in an active 53-year-old woman with a 5-year history of diabetes mellitus and peripheral neuropathy. She reported hearing a loud crack and feeling a sharp pain in the back of her right heel while walking in a hallway at work. Lateral radiographs revealed posterior and superior displacement of the posterior process of the calcaneus (Fig. 12-16). In addition to fracture, radiographs of her asymptomatic left foot revealed concentric resorption of the proximal phalanges, a cup-shaped proximal phalangeal base of the hallux, and fragmentation of the second metatarsal head.

Other classification systems, based on anatomic sites of involvement, have been described, but none of these schemes identify the stage of disease activity.[17,47,55,117–119] Several systems focus primarily on the midfoot and/or hindfoot,[17,117,119] while the classification system illustrated in this chapter includes the forefoot, midfoot, and hindfoot.

Current Diagnostics

The diagnosis of the Charcot foot rests primarily on the physician's clinical suspicion of the disease. This disorder should be suspected when bone and joint abnormalities, sometimes very subtle, are noted in a diabetic patient with loss of protective sensation, absent deep tendon reflexes, and diminished vibratory sense. The most specific diagnostic tools for distinguishing between Charcot's osteoarthropathy and osteomyelitis in the diabetic foot are a detailed clinical history, physical examination of the foot/ankle, and radiographic studies. Although magnetic resonance imaging (MRI) is increasingly being utilized to evaluate for latent bone infection, differentiating osteomyelitis from Charcot's osteoarthropathy, even with contrast-enhanced MRI, is still equivocal. Diagnosis of osteomyelitis can be complicated because the signal changes that are seen with acute Charcot osteoarthropathy can be mistaken for infection.[120] The efficacy of MRI is further limited by the presence of fracture fixation hardware (screws and plates) because artifact formation prevents adequate MRI examination. Osteomyelitis should be presumed when there has been chronic soft tissue ulceration and infection contiguous to bone. However, in the case of Charcot's osteoarthropathy, noninfectious soft tissue inflammation frequently accompanies rapidly progressive destruction of bone and joints in a well-vascularized, neuropathic, nonulcerated foot.[66] Rarely are bone scans, computed tomography, or MRI necessary to establish the diagnosis. Bone biopsy should be reserved for those cases that are ambiguous, for example, when there is a chronic nonhealing wound or infection contiguous to bone. It is important to note that radiographs may be unremarkable during the earliest presentation of the Charcot foot (stage 0).[54,55] At this time, the foot may be only mildly inflamed and radiographic findings are consistent with incipient osteoarthritis or osteolysis. In cases in which there is a clear history of

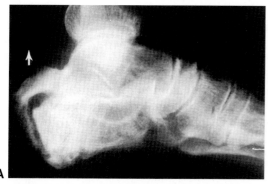

A

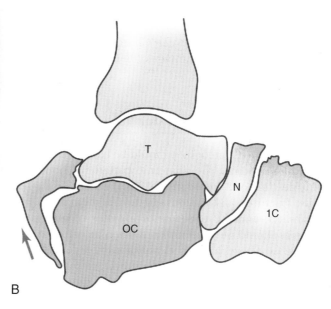

B

Figure 12–16   **A,** Lateral radiograph demonstrates an avulsion fracture of the posterior tubercle of the calcaneus. *Arrow* points in the direction of pull of the Achilles tendon. Early osteolytic changes are seen to affect the naviculocuneiform joint. **B,** Graphic illustration of radiographic findings. **N,** navicular; **OC,** calcaneous; **T,** talus; **1C,** medial cuneiform. *(From Sanders LJ, Frykberg RG: Diabetic neuropathic osteoarthropathy: The Charcot foot. In Frykberg RG [ed]: The High Risk Foot in Diabetes Mellitus. New York: Churchill Livingstone, 1991, with permission.)*

injury but the initial plain films are negative, radiographic studies should be repeated within 2 to 3 weeks to rule out stress fractures, fragmentation of bone, and periosteal new bone formation. During this time, a cautious approach to treatment should be taken, with a high index of suspicion. Affected limbs of neuropathic individuals should be immobilized and kept nonweight-bearing. Serial radiographs are useful in following the course of this disease through the stage of reconstruction.[11,12]

Computed tomography and MRI have been reported to be helpful adjuncts to the evaluation of the diabetic Charcot foot. Williamson and colleagues,[121] at the University of Virginia Medical School, reported that computed tomography scans correctly predicted the presence or absence of osteomyelitis in all of a series of seven patients. Nucleotide bone scans produced one false-positive result and one false-negative result. Beltran and colleagues[61] found MRI to be helpful in differentiating neuroarthropathy from osteomyelitis. They identified a distinctive pattern for Charcot's joints consisting of low signal intensity on T1- and T2-weighted images within the bone marrow space adjacent to the involved joint. Others[79,122] have made similar observations but question the ability of MR imaging to reliably distinguish rapidly progressing osteoarthropathy from osteomyelitis.

Positive technetium and gallium bone scans may be seen with osteomyelitis, but they may also be false-positive because of neuropathic bone disease.[63,123] Diffuse and focal uptake of technetium has been reported in neuropathic feet by several authors in areas of active bone turnover and increased bony blood flow, as seen in patients with osteoarthropathy.[84,124–126] Positive scans have been reported to sometimes precede radiographic changes.[125] Gallium-67 citrate, which accumulates in sites

of infection, has also been reported to localize in noninfected neuropathic bone.[127,128]

Leukocyte scanning with indium-111 (^{111}In) has been shown to have a high specificity and a very high negative predictive value for osteomyelitis.[123,129–132] Newman and colleagues[109] compared the results of radiographs, leukocyte scans with ^{111}In oxyquinolone, and bone scans with bone biopsy and culture results. Of all imaging tests, the leukocyte scan had the highest sensitivity, 89%. The specificity for osteomyelitis with ^{111}In has been reported to be from 78% to 89%.[129,130] compared with 38% to 75% for three-phase bone scans.[132] Schauwecker and colleagues[123,130] found that in the absence of infection, ^{111}In-labeled leukocytes do not usually accumulate in neuropathic bone. However, false-positive results do occur in the presence of noninfected osteoarthropathy, making this modality less specific in its ability to distinguish osteomyelitis from neuroarthropathy.[63,122,129] Although the utility of ^{99m}Tc hexamethyl propylenamine oxime–labeled leukocytes in this regard is still under investigation, one study reported no accumulation of the labeled white blood cells in subjects with noninfected Charcot joints.[62]

Hopfner and colleagues[65] recently reported that positron emission tomography (PET) scans could detect osteoarthropathy with 95% sensitivity and could reliably distinguish between Charcot neuroarthropathy and osteomyelitis even in the presence of metal implants.

In this small prospective study of 17 patients with type 2 diabetes, the investigators sought to determine the value of two types of PET in the preoperative evaluation of Charcot foot. They compared high-resolution ring PET and low-resolution hybrid PET with MRI. Of 39 lesions confirmed at surgery, 37 (95%) were successfully identified by ring PET. They concluded that PET has the ability to differentiate between inflammatory and infectious soft-tissue lesions and between Charcot lesions and osteomyelitis as well as the advantage of being unaffected by metal implants.

Treatment Recommendations

Management of the Charcot foot should be based on the acuteness of symptoms, the anatomic pattern of bone and joint destruction, the degree of involvement (e.g., deformity, fractures, dislocations, bone fragmentation, and instability), and the presence or absence of infection. Surgery should be contemplated when attempts at conservative care have failed to establish a stable, plantigrade foot or prevent plantar ulceration. As early as 1931, Steindler recognized the need for early detection of the neuropathic joint and the importance of immediate protection to prevent further deterioration of the articulation.[16] He believed that "early and adequate splinting, preservation of protecting musculature by physical therapy and, above all, earliest stabilization and alignment by conservative or operative means furnish the best prospects of extending the usefulness of these joints for many years." Johnson,[19] in his classic 1967 article, reiterated the need for protection sufficient enough to prevent further damage, ranging from a brace or plaster cast to complete bed rest. Healing would be indicated by lessened edema, reduced local temperature, and radiographic evidence of repair rather than resorption. Harris and Brand held a similar opinion, also recognizing the possible need for surgical stabilization should cast immobilization be ineffective in arresting the complete disintegration of the involved joints.[17]

An objective rationale of treatment based on the chronicity of injury, anatomic alignment, and associated degree of deformity was outlined by Lesko and Maurer[111] at the University of California, San Francisco. For acute injuries with acceptable alignment, they suggest immobilization and protective weight-bearing to prevent further progression of joint destruction. For acute dislocation with marked deformity and little bone fragmentation, reduction and surgical arthrodesis may be indicated. For chronic dislocation with severe deformity and bone fragmentation, surgical treatment is recommended only as a last resort if soft tissue breakdown cannot be prevented by therapeutic footwear and bracing. Armstrong and colleagues[44] reviewed the natural history of the Charcot foot and provided a treatment algorithm encompassing the aforementioned principles of management (Fig. 12-17).

Diabetic people with acute signs and symptoms of neuropathic osteoarthropathy, as evidenced by erythema, swelling, and bone and joint destruction, may be best treated by early hospitalization, bed rest, nonweight-bearing, and cast immobilization. Compliant patients with supportive family members or friends may be efficiently

managed on an outpatient basis. Hospitalization, although not often necessary, may be required to establish the diagnosis of the Charcot foot or to facilitate the treatment of poorly compliant or high-risk individuals. Unfortunately, in the current era of managed care, such admissions might not be deemed allowable.

Generally speaking, surgical intervention during the atrophic phase should be avoided, because it may accelerate the destructive process.[17,19] If the acute injury goes unnoticed and unprotected, luxation, fragmentation, architectural collapse, hypertrophic bone formation, and deformity will follow. The aim of treatment should be to obtain stability of the foot with no excessive pressure on the skin from a bony prominence.[14,19,48,49,52] The key to treatment is prevention of further trauma and deformity, thereby allowing the active process to convert to the reparative (quiescent) stage.

Progressive destruction of the neuropathic foot can be halted if recognized early enough.[17,24,49,67] The appropriate way to "treat" the Charcot foot is first to prevent its occurrence. Careful history and physical examination directed toward risk assessment and stratification will help to identify the individuals who are at greatest risk. Patients in their sixth or seventh decade who have had diabetes for more than 10 years and who demonstrate loss of protective sensation are prime candidates for the

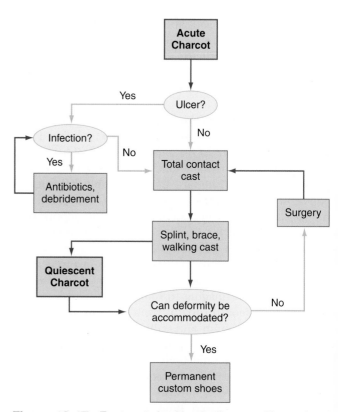

Figure 12–17 Treatment algorithm for the acute Charcot foot. *(From Armstrong DG, Todd WF, Lavery LA, et al: The natural history of acute Charcot's arthropathy in a diabetic foot specialty clinic. Diabet Med 14:357–363, 1997, with permission.)*

development of neuropathic osteoarthropathy. A stated history of trauma or suspicion of unrecognized injury completes this picture. Added risk factors include the presence of nephropathy and retinopathy.[41,45]

For early recognition of Charcot's osteoarthropathy, a high index of suspicion is essential. The physician and patient should be educated to look for areas of mild swelling, increased skin temperature, deformity, or instability of the foot and ankle. Local temperature assessment is valuable for monitoring tissue damage in the insensitive foot.[80,133] Areas of increased warmth correspond to areas of inflammation in the insensitive limb that are at risk for bony resorption and ulceration. A hand-held infrared digital thermometer is a useful tool to monitor the inflammatory response in insensate patients.[80,133] Any increase in skin temperature greater than 2°C should be considered a significant finding indicating impending osteoarthropathy or preulcerative inflammation. Degenerative changes in any foot with proven peripheral sensory impairment are indicative of neuropathic arthropathy.[81]

In contrast to Charcot's description of a painless arthropathy, pain is often an associated feature but appears to be less severe than would normally be expected in view of the pathologic changes that are present. One report indicated that 76% of patients with acute neuroarthropathy complained of pain on initial presentation.[44] Elevation of the limb to reduce edema, cessation of weight-bearing, prolonged cast immobilization, and comprehensive patient education are basic components of effective treatment.

Immobilization

Immobilization and reduction of weight-bearing stress are considered the mainstays of treatment for the acute Charcot foot. A general rule of thumb to follow in managing patients with neuropathic osteoarthropathy is that at least 8 to 12 weeks of nonweight-bearing cast immobilization is required to convert the active inflammatory arthritis to the quiescent phase. This period of immobilization could be much longer, depending on the anatomic pattern and extent of involvement as well as the presence of concomitant ulceration and infection. Involvement of the hindfoot, for example, often requires much more intensive treatment, often including surgical stabilization and/or a permanent ankle-foot orthosis (AFO). In general, however, patients may be weaned from cast immobilization to a removable cast walker and then to a therapeutic shoe with or without an AFO. The duration of immobilization is individualized and should be determined by assessment of skin temperature as well as by radiographic evidence of consolidation of fractures and fragmentation of bone. Warmth of the skin indicates persistent inflammation, which requires continued immobilization. Armstrong and colleagues[44] reported an average total-contact casting duration of 18.5 weeks in

their study of 55 patients with acute Charcot foot. No mention, however, is made of nonweight-bearing. After ambulatory total-contact casting, the patients were weaned into a removable cast walker prior to wearing accommodative footwear. Shaw and colleagues[134] found that approximately one third of the total load applied to the casted limb is transmitted to the leg via the walls of the cast. However, pressure was reduced least in the midfoot, while total force-time integral in the heel was actually increased in comparison to walking in shoes or barefoot. These findings suggest that ambulatory casting might not be as effective as was once thought and that nonweight-bearing should indeed be initially prescribed. Attention should also be directed to the "asymptomatic" limb with respect to the potential development of bilateral osteoarthropathy. Clohisy and Thompson[45] observed that when the patient with an affected limb was prevented from weight-bearing, involvement of the contralateral limb became evident after an average of 4.5 months.

Orthoses and Shoes

A patellar tendon-bearing (PTB) orthosis used together with therapeutic shoes can effectively decrease load on the foot.[45,111,135-137] Clohisy and Thompson[45] suggest short-term prophylactic protection of the "uninvolved" limb with a PTB cast or orthosis during the period of cast immobilization of the involved limb. For long-term protection of the affected limb, they prescribe a calf-containment PTB orthosis. Saltzman and colleagues,[136] measured mean peak force transmitted to the foot in six diabetic patients with neurotrophic arthropathy. They found that use of a properly fitted standard PTB orthosis with a free ankle and an extra-depth shoe reduced mean peak force to the entire foot by 15%. The addition of extra padding to the orthosis decreased the force by 32%. Interestingly, these investigators found that although load transmission was reduced in the hindfoot, it was not reduced in the midfoot or forefoot.

Pressure-reducing modalities alternative to casting or PTB bracing include prefabricated walking braces and custom-fabricated AFOs. Several studies have demonstrated that commercially available walking braces can be as effective as total-contact casting in reducing dynamic peak plantar pressures.[137-139] The greatest reductions were found in the forefoot, while pressure-time integrals, a measure of force and contact duration, were actually increased in the heel region compared to both cast and shoe.[138] Landsman and Sage reported on the use of a custom-fabricated padded AFO in a small series of patients with ulceration and midfoot Charcot osteoarthropathy.[140] The orthoses provided a reduction in peak pressure at the midfoot ulcer sites ranging from 70% to 92%, allowing ulcerations to heal in an average of 9 weeks. A variation on these modalities is the custom-fabricated Charcot restraint orthotic walker.[141] The authors describe this device as a custom, bivalved, total-contact

AFO, fully enclosing the foot, that consists of a polypropylene outer shell, a rocker sole, and a well-padded lining. The benefits of this modality, used after an initial period of nonweight-bearing, are stated to be edema control, effective ankle and foot immobilization, near-normal ambulation, and excellent patient satisfaction. Cost comparisons, including cost/benefit analyses between these various modalities, have yet to be made.

Prescription footwear and foot orthoses are essential for the management of individuals with diabetes, loss of protective sensation, and foot deformities. Cavanagh and colleagues[142] reported a significant reduction in the incidence of plantar lesions after the provision of special footwear to a group of high-risk neuropathic patients. Uccioli and colleagues[143] reported a reduction in the incidence of foot ulcer relapses in patients receiving therapeutic footwear. Ashry and colleagues[144] and Lavery and colleagues[145] confirmed the effectiveness of specially designed shoes with customized insoles in reducing elevated foot pressures.

Extra-depth, super-extra-depth, and thermal moldable shoes with soft leather uppers and well-molded insoles are cost-effective approaches to the management of patients with mild to moderate deformity. Shoes should be employed only after adequate initial conservative management with nonweight-bearing immobilization of the limb. Ulcers should be healed or very superficial before ambulation is allowed. An interim healing shoe can be fabricated by using a custom-molded orthosis in a surgical shoe as dictated by the patient's clinical circumstances.[48] More comprehensive coverage of this subject can be found in the chapter on footwear (Chapter 28).

Antiresorptive Pharmacologic Agents

The bisphosphonates (alendronate, ibandronate, and risedronate), calcitonin, estrogens, and raloxifene affect the bone remodeling cycle and are classified as antiresorptive drugs. These pharmacologic agents are currently approved by the U.S. Food and Drug Administration for the prevention and/or treatment of osteoporosis. However, at the present time, there are no approved indications for the use of these drugs for the prevention or treatment of the Charcot foot. Bisphosphonates are the most effective class of antiresorptive drugs available.[146] Bisphosphonates, as potent inhibitors of osteoclastic activity, have been most commonly used for the treatment of diseases typified by increased bone turnover such as osteoporosis, Paget's disease, hyperparathyroidism, and hypercalcemia. Structurally related to endogenous pyrophosphates, these analogues are selectively taken up on the skeletal surface at sites of bone resorption and become attached to exposed calcium hydroxyapatite crystals.[147] When ingested by migrating osteoclasts, the bisphosphonate molecules effectively inactivate the cells' ability to produce acid and proteolytic enzymes, thereby preventing bone absorption. At appropriate doses, the inhibition of osteoclastic activity has no effect on osteoblastic bone formation, which proceeds normally.[147] Risedronate, a potent nitrogen-containing bisphosphonate, has been shown effective in the treatment of Paget's disease of bone and other metabolic bone diseases. Harris and coinvestigators,[148] in a randomized, placebo-controlled clinical trial of 2458 postmenopausal women, demonstrated that treatment with 5 mg/day of risedronate decreased the cumulative incidence of new vertebral fractures by 41% over a 3-year period. The cumulative incidence of nonvertebral fractures over three years was reduced by 39%, and BMD increased significantly compared with placebo. Liberman and coinvestigators[149] studied the effects of oral alendronate on BMD and the incidence of fractures and height loss in 994 women with postmenopausal osteoporosis. The women receiving alendronate had significant, progressive increases in BMD at all skeletal sites. Overall, treatment with alendronate was associated with a reduction in the incidence of new vertebral fractures.

Interest has developed in the use of bisphosphonate compounds for the treatment of acute osteoarthropathy.[32,33,150] As was mentioned earlier, patients presenting with acute Charcot's osteoarthropathy have been found to have reduced bone density in their affected lower limb and elevated markers for osteoclastic activity.[62,135] Pitocco and coinvestigators[33] recently evaluated the efficacy of alendronate 70 mg by mouth once a week for 6 months in the treatment of acute Charcot neuroarthropathy. This study was a small randomized, placebo-controlled trial ($n = 20$). All patients received a total-contact cast boot for 2 months, followed by a pneumatic walker for 4 months. At the end of 6 months, there was a significant reduction in bone markers (ICTP and hydroxyprolin) and an increase in bone density in the test group. It is important to note that oral bisphosphonates have the potential to cause gastrointestinal irritation. Jude and coinvestigators,[32] studied the effects of bisphosphonate pamidronate in the treatment of acute Charcot neuroarthropathy. Pamidronate was administered in a single 90-mg infusion, in a randomized, double-blind placebo-controlled trial ($n = 39$) carried out at four centers in the United Kingdom. The investigators found that pamidronate given as a single dose led to a reduction in bone turnover, symptoms, and disease activity in diabetic patients with active Charcot neuroarthopathy. However, there was no mention of final outcome in terms of consolidation of bone or time to return to unrestricted ambulation.

Calcitonin is a hormone produced by the thyroid gland that acts directly on osteoclasts and inhibits bone resorption. It has been found to promote the cartilaginous phase of fracture healing. Calcitonin may speed up fracture repair and facilitate early mobilization of an injured limb.[151,152] Administration of salmon calcitonin, usually as a nasal spray, is approved for the treatment of osteoporosis and prevention of vertebral compression fractures in women who have been postmenopausal for 5 or more years. There is no evidence that calcitonin reduces the incidence of fractures anywhere else in the skeleton. Also, there have been no published reports to date on the efficacy of salmon calcitonin for the treatment of acute Charcot's osteoarthropathy.

Surgical Management

Surgical management of the Charcot foot remains a controversial issue. When conservative measures fail, surgical intervention may be indicated; however, complication rates are high,[153,154] especially in feet with chronic ulceration. Surgery should be contemplated only when attempts at conservative care have failed to obtain a stable, ulcer-free, and plantigrade foot.

Pinzur[155] reported on a retrospective study looking at 198 patients (201 feet) with Charcot osteoarthropathy treated over a 6-year period. At a minimum 1-year follow-up, 59.2% of the patients with midfoot involvement achieved the desired endpoint (long-term management with therapeutic footwear and orthoses) without surgical intervention, whereas 40% required surgery.

The unstable Charcot foot remains a surgical challenge. Instability, deformity, chronic ulceration, and progressive joint destruction, despite rest and immobilization, are the primary indications for surgical intervention in individuals with diabetes and Charcot's osteoarthropathy.[19,44,49,78,156] When the acute inflammatory stage has subsided, unstable joints and deformities that predispose to shearing stress and ulceration can be considered for surgical correction. This approach is fully discussed in Chapter 23.

Emerging Research

Osteoclastogenesis and the RANKL/OPG Signaling Pathway

The novel finding of the receptor activator for nuclear factor kappa B ligand (RANKL)/RANK signaling pathway is an important advance in our understanding of the mechanisms controlling osteoclastogenesis and metabolic bone disease.[56,57] RANKL may represent a key link between bone formation and resorption.[58] RANKL binds to RANK, inducing a signaling cascade leading to the differentiation of osteoclast precursor cells and stimulating the activity of mature osteoclasts.[56,57] The effects of RANKL are counteracted by osteoprotegerin (OPG), a recently recognized cytokine that acts as a decoy receptor. OPG has been shown to be an important inhibitor of osteoclast differentiation and activation in rodent models.[57] The RANKL/OPG pathway is also

believed to mediate the calcification of vascular smooth muscle cells of the arterial wall. The findings of vascular calcification and osteopenia are commonly associated with the acute Charcot foot.[59] Jeffcoate suggests that neuropathy might lead to increased expression of RANKL as a result of the loss of nerve-derived peptides, for example, calcitonin gene-related peptide, which normally exert a moderating influence on the pathway. He proposes that the unregulated activation of RANKL-mediated effects on bones and arteries may be triggered by the loss of nerve-derived peptides. Therefore, he suggests that in the short term, it might be more logical to consider treating the acute Charcot foot with calcitonin rather than bisphosphonates.

In a prospective population-based study of incident nontraumatic fractures, serum levels of RANKL and osteoprotegerin were assessed. A low level of RANKL emerged as a significant independent predictor of nontraumatic fracture.[58] The clinical value of serum OPG and soluble RANKL measurements as markers of disease activity requires additional study.[56]

The Role of Proinflammatory Cytokines

An intriguing hypothesis for the development of the acute Charcot foot has recently been proposed by William Jeffcoate and colleagues,[34] who theorize that the release of proinflammatory cytokines is the key to the development and perpetuation of the acute Charcot foot. Their theory is that an exaggerated inflammatory response to injury of the neuropathic foot is responsible for the cycle that results in fracture and/or subluxation or dislocation of the Charcot foot. The authors note that the acute inflammatory response to injury is mediated through increased expression of proinflammatory cytokines, primarily TNFα and interleukin 1β. These cytokines are believed to trigger increased expression of RANKL, leading to activation of NF-kB (RANK), inducing osteoclast differentiation and maturation. The implication of this theory is that TNFα and RANKL levels might be used as markers of disease activity or that inhibitors of these cytokines might be used to attenuate the inflammatory process.[34] However, this hypothesis has yet to be tested.

Summary

The Charcot foot continues to be a somewhat enigmatic challenge nearly 125 years after the condition was first described by Jean-Martin Charcot. Although his patients were afflicted with tertiary syphilis, previously the most common disease associated with this disorder, most of his observations and insights still hold true today. Indeed, Charcot osteoarthropathy remains a major complication of diabetes mellitus. Studies indicate that foot deformity, notably following osteoarthropathy, is a primary causal risk factor for subsequent ulceration and lower-limb amputation. Therefore, we must not only recognize this disorder early in its pathogenesis, but also fully appreciate the underlying pathophysiology that leads to its development. Only through such an understanding can we rationally approach the management of this difficult condition through both conservative and surgical means.

ACKNOWLEDGMENTS

We thank our wives, Debra Sanders and Heather Frykberg, for their lifelong support, encouragement, understanding, and sacrifices, which have enabled us to pursue our professional goals and achieve our dreams.

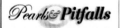 A high index of suspicion for this disorder will often lead to early diagnosis. Early diagnosis is crucial in order to prevent progressive deformity by prompt treatment.

Suspect Charcot's joint disease when a neuropathic patient presents with an inflamed and/or deformed foot, especially following a minor injury.

Most acute Charcot feet are *not* painless. They will usually have some degree of discomfort, though less than expected for the pathology present.

Always take three view plain radiographs when a neuropathic patient presents with a swollen foot.

If radiographs are negative but suspicion for the disease is high, repeat radiographs at 10 to 14 days. If still equivocal consider bone scan or MRI.

If initially unsure about the diagnosis, treat as for Charcot's joint disease by off-loading and total contact casting until osteoarthropathy is proven or disproven.

There is insufficient evidence to support the need for open surgical intervention for acute Charcot's joint disease.

The indications for surgical management of the chronic Charcot foot include unbraceable deformity, severe instability, recurrent ulceration, or inability to wear protective footwear.

Patients with Charcot foot are at risk for future pedal complications and contralateral involvement and therefore require lifelong surveillance.

Beware of the following:
- Failure to recognize the acute Charcot foot due to lack of awareness of this condition.
- Failure to obtain a detailed history or to believe the history obtained.
- Failure to adequately examine the patient in order to distinguish noninfective bone disease from osteomyelitis.
- Failure to obtain radiographs and correctly interpret them.
- Failure to respond promptly to the diagnosis with immediate immobilization and off-loading of the affected limb.
- Adopting a defeatist or cavalier attitude toward treatment of this disorder.
- Expecting a good result from a noncompliant patient.

References

1. Guillain G: J.-M. Charcot 1825–1893: His Life—His Work (edited and translated by Pearce Bailey). New York: Paul B. Hoeber, 1959.
2. Charcot J-M: Sur quelques arthropathies qui paraissent dépendre d'une lésion du cerveau ou de la moelle épinière. Arch Physio Norm Pathol 1:161–178, 1868.
3. Hoché G, Sanders LJ: On some arthropathies apparently related to a lesion of the brain or spinal cord, by Dr. J.-M. Charcot, January 1868. J Hist Neurosci 1(1):75–87, 1992.
4. Charcot JM: Lecture IV, on some visceral derangements in locomotor ataxia: Arthropathies of ataxic patients. In Sigerson G (ed, transl): Lectures on the Diseases of the Nervous System. New York: Hafner, 1962, pp 47–61.
5. Brower AC, Allman RM: The neuropathic joint: A neurovascular bone disorder. Radiol Clin North Am 19(4):571–580, 1981.
6. Brower AC, Allman RM: Pathogenesis of the neurotrophic joint: Neurotraumatic vs. neurovascular. Radiology 139(2):349–354, 1981.
7. Brower AC, Allman RM: Neuropathic osteoarthropathy in the adult. In Traveras JM, Ferrucci JT (eds): Radiology: Diagnosis—Imaging—Intervention, vol 5. Philadelphia: JB Lippincott, 1989, pp 1–8.
8. Delano PJ: The pathogenesis of Charcot's joint. Am J Roentgenol 56:189, 1946.
9. Soto-Hall R, Halderman KO: The diagnosis of neuropathic joint disease (Charcot joint): An analysis of 40 cases. JAMA 114:2076–2078, 1940.
10. Wartenberg R: Neuropathic joint disease. JAMA 111:2044, 1938.
11. Frykberg RG, Kozak GP: Neuropathic arthropathy in the diabetic foot. Am Fam Physician 17(5):105–113, 1978.
12. Frykberg RG: Osteoarthropathy. Clin Podiatr Med Surg 4(2):351–359, 1987.
13. Miller DS, Lichtman WF: Diabetic neuropathic arthropathy of feet: Summary report of seventeen cases. Arch Surg 70(4):513–518, 1955.
14. Norman A, Robbins H, Milgram JE: The acute neuropathic arthropathy: A rapid, severely disorganizing form of arthritis. Radiology 90(6):1159–1164, 1968.
15. Bruckner FE, Howell A: Neuropathic joints. Semin Arthritis Rheum 2(1):47–49, 1972.
16. Steindler A: The tabetic arthropathies. JAMA 96:250–256, 1931.
17. Harris JR, Brand PW: Patterns of disintegration of the tarsus in the anaesthetic foot. J Bone Joint Surg Br 48(1):4–16, 1966.
18. Wastie ML: Radiological changes in serial x-rays of the foot and tarsus in leprosy. Clin Radiol 26(2):285–292, 1975.
19. Johnson JT: Neuropathic fractures and joint injuries: Pathogenesis and rationale of prevention and treatment. J Bone Joint Surg Am 49(1):1–30, 1967.
20. Bjorkengren AG, Weisman M, Pathria MN, et al: Neuroarthropathy associated with chronic alcoholism. AJR Am J Roentgenol 51(4):743–745, 1988.
21. Mitchell SW, Morehouse GR, Keen WW: Gunshot Wounds and Other Injuries of Nerves. Philadelphia: JB Lippincott, 1864.
22. Kerwein G, Lyon WF: Neuropathic arthropathy of the ankle joint resulting from complete severance of the sciatic nerve. Ann Surg 115:267–278, 1942.
23. Newman JH: Non-infective disease of the diabetic foot. J Bone Joint Surg Br 63B(4):593–596, 1981.
24. Chantelau E: The perils of procrastination: Effects of early vs. delayed detection and treatment of incipient Charcot fracture. Diabet Med 22(12):1707–1712, 2005.
25. Jordan WR: Neuritic manifestations in diabetes mellitus. Arch Intern Med 57:307–366, 1936.
26. Kelly M: De arthritide symptomatica of William Musgrave (1657–1721): His description of neuropathic arthritis. Bull Hist Med J 37:372–377, 1963.
27. Mitchell JK: On a new practice in acute and chronic rheumatism. Am J Med Sci 8:55–64, 1831.
28. Goetz CG, Bonduelle M, Gelfand T: Charcot Constructing Neurology. New York: Oxford University Press, 1995.
29. MacCormac W, Klockmann JW: Transactions of the International Medical Congress: Seventh Session Held in London, August 2–9, 1881, vol 1. London: Balantyne, Hanson, 1881.
30. Charcot J-M: Demonstration of arthropathic affections of locomotor ataxy. BMJ 2:285, 1881.
31. Charcot J-M, Féré C: Affections osseuses et articulaires du pied chez les tabétiques (pied tabétique). Archives de Neurologie 6(18):305–319, 1883.
32. Jude EB, Selby PL, Burgess J, et al: Bisphosphonates in the treatment of Charcot neuroarthropathy: A double-blind randomised controlled trial. Diabetologia 44(11):2032–2037, 2001.
33. Pitocco D, Ruotolo V, Caputo S, et al: Six-month treatment with alendronate in acute Charcot neuroarthropathy: A randomized controlled trial. Diabetes Care 28(5):1214–1215, 2005.

34. Jeffcoate WJ, Game F, Cavanagh PR: The role of proinflammatory cytokines in the cause of neuropathic osteoarthropathy (acute Charcot foot) in diabetes. Lancet 366(9502):2058–2061, 2005.

35. Jeffcoate WJ: Abnormalities of vasomotor regulation in the pathogenesis of the acute charcot foot of diabetes mellitus. Int J Low Extrem Wounds 4(3):133–137, 2005.

36. Foster AV: Problems with the nomenclature of Charcot's osteoarthropathy. Diabetic Foot. 8(3), 2005.

37. Charcotian eponyms. South Med J 68(12):1592, 1975.

38. Bailey CC, Root HF: Neuropathic foot lesions in diabetes mellitus. N Engl J Med 236(11):397–401, 1947.

39. Forgacs S: Clinical picture of diabetic osteoarthropathy. Acta Diabetol Lat 3(3–4):111–129, 1976.

40. Pogonowska MJ, Collins LC, Dobson HL: Diabetic osteopathy. Radiology 89:265–271, 1967.

41. Sinha S, Munichoodappa CS, Kozak GP: Neuro-arthropathy (Charcot joints) in diabetes mellitus (clinical study of 101 cases). Medicine (Baltimore) 51(3):191–210, 1972.

42. Cofield RH, Morrison MJ, Beabout JW: Diabetic neuroarthropathy in the foot: Patient characteristics and patterns of radiographic change. Foot Ankle 4(1):15–22, 1983.

43. Lavery LA, Armstrong DG, Wunderlich RP, et al: Diabetic foot syndrome: Evaluating the prevalence and incidence of foot pathology in Mexican Americans and non-Hispanic whites from a diabetes disease management cohort. Diabetes Care 26(5):1435–1438, 2003.

44. Armstrong DG, Todd WF, Lavery LA, et al: The natural history of acute Charcot's arthropathy in a diabetic foot specialty clinic. J Am Podiatr Med Assoc 87(6):272–278, 1997.

45. Clohisy DR, Thompson RC Jr: Fractures associated with neuropathic arthropathy in adults who have juvenile-onset diabetes. J Bone Joint Surg Am 70(8):1192–1200, 1988.

46. Clouse ME, Gramm HF, Legg M, Flood T: Diabetic osteoarthropathy: Clinical and roentgenographic observations in 90 cases. Am J Roentgenol Radium Ther Nucl Med 121(1):22–34, 1974.

47. Sanders LJ, Mrdjenovich D: Anatomical patterns of bone and joint destruction in neuropathic diabetics. Diabetes 40(suppl 1): 529A, 1991.

48. Frykberg RG, Kozak GP: The diabetic Charcot foot. In Kozak GP, Campbell DR, Frykberg RG, Habershaw GM (eds): Management of Diabetic Foot Problems, 2nd ed. Philadelphia: WB Saunders, 1995, pp 88–97.

49. Sanders LJ, Frykberg RG: Diabetic neuropathic osteoarthropathy: The Charcot foot. In Frykberg RG (ed): The High Risk Foot in Diabetes Mellitus. New York: Churchill Livingstone, 1991, pp 297–338.

50. Schwarz GS, Berenyi MR, Siegel MW: Atrophic arthropathy and diabetic neuritis. Am J Roentgenol Radium Ther Nucl Med 106(3):523–529, 1969.

51. Gough A, Abraha H, Li F, et al: Measurement of markers of osteoclast and osteoblast activity in patients with acute and chronic diabetic Charcot neuroarthropathy. Diabet Med 14(7):527–531, 1997.

52. Newman JH: Spontaneous dislocation in diabetic neuropathy: A report of six cases. J Bone Joint Surg Br 61-B(4):484–488, 1979.

53. Eichenholtz SN: Charcot Joints. Springfield, IL: Charles C. Thomas, 1966.

54. Shibata T, Tada K, Hashizume C: The results of arthrodesis of the ankle for leprotic neuroarthropathy. J Bone Joint Surg Am 72(5):749–756, 1990.

55. Sella EJ, Barrette C: Staging of Charcot neuroarthropathy along the medial column of the foot in the diabetic patient. J Foot Ankle Surg 38(1):34–40, 1999.

56. Rogers A, Eastell R: Circulating osteoprotegerin and receptor activator for nuclear factor kappaB ligand: Clinical utility in metabolic bone disease assessment. J Clin Endocrinol Metab 90(11):6323–6331, 2005.

57. Rogers A, Saleh G, Hannon RA, et al: Circulating estradiol and osteoprotegerin as determinants of bone turnover and bone density in postmenopausal women. J Clin Endocrinol Metab 87(10):4470–4475, 2002.

58. Schett G, Kiechl S, Redlich K, et al: Soluble RANKL and risk of nontraumatic fracture. JAMA 291(9):1108–1113, 2004.

59. Jeffcoate W: Vascular calcification and osteolysis in diabetic neuropathy: Is RANK-L the missing link? Diabetologia 47(9): 1488–1492, 2004.

60. Treves F: Treatment of perforating ulcer of the foot. Lancet 2:949, 1884.

61. Beltran J, Campanini DS, Knight C, McCalla M: The diabetic foot: Magnetic resonance imaging evaluation. Skeletal Radiol 19(1): 37–41, 1990.

62. Blume PA, Dey HM, Daley LJ, et al: Diagnosis of pedal osteomyelitis with Tc-99m HMPAO labeled leukocytes. J Foot Ankle Surg 36(2):120–126, discussion 160, 1997.

63. Johnson JE, Kennedy EJ, Shereff MJ, et al: Prospective study of bone, indium-111-labeled white blood cell, and gallium-67 scanning for the evaluation of osteomyelitis in the diabetic foot. Foot Ankle Int 17(1):10–16, 1996.

64. Milgram JW: Osteomyelitis in the foot and ankle associated with diabetes mellitus. Clin Orthop Relat Res 296:50–57, 1993.

65. Hopfner S, Krolak C, Kessler S, et al: Preoperative imaging of Charcot neuroarthropathy in diabetic patients: Comparison of ring PET, hybrid PET, and magnetic resonance imaging. Foot Ankle Int 25(12):890–895, 2004.

66. Berendt AR, Lipsky B: Is this bone infected or not?: Differentiating neuro-osteoarthropathy from osteomyelitis in the diabetic foot. Curr Diab Rep 4(6):424–429, 2004.

67. Lippmann HI, Perotto A, Farrar R: The neuropathic foot of the diabetic. Bull N Y Acad Med 52(10):1159–1178, 1976.

68. Martin M: Charcot joints in diabetes mellitus. Proc R Soc Med 45:503–506, 1952.

69. Martin MM: Diabetic neuropathy: A clinical study of 150 cases. Brain 176:594, 1953.

70. Brooks AP: The neuropathic foot in diabetes: II. Charcot's neuroarthropathy. Diabet Med 3(2):116–118, 1986.

71. Young MJ, Marshall A, Adams JE, et al: Osteopenia, neurological dysfunction, and the development of Charcot neuroarthropathy. Diabetes Care 18(1):34–38, 1995.

72. Archer AG, Roberts VC, Watkins PJ: Blood flow patterns in diabetic neuropathy. Diabetologia 27:563, 1984.

73. Edelman SV, Kosofsky EM, Paul RA, Kozak GP: Neuro-osteoarthropathy (Charcot's joint) in diabetes mellitus following revascularization surgery: Three case reports and a review of the literature. Arch Intern Med 147(8):1504–1508, 1987.

74. Edmonds ME, Nicolaides KH, Watkins PJ: Autonomic neuropathy and diabetic foot ulceration. Diabet Med 3(1):56–59, 1986.

75. Lister J, Maudsley RH: Charcot joints in diabetic neuropathy. Lancet 2:1110, 1951.

76. El-Khoury GY, Kathol MH: Neuropathic fractures in patients with diabetes mellitus. Radiology 134: 313–316, 1980.

77. Grant WP, Foreman EJ, Wilson AS, et al: Evaluation of Young's modulus in Achilles tendons with diabetic neuroarthropathy. J Am Podiatr Med Assoc 95(3):242–246, 2005.

78. Banks AS, McGlamry ED: Charcot foot. J Am Podiatr Med Assoc 79(5):213–235, 1989.

79. Craig JG, Amin MB, Wu K, et al: Osteomyelitis of the diabetic foot: MR imaging-pathologic correlation. Radiology 203(3):849–855, 1997.

80. Lavery LA, Higgins KR, Lanctot DR, et al: Home monitoring of foot skin temperatures to prevent ulceration. Diabetes Care 27(11):2642–2647, 2004.

81. Kelly PJ, Coventry MB: Neurotrophic ulcers of the feet: Review of forty-seven cases. J Am Med Assoc 168(4):388–393, 1958.

82. Boulton AJ, Scarpello JH, Ward JD: Venous oxygenation in the diabetic neuropathic foot: Evidence of arteriovenous shunting? Diabetologia 22(1):6–8, 1982.

83. Cundy TF, Edmonds ME, Watkins PJ: Osteopenia and metatarsal fractures in diabetic neuropathy. Diabet Med 2(6):461–464, 1985.

84. Edmonds ME, Clarke MB, Newton S, et al: Increased uptake of bone radiopharmaceutical in diabetic neuropathy. Q J Med 57(224):843–855, 1985.

85. Edmonds ME: The neuropathic foot in diabetes: I. Blood flow. Diabet Med 3(2):111–115, 1986.

86. Forst T, Pfutzner A, Kann P, et al: Peripheral osteopenia in adult patients with insulin-dependent diabetes mellitus. Diabet Med 12(10):874–879, 1995.

87. Watkins PJ, Edmonds ME: Sympathetic nerve failure in diabetes. Diabetologia 25(2):73–77, 1983.

88. Radin EL: Mechanical aspects of osteoarthrosis. Bull Rheum Dis 26(7):862–865, 1976.

89. Arntz CT, Veith RG, Hansen ST Jr: Fractures and fracture-dislocations of the tarsometatarsal joint. J Bone Joint Surg Am 70(2):173–181, 1988.

90. Armstrong DG, Lavery LA: Elevated peak plantar pressures in patients who have Charcot arthropathy. J Bone Joint Surg Am 80(3):365–369, 1998.

91. Cavanagh PR, Sims DS Jr, Sanders LJ: Body mass is a poor predictor of peak plantar pressure in diabetic men. Diabetes Care 14(8):750–755, 1991.

92. Caputo GM, Cavanagh PR, Ulbrecht JS, et al: Assessment and management of foot disease in patients with diabetes. N Engl J Med 331(13):854–860, 1994.

93. Holmes GB, Jr., Hill N: Fractures and dislocations of the foot and ankle in diabetics associated with Charcot joint changes. Foot Ankle Int 15(4):182–185, 1994.

94. Cavanagh PR, Young MJ, Adams JE, et al: Radiographic abnormalities in the feet of patients with diabetic neuropathy. Diabetes Care 17(3):201–209, 1994.

95. Grant WP, Sullivan R, Sonenshine DE, et al: Electron microscopic investigation of the effects of diabetes mellitus on the Achilles tendon. J Foot Ankle Surg 36(4):272–278, discussion 330, 1997.

96. Frykberg RG: Biomechanical considerations of the diabetic foot. Lower Extremity 2:207–214, 1995.

97. Schoenhaus HD, Wernick E, Cohen R: Biomechanics of the diabetic foot. In Frykberg RG (ed): The High Risk Foot in Diabetes Mellitus. New York: Churchill Livingstone, 1991.

98. Brink SJ. Limited joint mobility as a risk factor for diabetes complications. Clin Diabetes 5:122, 1987.

99. Brownlee M, Cerami A, Vlassara H: Advanced glycosylation end products in tissue and the biochemical basis of diabetic complications. N Engl J Med 318(20):1315–1321.

100. Buckingham BA, Uitto J, Sandborg C, et al: Scleroderma-like changes in insulin-dependent diabetes mellitus: Clinical and biochemical studies. Diabetes Care 7(2):163–169, 1984.

101. Monnier VM, Glomb M, Elgawish A, Sell DR: The mechanism of collagen cross-linking in diabetes: A puzzle nearing resolution. Diabetes 45(suppl 3):S67–S72, 1996.

102. Monnier VM, Vishwanath V, Frank KE, et al: Relation between complications of type I diabetes mellitus and collagen-linked fluorescence. N Engl J Med 314(7):403–408, 1986.

103. Delbridge L, Perry P, Marr S, et al: Limited joint mobility in the diabetic foot: Relationship to neuropathic ulceration. Diabet Med 5(4):333–337, 1988.

104. Fernando DJ, Masson EA, Veves A, Boulton AJ: Relationship of limited joint mobility to abnormal foot pressures and diabetic foot ulceration. Diabetes Care 14(1):8–11, 1991.

105. Mueller MJ, Diamond JE, Delitto A, Sinacore DR: Insensitivity, limited joint mobility, and plantar ulcers in patients with diabetes mellitus. Phys Ther 69(6):453–459, discussion 459–462, 1989.

106. Jirkovska A, Kasalicky P, Boucek P, et al: Calcaneal ultrasonometry in patients with Charcot osteoarthropathy and its relationship with densitometry in the lumbar spine and femoral neck and with markers of bone turnover. Diabet Med 18(6):495–500, 2001.

107. Petrova NL, Foster AV, Edmonds ME: Calcaneal bone mineral density in patients with Charcot neuropathic osteoarthropathy: Differences between Type 1 and Type 2 diabetes. Diabet Med 22(6):756–761, 2005.

108. Herbst SA, Jones KB, Saltzman CL: Pattern of diabetic neuropathic arthropathy associated with the peripheral bone mineral density. J Bone Joint Surg Br 86(3):378–383, 2004.

109. Newman LG, Waller J, Palestro CJ, et al: Unsuspected osteomyelitis in diabetic foot ulcers. Diagnosis and monitoring by leukocyte scanning with indium in 111 oxyquinoline. J Am Med Assoc 266(9):1246–1251, 1991.

110. Kraft E, Spyropoulos E, Finby N: Neurogenic disorders of the foot in diabetes mellitus. Am J Roentgenol Radium Ther Nucl Med 124(1):17–24, 1975.

111. Lesko P, Maurer RC: Talonavicular dislocations and midfoot arthropathy in neuropathic diabetic feet: Natural course and principles of treatment. Clin Orthop Relat Res 240:226–231, 1989.

112. Thompson RC Jr, Havel P, Goetz F: Presumed neurotrophic skeletal disease in diabetic kidney transplant recipients. J Am Med Assoc 249(10):1317–1319.

113. Rubinow A, Spark EC, Canoso JJ: Septic arthritis in a Charcot joint. Clin Orthop Relat Res 147:203–206, 1980.

114. Kathol MH, el-Khoury GY, Moore TE, Marsh JL: Calcaneal insufficiency avulsion fractures in patients with diabetes mellitus. Radiology 180(3):725–729, 1991.

115. Coventry MB, Rothacker GW Jr: Bilateral calcaneal fracture in a diabetic patient: A case report. J Bone Joint Surg Am 61(3):462–464, 1979.

116. Biehl WC 3rd, Morgan JM, Wagner FW Jr, Gabriel R: Neuropathic calcaneal tuberosity avulsion fractures. Clin Orthop Relat Res 296:8–13, 1993.

117. Brodsky JW, Rouse AM: Exostectomy for symptomatic bony prominences in diabetic charcot feet. Clin Orthop Relat Res 296:21–26, 1993.

118. Schon LC, Easley ME, Cohen I, et al: The acquired midtarsus deformity classification system: Interobserver reliability and intraobserver reproducibility. Foot Ankle Int 23(1):30–36, 2002.

119. Schon LC, Weinfeld SB, Horton GA, Resch S: Radiographic and clinical classification of acquired midtarsus deformities. Foot Ankle Int 19(6):394–404, 1998.

120. Ledermann HP, Morrison WB: Differential diagnosis of pedal osteomyelitis and diabetic neuroarthropathy: MR imaging. Semin Musculoskelet Radiol 9(3):272–283, 2005.

121. Williamson BR, Teates CD, Phillips CD, Croft BY: Computed tomography as a diagnostic aid in diabetic and other problem feet. Clin Imaging 13(2):159–163, 1989.

122. Seabold JE, Flickinger FW, Kao SC, et al: Indium-111-leukocyte/technetium-99m-MDP bone and magnetic resonance imaging: Difficulty of diagnosing osteomyelitis in patients with neuropathic osteoarthropathy. J Nucl Med 31(5):549–556, 1990.

123. Schauwecker DS, Park HM, Burt RW, et al: Combined bone scintigraphy and indium-111 leukocyte scans in neuropathic foot disease. J Nucl Med 29(10):1651–1655, 1988.

124. Edmonds ME, Morrison N, Laws JW, Watkins PJ: Medial arterial calcification and diabetic neuropathy. Br Med J (Clin Res Ed) 284(6320):928–930, 1982.

125. Eymontt MJ, Alavi A, Dalinka MK, Kyle GC: Bone scintigraphy in diabetic osteoarthropathy. Radiology 140(2):475–477, 1981.

126. Hart TJ, Healey K: Diabetic osteoarthropathy versus diabetic osteomyelitis. J Foot Surg 25(6):464–468, 1986.

127. Glynn TP Jr: Marked gallium accumulation in neurogenic arthropathy. J Nucl Med 22(11):1016–1017, 1981.

128. Hartshorne MF, Peters V: Nuclear medicine applications for the diabetic foot. Clin Podiatr Med Surg 4(2):361–375, 1987.

129. Maurer AH, Millmond SH, Knight LC, et al: Infection in diabetic osteoarthropathy: Use of indium-labeled leukocytes for diagnosis. Radiology 161(1):221–225, 1986.

130. Schauwecker DS: Osteomyelitis: Diagnosis with In-111-labeled leukocytes. Radiology 171(1):141–146, 1989.

131. Zeiger LS, Fox IM: Use of indium-111-labeled white blood cells in the diagnosis of diabetic foot infections. J Foot Surg 29(1):46–51, 1990.

132. Keenan AM, Tindel NL, Alavi A: Diagnosis of pedal osteomyelitis in diabetic patients using current scintigraphic techniques. Arch Int Med 149:2262, 1989.

133. Armstrong DG, Lavery LA, Liswood PJ, et al: Infrared dermal thermometry for the high-risk diabetic foot. Phys Ther 77(2):169–175, discussion 176–167, 1997.

134. Shaw JE, Hsi WL, Ulbrecht JS,et al: The mechanism of plantar unloading in total contact casts: Implications for design and clinical use. Foot Ankle Int 18(12):809–817, 1997.

135. Guse ST, Alvine FG: Treatment of diabetic foot ulcers and Charcot neuroarthropathy using the patellar tendon-bearing brace. Foot Ankle Int 18(10):675–677, 1997.

136. Saltzman CL, Johnson KA, Goldstein RH, Donnelly RE: The patellar tendon-bearing brace as treatment for neurotrophic arthropathy: A dynamic force monitoring study. Foot Ankle 13(1):14–21, 1992.

137. Lavery LA, Vela SA, Lavery DC, Quebedeaux TL: Reducing dynamic foot pressures in high-risk diabetic subjects with foot ulcerations: A comparison of treatments. Diabetes Care 19(8):818–821, 1996.

138. Baumhauer JF, Wervey R, McWilliams J, et al: A comparison study of plantar foot pressure in a standardized shoe, total contact cast, and prefabricated pneumatic walking brace. Foot Ankle Int 18(1):26–33, 1997.

139. Fleischli JG, Lavery LA, Vela SA, et al: 1997 William J. Stickel Bronze Award: Comparison of strategies for reducing pressure at the site of neuropathic ulcers. J Am Podiatr Med Assoc 87(10):466–472, 1997.

140. Landsman AS, Sage R: Off-loading neuropathic wounds associated with diabetes using an ankle-foot orthosis. J Am Podiatr Med Assoc 87(8):349–357, 1997.
141. Morgan JM, Biehl WC 3rd, Wagner FW Jr: Management of neuropathic arthropathy with the Charcot Restraint Orthotic Walker. Clin Orthop Relat Res 296:58–63, 1993.
142. Cavanagh P, Sanders LJ, Sims DS Jr: The role of pressure distribution measurement in diabetic foot care: Rehabilitation R&D progress reports 1987. J Rehab Res Dev 25:53–54, 1988.
143. Uccioli L, Faglia E, Monticone G, et al: Manufactured shoes in the prevention of diabetic foot ulcers. Diabetes Care 18(10):1376–1378, 1995.
144. Ashry HR, Lavery LA, Murdoch DP, et al: Effectiveness of diabetic insoles to reduce foot pressures. J Foot Ankle Surg 36(4):268–271, discussion 328–269, 1997.
145. Lavery LA, Vela SA, Fleischli JG, et al: Reducing plantar pressure in the neuropathic foot: A comparison of footwear. Diabetes Care 20(11):1706–1710, 1997.
146. Rogers MJ: New insights into the molecular mechanisms of action of bisphosphonates. Curr Pharm Des 9(32):2643–2658, 2003.
147. Kirk JK, Spangler JG: Alendronate: A bisphosphonate for treatment of osteoporosis. Am Fam Physician 54:2053–2060, 1996.
148. Harris ST, Watts NB, Genant HK, et al: Effects of risedronate treatment on vertebral and nonvertebral fractures in women with postmenopausal osteoporosis: A randomized controlled trial. Vertebral Efficacy With Risedronate Therapy (VERT) Study Group. JAMA 282(14):1344–1352, 1999.
149. Liberman UA, Weiss SR, Broll J, et al: Effect of oral alendronate on bone mineral density and the incidence of fractures in postmenopausal osteoporosis: The Alendronate Phase III Osteoporosis Treatment Study Group. N Engl J Med 333(22):1437–1443, 1995.
150. Selby PL, Young MJ, Boulton AJ: Bisphosphonates: A new treatment for diabetic Charcot neuroarthropathy? Diabet Med 11(1):28–31, 1994.
151. Kaskani E, Lyritis GP, Kosmidis C, et al: Effect of intermittent administration of 200 IU intranasal salmon calcitonin and low doses of 1alpha(OH) vitamin D3 on bone mineral density of the lumbar spine and hip region and biochemical bone markers in women with postmenopausal osteoporosis: A pilot study. Clin Rheumatol 24(3):232–238, 2005.
152. Lyritis G, Boscainos PJ: Calcitonin effects on cartilage and fracture healing. J Musculoskelet Neuronal Interact 2(2):137–142, 2001.
153. Mendicino RW, Catanzariti AR, Saltrick KR, et al: Tibiotalocalcaneal arthrodesis with retrograde intramedullary nailing. J Foot Ankle Surg 43(2):82–86, 2004.
154. Jani MM, Ricci WM, Borrelli J Jr, et al: A protocol for treatment of unstable ankle fractures using transarticular fixation in patients with diabetes mellitus and loss of protective sensibility. Foot Ankle Int 24(11):838–844, 2003.
155. Pinzur M: Surgical versus accommodative treatment for Charcot arthropathy of the midfoot. Foot Ankle Int 25(8):545–549, 2004.
156. Kidd JG Jr: The Charcot joint: some pathologic and pathogenetic considerations. South Med J 67(5):597–602, 1974.

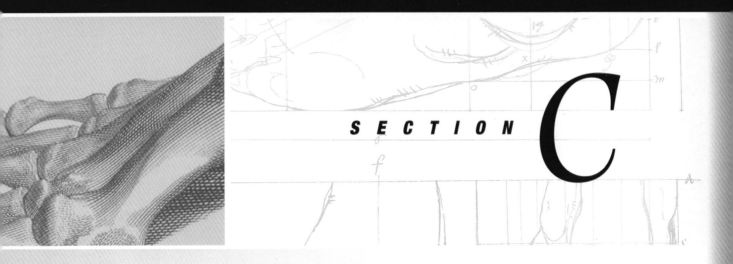

SECTION C

NONSURGICAL
MANAGEMENT

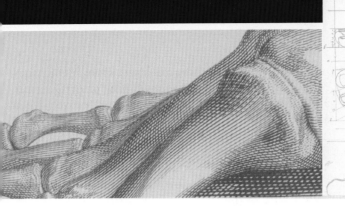

OFF-LOADING FOR DIABETIC FOOT DISEASE

DAVID R. SINACORE AND MICHAEL J. MUELLER ∎

Diabetic foot disease is a major long-term complication of poorly controlled diabetes mellitus and associated peripheral neuropathy. Sensory, motor, and autonomic neuropathy combine to predispose the feet to ulcers, fractures, deformity, high plantar stresses resulting in thick callus buildup, and dysregulation of pedal circulation leading to dry, fissured skin. The frequent result is limb-threatening infection that too often culminates in lower-limb amputation.[1]

Off-loading of unperceived (unfelt) areas of plantar stress is but one of several critical weapons in the foot specialist's arsenal for preventing and effectively treating clinical manifestations of diabetic foot disease, particularly neuropathic ulcers and fractures or acute inflammatory arthropathy.[2] This chapter describes several off-loading methods that can be used for the treatment of diabetic foot disease, including healing neuropathic plantar ulcers or immobilizing acute traumatic neuropathic pedal fractures or acute neuropathic (Charcot) osteoarthropathy. The major indications, contraindications, advantages, and disadvantages of each off-loading method as well as studies of each method's effectiveness are summarized. As in previous editions of this text, a basic method of total-contact casting (TCC) application is given in detail to allow the health care practitioner who is new to this technique to begin safely using therapeutic casting. Experienced diabetic foot care specialists will recognize that there are wide variations in casting methods in addition to several alternative commercially available pressure-relieving devices that can be selected in lieu of TCC under specific circumstances.

For example, alternative off-loading methods may be used when TCC is either unavailable or contraindicated or when certain patient characteristics are present. The authors present the reported effectiveness and expected outcomes of TCC and alternative off-loading methods, as well as some of the critical factors that may directly affect healing times and the eventual therapeutic outcome of each method.

Total-Contact Casting

TCC is unquestionably the gold standard off-loading method to most rapidly heal neuropathic plantar foot ulcers. Similarly, TCC is the optimal method to achieve maximal reduction of unperceived focal plantar stresses. Numerous clinical reports[3–16] and several randomized, controlled clinical trials[17–20] over the past several decades suggest that no other single treatment is as effective as TCC for rapidly healing Meggitt-Wagner (M-W) grade 1 or 2 neuropathic plantar ulcers.[21,22] Likewise, it has been reported that TCC can achieve maximal reduction in unperceived plantar stresses compared to therapeutic shoes with insoles or ankle-foot orthoses (AFOs).[23] Therefore, TCC and comparable alternative off-loading methods should be the cornerstone of treatment interventions and the first line of defense for healing neuropathic plantar ulcers. TCC can be used alone or in conjunction with other methods such as topical wound-healing agents that may act synergistically to accelerate ulcer closure.

History and Theory

TCC to heal neuropathic pedal ulcers is not a new method.[24] It has been time-tested and proven over many years, though there has been and still remains a general reluctance on the part of the medical community in the United States to embrace its use. The earliest reports of ambulatory casting for neuropathic pedal ulcers dates back to the 1930s. The technique was first used by Dr. Milroy Paul, an orthopedist working in Sri Lanka, who described an ambulatory technique for the treatment of neuropathic plantar ulcers occurring in patients with Hansen's disease (leprosy). One of the earliest written accounts was by Dr. Joseph Kahn in India, who described the use of casting as an off-loading alternative to prolonged, expensive periods of hospital bed rest for leprous ulcers.[25] Dr. Paul Brand, an orthopedic surgeon working in India in the 1950s, adopted this technique. Brand and his associates continued to refine and popularize the current casting technique in the early 1960s at the Gillis W. Long Hansen's Disease Center in Carville, Louisiana, for patients with diabetes and similar neuropathic foot ulcers.[26] TCC as a treatment for neuropathic plantar ulcerations has since been applied to a variety of conditions involving insensitivity of the feet, including patients with idiopathic peripheral neuropathy, myelodysplasia, Charcot-Marie-Tooth disease, tabes dorsalis, chronic alcoholism, and any other condition that results in sensory neuropathy.[27–29] More recently, immobilization with TCC has been used effectively for acute Charcot osteoarthropathy of the ankle or foot with or without accompanying pedal ulceration.[30–32]

It is well recognized that a primary factor in the cause of most diabetic plantar ulcers is the presence of peripheral neuropathy leading to diminished or absent sensation.[33] Pedal insensitivity allows unfelt excessive and prolonged stresses to occur in the foot, which ultimately result in tissue breakdown.[34,35] If the injury (ulcer) goes unnoticed or untreated, infection and major amputation are likely.[1]

The main purpose of treating a neuropathic plantar ulcer by TCC is to off-load it, thereby reducing the excessive mechanical stresses (both vertical pressure and horizontal shear) on the plantar surface of the foot as advocated by Brand and associates[26,28,29] while maintaining ambulation. The primary reason that TCC appears to be so effective at healing plantar wounds is that it reduces plantar pressures at the site of ulceration while walking by 84% to 92%.[23] The TCC is fabricated to reduce excessive forces at the ulcer site by spreading pedal pressure over an increased surface area of the foot and leg,[36,37] thus allowing the ulcer to heal rapidly. Two studies report that TCC can increase the plantar surface area of the foot by 15% to 24%.[38,39] These modest increases in plantar surface area result in dramatic reductions in overall peak plantar pressures. On average, these have been reduced 40% to 80% with TCC as compared to walking in thera-peutic footwear[23,38,39] or normal street shoes.[40] One study reported a 75% to 84% reduction in peak plantar pressure at the first and third metatarsal heads, respectively, when a person walked in a TCC compared to street shoes.[40]

Increasing the plantar surface area of the foot is not the only mechanism for the effectiveness of TCC. Shaw and colleagues determined that snug-fitting, well-molded casts extending to just below the knee transfer approximately 30% of the weight-bearing load to the cast wall, thereby decreasing pressure on the plantar aspect of the foot.[37] More recently, Leibner and colleagues confirmed this observation by removing the proximal shank portion of TCCs, increasing the average plantar force during walking by 31%.[36] Therefore, the utility of below-knee TCC consists in reducing peak plantar pressures through increasing the contact surface area throughout both the foot and the leg.[36,37]

Depending somewhat on the degree of foot deformity that is present, TCC provides the greatest and most consistent reductions in peak plantar pressures in the forefoot compared to the midfoot or hindfoot,[39–42] appearing to be least effective in the latter area.[39,42] This might help to explain why plantar ulcers that are located in the hindfoot take considerably longer to heal with casting than do either forefoot or midfoot ulcers.[42] Fortuitously, the metatarsal head region and great toe most frequently develop ulcers in the diabetic patient,[4] resulting in TCC being well suited for ulcers of the forefoot and midfoot by effectively reducing peak plantar pressures in these areas.

Effectiveness and Expected Outcomes of TCC

As was noted above, TCC is the most effective method for reducing excessive plantar pressures, making it the most effective method for healing neuropathic ulcers while allowing the patient limited ambulation.[43] Numerous studies report an average healing time of 36 to 43 days.[3–16,20,29,44] Several studies have reported rapid healing using TCC in patients who had plantar ulcers for widely varying periods (1 week to 13 years) despite other forms of treatment, including daily dressing changes, antibiotic therapy, frequent callus shaving, ulcer debridement, and multiple skin grafts.[8,14,20]

The authors conducted a prospective clinical trial that compared TCC to a control group receiving traditional treatment including daily wound care, dressing changes, and footwear modifications.[20] Nineteen of 21 ulcers (91%) that were treated with TCC healed in a mean time of 42 days compared to a healing rate of 32% (6 of 19 patients) in a mean time of 65 days in the control group. In addition, none of the casted ulcers developed an infection, while 26% (5 of 19 patients) in the traditional therapy group developed serious infections that required hospitalization. Of these, two required a subsequent forefoot amputation. The results of this study as well as results of other, more recent clinical trials confirm

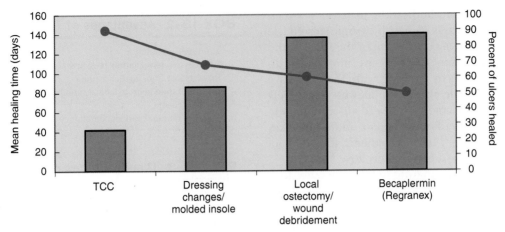

Figure 13-1 Comparison of mean healing times (in days) and average percentage of diabetic foot ulcers healed using various methods described. Bar heights correspond to the left ordinate; the solid curve corresponds to the right ordinate. Total-contact casting (TCC) represents the average from several studies.[3–6,8,11–14,16,20,50] Values for dressing changes and molded insoles are from Mueller and colleagues[20] and Holstein and colleagues[48] combined; values for local ostectomy and wound debridement are from Griffiths and Wieman[46] and Wieman and colleagues[49] combined; values for becaplermin (Regranex), a platelet-derived growth factor, are from Wieman and colleagues.[49]

earlier descriptive studies supporting the contention that TCC is superior to other treatment methods for maximal off-loading, greatest healing rate, quickest healing time, and prevention of serious infection.

Figure 13-1 shows the average healing time (in days) and the percentage of diabetic foot ulcers healed using each of several common treatment methods described in the literature. Clearly, TCC provides the most rapid healing time and consistently results in the greatest percentage of ulcers healed (mean = 90%). Other methods that do not maximize off-loading take longer than the average of 43 days for TCC and have a considerably greater percentage of ulcers that fail to heal.[45–49] Thus, comparisons of healing times and the percentage of ulcers healed among the various methods help to underscore the importance of maximizing pressure off-loading through casting to promote neuropathic ulcer healing.

Indications and Contraindications for TCC

The indications and contraindications for TCC are outlined in Box 13-1. The major indication for TCC is an M-W grade 1 or 2 plantar ulcer[21,50] in the presence of insensitivity. For the purposes of this chapter, we define insensitivity as the inability to feel a 5.07 (10-gram) Semmes-Weinstein monofilament in contact with any portion of the plantar surface of the foot. Some ulcers, though not technically on the plantar surface of the foot, may actually be weight-bearing ulcers and respond well to pressure off-loading therapy. For example, the patient who has an ulcer on the lateral border of the foot secondary to a severe varus deformity should respond well to TCC.[51] The other major indication for TCC is acute or subacute neuropathic (Charcot) osteoarthropathy of the foot or ankle with or without accompanying ulceration.[31,32]

Failure to observe the absolute and relative contraindications for TCC can either delay ulcer healing or

lead to a poor outcome.[52,53] Adherence to the guidelines listed in Box 13-1 will both maximize success and minimize potential side effects. A foot with deep soft tissue sepsis or osteomyelitis (M-W wound grades 3–5) should not be casted because complete ulcer closure is not possible over underlying infection.[50] Antibiotic therapy and bed rest until the acute infection has subsided have been recommended.[26]

A relative contraindication to TCC is an unfavorable area-to-depth ratio of the wound. If the ulcer's depth is greater than its width, it might be necessary to open the ulcer more widely prior to casting to prevent premature superficial closing. Packing the wound with loose-mesh gauze will help to ensure that its deeper layers heal before its surface closes over, thereby minimizing bacterial colonization.

BOX 13–1 Indications and Contraindications for TCC

INDICATIONS

1. M-W wound grade 1 or 2 plantar ulcers in the presence of insensitivity
2. Acute or subacute neuropathic (Charcot) osteoarthropathy

CONTRAINDICATIONS

Absolute

1. Active or acute deep infection, gangrene (M-W wound grades 3–5)

Relative

2. Ulcer depth greater than ulcer width
3. Fragile skin
4. Excessive leg or foot swelling
5. Patient unwilling to have cast on limb
6. Patient unable to comply with follow-up visits or wearing precautions
7. Patient unsafe in mobility while in cast
8. Doppler ABI < 0.4

Another relative contraindication to TCC is excessively fragile skin (e.g., as is seen with chronic steroid use or stasis ulcers) on the leg or dorsum of the foot. In the authors' experience, these patients are more likely to develop skin ulceration or abrasion with TCC than are patients with less fragile skin. Patients with excessively dry, cracked skin associated with severe autonomic neuropathy are also more susceptible to additional skin breakdown with casting.[53] In these patients, total-contact walking splints might be a better alternative.[27]

Excessive and/or fluctuating edema in the foot and/or lower leg presents another challenge for TCC. Because snug, uniform contact between the cast and the lower limb is essential to a successful outcome, the presence of edema should be noted prior to casting. Frequently, edema in the foot and leg will reduce rapidly after only a few days of TCC, causing the cast to loosen. This can allow excessive shearing as the cast moves on the skin and can both delay ulcer healing and cause additional skin breakdown. Therefore, patients who have significant lower-limb edema will require more frequent cast changes (every 3 to 7 days) until the edema has subsided or stabilized.

The authors recommend that any patient who is unable to keep regularly scheduled follow-up visits, is opposed to having a cast on the lower limb, or is unable to adhere to cast precautions and instructions should not be treated with TCC. For these patients, alternative off-loading methods, described later in this chapter, should be explored.

Advantages of TCC

The major advantages of TCC are outlined in Box 13-2. Above all, TCC allows the patient to remain ambulatory, avoiding the expense of lengthy hospital bed rest and frequent wound care. In many cases, TCC allows the patient to remain working, thereby minimizing loss of income.

The cast is fabricated to reduce excessive pressures on the plantar surface of the foot and to spread the peak forces uniformly throughout the entire foot and leg.[36,37] An even distribution of plantar pressure also helps to eliminate or reduce edema in the lower limb. Immobilization of the limb can help to localize any minor infection and prevent its spread to adjacent tissues.[20] The TCC also protects the insensitive foot from additional trauma during the healing process.

Finally, since there is no need for daily wound care with TCC, there is relatively little burden on the patient, family members, or the health care team to constantly care for the pedal ulcer. Weekly office visits for foot care or home visits for wound care are unnecessary. The cost of an entire period of casting (usually 6 to 8 weeks) is often less than the cost of one overnight admission to the hospital; one cast application is roughly equivalent to the cost of an office visit, including dressing supplies, topical antiseptic agents, or growth factor applications.

BOX 13-2 Advantages of TCC

1. Maintains ambulation
2. Reduces excessive plantar pressures
3. Protects foot from further trauma
4. Immobilization helps to localize and prevent spread of infection
5. Controls edema
6. Requires minimal patient compliance

BOX 13-3 Disadvantages of TCC

1. Impairs mobility (i.e., walking, basic and advanced activities of daily living, balance, coordination)
2. Joint stiffness, muscle atrophy, and bone loss if immobilization is prolonged
3. Possible skin abrasions or new ulcerations if cast is poorly applied or not monitored
4. Possible foul odor if ulcer drainage is excessive
5. Unable to inspect wound

Disadvantages of TCC

The major disadvantages of TCC for the patient are listed in Box 13-3. The biggest disadvantage of the cast is that it impairs patient mobility and makes it difficult to carry on the usual activities of daily living. The bulky nature of the below-knee cast, while allowing limited ambulation, can significantly impair balance and coordination, thereby placing the patient at greater risk for secondary injury due to falls. Combined with peripheral motor neuropathy, the sensory ataxia that is present in patients with chronic diabetes[54,55] can make walking in the cast difficult or unsafe. For all patients, the use of assistive devices such as a walker or crutches is recommended to prevent falls due to loss of balance.

If immobilization with a cast is prolonged, side effects such as joint stiffness and muscular atrophy can ensue. These side effects can be minimized with proper flexibility and strengthening exercises at each cast change and following its final removal. One study reported minimal change in ankle and subtalar joint range of motion measured before and after TCC immobilization.[6] Other side effects, such as bone demineralization and neuropathic (Charcot) osteoarthropathy, have been reported, although it is not clear whether these changes are consequent to prolonged immobilization or are osseous sequelae of diabetic neuropathy.[30,56] The authors and others have not observed any acute fractures or arthropathies following immobilization with TCC for pedal ulcers.[15,31]

Patients who do not limit their ambulation and remain fully weight-bearing seem to be more susceptible to skin abrasions from the cast. Similarly, if care is not taken in applying and removing the cast, skin breakdown and new ulcerations can occur, particularly around bony prominences or deformities. New skin abrasions from the cast can be minimized by its proper application and removal, by providing patients with precise cast-wearing instructions, and by patients' adherence to regularly scheduled follow-up visits. Even with optimal application of the cast and adherence to precautions by the patient, new skin abrasions and fungal infections can nonetheless develop.[5,20,52] In the author's experience, new abrasions as a result of TCC typically occur on non-weight-bearing areas and often heal quickly without cessation of casting. One study reported the complications of TCC observed in a single center over a 28-month period in 398 consecutive cast applications in 70 severely neuropathic patients.[52] Their overall temporary complication rate of new skin abrasions or ulcers was 5.5% per cast, while the incidence of permanent sequelae from cast-related injuries was only 0.25% per cast.[52] Thus, although minor complications are common with TCC in severely neuropathic diabetic patients, they do not appear to delay healing of the primary ulcer and rarely cause permanent sequelae.

Superficial fungal infections (most commonly *Trichophyton rubrum*) on the foot or leg occur in approximately 15% of casted patients.[57] They can be treated effectively with topical antifungal cream such as Lotrimin cream (Schering-Plough Healthcare Products, Inc., Kenilworth, NJ, www.lotrimin.com). In the presence of severe fungal infections, however, casting should be temporarily suspended until infection is controlled. Likewise, ulcers with even moderate amounts of drainage can have foul odors that are socially unacceptable during prolonged casting treatment. Delaying casting until drainage is minimal, or performing more frequent cast changes with ulcer cleansing (every 3 to 5 days) will minimize this problem.

Cast Application

Patient Preparation

A plantar ulcer must be thoroughly assessed by probing for any evidence of sinuses or penetration to bone. If the ulcer is deeper than it is wide, it may be opened to a width equal to or exceeding its depth to ensure adequate drainage and to encourage healing of the wound's deeper layers while preventing premature superficial healing. Alternatively, a deep ulcer can be packed loosely at its surface with wide-mesh gauze to prevent superficial healing. The ulcer should be thoroughly cleaned, including sharp removal of devitalized tissue. The value of shaving callus at the margins of the ulcer was shown by Young and colleagues, who demonstrated that callus removal can reduce dynamic plantar pressures in the forefoot by 30% during barefoot walking.[58]

Ulcer depth is measured by a millimeter rule or depth gauge. The perimeter of the ulcer may be traced onto clear radiographic film with an indelible ink marker, then placed in the patient's record for subsequent comparison measurements. The authors have found this a reliable method of quantifying changes in the size of the

ulcer[59] and very useful both in giving the patient visual feedback regarding the effectiveness of TCC and for convincing the reluctant patient to continue casting therapy.

After the ulcer has been evaluated, saline-soaked wide-mesh gauze can be placed over it, covered with a dry thin dressing, and secured with paper tape. The dressing should be kept as thin and small as possible to avoid excessive pressures from the dressing on the ulcer within the cast. If the ulcer is deep, loosely packed gauze can be used to fill it to the surface, after which the thin dressing is applied.

To apply a TCC, we advocate placing the patient in the prone position with the involved limb's knee and ankle flexed to 90 degrees and the plantar surface of the foot parallel to the floor. The authors believe that applying the cast with the patient prone is an important component of the procedure that contributes to comfort and walking stability and may limit abrasion from the cast. This position also relaxes the gastrocnemius and soleus muscles (triceps surae), allowing the foot to be held in position easily while the inner layers of the cast are setting, thus helping to prevent high-pressure areas such as dents in the cast. Many patients have tightness of the Achilles tendon/triceps surae musculotendinous unit, resulting in functional equinus deformity of the ankle.[60] A mild functional equinus deformity (<10 degrees of plantarflexion tightness) can be readily accommodated by adding plaster strips to the posterior plantar aspect of the cast to level the weight-bearing surface for walking.

Some patients are unable to comfortably assume the prone position because of hip flexor tightness or low back pain. It might be necessary to place pillows under their abdomen or pelvis to achieve comfort during casting. The authors typically have patients perform several slow stretches of the hip and knee flexors to temporarily loosen them immediately prior to TCC application. Adjustable tables, which allow half of the table to be lowered, to accommodate slight hip flexor tightness, can also provide a comfortable prone position during casting.

Casting Technique

A small amount of cotton padding is placed loosely between adjacent toes to prevent maceration by absorbing any moisture. A 3-inch-wide, close-fitting tubular cotton stockinette is rolled over the foot and leg up to the knee. The toe end of the stockinette should be sewn closed or can be folded into the toe sulcus and taped closed. The stockinette is pulled taut until it is wrinkle-free. The wrinkle that naturally occurs at the anterior ankle is cut transversely, and the edges are overlapped and taped to prevent an area of high pressure when the plaster is applied.

Next, a layer of 1/2-inch adhesive-backed Sifoam (DaysEnd Products, Temecula, CA) or felt is applied to cover and protect the toes. This foam layer, placed over

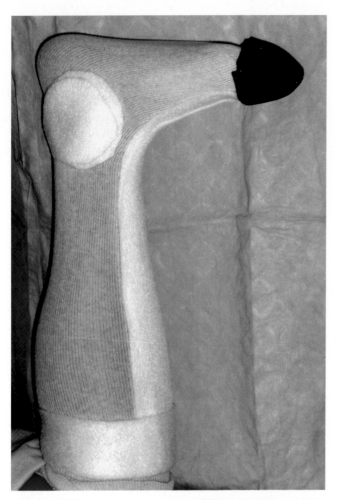

Figure 13-2   A foam layer covers the toes, which are enclosed for protection. Felt padding is applied over both the malleoli and tibial crest to protect the bony prominence. The felt strip along the tibia facilitates cast removal.

the closed stockinette, extends dorsally from the metatarsophalangeal joint level over the toe ends to the plantar toe sulcus (Fig. 13-2). The edges of the foam should be trimmed medially and laterally and beveled to minimize edge pressures. The insensitive toes are enclosed in plaster to protect them from striking obstructions and to prevent objects from becoming lodged in the cast. The leg should be supported by an assistant, and the foot and ankle should be held stable in the neutral position (90 degrees at the ankle), with the toes passively dorsiflexed slightly. Alternatively, the cast can be applied with the patient in the long-sitting position, although this is not ideal. When a TCC is applied in this position, it is paramount that the patient's knee be adequately flexed to relax the triceps surae and that the ankle be maintained in the 90-degree (neutral) position without a deforming position of the midfoot. Since many diabetic patients are unable to achieve the neutral ankle position secondary to joint or muscle limitations, attempts to achieve this position passively may produce abnormal midfoot pronation and a prominent talus or navicular bone medially,

resulting in areas of high pressure within the cast. Therefore, excessive pressure to achieve the neutral position is not recommended. As was noted above, a small amount of equinus can be accommodated in the cast by building up the posterior plantar portion of the cast with plaster strips to level the weight-bearing surface.

Next, two round pieces of 1/8- to 1/4-inch adhesive-backed felt, approximately 2 inches in diameter, are placed on the stockinette over the malleoli. Their edges should be beveled to reduce the edge pressure along the felt-to-plaster interface. Another felt pad, 18 to 20 inches long and 2 inches wide, is beveled and placed anteriorly along the tibial crest and onto the dorsum of the foot from just below the tibial tuberosity to the metatarsal heads (see Fig. 13-2). In addition to protecting the prominent tibial crest, this pad facilitates safe cast removal. Occasionally, additional bony prominences such as the styloid process of the fifth metatarsal bone or the talonavicular area might require padding, depending on the severity of foot deformity. Other additional padding is unnecessary.

One or two layers of fast-setting, creamy plaster bandage (Gypsona, BSN Medical, Inc., Charlotte, NC, www.bsnmedical.com) are then wrapped without tension around the leg and foot, commencing from 1 to 1 1/2 inches below the previously marked fibular head and continuing distally to beyond the metatarsal heads. Care must be taken to avoid any wrinkles in the plaster. The plaster bandage should be rolled quickly but without tension, leaving no gaps between wraps. The bandage is then rubbed continuously to conform to the shape of the foot and leg until it has set. The plaster is molded into every crevice and around all bony prominences and pads (Fig. 13-3). Particular attention should be given to molding the plaster to the contours of the sole of the foot. This thin layer of plaster is the most critical part of the total-contact cast. The patient should be instructed not to move the foot or leg once this "eggshell" layer has been applied. The assistant supporting the leg and foot should not move the foot or apply pressure to the plaster, which could distort it and cause potential areas of high pressure.

Once the inner eggshell layer of plaster has fully set (approximately 3 minutes), it is reinforced with plaster splints (five layers thick) approximately 30 inches long, applied anterior to posterior from the dorsal surface of the toes around the plantar surface of the foot and up the posterior aspect of the leg. A second set of splints is wrapped in a medial-to-lateral direction around the calcaneus and up both sides of the leg. These splints reinforce the plantar and posterior portions of the cast.

To complete the cast, one can add a rubber walking heel to the plantar surface of the cast. We typically use a 1/4-inch-thick plywood board between the walking heel and the cast to minimize the danger of cracks in the sole of the cast from pressure on the heel. The board should be cut slightly smaller than the length and width of the

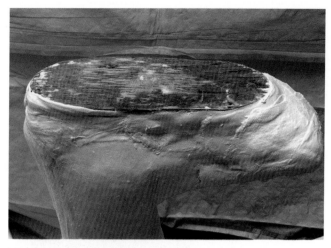

Figure 13-4   A 1/4-inch-thick plywood board is placed between the walking heel and the cast. The space between the board and the contoured cast sole is filled with plaster for support and to level the plantar surface for walking.

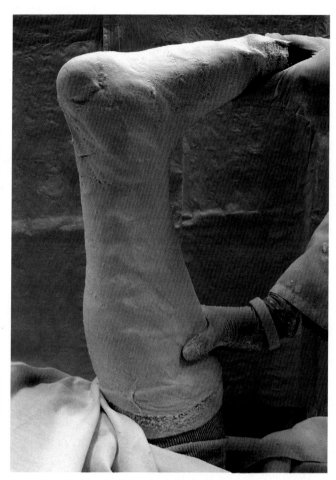

Figure 13-3   The first layer of fast-setting plaster is quickly applied and continuously molded (2 to 3 minutes) around bony prominences to conform to the foot and leg until it has set.

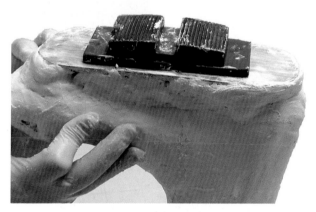

Figure 13-5   Note the placement of the walking heel on the board just behind the midline of the foot.

foot and should provide support from the posterior heelpad to the toe sulcus (Fig. 13-4). The space between the contoured sole of the cast and the board should be filled with a plaster roll to level the plantar surface. The position of the walking heel is critical for the patient's balance. It should be placed on the board just behind the midline of the foot viewed from the side (Fig. 13-5). Placing the heel too far forward on the foot will cause the patient to have difficulty with balance and can cause excessive movement of the foot and leg in the cast. Placing the heel too far back on the foot will cause the patient to roll forward onto the toe of the cast, contacting the ground and possibly breaking the toe of the cast. The walking heel is attached to the cast, and the toes are fully enclosed with an additional one or two rolls of plaster. Every attempt should be made to keep the anterior portion of the cast thin to facilitate removal. The authors use a fiberglass cast tape (Techform, Royce Medical, An Ossur Company, Camarillo, CA) to attach the heel and complete the outer layers (Fig. 13-6). This material is lightweight, durable, quick-setting, and water-resistant, although it is not as easily molded to the foot. The use of fiberglass tape is recommended, particularly

for patients who might need to bear weight soon after application.

In many cases, the rubber walking heel might not be appropriate because the patient's balance is poor or because casting causes acute back pain due to unequal limb lengths. In these cases, the authors prefer to use a postoperative cast boot for walking (Fig. 13-7). Boots with rigid, slightly rocker-bottom soles are most easily tolerated. Dhalla and colleagues found greater off-loading in the forefoot and midfoot with the combination of a TCC and a postoperative cast boot compared to a TCC with a rubber walking heel.[61] In contrast, they observed greater off-loading in the hindfoot using the rubber walking heel.[61] In all cases, it is advocated that the 1/4-inch-thick plywood board be used to strengthen the plantar aspect of the cast and prevent damage to its inner layers during weight-bearing. The board also helps to reduce localized plantar pressures by further increasing the plantar surface area. The completed cast should now be allowed to dry thoroughly. If plaster rolls and splints are used for reinforcement, the patient is instructed to limit weight-bearing for at least 24 hours after application to allow the inner plaster layers to harden. Before the patient is dis-

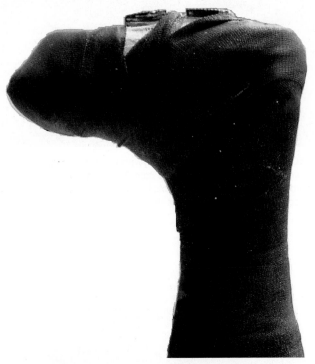

Figure 13–6 Completed cast. Weight-bearing should be delayed 24 hours to allow the inner layers to thoroughly set.

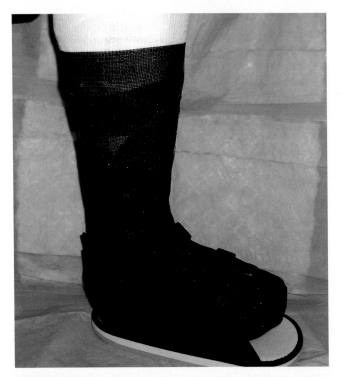

Figure 13–7 In this case, the postoperative cast boot covers the TCC in lieu of a rubber walking heel. The cast boot has a rigid rockered sole to assist walking.

missed, the cast should be checked for appropriate fit and the patient instructed in cast care and precautions.

Instructions to Patients

The patient with a total-contact cast should be given meticulous instruction in the care and monitoring of the cast, especially since the feet lack protective sensation. The authors routinely obtain written informed consent prior to casting to ensure that the patient understands the purpose of TCC and to explain the risks and precautions that are involved in this treatment. We have found that providing detailed, written instructions, including an explanation of the purpose of the TCC and how it differs from a more standard below-knee cast, has been useful. An emergency contact number is provided so that if problems occur, both severe complications as well as unnecessary and costly visits to the emergency room can be avoided. An example of these written instructions and some helpful reminders regarding the care of the cast are provided in Box 13-4. If the patient experiences any one or a combination of the following warning signs, the cast should be removed and the ulcer inspected immediately:

1. Excessive swelling of the leg or foot, causing the cast to become too tight
2. Overall cast loosening or excessive mobility of the foot in the cast
3. Deep cracks or soft spots in the cast
4. Drainage visible on the outside of the cast
5. Foul-smelling odor of cast
6. Sudden tenderness in the groin (inguinal lymph nodes)
7. Complaints of discomfort or pain.
8. Sudden increase in body temperature (fever) or chills

In addition to instruction in the warning signs, the patient should be taught proper ambulation. Both walking distance and walking frequency must be limited. The less a patient walks, the less the cumulative damage from pressure on the foot. In the absence of excessive pressure, the ulcer will heal quickly. The patient is also encouraged to shorten the stride length, reduce walking speed, and avoid excessive push-off in the late stance phase of the gait cycle and limit ambulation to one third of the normal daily amount.[62] The authors routinely advocate the use of crutches or a walker to help decrease weight-bearing and to improve balance. If patients develop low back pain or leg pain, a temporary lift may be added to the opposite shoe to level the pelvis. Alternatively, the walking heel may be removed and replaced with a postoperative cast boot.

Follow-up Visits

The initial cast is left on no more than 5 to 7 days. The cast should be changed earlier if excessive edema or drainage was present when the initial cast was applied.

BOX 13–4 Total-Contact Cast Instructions

You have a total-contact cast applied to your foot for the purpose of healing the ulcer (sore) on your foot. These ulcers do not heal, because of the extremely high pressures on the sole of the foot during walking. The cast is made to decrease the pressure on the ulcer, thereby allowing the ulcer to heal. In addition to the pressure relief, the cast is designed to be very snug-fitting with the toes enclosed for protection.

In order for the total-contact cast to be effective, you must know how to take care of your cast. The following is a list of what to **DO** and **NOT TO DO.**

- **DO NOT** bear weight or walk on your cast until you are told to do so by the person putting the cast on your foot. Usually, no weight-bearing is allowed for 24 hours after the cast is applied. This allows the inner layers of plaster to dry thoroughly.
- After 24 hours, you may resume walking. We recommend that you limit your walking to one third of the normal daily walking distance.
- Never use the cast to strike or hit objects. Dents, cracks, or softened areas of the cast may cause excessive pressure on your foot in the cast and should be reported immediately.
- Keep the cast dry at all times. Water will destroy your cast. Sponge bathing is recommended while your cast is on. **DO NOT** shower. If the cast does become wet, dry it immediately with a towel, or hair dryer set to "cool." If it rains, cover the cast with a plastic bag.
- Your cast may be inconvenient, and you may have difficulty sleeping. This is not uncommon. You may try wrapping your cast in a towel or placing it on a pillow while in bed. You may also want to wear a cotton athletic sock on your noncasted foot and leg to prevent the cast from causing abrasions or rubs.
- After you have worn the cast for several days, perspiration and dirt may cause itching of the skin inside the cast. This is common. You must ignore it. **DO NOT** stick pencils, coat hangers, or other objects in the cast to scratch the skin.
- Inspect the entire cast daily. Look and feel for deep cracks or soft spots on the cast. Use a small hand mirror to inspect the sole of the cast.
- Never attempt to remove your cast by yourself.

REMOVING YOUR CAST

We have a specially designed saw to remove the cast with little discomfort. The cast should be removed only by a health care professional. After removal, your skin may be flaky and dry, and your joints may feel stiff. Apply a thick cream or oil for several days to moisten and soften the skin. Your therapist will show you exercises to decrease the stiffness in your foot. You will need to have your specially made shoes ready to wear **immediately** after the cast is removed to prevent your foot from getting another ulcer. You should continue to use crutches or a walker for several weeks after the ulcer is healed to help protect your foot. Be sure to talk to your doctor or therapist about protecting the foot after the cast is removed.

WARNING SIGNS

If any of the following signs or symptoms occur call [phone number].
1. Excessive swelling of the leg or foot if the cast becomes too tight.
2. If the cast becomes too loose and your leg can move up or down in the cast more than 1/4".
3. If the cast has any deep cracks or soft spots.
4. Any drainage of pus or blood on the outside of the cast. This will appear brownish or dark yellow in color.
5. Any foul-smelling odor of the cast.
6. If you experience any excessive tenderness in your groin or the casted foot.
7. Any excessive leg pain or annoying pressure in the ankle or foot that will not go away.
8. If you notice any sudden onset of fever or increase in body temperature.

If any of the above conditions occur, **DO** the following:

1. Notify appropriate professional personnel as soon as possible at [phone number].
2. **DO NOT** walk on your cast. Keep your leg elevated.
3. Use crutches or a walker and keep the casted foot off the ground until seen by professional personnel.

The cast is removed by using a standard cast saw and spreaders. Cuts are made along the anterior surface of the leg and foot from proximal to distal along the felt strip, then medial to lateral at the level of the ankle. It should be remembered that the anterior wall of the cast is thin in comparison to the other walls, so caution must be taken to prevent injury to the skin from the saw.

At the first cast change, the ulcer is reevaluated, including retracing of its perimeter onto clear radiographic film to document any change in ulcer size. The first change also provides a chance to evaluate the patient's response to the cast.[44] Skin temperature checks will detect any local inflammation caused by cast rubbing so that modifications can be made to the next cast. Preparation for definitive footwear can also begin at this time because custom shoes and insole fabrication methods require a negative mold of the leg and foot. Since edema should now be resolved, the foot can be casted to allow adequate time for the fabrication of footwear. Although this practice is somewhat time-consuming, it will ultimately save time and expense and will provide immediate protection for the foot when the ulcer is healed. The cast is then reapplied as described previously

and may be left in place for up to 2 weeks. Of course, it should be changed more frequently in the presence of significant edema or drainage. At each visit, the cast is reapplied if healing is incomplete. For individuals whose compliance is dubious, more frequent monitoring and cast changes are recommended.

Once the ulcer is fully healed, the patient should be placed promptly into appropriate therapeutic footwear (see Chapter 28). Rigid rocker-bottom sole shoes with custom-molded insoles are recommended for forefoot ulcers.[28,34] In addition to supply of the appropriate footwear, the patient must be carefully instructed in monitoring the newly healed ulcer. Brand[26] noted that a newly healed ulcer is particularly susceptible to reulceration within the first month after healing because of the poor capacity of scar tissue to accommodate shear stress.[26] Several studies have documented that the recurrence rate after TCC is approximately 30%;[43] other studies have suggested that as many as 50% to 70% of ulcers recur.[9,13,63] Mueller and colleagues reported that 27% of foot ulcers recur within the first 3 months following transmetatarsal amputation and that 48% of these ulcers reopen within the first month.[64] These data underscore the critical nature of the period immediately following initial healing.[64] The diabetic patient with a newly healed ulcer should be instructed to increase weight-bearing activities slowly and to continue using ambulatory aids. Frequent checks of skin temperature are recommended to identify local warm spots on the feet that could indicate recurrent inflammation. Frequent follow-up visits after the cast is removed are mandatory to educate the patient and reinforce the roles of excessive pressure and insensitivity in recurrent ulceration.

Precautions

Although the methods of TCC application described in this chapter are detailed enough to replicate, caution is necessary. Thorough training and practice in this technique are requisite to ensure early success and to minimize the potential complications and sequelae of immobilizing an insensitive foot. The authors recommend visiting a local facility or medical center that regularly performs TCC to observe, learn, and practice the application of these casts before attempting this procedure. The TCC method described above is summarized at the U.S. Department of Health and Human Services, Bureau of Primary Health Care, National Hansen's Disease Program Website (http://www.hrsa.gov/hansens/publications.htm). The treatment of neuropathic ulcers by this method requires a strong commitment and willingness on the part of the diabetic foot care team members, including the individuals applying the cast, to respond quickly to patients' complaints or problems at any time.

In the authors' experience, the keys to successful management by this method, while minimizing potential complications and side effects, are close and frequent monitoring of the ulcer and the patient's tolerance of the lengthy casting program. Strict patient compliance with subsequent follow-up visits is paramount. If patients are unable or unwilling to return regularly as outpatients, the development of complications from the casts may be inevitable, and this method should not be employed.

Although the specific methodology of TCC has undergone several modifications and refinements[2,61,65] as the technique has gained popularity over the past several decades, its primary effectiveness can be attributed to two basic features: total contact with increased surface area achieved by carefully molding the plaster to the foot during application and the fact that cast removal by the patient is not readily possible. Currently, emphasis has been placed on utilizing newer materials or adapting commercially available cast walkers with improved technology to speed up the technically demanding and time-consuming application of TCC.[17,19] The continuing development of these technologies underscores the primary value of pressure off-loading as the mainstay in the rapid healing of neuropathic plantar ulcers.[17,19]

Compliance

TCC offers forced compliance, since the cast is not easily removed. Without doubt, this contributes to the high success rate and rapid healing times that are observed with TCC compared to removable devices, such as healing AFOs, despite similar reductions in plantar pressures.[23] If patients have the opportunity to remove the AFO while sitting or sleeping, they are more apt to stand or walk unprotected around their homes (e.g., night trips to the bathroom or standing in the shower), since their feet are insensitive.[66] Even these brief exposures to high plantar pressures are sufficient to delay or prevent wound healing. For these reasons, whenever compliance is dubious, TCC is the better treatment choice to ensure faster healing times.

The authors advocate the use of partial weight-bearing (PWB) on the casted limb, using a walker or bilateral crutches at all times during ambulation to help unload the casted limb and further reduce pedal stresses, thereby facilitating ulcer healing. Using PWB with these assistive devices decreases the ambulatory patient's walking speed and shortens the step length, thereby further reducing plantar pressures. However, compliance with PWB is a difficult, if not impossible, expectation, and not all authorities agree that PWB and assistive devices are necessary or even practical for diabetic patients with peripheral neuropathy and a pedal ulcer.[9,11] Although the major pressure off-loading afforded by the cast results from increasing the surface area of the foot, the authors nonetheless believe that further reduction in plantar pressures using an assistive device will likely promote a faster healing time.

In addition to strongly recommending PWB with assistive devices, the patient should be encouraged to reduce the amount of daily weight-bearing activity. The classic works of Kosiak[67] and Brand[28] indicate that ulcer formation and delayed wound healing are directly related to the magnitude and duration of peak plantar pressures as well as the number of repetitions. Even modest plantar pressures applied continuously throughout the day can delay ulcer healing. Therefore, any combination of strategies to limit plantar pressures should hasten healing time and reduce unnecessary complications, such as skin abrasions from the cast. Adherence to PWB instructions is problematic for patients with sensory neuropathy, and typically, only 30% of patients are compliant with instructions for PWB using assistive devices and in reducing their frequency of weight-bearing activities.[32] If they are compliant with PWB and reduced ambulation, significantly shorter healing times have been observed,[32] as well as fewer complications from casting and lower pedal pressures during walking. Additional research is needed, however, to conclusively determine whether adherence to PWB and limited ambulation in the cast contribute to faster healing times.

Alternative Off-Loading Methods

As was discussed above, effective off-loading must include adequate protection of the wound, although this protection must be balanced with other factors, such as ease of application, a need for frequent wound inspection, interference with mobility, cosmetic acceptability, safety, and overall compliance with wearing the device. TCC provides optimal protection to the wound from offending stresses and allows it to heal faster than occurs with any other treatment. Though TCC is optimal for protection, healing, and off-loading, it is seldom used in the clinic because of the factors cited above. The following section will review alternatives to TCC that attempt to provide the benefits of TCC while avoiding its limitations. For each device, its rationale, benefits and limitations, and outcomes are presented.

Removable Cast Walker

Removable cast walkers are commercially available devices that are designed to immobilize the lower leg, foot, and ankle and provide even pressure distribution on the plantar foot, while being relatively easy to apply and remove. In addition to providing good off-loading for the ulcer, they allow the wound to be inspected and treated as required. Two commonly used cast walkers are the XP Diabetic Walker System (Aircast, Summit, NJ, www.aircast.com) (Fig. 13-8A)[17] and the DH Pressure Relief Walker (Royce Medical, An Ossur Company, Camarillo, CA)[18] (Fig 13-8B). These devices typically have clamshell designs with Velcro straps that secure them to the lower leg. Soft or inflatable pads line the interior of the rigid shells; they help to distribute weight-bearing stresses and protect the skin from rubbing the rigid exoskeleton of these devices. A rigid rocker-bottom

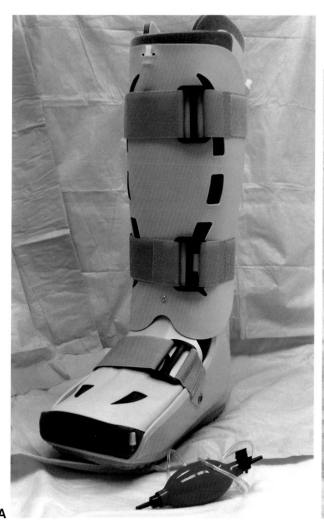 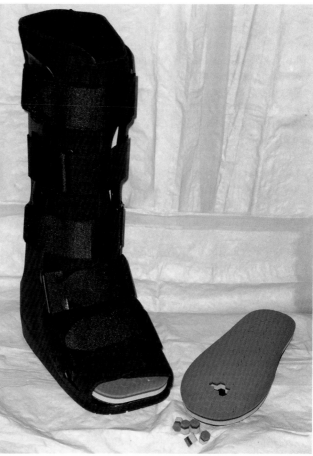

A **B**

Figure 13–8 **A,** The commercially available Aircast XP Diabetic Walker System has inflatable pads that line the interior of the walker, helping to distribute weight-bearing forces and protect the skin from rubbing against the rigid exoskeleton of the walker. **B,** The Royce Medical DH Pressure-Relief Walker has removable, multidensity rubber hexagonal plugs in the insole that can be customized to reduce pressures around the ulcer.

sole allows good rollover while keeping the entire sole of the foot in contact with the supporting device. The Aircast XP Diabetic Walker System has air cells inflated with a hand bulb, and a pressure gauge is provided to achieve the desired levels of inflation. The Royce Medical DH Pressure Relief Walker has a soft insole with removable hexagonal plugs that can help to unload specific areas on the plantar foot. Removal of the plugs should be performed with caution, however, since removal might allow increased edge stresses, and the wound site might "bottom out," that is, fall through to the rigid sole of the walker and cause increased stresses.

Some cast walkers show pressure reductions similar to those of TCC[33] but have demonstrated lower healing rates.[18] Armstrong and colleagues reported a 65% healing rate in a mean time of 50 days using one such device compared to a 90% healing rate in a mean time of 34 days using TCC.[18] These investigators reported that patients often removed the cast walker when at home. Patients wore activity monitors on their waist and on the cast walker, revealing that they wore the device only about 28% of the time.[66] It was concluded that the cast walker was not as effective as the TCC simply because patients were not compliant with wearing a removable device.

In summary, the advantages of the cast walker are that it is easy to apply and that the wound is easily accessible for adjunctive therapies and protected while the device is worn. The added convenience of easy removal, however, may also be its limitation, as patients may take the device off and walk with their ulcer unprotected. The clamshell design with adjustable Velcro closure allows for fluctuating edema in the lower leg, but the cast walker, unlike the TCC, might not provide sufficiently uniform compression to reduce edema. Another limitation of the cast walker compared to the TCC is that it is unable to accommodate severe bony deformities, particularly those in the frontal plane. The TCC, by contrast, is custom made for each patient and can be used to accommodate severe deformities, including those from acute and chronic Charcot osteoarthropathy.[31,32]

Irremovable Cast Walker

The irremovable cast walker is identical to a removable cast walker except that the device is made "irremovable" by wrapping it with a layer of cohesive or plaster bandage or fiberglass tape.[17,19] The rationale for making a cast walker irremovable is that it eliminates the compliance factor. In other words, patients are unable to easily remove the device and walk unprotected, thus continuing to reinjure the neuropathic ulcer.

Two randomized, controlled trials have compared ulcer healing times using the removable and irremovable cast walker or total contact cast. Armstrong and colleagues compared the irremovable cast walker to a removable cast walker,[17] and Katz and colleagues compared the irre-

movable cast walker to a total-contact cast.[19] In a 12-week follow-up, healing rates were 80% to 83% using the irremovable cast walker, 74% using TCC, and 53% using the removable cast walker. There were no differences in healing times between the irremovable cast walker and TCC, but the irremovable cast walker healed a significantly higher percentage of wounds (80% to 83% versus 53%) in a shorter time (42 ± 19 days versus 58 ± 15 days) compared to the removable cast walker. Katz and colleagues also reported that the irremovable cast walker took less time to apply and remove (39% and 36% reductions, respectively) and cost less than TCC.[19]

Given similar healing rates, the irremovable cast walker could have several advantages compared to TCC. Most important, the irremovable cast walker does not require extensive training to properly apply or remove. According to preliminary data, the irremovable cast walker takes less time to apply and remove and costs less than TCC.[19] However, similar to the removable cast walker, a limitation of the irremovable cast walker, compared to TCC, is that it is unable to accommodate severe frontal plane bony deformities and therefore might not be appropriate for patients with acute and chronic Charcot osteoarthropathy with significant deformity.[31,32] Because it is irremovable, all the precautions for patients that have been described for the TCC apply to patients using the irremovable cast walker (see Box 13-4). Furthermore, compared to some of the alternative methods listed below, the removable and irremovable cast walkers are bulky and expensive.

Felted Pads and Accommodative Dressing

As was noted above, limitations of TCC and cast walkers include bulkiness, excess weight, and relatively high expense. In addition, cast walkers are not custom-made to the patient's foot. Adhesive felt padding, sometimes called accommodative dressing or felted foam, can be used as an alternative to minimize these limitations. Adhesive felt padding is inexpensive, commonly used for custom off-loading of the metatarsal heads, and is usually combined with other simple footwear devices. Hissink and colleagues[68] described using 8-mm-thick adhesive felt padding, cut to the shape of the plantar surface, excluding the site of the ulcer and its dressing (Fig. 13-9). The foot is covered, and the shaped adhesive felt is added to a removable fiberglass shoe that allows free ankle movement. Birke and colleagues[69] used a similar 15-cm-long piece of 6-mm-thick adhesive felt attached to the forefoot with a cutout over the ulcer area. The foot and felt pad were covered with a Kling gauze dressing and placed in a surgical shoe modified with a wedged sole. Zimny and colleagues[70] described a similar approach except that they used a combination of 0.635-cm-thick rubber foam with a 0.158-cm-thick layer of felt adhered to the skin using rubber glue (Mastic-Verbandkleber; ASID Bonz und Sohn GmbH, Boeblingen, Germany).

They reported no skin irritations due to the rubber glue.

Noncontrolled studies using adhesive padding on carefully selected patients with localized forefoot wounds reported results comparable to those found by using TCC. Hissink and colleagues reported that 21 of 23 (91%) ulcers healed in a mean time of 34 days (7 to 75 days).[68] Birke and colleagues reported that 93% of the 26 patients treated with accommodative dressing healed in 36 ± 36 days compared to 92% of the wounds treated with TCC healing in 48 ± 32 days.[69] Zimny and colleagues[70] published a prospective, controlled trial comparing the felted foam technique to the use of standard care with off-loading by a half-shoe. The average healing time with the felted foam was 75 days (95% confidence interval [CI]: 67– to 84 days) and 85 days (95% CI: 79– to 92 days) in the conventional group that included a half shoe. Twenty-five percent of their subjects in the felted foam group and 23% in the conventional group developed soft-tissue infection, rates that are substantially higher than those reported from using other approaches. It was not clear whether an external shoe was used or how the foot with felted foam was otherwise protected in this study. The authors also stressed the need to change the felted foam every 3 to 4 days because the off-loading ability of the felted foam diminishes after that time.[70]

The advantage to using adhesive padding or accommodative dressing is that offending stresses can be off-loaded with minimal expense. Birke and colleagues[69] emphasized that these techniques can easily be used by those who typically manage foot ulcers, including nurses, physical therapists, and podiatrists. A cast boot is an inexpensive addition to the accommodative dressing and can quickly provide support and protection with off-loading to the patient with limited resources, as described below. When the foot is protected with additional footwear, healing outcomes appear to be comparable to those of TCC[68,69] but additional controlled clinical trials are required to verify these descriptive studies.

Cast Boot or Postsurgical Shoe

When time, expertise, or resources limit other off-loading options, minor modifications can be made to a cast boot or postsurgical shoe to provide some off-loading to the diabetic foot and protect it from most excessive stresses. A cast boot or postsurgical shoe is available in almost any clinic and costs about $10.00. These devices typically have a rigid sole and an adjustable, flexible upper that is secured with simple Velcro closures (Fig. 13-10). Without an insert, these devices have a rigid surface in contact with the plantar foot, so plantar pressures might be unacceptably high.[71] Therefore, the shoe should be used with some type of accommodative insole, such as the adhesive felt described above[69] or a simple half-inch layer of soft insole material (e.g., Plastazote #1, Alimed, Boston, MA, www.Alimed.com) cut to fit inside the boot or shoe.

Few data exist to describe outcomes for this commonly used treatment approach. Birke and colleagues,[71] however,

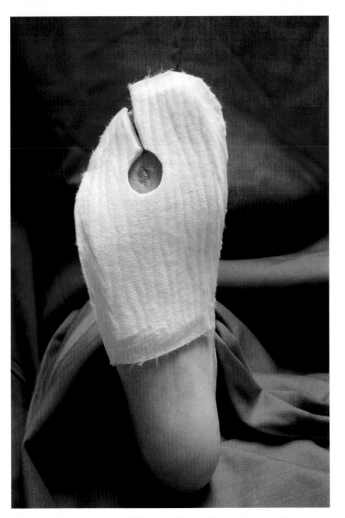

Figure 13–9   Eight-millimeter-thick adhesive felt padding cut to the shape of the plantar surface of the foot excluding the site of the ulcer and its dressing. *(Photo courtesy of James A. Birke, PT, PhD, CPed.)*

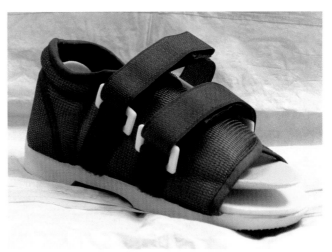

Figure 13–10   Postoperative surgical shoe with a rigid sole and a Plastazote #1 insert. The adjustable, flexible upper is secured with hook and loop (Velcro) closures.

described excellent wound-healing rates using a surgical shoe with an accommodative felt pad or a quarter-inch nonpolyethylene foam inlay with a relief cut under the ulcer area and a half-inch wedged sole. This group reported healing rates of 81% to 93%, comparable to those seen using TCC, in mean times of 36 to 41 days in groups of 26 and 57 patients.[69] In summary, a cast boot or postsurgical shoe is inexpensive, readily available, and easily modified to enhance off-loading, and if used properly, it can result in excellent healing rates. The limitations are that they are not very sturdy, can be difficult to walk in, and, if not adequately modified, can result in excessively high plantar pressures.

"Half-Shoe" or Wedged Forefoot Shoe

A "half-shoe" or wedged forefoot shoe is similar to a postsurgical shoe but is designed specifically to unload the forefoot. One common example is the Orthowedge® shoe (www.darcointernational.com) (Fig. 13-11). These shoes typically have a large (~4 cm) heel wedge that places the ankle in 10 to 15 degrees of dorsiflexion. Because there is no support under the forefoot, plantar pressures are greatly reduced in the forefoot beyond the apex of the wedge. Birke and colleagues[71] reported that forefoot pressures were 45% lower in a wedged shoe than in a postsurgical shoe in a group ($n = 12$) of patients with previous great toe ulceration. Pressures were reduced 54% if a soft insert was included in the wedge shoe. Healing rates generally are better than those with standard care, which is considered to be about 31%[72], but not as good as those with TCC or cast walkers. Several groups have investigated using the half-shoe and indicate that about 58% to 96% of wounds heal in mean times of 61 to 134 days.[18,59,73,74]

The greatest advantages of half-shoes are that they provide excellent off-loading to the forefoot, are relatively inexpensive, and are easy to apply. The greatest limitation of these devices is that they are not tolerated well by most patients with diabetic neuropathy and a plantar ulcer. This group often has limited ankle dorsiflexion range, with functional equinus and poor mobility and balance.[54,75] Their limited ankle dorsiflexion range makes them unable to tolerate the negative heel. Additionally, the relatively small base of support at the heel can make walking difficult. Patients who use a half-shoe will also likely require an assistive device such as a cane, a walker, or crutches for stability during walking. These limitations in comfort and mobility are likely to lessen compliance with these devices, which could account for their modest healing rates despite excellent off-loading characteristics.

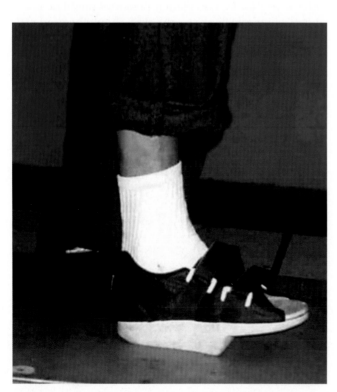

Figure 13–11   A wedged forefoot shoe ("half-shoe") is used to unload the forefoot. Because there is no support beyond the apex of the wedge, plantar pressures are greatly reduced in the forefoot.

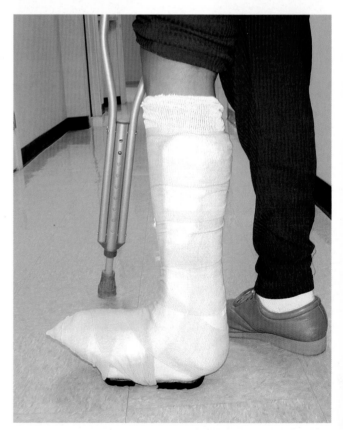

Figure 13–12   A custom-made walking splint similar to TCC, except that the cast is bivalved and its halves are secured with an elastic bandage. *(Photograph courtesy of James A. Birke, PT, PhD, CPed.)*

Custom Devices: Walking Splint and Ankle-Foot Orthosis

Some patients with severe foot or ankle deformity and a large wound complicated by infection might not be able to fit their leg into a commercial cast walker and might not tolerate a TCC. Patients who require both a custom approach and wound accessibility might benefit from a custom walking splint or an AFO. A walking splint is made in a manner similar to that of a TCC, after which the cast is bivalved. The anterior shell is either secured to the posterior shell with an elastic bandage or removed completely.[69] A custom AFO is constructed by taking a cast of the lower leg and foot and making a positive plaster mold from the cast. The positive mold of the leg and foot can then be modified before fabrication of the AFO to provide pressure relief over areas of ulceration or bony prominences[45] (Fig. 13-12).

Healing rates using this type of device might not be comparable to those of other approaches because patients who require this type of custom-made device may have additional complications, such as bony defor-

mity or infection. Despite this concern, Birke and colleagues report that 83% of their group of 18 patients healed in an average time of 50 days.[69] Boninger and Leonard reported on a group of 16 neuropathic ulcer patients with or without associated Charcot joint changes.[45] Their healing times were quite long (an average of 10 months) in this group of subjects with severe foot disease. They reported that patients with Charcot joint changes or neuropathic ulcers were able to tolerate the device for 45 and 66 months, respectively, before healing (Figs. 13-13A, 13-13B).

The primary indication for the custom walking splint or custom AFO is severe bony deformity or unusually large wounds with or without infection. The main limitations are that either device requires special expertise to fabricate and that the custom AFO can be relatively expensive, although it can be used again for recurrent ulcers. The authors have found the calf lacer well suited for off-loading in individuals with severe fixed deformities of the midfoot and hindfoot.[76] These devices offer maximal pressure relief and can be used with a variety of therapeutic footwear (Fig. 13-14).

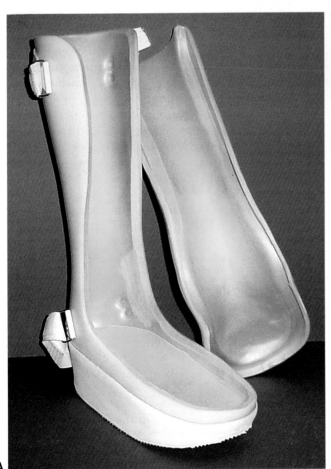
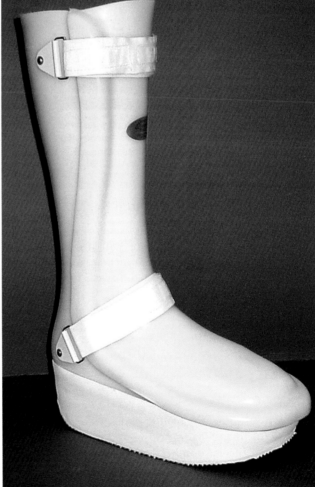

Figure 13-13   **A,** A custom-made Charcot restraint orthotic walker (CROW) with Plastazote liner. **B,** Halves of the CROW secured with Velcro straps.

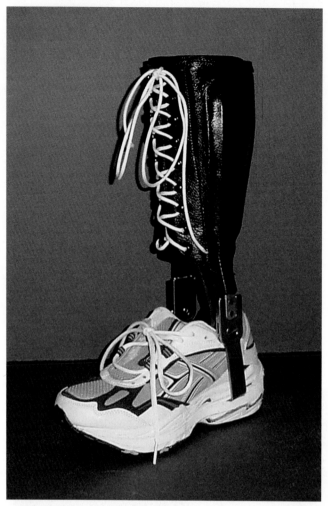

Figure 13-14   A calf-lacer with metal uprights, which can be affixed to almost any type of therapeutic footwear, offers maximal pressure off-loading for severe deformities of the ankle, hindfoot, or midfoot.

Therapeutic Footwear for Wound Healing

Traditionally, therapeutic footwear with several modifications has been used as a standard off-loading treatment for neuropathic plantar ulcers. As such, therapeutic footwear was long included in early clinical trials as a comparison treatment for the control group of patients.[20,22,50] The rationale for using therapeutic shoes for the treatment of neuropathic ulcers is that the shoes provide some off-loading and protection to the foot while generally allowing patients to walk unimpeded. Evidence confirms, however, that off-loading and pressure reduction in shoes are minimal in comparison to those in TCC.[23]

In early studies, therapeutic shoes were considered the standard for off-loading and good care practice for diabetic foot ulcers, despite the fact that overall documented healing rates were only 30% in 20 weeks.[72] More specifically, Mueller and colleagues[20] provided therapeutic shoes and conventional wound care to a control group of diabetic subjects with foot ulcers. They reported

that only 32% of ulcers healed in a mean time of 65 ± 29 days. Steed and colleagues[22] found that only 8% (2 of 25 patients) healed within 10 weeks when wet-to-dry saline dressings and therapeutic shoes were used compared to 35% (14 of 40) of patients who wore therapeutic shoes and applied an arginine-glycine-aspartic acid peptide matrix to their wounds. In short, wound healing rates with use of therapeutic shoes are considerably lower than those reported with use of other forms of off-loading.[17–20,65]

Although the benefits of therapeutic shoes for the treatment of neuropathic wounds include their easy availability and limited inconvenience, wound healing outcomes are unacceptably poor in comparison to those of other forms of off-loading.[72] The most likely basic reason that therapeutic footwear is associated with relatively low healing rates is that pressure reduction is not adequate to allow rapid ulcer healing to occur.[23,41,77] The authors conclude that therapeutic footwear can play an important role in preventing recurrence of plantar ulcers once the wound is healed (see Chapter 28) but should not be used as the primary off-loading strategy for healing neuropathic plantar ulcers.

Summary

Unnoticed, unfelt excessive plantar pressures have clearly been shown to be a prime contributing factor to neuropathic plantar ulcer formation. Off-loading the offending stresses from the ulcer area during walking should be the cornerstone of every management strategy. Though off-loading is the mainstay of every comprehensive treatment regimen for neuropathic plantar wounds, there is no single device or method that provides optimal healing for all patients. Health care practitioners should understand the benefits and limitations of the broad range of devices described in this chapter to best match their individual patients' impairments with the optimal off-loading strategy. If properly and maximally off-loaded, most (>90%) uncomplicated, nonischemic neuropathic ulcers should heal in 6 to 8 weeks. Research on TCC consistently report this range of healing rates, while those using alternative devices typically are slower. The benefits and limitations of the most appropriate options should be discussed with each patient, and the optimal off-loading strategy should be selected. This must be integrated with patient education and a comprehensive management approach to prevent ulcer recurrence.

TCC is an effective, rapid, and ambulatory therapy for healing diabetic neuropathic plantar ulcers. Though laborious to learn and time-consuming to apply, the methods of cast application are well worth mastering, since the reported healing benefits greatly outweigh potential complications. Given the persistent emphasis placed on shortened hospital stays, TCC and comparable off-loading methods provide effective and cost-prudent alternatives to prolonged, expensive periods of bed rest in the hospital.

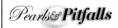

Pearls

- Off-loading is the key component of the overall management strategy for all patients with a plantar (weight-bearing) neuropathic ulcer.
- The optimal off-loading device will depend on several patient-related characteristics and environmental factors. No single off-loading device is optimal for all patients and situations. The patient and health care team members should discuss the benefits and limitations of each appropriate off-loading device to decide on the optimal approach for each individual.
- Patients should be instructed to transition slowly from off-loading devices throughout the ulcer-healing phase. For example, once an ulcer appears to be healed following TCC or another form of off-loading, the patient should be transitioned to a less restrictive form of off-loading and/or therapeutic footwear. Weight-bearing activity levels should be increased very slowly. Patients are at highest risk of skin breakdown in the first 4 to 8 weeks following initial healing of a full-thickness ulcer.

Pitfalls

- No off-loading device will be effective if it is not consistently used as prescribed. In general, irremovable off-loading devices (e.g., TCC or walker boot made irremovable) have faster healing times than do removable devices (e.g., therapeutic shoes or orthowedge shoes), which depend on patient compliance.
- An ill-fitting off-loading device can delay ulcer healing by excessive pressure or shear stresses, causing new skin breakdown. Patients must be educated on proper application and wearing schedules. Any new lesion, regardless of size or seeming insignificance, should be reported to the health practitioner immediately.
- Topical ointments, gels, growth factors, or dressing applications can be effective only if off-loading is a part of treatment. For example, a topical medicine may be effective at accelerating wound healing, but if a patient continues to walk with full weight-bearing on the ulcer location, healing cannot occur.

References

1. Pecoraro RE, Reiber GE, Burgess EM: Pathways to diabetic limb amputation: Basis for prevention. Diabetes Care 13:513–521, 1990.
2. American Diabetes Association: Consensus Development Conference on Diabetic Wound Care. Diabetes Care 1999; 22:1354–1360.
3. Baker RE: Total contact casting. J Am Pod Med Assoc 85(3): 172–176, 1995.
4. Birke JA, Novick A, Patout CA, Coleman WC: Healing rates of plantar ulcers in leprosy and diabetes. Lep Rev 63:365–374, 1992.
5. Boulton AJM, et al: Use of plaster casts in the management of diabetic neuropathic foot ulcers. Diabetes Care 9:149–152, 1986.
6. Diamond JE, Mueller MJ, Delitto A: Effect of total contact cast immobilization of subtalar and talocrural joint motion in patients with diabetes mellitus. Phys Ther 73:310–315, 1993.
7. Diamond JE, Sinacore DR, Mueller MJ: Molded double-rocker plaster shoe for healing a diabetic plantar ulcer. Phys Ther 67: 1550–1552, 1987.
8. Helm PA, Walker SC, Pullium G: Total contact casting in diabetic patients with neuropathic foot ulcerations. Arch Phys Med Rehabil 65:691–693, 1984.
9. Laing PW, Cogley DJ, Klenerman L: Neuropathic foot ulceration treated by total contact casts. J Bone Joint Surg (Br) 74-B:133–136, 1992.
10. Lee EH, Bose K: Orthopedic management of diabetic foot lesions. Ann Acad Med 14:331, 1985.
11. Myerson M, Papa J, Eaton K, Wilson K: The total contact cast for management of neuropathic plantar ulceration of the foot. J Bone Joint Surg 74-A:261–269, 1992.
12. Nawoczenski DA, Birke JA, Graham SL, Koziatek E: The neuropathic foot—A management scheme: A case report. Phys Ther 69:287–291,1989.
13. Pollard JP, LeQuesne LP: Method of healing diabetic forefoot ulcers. Br Med J 286:436–437, 1983.
14. Sinacore DR, Mueller MJ, Diamond JE, et al: Diabetic neuropathic ulcers treated by total contact casting. Phys Ther 67:1543–1549,1987.
15. Sinacore DR: Healing times of diabetic foot ulcers in the presence of fixed foot deformities using total contact casting. Foot Ankle Int 19(9):613–618, 1998.
16. Walker SC, Helm PA, Pullium G: Total contact casting and chronic diabetic neuropathic foot ulcerations: Healing rates by wound location. Arch Phys Med Rehabil 68:217–221, 1987.
17. Armstrong DG, Lavery LA, Wu S, Boulton AJM: Evaluation of removable and irremovable cast walkers in the healing of diabetic foot wounds: A randomized controlled trial. Diabetes Care 28(3):551–554, 2005.
18. Armstrong DG, Nguyen HC, Lavery LA, et al: Off-loading the diabetic foot wound: A randomized clinical trial. Diabetes Care 24(6):1019–1022, 2001.
19. Katz IA, Harlan A, Miranda-Palma B, et al: A randomized trial of two irremovable off-loading devices in the management of plantar neuropathic diabetic foot ulcers. Diabetes Care 28(3):555–559, 2005.
20. Mueller MJ, Diamond JE, Sinacore DR, et al: Total contact casting in treatment of diabetic plantar ulcers: Controlled clinical trial. Diabetes Care 12:384–388, 1989.
21. Lavery LA, Armstrong DG, Harkless LB: Classification of diabetic foot wounds. J Foot Ankle Surg 35(6):528–531, 1996.
22. Steed DL, Ricotta JJ, Prendergast JJ, et al: Promotion and acceleration of diabetic ulcer healing by arginine-glycine-aspartic acid (RGD) peptide matrix. RGD Study Group. Diabetes Care 18(1): 39–46, 1995.
23. Lavery LA, Vela SA, Lavery DC, Quebedaux TL: Reducing dynamic foot pressures in high risk diabetics with foot ulcerations: A comparison of treatments. Diabetes Care 19:818–821, 1996.
24. Sinacore DR: TCC: An old therapy with new indications. Biomechanics 3:71–74, 1996.
25. Kahn JS: Treatment of leprous trophic ulcers. Lepr India 11:19, 1939.
26. Brand PW: The diabetic foot. In Ellenberg M, Rifkin H (eds): Diabetes Mellitus. Garden City, NY, Medical Examination Publishing, 1983.
27. Birke JA, Novick A, Graham SL, et al: Methods of treating plantar ulcers. Phys Ther 71:116–122, 1991.
28. Brand PW: The insensitive foot. In Jahss MM (ed): Disorders of the Foot, vol. 2. Philadelphia, WB Saunders, 1982.
29. Coleman WC, Brand PW, Birke JA: The total contact cast: A therapy for plantar ulceration on insensitive feet. J Am Podiatry Assoc 74:548–552, 1984.
30. Armstrong DG, Todd WF, Lavery LA, et al: The natural history of acute Charcot's arthropathy in a diabetic foot specialty clinic. Diabet Med 14:357–363, 1997.
31. Lavery LA, Armstrong DG, Walker SC: Healing rates of diabetic foot ulcers associated with midfoot fracture due to Charcot's arthropathy. Diabet Med 14:46–49, 1997.
32. Sinacore DR: Acute neuropathic (Charcot) arthropathy in patients with diabetes mellitus: Healing times by foot location. J Diabetes Complications 12(5):287–293, 1998.
33. Boulton AJM, Kirsner RS, Vileikyte L: Neuropathic diabetic foot ulcers. New Engl J Med 351:48–55, 2004.
34. Bauman JH, Girling JP, Brand PW: Plantar pressures and trophic ulceration: An evaluation of footwear. J Bone Joint Surg 45:652–673, 1963.
35. Ctercteko GC, Dhanendran M, Hutton WC, LeQuesne LP: et al: Vertical forces acting on the feet of diabetic patients with neuropathic ulceration. Br J Surg 68:608, 1981.
36. Leibner ED, Brodsky JW, Pollo FE, et al: Unloading mechanism in the total contact cast. Foot Ankle Int 27(4): 281–285, 2006.

37. Shaw JE, His WL, Ulbrecht JS, et al: The mechanism of plantar unloading in total contact casts: Implications for design and clinical use. Foot Ankle Int 18(12):809–817, 1997.
38. Conti SF, Martin RL, Chaytor ER, et al: Plantar pressure measurements during ambulation in weight bearing conventional short leg casts and total contact casts. Foot Ankle Int 17:464–469, 1996.
39. Martin RL, Conti SF: Plantar pressure analysis of diabetic rocker bottom deformity in total contact casts. Foot Ankle Int 17:470–472, 1996.
40. Birke JA, Sims DA, Buford WL: Walking casts: Effect of plantar foot pressures. J Rehabil Res Dev 22:18–22, 1985.
41. Beuker BJ, Van Deursen RW, Price P, et al: Plantar pressure in off-loading devices used in diabetic ulcer treatment. Wound Rep Reg 13:537–542, 2005.
42. Hartsell HD, Fellner C, Saltzman CL: Pneumatic bracing and total contact casting have equivocal effects on plantar pressure relief. Foot Ankle Int 22(6):502–506, 2001.
43. Sinacore DR: Total-contact casting for diabetic neuropathic ulcers. Phys Ther 76:296–301, 1996.
44. Brenner MA: An ambulatory approach to the neuropathic ulceration. J Am Podiatry Assoc. 64:862, 1974.
45. Boninger ML, Leonard JA: Use of bivalved ankle foot-orthosis in neuropathic foot and ankle lesions. J Rehabil Res Dev 33:16–22, 1996.
46. Griffiths GD, Wieman TJ: Meticulous attention to foot care improves the prognosis in diabetic ulceration of the foot. Surg Gynecol Obstet 174:49–51, 1992.
47. Wieman TJ, Becaplermin Gel Studies Group: Clinical efficacy of Becaplermin (rh PDGF-BB) gel. Am J Surg 176(suppl 2A): 74S–79S, 1998.
48. Holstein P, Larsen K, Sager P: Decompression with the aid of insoles in the treatment of diabetic neuropathic ulcers. Acta Orthop Scand 47:463–468, 1976.
49. Wieman TJ, Griffiths GD, Polk HC: Management of diabetic midfoot ulcers. Ann Surg 215:627–632, 1992.
50. Wagner FW: Treatment of the diabetic foot. Compr Ther 10:29–38, 1984.
51. Sinacore DR: Neuropathic plantar ulcers in patients with diabetes mellitus. PT: Magazine Phys Ther 6:58–66, 1998.
52. Guyton GP: An analysis of iatrogenic complications from the total contact cast. Foot Ankle Int 26(11):903–907, 2006.
53. Sinacore DR, Mueller MJ: Total-contact casting for wound management. In Gogia PP (ed): Clinical Wound Management. Thorofare NJ, Slack, 1995, pp 147–162.
54. Cavanagh PR, Derr JA, Ulbrecht JS, et al: Problems with gait and posture in neuropathic patients with insulin-dependent diabetes mellitus. Diabet Med 9(5):469–474, 1992.
55. Simoneau GG, Ulbrecht JS, Derr JA, et al: Postural instability in patients with diabetic sensory neuropathy. Diabetes Care 17: 1411–1421, 1994.
56. Hastings MK, Sinacore DR, Fielder FA, Johnson JE: Bone mineral density during total contact cast immobilization for a patient with neuropathic (Charcot) arthropathy. Phys Ther 85(3):249–256, 2005.
57. Ha VG, Siney H, Hartmann-Heurtier A, et al: Nonremovable, windowed, fiberglass cast boot in the treatment of diabetic plantar ulcers: Efficacy, safety, and compliance. Diabetes Care 26(10): 2848–2852, 2003.
58. Young MJ, Cavanagh PR, Thomas G, et al: The effect of callus removal on dynamic plantar foot pressures in diabetic patients.

59. Diamond JE, Mueller MJ, Delitto A, Sinacore DR: Reliability of a diabetic foot evaluation. Phys Ther 69:797–802, 1989.
60. Armstrong DG, Lavery LA: Elevated peak pressure in patients with Charcot arthropathy. J Bone J Surg Am 80:365–369, 1998.
61. Dhalla R, Johnson JE, Engsberg J: Can the use of a terminal device augment plantar pressure reduction with a total contact cast? Foot Ankle Int 24(6):500–505, 2003.
62. Kelly VE, Mueller MJ, Sinacore DR: Gait characteristics associated with peak plantar pressures. Phys Ther 78:S38–39, 1998.
63. Matricali GA, Deroo K, Dereymaeker G: Outcome and recurrence rate of diabetic foot ulcers treated by a total contact cast: Short-term follow-up. Foot Ankle Int 24(9):680–684, 2003.
64. Mueller MJ, Allen BT, Sinacore DR: Incidence of skin breakdown and higher amputation following transmetatarsal amputation: Implications for rehabilitation. Arch Phys Med Rehabil 76:50–54, 1995.
65. Caravaggi C, Faglia E, De Giglio R, et al: Effectiveness and safety of a non-removable fiberglass off-bearing cast versus a therapeutic shoe in the treatment of neuropathic foot ulcers: A randomized study. Diabetes Care 23(12):1746–1751, 2000.
66. Armstrong DG, Lavery LA, Kimbriel HR, et al: Activity patterns of patients with diabetic foot ulceration: Patients with active ulceration may not adhere to a standard pressure off-loading regimen. Diabetes Care 26(9):2595–2597, 2003.
67. Kosiak M: Etiology and pathology of ischemic ulcers. Arch Phys Med Rehabil 40:62–69, 1959.
68. Hissink RJ, Manning HA, van Baal JG: The MABAL shoe, an alternative method in contact casting for the treatment of neuropathic diabetic foot ulcers. Foot Ankle Int 21(4):320–323, 2000.
69. Birke JA, Pavich MA, Patout CA Jr, Horswell R: Comparison of forefoot ulcer healing using alternative off-loading methods in patients with diabetes mellitus. Adv Skin Wound Care 15(5):210–215, 2002.
70. Zimny S, Reinsch B, Schatz H, Pfohl M: Effects of felted foam on plantar pressures in the treatment of neuropathic diabetic foot ulcers. Diabetes Care 24(12):2153–2154, 2001.
71. Birke JA, Lewis K, Penton A, et al: The effectiveness of a modified wedge shoe in reducing pressure at the area of previous great toe ulceration in individuals with diabetes mellitus. Wounds 16:109–114, 2004.
72. Margolis DJ, Kantor J, Berlin JA: Healing of diabetic neuropathic foot ulcers receiving standard treatment: A meta-analysis. Diabetes Care 22(5):692–695, 1999.
73. Chantelau E, Breuer U, Leisch AC, et al: Outpatient treatment of unilateral diabetic foot ulcers with "half shoes." Diabet Med 10(3):267–270, 1993.
74. Zimny S, Meyer MF, Schatz H, Pfohl M: Applied felted foam for plantar pressure relief is an efficient therapy in neuropathic diabetic foot ulcers. Exp Clin Endocrinol Diabetes 110(7):325–328, 2002.
75. Mueller MJ, Diamond JE, Delitto A, Sinacore DR: Insensitivity, limited joint mobility, and plantar ulcers in patients with diabetes mellitus. Phys Ther 69(6):453–459, 1989.
76. Carlson JM, Hollerbach F, Day B: A calf corset weightbearing ankle-foot orthosis design. J Prosthet Orthot 4(1):41–44, 1991.
77. Raspovic A, Newcombe L, Lloyd J, Dalton E: Effect of customized insoles on vertical plantar pressures in site of previous neuropathic ulceration in the diabetic foot. The Foot 10:133–138, 2000.

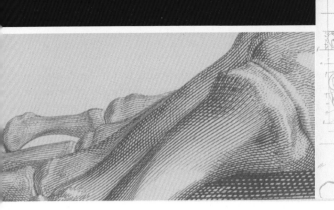

INFECTIOUS PROBLEMS OF THE FOOT IN DIABETIC PATIENTS

BENJAMIN A. LIPSKY ∎

Infections of various types may be more common and are often more severe in patients with diabetes mellitus.[1–4] On the basis of results of a large retrospective cohort study in Canada, nearly half of all people with diabetes have at least one hospitalization or physician visit for an infectious disease each year.[5] The risk ratio for diabetic versus nondiabetic people for infection was 1.21, that for infectious disease-related hospitalization was up to 2.17, and that for death attributable to infection was up to 1.92. Many types of infections, especially serious bacterial infections, were more common in people with diabetes.[5] Foot infections are probably the most common and important of these infections. Diabetic foot infections range in severity from relatively mild to limb-threatening (or even life-threatening). Most require immediate medical attention, including appropriate diagnostic evaluations, various therapeutic modalities, and sometimes hospitalization. Diabetic foot infections and their sequelae are associated with acute, and often long-term, morbidity, including the need for surgical resections and amputations. Almost all infections begin in a wound, often a neuropathic ulceration or traumatic break in the skin envelope. Infections that begin as a minor problem may progress to involve deep soft tissue, joints, or bone, especially if not managed properly.

Because of the substantial morbidity and occasional mortality caused by foot infections, several authoritative groups have recently developed guidelines for assessing and treating these lesions. These guidelines were made possible by studies conducted in the past two decades that have provided data useful for developing a rational approach to dealing with diabetic foot infections. Committees comprising various types of specialists from different countries have now largely agreed on what constitutes the proper approach to diabetic foot infections.[6–12] This chapter reviews the epidemiology, pathophysiology, microbiology, diagnosis and clinical presentation, and treatment of these complex infections.

Epidemiology

Clinical experience and some retrospective reviews have identified several types of infections that occur more frequently in diabetic patients. Soft tissue and foot infections are among the few types that have been shown by controlled observational studies to be significantly associated with diabetes.[1] The relative frequency of foot cellulitis is more than nine times greater in diabetic people than in nondiabetic people.[1] Similarly, osteomyelitis of the foot and ankle account for a greater proportion of hospitalizations of diabetic patients than do bone infections of other locations. Furthermore, the relative proportion of hospitalization for foot osteomyelitis is almost 12 times greater in diabetic people than in nondiabetic people.[1]

As many as a quarter of diabetic patients will develop a foot ulceration at some time in their lives, and depending on the definitions used, perhaps 40% to 80% of these will become infected. In light of the great frequency of foot infections, it is surprising that only recently have two prospective studies investigated the problem. A study from Texas found that among 1666 people with diabetes enrolled in a two-year longitudinal outcomes study in a managed-care–based outpatient clinic, 151 patients (9.1%) developed 199 foot infections.[13] All but one of these infections involved a wound or penetrating injury. Most patients had infections involving only the soft tissue, but 20% had osteomyelitis. The risk of hospitalization and lower-limb amputation was dramatically higher in those who developed a foot infection compared to the diabetic individuals who did not. Significant independent risk factors for foot infection from a multivariate analysis included wounds that penetrated to bone, had a duration of >30 days, were recurrent, or had a traumatic etiology, as well as the presence of peripheral vascular disease.[13] Another study examined the influence of physical, psychological, and social factors on the risk of foot infection. Using a case-control study of 112 people with diabetes, the authors compared those who were hospitalized with a severe foot infection with those who were admitted for a nonemergent medical or surgical cause.[14] Variables that were found to be significant risk factors for severe foot infection were a history of previous amputation, peripheral vascular disease, and peripheral neuropathy, but not social and economic factors.[14]

Fortunately, most foot infections are superficial, but about a quarter will spread contiguously from the skin to the deeper subcutaneous tissues, including bone. Up to half of diabetic individuals who have one foot infection will have another within a few years. Foot ulcerations and infections are now the most common diabetes-related cause of hospitalization in the United States, accounting for almost half of all hospital days. Clinical studies (most of which are retrospective) have reported that 25% to 50% of diabetic foot infections lead to a minor (i.e., foot-sparing) amputation, while 10% to 40% have required major amputations.[8] Other chapters in this textbook deal with the epidemiology of foot ulceration; of importance here is that about 10% to 30% of patients with a diabetic foot ulcer will eventually progress to an amputation, and about 60% of amputations are preceded by an infected foot ulcer. Thus, infection is often the proximate cause leading to this tragic outcome.[15,16]

Pathophysiology

A variety of physiologic and metabolic disturbances conspire to place diabetic patients at high risk for foot wounds. The various predisposing factors, including metabolic derangements, faulty wound healing, neuropathy, and vasculopathy, are covered in other chapters of this text. Microbial colonization of wounds is inevitable, usually with endogenous bacteria, but these are potentially pathogenic in the wound environment.[17] The risk of wound infection increases when local conditions favor bacterial growth rather than host defense. Avoiding infection in a wound is most effectively achieved by clearing devitalized tissue and foreign bodies and ensuring adequate tissue perfusion.[17,18]

Immunologic disturbances are also an important predisposing factor for infections. Among the defects in host immune defenses associated with diabetes are impairments of polymorphonuclear leukocyte functions; these include abnormalities of migration, phagocytosis, intracellular killing, and chemotaxis. Many of these immunodeficiencies are directly related to the metabolic perturbations caused by poorly controlled diabetes. The prevalence of these defects appears to be correlated, at least in part, with the adequacy of glycemic control.[19] Ketosis in particular impairs leukocyte function.[20] Some evidence suggests that in diabetic patients, cellular immune responses and monocyte function are reduced as well.[20] Hyperglycemia also appears to worsen complement function, at least in experimental situations.

Poor granuloma formation, prolonged persistence of abscesses, and impaired wound healing are further accompaniments of diabetes that may predispose to infectious complications. Diabetic patients also appear to have a higher rate of carriage of *Staphylococcus aureus* in their anterior nares and subsequently on the skin.[21] This colonization may predispose to skin infections with this virulent pathogen when there is a break in the protective dermal surface. In addition, several types of skin disorders, as well as skin and nail fungal (tenia) infections, disproportionately plague diabetic patients. In one study, evidence of pedal fungal infection was found in over 80% of people with long-term type 1 diabetes.[22] Fungal infections provide breaks in the cutaneous envelope that then offer potential sites for bacterial invasion.

The unique anatomy of the foot is among the reasons that infection is potentially so serious in this location.[23–25] The structure of the various compartments, tendon sheaths, and neurovascular bundles tends to favor the proximal spread of infection. The deep plantar space of the foot is divided into medial, central, and lateral compartments. Because rigid fascial and bony structures bound these compartments, edema associated with an acute infection may rapidly elevate compartment pressures, causing ischemic necrosis of the confined tissues.[26] Infection may spread from one compartment to another at their proximal calcaneal convergence or by direct perforation of septae, but lateral or dorsal spread is a late sign of infection.[26]

Microbiologic Considerations

Definitions

The skin is coated with bacteria present in a harmless association known as *colonization*; many of these organisms are present permanently, but some may be transient. Bacteria that are most often isolated from skin and soft tissue infections, such as *S. aureus* or β-hemolytic streptococci, are rarely resident on intact skin but may be present transiently and will rapidly colonize disrupted epithelium. When microbial multiplication ensues, with local tissue destruction and release of bacterial toxins inciting a host response, the wound is defined as *infected*. Infection may either follow colonization or occur as a primary event, for example, in the setting of acute trauma. Infection involves the invasion of host tissues by microorganisms (*pathogens*), with a subsequent host inflammatory response (erythema, induration, pain or tenderness, warmth, loss of function, purulent secretions). Some believe that findings such as foul odor, tissue friability, and lack of granulation tissue also suggest infection. In a wound, factors such as the number and types of microorganisms, their interactions with each other and with the wound environment, vascular status, and host resistance collectively influence whether or not the wound heals or becomes infected.[27] Superficial infection is confined to soft tissues external to the fascia (i.e., skin and subcutaneous fat), while deep infection involves invasion of fascia, muscle, tendon, joint, or bone. Infection may be due to a single organism (monomicrobial) or more than one (polymicrobial).

Bacteria are broadly divided into groups defined by their cell wall reaction with Gram's stain (positive or negative), their requirement for oxygen (aerobes or obligate anaerobes), and their morphology (bacilli [or rods] or cocci). The predominant bacteria of normal skin are gram-positive aerobes, particularly the low-virulence coagulase-negative staphylococci, α-hemolytic streptococci, and corynebacteria (short rods). When skin is abnormal (e.g., with eczema or psoriasis) or when the patient has certain underlying diseases (e.g., diabetes), the colonizing flora become more complex; virulent aerobic gram-positive cocci, notably *S. aureus* and β-hemolytic streptococci, may flourish. Antibiotic therapy can also alter the colonizing flora of skin or wounds, favoring organisms that are resistant to the agent administered. Lesions that have been infected for a short time tend to be monomicrobial and to be caused by gram-positive pathogens.[28,29] Chronic wounds develop complex flora, with aerobic gram-negative rods, anaerobes (gram-positive and negative), and enterococci, in addition to the gram-positive aerobes.[30] Fungi (including *Candida* and *Tenia* species) also appear to disproportionately colonize the skin of diabetic patients.[31]

Wound Cultures

Culturing a clinically uninfected wound is unnecessary unless the purpose is to seek the presence of an epidemiologically significant organism (e.g., methicillin-resistant *S. aureus*). When a wound is clinically infected, defining the microbiological cause(s) will usually assist in subsequent management. A culture will identify the etiologic agent(s), but only if specimens are collected and processed properly. Since it is necessary to traverse the skin or superficial layers of a wound to obtain wound samples, they may become contaminated with colonizers. Therefore, some argue that culturing a diabetic foot infection is futile, as "mixed flora" usually grow. Such a report, however, generally reflects a poorly obtained specimen. Cleansing and debriding the wound before obtaining a tissue specimen (see below) will lessen the likelihood of an unhelpful microbiology report. Certainly, patients with severe, long-standing, or complicated infections or who have already received antibiotic therapy may have polymicrobial infections. Even in this situation, however, culture and sensitivity results generally help to tailor (and in many cases constrain) antibiotic regimens. In antibiotic-naive patients with an uncomplicated infection, growth of staphylococci, streptococci, or both is the rule. But even in this situation, the rising prevalence of antibiotic-resistant organisms (especially methicillin-resistant *S. aureus*) makes obtaining antibiotic sensitivity results potentially useful.

Culture specimens are sometimes defined by how likely the results are to be reliable.[32] Deep tissue specimens that are obtained aseptically at surgery are more likely to contain only the true pathogens than cultures of superficial lesions.[33] Clinicians frequently culture superficial wounds by rolling a cotton swab across the surface, often without prior cleansing or debriding. This lesion will contain the total colonizing flora from which the infecting organisms originated, lowering the culture's specificity. Furthermore, the hostile environment of the air-filled cotton swab inhibits growth of anaerobes and fastidious organisms, lowering sensitivity. A curettage or tissue scraping from the base of a debrided ulcer provides more accurate results than a swab.[28,34] Specimens should be promptly submitted to the microbiology laboratory and cultured for both aerobes and anaerobes. Interpreting culture results requires clinical correlation and judgment.[10] Therapy directed against organisms grown from a swab culture is likely to be unnecessarily broad and may occasionally miss key pathogens. If multiple organisms are isolated, the clinician must decide which require specifically targeted therapy. Less virulent bacteria, such as enterococci, coagulase-negative staphylococci, or corynebacteria, can sometimes be ignored, although they may also represent infecting organisms. In general, organisms isolated from reliable specimens that are the sole or predominant pathogens on both the

Gram-stained smear and culture are likely to be true pathogens.

Mild infections occurring in patients who have not previously received antibiotic therapy are usually caused by only one or two species of bacteria, almost invariably aerobic gram-positive cocci. *S. aureus* is by far the most important pathogen in diabetic foot infections; even when it is not the sole isolate, it is usually a part of a mixed infection. Serious infections in hospitalized patients are often caused by three to five bacterial species, including both aerobes and anaerobes.[29,34] Gram-negative bacilli, mainly Enterobacteriaceae, are found in many patients with chronic or previously treated infections. *Pseudomonas* species are often isolated from wounds that have been soaked in water or treated with wet dressings, while enterococci are commonly cultured from patients who have previously received a cephalosporin, a class of antibiotics to which they are inherently resistant. Some data suggest that directing therapy at either of these organisms in diabetic foot infections might be unnecessary.[35] Obligate anaerobic species are most frequent in ischemic wounds with necrosis or that involve deep tissues. Anaerobes are rarely the sole pathogen but most often participate in a mixed infection with aerobes. Antibiotic-resistant organisms, especially methicillin-resistant *S. aureus*, are frequent in patients who have previously received antibiotic therapy; they are often (but not always) acquired during previous hospitalizations or at chronic care facilities.[36-38]

Diagnosis and Clinical Presentation

Diagnosing Infection

Because all skin wounds will be colonized with microorganisms, infection is diagnosed clinically (i.e., by the presence of purulent secretions or two or more signs or symptoms of inflammation), not microbiologically. Infection should be suspected at the first appearance of a local foot problem (e.g., pain, swelling, ulceration, sinus tract formation, or crepitation), a systemic infection (e.g., fever, rigors, vomiting, tachycardia, confusion, malaise), or a metabolic disorder (severe hyperglycemia, ketosis, azotemia). It should be considered even when the local signs are less severe than might be expected.[39] In some instances, inflammatory signs may be caused by such noninfectious disorders as gout or acute Charcot disease.[40] On the other hand, some uninflamed ulcers may be associated with underlying osteomyelitis.[41] Signs of systemic toxicity, including fever and leukocytosis, generally do not accompany diabetic foot infections,[42] even in patients with limb-threatening infections.[43]

Properly evaluating a diabetic foot infection requires a methodical approach, including the elements listed in Table 14-1. It is distressing that even in university-affiliated teaching hospitals, the great majority of dia-

TABLE 14-1   Recommended Evaluation of a Diabetic Patient with a Foot Infection*

Describe the lesion (cellulitis, ulcer, etc.) and any drainage (serous, purulent, etc.).
Enumerate the presence or absence and degree of various signs of inflammation.
Define whether or not infection is present and attempt to determine probable cause.
Examine the soft tissue for evidence of crepitus, abscesses, sinus tracts, foreign bodies.
Probe any skin breaks with sterile metal probe to see whether bone is exposed or palpable.
Measure the wound (length × width; estimate depth); consider taking photograph.
Palpate and record pedal pulses; use Doppler instrument if necessary.
Evaluate neurological status: protective sensation, motor and autonomic function.
Cleanse and debride the wound; remove any foreign material, eschar, or callus.
Culture the cleansed wound (preferably by curettage, aspiration, rather than swab).
Order plain radiographs of the infected foot in most cases; consider other imaging as needed.
Consider which consultants might need to see the patient and how quickly.

* Listed in the approximate order in which they are to be done; not all procedures are necessary in all patients.

betic patients with acute foot infection do not have even a minimally acceptable evaluation.[44] When infection is considered, the diagnosis should be pursued aggressively, as these infections can worsen quickly, sometimes in a few hours. While infection is diagnosed largely on clinical grounds, it can be aided by laboratory investigations. The latter may include hematologic, serologic, imaging, or other tests. The most important of the laboratory tests involve visualizing (on Gram-stained smear) and culturing microorganisms from samples of tissue, blood, body fluids, or pus.

Clinical Presentation

The clinical characteristics of patients with diabetic foot infections are similar in most reported series.[10] Their average age is about 60 years, and most have had diabetes for 15 to 20 years. Almost two thirds of patients have evidence of peripheral vascular disease (absence of pedal pulses), and about 80% have lost protective sensation in the feet. Infections most often involve the forefoot, especially the toes and metatarsal heads, particularly the plantar surface. About half of the patients in reported series have received antibiotic therapy for the foot lesion by the time they present, and up to one third have had their foot lesion for over a month. Many patients do not report pain with an infection because of their sensory neuropathy, but the new onset of pain in a previously neuropathic foot is ominous. More than half of all patients, including those with serious infections, lack a fever, elevated white blood cell count, or elevated erythrocyte sedimentation rate.[42,45]

Assessing Severity

Several classification systems have been proposed for diabetic foot lesions, none of which is universally accepted.[46,47] While the Wagner system has been the most used, it is imprecise, and only grade 3 addresses infection. The key factors in classifying a foot infection are assessing the depth of the wound (by both visually inspecting the tissues involved and estimating depth in millimeters), the presence of ischemia (absent pulses or diminished blood pressure in the foot), and the presence of infection.[48] The University of Texas system incorporates these features and has been validated in prospective studies.[49] A simple clinical classification of infections is shown in Table 14-2. Moderately severe infections may be limb-threatening, while severe infections may be life-threatening.

Assessing infection severity is essential in selecting an antibiotic regimen. This influences the route of drug administration and need for hospitalization. Severity also helps in assessing the potential necessity and timing of surgery. The wound should be carefully explored to determine its depth and to seek foreign or necrotic material, and it should be probed with a sterile metal instrument. Because of the anatomy of the foot, deep space infections often have deceptively few signs in the plantar or dorsal aspects. On the contrary, the presence of dorsal foot swelling or erythema in a patient with a plantar foot lesion should suggest that the infection involves the intervening deep tissues. Therefore, it is cru-cial that a patient with even mild swelling of the foot but with systemic toxicity be evaluated by a knowledgeable surgeon for an occult deep space infection.[26] Evidence of systemic toxicity or metabolic instability generally signifies a serious infection. In these instances, one should consider the possibility of potentially life-threatening necrotizing soft tissue infection. Clinical features that help to define the severity of infection are shown in Table 14-3.

One of the first decisions the clinician must make is determining which patients with a diabetic foot infection should be hospitalized. Virtually all patients with a severe infection, as well as most of those who need parenteral therapy, should be admitted. They might require special diagnostic studies, surgical interventions, fluid resuscitation, and control of metabolic derangements. Hospitalization should also be considered if the patient is unable or unwilling to perform proper wound care or if the patient cannot or will not be able to off-load the affected area. Furthermore, patients who are thought to be unlikely to comply with antibiotic therapy or who need close monitoring of response to treatment might need hospitalization. In the absence of these factors, most patients can be treated cautiously on an outpatient basis, with frequent reevaluation (i.e., every few days initially). Wound care (debridement, dressings, etc.) and glycemic control should be optimized; antibiotics will not overcome poor foot care. This is also an opportune time to review with the patient how to prevent future foot complications.

TABLE 14-2   Simple Clinical Classification of Severity of Diabetic Foot Infections

	Superficial Ulcer or Cellulitis Present	Deep Soft Tissue or Bone Involved	Tissue Necrosis or Gangrene Present	Systemic Toxicity or Metabolic Instability Present
Mild	√	—	±	—
Moderate	√	± (No gas or fasciitis)	± (Minimal)	—
Severe	√	±	±	√

√ = present; ± = may or may not be present; — = not present.

Bone Infection

Diabetic patients may have destructive bone changes caused by peripheral neuropathy that are called neuroarthropathy, osteoarthropathy, or Charcot disease. These disorders can be difficult to distinguish from those caused by bone infection. Bone infection generally results from contiguous spread of a deep soft tissue infection through the cortex (osteitis) to the bone marrow (osteomyelitis). While many diabetic patients with foot osteomyelitis have peripheral vascular insufficiency, this is not the major pathophysiologic issue in their infection. About 50% to 60% of serious foot infections are

TABLE 14-3   Clinical Characteristics That Help to Define the Severity of an Infection

Feature	Mild Infection	Serious Infection
Presentation	Slowly progressive	Acute or rapidly progressive
Ulceration	Involves skin only	Penetrates to subcutaneous tissues
Tissues involved	Epidermis and dermis	Fascia, muscle, tendon, joint, bone
Cellulitis	Minimal (<2-cm rim)	Extensive, or distant from ulceration
Local signs	Slight inflammation	Severe inflammation, crepitus, bullae
Systemic signs	None or minimal	Fever, chills, hypotension, confusion, volume depletion, leukocytosis
Metabolic control	Mildly abnormal (hyperglycemia)	Severe hyperglycemia, acidosis, azotemia, electrolyte abnormalities
Foot vasculature	Minimally impaired (normal/reduced pulses)	Absent pulses, reduced ankle or toe blood pressure
Complicating features	None or minimal (callus, ulcer)	Gangrene, eschar, foreign body, abscess, marked edema, osteomyelitis

complicated by osteomyelitis.[50,51] The proportion of apparently mild to moderate infections that have bone involvement is probably in the range of 10% to 20%. There are no validated or well-accepted guidelines for diagnosing or treating diabetic foot osteomyelitis. Among the important considerations are the anatomic site of infection (i.e., forefoot, midfoot, or hindfoot), the vascular supply to the area, the extent of soft tissue involvement, the presence of bone necrosis, the degree of systemic illness, and the patient's preferences.

All patients with a deep or long-standing ulcer or infection (especially if it is located over a bony prominence) should be clinically evaluated for possible osteomyelitis. Larger (>2 cm) and deeper (>3 mm) ulcers are more often associated with underlying osteomyelitis. Similarly, a swollen, erythematous digit ("sausage toe") suggests underlying osteomyelitis.[52] A substantially elevated erythrocyte sedimentation rate (>70 mm/hour) increases the likelihood of bone infection.[53,54] Clinical evaluation should include probing to bone.[55] Contacting a bony surface with a sterile metal probe has a high positive predictive value for osteomyelitis, at least in patients with a high pretest probability of disease.

Various imaging modalities can be used to assess for the presence of osteomyelitis.[56] Plain radiographs should be ordered for most patients with a diabetic foot infection except perhaps those with just cellulitis or an acute superficial ulcer. Roentgenographic changes generally take at least 2 weeks after bone infection to be evident, giving them a sensitivity of only about 55%.[57,58] The specificity of plain radiographs is about 75%, the characteristic changes including focal osteopenia, cortical erosions, or periosteal reaction early and sequestration of sclerotic bone late. When there is doubt about bone infection but the patient is stable, repeating a plain radiograph in a couple of weeks is probably more cost-effective than scanning procedures.

If clinical and plain radiographic findings do not confidently diagnose or exclude osteomyelitis, other imaging procedures can be useful.[59,60] Bone (e.g., technetium-99) scans are sensitive (~85%), but because they show increased uptake with noninfectious bone disorders they are too nonspecific (~45%). Leukocyte (e.g., indium-111 or ^{99m}Tc-hexamethyl propylenamine oxime) scans are similarly sensitive but more specific (~75%). Unlike bone scans, leukocyte scans may be useful for defining when infection has been arrested, but they are complicated and time consuming. Combining bone and leukocyte scans increases the accuracy and the localization of infection but also the cost. Radiolabeled antigranulocyte fragments (e.g., sulesomab) and ^{99m}Tc-dextran scintigraphy are newer techniques that may increase the accuracy of scanning.[61,62] Other newer diagnostic techniques that show promise are high-resolution ultrasound and positron emission tomography.[63] However, magnetic resonance imaging is probably now the diagnostic procedure of choice, with a sensitivity of over 90% and a specificity of over 80%.[64–66] Magnetic resonance imaging has the advantage of offering high-resolution views of not only bone but also soft tissue, allowing observation of sinus tracts and abscesses. Its limitations include the fact that early cortical infection may be missed and the fact that marrow edema or evolving neuropathic osteoarthropathy can cause false-positive results. The diagnostic test characteristics of all of these procedures exhibit high variation across studies, and their interpretation is greatly influenced by the pretest probability of disease.[60]

While clinical observations and imaging tests are useful, definitively diagnosing osteomyelitis and identifying the etiologic agent require obtaining bone for culture and histology. Several recent studies have shown that soft tissue specimens do not accurately reflect the pathogens in the bone.[67–71] Bone specimens may be obtained by open (e.g., at the time of debridement or surgery) or percutaneous (usually image-guided) biopsy. These procedures are both easy to perform and safe in experienced hands, although somewhat expensive. To avoid contamination, specimens must be obtained without traversing an open wound. Patients who are receiving antibiotic therapy may have a negative culture, but the presence on histopathology of inflammatory cells or necrosis can help to diagnose infection. Bone biopsy is most often needed if doubt remains after other diagnostic tests have been performed or if the etiologic agent(s) cannot be predicted because of confusing culture results or previous antibiotic therapy. Microbiologic studies of diabetic foot osteomyelitis have uniformly found that *S. aureus* is the most common etiologic agent (isolated in about 40% of infections); *S. epidermidis* (~25%), streptococci (~30%), and Enterobacteriaceae (~40%) are also common isolates in osteomyelitis, and some studies have found that the majority of cases are polymicrobial.[59]

Treatment

Debridement and Surgery

Minor

Almost all infected foot lesions (other than primary cellulitis) must be debrided.[72,73] Any appropriately trained health care professional should be able to perform this task safely. Debridement is aimed at removing any eschar (full-thickness dead skin), other necrotic tissue or foreign material, or surrounding callus. This procedure helps to fully evaluate the wound, prepare the wound for more accurate cultures, allow penetration of any topical agents applied, and hasten wound healing. It also serves to turn a chronic wound into an acute wound, which is more likely to heal.[6] Debridement is best done mechanically (i.e., with instruments) rather than with enzymatic or chemical agents. Sharp debridement for minor foot wounds can usually be done in the clinic or at the bedside; most patients are sufficiently neuropathic that local anesthesia is not required. Use a scalpel or scissors to progressively pare away callus and remove all undermining or to saucerize the wound. Some use tissue nippers for more aggressive debridement, sometimes including removing exposed bone. Definitive debridement will often require more than one session or need to be repeated at follow-up visits. One form of debridement therapy that is used in some patients with diabetic foot wounds is so-called larval (or maggot) biotherapy.[74,75] Studies have generally found this form of therapy to be safe and effective. One study even demonstrated that fewer days of antibiotic therapy were required in patients who were treated with maggot debridement.[76] It is important that clinicians caring for diabetic foot wounds understand that failure to adequately debride a wound is a common cause of persistent infection and lack of healing.

Surgical

Patients with deeper infections often need surgical debridement. Early surgical intervention can reduce the duration of antibiotic therapy, decrease the need for major amputations, and more quickly restore full ambulation.[77] The presence of pus in an enclosed space requires drainage. Similarly, fulminant soft tissue infections, such as gas gangrene or necrotizing fasciitis, require urgent debridement of involved tissue. Conditions within an abscess hamper the effectiveness of both polymorphonuclear leukocytes and antibiotics. Ischemic tissue cannot receive leukocytes or systemic antibiotics. Finally, dead tissue (especially bone) that cannot be quickly resorbed or remodeled provides a surface to which bacteria can adhere. There, they can establish complex communities of organisms enmeshed in an exocellular glycocalyx (a biofilm), which is remarkably resistant to most antibiotics.

The extent of the tissue destruction might not be apparent at first inspection. All deep compartments that are involved by infection must be opened. Necrotizing infections of the superficial or deeper tissues require rapid, thorough surgical debridement. Diabetic patients tolerate surgical excisions and drainage much better than they do undrained pus.[78] In the appropriate treatment setting, a surgeon with knowledge of foot anatomy should drain any areas of suspected infection, regardless of the patient's circulatory status. Patients with systemic toxicity will not improve until the wound has been adequately surgically debrided and thoroughly drained. While attempts should be made to conserve healthy tissue for later reconstruction, small stab wounds or inserting drains cannot usually accomplish adequate debridement and drainage.[78] Unfortunately, in some cases, limb salvage or reconstruction is not feasible, and amputation might be the only option. Experienced surgeons stress that amputation surgery should be the first step in the rehabilitation of a patient with a nonfunctional limb rather than the final step in treatment.[79]

Antibiotic Therapy

A recent systematic review undertook an extensive search for the evidence for antimicrobial interventions for treating diabetic foot ulcers as of the end of 2002.[80] The authors found 23 randomized controlled trials or controlled clinical trials of the effectiveness of various parenteral, oral, and topical agents, but these trials were small and too dissimilar to be pooled. The authors concluded that there was no strong evidence supporting any particular antimicrobial agent for resolving infection, healing an ulcer, or preventing amputation. While awaiting the large studies of effectiveness of antimicrobial interventions that the authors of this review called for, clinicians must make choices for treating diabetic foot infections.

Indications for Therapy

About 40% to 60% of diabetic patients who are treated for a foot ulcer receive antibiotic therapy.[81] Although some practitioners believe that any foot ulcer requires administering antibiotics, either for therapy or for prophylaxis, available data do not generally support this view. In most of the published clinical trials, antibiotic therapy did not improve the outcome of uninfected lesions.[82] One unpublished study, however, reported that in a small randomized trial, antibiotic therapy of uninfected foot ulcers increased the likelihood of healing and reduced the incidence of clinical infection, hospitalization, and amputation.[83] While provocative, this work would need to be replicated before this strategy is adopted. Antibiotic therapy is associated with frequent adverse effects, substantial financial costs, and potential harm to the local and global microbial ecology. In view of these undesirable outcomes, for now, antibiotic therapy should probably be used only to treat established infection.

Route of Therapy

Antibiotics should usually be given intravenously for patients who are systemically ill, have a severe infection, are unable to tolerate oral agents, or are known or suspected to have pathogens that are not susceptible to available oral agents. After the patient has been stabilized and the infection is responding, usually in about 3 to 5 days, most patients can be switched to oral therapy. Patients who require more prolonged intravenous therapy (e.g., for bacteremia, osteomyelitis, or infections that are resistant to oral agents) can often be treated on an outpatient basis when a program to provide ambulatory parenteral therapy is available.[84]

Of note is that in patients with peripheral vascular disease, therapeutic antibiotic concentrations with many agents are often not achieved in the infected tissues, even when serum levels are adequate.[85–87] These observations have led to experimentation with novel methods of antibiotic therapy. In one procedure, called retrograde venous perfusion, antibiotic solutions are injected under pressure into a foot vein while a sphygmomanometer is inflated on the thigh. High local antibiotic concentrations have been observed in anecdotal and uncontrolled reports. Some clinicians have also tried lower-limb intraarterial antibiotic administration. For infections that have undergone surgical tissue resection, antibiotic (usually an aminoglycoside)-loaded beads or cement have been used in some instances to fill the dead space and to supply high local antibiotic concentrations. More recently, some clinicians have used antibiotic-laden calcium sulfate beads.[88] None of these therapies has been adequately evaluated and cannot currently be routinely recommended.

Oral antibiotic therapy is less expensive and more convenient than parenteral therapy, and for patients who do not meet the criteria listed above, it is usually sufficient. Several newly licensed agents, particularly fluoroquinolones[89,90] and linezolid,[91] expanded the spectrum of organisms that can be treated. The bioavailability of oral antibiotics is variable, and diabetic patients may absorb oral medications poorly. Fortunately, some drugs (e.g., clindamycin, metronidazole, linezolid, and the fluoroquinolones) are well absorbed on oral dosing. Fluoroquinolones in particular usually achieve high tissue concentrations in diabetic foot infections when administered orally, even in patients with gastroparesis.

For mildly infected foot ulcers, an additional option is topical therapy. This approach has several theoretical advantages, including high local drug levels, avoidance of systemic antibiotic adverse effects, and the possibility of using novel agents not available for systemic use.[92] Furthermore, this route draws the attention of both the patient and physician to the foot and to the need for good wound care. Antiseptics (e.g., povidone-iodine or chlorhexidine) are generally not recommended, as they might be too harsh on the host tissues. Topical antibiotics, however, might have a role. Several agents, including silver sulfadiazine, neomycin, polymixin B, gentamicin, and mupirocin, have been used for soft tissue infections in other sites, but there are no published data on their efficacy in diabetic foot infections. Silver compounds have been incorporated into several preparations and dressings for the treatment of diabetic foot wounds, but to date, there have been no randomized or controlled clinical trials evaluating their clinical effectiveness.[93] An investigational peptide antibiotic, pexiganin acetate 1% cream (MSI-78), has been shown, in two large phase III randomized trials, to be safe and nearly as effective (about 85% to 90% clinical response rate) as oral ofloxacin for mildly infected diabetic foot ulcers.[94] These results are encouraging, and other novel topical antimicrobial therapies are being explored, including an antibiotic-impregnated bovine collagen sponge.

Choice of Antibiotic Agents

Most patients will begin antibiotic therapy with an empiric regimen, pending the results of wound cultures. This therapy should aim to cover the most common pathogens, with some modification according to infection severity.[10] Relatively narrow-spectrum agents may be used for mild infections, as there is likely to be time to modify treatment if there is no clinical response. Regimens for severe infection should generally be broader spectrum and most often intravenously administered, because the stakes are higher. Empiric regimens must also take into consideration such factors as patient allergies, renal dysfunction, previous antibiotic therapy, and known local antibiotic sensitivity patterns.

The selected antibiotic regimen should almost always include an agent that is active against staphylococci and streptococci. Previously treated or severe cases might need extended coverage that also includes gram-negative bacilli and *Enterococcus* species. Necrotic, gangrenous, or foul-smelling wounds usually require anti-anaerobic therapy. When culture and sensitivity results are available, more specific therapy should be chosen. Narrowerspectrum agents are preferred, but it is important to assess how the infection has been responding to the empiric regimen. If the infection is improving and the patient is tolerating therapy, there might be no reason to change, even if some or all of the isolated organisms are resistant to the agents being used. On the other hand, if the infection is not responding, treatment should be changed to cover all the isolated organisms. If the infection is worsening despite susceptibility of the isolated bacteria to the chosen regimen, reconsider the need for surgical intervention or the possibility that fastidious organisms were missed.

While theoretical and pharmacokinetic considerations are important, the proof of an antibiotic's efficacy is the clinical trial. Agents that have demonstrated clinical effectiveness in prospective studies of diabetic foot infections include the following:

- Penicillin/β-lactamase inhibitor congeners (amoxicillin/clavulanate orally; ampicillin/sulbactam, piperacillin/tazobactam,* and ticarcillin/clavulanate parenterally)
- Cephalosporins (cephalexin orally; cefoxitin and ceftizoxime parenterally)
- Clindamycin (orally and parenterally)
- Fluoroquinolones (ciprofloxacin, ofloxacin, trovafloxacin,* levofloxacin, and moxifloxacin, all both orally and parenterally)
- Carbapenems (imipenem/cilastatin and ertapenem* parenterally)
- Linezolid* (orally and parenterally)
- Daptomycin (parenterally)

---

*Agents with a specific U.S. Food and Drug Administration indication for treating diabetic foot infection.

Overall, the clinical and microbiologic response rates have been similar in trials with the various antibiotics, and no one agent or combination has emerged as most effective. New antibiotics are introduced, and some older ones are made obsolete by the emergence of resistance. Understanding the principles of antibiotic therapy is therefore more important than knowing the specific agents that are currently in vogue. The antimicrobial spectra of several antibiotics, grouped by class, are shown in Table 14-4. While all of the above agents (and others) are approved by the U.S. Food and Drug Administration for treating complicated skin and soft tissue infections, the only drugs that have been specifically approved for diabetic foot infections are shown with asterisks. Unfortunately, problems with hepatotoxicity have led to trovafloxacin being reserved for serious infections in hospitalized or institutionalized patients.

Cost of therapy is also an important factor in selecting an antibiotic regimen. A large prospective study of deep foot infections in Sweden found that antibiotics accounted for only 3% to 5% of the total costs of treatment; costs for topical wound treatments were considerably higher.[95] Variables that explained 95% of the total

treatment costs were the time between diagnosis, the final required procedure and wound healing, and the number of surgical procedures performed.[95] One American study demonstrated that therapy with ampicillin/sulbactam was significantly less expensive than was therapy with imipenem/cilastatin for limb-threatening diabetic foot infections, primarily because of the lower drug and hospitalization costs and less severe side effects associated with the former.[96] Regimens with parenteral agents that can be administered less frequently are likely to be cost-effective and more convenient than those requiring multiple daily doses. We need more comparative trials and economic analyses to further analyze this issue. Published suggestions on specific antibiotic regimens for diabetic foot infections vary but are more alike than different. My recommendations, by type of infection, are given in Table 14-5.

Duration of Therapy

The necessary duration of antibiotic therapy for diabetic foot infections has not been well studied. For mild to moderate infections, a 1- to 2-week course has been

TABLE 14-4 Selected Characteristics of Antibiotics That May Be Used for Diabetic Foot Infections

Antibiotic	Formulation		Relative Activity Against Likely Infection Pathogens			
	Oral	IM/IV	S. aureus[†]	Streptococci	Enterobacteriaceae	Anaerobes
Penicillins						
Penicillin G/V	Yes	Yes	+	++++	+	++
Cloxacillin, dicloxacillin	Yes	No	++++	+++	0	++
Nafcillin, oxacillin, methicillin	No	Yes	++++	+++	0	++
Ampicillin, amoxicillin	Yes	Yes	+	++++	++	++
Mezlocillin, ticarcillin, azlocillin, piperacillin	No	Yes	+	+++	+++	+++
Ampicillin/sulbactam, piperacillin/tazobactam, ticarcillin/clavulanate,	No	Yes	++++	++++	+++	++++
amoxicillin/clavulanate	Yes	No	++++	++++	++	+++
Cephalosporins						
Cephapirin, cefazolin, cefuroxime	No	Yes	++++	++++	++	++
Cephalexin, cefaclor, cephradine	Yes	No	++++	++++	++	++
Cefoxitin, cefotetan, ceftizoxime,	No	Yes	+++	+++	+++	+++
cefotaxime, cefoperazone, ceftriaxone, ceftazidime	No	Yes	+++	+++	++++	++
Aminoglycosides						
Gentamicin, tobramycin, amikacin, netilmicin	No	Yes	+++	0	++++	0
Fluoroquinolones						
Ciprofloxacin, ofloxacin	Yes	Yes	+++	++	++++	0
Levofloxacin	Yes	Yes	+++	+++	++++	+
Moxifloxacin, gatifloxacin	Yes	Yes	++++	++++	++++	+++
Others						
Doxycycline	Yes	Yes	+++	++	++	++
Trimethoprim/sulfamethoxazole	Yes	Yes	+++	++	+++	+
Rifampin	Yes	No	++++	++	0	0
Vancomycin	No	Yes	++++*	+++	0	++
Imipenem/cilastatin, ertapenem	No	Yes	++++	++++	++++	+++
Aztreonam	No	Yes	0	0	++++	0
Linezolid	Yes	Yes	++++*	++++	0	++
Daptomycin	No	Yes	++++*	++++	0	0
Anaerobic agents						
Clindamycin	Yes	Yes	+++	+++	0	++++
Metronidazole	Yes	Yes	0	0	0	++++

Activity: ++++, high = +++, moderate = ++, some = +, little = 0, none.
* = Covers methicillin-resistant staphylococci.
[†] = Methiallin (oxacillin) sensitive strains.

TABLE 14-5 Suggested Antibiotic Regimens for Treating Diabetic Foot Infections*

Severity of Infection	Recommended[†]	Alternative[‡]
Mild/moderate (oral for entire course)	Cephalexin (500 mg qid); or Amoxicillin/clavulanate (875/125 mg bid); or Clindamycin (300 mg tid)	Levofloxacin (500 mg po qd) ± clindamycin (300 mg po tid); or TMP/SMX (2 DS po bid)
Moderate/severe (intravenous until stable, then switch to oral equivalent)	Ampicillin/sulbactam (2.0 gm qid); or Clindamycin (450 mg po qid) + ciprofloxacin (750 mg bid)	Ertapenem (1gm qd); or Linezolid (600 mg bid) ± aztreonam (2 gm tid)
Life-threatening (prolonged intravenous)	Imipenem/cilastatin (500 mg qid)[§] Clindamycin (900 IV mg tid) + tobramycin[§] (5.1 mg/kg/day) + ampicillin (50 mg/kg IV qid)	Vancomycin (15 mg/kg bid) + ceftazidime (1 gm tid) + metronidazole (7.5 mg/kg IV qid)

* Given at usual recommended doses for serious infections; modify for azotemia, etc.
[†] Based on theoretical considerations and available clinical trials.
[‡] Prescribed in special circumstances (e.g., patient allergies, recent treatment with recommended agent, cost considerations).
[§] A similar agent of the same class or generation may be substituted.
TMP/SMX, trimethoprim/sulfamethoxazole.

found to be effective,[28] while for more serious infections, treatment has usually been given for 2 to 4 weeks. Adequate debridement, resection, or amputation of infected tissue can shorten the necessary duration of therapy. In the few patients with diabetic foot infection who develop bacteremia, therapy for at least 2 weeks seems prudent. Antibiotic therapy can generally be discontinued when all signs and symptoms of infection have resolved, even if the wound has not completely healed. Healing of an ulcer is a separate, albeit important, issue in treating diabetic foot infections. Some patients who cannot or will not undergo surgical resection, or who have surgical metalwork at the site of infection, might require prolonged suppressive antibiotic therapy.

Therapy of Osteomyelitis

Antibiotic choices should be based on bone culture results when possible, especially because of the need for long-duration therapy.[97] Soft tissue or sinus tract cultures probably do not accurately predict bone pathogens. If empirical therapy is necessary, the microbiology of osteomyelitis suggests that one should always cover *S. aureus.* Because mixed infections are relatively common, broader coverage should be considered if the history or soft tissue cultures suggest that it is needed. Antibiotics generally do not penetrate well to infected bone, and the number and function of leukocytes in this environment are suboptimal. Thus, treatment of osteomyelitis should usually be parenteral (at least initially) and prolonged (at least 6 weeks). Few data inform the choice of a specific agent for treating osteomyelitis.[98] Cure of chronic osteomyelitis has generally been thought to require removing the infected bone by debridement or resection. Several recent retrospective series have shown, however, that diabetic foot osteomyelitis can be arrested for at least 2 years with antibiotic therapy alone in about two thirds of cases.[99–101] Furthermore, oral antibiotics with good bioavailability (e.g., fluoroquinolones and clindamycin) may be adequate for most, or perhaps all, of

the therapy. Some dispute the view that this form of chronic osteomyelitis can be treated without surgical debridement. A recent large retrospective review found that aggressive surgical debridement and digit amputation and selected use of arterial bypass improved wound healing and limb salvage, while antibiotic therapy alone was associated with worsened outcomes.[102] If all of the infected bone is removed, a shorter course of antibiotic therapy (e.g., 2 weeks) might be sufficient. In some patients, long-term suppressive therapy or intermittent short courses of treatment for recrudescent symptoms are the most appropriate approaches. With a team approach and appropriately applying the principles discussed, some investigators have reported high cure rates in chronic osteomyelitis.[50,51,103]

Adjunctive Therapies

An essential question in managing most diabetic foot infections is "Does the patient need an operation?" This may be incision and drainage, removal of dead tissue, revascularization, or a procedure to alter the mechanics and pressure distribution of the foot. These maneuvers improve the physiologic perturbations, permitting antibiotics and normal host defenses to work together to arrest infection and heal ulceration. Several additional measures have been employed to improve infection resolution, wound healing, and host response. Those for which there are published data are briefly reviewed here.

Recombinant Granulocyte Colony-Stimulating Factor (G-CSF)

A recent meta-analysis found that there are five published randomized controlled studies, with a combined total of 167 patients, of the effect of adding (to usual care, including antibiotic therapy) subcutaneous injections of granulocyte colony-stimulating factor (G-CSF).[104] Adjunctive G-CSF treatment did not appear to hasten the clinical resolution of diabetic foot infection or ulceration, but it was associated with a reduced rate of amputation and other surgical procedures. The small number of patients who needed to be treated to gain these benefits suggests that using G-CSF should be considered, especially in patients with a limb-threatening infection. This expensive drug represents one of several growth factors that are now likely to emerge through biotechnology. Larger trials are needed to define whether, and for whom, these promising compounds can be recommended.

Hyperbaric Oxygen

This treatment is designed to increase oxygen delivery to ischemic tissue, which can help to fight infection and improve wound healing in the high-risk foot. For years, anecdotal and uncontrolled reports have suggested benefit in diabetic foot infections, especially osteomyelitis.[105,106] A meta-analysis of four prospective studies with a combined total of 147 patients concluded that hyperbaric oxygen therapy significantly reduced the risk of major amputation and can improve the chance of healing at 1 year.[107] The authors cautioned, however, that because of the small number of patients, methodologic shortcomings, and poor reporting, these results should be interpreted cautiously. Hyperbaric oxygen is a high-technology, expensive, and limited resource that will remain reserved for severe cases, even if it is further confirmed as effective.

Revascularization

Over the past decade, lower-limb vascular procedures, including angioplasty and bypass grafting, have been shown to be safe and effective for patients with diabetic foot infections. Feet with critical ischemia that once required amputation can now often be saved with these techniques. Improving blood flow may also be crucial to controlling infection in an ischemic foot. While initial debridement must be performed even in the face of poor arterial circulation, revascularization is generally postponed until sepsis is controlled.[108] Waiting for more than a few days in hopes of sterilizing the wound is inappropriate, however, and can result in further tissue loss. Several studies suggest that early recognition and aggressive surgical drainage of pedal sepsis followed by surgical revascularization are critical to achieving maximal limb salvage.[109] Long-term follow-up studies have shown that the presence of diabetes does not influence late mortality, graft patency, or limb salvage rates after lower-limb arterial reconstruction.[110]

Outcome of Treatment

A good clinical response for mild to moderate infections can be expected in 80% to 90% of appropriately treated patients and in 50% to 60% of deeper or more extensive infections. When infection involves deep soft tissue structures or bone, more thorough debridement is usually needed. Bone resections or partial amputations are required in about two thirds of these patients. Most of these amputations can be foot-sparing,[111] and long-term control of infection is achieved in over 80% of cases.[24,112] Many above-ankle amputations can be avoided and the length of hospitalization substantially reduced by aggressive early minor surgical procedures and appropriate antibiotic use.[77] Infection recurs in 20% to 30% of patients, many of whom have underlying osteomyelitis. Factors that predict healing include the absence of exposed bone, a palpable popliteal pulse, a toe pressure of more than 45 mm Hg or an ankle pressure of more than 80 mm Hg, and a peripheral white blood cell count of less than $12,000/mm^3$.[42] The presence of edema or atherosclerotic cardiovascular disease increases the likelihood of an amputation. Patients with combined soft tissue and bone infection might require amputation more often than either type of infection alone.[113] Patients who have had one infection are at substantial risk of having another within a few years; therefore, educating them on prevention techniques and prompt consultation for foot problems is critical.

Summary

Diabetic foot infections are a common, complex, and serious problem with dire financial and medical consequences. Fortunately, we have made much progress in this field in the past two decades. Prospective comparative trials have clarified the proper culture techniques, defined the differences in milder versus more severe infections, delineated the microbiology of these wounds, and shown the effectiveness of several specific antibiotic regimens in treating these infections. Careful prospective studies have shown that patients with mild, non–limb-threatening infections can be treated as outpatients with oral antibiotic therapy. The importance of debridement, surgical interventions, weight off-loading, and local foot care has been confirmed. Methods for diagnosing and treating osteomyelitis have been refined. Vascular surgical procedures have been developed, and their proper role has been defined. Adjunctive therapies are being added to the standard ones previously available. Accumulating evidence suggests that with proper wound care, optimal metabolic control, and early, aggressive, appropriate surgical and antibiotic therapy, infection can be controlled and a functional foot can be preserved in the great majority of patients. The current challenge is not only to continue to develop new treatments but also to marshal existing ones in a seamless, cost-effective, evidence-based, and multidisciplinary manner.

References

1. Boyko EJ, Lipsky BA: Infection and diabetes mellitus. In Harris MI (ed): Diabetes in America, 2nd ed. NIH publication No 95-1468. Bethesda, MD: National Institutes of Health. 1995, pp 485–499.
2. Gleckman RA, Al-Wawi M: A review of selective infections in the adult diabetic. Compr Ther 25:109–113, 1999.
3. Jackson LA: Evaluating diabetes mellitus as a risk factor for community-acquired infections. Clin Infect Dis 41(3):289–290, 2005.
4. Muller LM, Gorter KJ, et al: Increased risk of common infections in patients with type 1 and type 2 diabetes mellitus. Clin Infect Dis 41(3):281–288, 2005.
5. Shah BR, Hux JE: Quantifying the risk of infectious diseases for people with diabetes. Diabetes Care 26(2):510–513, 2003.
6. Cavanagh PR, Buse JB, Frykberg RG, et al, for the American Diabetes Association: Diabetic foot wound care. Census Development Conference. Diabetes Care 22:1354–1360, 1999.
7. Fong IW, for the Committee on Antimicrobial Agents: Management of diabetic foot infection: A position paper. Can J Infect Dis 7:361–365, 1996.
8. International Working Group on the Diabetic Foot: International Consensus on the Diabetic Foot. Amsterdam, May 1999, pp 1–96.
9. Lipsky BA: A report from the international consensus on diagnosing and treating the infected diabetic foot. Diabetes Metab Res Rev 20(suppl 1):S68–S77, 2004.
10. Lipsky BA, Berendt AR, et al: IDSA Guidelines: Diagnosis and treatment of diabetic foot infections. Clin Infect Dis 39:885–910, 2004.
11. Frykberg RG: A summary of guidelines for managing the diabetic foot. Adv Skin Wound Care 18(4):209–214, 2005.
12. Pinzur MS, Slovenkai MP, et al: Guidelines for diabetic foot care: Recommendations endorsed by the Diabetes Committee of the American Orthopaedic Foot and Ankle Society. Foot Ankle Int 26(1):113–119, 2005.
13. Lavery LA, Armstrong DG, Wunderlich RP, et al: Risk factors for foot infection in persons with diabetes. Diabetes Care 6:1288–1293, 2006.
14. Peters EJ, Lavery LA, et al: Diabetic lower extremity infection: Influence of physical, psychological, and social factors. J Diabetes Complications 19(2):107–112, 2005.
15. Pecoraro RE, Ahroni JH, Boyko EJ, Stencil VL: Chronology and determinants of tissue repair in diabetic lower-extremity ulcers. Diabetes 40:1305–1313, 1991.
16. Reiber GE, Pecoraro RE, Koepsell TD: Risk factors for amputation in patients with diabetes mellitus: A case control study. Ann Intern Med 117:97–105, 1992.
17. Bowler PG: Wound pathophysiology, infection and therapeutic options. Ann Med 34(6):419–427, 2002.
18. Levin M: Diabetic foot wounds: Pathogenesis and management. Adv Wound Care 10(2):24–30, 1997.
19. McMahon MM, Bistrian BR: Host defenses and susceptibility to infection in patients with diabetes mellitus. Infect Dis Clin North Am 9:1–10, 1995.
20. Sentochnik DE, Eliopoulos GM: Infection and diabetes. In Kahn CR, Weir GC (eds): Joslin's Diabetes Mellitus, 13th ed. Philadelphia: Lea & Febiger, 1994, pp 867–888.
21. Breen JD, Karchmer AW: Staphylococcus aureus infections in diabetic patients. Infect Dis Clin North Am 9:11–24, 1995.
22. Mayser P, Hensel J, et al: Prevalence of fungal foot infections in patients with diabetes mellitus type 1: Underestimation of moccasin-type tinea. Exp Clin Endocrinol Diabetes 112(5):264–268, 2004.
23. Rauwerda JA: Foot debridement: anatomic knowledge is mandatory. Diabetes Metab Res Rev 16(suppl 1):S23–S26, 2000.
24. Armstrong DG, Lipsky BA: Advances in the treatment of diabetic foot infections. Diabetes Technol Ther 6(2):167–177, 2004.
25. van Baal JG: Surgical treatment of the infected diabetic foot. Clin Infect Dis 39(suppl 2):S123–S128, 2004.
26. Bridges RM, Deitch EA: Diabetic foot infections: Pathophysiology and treatment. Surg Clin North Am 74:537–555, 1994.
27. Bowler PG: The 10(5) bacterial growth guideline: Reassessing its clinical relevance in wound healing. Ostomy Wound Manage 49(1):44–53, 2003.
28. Lipsky BA, Pecoraro RE, Larson SA, Ahroni JH: Outpatient management of uncomplicated lower-extremity infections in diabetic patients. Arch Intern Med 150:790–797, 1990.
29. Lipsky BA, Pecoraro RE, Wheat JL: The diabetic foot: Soft tissue and bone infection. Infect Dis Clin North Am 4:409–432, 1990.
30. Bowler PG, Duerden BI, et al: Wound microbiology and associated approaches to wound management. Clin Microbiol Rev 14(2):244–269, 2001.
31. Tan JS, Joseph WS: Common fungal infections of the feet in patients with diabetes mellitus. Drugs Aging 21(2):101–112, 2004.
32. Wheat LJ, Allen SD, Henry M, et al: Diabetic foot infections: Bacteriologic analysis. Arch Intern Med 146:1935–1940, 1986.
33. Pellizzer G, Strazzabosco M, et al: Deep tissue biopsy vs. superficial swab culture monitoring in the microbiological assessment of limb-threatening diabetic foot infection. Diabet Med 18(10):822–827, 2001.
34. Sapico FL, Witte JL, Canawati HN, et al: The infected foot of the diabetic patient: Quantitative microbiology and analysis of clinical features. Rev Infect Dis 6(suppl 1):171–176, 1984.
35. Lipsky BA, Armstrong DG, et al: Ertapenem versus piperacillin/tazobactam for diabetic foot infections (SIDESTEP): Prospective, randomised, controlled, double-blinded, multicentre trial." Lancet 366(9498):1695–1703, 2005.
36. Dang CN, Prasad YD, et al: Methicillin-resistant Staphylococcus aureus in the diabetic foot clinic: A worsening problem. Diabet Med 20(2):159–161, 2003.
37. Eady EA, Cove JH: Staphylococcal resistance revisited: Community-acquired methicillin resistant Staphylococcus aureus—An emerging problem for the management of skin and soft tissue infections. Curr Opin Infect Dis 16(2):103–124, 2003.
38. Tentolouris N, Petrikkos G, et al: Prevalence of methicillin-resistant Staphylococcus aureus in infected and uninfected diabetic foot ulcers. Clin Microbiol Infect 12(2):186–189, 2006.
39. Williams DT, Hilton JR, et al: Diagnosing foot infection in diabetes. Clin Infect Dis 39(suppl 2):S83–S836, 2004.
40. Pakarinen TK, Laine HJ, et al: Charcot arthropathy of the diabetic foot: Current concepts and review of 36 cases. Scand J Surg 91(2):195–201, 2002.
41. Newman LG, Waller J, Palestro CJ, et al: Unsuspected osteomyelitis in diabetic foot ulcers: Diagnosis and monitoring by leukocyte scanning with indium 111 oxyquinoline. JAMA 266:1246–1251, 1991.
42. Eneroth M, Apelqvist J, Stenstrom A: Clinical characteristics and outcome in 223 diabetic patients with deep foot infections. Foot Ankle Int 18:716–722, 1997.
43. Armstrong DG, Lavery LA, et al: Leukocytosis is a poor indicator of acute osteomyelitis of the foot in diabetes mellitus. J Foot Ankle Surg 35(4):280–283, 1996.
44. Edelson GW, Armstrong DG, Lavery LA, Caicco G: The acutely infected diabetic foot is not adequately evaluated in an inpatient setting. Arch Intern Med 156:2373–2378, 1996.
45. Armstrong DG, Perales TA, Murff RT, et al: Value of white blood cell count with differential in the acute diabetic foot infection. J Am Podiatr Med Assoc 86:224–227, 1996.
46. Pecoraro RE: Diabetic skin ulcer classification for clinical investigations. Clin Mater 8:257–262, 1991.
47. Foster A, Edmonds, ME: Simple staging system: A tool for diagnosis and management. Diabetic Foot 3(2):56–62, 2000.
48. Armstrong DG, Lavery LA, Harkless LB: Validation of a diabetic wound classification system: The contribution of depth, infection, and ischemia to risk of amputation. Diabet Med 21:855–859, 1998.
49. Oyibo SO, Jude EB, et al: A comparison of two diabetic foot ulcer classification systems: The Wagner and the University of Texas wound classification systems. Diabetes Care 24(1):84–88, 2001.
50. Snyder RJ, Cohen MM, et al: Osteomyelitis in the diabetic patient: Diagnosis and treatment. Part 1: Overview, diagnosis, and microbiology. Ostomy Wound Manage 47(1):18–22, 25–30; quiz 31–32, 2001.
51. Snyder RJ, Cohen MM, et al: Osteomyelitis in the diabetic patient: Diagnosis and treatment. Part 2: Medical, surgical, and alternative treatments. Ostomy Wound Manage 47(3):24–30, 32–41; quiz 42–43, 2001.
52. Rajbhandari SM, Sutton M, et al: "Sausage toe": A reliable sign of underlying osteomyelitis. Diabet Med 17(1):74–77, 2000.
53. Kaleta JL, Fleischli JW, et al: The diagnosis of osteomyelitis in diabetes using erythrocyte sedimentation rate: A pilot study. J Am Podiatr Med Assoc 91(9):445–450, 2001.

54. Karr JC: The diagnosis of osteomyelitis in diabetes using erythrocyte sedimentation rate. J Am Podiatr Med Assoc 92(5):314; author reply 314–315, 2002.

55. Grayson ML, Gibbons GW, Balogh K, et al: Probing to bone in infected pedal ulcers: A clinical sign of underlying osteomyelitis in diabetic patients. JAMA 273:721–723, 1995.

56. Sella EJ, Grosser DM: Imaging modalities of the diabetic foot. Clin Podiatr Med Surg 20(4):729–740, 2003.

57. Newman LG: Imaging techniques in the diabetic foot. Clin Podiatr Med Surg 12(1):75–86, 1995.

58. Bonham P: A critical review of the literature: I. Diagnosing osteomyelitis in patients with diabetes and foot ulcers. J Wound Ostomy Continence Nurs 28(2):73–88, 2001.

59. Lipsky BA: Osteomyelitis of the foot in diabetic patients. Clin Infect Dis 25:1318–1326, 1997.

60. Wrobel JS, Connolly JE: Making the diagnosis of osteomyelitis: The role of prevalence. J Am Podiatr Med Assoc 88:337–343, 1998.

61. Harwood SJ, Valdivia S, Hung G-L, Quenzer RW: Use of sulesomab, a radiolabeled antibody fragment, to detect osteomyelitis in diabetic patients with foot ulcers by leukoscintigraphy. Clin Infect Dis 28:1200–1205, 1999.

62. Sarikaya A, Aygit AC, et al: Utility of 99mTc dextran scintigraphy in diabetic patients with suspected osteomyelitis of the foot. Ann Nucl Med 17(8):669–676, 2003.

63. Keidar Z, Militianu D, et al: The diabetic foot: Initial experience with 18F-FDG PET/CT. J Nucl Med 46(3):444–449, 2005.

64. Craig JG, Amin MB, Wu K, et al: Osteomyelitis of the diabetic foot: MR imaging-pathological correlation. Radiology 203:849–855, 1997.

65. Schweitzer ME, Morrison WB: MR imaging of the diabetic foot. Radiol Clin North Am 42(1):61–71, vi, 2004.

66. Chatha DS, Cunningham PM, et al: MR imaging of the diabetic foot: Diagnostic challenges. Radiol Clin North Am 43(4):747–759, ix, 2005.

67. Khatri G, Wagner DK, et al: Effect of bone biopsy in guiding antimicrobial therapy for osteomyelitis complicating open wounds. Am J Med Sci 321(6):367–371, 2001.

68. Zuluaga AF, Galvis W, et al: Lack of microbiological concordance between bone and non-bone specimens in chronic osteomyelitis: An observational study. BMC Infect Dis 2(1):8, 2002.

69. Kessler L, Piemont Y, et al: Comparison of microbiological results of needle puncture vs. superficial swab in infected diabetic foot ulcer with osteomyelitis. Diabet Med 23(1):99–102, 2006.

70. Senneville E, Melliez H, et al: Culture of percutaneous bone biopsy specimens for diagnosis of diabetic foot osteomyelitis: Concordance with ulcer swab cultures. Clin Infect Dis 42(1):57–62, 2006.

71. Zuluaga AF, Galvis W, et al: Etiologic diagnosis of chronic osteomyelitis: A prospective study. Arch Intern Med 166(1):95–100, 2006.

72. Jones V: Debridement of diabetic foot lesions. Diabet Foot 3:88–94, 1998.

73. Smith J, Thow J: Update of systematic review on debridement. Diabetic Foot 6(1):12–16, 2003.

74. Armstrong DG, Mossel J, et al: Maggot debridement therapy: A primer. J Am Podiatr Med Assoc 92(7):398–401, 2002.

75. Claxton MJ, Armstrong DG, et al: 5 questions—and answers—about maggot debridement therapy. Adv Skin Wound Care 16(2):99–102, 2003.

76. Armstrong DG, Salas P, et al: Maggot therapy in "lower-extremity hospice" wound care: Fewer amputations and more antibiotic-free days. J Am Podiatr Med Assoc 95(3):254–257, 2005.

77. Tan JS, Friedman NM, Hazelton-Miller C, et al: Can aggressive treatment of diabetic foot infections reduce the need for above-ankle amputation? Clin Infect Dis 23:286–291, 1996.

78. Gibbons GW, Habershaw GM: Diabetic foot infections: Anatomy and surgery. Infect Dis Clin North Am 9:131–142, 1995.

79. Pinzur MS, Pinto MA, et al: Controversies in amputation surgery. Instr Course Lect 52:445–451, 2003.

80. Nelson EA, O'Meara S, Golder S, et al: Systematic review of antimicrobial treatments for diabetic foot ulcers. Diabet Med (in press), 2006.

81. Jaegeblad G, Apelqvist J, Nyberg P, Berger B: The diabetic foot: From ulcer to multidisciplinary team approach. A process analysis. In Abstracts of the 3rd International Symposium of the Diabetic Foot, Noordwijkerhout, The Netherlands, May 6, 1998, Abstract p87, p 149.

82. Chantelau E, Tanudjaja T, Altenhöfer F, et al: Antibiotic treatment for uncomplicated neuropathic forefoot ulcers in diabetes: A controlled trial. Diabet Med 13:156–159, 1996.

83. Edmonds M, Foster A: The use of antibiotics in the diabetic foot. Am J Surg 187(5A):25S–28S, 2004.

84. Tice A, Hoaglund P, et al: Outcomes of osteomyelitis among patients treated with outpatient parenteral antimicrobial therapy. Am J Med 114(9):723–728, 2003.

85. Raymakers JT, Houben AJ, et al: The effect of diabetes and severe ischaemia on the penetration of ceftazidime into tissues of the limb [online abstract & ms]. Diabetic Medicine 18(3):229–234, 2001.

86. Legat FJ, Maier A, et al: Penetration of fosfomycin into inflammatory lesions in patients with cellulitis or diabetic foot syndrome. Antimicrob Agents Chemother 47(1):371–374, 2003.

87. Oberdorfer K, Swoboda S, et al: Tissue and serum levofloxacin concentrations in diabetic foot infection patients. J Antimicrob Chemother 54(4):836–839, 2004.

88. Armstrong DG, Stephan KT, et al: What is the shelf-life of physician-mixed antibiotic-impregnated calcium sulfate pellets? J Foot Ankle Surg 42(5):302–304, 2003.

89. Greenberg RN, Newman MT, et al: Ciprofloxacin, lomefloxacin, or levofloxacin as treatment for chronic osteomyelitis. Antimicrob Agents Chemother 44(1):164–166, 2000.

90. Edmiston CE, Krepel CJ, et al: In vitro activities of moxifloxacin against 900 aerobic and anaerobic surgical isolates from patients with intra-abdominal and diabetic foot infections. Antimicrob Agents Chemother 48(3):1012–1016, 2004.

91. Lipsky BA, Itani K, et al: Treating foot infections in diabetic patients: A randomized, multicenter, open-label trial of linezolid versus ampicillin-sulbactam/amoxicillin-clavulanate. Clin Infect Dis 38(1):17–24, 2004.

92. Sibbald RG: Topical antimicrobials. Ostomy Wound Manage 49(5A suppl):14–18, 2003.

93. Bergin S, Wraight P: Silver based wound dressings and topical agents for treating diabetic foot ulcers. Cochrane Database Syst Rev 1:CD005082, 2006.

94. Lipsky BA, McDonald D, Litka PA: Treatment of infected diabetic foot ulcers: Topical MSI-78 vs. oral ofloxacin [abstract]. Diabetologia 40(suppl 1):482, 1997.

95. Ragnarson Tennvall G, Apelqvist J, Eneroth M: Costs of deep foot infections: An analysis of factors determining treatment costs. Abstracts of the 3rd International Symposium of the Diabetic Foot. Noordwijkerhout, The Netherlands, May 5–8, 1999, Abstract p 101, p 163.

96. McKinnon PS, Paladino JA, Grayson ML, et al: Cost effectiveness of ampicillin/sulbactam versus imipenem/cilastatin in the treatment of limb-threatening foot infections in diabetic patients. Clin Infect Dis 24:57–63, 1997.

97. Senneville E: Antimicrobial interventions for the management of diabetic foot infections. Expert Opin Pharmacother 6(2):263–273, 2005.

98. Lazzarini L, Lipsky BA, et al: Antibiotic treatment of osteomyelitis: What have we learned from 30 years of clinical trials? Int J Infect Dis 9(3):127–138, 2005.

99. Pittet D, Wyssa B, Herter-Clavel C, et al: Outcome of diabetic foot infections treated conservatively: A retrospective cohort study with long-term follow-up. Arch Intern Med 159:851–856, 1999.

100. Venkatesan P, Lawn S, Macfarlane RM, et al: Conservative management of osteomyelitis in the feet of diabetic patients. Diabetic Med 14:487–490, 1997.

101. Jeffcoate WJ, Lipsky BA: Controversies in diagnosing and managing osteomyelitis of the foot in diabetes. Clin Infect Dis 39(suppl 2):S115–S122, 2004.

102. Henke PK, Blackburn SA, et al: Osteomyelitis of the foot and toe in adults is a surgical disease: Conservative management worsens lower extremity salvage. Ann Surg 241(6): 885–892; discussion 892–894, 2005.

103. Salvana J, Rodner C, et al: Chronic osteomyelitis: Results obtained by an integrated team approach to management. Conn Med 69(4):195–202, 2005.

104. Cruciani M, Lipsky BA, et al: Are granulocyte colony-stimulating factors beneficial in treating diabetic foot infections?: A meta-analysis. Diabetes Care 28(2):454–460, 2005.

105. Chen CE, Shih ST, et al: Hyperbaric oxygen therapy in the treatment of chronic refractory osteomyelitis: A preliminary report. Chang Gung Med J 26(2):114–121, 2003.

106. Stone JA, Cianci P: The adjunctive role of hyperbaric oxygen in the treatment of lower extremity wounds in patients with diabetes. Diabetes Spectrum 10:118–123, 1997.

107. Kranke P, Bennett M, et al: Hyperbaric oxygen therapy for chronic wounds. Cochrane Database Syst Rev 2:CD004123, 2004.

108. Caputo GM, Cavanaugh PR, Ulbrecht JS, et al: Assessment and management of foot disease in patients with diabetes. N Engl J Med 331:854–860, 1994.

109. Sumpio BE, Lee T, et al: Vascular evaluation and arterial reconstruction of the diabetic foot. Clin Podiatr Med Surg 20(4):689–708, 2003.

110. Akbari CM, Pomposelli FB Jr, et al: Lower extremity revascularization in diabetes: late observations. Arch Surg 135(4):452–456, 2000.

111. Van Damme H, Rorive M, et al: Amputations in diabetic patients: A plea for footsparing surgery. Acta Chir Belg 101(3):123–129, 2001.

112. Rauwerda JA: Surgical treatment of the infected diabetic foot. Diabetes Metab Res Rev 20(suppl 1):S41–S44, 2004.

113. Eneroth M, Larsson J, Apelqvist J: Deep foot infection in diabetes mellitus: An entity with different characteristics, treatment and prognosis. J Diabetic Complications 13:254–263, 1999.

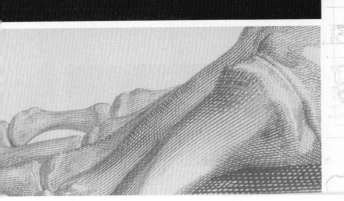

WOUND HEALING IN THE DIABETIC FOOT

KEVIN P. CONWAY AND K. G. HARDING ■

Introduction

Diabetes mellitus results in many complications to the individual, foot ulceration taking the greatest toll. Diabetic foot ulceration precedes lower-limb amputations in 85% of patients. Lower-limb amputation is associated with diabetes in 40% to 90% of cases. In the United States, in excess of 50,000 lower-limb amputations are performed annually in diabetic patients. Diabetic foot complications result in huge costs for both society and individual patients worldwide; in the United States alone, the cost has been estimated to be 4 billion dollars a year.[1] Lower-limb amputation represents a significant economic problem, particularly if amputation results in prolonged hospitalization. The average cost at 3 years for an initial lower-limb amputation has been estimated to be from $43,100 to $63,100.[2] The corresponding cost for individuals with primary healing has been estimated to be $17,500.[3]

The factors related to the development of foot ulcers are peripheral neuropathy, minor foot trauma, and foot deformities.[4] Sixty percent to 70% of diabetic foot ulcers are purely due to peripheral neuropathy, 15% to 20% to peripheral vascular disease, and the remainder to a combination (neuroischemia).[5] Peripheral neuropathy affects all fibers: sensory, motor, and autonomic. Sensory neuropathy leads to a loss of pain, pressure, temperature, and proprioception awareness in the foot. Motor neuropathy affects the nerves to muscles that control

motion of the foot. Autonomic neuropathy impairs the sweat and sebaceous glands, leading to excessive dryness and fissuring of the skin. The areas beneath the first and fifth metatarsal heads are the commonest sites of plantar ulceration in diabetic patients (Fig. 15-1).

Diabetic patients are more prone to complicated foot ulceration owing to thinning of the plantar skin and a reduced ability to withstand infection (Fig. 15-2). Peripheral vascular disease causing arterial insufficiency results in a poor outcome in patients with diabetic foot ulcers (Fig. 15-3). Peripheral vascular disease is present to some degree in most patients with long-standing diabetes. Other risk factors for the development of atherosclerosis are smoking, hyperlipidemia, and hypertension. Diabetic patients are at increased risk for atypical atherosclerosis, the tibial arteries being more commonly affected. Midfoot collapse from Charcot osteoarthropathy often results in a rocker-bottom foot, subject to plantar ulceration.

Wound Healing

Wound healing is an intricately regulated sequence of cellular and biochemical events orchestrated to restore tissue integrity after injury (Fig. 15-4).[6] The wound-healing response involves three distinct but overlapping phases: (1) hemostasis and inflammation, (2) proliferation, and (3) maturation or remodeling (see Fig. 15-4).[7]

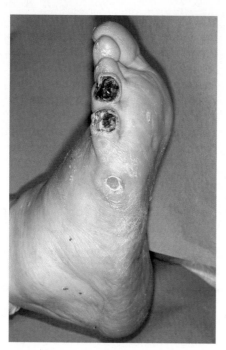

Figure 15–1   Plantar ulcer overlying the lateral aspect of the fifth metatarsal head.

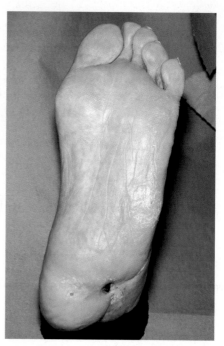

Figure 15–2   Long-standing diabetic foot ulcer of the left lateral heel with thinning of the surrounding plantar skin, complicated by osteomyelitis of the underlying bone.

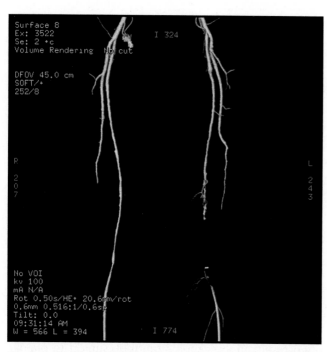

Figure 15–3   Arteriogram of a patient presenting with diabetic foot ulceration. The arteriogram shows a large atherosclerotic plaque occluding the left femoral artery.

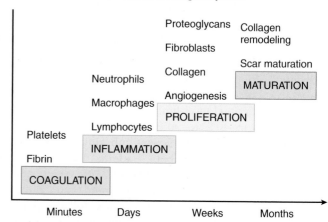

Normal Wound Healing Response

Figure 15–4   Normal wound healing is an intricately regulated sequence of cellular and biochemical events orchestrated to restore tissue integrity after injury.

Each of these phases is controlled by biologically active substances called growth factors.[8] Growth factors are hormone-like polypeptides present in only small amounts in the body that control the growth, differentiation, and metabolism of cells.[9] They interact with specific cell surface receptors to control the process of tissue repair (Fig. 15-5).[10]

Hemostasis and Inflammation Phase

Hemostasis follows the traumatic rupture of blood vessels that exposes subendothelial collagen to platelets, resulting in their aggregation and activation of the intrinsic part of the coagulation cascade.[11] Inflammation is characterized by increased vascular permeability, chemotaxis of cells (e.g., polymorphonuclear cells) from the circulation into the wound milieu, local release of cytokines and growth factors, and activation of migrating cells. The locally formed fibrin clot serves as a scaffolding for invading

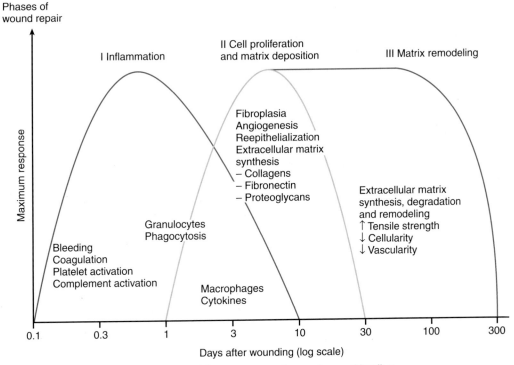

Figure 15-5 Time sequence of normal wound healing.

cells such as neutrophils, monocytes, fibroblasts, and endothelial cells.[12] Neutrophils are the first immune cells to arrive at the wound site, appearing approximately 24 hours after injury.[13] Neutrophil migration is stimulated by the increased vascular permeability and release of prostaglandins together with a concentration gradient of chemotactic substances. The roles of the neutrophil are primarily phagocytosis and wound debridement. Neutrophils are also a source of proinflammatory cytokines that probably serve as early signals to activate local fibroblasts and keratinocytes.[14] Although neutrophils decrease the likelihood of infection in the wound,[15] they are not essential, as their role in phagocytosis and antimicrobial defense may be taken over by macrophages.

Circulating monocytes are attracted to the site of injury by chemotactic factors.[16] There, monocytes differentiate into macrophages.[17] Macrophages migrate into the wound 48 to 96 hours after injury, becoming the predominant cell population prior to fibroblast migration and replication. Macrophages participate in and conclude the inflammatory processes. Their antimicrobial functions include phagocytosis and the generation of reactive free radicals, such as nitric oxide, oxygen, and peroxide. Chemotaxis of cells into the wound milieu is followed by functional activation, that is, a phenotypic alteration of cellular biochemical and functional properties induced by local mediators. The activation of macrophages is due initially to the brief release of growth factors from platelets. Macrophages develop functional complement receptors and undertake similar operations to the neutrophils.[18] However, further interactions

with interferons and subsequently with bacterial or viral products induce further differentiation into a fully active phenotype.[19] Interferons enhance endocytosis and phagocytosis and modulate the surface receptor function of newly migrated macrophages. Wound healing is severely impaired if macrophage infiltration of the wound is prevented.

Proliferation Phase

Early in the healing process, there is no vascular supply to the injured area. Angiogenesis or neovascularization, which is the formation of new blood vessels from existing vessels, and the proliferative phase occur simultaneously.[20] The new tissue matrix is essential to physically support the branching blood vessels arising from the intact vasculature in the surrounding dermis, and angiogenesis is essential to provide the oxygen and nutrients needed for synthesis of collagen and other connective tissues. Therefore, collagen and capillary proliferation occur in a codependent manner.

Fibroblasts and endothelial cells are the primary cells that increase in numbers during this phase. Fibroblasts are responsible for replacing the fibrin matrix (clot) with collagen-rich new matrix for the developing granulation tissue. In addition, fibroblasts produce and release proteoglycans and glycosaminoglycans, which are also important components of the extracellular matrix of granulation tissue. Once sufficient collagen matrix has been deposited in the wound, the fibroblasts stop producing collagen.

Angiogenesis is a fundamental biological mechanism that is reactivated during wound healing and repair.[21] This process is characterized by the invasion, migration, and proliferation of endothelial cells. Endothelial cells from the side of the vessel closest to the wound begin to migrate in response to angiogenic stimuli. Cytoplasmic pseudopods sprout into the wound space, and subsequently, the entire endothelial cell migrates into the perivascular space. Eventually, their tips join to form a new capillary plexus within the granulation tissue. Endothelial cells remaining in the original vessel also proliferate, adding to the numbers of migrating cells.[22] The growing endothelial cells produce a degradation enzyme, plasminogen activator, and hence are able to carve their way through the matrix (Fig. 15-6).[23]

Several biological stimuli for angiogenesis have been identified. Platelet, macrophage, lymphocyte, and keratinocyte products including fibroblast growth factors a and b (aFGF, bFGF), transforming growth factors α and β (TGF-α and TGF-β), epidermal growth factor, hepatocyte growth factor, and interleukin-1 have all been shown to be potent stimuli for new vessel formation.[24,25]

Hypoxia following injury creates an oxygen gradient between the vascularized periphery and the wound bed center, encouraging proliferation as well as stimulating the release of angiogenic factors from macrophages.[26] Lactate and the extracellular matrix proteins laminin and fibrinogen also mediate endothelial cell growth and chemotaxis.[27]

To migrate during wound healing, the basement membrane zones of blood vessels express several adhesive proteins, including von Willebrand factor, fibronectin, and fibrin. Endothelial cells upregulate the expression of $\alpha_v\beta_3$ integrin adhesion receptor for von Willebrand factor, fibrinogen, and fibronectin.[28] This integrin initiates a calcium-dependent signaling pathway leading to endothelial cell migration.[29]

T-lymphocytes migrate into the wound after inflammatory cells and macrophages on the fifth day following injury during the proliferative stage and peak at day 7.[30] The function of T-lymphocytes is still unclear; a recent study has postulated that they might bracket control of the proliferation phase of wound healing.[13] Once the wound is filled with new granulation tissue, angiogenesis

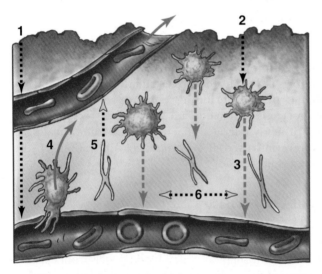

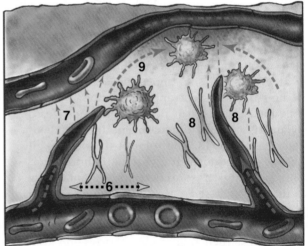

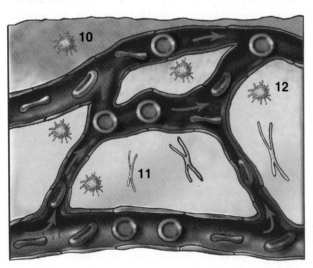

Figure 15–6   Angiogenesis is the formation of new blood vessels from existing vessels. This process requires a number of different features, such as proliferation and migration of endothelial cells and the appropriate regulation of endothelial cell to cell and cell to matrix adhesions. Following wounding, there is no blood supply to the injured area. Angiogenesis results from various stimuli present in the injured tissue, namely, (1) low oxygen tension creating an oxygen gradient from the vascularized periphery of the wound bed center; (2) this relative hypoxia also stimulates the release of angiogenic factors from macrophages, (3) which in turn act on preexisting capillaries, (4) recruiting more circulating monocytes to the wound. (5) The released growth factors also result in fibroblast proliferation, (6) causing the release of proteoglycans and glycosaminoglycan into the extracellular matrix. (7) The released growth factors act on the basement membrane to enable migration and proliferation of the endothelium (budding), (8) while further release of growth factors from macrophages and fibroblast causes endothelial sprouting. The endothelial cells (9) eventually arch and join. (10) Further sprouting results in (11) capillary loops produced under (12) the influence of growth factors, which ultimately result in a capillary network.

ceases, and many of the blood vessels disintegrate as a result of apoptosis.

Maturation and Remodeling Phase

The main feature of the maturation phase is the deposition of collagen in the wound space. The rate, quality, and total amount of matrix deposition determine the strength of the scar.[11] Wound matrix composition changes as the healing process progresses. Initially, it is composed of fibrin and fibronectin originating from hemostasis and macrophages. Glycosaminoglycans and proteoglycans are synthesized next, to support future matrix deposition and remodeling. Following this, collagens become the predominant scar protein. Extracellular matrix components are remodeled by matrix metalloproteinases and the tissue inhibitors of metalloproteinases.

Healthy skin is composed predominantly of collagen type I. Type III collagen is more common in granulation tissue, decreasing in amount as healing progresses.[31] Normal dermis shows a basket-weave pattern, whereas in scar, the thinner collagen fibers are arranged parallel to the skin. These fibers gradually thicken and organize along the stress line of the wound. This change is accompanied by increased scar tensile strength, indicating a positive correlation of fiber thickness and orientation with tensile strength. Despite a remodeling phase that lasts up to 1 year, the collagen fibers in scar tissue never become as organized as those in intact dermis. Collagen breakdown during healing begins early and is very active during the inflammatory phase. Sources of collagenases in the wound are the inflammatory cells and endothelial cells as well as fibroblasts and keratinocytes. Collagens are almost exclusively digested extracellularly by specific collagenases. These enzymes are able to degrade the normally very stable triple helical structure of collagen at specific sites, rendering the molecule more susceptible to degradation by other proteases. The activity of collagenases is tightly controlled by cytokines.

Wound Contraction

Wound contraction is the spontaneous approximation of the wound edges during healing, and wound contracture is the shortening of the scar itself. Several theories have been proposed for the mechanism of wound contracture. One proposes that a special cell, the myofibroblast, is responsible for contracture; another theory suggests that the locomotion of all fibroblasts leads to a reorganization of the matrix and therefore contraction (Fig. 15-7).[32,33]

Reepithelialization

Reepithelialization results in mature skin covering the wound and occurs only after granulation tissue is established. This process requires migration of keratinocytes from the edge of the wound over the collagen-fibronectin

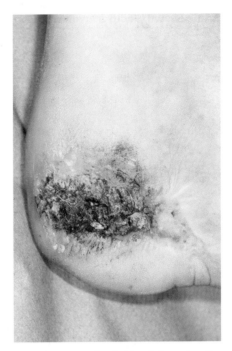

Figure 15–7 Long-standing left heel ulcer showing wound contraction proximally.

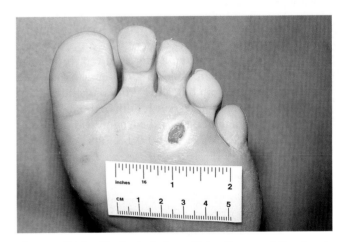

Figure 15–8 Plantar foot ulcer with healthy granulation tissue in the base with reepithelialization of the periphery.

surface and is necessary for the formation of a protective barrier over the wound. Reepithelialization represents a sequence of steps involving mobilization, migration, mitosis, and cellular differentiation of epithelial cells (Fig. 15-8).

Growth Factors Related to Wound Healing

Growth factors are polypeptides that control the wound-healing process by binding to specific high-affinity receptors on the cell surface. They have the ability to stimulate mitosis of quiescent cells. Various cell types produce them, including platelets, macrophages, epithelial cells, fibroblasts, and endothelial cells. Their effects occur by endocrine, paracrine, and autocrine action. The growth

TABLE 15-1 Growth Factors Involved in Wound Healing

Growth Factor	Abbreviation	Principal Source	Action
Epidermal growth factor	EGF	Platelets	↑ Collagen synthesis ↑ Epithelialization
Fibroblast growth factor	FGF	Fibroblasts, endothelium, smooth muscle, chondrocytes	↑ Angiogenesis ↑ Fibroblast proliferation ↑ Keratinocyte proliferation
Hepatocyte growth factor	HGF	Macrophages, fibroblasts	↑ Angiogenesis ↑ Fibroblast proliferation ↑ Keratinocyte proliferation
Insulin-like growth factors (somatomedins)	IGF-1	Hepatocytes	↑ Fibroblast proliferation ↑ Collagen synthesis ↑ Epithelialization
	IGF-2	Primarily of fetal origin	↑ Promotes proliferation of many cell types
Keratinocyte growth factor	KGF	Fibroblasts	↑ Keratinocyte proliferation
Platelet-derived growth factor	PDGF	Platelets, macrophages, smooth muscle, endothelium, fibroblasts	↑ Macrophages, fibroblast and smooth muscle cell migration ↑ Collagen synthesis
Transforming growth factors	TGF-α	Macrophages, keratinocytes, hepatocytes, eosinophils	↑ Keratinocyte and fibroblast proliferation
	TGF-β1 TGF-β2 TGF-β3	Platelets, macrophages, fibroblasts, keratinocytes, lymphocytes	↑ Angiogenesis ↑ Fibroblast proliferation ↑ Collagen synthesis ↓ Cell division
Vascular endothelial growth factor	VEGF	Endothelium	↑ Angiogenesis

factors that are most commonly involved in wound healing are described in Table 15-1. Other cytokines that are involved in the wound-healing process include tumor necrosis factor α and interleukin-1. Both of these cytokines are involved in angiogenesis and collagen synthesis.

The Effects of Diabetes on Wound Healing

Diabetes has been shown to influence many of the normal wound-healing responses. Trauma results in an acute diabetic foot wound, which may then progress to a chronic wound that is often difficult or slow to heal. The progression to a chronic wound is influenced by both extrinsic and intrinsic factors. Specific extrinsic factors that impair wound healing in diabetic patients include neuropathy, ischemia, and infection. Wound repair in diabetes is also impaired by intrinsic factors such as abnormalities of growth factor production, reduced neutrophil activity, and reduced expression of extracellular matrix.[34]

Growth Factors

A recent study of skin biopsies obtained from the edge of diabetic foot ulcers showed increased expression of TGF-β3 compared with skin biopsies of nondiabetic patients. Expression of TGF-β1 was not increased in any

of these biopsies.[35] A reduced expression of insulin-like growth factor 1 in the basal keratinocyte layer of diabetic skin has also been noted.[36] Glycation of bFGF significantly reduces its activity in vitro. Glycation causes significant reduction in the ability of bFGF to bind to its tyrosine kinase receptor and activate the signal transduction pathways. These growth factor abnormalities may play a role in delaying wound healing in patients with diabetes.

Extracellular Matrix and Protease Activity

Dermal wounds in nondiabetic patients heal by granulation tissue formation and contraction. In diabetic patients, wound closure is predominantly the result of granulation formation and reepithelialization.[37] Although simple epithelial repair in superficial wounds is not hindered in diabetes, the ability to form collagen in the repair of deeper wounds is severely impaired. Extracellular matrix components are remodeled by both matrix metalloproteinases and their tissue inhibitors (TIMPs). It has been demonstrated that there is an increased concentration of matrix metalloproteinases and a decreased concentration of TIMP-2 in diabetic patients.[38] Diabetes can also delay wound healing by insufficient granulation tissue formation, possibly due to a defect in fibroblast function.[39] Fibroblasts derived from chronic diabetic foot ulcers have impaired proliferative capacity compared with those from uninjured skin.[40]

Therapeutics in Wound Healing

The efficacy of many advanced therapeutic agents in chronic wounds has been less than what had been predicted from in vitro studies or from animal models and human acute wounds. This is due to the underlying pathophysiology and complicating features of chronic wounds. Initiation of the healing process in diabetes may be impaired by the excessive bacterial burden and possibly by the phenotypically abnormal cells present in and around the wound. The healing process of diabetic foot ulcers therefore becomes more than simply the surgical debridement of necrotic tissue. Chronic wound fluid has been shown to be deleterious to resident cells and may enhance bacterial colonization; therefore, removal of edema may also be critical in the management of diabetic ulcers.

Wound bed preparation implies optimizing the readiness of the wound bed to allow the normal endogenous process of wound healing to occur.[41] It is important to note that wound bed preparation is more than just debridement of necrotic tissue in chronic wounds; rather, it is a very comprehensive approach aimed at reducing edema and exudate, eliminating or reducing the bacterial burden, and, importantly, correcting the abnormalities that contribute to impaired healing. There are both basic and more advanced approaches to wound bed preparation and optimization of healing. Basic aspects, as with compromised acute wounds, include debridement, infection control, edema removal, and surgical correction of underlying defects[42,43] (Fig. 15-9). More advanced aspects, for which we might not have all the answers yet, include attempts at dermal reconstitution, as with the use of biological agents.

Therapeutic Growth Factors

Several recombinant growth factors have been tested for their ability to accelerate the healing of chronic wounds. Among others, some promising results have been obtained with the use of epidermal growth factor[44] and keratinocyte growth factor 2[45] for venous ulcers and fibroblast growth factor[46] and platelet-derived growth factor[47] for pressure ulcers. However, the only topically applied growth factor that is commercially approved for use is platelet-derived growth factor. In randomized, controlled clinical studies, platelet-derived growth factor has been shown to accelerate the healing of neuropathic diabetic foot ulcers by approximately 15%.[48]

Bioengineered Skin Products

A number of bioengineered skin products or skin equivalents have become available for the treatment of acute and chronic wounds, as well as for burns. Since the initial use of keratinocyte sheets,[49,50] several more complex constructs have been developed and tested in human wounds. Skin equivalents may contain living cells, such as fibroblasts or keratinocytes or both, while other products are made of acellular materials or extracts of living cells. Bioengineered skin may work by delivering living cells that are capable of adapting to their environment. There is evidence that some of the living constructs are able to release growth factors and cytokines,[51,52] but this cannot as yet be interpreted as being their mechanism of action. These allogeneic constructs do not survive for more than a few weeks when placed in a chronic wound.[53] Allogeneic constructs consisting of living cells derived from neonatal foreskin have been shown to accelerate the healing of neuropathic diabetic foot ulcers in randomized controlled trials and are available for clinical use.[54,55] The clinical effect of these constructs is improved healing times of 15% to 20% over conventional "control" therapy.

Gene Therapy

The technology now exists for introducing certain genes into wounds by a variety of physical means or biological vectors, including viruses. There are ex vivo approaches, in which cells are manipulated before reintroduction into the wound, and more direct in vivo techniques, which rely on simple injection or the use of the gene gun.[56,57] Inability to achieve stable and prolonged expression of a gene product, which has been a problem in the gene therapy of systemic conditions, can actually be an advantage in the context of nonhealing wounds, in which only transient expression is required. Most of the work with gene therapy of wounds has been performed

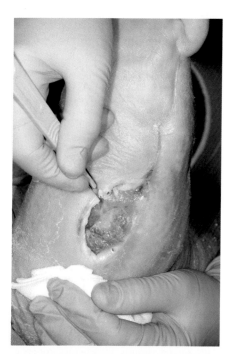

Figure 15–9   Basic preparation of the wound bed.

in experimental animal models. However, there are promising indications that certain approaches may work in human wounds. For example, the introduction of naked plasmid DNA encoding the gene for vascular endothelial growth factor has been reported to enhance healing and angiogenesis in selected patients with ulcers from arterial insufficiency.[58]

Stem Cell Therapy

Pluripotential stem cells are hypothesized to offer greater advantages than specific genes delivered to wounds because they are capable of differentiating into a variety of cell types, including fibroblasts, endothelial cells, and keratinocytes, which are critical cellular components required for healing. However, stem cell research remains controversial.

Antioxidant Therapy

An alternative approach to correcting abnormalities in healing seen in diabetic patients is to reduce the amount of free radical production. Raxofelast, a protective membrane antioxidant agent, significantly improves impaired wound healing in diabetic mice through stimulation of angiogenesis.[59] There remains considerable potential for this and other free radical scavenging agents to influence healing in patients with diabetes.

Summary

Management of diabetic foot ulcers requires an understanding of the clinical factors involved as well as the pathophysiologic components that underlie their impaired healing. Greater therapeutic innovation is required as well. For example, existing advanced therapeutic products tested in diabetic foot ulcers, such as growth factors and skin equivalents, have focused entirely on neuropathic ulcers of the metatarsal heads. Ischemic ulcers due to arterial insufficiency and more complex ulcers seen over the heel area have been exclusion criteria in those trials. Nonetheless, considerable progress has been made, and a number of therapeutic approaches are now available.

References

1. Reiber GE, Lipsky BA, Gibbons GW: The burden of diabetic foot ulcer. Am J Surg 176(suppl 2a):5–10, 1998.
2. Apelqvist J, Larsson J, Ragnarsson-Tennvall G, Persson U: Long term costs in diabetic patients with foot ulcers. Foot and Ankle 16:388–394, 1995.
3. Ragnarson Tennvall G, Apelqvist J: Health-economic consequences of diabetic foot lesions. Clin Infect Dis 39(suppl 2):S132–S139, 2004.
4. de Sonnaville JJJ, Colly LP, Wijkel D, Heine RJ: The prevalence and determinants of foot ulceration in type 2 diabetic patients in a primary health care setting. Diabetes Res Clin Pract 35:149–156, 1997.
5. Kumar S, Ashe HA, Parnell LN: The prevalence of foot ulceration and its correlates in type 2 diabetic patients: A population based study. Diabetic Med 11:480–484, 1994.
6. Park JE, Barbul A: Understanding the role of immune regulation in wound healing. Am J Surg 187:11S–16S, 2004.
7. Schilling JA: Wound healing. Surg Clin North Am 56:859–874, 1976.
8. Steed DL: The role of growth factors in wound healing. Surg Clin North Am 77:575–586, 1997.
9. Hunt TK, La Van FB: Enhancement of wound healing by growth factors. N Engl J Med 321:111–112, 1989.
10. Davidson J: Growth factors in wound healing: Wounds 7(suppl A):53A–64A, 1995.
11. Witte MB, Barbul A: General principles of wound healing. Surg Clin North Am 77:509–528, 1997.
12. Kurkinen M, Vaheri A, Roberts PJ, Stenmans S: Sequential appearance of fibronectin and collagen in experimental granulation tissue. Lab Invest 43:47–51, 1980.
13. Park JE, Barbul A: Understanding the role of immune regulation in wound healing. Am J Surg 187:11S–16S, 2004.
14. Hubner G, Brauchle M, Smola H, et al: Differential regulation of pro-inflammatory cytokines during wound healing in normal and glucocorticoid-treated mice. Cytokine 8:548–556, 1996.
15. Simpson DM, Ross R: The neutrophilic leukocyte in wound repair: A study with antineutrophil serum. J Clin Invest 51:2009–2023, 1972.
16. Martin P: Wound healing: Aiming for perfect skin regeneration. Science 276:75–81, 1997.
17. Leibovich SJ, Ross R: The role of the macrophage in wound repair: A study with hydrocortisone and antimacrophage serum. Am J Pathol 78:71–100, 1975.
18. Cherry GC, Hughes MA, Ferguson MWJ, Leaper DJ: Wound healing. In Morris PJ, Wood WC (eds): Oxford Textbook of Surgery. Oxford, UK: Oxford University Press, 2000, pp 131–159.
19. Beezhold DH, Personius C: Fibronectin fragments stimulate tumor necrosis factor secretion by human monocytes. J Leukoc Biol 51:59–64, 1992.
20. Risau W: Mechanisms of angiogenesis. Nature 386:671–674, 1997.
21. Carmeliet P: Angiogenesis in life, disease and medicine. Nature. 438:932–936, 2005.
22. Folkman J, Shing Y: Angiogenesis. J Biol Chem 267:10931–10934, 1992.
23. Clark RAF: Wound repair: Overview and general considerations. In Clark RAF (ed): The Molecular and Cellular Biology of Wound Healing. New York: Plenum Press, 1996, pp 3–50.
24. Lynch SE, Colvin RB, Antoniades HN: Growth factors in wound healing: Single and synergistic effects on partial thickness porcine skin wounds. J Clin Invest 84:640–646, 1989.
25. Grant DS, Kleinmann HK, Goldberg ID, et al: Scatter factor induces blood vessel formation in vivo. Proc Natl Acad Sci U S A 90:1937–1941, 1993.
26. Knighton DR, Hunt TK, Scheuenstuhl H, et al: Oxygen tension regulates the expression of angiogenesis factor by macrophages. Science 221:1283–1285, 1983.
27. Knighton DR, Fiegel VD: Macrophage-derived growth factors in wound healing: Regulation of growth factor production by the oxygen microenvironment. Am Rev Respir Dis 140:1108–1111, 1989.
28. Cheresh DA: Human endothelial cells synthesize and express an Arg-Gly-Asp-directed adhesion receptor involved in attachment to fibrinogen and von Willebrand factor. Proc Natl Acad Sci U S A 84:6471–6475, 1987.
29. Leavesley DI, Schwartz MA, Rosenfeld M, Cheresh DA: Integrin beta 1- and beta 3-mediated endothelial cell migration is triggered through distinct signaling mechanisms. J Cell Biol 12:163–170, 1993.
30. Fischel RS, Barbul A, Beschorner WE, et al: Lymphocyte participation in wound healing: Morphological assessment using monoclonal antibodies. Ann Surg 206:25–29, 1987.
31. Ehrlich PH; Krummel TM: Regulation of wound healing from a connective tissue perspective. Wound Repair Regen 4:203–210, 1996.
32. Schmitt-Graff A, Desmouliere A, Gabbiani G: Heterogeneity of myofibroblast phenotypic features: An example of fibroblastic cell plasticity [review]. Virchows Archiv 425:3–24, 1994.
33. Ehrlich HP: Wound closure: Evidence of cooperation between fibroblasts and collagen matrix. Eye 2:149–57, 1988.

34. International Working Group on the Diabetic Foot: Progress report: Wound Healing and Treatments for People with Diabetic Foot Ulcers. 2003.

35. Jude EB, Blakytny R, Bulmer J, et al: Transforming growth factor-beta 1, 2, 3 and receptor type I and II in diabetic foot ulcers. Diabet Med 19:440–447, 2002.

36. Blakytny R, Jude EB, Martin Gibson J, et al: Lack of insulin-like growth factor 1 (IGF1) in the basal keratinocyte layer of diabetic skin and diabetic foot ulcers. J Pathol 190:589–594, 2000.

37. Albertson S, Hummel RP 3rd, Breeden M, Greenhalgh DG: PDGF and FGF reverse the healing impairment in protein-malnourished diabetic mice. Surgery 114:368–372, 1993.

38. Lobmann R, Ambrosch A, Schultz G, et al: Expression of matrix-metalloproteinases and their inhibitors in the wounds of diabetic and non-diabetic patients. Diabetologia 45:1011–1016, 2002.

39. Yue DK, Swanson B, McLennan S, et al: Abnormalities of granulation tissue and collagen formation in experimental diabetes, uraemia and malnutrition. Diabet Med 3:221–225, 1986.

40. Hehenberger K, Kratz G, Hansson A, Brismar K: Fibroblasts derived from human chronic diabetic wounds have a decreased proliferation rate, which is recovered by the addition of heparin. J Dermatol Sci 16:144–151, 1998.

41. Falanga V: Classifications for wound bed preparation and stimulation of chronic wounds. Wound Repair Regen 8:347–352, 2000.

42. Barwell JR, Taylor M, Deacon J, et al: Surgical correction of isolated superficial venous reflux reduces long- term recurrence rate in chronic venous leg ulcers. Eur J Vasc Endovasc Surg 20:363–368, 2000.

43. Gloviczki P, Bergan JJ, Menawat SS, et al: Safety, feasibility, and early efficacy of subfascial endoscopic perforator surgery: a preliminary report from the North American registry. J Vasc Surg 25:94–105, 1997.

44. Falanga V, Eaglstein WH, Bucalo B, et al: Topical use of human recombinant epidermal growth factor (h-EGF) in venous ulcers. J Dermatol Surg Oncol 18:604–606, 1992.

45. Robson MC, Phillips TJ, Falanga V, et al: Randomized trial of topically applied repifermin (recombinant human keratinocyte growth factor-2) to accelerate wound healing in venous ulcers. Wound Repair Regen 9:347–352, 2001.

46. Robson MC, Phillips LG, Lawrence WT, et al: The safety and effect of topically applied recombinant basic fibroblast growth factor on the healing of chronic pressure sores. Ann Surg 216:401–406, 1992.

47. Pierce GF, Tarpley JE, Allman RM, et al: Tissue repair processes in healing chronic pressure ulcers treated with recombinant platelet-derived growth factor BB. Am J Pathol 145:1399–1410, 1994.

48. Smiell JM, Wieman TJ, Steed DL, et al: Efficacy and safety of becaplermin (recombinant human platelet-derived growth factor-BB) in patients with nonhealing, lower extremity diabetic ulcers: A combined analysis of four randomized studies. Wound Repair Regen 7:335–346, 1999.

49. Gallico GG, 3rd: Biologic skin substitutes. Clin Plast Surg 17:519–526, 1990.

50. Phillips TJ, Gilchrest BA: Clinical applications of cultured epithelium. Epithelial Cell Biol 1:39–46, 1992.

51. Mansbridge J, Liu K, Patch R, et al: Three-dimensional fibroblast culture implant for the treatment of diabetic foot ulcers: Metabolic activity and therapeutic range. Tissue Eng 4:403–414, 1998.

52. Falanga V, Isaacs C, Paquette D, et al: Wounding of bioengineered skin: Cellular and molecular aspects after injury. J Invest Dermatol 119:653–660, 2002.

53. Phillips TJ, Manzoor J, Rojas A, et al: The longevity of a bilayered skin substitute after application to venous ulcers. Arch Dermatol 138:1079–1081, 2002.

54. Gentzkow GD, Iwasaki SD, Hershon KS, et al: Use of dermagraft, a cultured human dermis, to treat diabetic foot ulcers. Diabetes Care 19:350–354, 1996.

55. Veves A, Falanga V, Armstrong DG, Sabolinski ML: Graftskin, a human skin equivalent, is effective in the management of noninfected neuropathic diabetic foot ulcers: A prospective randomized multicenter clinical trial. Diabetes Care 24:290–295, 2001.

56. Badiavas EV, Falanga V: Gene therapy. J Dermatol 28:175–192, 2001.

57. Eming SA, Medalie DA, Tompkins RG, et al: Genetically modified human keratinocytes overexpressing PDGF-A enhance the performance of a composite skin graft. Hum Gene Ther 9:529–539, 1998.

58. Isner JM, Baumgartner I, Rauh G, et al: Treatment of thromboangiitis obliterans (Buerger's disease) by intramuscular gene transfer of vascular endothelial growth factor: Preliminary clinical results. J Vasc Surg 28:964–973, 1998.

59. Galeano M, Torre V, Deodato B, et al: Raxofelast, a hydrophilic vitamin E-like antioxidant, stimulates wound healing in genetically diabetic mice. Surgery 2001, 129:467–477, 2001.

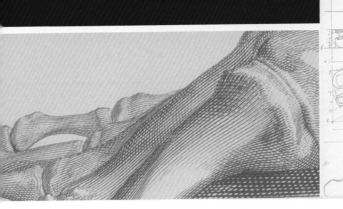

RADIOLOGIC INTERVENTION IN DIABETIC PERIPHERAL VASCULAR DISEASE

HANNO HOPPE AND JOHN A. KAUFMAN ∎

Introduction

Diabetes mellitus predisposes to peripheral vascular disease with an odds ratio between 2 and 3.[1] In 46% of patients with stenoses of the superficial femoral artery (SFA) and popliteal artery, the iliac arteries are simultaneously diseased. In almost 80% of patients, the distribution of lower-limb atherosclerosis is symmetric. Commonly, adjacent segments are involved with combined iliac artery and SFA disease in 46% and with femoropopliteal and tibial disease in 38%. Patients with diabetes mellitus frequently present with arterial stenosis or occlusion limited to an infrainguinal or infrageniculate distribution.[2] One of the most clearly defined measures of outcome in treatment of peripheral vascular disease is amputation. Population-based surveys estimate that people with diabetes require amputations about 10 times more frequently than do nondiabetic patients with peripheral vascular disease and at a younger age.

Although noninvasive vascular imaging is increasingly used for the evaluation of peripheral vascular disease, conventional angiography remains crucial in the evaluation of patients with symptomatic peripheral vascular disease.[3,4] Furthermore, angiography is necessary when a noninvasive study shows discrepant results or when percutaneous interventional treatment is extremely likely. Dotter first described percutaneous revascularization of a focal stenosis in the popliteal artery of a patient with peripheral vascular disease in 1964.[5] In 1974, Gruentzig had developed a balloon catheter for dilation of vascular lesions.[6] Percutaneous transluminal angioplasty (PTA) is recognized as a safe and effective alternative to surgery for the treatment of peripheral vascular disease in selected patients. In addition to the general efficacy of PTA, which is comparable to that of bypass surgery for selected lesions, angioplasty offers several distinct advantages over surgery. It is performed under local anesthesia, making it feasible to treat patients who are at high risk for general anesthesia. When compared to surgical revascularization, the morbidity from angioplasty is low, generally related to problems at the vascular access site, and mortality is extremely rare. Unlike vascular surgery, there is no recovery period after angioplasty, and most patients can return to normal activity within 24 to 48 hours of an uncomplicated procedure. Finally, angioplasty can be repeated if necessary, usually without increased difficulty or increased patient risk compared to the first procedure, and does not preclude surgery as adjunctive or definitive therapy.[7]

Recently, besides PTA, a variety of newer devices and technologies have become available for endovascular intervention, including laser angioplasty, excisional atherectomy, self-expanding and balloon-expandable bare stents, stent grafts, drug-eluting stents, brachytherapy, cryotherapy, cutting balloons, drug-coated balloons, and biodegradable stents (Table 16-1). Therefore, the treatment options for peripheral vascular disease have undergone a rapid change. Clinicians nowadays have multiple

TABLE 16-1 Revascularization Techniques in Peripheral Vascular Disease

Revascularization Technique	Description
Percutaneous transluminal balloon angioplasty (PTA)	Basic revascularization technique
	Controlled fracturing of obstructing plaque and stretching of the media using a balloon
Cutting balloon angioplasty	Modification of conventional PTA using a balloon with cutting blades to reduce force needed to dilate vessel
Endovascular cryoplasty	Targeted delivery of cold thermal energy to the vessel wall to alter biologic response and enable a more benign healing process after balloon injury
Balloon coating	Conventional PTA in combination with drug application to the site of treatment to prevent restenosis
Endovascular brachytherapy	Afterloading of γ radiation to reduce intimal hyperplasia and restenosis
Subintimal angioplasty	Intentional creation of dissection around an occlusion to reenter the lumen distally
Excisional atherectomy	Debulking of atherosclerotic plaque using differential cutting with rotating blade
	Prevention of barotrauma and plaque displacement
Laser angioplasty	Use of laser energy to vaporize sclerotic material
Self-expandable nitinol stent	Intravascular scaffold for the vessel lumen
	Plaque and vessel wall are pushed aside to enlarge the lumen
Balloon-expandable stent	Precise placement, but potential deformation by extrinsic compression in superior femoral artery
PTFE-covered stent-graft	Coverage of dissections
	Prevention of acute vessel occlusion due to elastic recoil
	Prevention of intraluminal vascular smooth muscle cell proliferation
Drug-eluting stents	Drug application to the site of treatment and limitation of neointimal hyperplasia and restenosis
Biodegradable stents	Dissolve slowly after placement to reduce intimal hyperplasia

PTA, percutaneous transluminal balloon angioplasty; PTFE, polytetrafluoroethylene.

treatment options at their disposal. It is challenging to select the most appropriate therapy for each individual patient based on predicted safety and efficacy.

Percutaneous Transluminal Balloon Angioplasty

Percutaneous transluminal balloon angioplasty is considered the basic technique for femoropopliteal revascularization. Its underlying mechanism is controlled fracture of the obstructing plaque, resulting in formation of fissures in the plaque itself and tearing of the edges of the plaque away from the adjacent normal intima. In addition, the media is stretched by using proper oversizing of the balloon. A normal finding following PTA are "cracks" or small dissections, but they may remodel over time, and the lumen may resume a more normal appearance (Fig. 16-1). In the SFA, PTA is usually the treatment of choice for short-segment stenoses and occlusions. Longer stenoses and occlusions can also be attempted, but previous experiences demonstrated less acceptable results as the length and number of lesions increase.[8] In case of a secondary fresh thrombus, catheter-directed thrombolysis can be attempted prior to PTA to reduce the length of occlusion or convert it into a stenosis.[9] On the other hand, femoropopliteal or femorodistal bypasses may be surgical options for those patients, but bypass grafting is associated with disadvantages, including invasive therapy, longer hospitalization, limited run-off vessels that could be treated percutaneously together with SFA, and the need for warfarin

therapy in patients receiving femorodistal bypass with an anastomosis below the knee.[10] Restenosis due to early vessel recoil and neointimal proliferation is one major limitation of PTA. Six months after PTA of the SFA, patency rates between 30% and 80% were reported, which is low in comparison to rates for other vessels.[11,12] The restenosis rate ($>50\%$) was 20% to 35% in the coronary artery and 15% to 20% in the renal artery 6 months after PTA. In the iliac artery, the restenosis rate was only 5% to 9% 1 year after PTA.[13]

Compared to the iliac and femoral arteries, PTA in patients with stenoses or occlusions of the popliteal and tibial arteries is performed less often. The majority of patients undergoing tibial angioplasty are people with diabetes (63% to 91%), who have a twofold risk for gangrene and a fourfold risk for amputation.[2] Indications are usually limb salvage in patients with critical ischemia with impending or ongoing tissue loss, or preservation of runoff distal to a bypass graft.[14–16] Lesions at the origins of the tibial arteries can be angioplastied safely by using "kissing balloons" or a safety wire. Simultaneous inflation of two balloons sized to the smaller branch vessels prevents complications such as dissection of the vessel origin. A safety wire in the uninvolved vessel is frequently used to preserve access should a complication occur during PTA. Traditionally, infrapopliteal angioplasty is basically limited to short segment stenosis. Technical success has been reported as high as 97%.[2] PTA has been shown to yield a 75% to 83% limb salvage rate at 2-year follow-up in carefully selected patients with "straight-line flow" in one tibial vessel to the foot. Less favorable anatomy has led to patency rates of less than 15% and frequent early failures.[10,17]

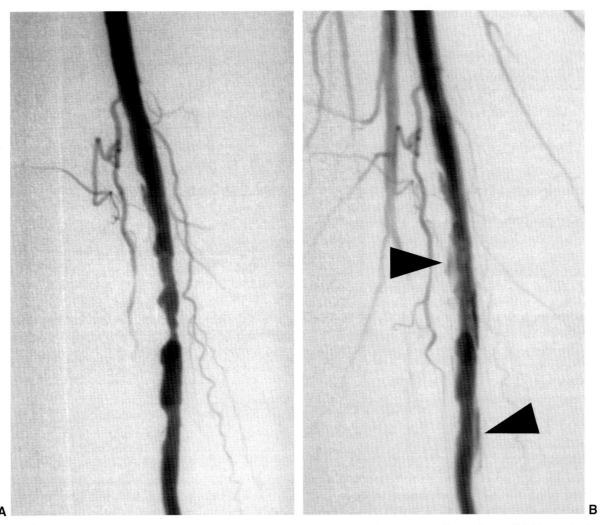

A   **B**

Figure 16–1   **A,** Appearance of a superficial femoral artery following angioplasty. Segment of a diseased superficial femoral artery demonstrating multiple stenoses of atherosclerotic origin. **B,** Fissuring of the atherosclerotic plaque (*arrowheads*) becomes apparent after angioplasty, which is a normal appearance post angioplasty not requiring further intervention. *(Reprinted from Kaufman JA: Vascular interventions. In Kaufman JA, Lee MJ. The requisites: Vascular and interventional radiology. Philadelphia: Mosby/Elsevier, 2004.)*

Cutting Balloon

Cutting balloon angioplasty basically represents a modification of conventional PTA.[18] The cutting blades of the balloon (Fig. 16-2) create controlled longitudinal incisions into the plaque of the stenotic lesion during the initial balloon inflation and consequently reduce the force needed to dilate the vessel, which is proposed to result in a lower rate of dissection and to trigger a more benign course of arterial healing as a result of limited stretch injury.[19] Although cutting balloon angioplasty has been positively evaluated in the coronary circulation, there are only a few reports on its efficacy in terms of reduction of neointimal hyperplasia in peripheral vessels. Preliminary results in infrainguinal bypass grafts indicate a technical success rate of 94% and cumulative patency rates of 84% and 67% at 6 months and at 12 to 18 months follow-up, respectively.[20] A larger study reported

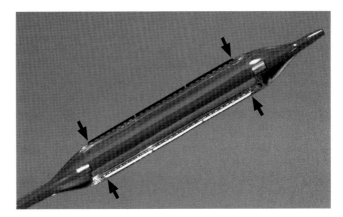

Figure 16–2   The Small Peripheral Cutting Balloon Flextome Device (Boston Scientific Inc., Natick, MA) is equipped with 1.5-cm-long atherotomes (*arrows*) to create controlled longitudinal incisions into the plaque of the stenotic lesion during balloon inflation.

a limb salvage rate of almost 90% after a mean follow-up of 1 year.[21]

Endovascular Cryoplasty

The technique of cryoplasty combines conventional balloon catheter dilation with cooling of the target lesion at the same time.[19] By inflating the balloon with nitrous oxide instead of saline solution and contrast medium, cold thermal energy is applied to the vessel, initiating an endothermal reaction with a heat sink of –10°C at the treatment position. Cryoplasty is an interesting novel technique that focuses on two major problems of conventional balloon angioplasty: initial technical failure by dissection or recoil and late restenosis formation caused by negative remodeling and neointima formation. The targeted delivery of cold thermal energy is proposed to alter the biological response of the vessel, potentially resulting in a more benign healing process after balloon injury.[22] Preliminary results show the potential of cryoplasty. The technical success rate was between 87% and 93%. At 6 months, the restenosis rate was 0%. On follow-up, patency was demonstrated in 85% of cases at 9 months and 83% at 14 months.[23,24]

Drug-Coated Balloon

Balloon coating, a novel method for prevention and therapy of restenosis, is currently under investigation. This technique uses a conventional angioplasty balloon to apply drugs to the site of treatment with a short contact time. The theory behind this method is that non-stent-based local delivery of antiproliferative drugs might offer additional flexibility and also reach vessel areas beyond the immediate stent coverage. Preclinical studies demonstrated the drug-coated balloon to be more effective in inhibiting the neointimal formation than a drug-eluting stent.[25] Clinical testing of this technique in patients with coronary artery in-stent restenosis underlined the preclinical results. Clinical study for femoral use is under way and should be reported shortly.[26]

Endovascular Brachytherapy

The issue of smooth muscle cell proliferation with consequent restenosis is directly addressed by brachytherapy using afterloading of γ radiation causing local inhibition of intimal hyperplasia at the treatment site. A pilot study using PTA plus brachytherapy showed a restenosis rate at 6 months of 28% compared to 54% with PTA alone.[27] Subsequent trials demonstrated significant reduction of the restenosis rate after femoral angioplasty of recurring lesions, but brachytherapy did not succeed in improving the rate of de novo lesions.[28] In contrast to the results

of PTA and brachytherapy, stenting combined with brachytherapy did not increase the patency rate at 6 months, according to a high incidence of early and late thrombotic occlusions.[29] Another multicenter study reported final results that did not show a significant difference between the treatment and control groups.[28] The results of this study and other factors such as problems coordinating the interdisciplinary cooperation between the interventionalist and radiation specialist, safety issues using radiation in a benign disease, and the availability of alternative treatment options result in a very limited use of this method.

Subintimal Angioplasty

Intentional subintimal angioplasty is an endovascular approach for the treatment of patients with vessel occlusion. The procedure involves intentionally creating a false channel or dissection around an arterial occlusion, then reentering the true lumen distally. The procedure has a relatively low incidence of complications and a high rate of technical success.[14] Primary technical success rates range from 76% to 90%. Extensive calcification can be a predictor for failure, particularly for missing spontaneous reentry. Complications are reported to be up to 5% and are exclusively related to the reentry site. The risk of perforation is minimal because there is no flow during the intervention in the occluded vessel. Preliminary results report a long-term patency of 71% at 1 year in femoropopliteal disease.[30] Inferior results were found in a more recent study with a patency rate of 37% on 1-year follow-up and a 6-month patency rate of 24% in patients with critical ischemia.[31] In patients who are poor candidates for bypass surgery, percutaneous intentional extraluminal recanalization proved to be useful for limb salvage.[32] However, subintimal recanalization causes extensive dissection, and stenting should be considered.

Laser Angioplasty

The inability to cross a vascular occlusion, which may occur in up to 30% of patients with femoropopliteal disease, led to the idea that debulking of obstructive material could transform an occlusion into a stenosis that could subsequently be treated with PTA. This was thought to cause limited damage to the arterial wall and, consequently, might reduce the stimuli causing restenosis. In the early 1980s, the innovative idea was brought up that laser energy can be used to vaporize sclerotic material, which led to the development of laser angioplasty as a clinical modality.[33] Laser angioplasty allows for step-by-step recanalization, using the ability to break molecular bonds directly by photochemical rather than thermal means.[34] Limitations of this technique include the need for additional angioplasty and a largest probe size of 2.5 mm, limiting its use in the SFA. Complications are vessel perforation and distal embolization. Technical success was achieved in 90.5% of patients in the SFA. One-year patency rates for the SFA range from 65% to 75%.[35] In a pilot study evaluating the use of laser angioplasty in combination with PTA including infrageniculate arteries in patients with critical limb ischemia, the success rate was 88%.[36] Almost 80% of the patients had diabetes mellitus as a risk factor. The limb salvage rate was 69%. For limbs that additionally received a stent, the 6-month limb salvage rate was 89%. Recent data from a multicenter trial indicate that laser angioplasty might be a viable treatment strategy for patients with chronic ischemic limb disease who are poor candidates for bypass surgery.[37]

Excisional Atherectomy

Historically, percutaneous excisional atherectomy has been associated with exorbitantly high restenosis rates, but newer designs recently gave reason for renewed enthusiasm. Excisional atherectomy (Fig. 16-3) is an alternative treatment option for peripheral artery stenosis to prevent barotrauma and plaque displacement occurring with PTA. This technique may be particularly useful in problematic subsets such as ostial disease and in the popliteal artery.[34] Limiting factors of this method are extensive vessel calcification and diffuse disease and the potential for distal embolization. Previous single-center studies on a predecessor device report high primary success rates and acceptable long-term results for treatment of femoral steno-occlusive disease.[38,39] However, another study found less enthusiastic results, and it was concluded that excisional atherectomy should not be used to replace PTA as routine treatment of short femoropopliteal lesions.[40] These outcomes in combination with the technically demanding procedure prevented the use of excisional atherectomy as a routine treatment method.

A recently introduced novel device is technically completely different from the previous devices and has demonstrated promising preliminary results with a restenosis rate of 32% after 6 months.[41,42] Lesions up to 8 cm in length of the femoropopliteal arteries could be treated successfully in most cases. In below-knee vessel lesions, the rates of restenosis (>70%) were 14% after 3 months and 22% after 6 months. The 3-month and 6-month cumulative patency rates were 98% and 94.1%, respectively.[43] Additional balloon angioplasty might be necessary in selected cases.

Bare Stents

Stents provide an intravascular scaffold for the vessel lumen. As the plaque and vessel wall are pushed aside by the stent to enlarge the lumen, the mechanism of action of stents is different from angioplasty. Many different stents are available. In the SFA, stainless-steel stents did not achieve a substantial reduction of the restenosis rate, and patency rates 1 year after placement range between 22% and 61%.[10] Because of mechanical limitations, only short lesions could be treated, and stents should have been placed only if PTA had failed to create a residual stenosis of less than 30% or a hemodynamically significant dissection had occurred. The introduction of a new alloy called nitinol for endovascular treatment raised hope, because nitinol stents exert a constant radial force on the arterial wall and are more flexible than metallic stents.[12] Nitinol stents are proposed to overcome the limitations of stainless-steel stents, and so far, several studies suggest higher patency rates compared to PTA or stainless-steel stents.[44] Self-expanding stents are advantageous in a superficial location that may be subject to external compression. Balloon-expandable stents (Fig. 16-4) are also available, but these stents may be deformed by extrinsic compression, which may lead to restenosis or reocclusion of the femoral or popliteal artery.[34] Initial results on the primary use of nitinol stents in patients with chronic limb ischemia are promising. For the SFA, the restenosis (>50%) rate is reported to be 11.6% at 6 months, 22% at 1 year, and 44% at 2 years after stent implantation.[12] Stenting of the infrapopliteal arteries may also improve the success of infrapopliteal interventions. Compared to PTA alone, the patency rate was

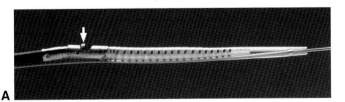

A

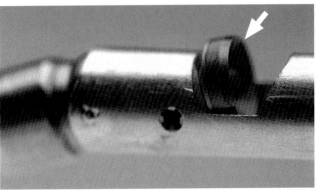

B

Figure 16–3   The SilverHawk system (FoxHollow Technologies, Redwood City, CA) for excisional atherectomy (**A**) is delivered through a catheter. **B,** A magnified view of the rotating blade (*arrow*), which is activated as the device is advanced through the vessel, shaving plaque from the artery walls as it moves forward. The plaque is collected in the tip of the catheter and can then be removed.

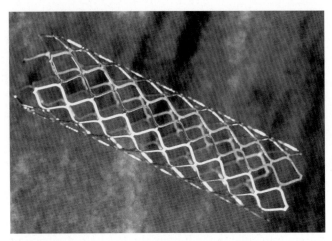

Figure 16–4   Example of a metallic balloon expandable stent (Cordis Corporation, New York, NY). *(Reprinted with permission from Kaufman JA. Vascular interventions. In Kaufman JA, Lee MJ. The requisites: Vascular and interventional radiology. Philadelphia, Mosby/Elsevier, 2004.)*

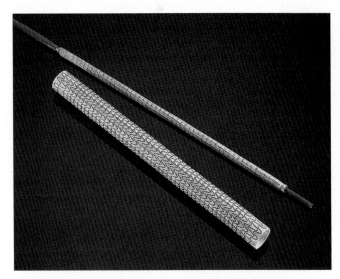

Figure 16–5   Example of a commercially available self-expanding stent graft and delivery system. The stent graft is constructed from nitinol metal and expanded PTFE and has an appropriate size for the superficial femoral artery (Viabahn, W.L. Gore, Flagstaff, AZ).

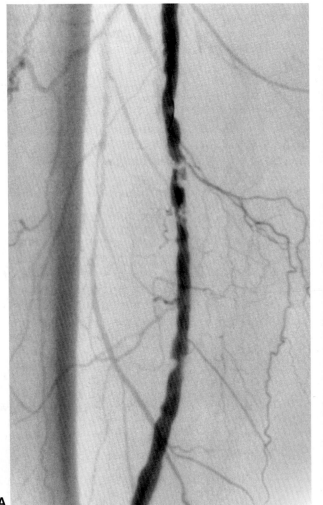

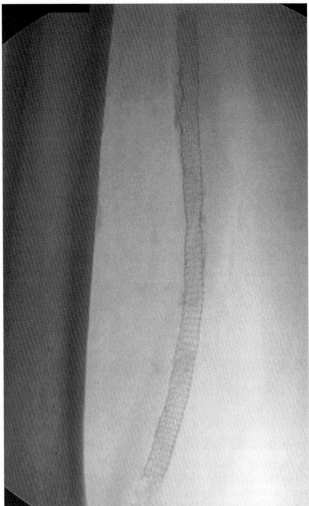

A   **B**

Figure 16–6   Treatment of long-segment SFA stenoses with ePTFE covered-stent graft. **A,** Angiography demonstrates multiple SFA stenoses with small muscular branches arising from the SFA. A stent graft (W.L. Gore, Flagstaff, AZ) was placed **(B),** and the multiple small branches are no longer seen on follow-up angiography **(C).** *(**A** and **C** reprinted with permission from Kaufman JA. Lower extremity arteries. In Kaufman JA, Lee MJ: The requisites: Vascular and interventional radiology. Philadelphia: Mosby/Elsevier, 2004.)*

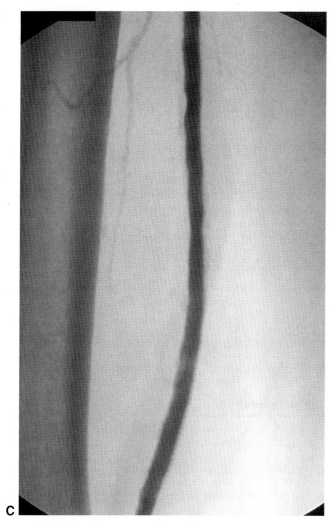

C

Figure 16–6, cont'd   See legend to C on opposite page.

significantly superior after stenting on 1-year follow-up: 53.4% and 83.6%, respectively.[45] The limb salvage rate after 1 year was 96% with PTA alone and 98.3% after stenting.

Another issue is fractures of nitinol stent struts that may occur after stent implantation across flexion points. On follow-up after SFA stent placement, stent fractures were observed in 18.2% of cases at 6 months and 24% at 2 years.[12] The risk of stent fracture was higher after long-segment artery stenting than after short-segment stenting, but no correlation between restenosis and stent fractures was found. One asymptomatic patient had to be rehospitalized owing to a stent fracture and received prophylactic placement of a covered stent graft for vessel ulceration at the site of a strut fracture.

Covered Stents

Covered stent grafts were initially developed to prevent acute vessel occlusion as a result of elastic recoil and an inhibition of vascular smooth muscle cell proliferation inside the lumen of the stent graft. Implantation of Dacron-covered stent-grafts for treatment of femoropopliteal lesions was disappointingly associated with a high early rethrombosis rate of 17% and a late 2-year patency rate of less than 50%. Furthermore, a considerable rate of complications, such as fever and pain, was observed in approximately 50% of patients.[46] Better results were achieved by using expanded polytetrafluoroethylene-covered stents (Figs. 16-5 and 16-6) demonstrating 79% primary and 93% secondary patency rates at 1 year and an 87% patency rate at 2-year follow-up.[47,48] On the one hand, the use of covered stents may improve the results of endovascular treatment for longer lesions; on the other hand, a larger sheath size is needed, and covered stents are more costly than uncoated nitinol stents.[49]

Drug-eluting Stents

Drug-eluting stents are novel implantable devices that release single or multiple bioactive agents into blood vessels after implantation.[50] One major purpose of drug-eluting stents is to limit neointimal hyperplasia. Drug-eluting stents implanted in the coronary arteries substantially improve long-term outcomes for restenosis.[51] The utility of these stents in peripheral atherosclerosis is currently under evaluation. To date, the Sirocco multicenter trail is the only study using drug-eluting, self-expanding nitinol stents in the SFA.[12] The results of this study showed inhibition of in-stent neointimal hyperplasia.[52] The rate of restenosis (>50%) was 0% with drug-eluting stents compared to 23.5% with uncoated stents. However, 2-year results indicate reduction of the benefit of drug elution. At this time, no significant differences between coated and bare nitinol stents were found.[26] First experiences with drug-eluting stents for infrapopliteal arteries are currently under way using a balloon-expandable coronary stent design, and data are currently pending.

Biodegradable Stents

Biodegradable stents are an innovative and potentially promising alternative technology.[53] Biodegradable stents might reduce intimal hyperplasia triggered after stent implantation by a foreign-body reaction to the stent itself. These stents provide optimal initial scaffolding and favorable initial luminal dimension but dissolve slowly after placement. Initial results from experimental and preliminary human studies exploring the utility of absorbable magnesium stents are encouraging. They indicate a significant corresponding decrease in intimal hyperplasia and complete reabsorption after 60 days.

Summary

Patients with diabetes mellitus are predisposed to peripheral vascular disease. For the treatment of vascular stenosis and occlusion, PTA is considered the basic technique for femoropopliteal angioplasty. Its underlying mechanism is based on controlled fracturing of the obstructing plaque and stretching of the media by using a balloon. PTA is a safe and effective alternative to surgery with an outcome comparable to that of bypass surgery for selected lesions. PTA is advantageous over surgery, as it is performed under local anesthesia and has a low morbidity and mortality rate. The recovery period after PTA is short. If necessary, PTA can be repeated without increased difficulty or increased patient risk compared to the first procedure, and it does not preclude surgery as adjunctive or definitive therapy.

Besides PTA, a diversity of newer techniques has recently become available for endovascular interventions challenging the clinician to select the most appropriate therapy for each individual patient based on predicted safety and efficacy. Cutting balloon angioplasty is a modification of conventional balloon dilation using a balloon with cutting blades to create longitudinal incisions into the plaque to reduce the force needed to dilate the vessel and lower the rate of dissections. Cryoplasty is based on a targeted delivery of cold thermal energy to the vessel wall to alter the biological response of the vessel and result in a more benign healing process after balloon injury. A novel technique, balloon coating, uses a conventional angioplasty balloon to apply drugs to the site of treatment. Brachytherapy uses afterloading of γ radiation to cause local inhibition of intimal hyperplasia at the treatment site, but it did not increase patency rates, according to a high incidence of thrombotic occlusions. When a vascular occlusion cannot be crossed, intentional subintimal angioplasty can be performed to intentionally create a false channel or dissection around an arterial occlusion to distally reenter the true lumen. Alternative debulking procedures are excisional atherectomy or laser angioplasty.

Stents are used for scaffolding of the vessel lumen, pushing plaque and vessel wall aside to enlarge the lumen. Different sorts of stents are available. Self-expandable nitinol stents are proposed to overcome the limitations of stainless-steel stents. Balloon-expandable stents are also available, but restenosis may be caused by its deformability by extrinsic compression, especially in the SFA. Covered stents may improve the results of endovascular treatment for longer lesions, but they are more costly than uncoated nitinol stents, and a larger sheath size is needed. Drug-eluting stents are proposed to limit restenosis caused by neointimal hyperplasia and are currently under evaluation in peripheral arteries. Another novel technique uses biodegradable stents that initially provide optimal intraluminal scaffolding and then dissolve slowly after placement to reduce intimal hyperplasia triggered by a foreign body reaction to the stent itself.

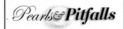

Pearls

- PTA is considered the basic technique for femoropopliteal angioplasty.
- Newer techniques for endovascular intervention include cutting balloon angioplasty, cryoplasty, and balloon drug coating.
- Subintimal angioplasty or alternative debulking procedures can be performed when a vascular lesion cannot be crossed.
- Stents are used for scaffolding of the vessel lumen.
- Covered stents may improve endovascular treatment of longer lesions.

Pitfalls

- Endovascular brachytherapy seems not to substantially increase patency rates.
- The use of balloon-expandable stents in the SFA may result in restenosis due to extrinsic compression.

References

1. Da SA, Widmer LK, Ziegler HW, et al: The Basle longitudinal study: Report on the relation of initial glucose level to baseline ECG abnormalities, peripheral artery disease, and subsequent mortality. J Chronic Dis 32:797–803, 1979.
2. Bakal CW, Cynamon J, Sprayregen S: Infrapopliteal percutaneous transluminal angioplasty: What we know. Radiology 200:36–43, 1996.
3. Rofsky NM, Adelman, MA: MR angiography in the evaluation of atherosclerotic peripheral vascular disease. Radiology 214:325–338, 2000.
4. Vogt FM, Ajaj W, Hunold P, et al: Venous compression at high-spatial-resolution three-dimensional MR angiography of peripheral arteries. Radiology 233:913–920, 2004.
5. Dotter CT, Judkins MP: Transluminal treatment of arteriosclerotic obstruction. Description of a new technic and a preliminary report of its application. Circulation 30:654–670, 1964.
6. Gruentzig A, Hopff H: Perkutane Rekanalisation chronischer arterieller Verschluesse mit einem neuen Dilatatonskatheter Modifikation der Dotter-Technik. Dtsch Med Wochenschr 99: 2502–2507, 1974.
7. Wiesinger B, Heller S, Schmehl J, et al: Percutaneous vascular interventions in the superficial femoral artery: A review. Minerva Cardioangiol 54:83–93, 2006.
8. White CJ: Non-surgical treatment of patients with peripheral vascular disease. Br Med Bull 59:173–192, 2001.
9. Drescher P, McGuckin J, Rilling WS, Crain MR: Catheter-directed thrombolytic therapy in peripheral artery occlusions: Combining reteplase and abciximab. AJR Am J Roentgenol 180:1385–1391, 2003.
10. Dormandy JA, Rutherford RB: Management of peripheral arterial disease (PAD). TASC Working Group. TransAtlantic Inter-Society Concensus (TASC). J Vasc Surg 31:S1–S296, 2000.
11. Duda SH, Poerner TC, Wiesinger B, et al: Drug-eluting stents: Potential applications for peripheral arterial occlusive disease. J Vasc Interv Radiol 14:291–301, 2003.
12. Duda SH, Bosiers M, Lammer J, et al: Sirolimus-eluting versus bare nitinol stent for obstructive superficial femoral artery disease: The SIROCCO II trial. J Vasc Interv Radiol 16:331–338, 2005.
13. Minar E, Ahmadi RA, Ehringer H, et al: [Percutaneous transluminal angioplasty (PTA) in peripheral arterial occlusive disease of the lower extremities]. Wien Klin Wochenschr 98:33–40, 1986.

14. Treiman GS, Whiting JH, Treiman RL, et al: Treatment of limb-threatening ischemia with percutaneous intentional extraluminal recanalization: a preliminary evaluation. J Vasc Surg 38:29–35, 2003.

15. Treiman GS, Treiman RL, Ichikawa L, Van AR: Should percutaneous transluminal angioplasty be recommended for treatment of infrageniculate popliteal artery or tibioperoneal trunk stenosis? J Vasc Surg 22:457–463, 1995.

16. Varty K, Bolia A, Naylor AR, et al: Infrapopliteal percutaneous transluminal angioplasty: A safe and successful procedure. Eur J Vasc Endovasc Surg 9:341–345, 1995.

17. Parsons RE, Suggs WD, Lee JJ, et al: Percutaneous transluminal angioplasty for the treatment of limb threatening ischemia: Do the results justify an attempt before bypass grafting? J Vasc Surg 28:1066–1071, 1998.

18. Rabbi JF, Kiran RP, Gersten G, et al: Early results with infrainguinal cutting balloon angioplasty limits distal dissection. Ann Vasc Surg 18:640–643, 2004.

19. Jahnke T: Cryoplasty for the treatment of femoropopliteal arterial disease: Will freezing solve the problem of cold feet? J Vasc Interv Radiol 16:1051–1054, 2005.

20. Engelke C, Sandhu C, Morgan RA, Belli AM: Using 6-mm cutting balloon angioplasty in patients with resistant peripheral artery stenosis: Preliminary results. AJR Am J Roentgenol 179:619–623, 2002.

21. Ansel GM, Sample NS, Botti IC Jr., et al: Cutting balloon angioplasty of the popliteal and infrapopliteal vessels for symptomatic limb ischemia. Catheter Cardiovasc Interv 61:1–4, 2004.

22. Grassl ED and Bischof, JC: In vitro model systems for evaluation of smooth muscle cell response to cryoplasty. Cryobiology 50:162–173, 2005.

23. Fava M, Loyola S, Polydorou A, et al: Cryoplasty for femoropopliteal arterial disease: Late angiographic results of initial human experience. J Vasc Interv Radiol 15:1239–1243, 2004.

24. Laird J, Jaff MR, Biamino G, et al: Cryoplasty for the treatment of femoropopliteal arterial disease: Results of a prospective, multicenter registry. J Vasc Interv Radiol 16:1067–1073, 2005.

25. Scheller B, Speck U, Abramjuk C, et al: Paclitaxel balloon coating, a novel method for prevention and therapy of restenosis. Circulation 110:810–814, 2004.

26. Tepe G, Schmehl J, Heller S, et al: Superficial femoral artery: Current treatment options. Eur Radiol 16:1316–1322, 2006.

27. Pokrajac B, Potter R, Wolfram RM, et al: Endovascular brachytherapy prevents restenosis after femoropopliteal angioplasty: Results of the Vienna-3 randomised multicenter study. Radiother Oncol 74:3–9, 2005.

28. Wolfram RM, Budinsky AC, Pokrajac B, et al: Endovascular brachytherapy: restenosis in de novo versus recurrent lesions of femoropopliteal artery: The Vienna experience. Radiology 236:338–342, 2005.

29. Wolfram RM, Budinsky AC, Pokrajac B, et al: Vascular brachytherapy with 192Ir after femoropopliteal stent implantation in high-risk patients: Twelve-month follow-up results from the Vienna-5 trial. Radiology 236:343–351, 2005.

30. London NJ, Srinivasan R, Naylor AR, et al: Subintimal angioplasty of femoropopliteal artery occlusions: The long-term results. Eur J Vasc Surg 8:148–155, 1994.

31. Laxdal E, Jenssen GL, Pedersen G, Aune S: Subintimal angioplasty as a treatment of femoropopliteal artery occlusions. Eur J Vasc Endovasc Surg 25:578–582, 2003.

32. Spinosa DJ, Leung DA, Matsumoto AH, et al: Percutaneous intentional extraluminal recanalization in patients with chronic critical limb ischemia. Radiology 232:499–507, 2004.

33. Cumberland DC, Sanborn TA, Tayler DI, et al: Percutaneous laser thermal angioplasty: Initial clinical results with a laser probe in total peripheral artery occlusions. Lancet 1:1457–1459, 1986.

34. Lyden SP, Shimshak TM: Contemporary endovascular treatment for disease of the superficial femoral and popliteal arteries: An integrated device-based strategy. J Endovasc Ther 13(suppl 2):II41–II51, 2006.

35. Scheinert D, Laird JR Jr, Schroder M, et al: Excimer laser-assisted recanalization of long, chronic superficial femoral artery occlusions. J Endovasc Ther 8:156–166, 2001.

36. Gray BH, Laird JR, Ansel GM, et al: Complex endovascular treatment for critical limb ischemia in poor surgical candidates: A pilot study. J Endovasc Ther 9:599–604, 2002.

37. Laird JR, Zeller T, Gray BH, et al: Limb salvage following laser-assisted angioplasty for critical limb ischemia: Results of the LACI multicenter trial. J Endovasc Ther 13:1–11, 2006.

38. Dorros G, Iyer S, Lewin R, et al: Angiographic follow-up and clinical outcome of 126 patients after percutaneous directional atherectomy (Simpson AtheroCath) for occlusive peripheral vascular disease. Cathet Cardiovasc Diagn 22:79–84, 1991.

39. Kim D, Gianturco LE, Porter DH, et al: Peripheral directional atherectomy: 4-year experience. Radiology 183: 773–778, 1992.

40. Tielbeek AV, Vroegindeweij D, Buth J, Landman GH: Comparison of balloon angioplasty and Simpson atherectomy for lesions in the femoropopliteal artery: Angiographic and clinical results of a prospective randomized trial. J Vasc Interv Radiol 7:837–844, 1996.

41. Zeller T, Krankenberg H, Reimers B, et al: Initial clinical experience with a new percutaneous peripheral atherectomy device for the treatment of femoro-popliteal stenoses. Rofo 176:70–75, 2004.

42. Kandzari DE, Kiesz RS, Allie D, et al: Procedural and clinical outcomes with catheter-based plaque excision in critical limb ischemia. J Endovasc Ther 13: 12–22, 2006.

43. Zeller T, Rastan A, Schwarzwalder U, et al: Midterm results after atherectomy-assisted angioplasty of below-knee arteries with use of the Silverhawk device. J Vasc Interv Radiol 15:1391–1397, 2004.

44. Grenacher L, Saam T, Geier A, et al: [PTA versus Palmaz stent placement in femoropopliteal artery stenoses: results of a multicenter prospective randomized study (REFSA)]. Rofo 176:1302–1310, 2004.

45. Scheinert D, Biamino G: Recanalization techniques in popliteal and tibial occlusive disease. In Euro PCR, Paris, 2004, pp 452–459. Accessed at www.congrhealth.com.

46. Ahmadi R, Schillinger M, Maca T, Minar E: Femoropopliteal arteries: Immediate and long-term results with a Dacron-covered stent-graft. Radiology 223:45–350, 2002.

47. Bray PJ, Robson WJ, Bray AE: Percutaneous treatment of long superficial femoral artery occlusive disease: efficacy of the Hemobahn stent-graft. J Endovasc Ther 10:619–628, 2003.

48. Saxon RR, Coffman JM, Gooding JM, et al: Long-term results of ePTFE stent-graft versus angioplasty in the femoropopliteal artery: Single center experience from a prospective, randomized trial. J Vasc Interv Radiol 14:303–311, 2003.

49. Saxon RR, Coffman JM, Gooding JM, Ponec DJ: Endograft use in the femoral and popliteal arteries. Tech Vasc Interv Radiol 7:6–15, 2004.

50. Boccara F, Teiger E, Cohen A: Role of drug eluting stents in diabetic patients. Heart 92:543–544, 2006.

51. Schwartz RS, Edelman ER, Carter A, et al: Preclinical evaluation of drug-eluting stents for peripheral applications: recommendations from an expert consensus group. Circulation 19;110:2498–2505, 2004.

52. Duda SH, Pusich B, Richter G, et al: Sirolimus-eluting stents for the treatment of obstructive superficial femoral artery disease: Six-month results. Circulation 106:1505–1509, 2002.

53. Heublein B, Rohde R, Kaese V, et al: Biocorrosion of magnesium alloys: A new principle in cardiovascular implant technology? Heart 89:651–656, 2003.

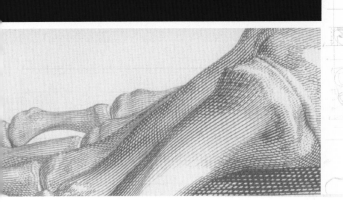

ADJUNCTIVE HYPERBARIC OXYGEN THERAPY IN THE TREATMENT OF THE DIABETIC FOOT

PAUL CIANCI AND THOMAS K. HUNT ■

Introduction

Diabetes mellitus affects 5% to 6% of the population (it is estimated that half are undiagnosed). The annual cost of care exceeds $132 billion.[1] Recent data from a study at a major health maintenance organization involving more than 175,000 patients showed that diabetic patients consumed 2.4 times more health care dollars than did nondiabetic controls ($480,660,718 versus $197,948,887).[2] The federal government is increasingly aware of this problem. "Diabetics account for 27% of the federal medical budget" (Newt Gingrich, Speaker of the House of Representatives, in an address to the AMA, March 9, 1998). At any given time, approximately 1 million diabetic patients have lower-limb ulcers. Twenty percent of hospital admissions of diabetic patients are due to lower-limb problems.[3] The incidence of amputation is 6 per 1000. Diabetic patients accounted for 50% to 70% of the 118,000 amputations performed in the United States in 1983. From 1993 to 1995, about 67,000 amputations were performed yearly among people with diabetes.[4] Nine percent required amputation of a foot, 31% required amputation of the lower leg, and 30% required amputation at or above the knee.[5] The cost of a primary amputation in 1986 was reported to be in excess of $40,000.[6] In 1995, private reimbursement for diabetic ulcers averaged $8988 per case with an 11.4-day average length of stay. Medicare reimbursement averaged $4862 per case with an average 8.8-day stay.[7] Medicare reimbursement for primary amputation is approximately $12,500.[8]

The morbidity and mortality associated with amputation are significant. Ipsilateral, often higher amputation will occur in 22% of cases. Contralateral amputation occurs at a rate of approximately 10% a year. Sixty-eight percent of elderly amputees will be alive at 4 years.[9] Only 40% to 50% of elderly amputees will be rehabilitated.[10] The length of hospital stay for primary amputation varies widely but has been reported to average 22 days.[11,12] Six to nine months may be necessary to maximize walking ability.[13] In 1997 dollars, the cost of amputation was in excess of $2.7 billion yearly.[14] Readmission within 2 years for stump modification or reamputation accounts for an additional $1.5 billion expenditure.[12] The perioperative mortality rate associated with amputation at a major teaching hospital was reported to be 4%. The morbidity rate, including myocardial infarction, arrhythmia, or congestive heart failure requiring therapy, was 14%.[11]

Many surgeons are quick to amputate, citing the traditionally long recovery time for diabetic foot wounds. Clearly, these data show that hasty amputation is far from an expeditious solution to the problem of foot wounds in diabetic patients. Apelquist, in a series of 314 patients, reported primary healing of ulcers in 63% of cases, healing after amputation of 24%, and death of 13%.[15] He later reported that total costs for patients who achieved primary healing and did not have critical ischemia were $16,000 compared to $63,000 for patients who had required major amputation.[16] The data of Holzer and colleagues, in a large retrospective series, are similar and demonstrate the increased cost of amputation.[17] An aggressive, multidisciplinary team approach to diabetic foot management can result in improved salvage and significant cost savings.[5,8,11,18,19] We have utilized this regimen at our community hospital since 1983. Patients are quickly evaluated, are revascularized aggressively, and, when indicated, receive hyperbaric oxygen (HBO) therapy as an adjunct to their medical and surgical care. This chapter comments on this experience.

Pathophysiology of the Diabetic Foot

The "diabetic foot" is characterized by sensory, motor, and autonomic neuropathy and macrovascular disease. These may lead to ulceration, infection, gangrene, and amputation. Motor neuropathy causes alteration of pressure distribution. Foot deformities and altered sensation result in ulceration. These wounds can occur in the absence of ischemia and frequently heal with conservative measures such as unweighting and aggressive wound management. Primary effort is directed toward patient education and foot care. Autonomic neuropathy may cause alterations in circulation and diversion of nutritive flow, resulting in cutaneous ischemia.[20] Ischemic ulcers may be associated with pathophysiologic alterations involving small cutaneous vessels in addition to the contribution of arterial insufficiency. Many diabetic patients have areas of low flow and hypoxia in their feet and ankles, even in the presence of palpable pulses. Contributing factors may be increased blood viscosity, platelet aggregation, excessive adherence of leukocytes to capillary endothelial cells, and accelerated capillary endothelial growth.[21-23] Surgical revascularization can often provide the necessary substrate for wound healing. Some wounds, however, fail to heal in the presence of restored circulation even when tissue perfusion appears adequate.[24] This dilemma may in part be explained by the phenomenon that was recently reported by Caselli and colleagues, whereby transcutaneous oxygen values took 3 to 4 weeks to reach levels optimal for healing after successful revascularization.[25] The diabetic responses to local tissue stresses are thrombosis and necrosis as opposed to an inflammatory response in nondiabetic patients.[26] There is now ample evidence that tight control of plasma glucose can delay the onset or prevent the progression of microvascular complications.[27-30] Indeed, there is a direct correlation between amputation and increased glycosylated hemoglobin (Fig. 17-1).[31]

The crucial role of the endothelium in the regulation of local microvascular hemodynamics is now apparent. Injury to the endothelium due to high glucose, high lac-

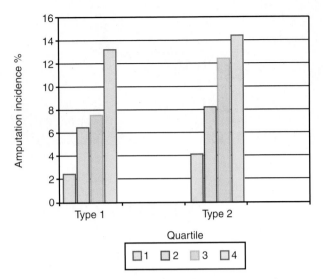

Figure 17-1 Glycosylated hemoglobin was measured at baseline, and the cohort was followed for 14 years with ascertainment of amputation. *(Data from the Wisconsin Epidemiologic Study of Diabetic Retinopathy.)*

tate, and increased pressure and flow due to neurogenic factors ultimately leads to sclerosis.[32-34] Whereas lipids were once the focus of diabetic arterial disease, recent studies have led attention toward redox regulation of endothelial cell function and the "toxic" effects of glucose and its derivative, lactate. Glucose itself is a mild oxidant. Lactate, made mostly by glycolysis, is a strong pro-oxidant that activates a variety of cytokines that cause endothelium to leak, to replicate, and to produce collagen. This mechanism acts at least partly through an ubiquitous set of enzymes, the nicotinamide adenine dinucleotide phosphate hydroxylate (NADPH)-linked oxidases that add an electron to oxygen, converting it to superoxide and thus hydrogen peroxide and other derivates. In excess, oxidants direct endothelial cells to produce and release vascular endothelial growth factor (VEGF), which causes them to become hyperpermeable, to become motile beyond normal expectations, and to deposit subintimal connective tissue.

The role of nitric oxide (NO) is closely allied. NO, like lactate, performs essential normal functions; but in excess, it interacts with the oxidants produced by the NADPH-linked oxidases. The reaction $NO + O_2^- \rightarrow NOOO$ (nitrogen peroxide) is well known to be a source of oxidative damage. In short, hyperglycemia, through lactate and NO, is toxic to arterial endothelium and the cells immediately adjacent. This effect is mediated, in part, through increased levels of endothelial NO.[35-40] Regardless of mechanisms, the net result of arterial damage is tissue hypoxia that involves focal regions of the foot or ankle, often toes, or the lateral side of the foot. Ironically, the same oxidant damage that leads to the problem is an essential part of the solution, that is, healing.

Role of Oxygen in Healing the Diabetic Foot

The central problem in the diabetic foot is that even minor injuries become infected and fail to heal owing to hyperglycemia, lack of blood flow, and, in particular, too little oxygen.[41] The reasons are complex. The combined animal and human data record retarded development of tensile strength, contraction, angiogenesis, and epithelialization in acute wounds. Resistance to infection is impaired in all wounds in diabetic patients. Behind these defects there are issues of growth factor production, collagen deposition, and angiogenesis. Most of these problems are the direct result of hyperglycemia and often can be overcome simply by tight management of plasma glucose. However, after diabetes has been present for some time, the major issue becomes the lack of blood and oxygen supply due to diabetic vascular disease. Other long-term problems include chronic reinjury and failed inflammation due to diabetic neuropathy, and an ill-defined abnormality of the arterial endothelial cell. Within these categories, there are multiple overlapping subissues. A number of these impediments are at least partly corrected by supplementing the oxygen supply by HBO therapy.

Oxygen, and the lack of it, are recurring themes in wound healing. Experimental studies long ago predicted the value of high-dose oxygen, even in diabetes-retarded wounds. However, the clinical value of HBO was at first obscured by the complexity of the issues.[42] As the detrimental effects of hyperglycemia have become known, improved plasma glucose control has made it easier to isolate and appreciate the effects of oxygen. Similarly, exaggerated levels of sympathetic nervous tone due to dehydration, pain and hypothermia, limited ability to assess the degree of local hypoxia in arterial insufficiency, and the inhibitory effects of established infection have also tended to confuse the results of clinical studies.[43] These impediments can be controlled. Clinical trials in which they are controlled are ongoing and are demonstrating the clinical importance of high-dose oxygen. If these issues are ignored and not corrected in the individual patient, as has often been the case, oxygen therapy is not likely to be effective. Therefore, a working knowledge of how oxygen acts and the circumstances that govern its availability in wounded tissue is needed for optimal care, especially of the diabetic foot.

A Modern View of Wound Healing

As a result of recent discoveries, we can now define wound healing as the result of a changed tissue redox environment induced by injury and the lactate and hydrogen peroxide accumulation that follows.[44] This,

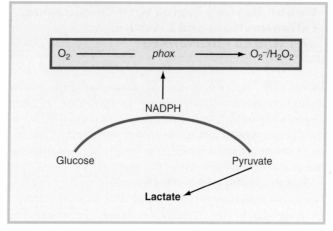

Figure 17-2   Activation of *phox* consumes NADPH and as a result also activates the hexose monophosphate shunt. This leads to a large increase in oxygen consumption and lactate production. Note that the lactate (that rises as much as fivefold when leukocytes are fully activated) is not an effect of hypoxia. Some glucose is required, but bactericidal oxidant production falls 50% as glucose rises above normal. Loss of *phox* function retards wound healing as well as resistance to infection. There are at least four similar enzymes that produce lactate and oxidants and perform signaling functions. These in turn require at least five separate proteins to activate the enzyme. This area of regulating wound healing and infection risk will take many years to work out.

together with the continued presence of oxygen, albeit at somewhat low levels, leads to expression of a variety of growth factors and cytokines.[45] The problem with diabetes is that hyperglycemia impairs these mechanisms.

It is now apparent that lactate redirects the use of oxygen into reparative and defensive functions and that these functions are increasingly better served as the local oxygen concentration rises, at least intermittently. For instance, accumulated lactate, acting as a sort of "pseudo-hypoxia," increases the presence of the so-called hypoxia-inducible genes that include hypoxia-inducible factor (hif-1α), vascular endothelial growth factor (VEGF), and others, even in the presence of oxygen.[46–48] The cells that surround the area of injury can obey these signals, deposit collagen, start growth of new microvasculature, kill bacteria, and so forth only when molecular oxygen is present in fairly large quantities. It is therefore important to realize that lactate production is aerobic, not anaerobic[49] (Fig. 17-2).

Wound healing in general does not occur when local PO_2 in the region is below about 15 mm Hg. It accelerates rapidly in the range of 30 to about 150 mm Hg and then more slowly to its peak rate that, by extension of known data, should occur at about 200 mm Hg. The implied paradox of lactate accumulating in the presence of increased oxygen has been resolved by the demonstration that activated inflammatory cells produce large amounts of lactate and hydrogen peroxide even in the presence of oxygen, thus redirecting the flux of oxygen and its reactive oxygen species to sites in the cell that, in turn, stimulate the expression of VEGF and hif-1α.

Wound Healing Begins with Coagulation, Inflammation, and Creation of a Wound Environment

Blood with platelets and coagulation proteins enters wounds immediately after injury. In this sense, healing begins with an infusion of platelet-derived growth factor, insulin-like growth factor, fibrin, and fibrin split products, all of which are transported in relatively high amounts in the blood that is spilled into the wound.

Polymorphologic leukocytes (granulocytes) are the first nucleated cells to enter the wound. The journey activates them to initiate the "respiratory burst," in which they consume large amounts of oxygen; produce bactericidal oxidants, hydrogen peroxide, and superoxide; and release lactate by action of the phagocytic NADPH-linked oxidase (*phox*) (see Fig. 17-2).

Within a day or two of injury, macrophages enter the injury site. They, too, produce lactate as a consequence of their respiratory burst; but in contrast to granulocytes, macrophages have the capacity to respond to the developing "healing environment," and they produce the various signals for angiogenesis, such as VEGF. Lactate quickly rises to an equilibrium value within the first 12 hours or so, but hypoxia does not develop until about the second day.[50] VEGF, thought to be the most powerful of the signals for angiogenesis, is instigated after the lactate rises and prior to the emergence of hypoxia. This is testimony to the important role of lactate.

Lactate accumulates in the cytoplasm of macrophages, where, chelated with iron and in the presence of H_2O_2, it stimulates the production of a number of growth factors and transcriptional proteins, particularly VEGF and hif-1α.[46] Although these are also known as hypoxia-inducible factors because hypoxia activates their gene expressions, their functions, that is, collagen deposition and angiogenesis, depend on the presence of molecular oxygen and accumulated lactate.

The lactate flux from inflammatory cells is so great as to overflow into the extracellular fluid from where it enters surrounding cells and the bloodstream at will, thereby stimulating adjacent or even distant fibroblasts and endothelial cells to migrate, to synthesize and deposit collagen, and to stimulate the formation of new vessels. The extraordinary mobility of lactate also plays a role in the body economy of large injuries—burns, for instance. Excess lactate spills into the blood and is transported to the liver, where it is recycled into glucose, which then returns to the wound.[51] Lactate accumulates because *phox* (and other sources) stimulate glycolysis and generate huge amounts of pyruvate, far greater than the relatively few mitochondria can process. Thus, the excess pyruvate is mainly converted to lactate via lactate dehydrogenase.

Lactate stimulates production of such growth factors as VEGF and transforming growth factor β by yet another

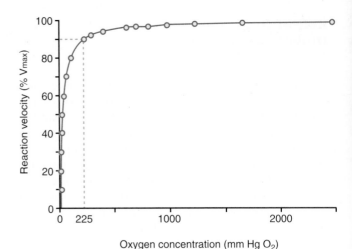

Figure 17-3   Kinetics of prolyl hydroxylase (K_m = 25 mm Hg). Reaction velocity of prolyl hydroxylase depends on the concentration of oxygen in the endoplasmic reticulum, with half maximal velocity (K_m) at about 20 mm Hg. Normally, the PO_2 there varies between a few to perhaps 50 mm Hg. Normal mean probably is in the region of 30 to 40 mm Hg. In foot lesions in diabetic patients, the number of focal areas at which PO_2 is zero increases markedly, and the mean may fall close to zero. Clearly, there is better collagen deposition at higher levels.

mechanism: regulation of ADP ribosylation.[48,52] It also stimulates collagen synthesis and deposition by tilting the balance of NAD^+/NADH in favor of NADH.[53] The loss of NAD^+ necessarily reduces the substrate for ADP ribosylation (the enzyme is polyadenosyl phosphorylase) that, when plentiful, ribosylates the transcription factor known as SP-1, preventing its binding to the collagen and VEGF gene promoters. Reduction of NAD^+ and consequently of SP-1 ribosylation as a result of high lactate frees a transcription factor to bind to the promoter and to enhance transcription of the collagen and VEGF genes (and probably others such as transforming growth factor β).[45] As a result, connective tissue deposition and angiogenesis are increased by two major mechanisms: reactive oxygen species and ADP ribosylation.

No matter how important lactate might be, however, neither the molecular events leading to gene transcription nor the deposition of connective tissue and angiogenesis themselves can occur without oxygen.[47,54] Oxygen is required to hydroxylate certain prolines in the nascent collagen molecule so that mature collagen can be exported from the cell. Ascorbic acid, essential for healing in humans, is a component of the reactive oxygen species formation that are central to this mechanism. Without this step, healing cannot occur. Collagen deposition in wounds is proportional to oxygen tension from zero to about 200 mm Hg (Fig. 17-3).[54]

The addition of lactate to experimental, primarily closed wounds enhances wound healing without changing the oxygen tension.[45] The common assumption that hypoxia initiates healing has been disproved.[50] The addition of oxygen to wounds in which lactate has been

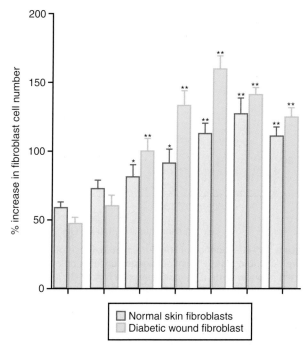

Figure 17–4 Percentage increase in fibroblast cell number, DNA content, 24 hours after a 1-hour treatment at multiple oxygen pressures as compared with untreated cells. Normal skin (*purple bars*) and chronic diabetic wounds (*orange bars*). Values represent the mean ± standard deviation of five different patients, each assayed in triplicate. Significant difference (*$p < .05$, **$p < .01$) compared with 21 kPa (untreated cells). *(Redrawn with permission from Hehenberger K, et al: Dose-dependent hyperbaric oxygen stimulation of human fibroblast proliferation. Wound Repair Regen 5:147–150, 1997.)*

exogenously elevated enhances healing still further. Transforming growth factor β and interleukin 1 are similarly elicited.[45]

Other molecules that, like lactate, enter the cell before exerting their oxidant effect have also elicited VEGF in vitro. Therefore, it is probably safe to say that lactate is not unique in its effects and that whatever can be said for lactate/H_2O_2 can probably be said to a degree about NO and other oxidants as well.

Cell replication also requires oxygen. Fibroblasts and endothelial cells ordinarily replicate most rapidly at a PO_2 of about 40 to 60 mm Hg.[55] The implication of many studies is that the most favorable PO_2 for cell replication is depressed in hyperglycemia and presumably influenced toward normal by a higher PO_2 (Fig. 17-4).

Resistance to Infection, a Function of Granulocytes That Depends on Oxygen

Polymorphonuclear leukocytes, the first inflammatory cells to appear at the site, marginate, penetrate the endothelium, and migrate into the injured space where they start the healing sequence and remove tissue debris while ingesting and killing contaminating bacteria. They are

the major source of innate resistance to bacterial infection. They ingest bacteria and in that process activate a complex and critical enzyme, the phagocytic NADPH-linked oxidase (also known as *phox*) (see Fig. 17-2).

Activation of *phox* increases the cellular oxygen consumption 25-fold or more in the so-called respiratory burst.[56] As is noted in Figure 17-2, *phox* converts almost all of this oxygen to the bactericidal oxidants superoxide and hydrogen peroxide (H_2O_2) and inserts them mainly into the phagosome.* The rate of oxidant formation and thus killing capacity is half-maximal at 60 mm Hg PO_2, which is about as high as occurs in wounds, even in ideal wounds in normal individuals breathing air.[56] The implication of this high K_m is that bacterial killing is not as effective during air breathing as it is in hyperoxia, even in ideal wounds. If the oxygen supply is insufficient to maintain PO_2 at a reasonable level, bacterial killing fails, and the probability of infection rises (Fig. 17-5). Theoretically, the maximum bactericidal potential is reached at a PO_2 of about 500 mm Hg. The difference between bacterial killing at a PO_2 of 40 (a common level) and 300 mm Hg (often reachable with hyperbaric oxygen therapy) is on the order of fivefold![56] The rewards of added oxygen, however, become progressively less as PO_2 rises into the higher ranges above 200 mm Hg (Fig. 17-6).

Several separate prospective, blinded, clinical studies have shown that attending to the "details" of maintaining the PO_2 of wounds, even by administering oxygen at sea level, has reduced postoperative wound infection rates by about 45%.[57–59] These "details" are critical.[60] They involve administering high-oxygen breathing mixtures but also require maintaining euthermia (total body and wound site), an adequate blood volume (though not necessarily a high red cell level), and pain control.

Unfortunately, *phox* is not entirely reliable. In a rare disorder, chronic granulomatous disease, the absence of one or more of the genes that encode any of its several proteins confers a profound, often fatal susceptibility to infection as well as poor healing. Hypoxia, that is, loss of its substrate, oxygen, confers the same problem. Glucose is necessary for production of NADPH on which this enzyme relies. However, even modest hyperglycemia impairs the enzyme (glucose 6 phosphate dehydrogenase) that supplies the needed NADPH (see Fig. 17-2).[61] The effect is so large that a glucose level of 15 mM reduces the effectiveness of *phox* by half and increases the incidence of wound infection in surgical patients by about twofold! Maintaining glucose levels in the normal range and oxygen in the high range are the most important means of ensuring normal healing and resistance to infection in diabetic patients. The effects of high-dose oxygen are then supplementary. Maintaining

---

*There are at least five such enzymes. *Phox* is mostly important to resistance to infection and produces the most bactericidal oxidants. Other "nonphagocytic" forms are ubiquitous and important in redox-related cell signaling.

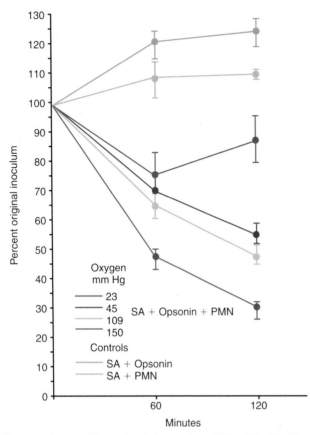

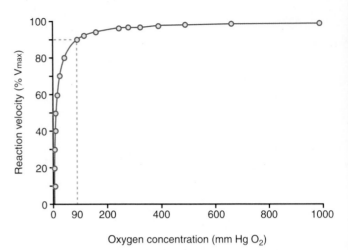

Figure 17–6 Kinetics of NADPH-linked oxidase of leukocytes. Curve describing NADPH-linked oxidase conversion of molecular oxygen of superoxide (O_2) (compare with Fig. 17-3). K_m is variously estimated at 8 and 25 mm Hg. Thus, the V_{max} will vary from approximately 80 to 250 mm Hg. The oxidative antibacterial system is particularly directed at the usual wound pathogens, such as *Staphylococcus*, *Streptococcus*, and *Escherichia coli*.

Figure 17–5 This study reinforces the validity of the kinetic approach noted in Figure 17-3. Mean (± SE [brackets]) phagocytic killing of *Staphylococcus aureus* (SA) under different oxygen tensions. SA, rabbit peritoneal leukocytes (PMN), and opsonin (10% normal human serum) were tumbled for 30 minutes at 40° C in a total volume of 1 mL. Each tube was decanted into a culture dish so that the suspension was 1 mm thick; an aliquot was removed for determination of the number of colony-forming units (CFUs) of SA. Dishes were placed under different oxygen tensions at 37° C and were removed after 60 or 120 minutes, at which time the number of CFUs of the initial inoculum was counted. At least six separate experiments at each oxygen tension were performed, each in duplicate. As oxygen tension increases, staphylococcal survival decreases, reflecting increased killing by PMNs.
(Courtesy of Jon Mader, M.D.)

Angiogenesis

Inflammatory angiogenesis occurs when lactate accumulates in the presence of oxygen. The mechanism is as noted above. Lactate, iron, and oxygen lead to a redirection of oxygen into redox regulation of growth factors. The result is transcription of VEGF and collagen genes in addition to the posttranslational modification (hydroxylation) of collagen. These events are also proportional to local oxygen concentration and are most accelerated when local PO_2 reaches several hundred mm Hg, although most of the change occurs in the range of 0 to 100 mm Hg. Angiogenic progenitor cells are mobilized into the blood by hyperbaric oxygen therapy[63] and seem to find a favorable home in the presence of high lactate.[64] In addition, redox changes due to lactate increase the migratory activity of endothelial cells. Their ability to produce collagen and hence provide support for themselves is again proportional to oxygen just as it is in fibroblasts. Hyperbaric oxygen therapy increases both VEGF and angiogenesis.[65,66]

The development of angiogenesis takes time. After successful vascular surgery, tissue PO_2 in the foot rises to its peak at about 3 weeks.[25] This effect promises a great future for elevating oxygen tensions in ischemic tissues. From both clinical observation and laboratory experiment, there is no longer any doubt that angiogenesis occurs most rapidly in well-oxygenated animals and that hyperbaric oxygen can produce clinically significant angiogenesis. In the latest of these, anti-VEGF antibody abrogated the effects of hyperbaric oxygen on angiogenesis in a Matrigel model.[66] HBO therapy stimulates angiogenesis and leads to an increase in new, mature vessels.[65] As this occurs, $TcPO_2$ increases. This increase seems to be

normoglycemia also helps to support blood volume by preventing osmotic diuresis. Euthermia, normoglycemia, pain relief, and whatever else that can inhibit vasoconstriction in the individual patient have additional value and are now standard practice whenever bacterial infection is a risk.* The level of oxygen also affects adherence molecules such as integrins that facilitate leukocyte adherence.[62] Hyperbaric oxygen tends to preserve this function. There are probably other effects of HBO that pertain to infection.

---

*Staphylococcus aureus, the major wound-infecting bacterium, is particularly susceptible to oxidative killing. Unfortunately, no serious attempt has been made to determine whether any other species of bacteria are or are not susceptible to enhanced oxidative killing.

long-lasting, perhaps "permanent." (See the case study at the end of the chapter.)

Epithelialization

Healing of epithelium has been surprisingly difficult to study. The epithelial layer is inescapably dependent on healing of the deeper tissues. The beneficial effects of retained moisture are so dominant that the clash between the external and internal environments leaves a bewildering array of gradients and transients. In general, studies have shown that oxygen administration accelerates coverage of epithelium over superficial burns after removal of eschar. Both topical and systemic therapies have been reported to be effective,[67] but clinicians disagree about the effectiveness of topical treatment. The migration of epithelial cells in culture is accelerated by oxidant generation due to the NADPH oxidases.[68] This subject is likely to remain controversial.

Healing of Chronic Wounds

Diabetes imposes a great deal of extra complexity on wound healing in general and especially on the healing of chronic wounds. Although healing of acute wounds in diabetic patients is impaired only by hyperglycemia and neuropathy, provided that oxygen supply is sufficient (i.e., there is no local ischemia), healing of chronic wounds is impaired by infection, chronic scarring, repeated trauma, and the neuropathy that impairs the neurogenic component of healing. Hehenberger and colleagues have reported that diabetes diminishes fibroblast replication, whereas hyperbaric oxygen dramatically increases it. The maximal effect was at 2.5 atmospheres.[55]

Ironically, even as hyperglycemia impairs the respiratory burst in stimulated phagocytes, it increases resting (i.e., unstimulated) *phox* activity. The consequent increased oxidant production is thought to damage endothelium when repeated day after day and month after month. The net conclusion is that the inevitable periods of hyperglycemia and accumulated tissue lactate that all of us incur after eating must be as short as possible to avoid chronic arterial damage.

There is no doubt, however, that people with diabetes do incur problems with healing of wounds that stay open long enough to develop characteristics of chronicity, that is, scarring of the surrounding tissues, surface or deep infection, periwound erythema, and edema. There are three major causes of this state: repetitive reinjury due to the insensitivity of diabetic neuropathy, local ischemia due to diabetic vascular disease, and hyperglycemia.

Chronic diabetic wounds take on their own character, and repetitive and prolonged episodes of excessively high glucose and lactate are part of it. One characteristic is severe scarring and inflammation at the wound edges

due to the long-term effects of frustrated healing and excessive oxidant production. This scarred tissue, like all scars, becomes ischemic in time. The wound will not heal in most cases until this ischemic scar is excised back to bleeding tissue so that the wound can be given a new start, presumably with the patient's glucose under tightened control. For diabetic neuropathic ulcers, physical protection for the insensate skin must also be provided. One of the most important lessons of the last few decades is that radical debridement can restore circulation to the wound edge. Even though debridement initially enlarges the wound, it makes healing possible.

But can one do anything about the regional ischemia? One of the most tantalizing findings is that intermittent hyperoxia, that is, hyperbaric oxygenation, is angiogenic.[65] This is proved in animals, and there is excellent evidence that it works in humans as well and that it may be permanent (see the case study at the end of the chapter).[65] In this case, the angiogenesis appears to occur in ischemic or inflamed, though not necessarily injured, tissue. To the best of current knowledge, it does not occur in tissues that are not producing excess lactate.

Chronic wounds in diabetic patients are ischemic, infected, and impaired. A short period (90 to 120 minutes once or twice daily) of increased leukocyte killing can go a long way, just as a short period of a twice daily antibiotic can. When infection is cleared, oxygen demands fall, and healing can proceed.

In summary, diabetes complicates wound healing. A special knowledge of healing and how it is affected is required to ensure optimal treatment of wounds in the diabetic foot. Enhancement of impaired healing by HBO has been controversial, largely because the method has been abused; and third-party payers have been reluctant to pay for it on the grounds that sufficient numbers of prospective studies have not been done! Because of their complexity, it has turned out to be difficult to demonstrate the efficacy of any method of treating wounds in humans. The proof of principle in animals is plentiful. The "proof" that enhancing oxygen tension is critical in diabetic wounds is so well based in theory and experimental fact derived in vitro, in animals, and in human wounds that it cannot be denied. The problem that remains in obtaining the proof in humans is learning how to select a homogeneous group of patients whose glucose and oxygen levels can be controlled and who are likely to benefit, that is, those whose wound PO_2 can be changed by HBO. This will not be easy; but when it happens, the conclusion will be favorable to the principle.

Hyperbaric Oxygen Therapy

The Undersea and Hyperbaric Medical Society, an international scientific organization and the leading authority for diving and hyperbaric medicine in the United States, defines HBO therapy as the intermittent administration

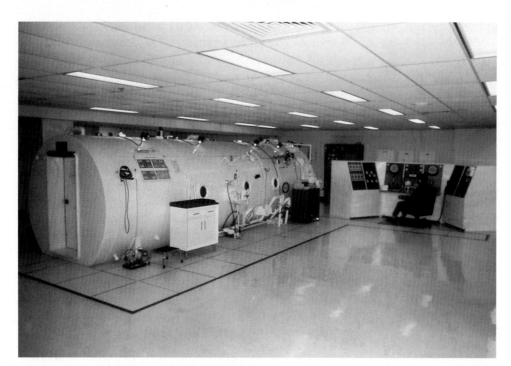

Figure 17–7   Multiplace chamber with capacity for concurrent treatment of multiple patients. Hands-on capability and provision of critical care are advantages of this type of unit. *(Courtesy of Dean Heimbach, M.D., Ph.D., San Antonio, TX.)*

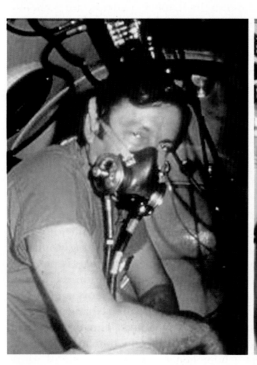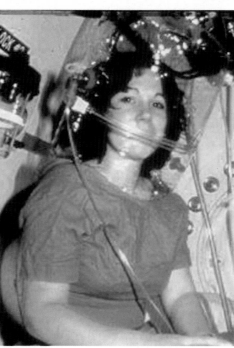

Figure 17–8   In multiplace chambers, patients breathe 100% oxygen through a mask, head tent, or endotracheal tube. The chamber is pressurized to treatment depth with compressed air.

of 100% oxygen inhaled at pressure greater than sea level. The technique may be implemented in a walk-in (multiplace) chamber (Fig. 17-7) compressed to depth with air while the patient breathes 100% oxygen via head tent, face mask, or endotracheal tube (Fig. 17-8). Alternatively, the patient may be treated in a one-person (monoplace) chamber (Fig. 17-9) pressurized to depth with oxygen. In either case, the arterial partial pressure of oxygen will approach 1500 mm Hg at the pressure equivalent of 33 feet of seawater (2 atmospheres absolute [ATA], 10 m).

HBO therapy is not new, having been used since 1943.[69] Modern therapy dates to the early 1960s, when Dutch investigators demonstrated the efficacy of HBO therapy in gas gangrene and anemic states.[70,71] Hyperbaric oxygen therapy is currently used as the primary treatment for decompression sickness (the bends), air embolism, and severe carbon monoxide poisoning.[72–75] Adjunctive indications include clostridial myonecrosis,[71,76,77] crush injury and traumatic ischemia,[78–80] enhancement of healing in selected problem wounds,[81] necrotizing soft tissue infections,[82–84] refractory osteomyelitis,[85–89] radia-

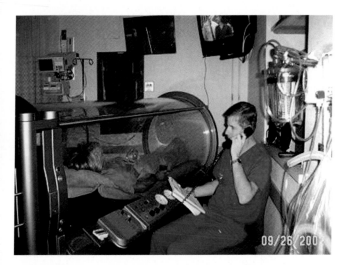

Figure 17–9   Patient being treated in a monoplace chamber pressurized with 100% oxygen. No mask or head tent is necessary.

tion damage to soft or hard tissue,[90–95] compromised skin grafts or flaps,[80,96,97] and burns.[99–102] All of these conditions have focal hypoperfusion or hypoxia, or both, in common.

Mechanisms of Action

Oxygen inhaled at pressure dissolves in plasma. At the pressure equivalent of 3 atmospheres (66 feet of seawater), an arterial PO_2 of nearly 2200 mm Hg may be achieved. Up to 6.9 volume % of oxygen may be forced into solution, a quantity sufficient to maintain life in the absence of hemoglobin.[70]

With HBO therapy, tissue oxygen tensions can often be raised to the relatively moderate levels necessary for fibroblast replication, development of a collagen matrix, and the ingress of capillaries into avascular areas. This can occur because wounds actually consume relatively little oxygen. Diffusion of oxygen away from functional capillaries is mainly a function of PO_2, independent of hemoglobin, and is increased twofold to fourfold at the pressure equivalent of 3 ATA. This may be of vital importance in preserving marginally viable tissue, enhancing

collagen deposition, angiogenesis, and the killing of bacteria in wounds. A marked increase in tissue oxygen tension may be achieved only with HBO therapy (Table 17-1).[87,103–106]

Topical Oxygen Therapy

Topical oxygen therapy rendered in limb-encasing devices is not HBO therapy.[107–109] Although some investigators consider it useful, the benefits of topical oxygen are disputed.[110]

Neovascularization

Restoration of abnormally low tissue oxygen tensions to physiologic values assists in capillary proliferation and advancement into the wound space. The reasons are not entirely clear. The effect may be due to oxidant-induced VEGF production and/or support of endothelial growth and/or migration[111] (Fig. 17-10).

Enhancement of White Cell Killing Ability

Any interference with oxygen delivery to wounds also increases susceptibility to infection. Wounds of the limbs are often infected, whereas those of tissues that have higher blood flow and thus higher tissue oxygen tensions, such as the tongue or face, are rarely infected. Leukocytes kill bacteria most effectively when supplied with abundant oxygen (see Fig. 17-5).[87] Phagocytosis stimulates a huge, often 25-fold, increase in oxygen consumption, the so-called respiratory burst. At least 98% of this oxygen is converted to superoxide anion, peroxide, and other reactive oxygen species (oxygen radicals) which, when released into phagosomes, are lethal to many bacteria. This oxidative mechanism is most effective in high PO_2, even up to several hundred millimeters of mercury.[112] The K_m of the key *phox* enzyme that converts oxygen to superoxide is even higher than prolyl hydroxylase, meaning that its dependence on oxygen is

TABLE 17-1   Tissue Oxygen Tension with Increasing Inspired Oxygen Pressure

		Subject				
		Rabbit Tibia		Man (Clostridial Myonecrosis)	Man (Subcutaneous)	
ATA O_2 (mm Hg)	Rat Brain	Normal	Osteo	Phlegmon	Muscle	Tissue
0.2	34	45	21	50	29 + 3	37 + 6
1.0	90	—	—	110	59 + 13	53 + 10
2.0	244	321	104	250	221 + 72	221 + 72
3.0	452	—	—	330	—	—

ATA, 1 atmosphere; O_2, oxygen.
Data from Thom SR, Stephen R: Hyperbaric oxygen therapy. J Intensive Care Med 4:58–74, 1989.

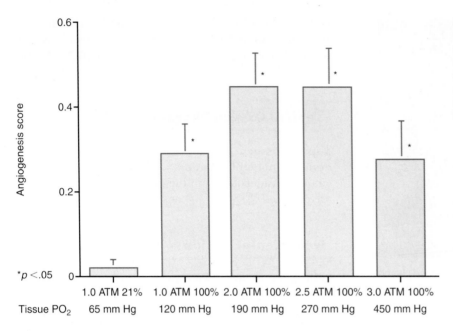

Figure 17-10 Angiogenesis score with nonsupplemented Matrigel under increasing oxygen tensions. *$p < .05$ compared to control at 1 atmosphere (1.0 ATA), 21% oxygen. Fisher's LSD Mean ± SE. *(Redrawn with permission from Gibson JJ, Angeles AP, Hunt TK: Increased oxygen tension potentiates angiogenesis. Surg Forum 48:696–699, 1997.)*

even greater (see Fig. 17-6). Bacterial killing fails most rapidly as tissue PO_2 falls to less than 30 to 40 mm Hg. Hunt and colleagues showed that oxidative and antibiotic killing of bacteria are independent mechanisms and are additive in wounds.[113,114] Several investigators have also demonstrated that random soft tissue flaps, which have low distal oxygen tensions analogous to those measured near diabetic foot ulcers, are susceptible to infection and suffer a high degree of necrosis[115–118] and that oxygen administration to elevate PO_2 values to more than 100 mm Hg minimizes infection/necrosis. Borer[119] has seen significant improvement in diabetic white cell function when the cells are exposed to elevated doses of oxygen. This effect seems to be mediated by both adherence molecules, such as intercellular adhesion molecules, and increased levels of nitric oxide (NO). We are also beginning to elucidate the vital role of reactive oxygen species on cell signaling and stimulation of growth factors in support of wound healing.[120–131] Control of infection is a critical aspect of caring for diabetic foot ulcers. When HBO therapy is effective, diminution of inflammation is an early feature. Doctor and colleagues[132] have shown rapid sterilization of diabetic wounds using HBO and appropriate antibiotics. Interestingly, the actual spectrum of bacteria that are sensitive to oxidative killing has not been elucidated. Indications are that sensitivity is widespread but variable among species.

Vasoconstriction

Exposure to oxygen at pressure results in a 20% reduction in blood flow in normal tissue. This effect is offset by the tenfold to fifteenfold increase in the oxygen content of plasma. This vasoconstriction may favorably affect the neurogenic edema that is seen in the feet of diabetic patients.[133] Hyperoxia probably does not cause vasoconstriction in ischemic or hypoxic tissues.[115]

Oxygen Toxicity and Other Side Effects

Risks involved in the use of HBO therapy are related to pressure changes and the toxic effects of oxygen. They include barotrauma to the ears or sinuses, pulmonary overpressure accidents with pneumothorax, and pulmonary toxicity. Sinus or ear barotrauma can be averted by slow compression, the use of decongestants, and patient education. Occasionally, myringotomy is necessary. Pulmonary overpressure accidents are very rare, perhaps 1 in 50,000 treatments (P. Cianci, personal survey), and can be avoided by careful pretreatment screening for pulmonary blebs, air trapping caused by bronchospasm or secretions, and the presence of preexisting pneumothorax secondary to chest compression, central lines, ventilatory support, or other forms of trauma.[134] An undetected pneumothorax at sea level can be converted to a tension pneumothorax on ascent from a hyperbaric treatment as ambient pressure decreases. Treatment is immediate insertion of a chest tube.

Oxygen has definite toxic effects as a result of overdosage, usually affecting the brain or lungs. Exposure to oxygen at depth can cause grand mal seizures, possibly related to interference with γ-aminobutyric acid (GABA) metabolism.[135–137] Susceptibility varies widely. As the PO_2 value rises, so does the risk of seizures. For this reason, oxygen treatments are usually limited to a maximum depth of 2.8 ATA (60 ft of seawater, 18.2 m) (Fig. 17-11). Fever and certain medications can predispose one to this complication, and careful attention to potential drug enhancement is mandatory. Oxygen seizures are, in fact, rare, occurring in perhaps 1 in 10,000 to 12,000 treat-

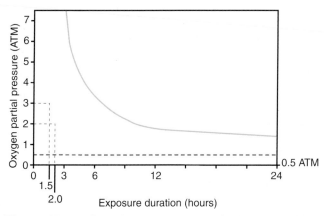

Figure 17-11   Central nervous system and pulmonary toxicity as a function of depth and time of exposure. Treatment protocols are designed to stay within acceptable limits of tolerance. Oxygen is not administered at depths greater than 66 feet. Most clinical exposures are 2 to 2.4 atmospheres for 90 minutes once or twice daily.

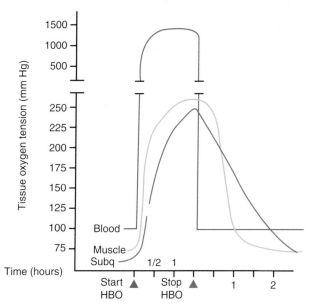

Figure 17-12   Rapidity of rise of oxygen tension after the onset of HBO is proportional to the capillary density of the organ at which the oxygen is transferred, either in the blood or to the peripheral tissue. The decline also is proportional to the height of the peak and to the rate of oxygen consumption. Subcutaneous tissue consumes little oxygen. The height of the peak is lower and the decline rather more rapid in inflamed tissue. *(Courtesy of George Hart, M.D.)*

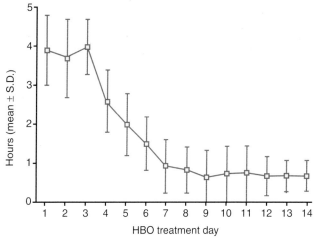

Figure 17-13   Time required for the $PscO_2$ to return to baseline after termination of each hyperbaric oxygen treatment (*n* = 22 ears). Of note, the mean value for day 14 was 3.4 ± 0.8 hours compared with 0.7 ± 0.6 hour for the treatment group (*p* <.005). *(Redrawn with permission from Siddiqui A, Davidson JD, Mustoe TA: Ischemic tissue oxygen capacitance after hyperbaric oxygen therapy: A new physiologic concept. Plast Reconstr Surg 99:148–155, 1997.)*

ments.[138] They are self-limited and treated by cessation of oxygen therapy. Hyperbaric oxygen treatment may be reestablished after seizure activity has ceased.

Damage to lung tissue, manifested by irritation to the large airways and a decrement in vital capacity, is a predictable complication of oxygen exposure at depth. The mechanism is believed to be loss of surfactant and changes in the pulmonary macrophages.[72,139] Because toxicity is related to the depth and duration of exposure, treatment protocols are designed to use the shallowest depth that is consistent with the desired results (see Fig. 17-11). In practice, pulmonary toxicity from currently used wound-healing protocols is virtually unheard of.[69,140,141] An additional minor side effect is a transient change in visual acuity that usually reverts to baseline within a few weeks to months after treatment. There is no evidence that the protocols currently used in the United States predispose to cataract formation.[142–144]

Confinement Anxiety

Although not a complication of treatment, confinement anxiety may be a problem for patients being treated in hyperbaric chambers. Sedation and reassurance are usually effective. A small percentage of patients cannot tolerate treatment.

Use of Hyperbaric Oxygen Therapy in the Treatment of the Diabetic Foot

Restoration of $TcPO_2$ to normal or slightly raised levels enhances epithelialization, fibroplasia, collagen deposition, angiogenesis, and bacterial killing. Controversy remains as to whether specific cellular immunity is diminished in diabetic people in the absence of hyperglycemia,

but no one argues that hypoxia increases the severity of infection, resulting in sepsis, loss of life or limb, or both.

Hyperbaric oxygen greatly increases tissue oxygen levels; and even though treatment is brief (90 to 120 minutes once or twice daily), oxygen tension values may remain elevated for some time after the cessation of therapy (Fig. 17-12).[106,145] Siddiqui and colleagues have demonstrated elevation of subcutaneous tissue oxygen tensions for several hours after exposure (Fig. 17-13).[123] The extent of change will depend on the degree of tissue hypoxia. HBO elevates normal tissue PO_2 strikingly but much less at the wound edge.

In the long run, the effect on angiogenesis might be the fundamental one. Sheffield[115] has elegantly demonstrated the improvement in capillarity, measuring transcutaneous oxygen levels over healing tissue in diabetic feet. His experience clearly documents the slow improvement in blood flow over the first 3 weeks of therapy as evidenced by rising oxygen tensions in the tissue, especially during HBO therapy sessions. Faglia and colleagues have also shown a highly significant and apparently permanent increase in transcutaneous oxygen values in diabetic patients who benefited from hyperbaric oxygen therapy to an average of 30 mm Hg ($p <.016$).[65] Marx and colleagues[94] have demonstrated similar changes in ischemic, irradiated tissues.

Clinical Experience

Several groups have reported increased limb salvage with HBO.[146–148] Baroni and colleagues[133] reported a statistically significant reduction in morbidity (amputation) in HBO-treated patients. Sixteen of 18 patients in their hyperbaric-treated group completely healed, whereas only one in ten in the control group did. The amputation rate was 40% in the control group versus 12.5% in the treated group ($p < .001$). HBO-treated patients were improved sufficiently to be discharged in 62 days. Nine of ten of the control patients had not healed 82 days later. In a later randomized study, Oriani and colleagues[147] compared 62 patients who were treated with good wound care and hyperbaric oxygen with 18 controls who received comparable wound care. A 95% salvage rate was achieved in the HBO-treated group with only three amputations required (4.8%). The control group suffered six amputations (33%, $p < .001$). The incidence of amputation in the untreated group was essentially unchanged from a historical control group of patients treated nearly 10 years earlier without adjunctive HBO therapy. There were no statistical differences in any of the groups relating to age, glycemic control, or diabetic complications. In 1988, our group[12] reported a series of 19 diabetic patients as a subset of 39 patients with lower-limb lesions. We attained a salvage rate of 89%. Forty-two percent of these patients had undergone successful revascularization and were referred to us because of continuing infection or nonhealing wounds. Salvage was defined as bipedal ambulation (if two limbs were originally present) and wound coverage for at least 1 year. Hyperbaric oxygen costs were $12,668 and were reflected in total hospital charges of $34,370, with an average stay of 35 days. The authors have additionally reported a longitudinal outcome study of 41 diabetic patients averaging 63.1 years in age. All patients had limb-threatening lesions. Twenty patients (49%) had

undergone revascularization. The average Wagner grade was 4 (gangrene of the toes or forefoot). Thirty-five patients' limbs were salvaged (85%). Hyperbaric charges were $15,000, total hospital charges were $31,264, and the average length of stay was 27 days (Table 17-2).[8] These costs compare favorably with the cost of primary amputation, which had been reported as more than $40,000 at the time of the study in 1986.[6] Avoidance of perhaps another $40,000 to $50,000 in rehabilitation costs,[12] the costs involved in reamputation or stump revision, and the lifelong provision of prostheses were additional savings. In the author's study, follow-up in 1991 and 1993 demonstrated that the effect persisted at 32 and 55 months, respectively (Tables 17-3 and 17-4). Even in the patients who had died, the average durability of repair was 42 months.[8]

Stone has reported a large series showing 70% salvage in hyperbaric-treated patients compared to 53% in con-

TABLE 17-2   Initial Patient Profile

Average age	63.6 years
Average Wagner score	4
Patients with limb-threatening lesions	41 (100%)
Patients undergoing vascular surgery	20 (49%)
Average length of stay	27 days
Mean hospital charges (including HBO charges)	$31,264
HBO charges	$15,000
Patients with salvaged limbs, initially	35 (85%)

Values determined from a patient population of 41.
Data from Cianci P, Hunt TK: Long-term results of aggressive management of diabetic foot ulcers suggest significant cost effectiveness. Wound Repair Regen 5:141–146, 1997.

TABLE 17-3   Summary of 1991 Follow-up of the Original 41 Patients with Diabetes

Patients contacted	28 (80%)
Average age	67.3 years
Patients with limb intact	27 (96%)
Patients with transtibial amputation	1 (4%)
Mean durability of repair	2.63 years (32 months)

Values based on a patient population of 35.
Data from Cianci P, Hunt TK: Long-term results of aggressive management of diabetic foot ulcers suggest significant cost effectiveness. Wound Repair Regen 5:141–146, 1997.

TABLE 17-4   Summary of the 1993 Follow-up of Initial Patient Population

Follow-up obtained	22 (81%)
Patients deceased	6 (27%)
Average age of deceased patients	72.6 years
Average duration of repair of deceased patients	3.4 years (42 months)
Patients still living	16 (73%)
Average age	68.3 years
Patients with transtibial amputation	1 (6%)
Patients with limb intact	15 (94%)
Duration of repair	4.6 years (55 months)

Values are based on a patient population of 27.
Data from Cianci P, Hunt TK: Long-term results of aggressive management of diabetic foot ulcers suggest significant cost effectiveness. Wound Repair Regen 5:141–146, 1997.

trol patients with similar wounds who did not receive HBO ($p < .002$).[149] Faglia and colleagues, in a prospective, randomized, and blinded study, showed an 8.6% amputation rate in HBO-treated patients versus 33.3% in the controls ($p < .016$).[65] Transcutaneous oxygen measurements significantly improved in the treated group (14.0 ± 11.8 versus 5.0 ± 5.4) compared to the nontreated group ($p < .0002$). An example of this phenomenon is shown in the case study presented at the end of this chapter. The authors concluded that hyperbaric oxygen therapy in conjunction with an aggressive multidisciplinary protocol is effective in severe, ischemic diabetic foot lesions.[65] In a prospective study, Zamboni reported more rapid healing of diabetic wounds in comparison to non-hyperbaric treated controls (Table 17-5 and Fig. 17-14).[150] In a randomized controlled study, Abidia and colleagues showed complete epithelialization in 13 of 19 hyperbaric patients compared to only 4 of 14 in the control group.[151]

TABLE 17-5   Baseline Patient Characteristics (Mean ± SEM)

Characteristics	Control (*N* = 5)	HBO Therapy (*N* = 5)
Age (years)	53.8 ± 3.50	63.6 ± 3.96
Gender: male/female	4 : 1	4 : 1
Baseline wound area (cm²)	4.4 ± 1.50	6.02 ± 1.73
TcPo₂ (mm Hg)		
Reference (room air)	60.0 ± 2.12	53.4 ± 4.35
Wound at:		
Room air	35.3 ± 2.30	12.0 ± 2.91
100% mask O₂	80.0 ± 16.34	71.2 ± 25.23
HBO 2.0 ATA	N/A	562.4 ± 55.79
Osteomyelitis	60% (3/5)	80% (4/5)

TcPo₂, transcutaneous oxygen tension; mm Hg, millimeters of mercury; HBO, hyperbaric oxygen; ATA, atmospheres absolute.
Data from Zamboni WA, Wong HP, Stephenson LL, Pfeifer MA: Evaluation of hyperbaric oxygen for diabetic wounds: A prospective study. J Hyperbar Med 24:175–179, 1997.

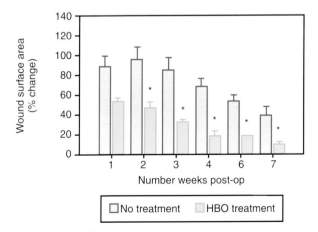

Figure 17-14   Weekly mean wound area as a percentage of the initial baseline pretreatment wound area for control and hyperbaric oxygen (HBO) patient treatment groups (**p <.05 versus controls*). *(Redrawn with permission from Zamboni WA, Wong HP, Stephenson LL, Pfeifer MA: Evaluation of hyperbaric oxygen for diabetic wounds: A prospective study. J Hyperbar Med 24:175–179, 1997.)*

The decrease in wound size was 96% in the treatment group compared to 41% in the controls ($p = .043$). The Karolinska Institute[152] reported a randomized study that demonstrated hyperbaric oxygen–treated patients had a 76% healing rate and intact skin at 3 years, whereas only 48% of controls were healed. Amputations were required in 12% of the treatment group versus 33% in the controls (note the similarity to the earlier reports of Baroni and Faglia). Kessler and colleagues[153] conducted a prospective, randomized study that demonstrated an improvement in the healing rate of the HBO-treated group with a 41.8% reduction in wound size compared to 21.7% in controls ($p = .037$). Despite more serious wounds in the hyperbaric group, Lee and colleagues[154] in a double-blinded, randomized, prospective study, reported earlier healing ($p < .03$) and fewer amputations ($p < .005$) in the oxygen-treated group. Strauss, in an evidence-based review, reported an overall wound healing improvement of 48% to 76% and a reduction of amputation rate from 45% to 19%.[155]

These studies are encouraging; but as with all other therapeutic interventions in the diabetic foot, adequacy of control data remains a problem.[156,157] One cannot escape the reality, however, that there is no such thing as a "control chronic wound" in humans. Fortunately, the large number of controlled studies and firm mechanistic data in animals are convincing, and the recent clinical reports confirm these animal data.

Patient Selection

Shallow ulcers, particularly of neuropathic origin, unless grossly infected, will usually respond to more conservative treatment. Patients with Wagner grade 3, 4, or 5 lesions are considered for treatment on the basis of assessment of blood flow. Patients without adequate arterial flow are referred for angiograms and revascularization as indicated.

TcPO₂ values are increasingly recognized as the most reliable, useful, noninvasive method for evaluation of perfusion and selecting patients for vascular referral.[158–161] This measurement is widely available and can be helpful in patient selection for HBO therapy. Pecoraro and Reiber have shown that low TcPO₂ confers a high risk of amputation.[157,162] Patients with transcutaneous peri-wound TcPO₂ values greater than 30 to 40 mm Hg on room air may heal without intervention. Patients with readings less than 20 mm Hg while breathing air have a poor prognosis.[163] An increase to 40 mm Hg or greater while breathing 100% oxygen by tight-fitting mask or while in the hyperbaric chamber at 1 atmosphere indicates that perfusion is adequate for oxygen therapy to benefit.[115] If periwound TcPO₂ levels are low and unresponsive, angiography might be helpful in selecting patients who might benefit from revascularization. In cases in which the TcPO₂ level is low and revascularization

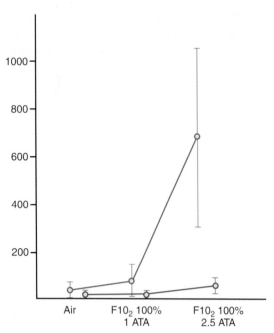

Figure 17–15   Measurement of periwound transcutaneous oxygen level while breathing 100% oxygen in a hyperbaric chamber appears to be a good predictor of healing. Patients showing increase (*purple circles*) would be expected to benefit from hyperbaric oxygen therapy. *(Redrawn with permission from Wattel F, Mathieu D, Coget J-M, Billard V: Hyperbaric oxygen therapy in chronic vascular wound management. Angiology 41:59–65, 1990.)*

is not possible, the prognosis is very guarded. In these instances, a trial of therapy might be indicated on a case-by-case basis if limb loss is the only alternative. Wattel and colleagues[164] have reported that patients who show transcutaneous oxygen values of 100 mm Hg in the vicinity of the wound while breathing pure oxygen at 2.5 ATA heal 75% of the time, whereas patients with lower values will go on to amputation (Fig. 17-15). Hart and colleagues[165] have reported data that support this hypothesis. In a multicenter study involving more than 1100 patients, Fife[166] showed the predictive healing value of a $TcPO_2$ measurement of 200 mm Hg or higher while in the hyperbaric chamber breathing 100% O_2. Strauss[155] and Niinikosi[167] have reported similar findings. Transcutaneous oxygen measurements can be valuable in determining when a patient may have obtained maximum benefits of therapy with normalization of periwound $TcPO_2$ values.[168] As more data become available, patient selection criteria will become even more precise; but clearly, response to oxygen challenge has become an important assessment tool.

Treatment Protocols

Treatment protocols vary depending on the severity of the problem and the type of chamber that is used. In larger, multiplace chambers that are compressed to depth with air, treatments are rendered at 2 to 2.4 atmospheres (equivalent to 33 to 45 feet of seawater) for 90 to 120 minutes once or twice daily. In monoplace, single-person configurations that are compressed to depth with oxygen, most centers treat at 2 atmospheres of pressure for 90 to 120 minutes at depth.

Patients with serious infections are hospitalized for intravenous antibiotics and tight diabetes control. Hyperbaric oxygen treatment in such cases is usually rendered twice daily for 90 minutes. As soon as is feasible, patients are transferred to an in-house skilled nursing facility or to home health care, where daily wound care, debridement, and HBO treatments can be continued in an outpatient setting. In such instances, HBO is administered once daily for 2 hours, usually right after wound care has been provided.

After a suitable capillary bed has been established, split-thickness meshed skin grafts or other plastic techniques are used to effect rapid wound closure. In our experience, early application of such grafts, when appropriate, can significantly shorten morbidity, hospital stay, and cost of care. With proper coordination, this program has proved cost-effective, even in this era of severe fiscal constraint.[8,12,169] Guo, in a recent technology assessment and cost analysis, determined that adjunctive hyperbaric therapy was cost-effective, particularly when viewed from a long-term perspective.[170] It is ironic that the federal reimbursement for amputation, which involves a much greater long-term cost, is 30% greater than that provided for attempts at limb salvage.[8,171,172]

Evidence-Based Assessment

An objective evaluation of the data currently available concludes that HBO is effective in the treatment of severe diabetic foot ulcers and should be utilized if available. Indeed, the Consensus Development Conference of the American Diabetes Association has recognized the value of adjunctive hyperbaric oxygen in difficult cases, stating that "It is reasonable to use this modality to treat severe or limb-threatening wounds that have not responded to other treatments, particularly if ischemia that cannot be corrected by vascular procedures is present."[173] The European Consensus Conference determined in 2000 that "In diabetic patients the use of HBOT (hyperbaric oxygen therapy) is recommended in the presence of chronic critical ischemia (as defined by the European Consensus Conference on critical ischemia) if transcutaneous oxygen pressure readings under hyperbaric conditions (2.5 ATA, 100% oxygen) are higher than 100 mmHg."[174] The *British Journal of Medicine* clinical reference review[175] categorized hyperbaric oxygen treatment for the diabetic foot ulcer as likely to be beneficial. The Center for Medicare Services analyzed the data available in 2002 and concluded that "CMS believes that the evidence supports the use of HBO therapy in the treatment of diabetic lower-limb wounds that are limb threatening and are Wagner III or greater."[176] The Cochrane Collaboration in 2005 reported: "The review of trials found that HBOT (hyperbaric oxygen therapy) seems to reduce the number of amputations in people with diabetes who have chronic foot ulcers."[177] Roeckl-Wiedmann and colleagues[178] in 2005 reported similar findings in a pooled analysis of randomized studies: "The risk of major amputation was significantly reduced in the HBOT (RR: 0.31; 95% c.i. 0.13 to 0.71). Sensitivity analyses did not affect the result. The NNT to avoid one amputation was four (95% c.i. 3 to 11)."

Future Trends

Recent data suggest that in selected cases, wound growth factors and HBO therapy might be synergistic and lead to even further shortening of healing times (J. Dunn et al., personal communication, 1992).[179] Zhao and colleagues[124] have demonstrated synergism when used in conjunction with hyperbaric oxygen therapy. Two additional recent studies are worthy of comment. Uhl and colleagues showed markedly improved healing in a well-designed ischemic animal model. Hyperbaric-treated animals healed faster than nontreated ischemic controls and also faster than nonischemic controls![180] Hammarlund and colleagues have shown in a randomized, double-blinded,

controlled clinical study that HBO increased healing (decreased wound sizes over time) when compared to nontreated controls.[181]

Summary

Hyperbaric oxygen therapy rendered in specially designed chambers is an adjunct to current medical and surgical treatment of discouraging and difficult problems of healing failure in people with diabetes. Recent investigations have demonstrated that adequate tissue oxygen tension is an essential factor in wound healing. Frequently, adequate levels can be reached only through adjunctive HBO treatment. This results in more normal fibroblast proliferation, angiogenesis, collagen deposition, epithelialization, and enhancement of bacterial killing. Although HBO therapy can be costly, the ability to preserve a durable, functional limb can reduce the high cost of disability resulting from amputation. Additionally, the shortened healing time for chronic wounds can reduce the cost of frequent, repeated surgical procedures. As part of a multidisciplinary program of wound care, it is cost-effective and durable.[8] (See Figs. 17-16 to 17-21 for case illustrations.)

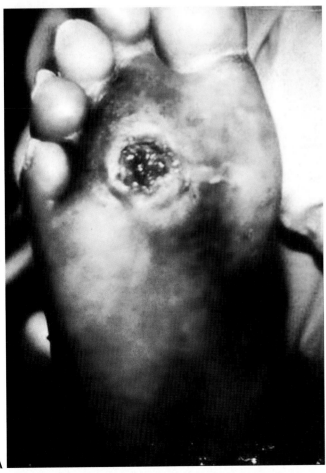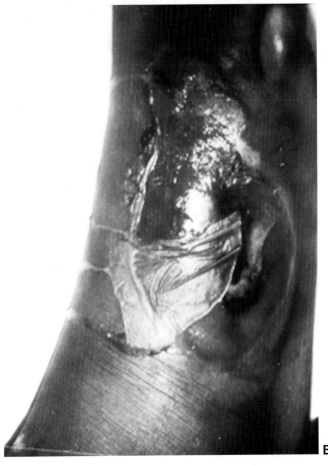

Figure 17-16 **A,** Mal perforans ulcer in a 57-year-old insulin-dependent diabetic. **B,** Dorsum view showing cellulitis and desquamation of overlying skin.

Illustration continued on following page.

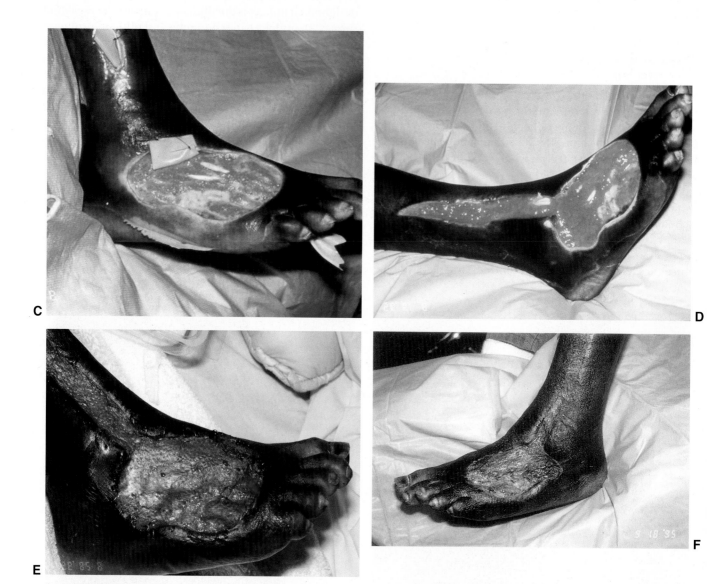

Figure 17–16, cont'd   C, Wound has been debrided and drained; patient has received 1 week of hyperbaric oxygen therapy. **D,** Eleven days later with further debridement and hyperbaric oxygen therapy; note the exuberant granulation tissue, even over exposed tendons. **E,** Patient 9 days later shows excellent take of split-thickness mesh graft. **F,** Patient 21 days later; excellent coverage; intact foot.

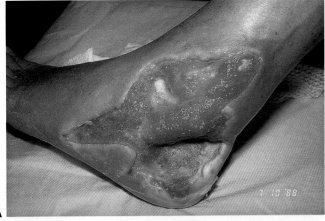

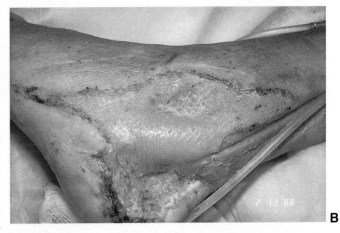

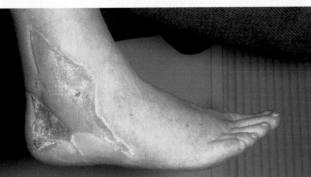

Figure 17–17 **A,** Infection of several tarsal joint spaces, and lateral skin necrosis. In the subsequent debridement, these spaces were opened and expanded. Cartilage was not debrided. **B,** Much of this wound healed during a period in which the patient breathed oxygen at sea level pressure. After several weeks of HBO therapy, skin grafts were placed. **C,** Wound remained healed, and the patient ambulant 20 months later.

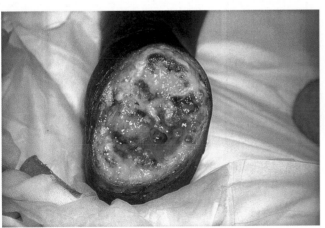

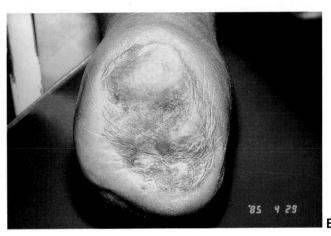

Figure 17–18 **A,** Unhealed transmetatarsal wound in a 55-year-old man 5 weeks after extensive debridement and successful revascularization of viable tissue. Standard wound care was provided, but wound failed to heal **B,** Angiogenesis after 10 days of wound care and HBO treatment. **C,** Wound remained healed after split-thickness mesh grafting at 27 months' follow-up. The contralateral limb was paralyzed.

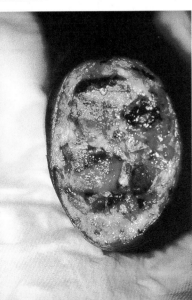

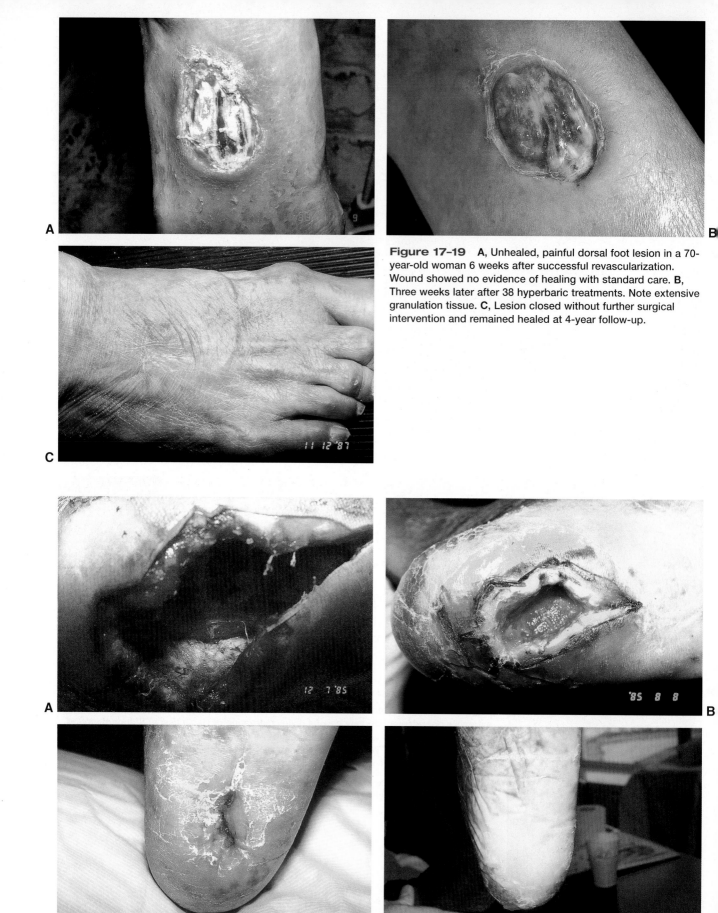

Figure 17-19 **A,** Unhealed, painful dorsal foot lesion in a 70-year-old woman 6 weeks after successful revascularization. Wound showed no evidence of healing with standard care. **B,** Three weeks later after 38 hyperbaric treatments. Note extensive granulation tissue. **C,** Lesion closed without further surgical intervention and remained healed at 4-year follow-up.

Figure 17-20 **A,** Deep calcaneal lesion 2 days after successful revascularization and debridement of necrotizing heel lesion. Because of infection, compromised host, and a limb-threatening lesion, adjunctive HBO therapy was initiated early. **B,** Fifty percent reduction of wound diameter and volume after 27 days of wound care and adjunctive HBO treatment. **C,** Healed lesion after 28 HBO treatments. **D,** At 4-year follow-up, the lesion remained healed. Patient lost opposite limb during interim.

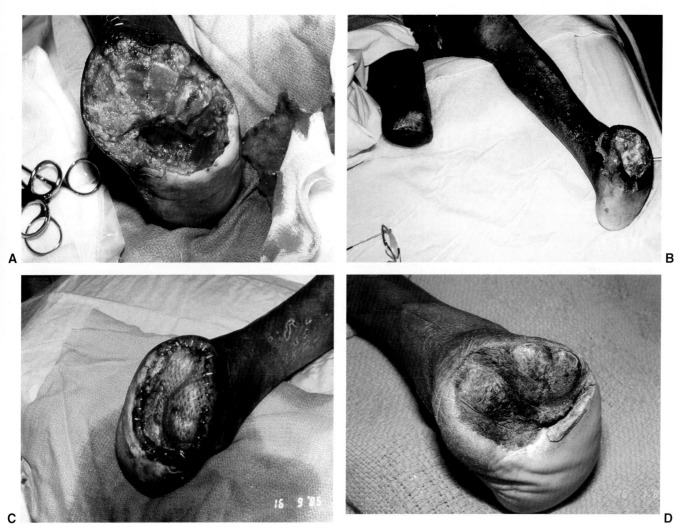

Figure 17–21   **A**, Forefoot amputation status after revascularization in a 70-year-old man with diabetes mellitus, renal failure, and necrotizing infection. Because of a limb-threatening lesion and prior contralateral limb amputation, adjunctive HBO therapy was initiated in the postoperative period. **B**, Lesion 3 weeks later, after 21 HBO treatments and aggressive wound care. Note extensive healing. **C**, Lesion 50 days after radical debridement and split-thickness mesh graft was placed. **D**, Foot remained healed at 1-year follow-up.

CASE STUDY (Fig. 17-22)

Transcutaneous oxygen values over course of therapy in severe (Wagner grade 4) foot lesion. Note the marked improvement as angiogenesis proceeds and the wound heals.

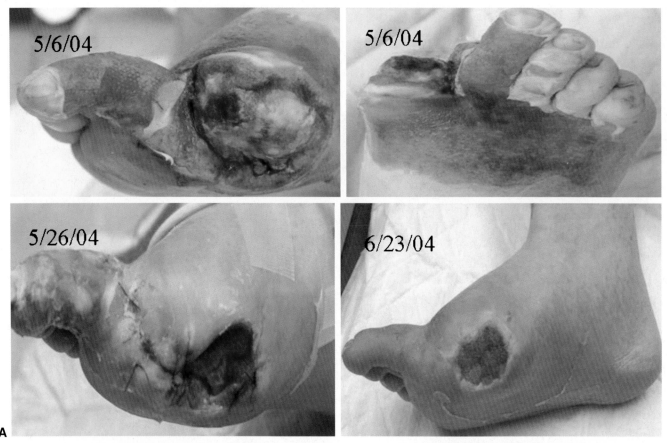

Figure 17–22 **A,** 47-year-old NIDD male with grade 4 Wagner lesion and osteomyelitis status after amputation of gangrenous toe. Note exposed bone.

Patient name:
HBO physician:

Date: 5/6/04 Transcutaneous Oximetry Evaluation
TCOM TECHNICIAN: Ross

Patient history/comments: Progressive necrotizing infection, right foot. Diabetic male. 3 completed
treatments at time of this transcutaneous oximetry.
SITE #1: Dorsum of mid right foot, medial aspect
SITE #2: Dorsum of mid right foot, lateral aspect

(mm Hg)	Ground level air	1 min	2	3	4	5	6	7	8	9	10 min	% *Change*
SITE #1	16	30	62	83	*90*	89	87	80	82	81	80	*400%*
SITE #2	24	32	46	57	61	*62*	61	59	59	59	59	*146%*

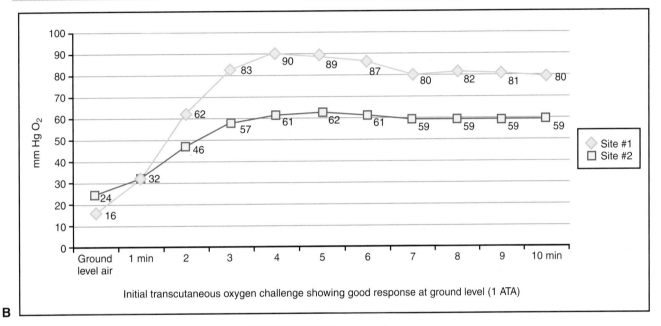

Initial transcutaneous oxygen challenge showing good response at ground level (1 ATA)

B

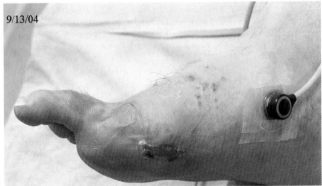

C

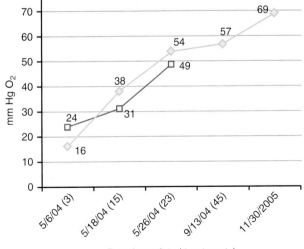

D

Figure 17–22, cont'd   B, Initial transcutaneous oxygen
challenge showing good response at ground level (1 ATA).
C, Medial wound 3 months after hyperbaric oxygen completed;
amputation site completely healed. **D,** Transcutaneous oxygen
values, foot, 14.5 months after amputation, showing continuing
normal value.

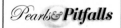

Pearls

- Use of transcutaneous oxygen measurements can help to select patients who might benefit.
- A proper vascular evaluation to determine blood flow is critical.
- Correction of ischemia by bypass or angioplasty should always be done prior to HBO therapy except for those instances in which concurrent therapy can prevent limb loss.
- Many wounds "stall out" after revascularization despite restoration of blood flow. HBO can provide the critical bridge necessary to promote healing in these instances.
- Aggressive surgical management, including sharp debridement to viable tissue, and aggressive use of grafts will significantly affect outcome and length of stay.
- Keep the affected area and the patient warm.
- Sedation for claustrophobic patients can be accomplished by utilizing sublingual Ativan, not its generic equivalent.

Pitfalls

- Improper patient selection: Patients who have little or no chance of success or have dead digits or limbs are not candidates for HBO therapy. It will not resurrect necrotic tissue.
- Ineffective pain control: The effect of catecholamines stimulated by pain can result in vasoconstriction and delayed wound healing.
- Insulin requirements may decrease with hyperbaric oxygen therapy. Therefore, carefully monitor serum glucose in diabetics to avoid hypoglycemia.
- Isolated hyperbaric oxygen therapy in the absence of proper medical and surgical management is not effective. An aggressive coordinated approach is mandatory to ensure the best chance for success.

References

1. Hogan P, Dall T, Nikolov P: Economic costs of diabetes in the US in 2002. Diabetes Care 26(3):917–932, 2003.
2. Selby JV, Ray GT, Zhang D, Colby C: Excess costs of medical care for patients with diabetes in a managed care population. Diabetes Care 20(9):1396–1402, 1997.
3. Block P: The diabetic foot ulcer: a complex problem with a simple treatment approach. Mil Med 146(9):644–646, 1981.
4. U.S. Department of Health and Human Services: National Diabetes Fact Sheet. Washington, DC: U.S. Government Printing Office, 1997.
5. Knighton DR, Fylling CP, Fiegel VD, Cerra F: Amputation prevention in an independently reviewed at-risk diabetic population using a comprehensive wound care protocol. Am J Surg 160(5):466–471; discussion 471–472, 1990.
6. Mackey WC, McCullough JL, Conlon TP, et al: The costs of surgery for limb-threatening ischemia. Surgery 99(1):26–35, 1986.
7. Reiber GE, Lipsky BA, Gibbons GW: The burden of diabetic foot ulcers. Am J Surg 176(2A suppl):5S–10S, 1998.
8. Cianci P, Hunt TK: Long-term results of aggressive management of diabetic foot ulcers suggest significant cost effectiveness. Wound Repair Regen 5:141–146, 1997.
9. Ebskov B, Josephsen P: Incidence of reamputation and death after gangrene of the lower extremity. Prosthet Orthot Int 4(2):77–80, 1980.
10. Couch NP, David JK, Tilney NL, Crane C: Natural history of the leg amputee. Am J Surg 133(4):469–473, 1977.
11. Gibbons GW: Improved quality of diabetic foot care, 1984 vs 1990. Arch Surg 1128:576–578, 1993.
12. Cianci P, Petrone G, Drager S, et al: Salvage of the problem wound and potential amputation with wound care and adjunctive hyperbaric oxygen therapy: An economic analysis. J Hyperbar Med 3(3):127–141, 1988.
13. Kihn RB, Warren R, Beebe GW: The "geriatric" amputee. Ann Surg 176(3):305–314, 1972.
14. Levin ME: Diabetic foot lesions: Pathogenesis and management. J Enterostomal Ther 17(1):29–34, 1990.
15. Apelqvist J, Ragnarson-Tennvall G, Persson U, Larsson J: Diabetic foot ulcers in a multidisciplinary setting: An economic analysis of primary healing and healing with amputation. J Intern Med 235(5):463–471, 1994.
16. Apelqvist J, Ragnarson-Tennvall G, Larsson J, Persson U: Long-term costs for foot ulcers in diabetic patients in a multidisciplinary setting. Foot Ankle Int 116(7):388–394, 1995.
17. Holzer SE, Camerota A, Martens L, et al: Costs and duration of care for lower extremity ulcers in patients with diabetes. Clin Ther 20(1):169–181, 1998.
18. Larsson J, Apelqvist J, Agardh CD, Stenstrom A: Decreasing incidence of major amputation in diabetic patients: A consequence of a multidisciplinary foot care team approach? Diabet Med 12(9):770–776, 1995.
19. Stone JA, Cianci P: The adjunctive role of hyperbaric oxygen therapy in the treatment of lower extremity wounds in patients with diabetes. Diabetes Spectrum 10:118–123, 1997.
20. Edmonds ME, Blundell MP, Morris ME, Thomas EM, et al: Improved survival of the diabetic foot: The role of a specialized foot clinic. Q J Med 60(232):763–771, 1986.
21. Aagenaes O, Moe H: Light- and electron-microscopic study of skin capillaries of diabetics. Diabetes 10:253–259, 1961.
22. Arenson DJ, Sherwood CF, Wilson RC: Neuropathy, angiopathy, and sepsis in the diabetic foot: II. Angiography. J Am Podiatry Assoc 71(12):661–665, 1981.
23. McMillan DE, Breithaupt DL, Rosenau W, et al: Forearm skin capillaries of diabetic, potential diabetic and nondiabetic subjects: Changes seen by light microscope. Diabetes 15(4):251–257, 1966.
24. Wyss CR, Robertson C, Love SJ, et al: Relationship between transcutaneous oxygen tension, ankle blood pressure, and clinical outcome of vascular surgery in diabetic and nondiabetic patients. Surgery 101(1):56–62, 1987.
25. Caselli A, Latini V, Lapenna A, et al: Transcutaneous oxygen tension monitoring after successful revascularization in diabetic patients with ischaemic foot ulcers. Diabet Med 22(4):460–465, 2005.
26. Joseph WS, LeFrock JL: The pathogenesis of diabetic foot infections: Immunopathy, angiopathy, and neuropathy. J Foot Surg 26(1 suppl):S7–S11, 1987.
27. Ohkubo Y, Kishikawa H, Araki E, et al: Intensive insulin therapy prevents the progression of diabetic microvascular complications in Japanese patients with non-insulin-dependent diabetes mellitus: A randomized prospective 6-year study. Diabetes Res Clin Pract 28(2):103–117, 1995.
28. Reichard P, Nilsson BY, Rosenqvist U: The effect of long-term intensified insulin treatment on the development of microvascular complications of diabetes mellitus. N Engl J Med 329(5):304–309, 1993.
29. The Diabetes Control and Complications Trial Research Group: The effect of intensive treatment of diabetes on the development and progression of long-term complications in insulin-dependent diabetes mellitus. N Engl J Med 329(14):977–986, 1993.
30. Reiber GE, Boyko EJ, Smith DG: Lower extremity foot ulcers and amputations in diabetes. In Harris MI (ed): Diabetes in America. Bethesda, MD: National Institutes of Health, 1995, pp 409–427.
31. Klein R: Hyperglycemia and microvascular and macrovascular disease in diabetes. Diabetes Care 18(2):258–268, 1995.
32. Flynn MD, Tooke JE: Diabetic neuropathy and the microcirculation. Diabet Med 112(4):298–301, 1995.
33. Tooke JE: Microvascular function in human diabetes: A physiological perspective. Diabetes 44(7):721–726, 1995.
34. Skalak TC, Price RJ: The role of mechanical stresses in microvascular remodeling. Microcirculation 3:143–165, 1996.
35. Borer RC, Gamble JR: Hyperbaric oxygen therapy (HBO) corrects impaired neutrophil adhesion in patients with non-insulin dependent diabetes mellitus (NIDDM). Undersea Hyperb Med 24(suppl):15, 1997.
36. Boykin JV Jr: The nitric oxide connection: Hyperbaric oxygen therapy, becaplermin, and diabetic ulcer management. Adv Skin Wound Care 13(4 pt 1):169–174, 2000.

37. Buras J: HBO regulation of ICAM 1 in an endothelial cell model of ischemia/reperfusion injury. Presented at Hyperbaric Medicine 1998 Advanced Symposium, University of South Carolina School of Medicine, 1998.

38. Buras J, Reenstra WR, Svoboda KKH: Hyperbaric oxygen down-regulates hypoxia/hypoglycemia-stimulated endothelial cell surface ICAM-1 protein expression. Mol Biol Cell 8:230A, 1997.

39. Buras J, Reenstra WR, Svoboda KS: HBO decreases endothelial cell intercellular adhesion molecule-1 (ICAM-1) protein expression and neutrophil adhesion in an in-vitro model of ischemia/reperfusion. Undersea Hyperb Med 25(suppl):51, 1998.

40. Martindale VE: Nitric oxide as therapeutic mechanism in HBO therapy? Presented at Hyperbaric Medicine 1998 Advanced Symposium, University of South Carolina School of Medicine, 1998.

41. Falanga V: Wound healing and its impairment in the diabetic foot. Lancet 366(9498):1736–1743, 2005.

42. Kranke P, Bennett M, Roeckl-Wiedmann I, Debus S: Hyperbaric oxygen therapy for chronic wounds. CD 2004.

43. Hunt TK, Hopf HW: Wound healing and wound infection: What surgeons and anesthesiologists can do. Surg Clin North Am 77(3):587–606, 1997.

44. Roy S, Khanna S, Nallu K, et al: Dermal wound healing is subject to redox control. Mol Ther 13(1):211–220, 2006.

45. Trabold O, Wagner S, Wicke C, et al: Lactate and oxygen constitute a fundamental regulatory mechanism in wound healing. Wound Repair Regen 11(6):504–509, 2003.

46. Ali MA, Yasui F, Matsugo S, Konishi T: The lactate-dependent enhancement of hydroxyl radical generation by the Fenton reaction. Free Radic Res 32(5):429–438, 2000.

47. Hopf HW, Gibson JJ, Angeles AP, et al: Hyperoxia and angiogenesis. Wound Repair Regen 13(6):558–563, 2005.

48. Constant JS, Feng JJ, Zabel DD, et al: Lactate elicits vascular endothelial growth factor from macrophages: A possible alternative to hypoxia. Wound Repair Regen 8:353–360, 2000.

49. Gladden LB: Lactate metabolism: A new paradigm for the third millennium. J Physiol 558(pt 1):5–30, 2004.

50. Albina JE, Reichner JS: Oxygen and the regulation of gene expression in wounds. Wound Repair Regen 11(6):445–451, 2003.

51. Wilmore DW: Carbohydrate metabolism in trauma. Clin Endocrinol Metab 5(3):731–745, 1976.

52. Jensen JA, Hunt TK, Scheuenstuhl H, Banda MJ: Effect of lactate, pyruvate, and pH on secretion of angiogenesis and mitogenesis factors by macrophages. Lab Invest 54:574–578, 1986.

53. Ghani QP, Wagner S, Hussain MZ: Role of ADP-ribosylation in wound repair: The contributions of Thomas K. Hunt, MD. Wound Repair Regen 11(6):439–444, 2003.

54. Attard JA, Raval MJ, Martin GR, et al: The effects of systemic hypoxia on colon anastomotic healing: An animal model. Dis Colon Rectum 48(7):1460–1470, 2005.

55. Hehenberger K, Brismar K, Lind F, Kratz G: Dose-dependent hyperbaric oxygen stimulation of human fibroblast proliferation. Wound Repair Regen 5:147–150, 1997.

56. Allen DB, Maguire JJ, Mahdavian M, et al: Wound hypoxia and acidosis limit neutrophil bacterial killing mechanisms. Arch Surg 132(9):991–996, 1997.

57. Belda FJ, Aguilera L, Garcia de la Asuncion J, et al: Supplemental perioperative oxygen and the risk of surgical wound infection: A randomized controlled trial. JAMA 294(16):2035–2042, 2005.

58. Dellinger EP: Increasing inspired oxygen to decrease surgical site infection: Time to shift the quality improvement research paradigm. JAMA 294(16):2091–2092, 2005.

59. Greif R, Akca O, Horn EP, et al: Supplemental perioperative oxygen to reduce the incidence of surgical-wound infection. Outcomes Research Group. N Engl J Med 342(3):161–167, 2000.

60. Ueno C, Hunt TK, Hopf HW: Using physiology to improve surgical wound outcomes. Plast Reconstr Surg 117(7 suppl):59S–71S, 2006.

61. Perner A, Nielsen SE, Rask-Madsen J: High glucose impairs superoxide production from isolated blood neutrophils. Intensive Care Med 29(4):642–645, 2003.

62. Thom SR: Effects of hyperoxia on neutrophil adhesion. Undersea Hyperb Med 31(1):123–131, 2004.

63. Thom SR, Bhopale VM, Velazquez OC, et al: Stem cell mobilization by hyperbaric oxygen. Am J Physiol Heart Circ Physiol 290:H1378–H1386, 2005.

64. Aslam R, Hunt TK: The Mechanism of the Lactate Effect on Wound Healing. San Francisco: University of California, 2006.

65. Faglia E, Favales F, Aldeghi A, et al: Adjunctive systemic hyperbaric oxygen therapy in treatment of severe prevalently ischemic diabetic foot ulcer: A randomized study. Diabetes Care 19(12):1338–1343, 1996.

66. Sheikh AY, Rollins MD, Hopf HW, Hunt TK: Hyperoxia improves microvascular perfusion in a murine wound model. Wound Repair Regen 2005;13(3):303–308, 2005.

67. Kalliainen LK, Gordillo GM, Schlanger R, Sen CK: Topical oxygen as an adjunct to wound healing: A clinical case series. Pathophysiology 9(2):81–87, 2003.

68. Sen CK, Khanna S, Babior BM, et al: Oxidant-induced vascular endothelial growth factor expression in human keratinocytes and cutaneous wound healing. J Biol Chem 277(36):33284–33290, 2002.

69. Foreman C: The FDA and HBO. Presented at Hyperbaric Medicine 1998 Advanced Symposium, University of South Carolina School of Medicine, 1998.

70. Cotto-Cumba C, Velez E, Velu SS, et al: Transcutaneous oxygen measurements in normal subjects using topical HBO control module. Undersea Biomed Res 1991;18(suppl):109.

71. Leslie CA, Sapico FL, Ginunas VJ, Adkins RH: Randomized controlled trial of topical hyperbaric oxygen for treatment of diabetic foot ulcers. Diabetes Care 11(2):111–115, 1998.

72. Feldmeier JJ, Hopf HW, Warriner RA, et al: UHMS position statement: Topical oxygen for chronic wounds. Undersea Hyperbaric Med 32(3):157–168, 2005.

73. Davis JC: Refractory osteomyelitis. In Davis JC, Hunt TK (eds): Problem Wounds: The Role of Oxygen. New York: Elsevier, 1988, pp 125–142.

74. Boerema I, Meyne NG, Brummelkamp WH, et al: [Life without blood.]. Ned Tijdschr Geneeskd 104:949–954, 1960.

75. Brummelkamp WH: Considerations on hyperbaric oxygen therapy at three atmospheres absolute for clostridial infections type welchii. Ann N Y Acad Sci 117:688–699, 1965.

76. Goodman MW, Workman RD: Minimal recompression, oxygen breathing approach to treatment of decompression sickness in divers and aviators. Washington, DC: U.S. Navy Experimental Diving Unit, 1965.

77. Kindwall E: Carbon monoxide and cyanide poisoning. Hyperb Oxygen Rev 1:115–122, 1980.

78. Thom SR, Taber RL, Mendiguren, II, et al: Delayed neuropsychologic sequelae after carbon monoxide poisoning: Prevention by treatment with hyperbaric oxygen. Ann Emerg Med 25(4):474–480, 1995.

79. Yarborough OD, Behnke AR: The treatment of compressed air illness utilizing oxygen. J Ind Hyg Tox 21(6):213–218, 1939.

80. Hart GB, Lamb RC, Strauss MB: Gas gangrene. J Trauma 23(11):991–1000, 1983.

81. Heimbach RD: Gas gangrene: Review and update. Hyperb Oxygen Rev 1:41–61, 1980.

82. Bouachour G, Cronier P, Gouello JP, et al: Hyperbaric oxygen therapy in the management of crush injuries: A randomized double-blind placebo-controlled clinical trial. J Trauma 41(2):333–339, 1996.

83. Strauss MB, Hart GB: Crush injury and the role of hyperbaric oxygen. Top Emerg Med 6:9–24, 1984.

84. Tan CM, Im MJ, Myers RA, Hoopes JE: Effects of hyperbaric oxygen and hyperbaric air on the survival of island skin flaps. Plast Reconstr Surg 73(1):27–30, 1984.

85. Hunt TK, Niinikoski J, Zederfeldt BH, Silver IA: Oxygen in wound healing enhancement: cellular effects of oxygen. In Davis JC, Hunt TK (eds): Hyperbaric Oxygen Therapy. Bethesda, MD: Undersea Medical Society, 1988, pp 111–122.

86. Bakker DJ: Pure and mixed aerobic and anaerobic soft tissue infections. Hyperb Oxygen Rev 6:65–96, 1985.

87. Gozal D, Ziser A, Shupak A, et al: Necrotizing fasciitis. Arch Surg 121(2):233–235, 1986.

88. Riseman JA, Zamboni WA, Curtis A, et al: Hyperbaric oxygen therapy for necrotizing fasciitis reduces mortality and the need for debridements. Surgery 108(5):847–850, 1990.

89. Davis JC: Hyperbaric oxygen therapy. Intensive Care Med 4:55–57, 1989.

90. Davis JC: Chronic non-hematogenous osteomyelitis treated with adjuvant hyperbaric oxygen. J Bone Joint Surg 68A:1210–1217, 1986.

91. Mader JT, Brown GL, Guckian JC, et al: A mechanism for the amelioration by hyperbaric oxygen of experimental staphylococcal osteomyelitis in rabbits. J Infect Dis 142(6):915–922, 1980.

92. Morrey BF, Dunn JM, Heimbach RD, Davis J: Hyperbaric oxygen and chronic osteomyelitis. Clin Orthop Relat Res 144:121–127, 1979.

93. Slack WK, Thomas DA, Perrins D: Hyperbaric oxygenation chronic osteomyelitis. Lancet 14:1093–1094, 1965.

94. Feldmeier JJ, Heimbach RD, Davolt DA, Brakora MJ: Hyperbaric oxygen as an adjunctive treatment for severe laryngeal necrosis: A report of nine consecutive cases. Undersea Hyperb Med 20(4): 329–335, 1993.

95. Feldmeier JJ, Heimbach RD, Davolt DA, et al: Hyperbaric oxygen as an adjunctive treatment for delayed radiation injury of the chest wall: A retrospective review of twenty-three cases. Undersea Hyperb Med 22(4):383–393, 1995.

96. Feldmeier JJ, Jelen I, Davolt DA, et al: Hyperbaric oxygen as a prophylaxis for radiation-induced delayed enteropathy. Radiother Oncol 35(2):138–144, 1995.

97. Feldmeier JJ, Heimbach RD, Davolt DA, et al: Hyperbaric oxygen an adjunctive treatment for delayed radiation injuries of the abdomen and pelvis. Undersea Hyperb Med 23(4):205–213, 1996.

98. Marx RE, Ehler WJ, Tayapongsak P, Pierce LW: Relationship of oxygen dose to angiogenesis induction in irradiated tissue. Am J Surg 160(5):519–524, 1990.

99. Myers RAM, Marx RE: Use of hyperbaric oxygen in postradiation head and neck surgery. In Fox PC, Janson CC, Redmond JB (eds): National Institutes of Health Consensus Development Conference on Oral Complications of Cancer Therapies: Diagnosis, Prevention, and Treatment. Bethesda, MD: US Department of Health and Human Services, 1989, pp 151–157.

100. Kaelin CM, Im MJ, Myers RA, et al: The effects of hyperbaric oxygen on free flaps in rats. Arch Surg 125(5):607–609, 1990.

101. Zamboni WA, Roth AC, Russell RC, et al: The effect of acute hyperbaric oxygen therapy on axial pattern skin flap survival when administered during and after total ischemia. J Reconstr Microsurg 5(4):343–347; discussion 349–350, 1989.

102. Zatz R, Brenner BM: Pathogenesis of diabetic microangiopathy: The hemodynamic view. Am J Med 80(3):443–453, 1986.

103. Cianci P, Lueders H, Lee H, et al: Adjunctive hyperbaric oxygen reduces the need for surgery in 40–80% burns. J Hyperbar Med 3(2):97–101, 1988.

104. Cianci P, Lueders HW, Lee H, et al: Adjunctive hyperbaric oxygen therapy reduces length of hospitalization in thermal burns. J Burn Care Rehabil 10(5):432–435, 1989.

105. Cianci P, Williams C, Lueders H, et al: Adjunctive hyperbaric oxygen in the treatment of thermal burns: An economic analysis. J Burn Care Rehabil 11(2):140–143, 1990.

106. Hart GB, O'Reilly RR, Broussard ND, et al: Treatment of burns with hyperbaric oxygen. Surg Gynecol Obstet 139(5):693–696, 1974.

107. Brummelkamp WH, Hoogendijk J, Boerema I: Treatment of anaerobic infections (clostridial myositis) by drenching the tissues with oxygen under high atmospheric pressure Surgery 49:299–302, 1961.

108. Jamieson D, Vandenbrenk HA: Measurement of oxygen tensions in cerebral tissues of rats exposed to high pressures of oxygen. J Appl Physiol 18:869–876, 1963.

109. Thom SR: Hyperbaric oxygen therapy. J Intensive Care Med 4:58–74, 1989.

110. Wells CH, Goodpasture JE, Horrigan DJ, Hart GB: Tissue gas measurements during hyperbaric oxygen exposure. In Smith G (ed): Proceedings of the 6th International Conference on Hyperbaric Medicine. Aberdeen, Scotland: Aberdeen University Press, 1977, pp 118–124.

111. Gibson JJ, Angeles AP, Hunt TK: Increased oxygen tension potentiates angiogenesis. Surg Forum 1997;48:696–699.

112. Rabkin J, Hunt TK: Infection and oxygen. In Davis JC, Hunt TK (eds): Problem Wounds: The Role of Oxygen. New York: Elsevier, 1988, pp 1–16.

113. Hunt TK: The physiology of wound healing. Ann Emerg Med 17(12):1265–1273, 1988.

114. Knighton DR, Halliday B, Hunt TK: Oxygen as an antibiotic: The effect of inspired oxygen on infection. Arch Surg 119(2):199–204, 1984.

115. Sheffield PJ: Tissue oxygenation measurements. In Davis JC, Hunt TK (eds): Problem Wounds: The Role of Oxygen. New York: Elsevier, 1988, pp 17–51.

116. Chang N, Mathes SJ: Comparison of the effect of bacterial inoculation in musculocutaneous and random-pattern flaps. Plast Reconstr Surg 70(1):1–10, 1982.

117. Gottrup F, Firmin R, Hunt TK, Mathes SJ: The dynamic properties of tissue oxygen in healing flaps. Surgery. 95(5):527–536, 1984.

118. Johnsson K, Hunt TK, Mathes SJ: Effect of environmental oxygen on bacterial-induced tissue necrosis in flaps. Surg Forum 35:589–591, 1984.

119. Borer RC: Neutrophil adhesion and the diabetic. Presented at Hyperbaric Medicine 1998 Advanced Symposium, University of South Carolina School of Medicine, 1998.

120. Davis JC, Hunt TK: Problem Wounds: The Role of Oxygen. New York: Elsevier, 1988.

121. Niinikoski J, Heughan C, Hunt TK: Oxygen tensions in human wounds. J Surg Res 12:77–82, 1972.

122. Sheffield PJ: Tissue oxygen measurements with respect to soft tissue wound healing with normobaric and hyperbaric oxygen. HBO Rev 6:18–46, 1985.

123. Siddiqui A, Davidson JD, Mustoe TA: Ischemic tissue oxygen capacitance after hyperbaric oxygen therapy: A new physiologic concept. Plast Reconstr Surg 99:148–155, 1997.

124. Zhao LL, Davidson JD, Wee SC, et al: Effect of hyperbaric oxygen and growth factors on rabbit ear ischemic ulcers. Arch Surg 129(10):1043–1049, 1994.

125. Bonomo S, Davidson JD, Yu Y, et al: Hyperbaric oxygen as a signal transducer: Upregulation of platelet derived growth factor-beta receptor in the presence of HBO2 and PDGF. Undersea Hyperb Med 25:211–216, 1998.

126. Sen CI, Pack L, Hanninen O: Handbook of Oxidants and Antioxidants in Exercise. Amsterdam: Elsevier Science, 2000.

127. Halliwell B, Gutteridge JMC: Free Radicals in Biology and Medicine. Oxford, UK: Oxford Science Publications, 1999.

128. Hussain MZ, Ghani QP, Fend JJ, Hunt TK: Regulatory aspects of neovascularization: regulation of wound angiogenesis by metabolic alterations. In Teicher BA (ed): Angiogenic Agents in Cancer Therapy. Totowa, NJ: Humana Press, 1998, pp 143–150.

129. Gibson JJ, Sheikh AY, Rollins MD, et al: Increased oxygen tension and wound fluid vascular endothelial growth factor levels. Surg Forum 89:607–610, 1998.

130. Cho M, Hunt TK, Hussain MZ: Hydrogen peroxide stimulates macrophage vascular endothelial growth factor release. Am J Physiol 280:H2357–H2363, 2001.

131. Sheikh AY, Gibson JJ, Rollins MD, et al: Effect of hyperoxia on vascular endothelial growth factor in a wound model. Arch Surg 135:1293–1297, 2000.

132. Doctor N, Pandya S, Supe A: Hyperbaric oxygen therapy in diabetic foot. J Postgrad Med 38(3):112–114, 1992.

133. Baroni G, Porro T, Faglia E, et al: Hyperbaric oxygen in diabetic gangrene treatment. Diabetes Care 110(1):81–86, 1987.

134. Murphy DG, Sloan EP, Hart RG, et al: Tension pneumothorax associated with hyperbaric oxygen therapy. Am J Emerg Med 9(2):176–179, 1991.

135. Wood JD: GABA and oxygen toxicity: A review. Brain Res Bull 6:777–780, 1980.

136. Wood JD, Peesker SJ, Rozdilsky B: Sensitivity of GABA synthesis in human brain to oxygen poisoning. Aviat Space Environ Med 146(9):1155–1156, 1975.

137. Yoneda Y, Kuriyama K, Takahashi M: Modulation of synaptic GABA receptor binding by membrane phospholipids: Possible role of active oxygen radicals. Brain Res 333(1):111–122, 1985.

138. Clark J: Side Effects and Complications. Kensington, MD: Undersea and Hyperbaric Medical Society, 2003.

139. Armbruster S, Klein J, Stouten EM, et al: Surfactant in pulmonary oxygen toxicity. Adv Exp Med Biol;215:345–34, 1987.

140. Hart GB, Strauss MB, Riker J: Vital capacity of quadriplegic patients treated with hyperbaric oxygen. J Am Paraplegia Soc 7(1):8–9, 1984.

141. Pott F, Westergaard P, Mortensen J, Jansen EC: Hyperbaric oxygen treatment and pulmonary function. Undersea Hyperb Med 26(4):225–228, 1999.

142. Butler FK Jr: Diving and hyperbaric ophthalmology. Surv Ophthalmol 39(5):347–366, 1995.

143. Kindwall E: Contraindications and side effects to hyperbaric oxygen treatment. In Kindwall EP (ed): Hyperbaric Medicine Practice, 2nd ed. Flagstaff, AZ: Best Publishing Company, 1999, pp 83–97.
144. Palmquist BM, Philipson B, Barr PO: Nuclear cataract and myopia during hyperbaric oxygen therapy. Br J Ophthalmol 68(2):113–117, 1984.
145. Niinikoski J, Aho AJ: Combination of hyperbaric oxygen, surgery, and antibiotics in the treatment of clostridial gas gangrene. Infect Surg 2:23–37, 1983.
146. Cianci P: Adjunctive hyperbaric oxygen in the treatment of problem wounds: An economic analysis. In Kindwall E (ed): Proceedings of the Eighth International Congress on Hyperbaric Medicine, 1984. San Pedro, CA: Best Publishing Company, 1984, pp 213–216, 1984.
147. Oriani G, Meazza D, Favales F, et al: Hyperbaric oxygen therapy in diabetic gangrene. J Hyperbar Med 5:171–175, 1990.
148. Strauss MB, Villavicencio P, Hart GB, Benge C: Salvaging the difficult wound through a combined management program. In Kindwall E (ed): Proceedings of the Eighth International Conference on Hyperbaric Medicine, 1984. San Pedro, CA: Best Publishing Company; 1984, pp 207–212.
149. Stone JA, Scott RG, Brill LR, Levine BD: The role of hyperbaric oxygen therapy in the treatment of the diabetic foot. Diabetes 44(suppl 1):71A, 1995.
150. Zamboni WA, Wong HP, Stephenson LL, Pfeifer MA: Evaluation of hyperbaric oxygen for diabetic wounds: A prospective study. Undersea Hyperb Med 24(3):175–179, 1997.
151. Abidia A, Laden G, Kuhan G, et al: The role of hyperbaric oxygen therapy in ischaemic diabetic lower extremity ulcers: A double-blind randomised-controlled trial. Eur J Vasc Endovasc Surg 25(6):513–518, 2003.
152. Kalani M, Jorneskog G, Naderi N, et al: Hyperbaric oxygen (HBO) therapy in treatment of diabetic foot ulcers: Long term follow-up. J Diabetes Complications 16:153–158, 2002.
153. Kessler L, Bilbault P, Ortega F, et al: Hyperbaric oxygenation accelerates the healing rate of nonischemic chronic diabetic foot ulcers: A prospective randomized study. Diabetes Care 26(8):2378–2382, 2003.
154. Lee CT, Ramiah R, Choong SK, et al: Adjunctive hyperbaric oxygen in diabetic foot ulcers: A randomized, prospective double-blind study. Undersea Hyperb Med 31(3):310, 2004.
155. Strauss MB, Bryant BJ, Hart GB: Transcutaneous oxygen measurements under hyperbaric oxygen conditions as a predictor for healing of problem wounds. Foot Ankle Int 23(10):933–937, 2002.
156. Grunfield C: Diabetic foot ulcers: Etiology, treatment, and prevention. In Stollerman GH (ed): Advances in Internal Medicine. St. Louis: Mosby Year Book, 1991, pp 103–132.
157. Pecoraro RE, Ahroni JH, Boyko EJ, Stensel VL: Chronology and determinants of tissue repair in diabetic lower-extremity ulcers. Diabetes 40(10):1305–1313, 1991.
158. Ballard JL, Eke CC, Bunt TJ, Killeen JD: A prospective evaluation of transcutaneous oxygen measurements in the management of diabetic foot problems. J Vasc Surg 22(4):485–490; discussion 490–492, 1995.
159. Bunt TJ, Holloway GA: TcPO2 as an accurate predictor of therapy in limb salvage. Ann Vasc Surg 10(3):224–227, 1996.
160. Hanna GP, Fujise K, Kjellgren O, et al: Infrapopliteal transcatheter interventions for limb salvage in diabetic patients: Importance of aggressive interventional approach and role of transcutaneous oximetry. J Am Coll Cardiol 30(3):664–669, 1997.
161. Hauser CJ, Klein SR, Mehringer CM, et al: Assessment of perfusion in the diabetic foot by regional transcutaneous oximetry. Diabetes 33(6):527–531, 1984.
162. Reiber GE, Pecoraro RE, Koepsell TD: Risk factors for amputation in patients with diabetes mellitus: A case-control study. Ann Intern Med 117(2):97–105, 1992.
163. Pecoraro RE: The nonhealing diabetic ulcer: A major cause for limb loss. Prog Clin Biol Res 365:27–43, 1991.
164. Wattel F, Mathieu D, Coget JM, Billard V: Hyperbaric oxygen therapy in chronic vascular wound management. Angiology 41(1):59–65, 1990.
165. Hart GB, Meyer GW, Strauss MB, Messina VJ: Transcutaneous partial pressure of oxygen measured in a monoplace hyperbaric chamber at 1, 1.5, and 2 atm abs oxygen. J Hyperbar Med 5(4):223–229, 1990.
166. Fife CE, Buyukcakir C, Otto GH, et al: The predictive value of transcutaneous oxygen tension measurement in diabetic lower extremity ulcers treated with hyperbaric oxygen therapy: A retrospective analysis of 1,144 patients. Wound Repair Regen 10(4):198–207, 2002.
167. Niinikoski J: Hyperbaric oxygen therapy of diabetic foot ulcers, transcutaneous oxymetry in clinical decisiion making. Wound Repair Regen 11:458–461, 2003.
168. Clarke D: Transcutaneous oxygen: Interpretation and reporting. Presented at Hyperbaric Medicine Symposium, University of South Carolina School of Medicine, 1994.
169. Cianci P, Petrone G, Green B: Adjunctive hyperbaric oxygen in the salvage of the diabetic foot. Undersea Biomed Res 18(suppl):108, 1991.
170. Guo S, Counte MA, Gillespie KN, Schmitz H: Cost-effectiveness of adjunctive hyperbaric oxygen in the treatment of diabetic ulcers. Int J Technol Assess Health Care 19(4):731–737, 2003.
171. Gupta SK, Veith FJ: Inadequacy of diagnosis related group (DRG) reimbursements for limb salvage lower extremity arterial reconstructions. Ad hoc committee of the Joint Council of the Society for Vascular Surgery and the North American Chapter of the International Society for Cardiovascular Surgery. J Vasc Surg 11(2):348–356; discussion 356–357, 1990.
172. Lorenz EW: The Physician's DRG Working Guidebook 1988. St. Anthony's Publications, 1988.
173. Assoc AD: Consensus Development Conference on Diabetic Foot Wound Care. Diabetes Care 22(8):1354–1360, 1999.
174. Wattel F, Marroni A, Mathieu D: European Committee for Hyperbaric Medicine (ECHM) to coordinate, promote and study the development of clinical hyperbaric medicine in Europe. Minerva Anestesiol 66(10):733–748, 2000.
175. Care of diabetic foot ulcer. Br J Med (Clinical Evidence Issue 5) 2001.
176. Shuren J, Dei Cas R, Kucken L, Tillman K: Coverage decision memorandum for hyperbaric oxygen therapy in the treatment of hypoxic wounds and diabetic wounds of the lower extremities. Centers for Medicare and Medicaid, 2002, pp 1–29.
177. Kranke P, Bennett M, Roeckl-Wiedmann I, Debus S: Hyperbaric oxygen therapy for chronic wounds [review]. In The Cochrane Library 2005. John Wiley & Sons Ltd, 2005, pp 1–34.
178. Roeckl-Wiedmann I, Bennett M, Kranke P: Systematic review of hyperbaric oxygen in the management of chronic wounds. Br J Surg 92:24–32, 2005.
179. Zhao LL, Davidson JD, Wu L, Mustoe TA: Total reversal of hypoxic wound healing deficit by hyperbaric oxygen plus growth factors. Surg Forum 43:711–714, 1992.
180. Uhl E, Sirsjo A, Haapaniemi T, et al: Hyperbaric oxygen improves wound healing in normal and ischemic skin tissue. Plast Reconstr Surg 93(4):835–841, 1994.
181. Hammarlund C, Sundberg T: Hyperbaric oxygen reduced size of chronic leg ulcers: A randomized double-blind study. Plast Reconstr Surg 93(4):829–833; discussion 834, 1994.

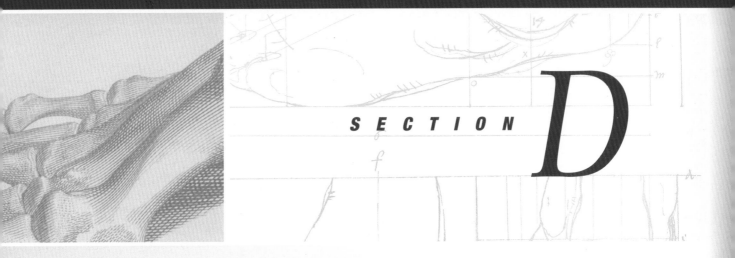

SECTION *D*

SURGICAL ASPECTS

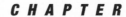

CHAPTER

18

SURGICAL PATHOLOGY OF THE FOOT AND CLINICOPATHOLOGIC CORRELATIONS

LAWRENCE W. O'NEAL ■

K nowledge of anatomy is essential so that the progression of pathologic changes in the diabetic foot
can be understood and proper surgical treatment can
be applied. Effective clinical evaluation and surgery are
based on an understanding of gross anatomy and of the
alterations produced by disease. In the treatment of diabetic foot problems, success is often uncertain, limited,
and temporary even under the care of the most knowledgeable and diligent physician. Close attention to detail
is necessary to obtain optimal results.

Anatomy of the Foot

Some of the easily visible landmarks of the foot are
shown in Figure 18-1.

Skin

The dorsal skin of the foot is flexible and unspecialized.
It is about 2 mm thick and contains hair follicles, sweat
glands, and scanty sebaceous glands. Only a few fibrous
septa attach the dermis to deeper fascial structures
except in the creases overlying the metatarsophalangeal
(MTP) joints and the interphalangeal (IP) joints,
making the skin at these sites relatively more fixed. The
plantar skin is 4 to 5 mm thick, with the heaviest areas
over the heel and the distal metatarsals. The skin of the
plantar surface is richly innervated; it has numerous

sweat glands but no sebaceous glands or hair follicles.
Throughout the plantar skin, the collagenous fibers of
the dermis are connected to the deep fascia by heavy
fibrous septa, which separate the subcutaneous fat into
firm, partly discontinuous lobules. These septa are
particularly heavy at the creases. Because of this firm
dermal fixation to deep fascia, the skin of the sole is
relatively fixed, moving only 1 cm or less over deeper
structures, compared to the dorsal skin, which will glide
2 or 3 cm.

Nails

The nails are specialized skin appendages, composed of
keratinous, flattened epithelial cells derived from the
generative areas of the nailfold and nailbed (Fig. 18-2).
The adult nail is composed of three ill-defined layers:
dorsal, intermediate, and ventral.[1] The dorsal nail arises
from the nailfold in the proximal half of its roof and
from the most proximal part of its floor. The intermediate nail originates from the distal part of the nailfold
and from the proximal nailbed up to the distal margin
of the lunula. The ventral nail arises from the distal half
to two thirds of the nailbed up to the hyponychium (Fig.
18-3). The nail is firmly attached to the epithelium of its
bed, which advances with nail growth, manifested by the
distal migration of small subungual hematomas. The
margins of the nail are overhung with skin folds called
the nail wall.

367

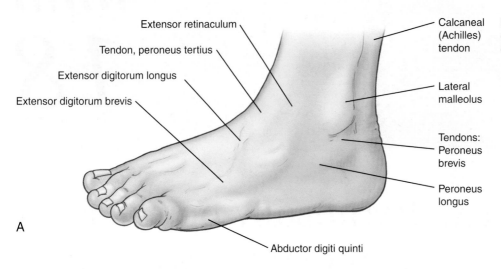

Extensor retinaculum

Tendon, peroneus tertius

Extensor digitorum longus

Extensor digitorum brevis

Calcaneal (Achilles) tendon

Lateral malleolus

Tendons: Peroneus brevis

Peroneus longus

Abductor digiti quinti

A

Figure 18–1   Surface anatomy of **(A)** lateral and **(B)** medial aspects of the foot.

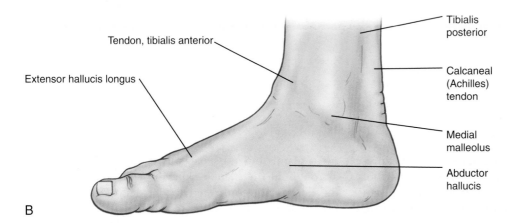

Tendon, tibialis anterior

Extensor hallucis longus

Tibialis posterior

Calcaneal (Achilles) tendon

Medial malleolus

Abductor hallucis

B

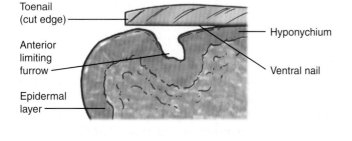

Toenail (cut edge)

Anterior limiting furrow

Epidermal layer

Hyponychium

Ventral nail

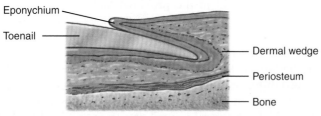

Eponychium

Toenail

Dermal wedge

Periosteum

Bone

Figure 18–2   Anatomy of the nails with longitudinal sections of the digits. *(Redrawn from Lewis BL: Microscopic studies of fetal and mature nail and surrounding soft tissue. Arch Dermatol Syph 70:732, 1954.)*

Nerves

The *sciatic nerve* divides into the common peroneal and tibial nerves in the posterior thigh. Elements of the sciatic nerve furnish the motor and sensory innervation of the foot with contributions from the fourth and fifth lumbar and first and second sacral segments (Fig. 18-4). The common peroneal nerve, the major lateral branch of the sciatic nerve, reaches the leg at the fibular head, then crosses anterior to the fibular neck deep to the origin of the peroneus longus muscle, where it divides into two main branches: the superficial peroneal (musculocutaneous) and the deep peroneal nerves. The superficial peroneal nerve enters the lateral (peroneal) compartment of the leg and supplies the peroneus longus and brevis muscles, then pierces the fascia in the lower third of the leg. A medial dorsal cutaneous (sensory) branch descends in front of the ankle joint to the medial side of the hallux and to the adjoining surfaces of the second and third toes. The intermediate dorsal cutaneous branch of the superficial peroneal nerve lies anterior to the lateral malleolus and innervates the skin of the third and fourth interdigital spaces and corresponding digital

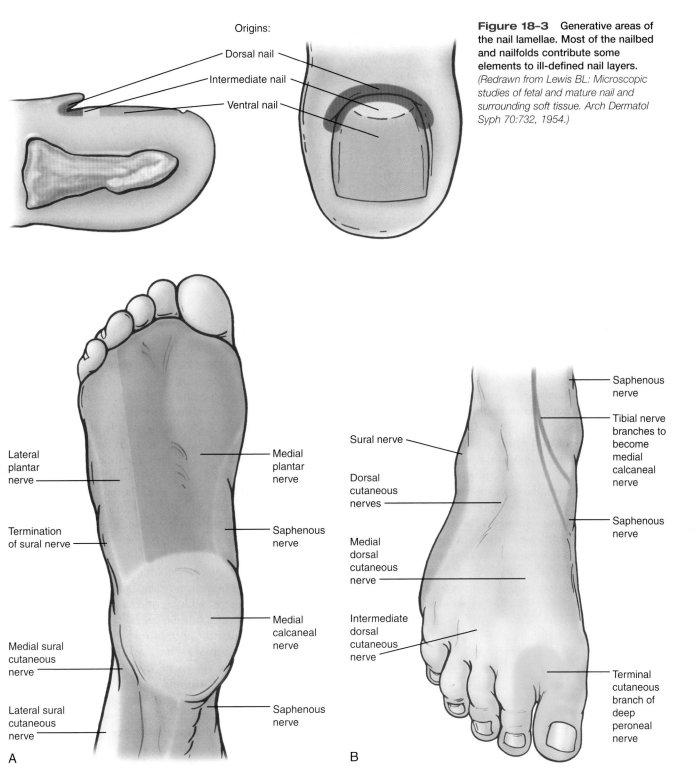

Origins:
- Dorsal nail
- Intermediate nail
- Ventral nail

Figure 18–3 Generative areas of the nail lamellae. Most of the nailbed and nailfolds contribute some elements to ill-defined nail layers. *(Redrawn from Lewis BL: Microscopic studies of fetal and mature nail and surrounding soft tissue. Arch Dermatol Syph 70:732, 1954.)*

Lateral plantar nerve

Termination of sural nerve

Medial sural cutaneous nerve

Lateral sural cutaneous nerve

Medial plantar nerve

Saphenous nerve

Medial calcaneal nerve

Saphenous nerve

Sural nerve

Dorsal cutaneous nerves

Medial dorsal cutaneous nerve

Intermediate dorsal cutaneous nerve

Saphenous nerve

Tibial nerve branches to become medial calcaneal nerve

Saphenous nerve

Terminal cutaneous branch of deep peroneal nerve

A

B

Figure 18–4 Cutaneous nerve distribution of (**A**) the sole and (**B**) the dorsum of the foot.

segments. The deep branch of the common peroneal nerve enters the anterior (extensor) compartment of the leg and is distributed to the dorsiflexor (extensor) muscles of the ankle and toes. It terminates in a dorsal digital nerve to the first interdigital web and adjoining aspects of the hallux and the second toe. The lateral margin of the foot derives its nerve supply from the sural nerve, which is known in the foot as the lateral dorsal cutaneous nerve. The saphenous nerve supplies the medial calf and ankle, ending distally at the medial side of the first MTP joint.

The tibial nerve divides into medial and lateral plantar branches deep to the plantar fascia. The cutaneous distribution of the medial plantar nerve includes the medial three and one half toes and the distal two thirds of the medial sole. Small interdigital twigs innervate the nailbeds of the medial three toes. The lateral plantar nerve supplies the lateral portion of the sole and the lateral one and one half toes. The heel receives its sensory innervation from the medial calcaneal branch of the tibial nerve.

Vessels

All the arterial supply of the foot is derived from the popliteal artery, which lies posteriorly on the knee joint capsule and popliteal muscle. At the lower border of the popliteal muscle, the popliteal artery divides into anterior and posterior tibial branches. The anterior tibial artery penetrates the upper part of the interosseous membrane and enters the anterior compartment of the leg. Distally, it lies between the tibialis anterior and toe extensor muscles. At the ankle, it lies more medially, crossing the ankle joint anteriorly to become the dorsalis pedis artery of the foot. It usually lies lateral to the extensor hallucis longus muscle. Small dorsal digital arteries arise from a variable dorsal arcuate branch. The posterior tibial artery accompanies the tibial nerve, lying between the tibialis posterior and flexor digitorum longus muscles and the soleus muscle and Achilles tendon. Near the medial malleolus, it sends a branch to the heel pad along with the medial calcaneal nerve. In the medial plantar space, the posterior tibial artery divides into medial and lateral plantar arteries, which course with the medial and lateral plantar nerves. The plantar arch is formed by anastomosis between the medial and lateral plantar arteries, with a contribution from the dorsalis pedis artery at the first intermetatarsal space.

The plantar digital arteries arise from the plantar arch, which is variable in detail but provides abundant collateral circulation to the distal foot. The arterioles to the skin form an internal vascular belt at the junction of the subcutaneous tissue and dermis. Intimately interconnected dermal plexuses arise from this belt, forming a reticular network of vessels of different sizes. From this network, arboreal terminal branches form a subpapillary plexus with capillary loops into the dermal papillae, integrating a number of papillae into vascular districts, which are also interconnected.

Muscles, Tendons, and Fascia

The foot and toe dorsiflexors, located in the anterior compartment of the leg, include the tibialis anterior, extensor hallucis longus, and extensor digitorum longus muscles. The peroneal muscles lie in the lateral compartment of the leg. Both the anterior and lateral muscle groups are innervated by the common peroneal nerve. The plantar flexors of the foot and toes lie in the posterior compartment of the leg behind the interosseous membrane and are innervated by the tibial nerve. The

deep muscular (crural) fascia encloses the muscles of the anterior and lateral compartments. At the anterior ankle, thickened areas of this fascia form the extensor retinacula (the transverse crural and cruciate crural ligaments), under which the extensor tendons course. This fascia is continuous with the thinner fascia over the dorsum of the foot and toes.

The gastrocnemius muscle bellies arise from medial and lateral origins on the posterior femur just proximal to the femoral condyles and together form the distal margin of the popliteal fossa. The soleus muscle arises deep to the gastrocnemius from the proximal tibia and fibula. It joins the gastrocnemius muscle to form the so-called triceps surae muscle, which in turn forms the Achilles (calcaneal) tendon inserted on the calcaneus. The small plantaris muscle arises from the lateral femoral condyle, then crosses between the soleus and the gastrocnemius to join the medial portion of the Achilles tendon. The gastrocnemius, soleus, and plantaris muscles are innervated by branches of the tibial nerve. Across the posterior ankle, the long tendons are held in position relative to each other by fascial condensations.

The plantar fascia (aponeurosis) is the most superficial fascia in the sole of the foot.[2] Its very thick central portion arises from the medial tubercle of the calcaneus. From there, the plantar fascia spreads fan-like toward the toes. Near the metatarsal heads, its fibers divide into five processes, which form bundles surrounding the metatarsal heads (Fig. 18-5). Distally, the plantar fascia joins the superficial transverse metatarsal ligament to anchor the dermis at the distal plantar crease. Some deeper fibers extend to the flexor sheaths near the MTP joints.

The flexor digitorum brevis muscle arises from the proximal portion of the plantar fascia in the central plantar space. Thinner portions of the plantar fascia cover the abductor hallucis muscle medially and the abductor digiti quinti muscle laterally. The strong central portion of the plantar aponeurosis forms the principal stay of the longitudinal arch.

Deep to the plantar fascia, the muscles in the sole of the foot are divided into four layers. The superficial *first layer* (Fig. 18-6)[2] consists of the flexor digitorum brevis, the abductor hallucis, and the abductor digiti quinti muscles. The flexor digitorum brevis originates from the medial tubercle of the calcaneus and from the deep surface of the plantar aponeurosis. Its four tendons insert into the middle phalanges of the four lateral toes. The abductor hallucis arises from the medial tubercle of the calcaneus and inserts medially on the base of the proximal phalanx of the great toe. The abductor digiti quinti arises from the medial and lateral tubercles of the calcaneus and inserts into the base of the proximal phalanx of the little toe.

The second layer is composed of the tendons of the flexor hallucis longus and flexor digitorum longus muscles. These tendons insert plantarly on the proximal por-

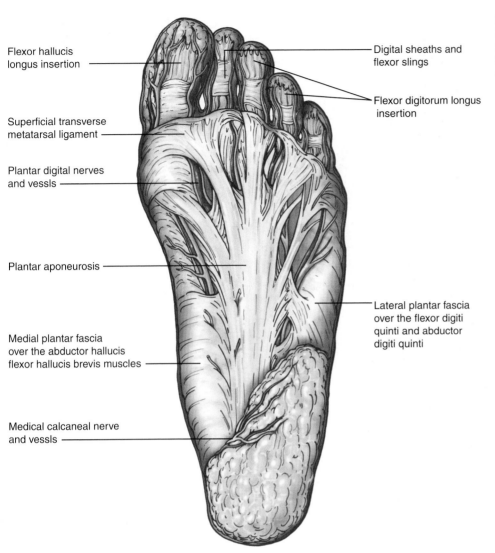

Flexor hallucis longus insertion

Superficial transverse metatarsal ligament

Plantar digital nerves and vessls

Plantar aponeurosis

Medial plantar fascia over the abductor hallucis flexor hallucis brevis muscles

Medical calcaneal nerve and vessls

Digital sheaths and flexor slings

Flexor digitorum longus insertion

Lateral plantar fascia over the flexor digiti quinti and abductor digiti quinti

Figure 18–5 Plantar fascia. Note bundles separating the near metatarsal heads. *(Redrawn from Grant JCB: An Atlas of Anatomy, 6th ed. Baltimore: Williams & Wilkins, 1972.)*

tion of the distal phalanges. The quadratus plantae muscle (accessory flexor) arises from the calcaneus and inserts on the flexor digitorum longus tendons. The four lumbrical muscles arise from the medial side of the tendons of the flexor digitorum longus muscle, pass to the medial side of each toe, and insert on the capsule of the MTP joint and on the dorsal expansion of the extensor tendon of the lateral four toes. The tendons of the lumbricals lie superficial to the deep transverse metatarsal ligament, allowing them to extend the proximal interphalangeal (PIP) joints and assist in flexion of the MTP joints.

The flexor hallucis brevis, the flexor digiti quinti, and the two heads of the adductor hallucis muscle, oblique and transverse, make up the third layer (Fig. 18-7).[2] The flexor hallucis brevis originates from the dense fibrous plantar tarsometatarsal ligaments and from the inferior aspect of the cuboid. It splits to form medial and lateral tendons, each of which encases a sesamoid bone under the first metatarsal head. At their insertion on the proximal phalanx of the hallux, they are joined by the tendon of the abductor hallucis muscle medially and the ten-

dons of the oblique and transverse heads of the adductor hallucis to form a composite tendon. The oblique head of the adductor hallucis arises from the bases of the second, third, and fourth metatarsal bones and from the fascial sheath of the peroneus longus. Its transverse head originates on the plantar aspect of the four lateral MTP joints and the deep transverse metatarsal ligament. The flexor digiti quinti arises from the base of the fifth metatarsal and inserts on the base of the proximal phalanx of the fifth toe.

The plantar and dorsal interosseus muscles and the tendons of the tibialis posterior and peroneus longus muscles lie in the fourth layer (Fig. 18-8).[2] The three plantar interossei arise from the third, fourth, and fifth metatarsal shafts and insert on the medial side of the bases of the corresponding proximal phalanges, acting as adductors to these toes. The four dorsal interossei arise from adjoining metatarsal surfaces in the first, second, third, and fourth intermetatarsal spaces and attach at the bases of the proximal phalanges of the second, third, and fourth toes. The dorsal interossei abduct from the axis of the second toe. The tendon of

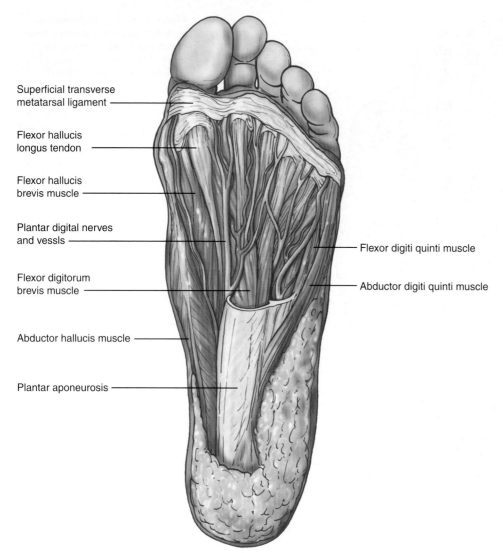

Superficial transverse metatarsal ligament

Flexor hallucis longus tendon

Flexor hallucis brevis muscle

Plantar digital nerves and vessls

Flexor digitorum brevis muscle

Abductor hallucis muscle

Plantar aponeurosis

Flexor digiti quinti muscle

Abductor digiti quinti muscle

Figure 18–6   First layer of plantar muscles. *(Redrawn from Grant JCB: An Atlas of Anatomy, 6th ed. Baltimore: Williams & Wilkins, 1972.)*

the peroneus longus lies in a groove on the inferior aspect of the cuboid, passes deep to the flexor hallucis brevis, and inserts on the lateral side of the bases of the first metatarsal and the medial cuneiform just opposite the insertions of the tibialis anterior on these same bones. Together, the two form a sling that everts and inverts the foot, respectively. The tibialis posterior inserts chiefly on the medial aspect of the navicular tubercle but also sends plantar fibrous attachments to the complex tarsal and tarsometatarsal ligaments. The extensor digitorum brevis and extensor hallucis brevis *muscles* are innervated by branches of the peroneal nerve. The short flexors of the lateral toes and hallux, the interossei, the lumbricals, and the abductor hallucis muscle are all innervated by the tibial nerve.

The collagenous structures of the distal foot intermingle to a degree that is difficult to convey by any description. In the 2 cm between the heads of the metatarsals proximally and the plantar metatarsophalangeal crease distally, the dermal collagen, plantar fascia, flexor sheaths, joint capsules, and periosteum of the sesamoids, metatarsals, and proximal phalanges are closely approximated and

attached more or less by common fibrous sheaths and septa. The superficial transverse metatarsal ligament is a local condensation of this fibrous tissue. The deep transverse metatarsal ligament is adjacent to the joint capsule and comingles with joint capsule fibers. The bones of the foot with some of the major tendon insertions are shown in Figure 18-9.

Plantar Spaces (Compartments) of the Foot

The medial plantar space is bounded by the inferior surface of the first metatarsal dorsally, an extension of the plantar aponeurosis medially, and the intermuscular septum laterally (Fig. 18-10).[3] This space contains the abductor hallucis and flexor hallucis brevis muscles and the flexor hallucis longus, peroneus longus, and posterior tibial tendons. The central plantar space is bounded by the plantar fascia inferiorly, intermuscular septa medially and laterally, and the tarsometatarsal structures dorsally. This space contains the flexor digitorum brevis muscle, flexor digitorum longus tendons, the lumbrical, quadratus plantae, and adductor hallucis muscles, the peroneal

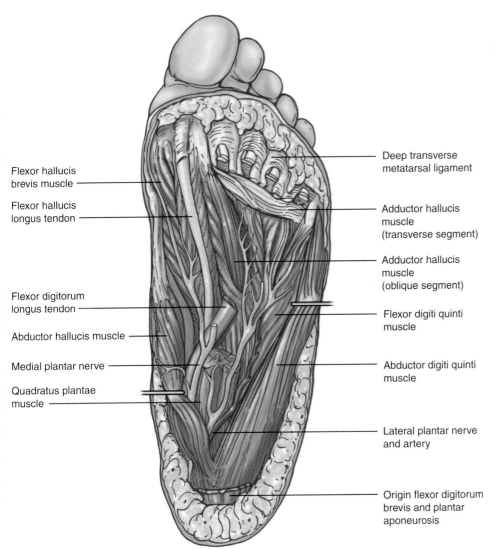

Figure 18–7 Third layer of plantar muscles. *(Redrawn from Grant JCB: An Atlas of Anatomy, 6th ed. Baltimore: Williams & Wilkins, 1972.)*

Deep transverse metatarsal ligament

Adductor hallucis muscle (transverse segment)

Adductor hallucis muscle (oblique segment)

Flexor digiti quinti muscle

Abductor digiti quinti muscle

Lateral plantar nerve and artery

Origin flexor digitorum brevis and plantar aponeurosis

Flexor hallucis brevis muscle

Flexor hallucis longus tendon

Flexor digitorum longus tendon

Abductor hallucis muscle

Medial plantar nerve

Quadratus plantae muscle

and posterior tibial tendons, and the plantar arterial arch. The lateral plantar space is bounded by the fifth metatarsal dorsally, an intermuscular septum medially, and the edge of the plantar aponeurosis laterally. It contains the abductor digiti quinti, flexor digiti quinti, and opponens muscles of the fifth toe. The interosseous compartment is bounded by the interosseous fascia of the metatarsals and contains the seven interosseous muscles.

The Vulnerable Foot in Diabetes Mellitus

The Role of Deformity

Foot deformities are common in diabetes of long duration. In a survey of diabetic patients at a Veteran's Affairs Hospital clinic, 50% had vascular insufficiency, neuropathy, and a coexisting foot deformity, indicating a high risk of morbidity.[4] The common deformities were angular, usually hallux valgus and claw toes. Less common but significant problems were submetatarsal head calluses, interdigital soft corns, and Charcot neuroarthopathy.

Several of these deformed feet were ulcerated; one patient had osteomyelitis and one had gangrene of the hallux. A Swedish study[5] showed that angular foot deformities were present in 68% of diabetic men, compared with 28% of men without diabetes. Some of the deformities in diabetic individuals may be old problems that are tolerated until neuropathy and/or vascular insufficiency ensue. Others are unique to diabetic people as the result of profound changes in the delicate muscle balance between flexors and extensors and between abductors and adductors.[6] A variety of angular deformities subject the insensitive foot to the risk of injury by the incessant friction of poorly fitting footwear.

The Role of Neuropathy

Although much emphasis has been rightly placed on the effect of sensory neuropathy on the feet, it should be noted that neuropathy of the motor nerves is also common in diabetic people.[7] Decreased motor nerve conduction velocity is a predictor of plantar ulceration and amputation in diabetic patients without significant

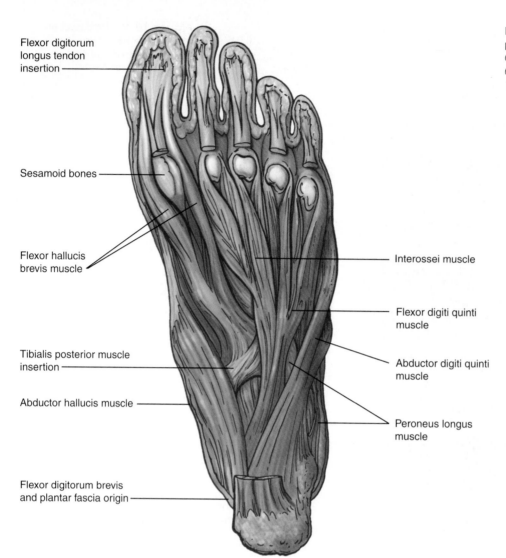

Flexor digitorum
longus tendon
insertion

Sesamoid bones

Flexor hallucis
brevis muscle

Tibialis posterior muscle
insertion

Abductor hallucis muscle

Flexor digitorum brevis
and plantar fascia origin

Interossei muscle

Flexor digiti quinti
muscle

Abductor digiti quinti
muscle

Peroneus longus
muscle

Figure 18–8   Fourth layer of
plantar muscles. *(Redrawn from
Grant JCB: An Atlas of Anatomy,
6th ed. Baltimore: Williams & Wilkins,
1972.)*

peripheral vascular disease.[8] Motor neuropathy, like sensory neuropathy, progresses from distal to proximal. The first motor nerves to be involved are those to the intrinsic muscles of the feet. With atrophy of the lumbricals, the opposing muscles, with more proximal innervation, extend the MTP joints and flex the PIP joints with resultant clawing of the toes and distal migration of the cushioning fat pads that lie under the metatarsal heads.[9] Atrophy of the distal dorsal foot muscles can be demonstrated early and is predictive of severe sensory neuropathy and foot ulceration.[6,10,11] Atrophy becomes apparent clinically as dorsal depressions between the metatarsal shafts but is not necessarily associated with toe deformity.[8,10] Conversely, diabetic foot ulceration is not always accompanied by muscle weakness.[6]

Early motor neuropathy affects not only the lumbricals, but all the distal foot muscles. Loss of abduction function of the dorsal interossei causes the toes to become crowded onto the axis of the second digit, accentuating the angular prominences at the first and fifth

MTP joints (bunion and bunionette, respectively). Limited joint mobility accompanies these deformities.[12] When circulation is adequate, prophylactic surgery to alleviate angular prominences can be cautiously considered.[13] The structural changes in the distal foot are accompanied by a decrease in sensation and evolving microangiopathy.[14–16] Intradermal nerve fiber density is decreased significantly after diabetes of 5 years' duration.[17] Sympathetic neuropathy results in loss of sweating and dry (xerotic) skin, which may contribute to the accumulation of interdigital detritus (Fig. 18-11).

The Role of End-Artery Disease

The rich collateral circulation in the foot allows major trauma, operations, and infections to be tolerated in the nondiabetic patient with little concern for circulation distal to the ankle. In the diabetic, however, multiple complete and partial arteriosclerotic blockades of large, medium, and small arteries result in a situation comparable to end-arteries in the heart or kidney, where opportunity for collateral circulation does not exist. In these organs, if an end-artery becomes blocked, there is no replacement for its function, and the tissue supplied by it dies (Fig. 18-12). A similar situation can be seen in plantar space abscesses. With penetrating wounds of the sole from a tack, pin, glass, or nail, a plantar space may be entered directly, and an abscess may form. In the nonexpansile central plantar space, infection can quickly obliterate the plantar arterial arch and its branches, to be followed by necrosis not only of tissue in the central plantar space but also of the second, third, and fourth toes, which receive most of their blood supply from the plantar arch (Fig. 18-13). The fifth toe and the hallux receive some of their circulation through the lateral and medial plantar spaces, respectively, and may survive central plantar space abscesses. Digital and web infections can produce localized gangrene that spreads by means of septic obliterative angiopathy until the digital arteries are reached. Occlusion of these will lead to gangrene of the adjoining digits if the neighboring small vessels are obstructed, creating an end-artery situation (Fig. 18-14).

Histologically, there are no clear-cut differences between the lower-limb arteriosclerosis of diabetic individuals and of nondiabetic individuals. In the diabetic limb, however, the obstructive disease tends to be more distal and in particular to involve the metatarsal and digital arteries. These findings have been amply confirmed and are often seen in lower-limb angiograms. The distinctive distal patchy atherosclerosis of the diabetic with multiple blockades in capillaries, arterioles, small arteries, and named larger arteries sometimes converts tissue that in healthy people is perfused by interlocking, alternate channels of blood flow into tissue that is supplied by only one artery, sometimes tenuously. The amount of tissue that is thus dependent on its single artery may vary from a few square millimeters of skin in a vascular district to the entire foot or leg.

Common Foot Abnormalities in Diabetic Patients

Isakov and colleagues[18] found that the initial anatomic site of lesions resulting in amputations in diabetic patients was as follows: digits, 62.2%; distal foot under metatarsal heads, 8.0%; midfoot and heel, 8.5%; dorsum of foot, 3.3%; and ankle or distal leg, 5.7%.

Nails

Nail deformities due to trauma, fungus infection, systemic disease, or poor care are common in the general population; in the ischemic, neuropathic foot of diabetic individuals, they appear to be universal (Box 19-1). The reduced vision and abdominal obesity of many diabetic patients make it very difficult for them to reach their nails for self-care; even then, they may cut the adjacent skin. With neglect, a nail will grow too long, often gouging the skin of its neighbor (Fig. 18-15). Also, with growth, a nail may incurve and partly encircle the distal nailbed (Fig. 18-16). Simply stubbing the toe or wearing new shoes can then break the skin. At times, excess keratin and debris accumulate beneath the nail and in the nailfolds, where bacteria can grow (Fig. 18-17).

Toes

Toe deformities are common in diabetic individuals (Fig. 18-18). Motor neuropathy results in atrophy of the lumbricals allowing the long toe extensors, with more proximal innervation, to extend the MTP joints while the long flexors flex the IP joints. The result is claw toes, with angular prominence at the PIP joints. Atrophy of the dorsal interossei causes the second, third, and fourth toes to become crowded. Angular prominences are susceptible to shoe-on-skin friction. As the toes extend at the MTP joints, they no longer share weight-bearing with the metatarsal heads, which become visibly and palpably more prominent.[11] The cushioning fat pad beneath the metatarsal heads migrates distally, leaving the metatarsal heads to press on thinner tissue unsuited to the stress of walking (Fig 18-19).[9,11,19,20] In claw toes, a corn (clavus) forms over the dorsal bony prominence of the PIP joint. When the clavus ulcerates, there is direct access to the joint (Fig. 18-20). Frequently, callus and an ulcer can develop on the tip of a toe with distal interphalangeal joint flexion contracture (mallet toe), which will rub on the inner sole of the shoe. Friction (shear) on these bony prominences produces blisters, calluses, and ulcers that are often ignored in the insensitive foot.

In cock-up deformity of the hallux, an imbalance between the flexor and extensor muscles causes the IP joint to flex and the MTP joint to extend, making the extensor tendon prominent. Ulceration of the resulting callus on the dorsum of the IP joint may result in penetration of the joint, causing infection. Adduction of the hallux with resultant toe crowding is common. Hammer toe is associated with ulceration of the distal toe tip.[21] Decreased joint mobility is found in all the toe deformities.[12] Varus deformity, in which the third, fourth, and fifth toes drift medially, may cause nails to gouge adjacent toes, producing small ulcers. Crowding, sometimes with overlap, causes friction of toe on toe.

Heloma Molle

Heloma molle (soft corn) between the toes is caused by crowding of the toes in tight shoes. The most common location is on the lateral base of the fourth toe from pressure and friction from the adjacent, prominent head

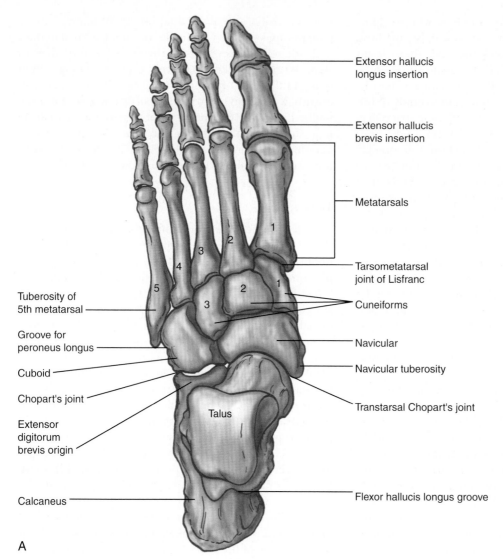

Figure 18–9   **A**, Bones of the foot from the dorsal aspect.

Extensor hallucis longus insertion

Extensor hallucis brevis insertion

Metatarsals

Tarsometatarsal joint of Lisfranc

Cuneiforms

Navicular

Navicular tuberosity

Transtarsal Chopart's joint

Flexor hallucis longus groove

Tuberosity of 5th metatarsal

Groove for peroneus longus

Cuboid

Chopart's joint

Extensor digitorum brevis origin

Calcaneus

Talus

A

of the proximal phalanx of the fifth toe. Heloma molle can also occur wherever a knobby joint of one toe crowds in on its neighbor and can lead to web space abscess (Fig. 18-21).

Hallux Valgus

Hallux valgus is a lateral deviation, at the MTP joint, of the great toe toward the second toe. A bony prominence (exostosis) is present on the metatarsal head medially, over which a thick-walled bursa forms. Ulceration of the skin over this medial bony prominence allows spread of infection into the bursa, then into the MTP joint and medial plantar space (Fig. 18-22).

Tailor's Bunion

Tailor's bunion (bunionette) is a prominence of the lateral part of the fifth metatarsal head, often associated with varus deformity of the fifth toe. As in hallux valgus, ulceration of the bursa over the lateral aspect of the fifth metatarsal head can occur, with bacteria entering the bursa and MTP joint or into the central plantar space via the short flexor and abductor muscles of the fifth toe.

Calluses

Distal foot calluses are highly predictive of ulceration in the diabetic patient[22] (Fig. 18-23). Ulceration of calluses leads to mal perforans, which is discussed later in this chapter. The majority of foot calluses occur under the metatarsal heads, the first, second, and fifth heads being most frequently involved, in that order. All patients with calluses and ulcers exert maximum loads at the site of the lesion. Distal migration of the fat pad cushion beneath the metatarsal heads allows pressure transfer to thinner, more proximal plantar skin that is unsuitable for weight-bearing, greatly contributing to ulceration.

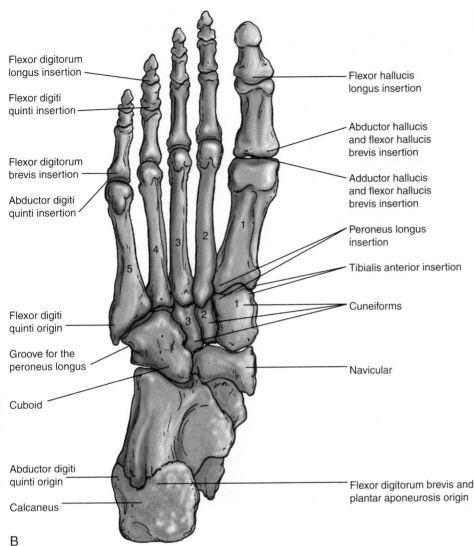

Figure 18–9, cont'd   B, Bones of the foot from the plantar aspect.

Flexor digitorum longus insertion

Flexor digiti quinti insertion

Flexor digitorum brevis insertion

Abductor digiti quinti insertion

Flexor digiti quinti origin

Groove for the peroneus longus

Cuboid

Abductor digiti quinti origin

Calcaneus

B

Flexor hallucis longus insertion

Abductor hallucis and flexor hallucis brevis insertion

Adductor hallucis and flexor hallucis brevis insertion

Peroneus longus insertion

Tibialis anterior insertion

Cuneiforms

Navicular

Flexor digitorum brevis and plantar aponeurosis origin

Midfoot

The midfoot is not as subject to calluses and ulcerations as is the forefoot, but the midfoot is frequently injured by penetrating objects. In the patient with advanced diabetes who cannot see well and cannot feel pain, infection following penetration of the midfoot spreads rapidly either directly to the central plantar space or along collagenous septa that connect the dermis to the plantar fascia. This process is hastened by inadequate circulation and failure to cease bearing weight on the foot. When a tarsometatarsal Charcot neuroarthropathy collapses into a rocker-bottom deformity, weight-bearing will be concentrated on the middle of the sole with a resultant ulcer.

Heel

The heel is sometimes the site of neurotrophic ulcers because of the bony prominences of the calcaneus.

Ulcers and patches of gangrene can develop on its posterolateral surface as the immobile patient lies supine on a mattress (Fig. 18-24). In contrast, lesions of the posterior heel usually indicate excessive walking on an insensitive foot (Fig. 18-25). When ulceration and gangrene occur in the heel, the foot might not be salvageable because debridement and amputations in this area can preclude functional weight-bearing. Transtibial or transfemoral amputation might be the only remedy.

Mechanisms of Onset of Foot Lesions

Initial Lesions

Although the end of the process may be loss of limb or life or both, the initial event is most often a break in the skin followed by penetration of bacteria. Ordinarily, most of the incidents leading to severe infection, gangrene,

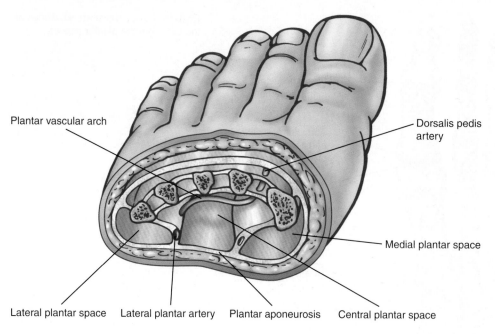

Figure 18–10 Plantar spaces in the distal foot.

Plantar vascular arch

Dorsalis pedis artery

Medial plantar space

Lateral plantar space   Lateral plantar artery   Plantar aponeurosis   Central plantar space

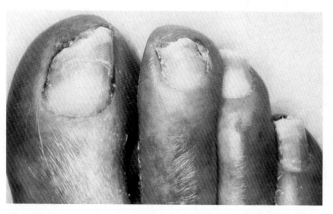

Figure 18–11 Foot in a patient with advanced diabetes shows shiny, thin, dry, hairless skin; dermal hemosiderin deposits; and irregular growth of nails, with evidence of poor care. This man, in his fifties, had had his left leg amputated and was nearly blind from retinopathy.

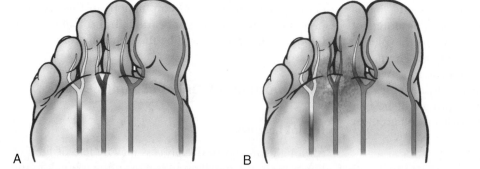

A   B   C

Figure 18–12 Schematic of mechanisms whereby advancing infection causes obliteration of small arteries that have been converted into end-arteries by arteriosclerotic disease process, with resultant gangrene. **A,** Early web space infection in a foot with patchy segmental arteriosclerotic occlusion of digital and metatarsal vessels. **B,** Thrombosis of arteries adjacent to web space infection. **C,** Gangrene of second and third toes.

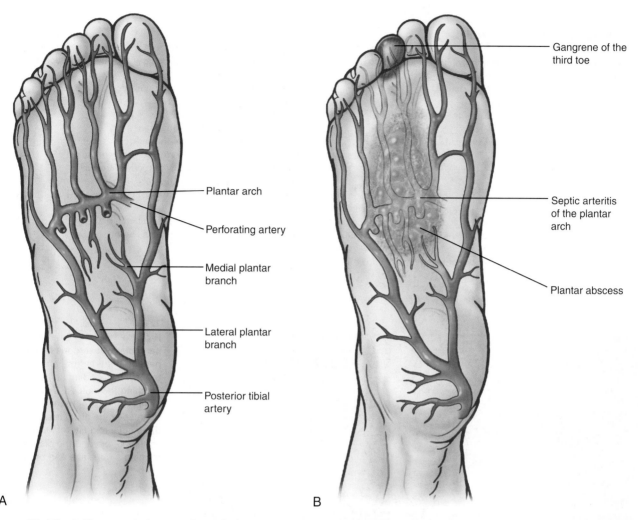

Plantar arch

Perforating artery

Medial plantar branch

Lateral plantar branch

Posterior tibial artery

Gangrene of the third toe

Septic arteritis of the plantar arch

Plantar abscess

A

B

Figure 18-13 **A,** The normal plantar arch receives contributions from the medial and lateral plantar branches of the posterior tibial artery and from the dorsalis pedis artery via a perforating artery or arteries. **B,** If a central plantar space abscess causes occlusion of the plantar arch, gangrene of the middle toe will result.

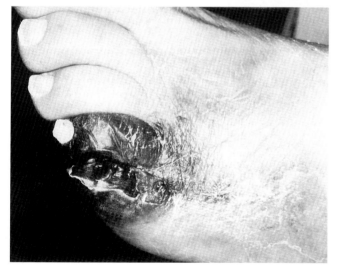

Figure 18-14 Tissue necrosis by both microangiopathy (fifth toe) and end-artery disease (fourth toe) in the same foot. After the fifth toe was stubbed, gangrene began in the injured tissue near the avulsed nail. When the infection reached the foot, the fourth toe became gangrenous as the lateral digital artery of the fourth toe became obliterated. Inflammatory change in the dorsum of the foot is called phlegmon. When photographed, the dorsalis pedis pulse could be felt.

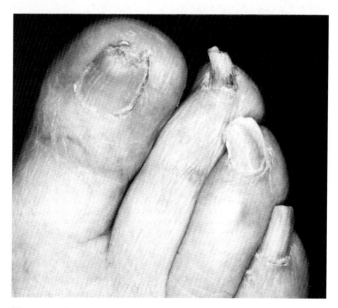

Figure 18-15 Toes of an obese diabetic patient with onychomycosis of the hallux and incurving distal growth of all nails. Nails have grown long because of neglect. Note that the nail of the third toe gouges the skin of the second toe.

BOX 18-1   Glossary of Nails

Onych-, onycho- Greek *Onyx*, meaning nail
Onychatrophy Atrophy of the nails
Onychauxis Marked overgrowth of the nails
Onychectomy Ablation of a nail
Onychia Inflammation of the matrix of the nail; onychitis
    O. lateralis Paronychia
    O. maligna Acute onychia in debilitated patients
    O. parasitica Onychomycosis
    O. periungualis Paronychia
    O. sicca Brittle nails
Onychitis Onychia
Onychodystrophy Dystrophy in the nails occurring as a congenital
    defect or due to any illness or injury that may cause a malformed nail
Onychogryposis Enlargement with increased curvature of the nails
    (Fig. 18-17)
Onycholysis Loosening of the nails, beginning at the free border and
    usually incomplete

Onychomadesis Complete shedding of the nails, usually with
    systemic disease
Onychomalacia Abnormal softness of the nails
Onychomycosis Fungus infection of the nails
    O. favus Favus of the nails
    O. trichophytina Tinea unguium
Onychonosus Any disease of the nails; onychopathy, onychosis
Onychophosis Growth of horny epithelium in the nailbed
Onychophyma Swelling or hypertrophy of the nails
Onychoptosis Falling off of the nails
Onychorrhexis Abnormal brittleness of the nails with splitting of free
    edge
Onychoschizia Loosening of the nail from the nailbed
Ungius incarnatus Ingrowing nail; onychocryptosis

Adapted from Sutton RL Jr: Diseases of the Skin, 11th ed. St. Louis: Mosby-Year Book, 1956, with permission.

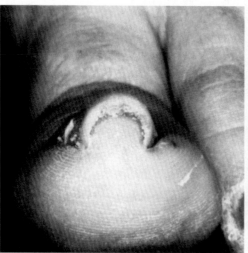 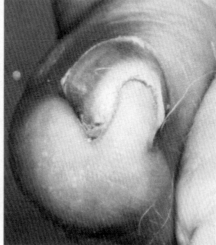

A   B

Figure 18-16 Type of nail that is particularly hazardous in the diabetic patient. It starts from a wide base at the nail root and incurves distally, pinching the nailbed. These two nails form arcs of more than 200 degrees at the distal toe. If neglected, the medial and lateral nail margins may meet beyond the distal toe, forming a full circle and brittle claw.

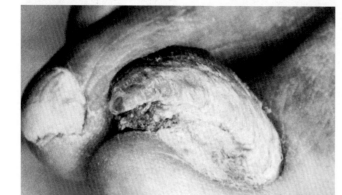

Figure 18-17 Onychogryposis. In a diabetic patient, infection may begin in debris covering the nailbed. This type of nail easily hooks bedding, socks, or furniture, causing avulsion of the nail and trauma to the proximal nailfold.

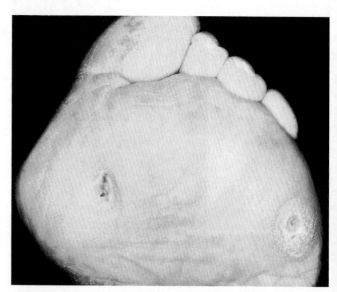

Figure 18-18 Diabetic foot with crowding of toes, hammer toes (note position of nails), bunion, and distal plantar calluses.

and amputation in the diabetic seem trivial and indeed would be so in most nondiabetic individuals. The diabetic person with severe neuropathy frequently does not even know how the injury happened. It might have been due to acute mechanical trauma in which skin was torn or punctured. Frequently, the poor vision and impaired balance of the diabetic patient contribute to toe-stubbing, stepping on sharp objects, or gouging the skin while trimming nails. Thermal trauma from foot baths and heating pads can also destroy skin in the neuropathic foot. Incessant friction over angular bony prominences is

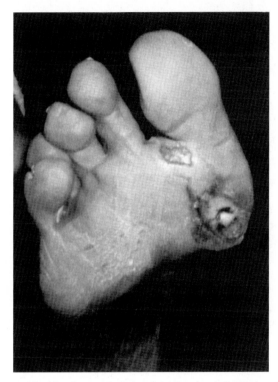

Figure 18–19 Concentrated weight-bearing in intrinsic minus foot with resultant ulcer under the first metatarsal head.

associated with improperly fitting shoes, with one brief episode of walking resulting in blistering and ulceration. If the circulation is adequate, healing usually occurs with consistent off-loading of the foot. Conversely, if circulation is inadequate to deliver the hyperemic response needed for healing, gangrene may follow.

Toes normally play an important role during walking by increasing the weight-bearing area of the foot. Several toe deformities, however, may cause concentration of weight-bearing under the metatarsal heads, leading to callus formation and ulceration. Areas of callus and ulceration correlate well with areas of maximum vertical and shear forces. In bedridden, immobile patients, the heel is vulnerable to ulceration due to the weight of the immobile foot on the mattress, obliterating blood perfusion in skin on the posterolateral side of the heel. The consequence of these initial events, which seem minor and are often ignored or minimized, may be transfemoral amputation when ulcers occur in a foot debilitated by diabetes. The greatly increased vulnerability of the diabetic foot is often not appreciated by the patient and/or family, who might have difficulty in understanding why "such a little thing" can result in tissue loss and progressive disability.

Local Progression

The progression to major infection with necrosis of tissue results from (1) arterial circulation inadequate to confine the infection; (2) neuropathy so profound that the patient does not voluntarily remove all weight from the foot as a person with normal sensation would, resulting in "milking" of the infection along fascial pathways by continued weight-bearing; and (3) more aggressive bacterial superinfection. Although the "ischemic" foot might follow a somewhat different pattern than the "neuropathic" foot and one pattern or the other might

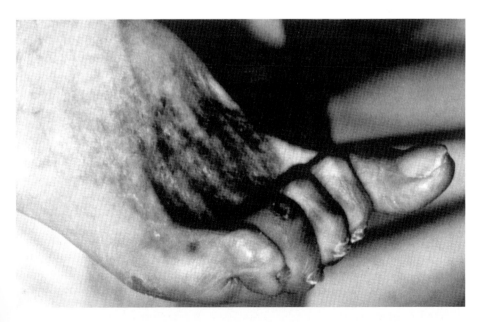

Figure 18–20 Intrinsic minus foot with claw toes and ulcer over the PIP joint of the fourth toe. Such ulcers can readily enter the joint.

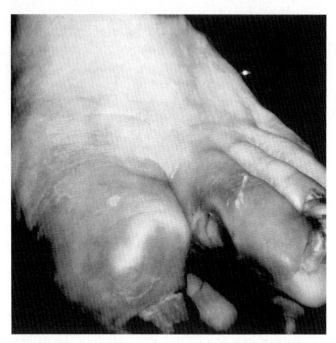

Figure 18-21   Heloma molle of the base of the second toe from pressure of the deformed adjacent interphalangeal joint of the hallux.

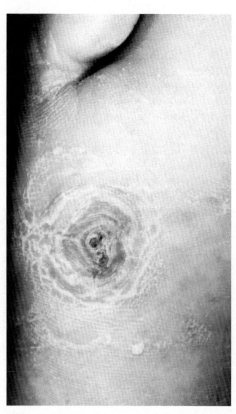

Figure 18-23   Callus of the distal part of the lateral sole. Fissuring allows the entry of bacteria.

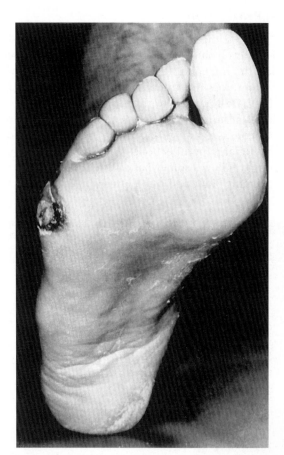

Figure 18-22   Ulcerated callus over bunionette. Amputation of the fifth ray was required because of penetration to the joint. Ulcerated bunionette is often associated with shoes that are too snug.

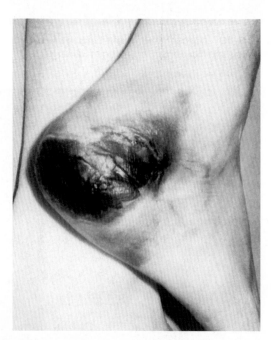

Figure 18-24   Gangrene of the heel in a bedridden diabetic patient caused by weight of the immobile neuropathic foot on the mattress.

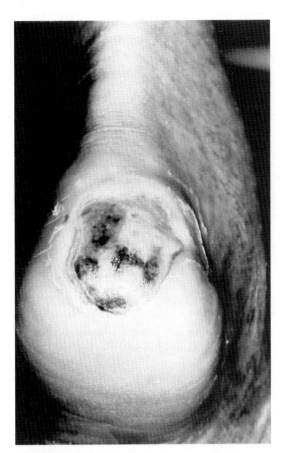

Figure 18-25 This heel ulcer began as a blister after one episode of excessive walking in a patient with severe neuropathy.

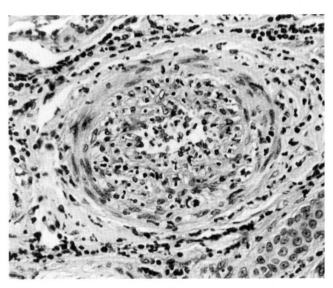

Figure 18-26 Obliteration of the lumen of a small dermal arteriole by intimal hyperplasia and septic thrombus. Note cellular evidence of inflammation in the areolar tissues near the arteriole, which was about 1 mm from the margin of dry gangrene.

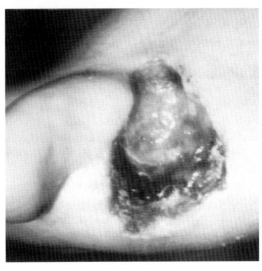

Figure 18-27 Creeping gangrene after amputation of the fifth toe. Small skin vessel thrombosis led to a patch of gangrenous skin inferior to base of toe.

predominate, both vascular lesions and neuropathy contribute to the problem.

Septic Arteritis and Tissue Necrosis

Small vessels in tissues adjoining an infected area develop thrombotic occlusion, which is partly responsible for the necrosis of tissue in these lesions and for the frequent chronicity of these infections. In tissues with otherwise normal small vessels, this process usually occurs only at the margin of the infection. After sloughing, draining, or other control of an infection, normal arterioles recanalize and form abundant granulation tissue, the first stage in wound healing. Partial recanalization of arterioles adjacent to foot ulcers can occur after healing of the ulcer.[23]

Numerous bacteria elaborate angiotoxic (necrotizing) substances. The alpha-toxin of staphylococci, for example, when injected into the skin, results in an impressive local necrotic lesion. Streptokinase and streptococcal hyaluronidase have also been implicated in the rapid extension of cellulitis by digestion of fibrin barriers and intracellular ground substance. In the mixed infections that are so common in the diabetic foot, necrotizing toxins following these spreading factors can produce a devastating lesion.

In the diseased small vessels of the diabetic patient,[16,23] the occlusive process is exaggerated, with paronychia, ingrown toenails, and minor injuries proceeding to ever enlarging areas of necrosis rather than being self-limited. As more arterioles and small arteries become occluded, infection and necrosis continue to progress (Fig. 18-26). Creeping advancement of this process of infective obliterative microangiopathy (Fig. 18-27) can occur until a plantar space, tendon sheath, or joint is reached into which bacteria will spread, augmented by continued weight-bearing.

The damage from infection arising in local lesions is greater in diabetes than in other neuropathic conditions such as paraplegia, syringomyelia, tabes dorsalis, and leprosy. This might indicate that the capillaries and arterioles of diabetic people are more likely to occlude when exposed to bacterial toxins. Many authors have taken a static view toward the role of microangiopathy in the progression of foot infections. It is apparent now that the maximum vasodilation capacity of the resistance vessels and the autoregulation of blood flow are reduced in long-term diabetic patients.[14,15,16] Consequently, when increased blood flow is needed to contain infection in the foot, it is not always readily available.

Major Foot Infections

Plantar Space Abscesses

Central plantar space abscesses, the most devastating infections in the foot, may arise in several ways. Direct penetration of the central plantar space foot by a sharp object might not be recognized in an insensitive foot until the abscess is well established and has produced swelling so pronounced that it can prevent donning shoes. Web space infections are particularly insidious because they may simply occur due to poor foot hygiene with accumulation of moist detritus or fungal infection in the interdigital webs, followed by fissuring of skin and entrance of bacteria, all without preexisting anatomic deformity. Dry skin from sympathetic neuropathy contributes to this scenario. Infections that begin in the webs are especially dangerous because of proximity to the digital arteries and to the deeper structures of the foot by way of the bursa of the lumbrical muscles, thence into the central plantar space.

Infections that begin in the nailbed, paronychium, or nail wall spread over the dorsal and lateral aspects of the toe to the dorsum of the foot by way of the lymphatics (Fig. 18-28). If the distal segment of the digit becomes necrotic, the flexor tendon sheath may be entered. After the initial break in the skin, the rate of spread of infection depends on the virulence of the pathogenic bacteria and the degree of ischemia. Indolent infections may be confined to the tissues adjacent to the nail for a long time. Relief of infections near the nails usually requires removal of a portion of the nail, which must be done cautiously to avoid further tissue damage. Infection anywhere in the toes may also spread into the central plantar space by means of suppurative tenosynovitis of the flexor tendon sheath.

Once the infection is established, the characteristic signs of central plantar space abscess appear. The longitudinal arch and the plantar skin creases disappear, and the area of the arch may bulge, the sole of the foot becoming edematous. In the diabetic patient, pain and tenderness are often absent, encouraging continued ambulation, thus adding foot dependency and the "milking" action of weight-bearing to other factors influencing spread of the infection. In a few days, dorsal edema of the foot appears. Thrombotic obliteration of small and

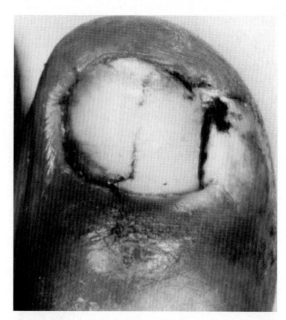

Figure 18-28   Ingrowing nail with infection and granulation tissue of the medial nail wall and cellulitis near the base of nail.

medium-sized vessels may result in progressive necrosis of the plantar fascia, tendons, and tendon sheaths. With adjacent infection, thrombotic occlusion of the plantar arch and the plantar digital arteries can follow, leading to necrosis of all or portions of the second, the fourth, and particularly the third toes. If extensive, this necrosis might prohibit salvage of the foot. The tendons lying posterior to the medial malleolus provide a route for infection to enter the lower leg, where they exit the plantar space. Central plantar space abscesses can also eventually rupture through the sole of the foot. Systemic signs of severe infection such as fever, malaise, and loss of diabetic control with ketoacidosis are usually present. Glucosuria is sometimes the first abnormality noted by the patient and may be the feature that precipitates a visit to the physician.

The medial and lateral plantar spaces contain the abductor and short flexor muscles of the first and fifth toes, respectively. In addition to direct penetrating trauma, infection may enter these spaces from infected bunions or bunionettes. These lesions frequently start with new shoes, which abrade the skin over the prominences of the first and/or fifth metatarsal heads. After ulceration through the bursa of a bunionette, infection may spread along the abductor hallucis and flexor digiti quinti brevis muscles, entering the lateral plantar space. Alternatively, an ulcer may erode the MTP joint capsule with resultant septic arthritis and osteomyelitis (Fig. 18-29). Medial and lateral plantar space abscesses seldom spread into the central plantar space.

Dorsal Cellulitis (Phlegmon) of the Foot

The extensor tendons of the toes are not encased in sheaths but lie in loose areolar tissue on the dorsum of

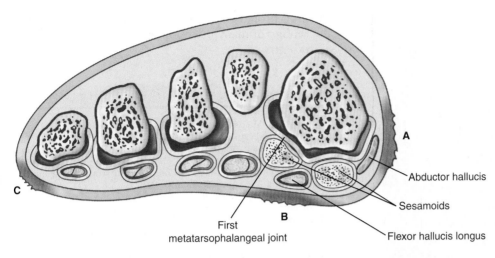

Figure 18-29   Common modes of spread of infection in the distal foot. **A,** Infection from an ulcerated bunion may enter the medial plantar space or first MTP joint fairly readily. Joint infection can then penetrate into the central plantar space. **B,** Mal perforans ulcer fixes the flexor tendons. With progression of infection, the central plantar space or joint may be entered. **C,** Ulcerated tailor's bunion finds a meager tissue barrier to entry into the fifth MTP joint.

Abductor hallucis

Sesamoids

First metatarsophalangeal joint

Flexor hallucis longus

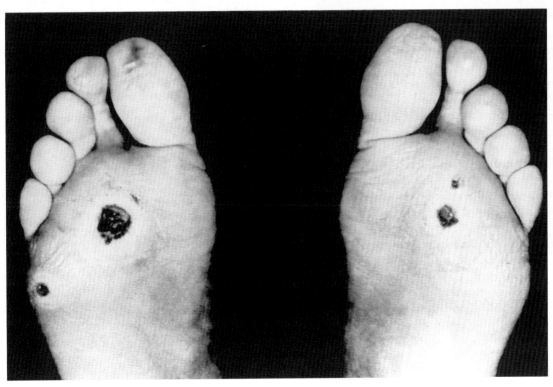

Figure 18-30   Mal perforans of both feet over the metatarsal heads.

the foot. Deep to the extensor tendons, a dense fascia overlies the interosseous muscles and metatarsal bones. The extensor tendons themselves are covered by a thin superficial fascia, which is continuous with the extensor retinaculum of the anterior ankle which serves to contain the tendons, preventing bowstringing. Spread of infection over the dorsum of the foot occurs via the lymphatics. The tissues of the dorsum first become red and edematous, the amount of pain and tenderness depending on the degree of neuropathy. Edema may be of impressive proportions in diabetic patients with neuropathy, whose lack of pain encourages limb dependency and weight-bearing. With infective occlusions of small vessels in the skin, the result is often extensive necrosis of the skin overlying the cellulitic area.

Mal Perforans

Mal perforans is a chronic, indolent ulcer of the insensitive sole, usually beneath the head of the first, second, or fifth metatarsal (Fig. 18-30). It forms by ulceration of skin beneath a preexisting callus over a bony prominence, often with limited joint mobility as a contributing factor.[12] Even after the ulcer occurs, an area of hyperkeratinization continues to surround the ulcer crater. Mal perforans is typically associated with severe neuropathy in the presence of adequate blood flow. Lateral spread of subcutaneous infection from mal perforans may be limited for a considerable time by the dense fibrous septa that partition the subcutaneous fat into lobules. Beneath a metatarsal head, where the fibers of the plantar

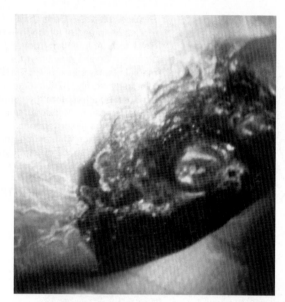

Figure 18-31   Gangrene spreading radially from mal perforans after superficial femoral artery thrombosis.

aponeurosis split and pass between the metatarsal heads, the flexor tendon may form the base of the ulcer. The tendon becomes fixed to its sheath and the underlying MTP joint capsule and periosteum. Ultimately, the tendon is eroded and the joint is entered, with subsequent septic arthritis and osteomyelitis. The referring physician often understimates the depth of penetration of the plantar ulcer. When bone is contacted by probing, specialized radiographic and radionuclide studies to identify osteomyelitis might be unnecessary. Radiographs and magnetic resonance imaging can be used to uncover clinically unsuspected osteomyelitis and tendon involvement.[24,25] Osteomyelitis and septic arthritis are most frequent in the first and fifth MTP joints. Infection can be carried via the tendon sheaths into the central plantar space. Episodes of quiescence in a mal perforans can alternate with flare-ups of infection. The arterial circulation is usually adequate; otherwise, this infection would not be contained for prolonged periods. Gangrene of the skin, spreading radially from the center of the mal perforans, can mean that occlusion of a major vessel (superficial femoral, popliteal) higher in the leg has occurred, indicating a need for angiography (Fig. 18-31).

Summary

In this chapter, normal foot anatomy has been presented as a prerequisite to understanding the structural, neurologic, and vascular changes produced in the foot over time by poorly controlled diabetes mellitus. The genesis of ulcers and infection and the well-defined anatomic paths for the spread of infection throughout the foot and into the leg have been described. Emphasis should be placed on effective clinical evaluation and surgical treatment based on a thorough grasp of these facts,

which, if properly and promptly applied, should lead to the salvage of many more lower limbs than is occurring at present.

References

1. Lewis BL: Microscopic studies of fetal and mature nail and surrounding soft tissue. Arch Dermatol Syph 70:7252, 1954.
2. Grant JCB: An Atlas of Anatomy, 6th ed. Baltimore: Williams & Wilkins, 1972.
3. Lee BY, Guerra J, Civelek B: Compartment syndrome in the diabetic foot. Adv Wound Care 8:36, 1995.
4. Spencer F, Sage R, Graner J: The incidence of foot pathology in a diabetic population. J Am Podiatr Assoc 75:590, 1985.
5. Bresäter L-E, Welin L, Romanus B: Foot pathology and risk factors for diabetic foot disease in elderly men. Diabetes Res Clin Pract 32:103, 1996.
6. van Schie CHM, Vermigli C, Carrington AL, Boulton A: Muscle weakness and foot deformity in diabetes. Diabetes Care 27:1668, 2004.
7. Anderson H, Gjerstad MD, Jakobsen J: Atrophy of foot muscles: A measure of diabetic neuropathy. Diabetes Care 27:2382, 2004.
8. Corrington AL, Shaw JE, van Schie CH, et al: Can motor nerve conduction velocity predict foot problems in diabetic subjects over a 6 year outcome period? Diabetes Care 25:2019, 2002.
9. Bus SA, Maas M, Cavanagh PR, et al: Plantar foot-pad displacement in neuropathic diabetic patients with toe deformity. Diabetes Care 27:2376, 2004.
10. Bus SA, Yang QX, Wang JH, et al: Intrinsic muscle atrophy and toe deformity in the diabetic neuropathic foot. Diabetes Care 25:1444, 2002.
11. Greenman RL, Khandhair L, Lima C, et al: Small muscle atrophy is present before the detection of clinical neuropathy. Diabetes Care 28:1425, 2005.
12. Zimny S, Schatz H, Pfohl M: The role of limited joint mobility in diabetic patients with an at-risk foot. Diabetes Care 27:942, 2004.
13. Armstrong DG, Frykberg RG: Classification of diabetic foot surgery: toward a rational definition. Diabetic Med 20:329, 2003.
14. Williams DT, Norman PE, Stacy M: Comparative roles of microvascular and nerve function in foot ulceration in type 2 diabetics. Diabetes Care 27:3026, 2004.
15. Krishnan STM, Baker NR, Carrington AL, Rayman G: Comparative roles of microvascular and nerve function in foot ulceration in type 2 diabetes. Diabetes Care 27:1343, 2004.
16. Chabbert-Buffet N, Le Devehat C, Khodabandhelou T, et al: Evidence for associated cutaneous mictoangiopathy in diabetic patients with neuropathic foot ulceration. Diabetes Care 23:960, 2003.
17. Pittenger GL, Ray M, Burrus NS, et al: Intraepithelial nerve fibers are indicators of small-fiber neuropathy in both diabetic and nondiabetic patients. Diabetes Care 27:1974, 2004.
18. Isakov E, Budoragin N, Shenhav S, et al: Anatomical sites of foot lesions resulting in amputation among diabetics and nondiabetics. Am J Phys Med Rehabil 74:130, 1995.
19. Gooding GAW, Stess RM, Graf PM, et al: Sonography of the sole of the foot: Evidence for loss of foot pad thickness in diabetes and its relationship to ulceration of the foot. Invest Radiol 21:45, 1986.
20. Bernstein RK: Physical signs of the intrinsic minus foot. Diabetes Care 26:1945, 2003.
21. Boffeli TJ, Bean JK, Natwick JR: Biomechanical abnormalities and ulcers of the great toe in patients with diabetes. J Foot Ankle Surg 41:359, 2002.
22. Murray HV, Young MJ, Hollis S, Boulton AJ: The association between callus formation, high pressures, and neuropathy in diabetic foot ulceration. Diabet Med 13:979, 1996.
23. Piaggesi A, Vicava P, Rizzo L, et al: Semiquantative analysis of the histopathological features of the neuropathic foot. Diabetes Care 26:3123, 2003.
24. Lederman HP, Morrison WB, Schweitzer ME: MRI image analysis of pedal osteomyelitis. Radiology 223:847, 2002.
25. Lederman HP, Morrison WB, Schweitzer ME, Raikin SM: Tendon involvement in pedal infection. Am J Roentg 179:939, 2002.

MEDICAL MANAGEMENT OF PATIENTS WITH DIABETES MELLITUS DURING THE PERIOPERATIVE PERIOD

JANET L. KELLY AND IRL B. HIRSCH ■

The Centers for Disease Control and Prevention estimate that there are 20.8 million people in the United States with diabetes mellitus, or 7.0% of the population.[1] While an estimated 14.6 million have been diagnosed, another 6.2 million people (or nearly one third the number with the disease) are unaware that they have diabetes. This is of special concern because they are unknowingly at risk for the microvascular and macrovascular complications of this disease.

About 60% to 70% of people with diabetes have some form of related nervous system damage. These include peripheral neuropathy with impaired sensation or pain in the feet or hands, gastroparesis with slowed digestion of food in the stomach, carpal tunnel syndrome, and other nerve problems. Among patients with diabetes, approximately 15% will develop a foot ulcer at some time in their life, and of these, 14% to 24% will subsequently require a lower-limb amputation.[2] More than 60% of all nontraumatic lower-limb amputations in the United States occur in patients with diabetes, despite their representing only 7.0% of the population.[1]

Historically, hyperglycemia has largely been ignored in the hospital setting because of fear of hypoglycemia and the belief that short-term hyperglycemia was harmless. Although the origins of the practice are unclear, routine sliding-scale insulin orders have long been a mainstay in the management of hospitalized patients. The use of these regimens is not supported by controlled clinical trials, and the practice fails to take into account interpatient variability in insulin sensitivity and the timing of blood glucose level in relation to nutritional intake. More recent data have shown that tight glycemic control is important in the hospital setting, and the use of sliding-scale insulin regimens is at odds with this goal.

Current Diagnosis

Classification of Diabetes Mellitus

In 1997, the American Diabetes Association set forth a new classification system for diabetes. The terms *insulin-dependent* and *non–insulin-dependent* were eliminated in favor of *type 1 diabetes* and *type 2 diabetes*, respectively. Type 1 diabetes is caused by autoimmune destruction of the pancreatic beta cells, resulting in an absolute insulin deficiency. Type 1 diabetes occurs most commonly in children and young adults, but its onset can occur at any age. It accounts for about 5% to 10% of the diagnosed diabetes population. If exogenous insulin is not administered to a patient with type 1 diabetes, hepatic lipolysis and ketogenesis may quickly develop into ketoacidosis.

In contrast, type 2 diabetes results from a combination of insulin resistance, a disorder in which body cells do not use insulin properly, and a relative insulin deficiency. The pancreatic beta cells initially compensate by secreting additional insulin. As insulin resistance increases, however, the pancreas gradually loses its ability to compensate, and many people with type 2 diabetes require exogenous insulin to maintain optimal glycemic control. Approximately 90% of the people with diabetes have type 2, and they frequently are not diagnosed until complications appear. Patients with type 2 diabetes rarely develop ketoacidosis: however, metabolic stresses associated with surgery and acute illness can result in a nonketotic hyperosmolar coma. The factors that are responsible for the general absence of ketoacidosis in nonketotic hyperosmolar coma are incompletely understood. One theory is that fat and glucose have differential sensitivities to insulin. Studies in humans have shown that the amount of insulin required to suppress lipolysis is one tenth the amount required to promote glucose utilization.[3]

Emerging Research/Evidence-Based Literature

Pathophysiology of Hyperglycemia

Hyperglycemia is not uncommon even in patients without diabetes in the hospital setting and has been linked to poor outcome. Capes and colleagues did a meta-analysis of 15 trials and found that hyperglycemia, defined as blood glucose greater than 110 mg/dL (6.1 mmol/L), with or without a prior diagnosis of diabetes, increased both hospital mortality and congestive heart failure in patients admitted for acute myocardial infarction.[4] Bolk and colleagues found similar results in a prospective study of 336 patients admitted for acute myocardial infarction.[5] Umpierrez and colleagues found that hyperglycemia, fasting blood glucose greater than 126 mg/dL (7.0 mmol/L), or random blood glucose greater than 200 mg/dL (11.1 mmol/L) in general medical and surgical units was associated with increased hospital mortality, a longer length of hospital stay, a greater risk of infection, and more need for subsequent nursing home care.[6] Furnary and colleagues evaluated various insulin regimens and target blood glucose levels in patients with diabetes having cardiac surgery and found that patients with hyperglycemia had greater mortality and increased incidence of deep sternal wound infections.[7,8] Further analysis of this cohort of patients revealed that hyperglycemia on the first and second postoperative days was the single most important predictor of serious infectious complications. A meta-analysis of 26 studies of stroke found increased hospital mortality in patients with admission blood glucose levels of 110 to 126 mg/dL (6.1 to 7.0 mmol/L). In addition, stroke survivors with admission blood glucose levels of 121 to 144 mg/dL (6.7 to 8 mmol/L) had poor functional recovery.[9] Patients with blood glucose levels greater than 140 mg/dL (7.8 mmol/L) had more severe strokes and greater mortality.

Although the data link hyperglycemia to poor patient outcomes, it is not clear whether good control of blood glucose improves outcomes. The first Diabetes Insulin Glucose in Acute Myocardial Infarction (DIGAMI) trial was a prospective interventional trial that found decreased mortality at 1 year in patients with diabetes admitted for acute myocardial infarction who received intensive therapy with insulin infusion followed by subcutaneous insulin for 3 or more months, compared to patients receiving conventional therapy (Fig. 19-1).[10] Follow-up at 3.4 years revealed continued benefit for intensive therapy compared to conventional therapy (mortality rate of 33% versus 44%).[11] Van den Berghe and colleagues found that intensive insulin therapy with a mean blood glucose of 103 ± 19 mg/dL reduced intensive care unit mortality as well as overall hospital mortality compared to conventional therapy with a mean blood glucose level of 153 ± 33 mg/dL in patients receiving mechanical ventilation.[12,13] Lazar and colleagues found that maintenance of blood glucose between 125 and 200 mg/dL (7.0 to 11.1 mmol/L) using glucose-insulin-potassium (GIK) infusion in patients with diabetes undergoing coronary artery bypass grafting reduced the incidence of atrial fibrillation (16.6% versus 42%) and decreased the length of hospital stay (6.5 days versus 9.2 days) compared to conventional treatment using intermittent subcutaneous insulin.[14] In addition, patients receiving GIK infusion had a survival advantage over the initial 2 years following surgery, had decreased episodes of recurrent ischemia (5% versus 19%, $p = .01$), and developed fewer recurrent wound infections (1% versus 10%, $p = .03$).

The second DIGAMI trial was designed to determine whether the mortality advantage that was seen in the first DIGAMI trial was the result of the acute GIK infusion or of the long-term insulin-based metabolic control or both.[15] It was a multicenter, prospective, randomized, open trial with blinded evaluation comparing three different metabolic control regimens. The regimens were a 24-hour GIK infusion followed by long-term subcutaneous insulin (group 1), a 24-hour GIK infusion followed by standard glucose control (group 2), and routine glucose control according to the local practice (group 3). Patients were recruited from January 1998 through May 2003. Recruitment was slow; therefore, the study closed after enrolling only 1253 patients rather than the planned 3000. Patients were followed for a median of 2.1 years, and there was no significant difference among the three treatment regimens with respect to metabolic control (fasting blood glucose or HbA1C) or mortality. Possible explanations for the lack of benefit in this study include better-than-expected blood glucose control in groups 2 and 3, poor adherence to the use of insulin in group 1 (this group did not

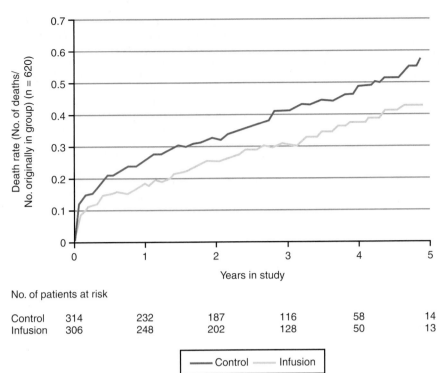

Figure 19–1 **Actuarial mortality curve for the long-term follow-up DIGAMI trial.** Actuarial mortality curves during long-term follow-up in patients receiving insulin-glucose infusion and in the control group among total DIGAMI cohort. The absolute reduction in risk was 11% relative risk 0.72 (confidence interval 0.55 to 0.92) with ***p* = .011.** *(Reprinted with permission from Malmberg K, for the DIGAMI Study Group: Prospective randomized study of intensive insulin treatment on long-term survival after acute myocardial infarction in patients with diabetes mellitus. BMJ 314:1512–1515, 1997.)*

No. of patients at risk

Control	314	232	187	116	58	14
Infusion	306	248	202	128	50	13

achieve the target glucose range of 90 to 180 mg/dL), and insufficient power due to slow patient recruitment and a lower-than-expected mortality rate. The actual 2-year mortality rate was 18.4%, which is the lowest presented long-term mortality rate in a cohort of patients with diabetes and myocardial infarction.

The mechanism by which hyperglycemia worsens clinical outcomes has not been fully elucidated. Studies have shown that hyperglycemia induces phagocyte dysfunction; impairs cardiac ischemic preconditioning with resultant increased infarct size; increases blood pressure; increases natriuretic peptide levels; prolongs the QT interval; increases thromboxane biosynthesis, causing platelet hyperactivity; increases several markers of inflammation (TNF-α, IL-6, IL-18); increases free fatty acid oxidation; and causes endothelial cell dysfunction.[16–32] Attempts to identify unifying basic mechanisms for many of the diverse effects of acute hyperglycemia point to the ability of hyperglycemia to produce oxidative stress (Fig. 19-2).[33] Acute experimental hyperglycemia, with blood glucose of 142 to 300 mg/dL (7.9 to 16.7 mmol/L), induces reactive oxygen species generation. Furthermore, acute hyperglycemia induces NF-κB, the nuclear transcription factor that regulates the inflammatory response.[34]

The data presented support the importance of preventing hyperglycemia; however, the threshold blood glucose that is associated with increased morbidity and mortality differs for each of the studies and patient populations; therefore, glycemic goals are not well established for hospitalized patients. The focus on in-hospital

glycemic control must also be mitigated by attention to the prevention of hypoglycemia. The American College of Endocrinology consensus conference on inpatient diabetes and metabolic control recommends the following glycemic targets: blood glucose less than or equal to 110 mg/dL (6.1 mmol/L) for critical care patients and preprandial blood glucose of less than or equal to 110 mg/dL (6.1 mmol/L) and maximal blood glucose levels of no greater than 180 mg/dL (10.0 mmol/L) for patients in noncritical care units.[35] The ADA supports these targets but suggests that more conservative targets might be appropriate for hospital systems that implement inpatient glucose protocols, although the ultimate goal should be to reach the original glycemic targets based on the consensus conference.[36]

Elevated blood glucose levels are caused by both (relative) insulin deficiency and insulin resistance.[37] Insulin secretion has consistently been found to be blunted with general anesthesia, and the increase in insulin resistance is presumed to be secondary to elevated counterregulatory hormone levels. The exact stress response is a function of the degree of trauma and can be modified by anesthesia. Therefore, declaring that surgery causes an increase in the principal counterregulatory hormones (glucagon, the catecholamines epinephrine and norepinephrine, growth hormone, and cortisol) is an oversimplification of a complex metabolic process. Studies to date have shown remarkable variations in the individual counterregulatory hormone response to surgery,[38,39] and this is likely the result of variations in surgical procedure, surgical technique, and type of anesthesia used.

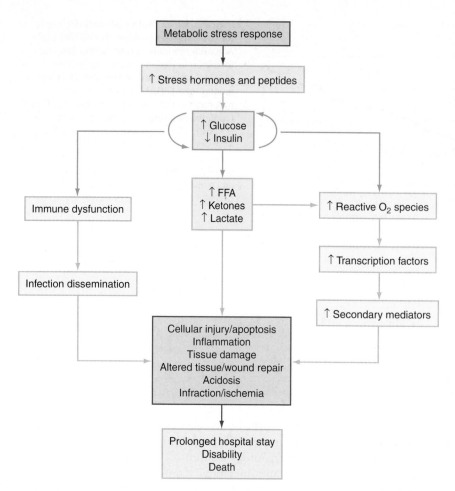

Figure 19–2   Plausible mechanism of the link between hyperglycemia and poor hospital outcome. Hyperglycemia and relative insulin deficiency caused by metabolic stress triggers immune dysfunction and release of fuel substrates and other mediators such as reactive oxygen species. Tissue and organ injury occur via the combined insults of infection, direct fuel-mediated injury, and oxidative stress and other downstream mediators. *(Reprinted with permission from Clement S, Braithwaite SS, Magee MF, et al: Management of diabetes and hyperglycemia in hospitals. Diabetes Care 27:553–591, 2004.)*

Treatment Recommendations

Preoperative Evaluation

Preoperative issues may be separated into two categories: the assessment of the acute metabolic status and the evaluation of the chronic complications of diabetes that may affect the surgical outcome. With regard to the former issue, because of the potential deleterious metabolic effects of surgery, significant preoperative hyperglycemia and electrolyte abnormalities should be corrected. Therefore, preoperative plasma glucose level and electrolyte concentrations, in addition to urinary ketone levels (patients with type 1 diabetes), should be assessed. Significant metabolic instability (e.g., ketosis, blood glucose levels greater than 400 mg/dL, hypokalemia) will require that surgery be delayed until metabolic control is improved.

The complete assessment of the various chronic complications should ideally be completed prior to admission. Cardiovascular disease is the most common cause of perioperative mortality among patients with diabetes. Patients with diabetes are two to five times as likely to report having heart disease as are their nondiabetic counterparts, and up to 80% of deaths in people with diabetes are caused by cardiovascular disease.[40,41] Although extremely common, heart disease in patients with diabetes can be difficult to diagnose because these patients frequently do not manifest classic cardiac symptoms.

The optimum preoperative cardiovascular assessment is controversial,[42–44] in part because of the high frequency of asymptomatic myocardial ischemia in this population[45] but also because of the relatively low predictive value of routine cardiovascular evaluation, especially in patients with renal disease. The updated American Heart Association guidelines on perioperative cardiac assessment of patients undergoing noncardiac surgery classifies patients with diabetes at a minimum of "intermediate cardiovascular risk" even without cardiac symptoms and "high cardiovascular risk" if they have symptoms of angina, arrhythmias, or decompensated congestive heart failure.[46,47] Cardiac evaluation for diabetic patients prior to a low-risk procedure (i.e., cataract surgery or superficial procedures) is usually not necessary. For intermediate-risk procedures (orthopedic, head and neck, intraperitoneal, and intrathoracic surgery) and high-risk procedures (peripheral vascular, aortic, and other major vascular surgery), the American Heart Association guidelines recommend a more thorough cardiac evaluation. This topic is too extensive to be covered in greater detail in this chapter, but excellent reviews are available.[42,46,47]

Preoperative evaluation also requires the assessment of diabetic nephropathy. A serum creatinine concentration is not a sufficient indicator for renal disease in patients with diabetes, because its level usually remains normal until nephropathy is advanced.[48] Nevertheless, it is now clear that some patients with type 2 diabetes may develop renal insufficiency without significant albuminuria; therefore, both serum creatinine and albuminuria should be measured yearly in all patients with type 2 diabetes.[34] Persistent albuminuria in the range of 30 to 299 mg per 24 hours (microalbuminuria) is the earliest stage of diabetic nephropathy in type 1 diabetes and continues to be a strong marker for the development of nephropathy in type 2 diabetes. Unfortunately, dipstick-positive proteinuria does not usually occur until urinary albumin excretion exceeds 250 to 300 mg per 24 hours. Therefore, the American Diabetes Association now recommends yearly assessments for microalbuminuria for all patients with diabetes.[48] The preoperative assessment of proteinuria/microalbuminuria is important for two reasons. First, any potential nephrotoxic agent should be avoided for the patient with proteinuria/microalbuminuria. Second, microalbuminuria is also a well-established marker of increased cardiovascular disease risk.[49,50]

The need for medical consultation will vary depending on the surgeon's and anesthesiologist's comfort with the various preoperative issues. To safely achieve the ACE/ADA glycemic goals in clinical practice, there must be collaboration among all medical professions caring for the patients, in the form of clinical pathways and treatment algorithms with a stepwise approach to glycemic goals, appropriate blood glucose monitoring of these patients, and open communication between the acute care and ambulatory providers.

Anesthesia and Hypoglycemia

Selection of the anesthetic modality is the prerogative of the anesthesiologist and is based on the type of surgery, the medical and surgical risks, and individual preferences without primary consideration of concomitant diabetes. Modern inhalation anesthesia has relatively little effect on metabolic regulation, while spinal, epidural, and peripheral nerve blocks produce the least disturbance in glycemic control.[37] Ankle block is preferred for most patients requiring foot surgery. The prudent use of preoperative medication, including sedation and muscle relaxants, facilitates anesthetic induction; however, any type of sedation can also impair symptomatic recognition of hypoglycemia. Fear of hypoglycemia and the altered ability of patients to self-report symptoms of hypoglycemia perioperatively have led to inadequate prescribing of insulin and inappropriate tolerance for hyperglycemia. Rapid and appropriate treatment of hypoglycemia prevents long-term sequelae; therefore, frequent blood glucose monitoring is imperative in the perioperative setting.

Treatment Modalities for Glycemic Control in the Perioperative Setting

Oral Agents

None of the oral agents used for type 2 diabetes mellitus have been studied for use during the perioperative period. There are five categories of oral agents: insulin secretagogues (sulfonylureas and meglitinides), alpha glucosidase inhibitors, biguanides, thiazolidinediones, and, most recently, the dipeptidyl peptidase-4 inhibitors. All have characteristics that limit their use for perioperative patients. In addition, they do not allow the necessary flexibility to treat patients with acutely changing needs. Of note, metformin has been associated with rare cases of lactic acidosis (fewer than 0.1 case per 1000 patient years).[51] Major risk factors for lactic acidosis with metformin include hypoperfusion states, including congestive heart failure, renal insufficiency, or hepatic insufficiency; therefore, metformin is inappropriate in the perioperative period. It should be discontinued the morning of surgery, withheld for 48 hours subsequent to any procedure anticipated to adversely affect renal function, and reinstituted only after renal function has been reevaluated and found to be normal.

Insulin

Insulin allows for the greatest flexibility and therefore is the preferred treatment modality for perioperative patients who require treatment of hyperglycemia. In addition, a growing body of literature suggests that insulin may have direct benefits that are independent of its effect on blood glucose.[52–55] To use insulin safely and effectively in hospitalized patients, it is imperative that providers have a thorough understanding of insulin physiology and the pharmacodynamics of exogenously administered insulin.

Continuous intravenous (IV) infusion of regular insulin provides the greatest flexibility for titration in perioperative patients. The onset of action is mere minutes with a pharmacodynamic half-life on the order of minutes rather than hours for subcutaneously administered insulin, which allows for rapid titration. Continuous intravenous insulin infusion is preferred in the following clinical situations: diabetic ketoacidosis or a nonketotic hyperosmolar condition; general preoperative, intraoperative, and postoperative care requiring general anesthesia; prolonged (more than 8 hours) fasting status; acute myocardial infarction; and critical illness in which insulin requirements are rapidly changing and the absorption of subcutaneous insulin may be unpredictable (Table 19-1).[33]

Several insulin infusion protocols have been validated in practice and published, and many more are in clinical use that have not been published.[10,12,56–59] Results of studies comparing different protocols are not available, and it is likely that different institutions will require different protocols based on their patient populations and staffing. Historically, insulin infusion protocols have

TABLE 19-1 Indications for Intravenous Insulin Infusion Among Nonpregnant Adults with Established Diabetes or Hyperglycemia

Indication	Strength of Evidence
Diabetic ketoacidosis and nonketotic hyperosmolar state	A
General preoperative, intraoperative, and postoperative care	C
Postoperative period following heart surgery	B
Organ transplantation	E
Myocardial infarction or cardiogenic shock	A
Stroke	E
Exacerbated hyperglycemia during high-dose glucocorticoid therapy	E
NPO status in type 1 diabetes	E
Critically ill surgical patient requiring mechanical ventilation	A
Dose-finding strategy, anticipatory to initiation or reinitiation of subcutaneous insulin therapy in type 1 or type 2 diabetes	C

Reprinted with permission from Clement S, Braithwaite SS, Magee MF, et al: Management of diabetes and hyperglycemia in hospitals. Diabetes Care 27:553–591, 2004.

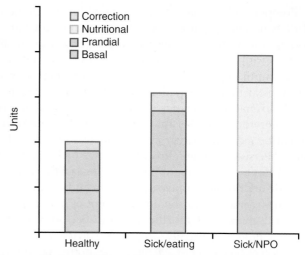

Figure 19–3 Insulin requirements in health and illness. Components of the insulin requirements are divided into basal, prandial or nutritional, and correction insulin. In writing insulin orders, the basal and prandial or nutritional insulin doses are written as programmed (scheduled) insulin, and correction-dose insulin is written as an algorithm to supplement the scheduled insulin. All components of the daily insulin requirement are increased in illness. *(Reprinted with permission from Clement S, Braithwaite SS, Magee MF, et al: Management of diabetes and hyperglycemia in hospitals. Diabetes Care 27:553–591, 2004.)*

been based solely on the patient's blood glucose, and the infusion was changed by a fixed increment for all patients.[60] An ideal insulin infusion protocol is based not only on the current blood glucose, but also on the rate of change in blood glucose and the patient's insulin sensitivity. Frequent blood glucose monitoring is necessary with insulin infusions, and most protocols recommend hourly monitoring initially until stability is achieved, after which the frequency can be reduced.

In the ambulatory setting, the daily insulin requirements can be divided into three categories: basal, prandial, and correction insulin. Perioperative patients frequently do not eat discrete meals; therefore, a better categorization is basal insulin, "nutritional insulin," and correction insulin requirements.[33] The term *basal insulin* requirement refers to the amount of exogenous insulin necessary to maintain euglycemia in the absence of nutrition. In physiologic terms, basal insulin refers to the insulin that is required to suppress hepatic glucose production overnight and between meals. The term *nutritional insulin requirement* refers to the amount of insulin that is necessary to cover intravenous dextrose, total parenteral nutrition, enteral feedings, or discrete meals. Nutritional insulin is the amount of insulin that is necessary for uptake of glucose by peripheral muscle. The correction insulin requirement refers to the additional insulin that is required as a result of insulin resistance secondary to counterregulatory hormone response to stress and/or the use of corticosteroids, vasopressor agents, and/or other medications. This classification of the various components of the daily insulin requirement is shown pictorially in Figure 19-3.

For most ambulatory patients, the daily insulin requirement is equally divided between basal and prandial insulin. In contrast, for hospitalized or perioperative

patients, the nutritional component of the daily insulin requirement may be substantially greater than the basal component. Parenterally administered glucose frequently requires more insulin than the same amount of glucose given enterally. The mechanisms underlying this observation are not clear, but there are likely gut-related, glucose-lowering peptides (such as glucagon-like peptide 1 and other incretins) as well as gut signaling that are important in pancreatic function for first-phase and total nutrient-related insulin secretion. In addition, glucocorticoids are frequently administered to perioperative patients and are well know to affect carbohydrate metabolism. They inhibit glucose uptake into muscle and, to a lesser extent, increase hepatic glucose production[60] and thus have the greatest effect on the nutritional component of the daily insulin requirement.

There are currently only three options for basal insulin therapy: NPH, glargine (Lantus[R]), or detemir (Levimer[R]). NPH has a pronounced peak, which can lead to hypoglycemia if a snack is not consumed or a meal is delayed, and insufficient duration of effect, requiring multiple daily injections. Using smaller, more frequent doses of NPH administered every 6 to 8 hours provides more consistent levels, with less of a peak effect.[61] Insulin glargine, the first long-acting insulin analogue, was approved in April 2000. Insulin glargine differs from native insulin in that the 21 amino acid residue on the A chain has been replaced by a glycine residue and two arginine residues have been added to the B chain. When injected into subcutaneous tissue, these structural alterations shift the isoelectric point making insulin glargine less soluble at physiologic pH, thus prolonging systemic absorption to approximately 24 hours in a majority of patients without a notable peak. Insulin detemir is another long-acting insulin analogue, which differs from human insulin in that the amino acid threonine in position B30 has been omitted and a C14 fatty acid chain has been attached to the amino acid B29. Insulin detemir has a fatty acid side chain that allows albumin binding, primarily resulting in association with tissue-bound albumin at the injection sites, which leads to prolongation of action and allows for once or twice daily administration without a notable peak.

The options for prandial insulin include regular insulin and the rapid-acting insulin analogues (lispro [Humalog], aspart [Novolog], and glulisine [Apidra]). The rapid-acting insulin analogues have a rapid onset of appearance of 5 to 20 minutes, attain peak blood levels in about 1 hour, and have a duration of action of 4 to 5 hours. This matches well, in contrast to regular insulin, with the absorption of glucose from low-fat meals. In addition, the rapid onset makes it possible to give the insulin immediately prior to eating. It should be noted, however, that ideally, even the rapid-acting analogues should be administered 10 to 15 minutes before eating. Even longer lag times are optimal if the patient has significant premeal hyperglycemia. In the hospital setting, optimal lag times are not always practical, and administering a rapid-acting analogue immediately before eating results in a smaller postprandial spike than occurs with regular insulin administered in a similar manner. The onset of action for regular insulin is 30 to 60 minutes, with a peak effect in 2 to 4 hours and a 6- to 8-hour duration of action. The slow onset makes it necessary to inject regular insulin 30 to 60 minutes before the meal is eaten, which is challenging for patients and health care professionals. In practice, most nurses have learned not to give insulin until the meal arrives on the nursing unit; thus, if regular insulin is used, there will be a rapid rise in blood glucose because the carbohydrate from the meal is absorbed before regular insulin starts to work. Given the prolonged duration of action of regular insulin, significant insulin is still on board from the previous mealtime injection, which results in "insulin stacking" and increases the risk of hypoglycemia. On the other hand, regular insulin may better match the absorption of carbohydrate from high-fat and high-protein meals, but typically, these are not provided in the health care setting. In addition, regular insulin may be the preferred prandial insulin in patients with gastroparesis. Patients with gastroparesis have markedly delayed absorption of food; therefore, the rapid-acting insulin analogues may cause hypoglycemia before the food is absorbed.

There are also premixed insulin preparations, which contain mixtures of prandial and basal insulin. NPH and regular insulin are available in a 70/30 mix, which contains 70% NPH and 30% regular insulin, as well as a 50/50 mix. Insulin aspart is available in a 70/30 mix with protamine insulin aspart, which is very similar to NPH in its onset, duration, and peak. Similarly, insulin lispro is available as a 75/25 and 50/50 mix with protamine insulin lispro. These premixed insulin preparations do not allow for independent titration of the prandial and basal components and therefore do not provide the flexibility of the individual components. However, they are a useful step in patients with type 2 diabetes who are reluctant to start insulin therapy.

Newer Hormone Therapies for Diabetes

Pramlintide is a stable analogue of amylin that was approved by the FDA in the spring of 2005 for adjunctive therapy in insulin-deficient patients (either type 1 or 2) not receiving adequate glycemic control despite the use of prandial insulin. Amylin is a peptide that is cosecreted with insulin by the pancreatic beta cells. Amylin slows gastric emptying without altering the overall absorption of nutrients. In addition, amylin suppresses glucagon secretion (not normalized by insulin alone), which leads to suppression of endogenous glucose output from the liver. Amylin also regulates food intake caused by centrally mediated modulation of appetite. Pramlintide increases the potential for hypoglycemia, and since its primary action is to minimize postprandial blood glucose excursions, it should be discontinued prior to surgery and restarted cautiously once the patient is able to tolerate a full diet. In addition, some clinicians prefer regular insulin over prandial insulin in patients receiving pramlintide, because pramlintide delays the absorption of carbohydrates. The rapid-acting analogues are preferred in the majority of patients for nutritional coverage and correction of hyperglycemia, however, during the perioperative period when pramlintide is held. Given the complexity of titrating insulin and pramlintide and the high risk of postprandial hypoglycemia with pramlintide in the surgical patient who is transitioning from a fasting status back to food, we recommend not restarting pramlintide until the patient is tolerating a full regular diet.

Exenatide is a synthetic glucagon-like peptide 1 (GLP-1) analogue that was approved in the spring of 2005 for use in patients with type 2 diabetes not adequately controlled with oral agents. GLP-1 is an enteric hormone secreted by the intestine in response to nutrient ingestion. Exenatide enhances glucose-dependent insulin secretion by pancreatic beta cells, suppresses inappropriately elevated glucagon secretion, and slows gastric emptying. In addition, animal models suggest that exenatide might promote neogenesis and proliferation of pancreatic beta cells and improve insulin resistance. Exenatide is given subcutaneously twice daily (breakfast and dinner) to minimize postprandial glucose excursions and therefore is not indicated in patients who will be fasting for a surgical procedure. Exenatide should be discontinued prior to surgery and reinitiated only after the patient is able to tolerate a full diet.

Perioperative Treatment for Patients with Type 1 Diabetes (Fig. 19-4)

There is general agreement that patients with type 1 diabetes receiving general anesthesia should receive their insulin as a continuous intravenous infusion.[33] For elective procedures, the basal insulin should be given at 80% to 100% of the usual dose the evening before surgery, with an insulin infusion initiated the morning of surgery. Even with normal basal insulin the night before, low-dose IV insulin will be required, and it is usually begun when the blood glucose level rises above 130 mg/dL. For shorter procedures, some institutions do not use IV infusions. In fact, if anesthesia will be required for just 1 to 2 hours, some authors recommend small doses of subcutaneous correction-dose insulin with a rapid-acting analogue, although this practice has never undergone a clinical trial. Usually, basal insulin should make up 40% to 50% of the total daily insulin dose. For safety reasons, we recommend using 80% of the usual basal insulin dose when the patient is taking more than half of his or her total daily insulin in the form of basal insulin. This suggests that the basal insulin is also being used to cover food, and therefore, a reduction in dose is necessary in a patient who will not be eating. Basal insulin should not be withheld the evening before surgery, as to do so would result in ketosis in patients with type 1 diabetes. Sufficient glucose is also required during the perioperative period for basal energy requirements and for the prevention of hypoglycemia. There are no data regarding the optimum quantity of glucose to be administered; however, most authors give 5 to 10 grams of glucose per hour.[37] Urine ketone levels should be routinely measured in type 1 patients who are fasting over 24 hours to identify starvation ketosis and the need for increased glucose and insulin administration. Some studies support the use of GIK infusions; however, in clinical practice, it is difficult to achieve optimal glycemic control with GIK infusions; therefore, we recommend using separate infusions for the glucose and insulin.

Recommendations for the perioperative management of the patient with type 1 diabetes receiving local anesthesia is less clear. While an intravenous insulin infusion would work, it complicates discharge in that it requires transition back to subcutaneous insulin, and it probably is not necessary. We recommend continuing the basal insulin regimen (glargine, detemir, or NPH insulin) and administering a rapid-acting analogue (lispro, aspart, or glulisine insulin) to correct stress hyperglycemia should it occur. Although formal studies have not been done, the rapid-acting insulin analogues are preferred for correction insulin because of their rapid onset and short duration of action. At our institution, we have developed standardized correction algorithms using lispro or aspart

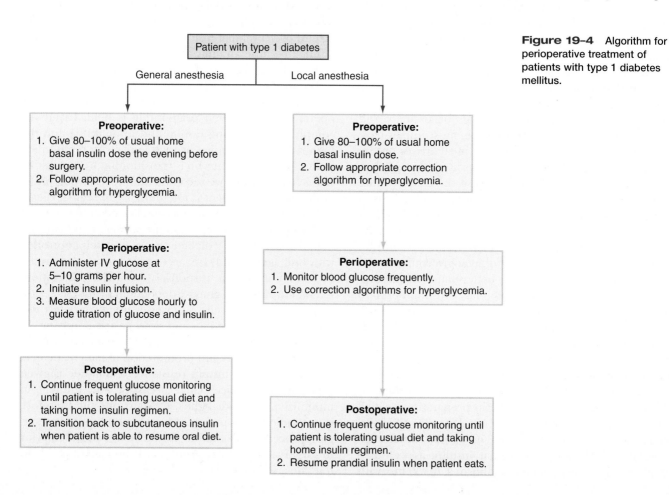

Figure 19–4 Algorithm for perioperative treatment of patients with type 1 diabetes mellitus.

Premeal algorithm for hyperglycemia: To be administered <u>in addition</u> to the scheduled insulin dose to correct premeal hyperglycemia
        ☐ Lispro (Humalog)
        ☐ Aspart (Novolog)
(Must specify algorithm below)

☐ LOW DOSE ALGORITHM
(For patients requiring less than 40 units of insulin/day)

Premeal BG	Additional Insulin
150–199	1 unit
200–249	2 units
250–299	3 units
300–349	4 units
>349	5 units

☐ MEDIUM DOSE ALGORITHM
(For patients requiring 40 to 80 units of insulin/day)

Premeal BG	Additional Insulin
150–199	1 unit
200–249	3 units
250–299	5 units
300–349	7 units
>349	8 units

☐ HIGH DOSE ALGORITHM
(For patients requiring more than 80 units of insulin/day)

Premeal BG	Additional Insulin
150–199	2 unit
200–249	4 units
250–299	7 units
300–349	10 units
>349	12 units

☐ INDIVIDUALIZED ALGORITHM

Premeal BG	Additional Insulin
150–199	
200–249	
250–299	
300–349	
>349	

Figure 19–5   Standardized correction algorithms using rapid-acting insulin analogues.   *(Adapted with permission from Trence DL, Kelly JL, Hirsch IB: The rationale and management of hyperglycemia for in-patients with cardiovascular disease: Time for change. J Clin Endocrinol Metab 88(6):2430–2437, 2003.)*

and the 1800 rule (Fig. 19-5).[62] Blood glucose should be monitored every hour during and immediately after discharge.

Perioperative Treatment of Patients with Type 2 Diabetes

Patients with type 2 diabetes make up the majority of individuals requiring lower-limb surgery. However, many patients with type 2 diabetes require insulin for optimal glycemic control and therefore can be managed perioperatively like patients with type 1 diabetes. Being similar to type 1 patients, these patients should receive a continuous insulin infusion for procedures requiring general anesthesia (Fig. 19-6) and can receive basal subcutaneous insulin (NPH, glargine, or detemir) for procedures with local anesthesia (Fig. 19-7). We have found that a greater number of patients with type 2 diabetes receive excessive basal insulin; therefore, we recommend giving only 60% to 80% of the usual dose the evening before surgery. Patients who are well controlled at home with diet alone require only hourly blood glucose monitoring during surgery; however, should blood glucose exceed 150 to 180 mg/dL, an intravenous insulin infusion should be implemented promptly. Fasting blood glucose levels exceeding 200 mg/dL indicate an absolute insulin deficiency,[63] while blood glucose levels exceeding 180 mg/dL

exceed the renal threshold and result in glucose spilling in the urine. It is not uncommon for previously well controlled patients to require insulin infusion therapy due to a hyperglycemic response to surgery. In addition, infection requiring lower-limb surgery contributes to insulin resistance and increases the propensity to insulin infusion therapy.

There is some disagreement regarding the management strategies for patients requiring general anesthesia whose diabetes is well controlled with oral agents. We agree with Alberti[64] and recommend withholding all oral therapies for diabetes the morning of surgery. An insulin infusion should be initiated if the blood glucose level rises above 130 to180 mg/dL. The threshold for initiating an insulin infusion is controversial in patients who are receiving oral therapy for their diabetes prior to surgery. Adherence to the ACE/ADA glycemic goals for hospitalized patients suggests implementing it at lower blood glucose levels, but this must also be balanced with the duration of the procedure and the likelihood that the patient will soon be able to resume a normal diet and oral therapy. The benefit of a few hours of improved glycemic control with an insulin infusion is unclear if the patient was well controlled previously and will be able to resume previous oral therapy within a matter of hours. However, if the patient was poorly controlled preoperatively and will likely require insulin postoperatively, the

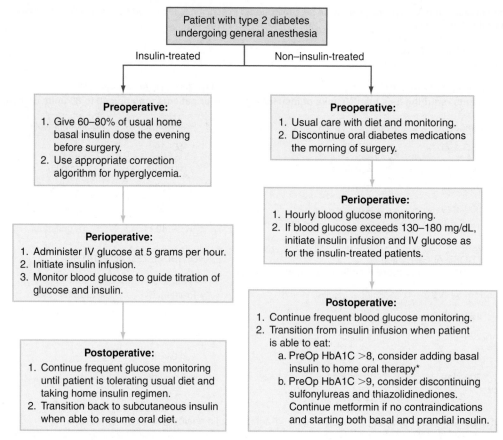

Figure 19-6   Algorithm for perioperative treatment of patients with type 2 diabetes mellitus receiving general anesthesia. *Following any procedure that alters renal function, metformin should be held for 48 hours and restarted only after normal renal function is confirmed.

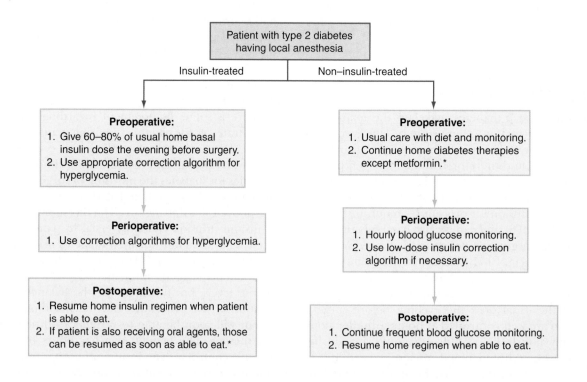

Figure 19-7   Algorithm for perioperative treatment of patients with type 2 diabetes mellitus receiving local anesthesia. *Following any procedure that alters renal function, metformin should be held for 48 hours and restarted only after normal renal function is confirmed.

use of an insulin infusion will provide useful information regarding the patient's insulin requirements, which makes transitioning to subcutaneous insulin easier.

Postoperative Management

The ideal time to transition from IV insulin to subcutaneous insulin depends on several factors: the presence of postoperative nausea and vomiting, a planned subcutaneous regimen, the meal schedule, and discharge considerations. In practice, the transition from IV to subcutaneous insulin is anything but ideal and requires clinical judgment, close monitoring, and dose titration. Recommendations and guidelines for this transition are detailed in Figure 19-8. We assumed that perioperative patients received little nutritional therapy (5 to 10 grams of glucose per hour) while receiving an insulin infusion; therefore, the estimated daily insulin requirement is really that for basal insulin.

For patients receiving an insulin infusion who were previously well controlled on oral agents, it is easiest to revert to their oral therapy in the morning with breakfast. The oral medication can be administered and 1 hour later the insulin infusion can be discontinued. Of note, metformin should not be restarted until 48 hours after the procedure and not until normal renal function has been confirmed. Alternatively, if the goal is to discharge the patient the same day, the insulin infusion can be discontinued postoperatively. However, patients must be instructed to check blood glucose at home every 2 hours until they are able to eat a full diet and have restarted their oral medications. These patients will also need to know whom to call and what to do should their blood glucose level exceed the established threshold.

For patients receiving an insulin infusion who are not well controlled on oral agents prior to admission or who are requiring more than two to three units of insulin per hour, we recommend a transition to subcutaneous insulin postoperatively. The total daily insulin requirement can be estimated by taking the infusion rate for the preceeding 4 to 8 hours and extrapolating this dose to a 24-hour amount. This should be reduced empirically by 40% to address the acute stress of surgery and thus avoid hypoglycemia. If the plan is to use a long-acting analogue for basal insulin and a rapid-acting analogue for meals, half of the total insulin requirement can be given as the long-acting analogue, the remaining half being divided and given as a rapid-acting analogue prior to each meal. Alternatively, NPH and regular insulin can be used in patients with type 2 diabetes who are reluctant to give themselves four daily injections and in whom the need for insulin therapy is anticipated to be for only a matter of a few weeks postoperatively. This sort of regimen should be viewed as temporary and is not appropriate for long-term use in type 2 diabetes or ever in type 1 diabetes. Using NPH and regular insulin, two thirds of the total daily insulin requirement is given in the morning, one third as regular and two thirds as NPH. The remaining one third is given at dinner, equally divided between regular and NPH insulin.

Postoperatively, patients who have received a local anesthetic and will be discharged the same day can resume prandial insulin with their next meal. Patients who are treated with oral agents can resume their oral agent the following day, with the exception of metformin as described previously. With the increasing emphasis on outpatient surgeries, it is imperative that patients with diabetes be instructed how to manage their diabetes postoperatively. Blood glucose monitoring should be done frequently, with hourly monitoring for the first few hours. Patients with type 1 diabetes should have the ability to measure urinary ketone levels at home, and any diabetic patient with nausea and vomiting should be screened for urinary ketones. In addition, patients who are treated with insulin should be given a correction algorithm to use for hyperglycemia. All patients should be given specific instructions about when and how to contact their providers.

Summary

Lower-limb surgery is a common occurrence for patients with diabetes, and there is now a wide body of evidence that hyperglycemia is linked to poor surgical outcome. Furthermore, large well-designed clinical trials have shown that improving glycemic control improves outcomes. Thus, the challenge to surgeons and other health care providers today is to facilitate improvement of glycemic control for our patients. First and foremost, we can no longer ignore hyperglycemia in the perioperative period.

Insulin misadministration accounts for up to 11% of medication errors in the hospital setting;[65] therefore, insulin has been identified as one of several high-alert medications.[66] How can we improve blood glucose control of our hospitalized patients and minimize insulin-related medication errors? Outcomes using standardized insulin treatment pathways and dose titration protocols are superior to those achieved with individualization of care.[66] A multidisciplinary team approach is needed to establish safe and effective diabetes care pathways for perioperative patients. The key to success is having a "champion" of each discipline available for questions about all aspects of diabetes care. Furthermore, when system-wide changes are being implemented, it is important to move slowly but persistently by setting reasonable and obtainable goals at each step.

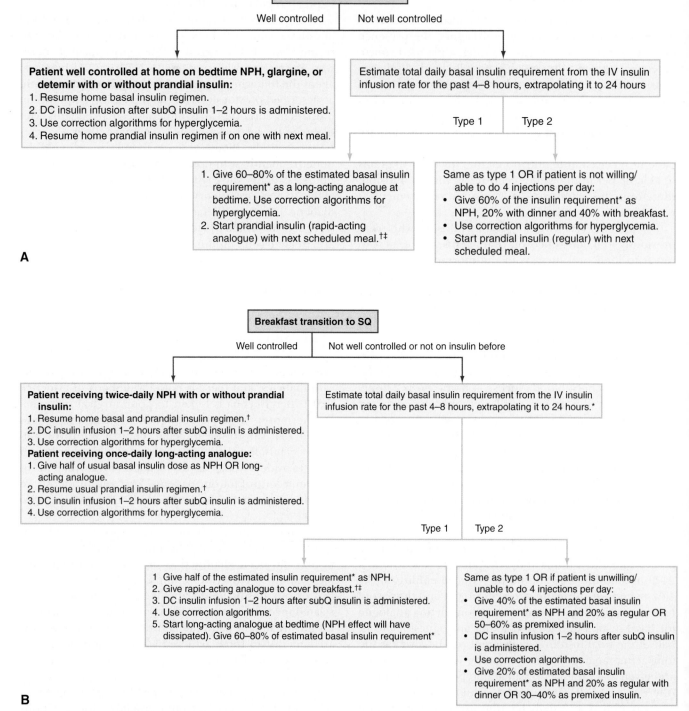

Figure 19–8 Transitioning from IV insulin infusion to subcutaneous insulin. *Assumes the patient was receiving little or no nutritional therapy while on the insulin infusion. †Adjust prandial doses down if patient is not able to tolerate a full diet. Withhold if patient refuses food. ‡Most patients will require about equal amounts of basal and prandial insulin once they are eating a full diet. The prandial insulin requirements should be divided among the number of meals a patient eats per day.

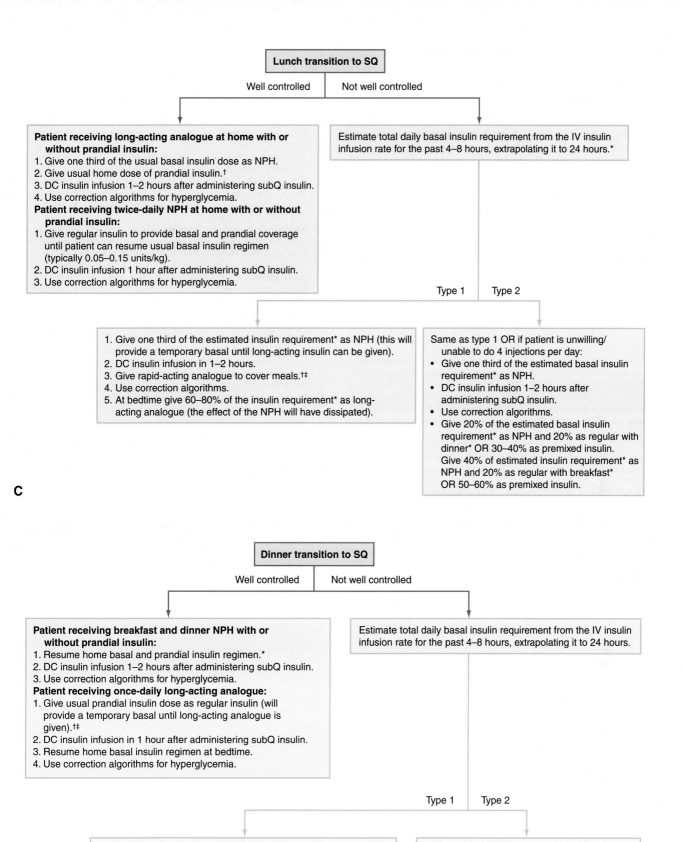

C

Lunch transition to SQ

Well controlled | Not well controlled

Patient receiving long-acting analogue at home with or without prandial insulin:
1. Give one third of the usual basal insulin dose as NPH.
2. Give usual home dose of prandial insulin.†
3. DC insulin infusion 1–2 hours after administering subQ insulin.
4. Use correction algorithms for hyperglycemia.

Patient receiving twice-daily NPH at home with or without prandial insulin:
1. Give regular insulin to provide basal and prandial coverage until patient can resume usual basal insulin regimen (typically 0.05–0.15 units/kg).
2. DC insulin infusion 1 hour after administering subQ insulin.
3. Use correction algorithms for hyperglycemia.

Estimate total daily basal insulin requirement from the IV insulin infusion rate for the past 4–8 hours, extrapolating it to 24 hours.*

Type 1 | Type 2

1. Give one third of the estimated insulin requirement* as NPH (this will provide a temporary basal until long-acting insulin can be given).
2. DC insulin infusion in 1–2 hours.
3. Give rapid-acting analogue to cover meals.†‡
4. Use correction algorithms.
5. At bedtime give 60–80% of the insulin requirement* as long-acting analogue (the effect of the NPH will have dissipated).

Same as type 1 OR if patient is unwilling/unable to do 4 injections per day:
• Give one third of the estimated basal insulin requirement* as NPH.
• DC insulin infusion 1–2 hours after administering subQ insulin.
• Use correction algorithms.
• Give 20% of the estimated basal insulin requirement* as NPH and 20% as regular with dinner* OR 30–40% as premixed insulin. Give 40% of estimated insulin requirement* as NPH and 20% as regular with breakfast* OR 50–60% as premixed insulin.

D

Dinner transition to SQ

Well controlled | Not well controlled

Patient receiving breakfast and dinner NPH with or without prandial insulin:
1. Resume home basal and prandial insulin regimen.*
2. DC insulin infusion 1–2 hours after administering subQ insulin.
3. Use correction algorithms for hyperglycemia.

Patient receiving once-daily long-acting analogue:
1. Give usual prandial insulin dose as regular insulin (will provide a temporary basal until long-acting analogue is given).†‡
2. DC insulin infusion in 1 hour after administering subQ insulin.
3. Resume home basal insulin regimen at bedtime.
4. Use correction algorithms for hyperglycemia.

Estimate total daily basal insulin requirement from the IV insulin infusion rate for the past 4–8 hours, extrapolating it to 24 hours.

Type 1 | Type 2

1. Give 20% of the estimated basal insulin requirement* as regular (this provides a temporary basal and covers the meal).
2. DC insulin infusion 1 hour after administering subQ insulin.
3. Use correction algorithms.
4. At bedtime give 60–80% of the estimated insulin requirement* as long-acting analogue (the effect from regular will have dissipated).
5. The next day start rapid-acting analogues for prandial coverage.†‡

Same as type 1 OR if patient is unwilling/unable to do 4 injections per day:
• Give 20% of the estimated insulin requirement as NPH and 20% as regular.† OR 30–40% as premixed insulin.
• DC insulin infusion 1 hour after administering subQ insulin.
• Use correction algorithms.
• The next morning give 40% of the estimated insulin requirement* as NPH and 20% as regular† OR 50–60% as premixed insulin.

Figure 19–8, cont'd

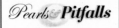

> ● Hypoglycemia is the primary complication of improved glycemic control. Appropriate patient monitoring, staff education, and standardized treatment pathways are important to minimize the incidence and impact of hypoglycemia.
> ● The keys to successful glycemic control in the perioperative period include:
>   ◆ Setting small achievable goals and building on your successes
>   ◆ Multidisciplinary team approach
>   ◆ Champions from each discipline

References

1. Centers for Disease Control: www.cds.gove/diabetes/pubs/pdf/ndfs_2005.pdf.
2. American Diabetes Association: Consensus development conference on diabetic foot wound care: Boston, Massachusetts 7–8 April 1999. Diabetes Care 22(8):1354–1360, 1999.
3. Zierler, KL, Rabinowitz, D: Effect of very small concentrations of insulin on forearm metabolism: Persistence of its action on potassium and free fatty acids without its effect on glucose. J Clin Invest 43:950, 1964.
4. Capes S, Hunt D, Malmberg K, et al: Stress hyperglycemia and increased risk of death after myocardial infarction in patients with and without diabetes: A systematic overview. Lancet 355:773–778, 2000.
5. Bolk J, van der Ploeg T, Cornel JH, et al: Impaired glucose metabolism predicts mortality after a myocardial infarction. Int J Cardiol 79:201–214, 2001.
6. Umpierrez GE, Isaacs SD, Bazargan N, et al: Hyperglycemia: An independent marker of inhospital mortality in patients with undiagnosed diabetes. J Clin Endocrinol Metab 87:978–982, 2002.
7. Furnary A, Zerr K, Grunkemeier G, et al: Continuous intravenous insulin infusion reduces the incidence of deep sternal wound infection in diabetic patients after cardiac surgical procedures. Ann Thorac Surg 67:352–362, 1999.
8. Furnary AP, Gao G, Grunkemeier GL, et al: Continuous insulin infusion reduces mortality in patients with diabetes undergoing coronary artery bypass grafting. J Thorac Cardiovasc Surg 125:1007–1021, 2003.
9. Capes S, Hunt D, Malmberg K, et al: Stress hyperglycemia and prognosis of stroke in nondiabetic and diabetic patients: A systematic overview. Stroke 32:2426–2432, 2001.
10. Malmberg K, Ryden L, Efendic S, et al: Randomized trial of insulin-glucose infusion followed by subcutaneous insulin treatment in diabetic patients with acute myocardial infarction (DIGAMI study): Effects on mortality at 1 year. J Am Coll Cardiol 26:57–65, 1995.
11. Malmberg K, for the DIGAMI Study Group: Prospective randomized study of intensive insulin treatment on long-term survival after acute myocardial infarction in patients with diabetes mellitus. BMJ 314:1512–1515, 1997.
12. Van den Berghe G, Wouters P, Weekers F, et al: Intensive insulin therapy in critically ill patients. N Engl J Med 345:1359–1367, 2001.
13. Van den Berghe G, Wouters PJ, Bouillon R, et al: Outcome benefit of intensive insulin therapy in the critically ill: Insulin dose versus glycemic control. Crit Care Med 31:359–366, 2003.
14. Lazar HL, Chipkin SR, Fitzgerald CA, et al: Tight glycemic control in diabetic coronary artery bypass graft patients improves perioperative outcomes and decreases recurrent ischemic events. Circulation 109:1497–1502, 2004.
15. Malmberg K, Ryden L, Wedel H, et al: Intense metabolic control by means of insulin in patients with diabetes mellitus and acute myocardial infarction (DIGAMI 2): Effects on mortality and morbidity. Eur Heart J 26:650–661, 2005.
16. Kersten J, Schmeling, T, Orth K, et al: Acute hyperglycemia abolishes ischemic preconditioning in vivo. Am J Physiol 275:H721–H725, 1998.
17. Marfella R, Nappo F, Angelis LD, et al: The effect of acute hyperglycaemia on QTc duration in healthy man. Diabetologia 43:571–575, 2000.
18. Cinar Y, Senyol A, Duman K: Blood viscosity and blood pressure: Role of temperature and hyperglycemia. Am J Hypertens 14:433–438, 2001.
19. McKenna K, Smith D, Tormey W, et al: Acute hyperglycaemia causes elevation in plasma atrial natriuretic peptide concentration in type 1 diabetes mellitus. Diabet Med 17:512–517, 2000.
20. Davi G, Catalano I, Averna M, et al: Thromboxane biosynthesis and platelet function in type II diabetes mellitus. N Engl J Med 322:1769–1774, 1990.
21. Knobler H, Savion N, Shenkman B, et al: Shear-induced platelet adhesion and aggregation on subendothelium are increase in diabetic patients. Thromb Res 90:181–190, 1998.
22. Davi G, Ciabattoni G, Consoli A, et al: In vivo formation of 8-iso-prostaglandin f2 alpha and platelet activation in diabetes mellitus: Effects of improved metabolic control and vitamin E supplementation. Circulation 99:224–229, 1999.
23. Sakamoto T, Ogawa H, Kawano H, et al: Rapid change of platelet aggregability in acute hyperglycemia: Detection by a novel laser-light scattering method. Thromb Haemost 83:475–479, 2000.
24. Gresele P, Guglielmini G, DeAngelis M, et al: Acute, short-term hyperglycemia enhances shear stress-induced platelet activation in patients with type II diabetes mellitus. J Am Coll Cardiol 41:1013–1020, 2003.
25. Morohoshi M, Fujisawa K, Uchimura I, et al: Glucose-dependent interleukin 6 and tumor necrosis factor production by human peripheral blood monocytes in vitro. Diabetes 45:954–959, 1996.
26. Esposito K, Nappo F, Marfella R, et al: Inflammatory cytokine concentrations are acutely increase by hyperglycemia in humans: Role of oxidative stress. Circulation 106:2067–2072, 2002.
27. Williams S, Goldfine A, Timimi F, et al: Acute hyperglycemia attenuates endothelium dependent vasodilation in humans in vivo. Circulation 97:1695–1701, 1998.
28. Kawano H, Motoyama T, Hirashima O, et al: Hyperglycemia rapidly suppresses flow mediated endothelium-dependent vasodilation of brachial artery. J Am Coll Cardiol 34:146–154, 1999.
29. Shige H, Ishikawa T, Suzukawa M, et al: Endothelium-dependent flow mediated vasodilation in the postprandial state in type 2 diabetes mellitus. Am J Cardiol 84:1272–1274, 1999.
30. Title LM, Cummings PM, Giddens K, et al: Oral glucose loading acutely attenuates endothelium-dependent vasodilation in healthy adults without diabetes: An effect prevented by vitamins C and E. J Am Coll Cardiol 36:2185–2191, 2000.
31. Beckman J, Goldfine A, Gordon M, et al: Ascorbate restores endothelium-dependent vasodilation impaired by acute hyperglycemia in humans. Circulation 103:1618–1623, 2001.
32. Giugliano D, Marfella R, Coppola L, et al: Vascular effects of acute hyperglycemia in humans are reversed by L-arginine: Evidence for reduced availability of nitric oxide during hyperglycemia. Circulation 95:1783–1790, 1997.
33. Clement S, Braithwaite SS, Magee MM, et al: Management of diabetes and hyperglycemia in hospitals. Diabetes Care 27:553–591, 2004.
34. Schiekofer S, Andrassy M, Chen J, et al: Acute hyperglycemia causes intracellular formation of CML and activation of ras, p42/44 MAPK, and nuclear factor kappaB in PBMCs. Diabetes 52:621–633, 2003.
35. www.aace.com/pub/ICC/inpatientStatement.php.
36. American Diabetes Association Position Statement: Standards of medical care in diabetes: 2006. Diabetes Care 29:S4–S42, 2006.
37. Hirsch IB, McGill JB, Cryer PE, et al: Perioperative management of surgical patients with diabetes mellitus. Anesthesiology 74:346–359, 1991.
38. Monk TG, Mueller M, White PF: Treatment of stress response during balanced anesthesia. Anesthesiology 76:39–45, 1992.
39. Domalik LJ, Feldman JM: Carbohydrate metabolism and surgery. In Bergman M, Sicard GA (eds): Surgical Management of the Diabetic Patient. New York: Raven Press, 1991.
40. Wingard DL, Barrett-Connor E: Heart Disease and Diabetes, Diabetes in America, 2nd ed. Bethesda, MD: National Institutes of Health, 1995.
41. Coursin DB, Connery LE, Ketzler JT: Perioperative diabetic and hyperglycemic management issues. Crit Car Med 32(suppl):S116–S125, 2004.

42. Eagle KA, Brundage BH, Chaitman BR, et al: Guidelines for perioperative cardiovascular evaluation for noncardiac surgery: Report of the American College of Cardiology/American Heart Association Task Force on Practice Guidelines (Committee on Perioperative Cardiovascular Evaluation for Noncardiac Surgery). J Am Coll Cardiol 27:910–948, 1996.

43. Freeman WK, Gibbons RJ, Shub C: Preoperative assessment of the cardiac patients undergoing non-cardiac surgical procedures. Mayo Clin Proc 64:1105–1117, 1989.

44. Heller GV: Evaluation of the patient with diabetes mellitus and suspected coronary artery disease. Am J Med 118(suppl 2):9S-14S, 2005.

45. Deluca AJ, Saulle LN, Aronow WS, et al: Prevalence of silent myocardial ischemia in persons with diabetes mellitus or impaired glucose tolerance and association of hemoglobin A1c with prevalence of silent myocardial ischemia. Am J Cardiol 95(12):1472–1474, 2005.

46. Eagle KA, Berger PB, Calkins H, et al: ACC/AHA Guideline Update for Perioperative Cardiovascular Evaluation for Noncardiac Surgery: Executive Summary. A report of the American College of Cardiology/American Heart Association Task Force on Practice Guidelines (Committee to Update the 1996 Guidelines on Perioperative Cardiovascular Evaluation for Noncardiac Surgery). Anesth Analg 94:1052–1064, 2002.

47. Mandoline C, Tornini A, Borgia MC: About cardiovascular risk in non-cardiac surgery. Ann Ital Med Int 19(4):262–268, 2004.

48. American Diabetes Association Position Statement: Standards of medical care in diabetes. Diabetes Care 28(suppl 1):S4–S36, 2005.

49. Garg JP, Bakris GL: Microalbuminuria: Marker of vascular dysfunction, risk factor for cadiovascular disease. Vasc Med 7:35–43, 2002.

50. Klausen K, Borch-Johnson K, Feldt-Rasmussen B, et al: Very low levels of microalbuminuria are associated with increased risk of coronary heart disease and death independently of renal function, hypertension and diabetes. Circulation 110:32–35, 2004.

51. Salpeter S, Greyber E, Pasternak G, et al: Metformin dose not increase fatal or nonfatal lactic acidosis or blood lactate levels in type 2 diabetes mellitus. Cochrane Database Syst Rev 2:CD002967, 2002.

52. Dandona P, Aljada A, Mohanty P. The anti-inflammatory and potential anti-atherogenic effect of insulin: A new paradigm. Diabetologia 45:924–930, 2002.

53. Dandona P, Aljada A, Bandyopadhyay A: The potential therapeutic role of insulin in acute myocardial infarction in patients admitted to intensive care and those with unspecified hyperglycemia. Diabetes Care 26:516–519, 2003.

54. Melidonis A, Stefanidis A, Tournis S, et al: The role of strict metabolic control by insulin infusion on fibrinolytic profile during an acute coronary event in diabetic patients. Clin Cardiol 23:160–164, 2000.

55. Das UN: Is insulin an endogenous cardioprotector? Crit Care 6:389–393, 2002.

56. Goldberg PA, Siegel MD, Sherwin RS, et al: Implementation of a safe and effective insulin infusion protocol in a medical intensive care unit. Diabetes Care 27:461–467, 2004.

57. Ku SY, Sayre CA, Hirsch IB, et al: New insulin infusion protocol improves blood glucose control in hospitalized patients without increasing hypolycemia. Jt Comm J Qual Saf 31:141–147, 2005.

58. Markovitz LJ, Wiechmann RJ, Harris N, et al: Description and evaluation of a glycemic management protocol for patients with diabetes undergoing heart surgery. Endocr Pract 8:10–18, 2002.

59. Krinsley JS: Effect of an intensive glucose management protocol on the mortality of critically ill adult patients. Mayo Clin Proc 79:992–1000, 2004.

60. Hirsch, IB, Paauw DS, Brunzell J. Inpatient management of adults with diabetes. Diabetes Care 18:870–878, 1995.

61. Lalli C, Ciofetta M, Del Sindaco P, et al: Long-term intensive treatment of type 1 diabetes with the short-acting insulin analogue lispro in variable combination with NPH insulin at mealtime. Diabetes Care 22:468–477, 1999.

62. Trence DL, Kelly JL, Hirsch IB: The rationale and management of hyperglycemia for in-patients with cardiovascular disease: Time for change. J Clin Endocrinol Metab 88(6):2430–2437, 2003.

63. Defronzo RA, Ferrannini E, Kovisto V: New concepts in the pathogenesis and treatment of non-insulin-dependent diabetes mellitus. Am J Med 74:52–81,1983.

64. Alberti KGMM: Diabetes and surgery [editorial]. Anesthesiology 74:209–211, 1991.

65. Cohen MR, Proulx SM, Crawford SY: Survey of hospital systems and common serious medication errors. J Health Risk Manage 18:16–27, 1998.

66. Cohen MR: Medication Errors. Washington, DC: Institute for Safe Medication Practices, American Pharmaceutical Association, 1999.

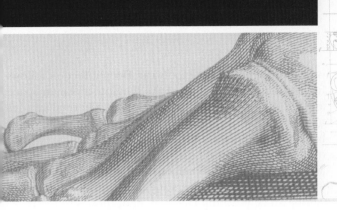

20

MINOR AND MAJOR LOWER-LIMB AMPUTATIONS AND DISARTICULATIONS IN PATIENTS WITH DIABETES MELLITUS

JOHN H. BOWKER ■

Any surgeon who is consulted regarding disorders of the foot and ankle in diabetic patients will inevitably need to perform an amputation of part or all of the foot. Most often, this situation arises emergently as a result of infection with or without ischemia and occasionally as a failure of nonsurgical or surgical treatment of Charcot neuroarthropathy. The real challenge to the surgeon is to regard an amputation or disarticulation as a reconstructive procedure on a par with any other limb reconstruction such as hip replacement, not to be treated offhandedly as a failure of salvage attempts. This latter attitude is exemplified by assigning the case to the most junior surgical trainee without adequate intraoperative supervision, often resulting in a poorly fashioned residual limb. Conversely, modern amputation techniques should result in the creation of a modified locomotor end-organ that will interface comfortably with a prosthesis, orthosis, or modified footwear, fulfilling the goal of amputation as the first step in restoring the diabetic's quality of life to an acceptable level. Descriptions of commonly utilized procedures are given, along with their expected functional outcomes. Evaluation and management of limb-threatening emergencies, with emphasis on decision making, are thoroughly discussed.

Historical Perspective

Until the last half of the 20th century, partial foot amputations and disarticulations were rarely done except in cases of trauma. When "wet" gangrene related to infection or "dry" gangrene due to critical limb ischemia occurred, the customary treatment was a major lower-limb amputation. More often than not, the transfemoral level was chosen, since the rationale was to amputate where primary healing could be safely anticipated. Failure of primary healing due to wound ischemia or infection posed a very real danger of death in the pre-antibiotic era, when the emphasis was on survival rather than functional rehabilitation. With improvements in vascular reconstruction, amputation surgery, and prosthetics, as well as convergent advances in diverse but interrelated fields such as plasma glucose control, nutrition, wound healing, the measurement of tissue oxygenation, and antibiotic therapy, the surgeon now has the opportunity to consider the foot rather than the tibia or femur as the level of choice for amputation in selected cases of diabetic infection, with or without peripheral vascular disease.[1]

Burden of the Problem

A crucial question is how to best utilize the advances noted above to conserve all tissue commensurate with the diagnosis and good ambulatory function. Unfortunately, many surgeons still consider a transverse ablation, such as a transmetatarsal amputation, to be the best solution for a forefoot infection, even if only a single ray (toe and metatarsal) is involved, analogous to the automatic selection of a transfemoral rather than transtibial level in the past. Happily, conservative surgical care of the diabetic foot has become a much more common part of the surgeon's repertoire in recent years as a result of a wider appreciation of the functional benefits that retention of a partial foot offers many patients.

Partial foot ablations offer two important advantages over transtibial or more proximal amputations. Perhaps the most cogent is preservation of end-weight-bearing along normal proprioceptive pathways. This is in sharp contrast to the situation of the person with a transtibial amputation, who must interpret an entirely new feedback system, originating from the stump-socket interface below the knee joint. The degree to which normal walking function can be restored to the partial foot amputee by means of footwear, orthosis, or prosthesis is related to the loss of forefoot lever length and associated muscles. This ranges from virtually normal gait in the case of a single lateral ray (toe and metatarsal) amputation to somewhat impaired gait in the case of a midtarsal (Chopart) disarticulation. Barefoot walking is difficult for most partial foot amputees owing to the loss of plantar foot surface, but retention of even the hindfoot can preserve far greater independence without a prosthesis in both transfer activities and household ambulation than either a transtibial or transfemoral amputation, both of which require a prosthesis for weight-bearing. The second advantage of these levels is that they result in the least alteration of body image of any lower-limb ablations, easily masked by the ambulatory aids noted above. It should be noted that these devices have been greatly improved in usefulness during recent decades owing to advances in material science. When the foot cannot be salvaged, however, every attempt should be made to retain the knee joint, because the transtibial level is the most proximal one at which near-normal walking function with a prosthesis can be expected for most patients.[2]

Current Diagnostics

Causal Conditions

The most common cause for amputations in people with diabetes mellitus is infection resulting in "wet" gangrene. The usual etiology is a combination of sensory neuropathy and direct or shear forces applied to the skin over a bony prominence by ill-fitting footwear. Deep infection follows full ulcerative penetration of the skin into a plantar space and/or the bones and joints of the foot. Thermal injuries to bare feet from hot soaks or baths, automobile floorboards or transmission tunnels, solar radiation, fireplaces, or floor-furnace grids are also common. Dysvascularity added to sensory neuropathy and any of these causal factors will result in ischemic ulcers and "dry" gangrene. Smoking can be an aggravating factor in all of these situations.

Determining the Level of Amputation

A number of factors influence level selection. First and foremost, amputation must be done proximal to an irreparably damaged or gangrenous body part. For example, an ablation distal to the ankle is unlikely to succeed if there are gangrenous changes of the heel pad. In the case of a foot abscess, its decompression by prompt incision and drainage in the emergency department will assist in controlling proximal spread of infection prior to definitive debridement, helping to achieve a more distal amputation level.

Tissue oxygen perfusion is a major determinant of level; if decreased, it can sometimes be improved by vascular surgery or enhanced with postoperative hyperbaric oxygen therapy. Before attempting the procedures described in this chapter, therefore, it is essential that a thorough evaluation of arterial blood flow be done. Lack of protective sensation, by itself, should not be considered a criterion for more proximal amputation through sensate skin, since the decrease in sensation can be compensated for by the skillful use of protective interface materials in prostheses, orthoses, and footwear. The bony level selected must match the skin available in terms of length and quality, both to ensure closure without tension and to permit placement of scar away from areas of direct weight-bearing forces. A lack of suitable skin in relation to bone therefore requires ablation at a level at which these criteria can be met.

Other factors related to level selection have strong behavioral overtones on the part of both the patient and the physician. The most obvious examples are patients with uncontrolled psychosis or a history of major noncompliance with foot care programs. In these situations, the surgeon may be deterred from performing a procedure that requires a high degree of patient compliance for success to be ensured, both in the immediate postoperative period and in the long term, such as a Syme ankle disarticulation. Other behavior-linked factors that are at least partially controllable and/or reversible include nicotine addiction and poor plasma glucose control. Although they should not dictate level selection, they do deserve adequate preoperative evaluation and assiduous correction. Because behavioral factors can profoundly affect outcome, the patient and family should fully participate in surgical decisions and follow-up to provide the best chance of optimum rehabilitation.[3]

Preoperative Assessment of Factors Affecting Wound Healing

Tissue Oxygen Perfusion

As was noted above, adequate oxygen perfusion of tissues at the proposed level of amputation is crucial to healing; therefore, a noninvasive evaluation of arterial circulation should be made before definitive surgical care is initiated. Although pedal pulses may be palpable, this does not automatically mean that distal forefoot and digital flow are adequate to support healing. Forefoot and toe pressures may be obtained by using Doppler devices; although these are widely available and quite portable, they are of limited use in determining foot amputation levels in diabetic patients. This is because artificially high "systolic" pressure values will be obtained from heavily calcified and hence incompressible vessels. In addition, arteriovenous shunting in the foot may provide adequate pressures at the ankle while depriving the distal forefoot and toes of sufficient oxygen.[4]

In contrast, pulse volume recordings can overcome these deficiencies by providing a visual waveform image of pulsatile flow to all limb segments, including the toes.[5] If pulsatile flow is not detectable, indirect determination of skin perfusion by transcutaneous oxygen measurements ($TcPO_2$) may be useful in evaluating healing potential. Although current technology does not allow $TcPO_2$ measurement at the toe level, it can be evaluated from the proximal thigh down to the distal dorsal metatarsal level. This test is useful in the logical selection of the small minority of patients who may benefit from perioperative hyperbaric oxygen therapy. Values greater than 30 to 40 mm Hg indicate that the wound should heal without the assistance of hyperbaric oxygen.[6] A value less than 20 mm Hg at a given location indicates that healing is unlikely to occur at that level.[7] The predictive value of this test can be significantly enhanced by an oxygen challenge in which 100% normobaric oxygen is administered via a snug mask for 20 minutes.[8–10] Sheffield found that an increase of $TcPO_2$ to 40 mm Hg or more indicated a sufficient enhancement of tissue perfusion for hyperbaric oxygen therapy to be of practical benefit.[10] Harward and associates found that an increase of just 10 mm Hg over the baseline value is predictive of wound healing.[11] If normobaric values on 100% O_2 are predictive of failure and vascular intervention is not feasible, with amputation remaining as the only option, $TcPO_2$ measurements may be repeated in the hyperbaric chamber with 100% oxygen at 2.5 atmospheres. Using this method, Wattel and associates demonstrated that healing will occur in 75% of patients in whom the $TcPO_2$ level adjacent to the wound rises to 100 mm Hg.[12]

Tissue oxygen perfusion may be profoundly decreased by the chronic use of vasoconstrictors. The use of nicotine and caffeine should therefore be actively discouraged.

Smoking is a risk factor of real significance, due not only to the short-term effects of vessel constriction, but also, over time, to enhanced development of atherosclerosis.[13,14] In smokers, healing is also retarded by decreased tissue oxygenation because of carbon monoxide binding to sites on hemoglobin that normally carry oxygen. This is clearly seen in lowered baseline transcutaneous oxygen levels in the hands and feet of smokers as compared to nonsmokers. Ricci and associates found that $TcPO_2$ levels fell significantly within 10 minutes after smoking one cigarette, reached their lowest point in 30 minutes, and were still below baseline at 60 minutes. The use of nicotine gum or patches resulted in levels intermediate between those of smokers and those of nonsmokers and was recommended as an aid to smoking cessation in patients with acute or chronic wounds.[15] A study by Lind and colleagues showed a marked increase in complications after primary amputations of the lower limb in those patients who continued to smoke cigarettes postoperatively. This group's rate of infection and reamputation was 2.5 times higher than that of cigar smokers and nonsmokers. The authors concluded that smoking should cease at least 1 week preoperatively to allow platelet function and fibrinogen levels to normalize.[16]

Laser Doppler velocimetry measures the mean velocity of red blood cells within skin capillaries. Karanfilian and associates compared the value of $TcPO_2$, laser Doppler velocimetry, and segmental Doppler ankle pressures in predicting the healing of ischemic ulcerations and amputations in the forefoot of 59 patients, 22 with and 37 without diabetes mellitus. The outcome was correctly predicted in 95% of the patients by $TcPO_2$, in 87% by laser Doppler velocimetry, but in only 52% by ankle systolic pressures.[17] When such studies indicate that perfusion is insufficient to support healing, a vascular surgeon should be consulted to determine whether vessel reconstruction or recanalization will permit limited amputation at the time of revascularization. No currently available test, whether invasive or noninvasive, can predict failure of healing with total accuracy.[18] Accordingly, these evaluations serve only as guides in the total assessment of the patient.

Nutritional Status

Another reversible and/or controllable factor influencing wound healing is nutritional status. This is reflected in serum albumin levels, which, when below 3.0 g/dL, can be indicative of starvation, severe renal disease with loss of protein in the urine, acute stress, or a combination of these factors. Wound-healing potential is also diminished in patients who are immunosuppressed, as indicated by a total lymphocyte count below 1500/mm^3. In a retrospective study, Dickhaut and associates reviewed the healing rate of 23 diabetic Syme ankle disarticulates who met Wagner's criteria for that level.[19,20] Serum albumin levels and total lymphocyte counts that had been obtained on admission were evaluated as possible additional screening criteria of wound-healing potential. Eighty-six percent of patients with a serum albumin level of at least 3.5 g/dL and a total lymphocyte count of 1500/mm^3 healed, in contrast to 43% of those who failed to meet these additional criteria. Of the two, serum albumin appeared to be the more significant.[19] A similar study by Pinzur and associates showed an 82% healing rate, but they concluded that a minimum serum albumin level of 3.0 g/dL was sufficient.[21] In this regard, it must be remembered that in attempting to improve the nutrition of diabetic patients by increasing their caloric intake, a matching increase in hypoglycemic agents will be required to avert iatrogenic hyperglycemia.

Plasma Glucose Control

Diffuse tissue glycation, which results from prolonged uncontrolled hyperglycemia, can be inferred from high levels of glycohemoglobin. Levels of 7% or more indicate poor adherence to plasma glucose control on the part of the patient and may be related to impaired wound healing. Although direct evidence of impaired wound healing in humans secondary to poor plasma glucose control is lacking, several studies implicating uncontrolled glucose levels in poor wound healing in rats have been published. These wounds exhibited decreased numbers of leukocytes and impaired neovascularization as well as decreased nitric acid synthesis, wound strength, collagen content, and granulation tissue mass.[22–25] Additionally, the dramatic decrease in complications affecting the eyes, kidneys, and nerves in diabetic humans, thoroughly documented by the Diabetes Control and Complications Trial, is sufficient to recommend tight plasma glucose control.[26]

Treatment Recommendations

Management of Limb-Threatening Emergencies

Ischemia

Ischemic necrosis of the foot often results from peripheral vascular disease associated with diabetes mellitus. As long as necrotic areas remain dry, there is often ample time to allow for complete demarcation between viable and dead tissue and for a thorough evaluation of vascular perfusion of the lower limbs. If arterial circulation proximal to the necrotic tissue is found to be significantly impaired, consultation with a vascular surgeon is advised regarding the feasibility of arterial bypass or recanalization with concomitant or delayed limited distal amputation. If blood flow cannot be restored, amputation at the next appropriate level should be done promptly to minimize deconditioning due to prolonged immobility.

In selected cases, maximum tissue preservation can be achieved by allowing autoamputation of the necrotic parts, especially if gangrene is limited to the digits. This approach is appropriate when the patient is not a candidate for limb bypass surgery because of health status yet has not developed critical limb ischemia requiring a major amputation. The entire process may take several months (Fig. 20-1). Regular outpatient observation is mandatory until the process is complete. If low-grade infection occurs at the boundary between necrotic and viable tissue, a regimen consisting of local application of a drying agent such as povidone-iodine, minor debridement, and a short course of oral antibiotics may avert conversion to wet gangrene. As each toe sloughs its necrotic portion, usually through a joint, the wound will have largely or completely closed. Most important, areas of dry gangrene must never be treated with soaks, whirlpool baths, wet dressings, or debriding agents. Moistening the junction of viable and gangrenous tissue by these methods encourages bacterial and fungal growth, converting a localized, fairly benign condition to limb-threatening wet gangrene.

Infection

Infective wet gangrene may spread along fascial planes and tendon sheaths with alarming rapidity, abetted by several factors. Continued walking, commonly seen in diabetic patients who lack protective sensation, causes dispersion of pus that has accumulated under pressure, along fascial planes (Fig. 20-2). Therefore, as soon as the patient is seen, all further weight-bearing should be prohibited. With presentation for definitive treatment often delayed by the patient because of denial associated with the loss of protective sensation, single-species infections rapidly become polymicrobial. The inciting wound should be probed with a sterile instrument or applicator. If bone is contacted, a presumptive diagnosis of osteomyelitis can be made, avoiding the need for expensive bone scans.[27] Confirmation is obtained by coned-down radiographs. Aerobic and anaerobic cultures should be taken at this time, allowing presumptive selection of antibiotics pending the results of cultures and antibiotic sensitivity tests. Because most diabetic foot infections are polymicrobial, broad-spectrum antibiotics should be administered intravenously. The antibiotics that are selected should be effective against staphylococci and streptococci as well as the commonly encountered gram-negative bacilli and anaerobes.[28–30]

Prior to definitive debridement in the operating suite, a thorough noninvasive vascular assessment and plain radiographs should be obtained. These will provide valuable guidance as to the options available for foot salvage. Nonetheless, at the beginning of debridement, the surgeon cannot be certain of the full proximal extent of the infective process or the viability of remaining tissues. The patient and family must be told that the procedure is somewhat exploratory in nature and that, on the basis of the operative findings, the surgeon will be as conservative

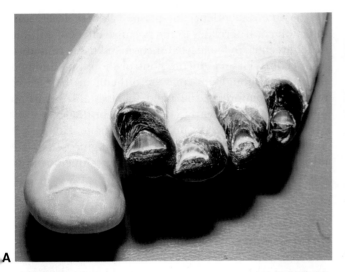

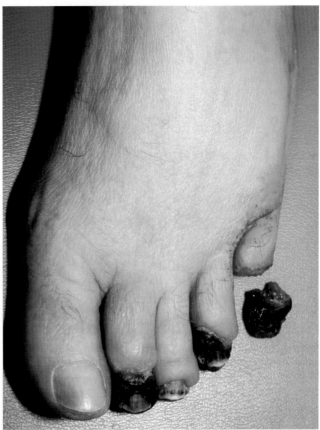

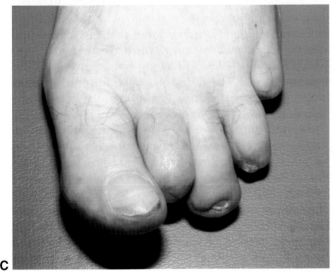

Figure 20–1   **A,** Foot of a 77-year-old diabetic male with a 30-year history of smoking. Note the dry gangrene of the four lateral toes. Vascular reconstruction was not feasible owing to cardiac status. **B,** Three months later, apparent gangrene had receded in all toes, and the fifth toe had partially sloughed. **C,** Final result at 6 months, showing considerable salvage of toe tissue by allowing completion of autoamputation without surgical interference. (**A** and **C** from Bowker JH, Poonekar PD: In Murdoch G, Wilson AB Jr [eds]: Amputation. Oxford, UK: Butterworth-Heinemann, 1996, with permission.)

as possible in the removal of tissue, even to the extent of leaving some skin with marginal perfusion in hopes that it may recover. If blood flow is not adequate, consultation with a vascular surgeon following debridement is advised.

Since the length of foot that can be salvaged is often profoundly affected by the temporal factors noted, surgical debridement must be undertaken promptly to avert further tissue loss. If definitive debridement must be delayed more than a few hours, the abscess should be drained in the emergency department to control further spread of infection. This can be done with or without ankle block anesthesia, depending on the severity of sensory neuropathy. Decompressive incisions must respect all normal weight-bearing skin surfaces, such as the heel pad, the lateral sole, and the surface directly plantar to the metatarsal heads. Also, they should be longitudinally oriented to avoid as many vascular and neural structures as possible. By unnecessarily extending an incision into the heel pad or proximal to the ankle joint, a more prox-

imal ablation, such as a Syme ankle disarticulation, can be severely compromised.

Both plantar and dorsal incisions might be required to fully drain all abscess pockets. The plantar spaces described by Grodinsky and later confirmed by Loeffler and Ballard can be opened by a single extensile plantar incision that begins posterior to the medial malleolus and ends distally between the first and second metatarsal heads.[31,32] The incision may be extended deeply into the first web space as well. Either part or all of this incision may be used, depending on the extent of the infection. Infections involving the fat pad beneath the metatarsal heads may track across the entire foot, requiring a transverse plantar incision at the base of the toes, its length depending on the extent of the infection. Full exposure of a dorsal infection may require two parallel longitudinal incisions, but they should be as widely separated as possible. Even with this precaution, the intervening skin bridge may necrose because of septic thrombosis of its small skin vessels. Following removal of patently necrotic

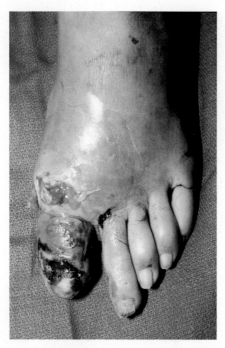

Figure 20–2 Infective (wet) gangrene of insensate foot that began in the great toe of this diabetic man and spread throughout the entire foot with continued weight-bearing.

tissue, the dorsal and plantar surfaces of the foot should be firmly stroked from proximal to distal to discover and empty pockets of pus. These recesses are then probed to their proximal end, widely opened, and thoroughly debrided. If an extensive infection involves the midfoot but spares the heel pad, an open Syme ankle disarticulation may be done. Spread of infection into the heel pad or ankle joint or along tendon sheaths proximal to the ankle joint generally precludes anything but an ankle disarticulation with opening of involved crural compartments and a delayed transtibial amputation as described in the section on transtibial amputation. Although it would seem that thorough exploration to fully determine the extent of involvement might be very time-consuming, it can be done efficiently and conservatively by applying basic anatomic knowledge, rarely adding significantly to the overall operative time.

In addition to obviously infected and necrotic tissue, all poorly vascularized tissues, such as articular cartilage, joint capsules, volar plates, and tendons, should be removed as part of a thorough debridement. Otherwise, the wound might remain open, often for months, with these tissues harboring residual infection by acting as foreign bodies until they eventually sequestrate. All visually uninvolved, well-vascularized tissue should be saved for secondary reconstruction. Since gangrenous areas vary so much in their configuration, the skin flaps that are preserved for immediate or delayed closure will frequently be nonstandard. The "guillotine" approach to amputation, in contrast, will preclude creative use of otherwise salvageable tissues in preserving forefoot length.

The interdependence of plasma glucose levels and infection control relates to the negative effect of chronic hyperglycemia on leukocyte function and tissue resistance to infection. Plasma glucose control should be initiated promptly, although this may be difficult in the face of infection, reinforcing the need for assistance from an internist as well as early complete debridement of all necrotic and infected tissue, including bone. However, it may be unsafe to strive for tight plasma glucose control until the patient is metabolically stable postoperatively to avoid iatrogenic hypoglycemia.

Partial Foot Amputations and Disarticulations

As was noted above, partial foot ablations have two important advantages over transtibial and higher levels: preservation of end-weight-bearing along normal proprioceptive pathways and a limited disruption of body image, which is easily masked with an orthosis, a prosthesis, or a modified shoe. These devices can restore near-normal walking function, relative to the loss of forefoot lever length and associated musculature.

If the criteria for level selection are met and the factors required for wound healing are correctly assessed, no amputation level in the foot need be excluded on the basis of sensory neuropathy alone. One should, however, consider the possibility that a forefoot or midfoot ablation that is too close to infected distal tissues can forfeit the chance for a Syme ankle disarticulation; therefore, the surgeon must be reasonably sure that a partial foot amputation is the logical initial procedure. Longitudinal instead of transverse amputation should be the goal whenever functionally feasible because by only narrowing rather than shortening the foot, postoperative fitting of footwear is greatly simplified.

Preventing ulceration of the insensate residual foot from the direct and shear forces generated during walking requires that the soft tissue envelope over most surfaces of the foot is mobile, that is, not adherent to underlying bone. Thus, coverage with split-thickness skin graft on the distal, medial, lateral, and plantar surfaces of the residual foot should be avoided whenever possible. Conversely, split-thickness grafts placed dorsally, even on bony surfaces covered only with granulation tissue, can last indefinitely with reasonable care (Fig. 20-3). Flaps are ideally formed of plantar skin, subcutaneous fat, and investing fascia, generously fashioned so that wound closure will not be under tension. To prevent further damage to skin that is ischemic from vascular disease or infection, never handle it with forceps during surgery. Also, proper contouring of all bone ends will prevent damage to the soft tissue envelope from within wherever it will be compressed between bone and the prosthesis, orthosis, or shoe.

Specific levels of amputation and disarticulation, starting with the toes, will now be considered.

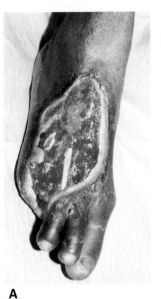
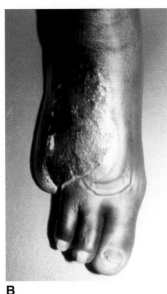

A   **B**

Figure 20–3   **A,** Foot of a 52-year-old diabetic woman following disarticulation of the fourth and fifth toes and excision of necrotic dorsal skin. The wound is well covered with granulation tissue and ready for split skin graft. **B,** Same foot 3 months after grafting. The graft has now tolerated shoe wear for many years. *(From Bowker JH: Partial foot amputations and disarticulations. Foot Ankle Clin 2:153, 1997, with permission.)*

within the flexor hallucis longus tendon at the level of the interphalangeal joint is removed by shortening the tendon. The proximal phalanx will continue to aid with standing balance owing to preservation of the windlass mechanism in contrast to disarticulation at the metatarsophalangeal (MTP) joint, where it is lost with removal of the flexor hallucis brevis/sesamoid complex. When a more radical resection of the proximal phalanx is required, Wagner recommends leaving its uninfected base to keep the sesamoid bones beneath the metatarsal head, again saving the windlass mechanism. The interphalangeal joint capsule is also left intact, helping to limit proximal spread of infection.[33]

If the entire proximal phalanx is infected, the MTP joint is the next site of election (Fig. 20-5). After release of the flexor hallucis brevis tendon insertions on the proximal phalanx, the sesamoid bones will displace proximally, exposing the crista on the plantar surface of the first metatarsal head. If the crista is prominent, it should be removed. The medial sesamoid, especially, may produce a bony prominence of its own just proximal to the metatarsal head. For this reason and to remove all avascular structures, the sesamoids, their fibrocartilaginous plate, and the articular cartilage should be excised. The metatarsal head is then smoothly rounded with a file.

Great Toe Disarticulations

In cases of osteomyelitis of the distal phalanx, sufficient skin can often be salvaged to permit closure of an interphalangeal disarticulation (Fig. 20-4). To close the wound without tension, it might be necessary to trim the condylar prominences of the proximal phalanx medially, laterally, and plantarly as well as to shorten it slightly by removing the articular cartilage. The sesamoid bone

Lesser Toe Disarticulations

Osteomyelitis of the distal phalanx of an insensate lesser toe often follows ulceration of a fixed mallet toe deformity. It is most commonly noted in the second toe in association with a long second metatarsal bone (Fig. 20-6). Removal of the infected distal phalanx shortens the toe so that it no longer projects beyond the adjacent toes, reducing the risk of future ulceration.

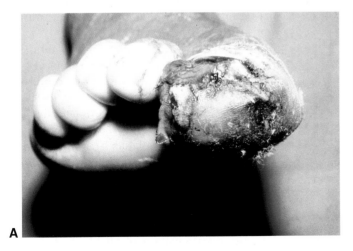

A

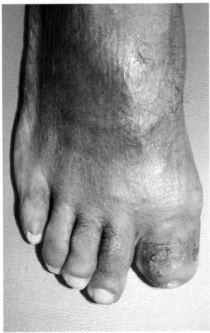

B

Figure 20–4   **A,** Foot of a 49-year-old diabetic male with necrosis of great toe and adequate perfusion proximally. **B,** Same case after interphalangeal disarticulation made possible by conservative debridement and primary closure over Kritter flow-through irrigation system. *(From Bowker JH: AAOS Instructional Course Lectures 39:355, 1990, with permission.)*

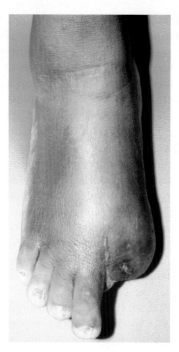

Figure 20–5 Disarticulation of great toe at MTP joint with excision of sesamoid bones. At this level, the windlass mechanism is lost.

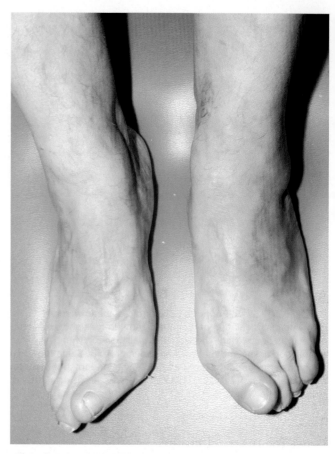

Figure 20–7 Result following bilateral MTP disarticulation of second toes in insensate feet of leprosy patient. Note hallux valgus deformities due to loss of lateral support provided by second toes.

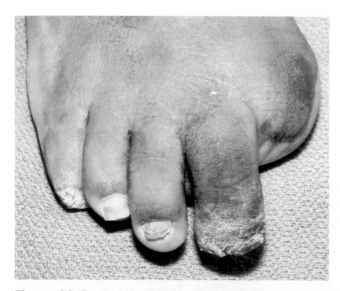

Figure 20–6 Foot of a diabetic patient with osteomyelitis of distal phalanx of insensate second mallet toe (DIP joint contracture). Disarticulation at DIP joint removed infective focus and shortened prominent toe. Previous MTP joint disarticulation of the great toe had exposed the second toe to distal trauma from a shoe.

Disarticulation of the second toe at the MTP joint may create a secondary problem by removing the lateral support that it provides to the great toe, resulting in a hallux valgus (bunion) deformity, which invites future ulceration over the prominent medial aspect of the first metatarsal head (Fig. 20-7). To avoid this iatrogenic bony prominence, it is better to remove the second metatarsal

through its proximal metaphysis along with the toe. Following this second ray amputation, the forefoot can then narrow as the first and third metatarsals approximate each other, giving a good cosmetic and functional result (Fig. 20-8).

If the third or fourth toe alone is disarticulated at the MTP joint, the adjacent ones will tend to close the gap, restoring a smooth contour to the distal forefoot (Fig. 20-9). Disarticulation of the fifth toe may leave its metatarsal head unduly prominent laterally. This can be narrowed by trimming its lateral condyle sagittally. Leaving a lesser toe isolated by removing the toes on either side should be avoided because of the increased susceptibility to injury of the isolated and functionless toe (Fig. 20-10).

Occasionally, dry gangrene will occur in all five toes without significant change in perfusion proximally. In this case, disarticulation of all five toes can be accomplished with primary coverage of the metatarsal heads, provided that the dorsal and plantar incisions are both made as far distally as possible, even into the web space dorsally. Removal of the articular cartilage and volar plates will increase the amount of skin available for closure.

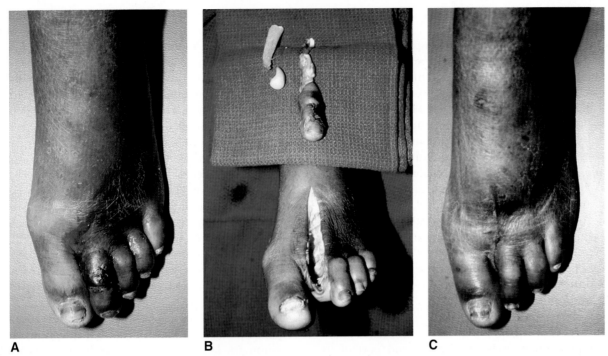

A   **B**   **C**

Figure 20–8   **Foot of a diabetic woman with osteomyelitis of second ray from a penetrating ulcer beneath the prominent metatarsal head.** A, Dorsal view demonstrates swelling centered over the second ray. B, Intraoperative view. Note dissolution of the metatarsal neck and other resected tissue. C, Postoperative view. Note forefoot narrowing with no significant hallux valgus because of lateral support provided by the third toe. *(Reproduced with permission from Bowker JH: Amputations and disarticulations within the foot: Surgical management. In Smith DG, Michael JW, Bowker JH [eds]: Atlas of Amputations and Limb Deficiencies, 3rd ed. Rosemont, IL: American Academy of Orthopaedic Surgeons, 2004.)*

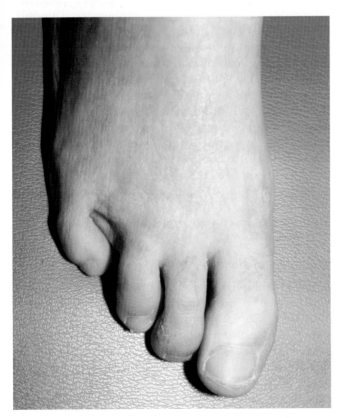

Figure 20–9   Medial shift of fifth toe closed the gap from earlier disarticulation of the fourth toe, restoring a smooth distal contour to the forefoot. No further ulcerations occurred during the 8.5-year follow-up period.

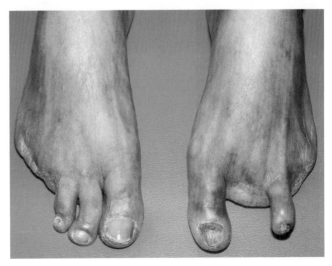

Figure 20–10   On the right foot, adjacent remaining lesser toes and great toe provide mutual protection from trauma and smooth distal contour. On the left foot, the remaining intact fourth toe is constantly exposed to minor trauma and does not contribute to foot length or rollover and propulsion during gait as the great toe does. The fourth toe should have been removed with the necrotic lesser toes at initial surgery.

Expected Functional Outcome

Following toe disarticulations, walking function should approach normal, provided that a shoe with a firm sole and a soft molded insert incorporating any required filler has been fitted. Function will be most affected by disarticulation of the great toe at the MTP joint. This is because the specialized function of the first ray in the final transfer of weight during late stance phase is lost. Mann and associates found that, following removal of the great toe, the end point of progression of the moving center of plantar pressure during stance shifted from the second metatarsal head to the third. This occurred because of loss of the great toe's stabilizing windlass mechanism associated with the flexor hallucis brevis complex, despite a dropping of the first metatarsal head. Removal of lesser toes, in contrast, appears to cause little clinical difficulty.[34]

Ray Amputations

A ray amputation is excision of a toe and part of its metatarsal. In regard to the first ray, as much metatarsal shaft length as possible should be left to allow for effective elevation of the medial arch with a custom-molded insert (Fig. 20-11). The insert should be fitted into a shoe with a rigid rocker bottom. Preservation of first metatarsal length is often simple because the usual cause

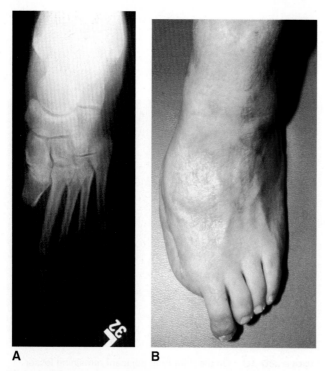

Figure 20–11   A, Radiograph of foot after a radical first-ray amputation for diabetic infection. Insufficient metatarsal shaft length remains to allow effective medial orthotic support. **B,** Note the planovalgus position of the foot secondary to loss of medial column length. *(From Bowker JH: J Prosthet Orthot 423, 1991, with permission.)*

of infection is a penetrating ulcer beneath the metatarsal head. In addition to the involved great toe, only a portion of the head might need to be removed to eradicate the infection, leaving all the unaffected portions of the head and shaft. The extent of osteomyelitis in a metatarsal can generally be determined visually. Curettage and culture of the marrow cavity are recommended. The bone should be beveled on the plantar aspect to avoid an area of increased pressure during latter stance phase.

A single amputation of ray 2, 3, or 4 affects only the width of the forefoot. Resection should be performed through the proximal metaphysis, where the involved ray intersects with the adjacent metatarsals, leaving the tarsometatarsal joints intact (Fig. 20-12). The fifth metatarsal should be transected obliquely with an inferolateral facing facet. The uninvolved half to three quarters of the shaft is left to enhance the weight-bearing area and to preserve the insertion of the peroneus brevis tendon (Fig. 20-13).

On occasion, multiple lateral ray resections are required in cases of massive forefoot infections. In this situation, the lateral metatarsals can be divided obliquely with an inferolateral-facing facet. Each affected metatarsal is cut somewhat longer as one progresses toward the first ray (Fig. 20-14). If all but the first ray are involved, it can be left as the only complete one (Fig. 20-15). This strategy retains both rollover function at the end of stance and full foot length in the shoe. With proper pedorthic fitting, this is far preferable to a transmetatarsal amputation. Removal of two or more central rays is to be avoided; here, it is better to include the uninvolved lateral ray(s) in the resection to obviate a poor functional and cosmetic result (Fig. 20-16). In all ray amputations, the full thickness of the inciting ulcer can be easily cored out with a #11 blade down to the underlying bone. Even when it is feasible to close the primary wound over a Kritter flow-through irrigation system, the ulcer wound can be left open to contract and heal secondarily from its depth to the surface. This is greatly assisted by twice-daily gentle packing of the ulcer wound with normal saline-moistened gauze dressings or other absorbent material, provided that it is nontoxic to granulation tissue.

Expected Functional Outcome

A first-ray amputation involving major removal of the first metatarsal is devastating because a long medial column is essential to proper foot function during both stance and forward progression. Therefore, the effectiveness of orthotic restoration of the medial arch is directly related to the length of first metatarsal shaft preserved. Single lesser ray amputation, in contrast, will provide an excellent result from both functional and cosmetic points of view. In these cases, only the width of the forefoot is affected, while rollover function during terminal stance appears to remain essentially normal. Removal of several lateral rays, if done as conservatively as possible,

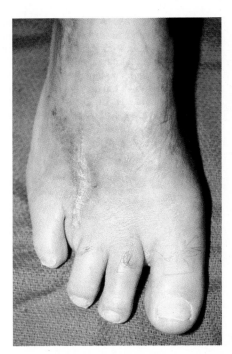

Figure 20–12 Foot of a diabetic male with a fourth-ray amputation that healed by secondary intention. Note narrowing of the forefoot and excellent distal forefoot contour. *(From Bowker JH, San Giovanni TP: Amputations and disarticulations. In Myerson M [ed]: Foot and Ankle Disorders. Philadelphia: WB Saunders, 2000, with permission.)*

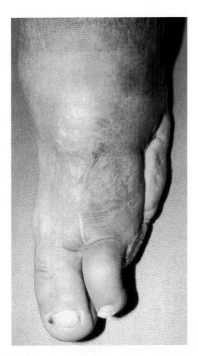

Figure 20–14 Foot of a diabetic male with third-, fourth-, and fifth-ray amputations. He functions well with a depth shoe and custom-molded insert with integral lateral filler.

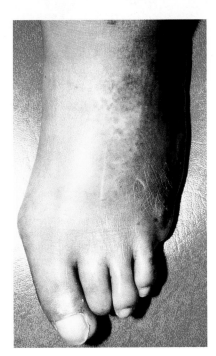

Figure 20–13 Foot of a diabetic female with a healed fifth-ray amputation. The proximal half of the shaft was left to retain insertion of the peroneus brevis tendon and as much forefoot width as possible.

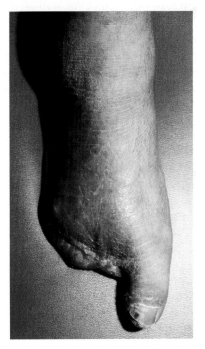

Figure 20–15 Foot of a diabetic male with the lateral four rays excised in an oblique fashion for a severe diabetic foot abscess. The first ray was left intact. Good walking function was achieved with a depth shoe with custom-molded insert with integral toe filler.

Excision of the First MTP Joint

When a penetrating ulcer destroys the first MTP joint, leaving the great toe viable and minimally infected, the joint alone can be removed through a medial longitudinal

can be adequately compensated for by a good pedorthic fitting. Barefoot walking appears to be markedly impaired in all but single lesser ray amputations.

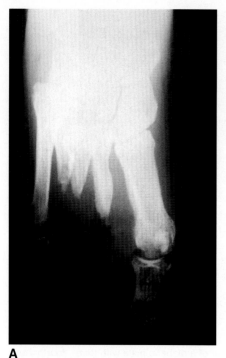

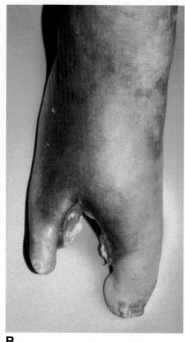

A

B

Figure 20–16 **A,** Radiograph of foot of diabetic male after excision of three central rays for abscess. **B,** Poor cosmetic and functional result. Transmetatarsal amputation was required to correct chronic plantar ulceration. Initial oblique removal of lateral rays might have averted this outcome. (**B** *from Bowker JH: Medical and surgical considerations in the care of patients with insensitive dysvascular feet. J Prosthet Orthot 4:23,1991, with permission.*)

incision in lieu of a first-ray amputation. The inciting ulcer as well as all avascular tissues, including the sesamoid complex, remaining articular cartilage, joint capsule, flexor tendons, and infected cancellous bone, should be excised (Fig. 20-17). The extensor hallucis longus tendon, if uninvolved, can usually be retained to provide active dorsiflexion (Fig. 20-18). If the wound appears clean at the conclusion of the procedure, it can be closed loosely over a Kritter flow-through irrigation system, which is described later in the chapter.[35] Temporary stabilization with Kirschner wires can be useful. The cosmetic and shoe-fitting result is much better than that following great toe amputation, although the stabilization of the MTP joint by the windlass mechanism is lost with the excision of the flexor hallucis brevis complex.

Transmetatarsal Amputation

Transmetatarsal amputation should be considered whenever two or more medial rays are infected. To ensure maximum function, it is important to save all metatarsal shaft length that can be covered distally with good plantar skin, avoiding the use of split skin grafts distally as well as plantarly (Fig. 20-19). In contrast, residual dorsal defects can be easily closed with split skin grafts. To assist in preserving forefoot length and in ensuring distal coverage of the metatarsal shafts with a durable soft tissue envelope, the initial transverse plantar and dorsal incisions are made at the base of the toes. To further preserve bone length, the shaft cuts should begin medially within the distal metaphysis of the first metatarsal, with each metatarsal shaft made slightly shorter as one proceeds laterally, taking off as little as possible while

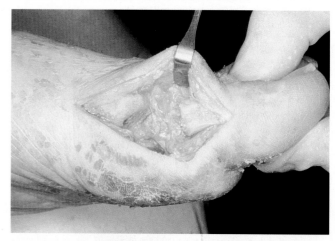

Figure 20–17 Intraoperative view of forefoot of a diabetic man with excision of chronically infected first MTP joint demonstrates plantar bevel of the distal metatarsal metaphysis. Joint infection followed penetration from a plantar ulcer beneath the sesamoids. The apparent excessive gap is due to traction on toe for photograph. *(From Bowker JH: Partial foot amputations and disarticulations. Foot Ankle Clin North Am 1997:153, with permission.)*

removing all involved bone. These cuts parallel the 15-degree angle formed by the intersection of the long axis of the foot with a line drawn along the MTP joints that represents the normal "toe break" of the shoe. The metatarsal shafts should also be beveled plantarly to reduce distal peak pressure during rollover. If a large necrotic plantar forefoot ulcer is present, it can be excised in a longitudinal elliptical manner and closed in a "T" fashion (Fig. 20-20). All flaps are trimmed to fit without tension or redundancy. With good local blood flow, healing should be uneventful. If no passive ankle

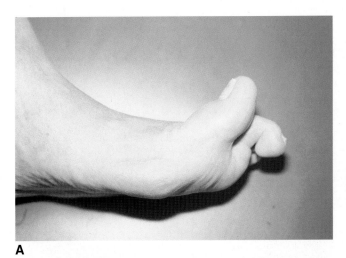
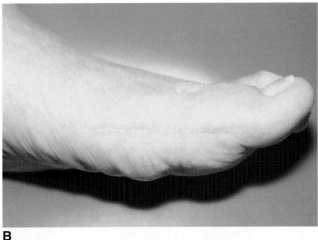

A

B

Figure 20-18 Foot of a diabetic man 14 months after excision of the first MTP joint for septic arthritis. **A,** Intact extensor hallucis longus tendon provided active dorsiflexion. **B,** When active plantar flexion is attempted, absence of extension contracture is evident. *(From Bowker JH, San Giovanni TP: Amputations and disarticulations. In Myerson MS [ed]: Foot and Ankle Disorders. Philadelphia: WB Saunders, 2000, with permission.)*

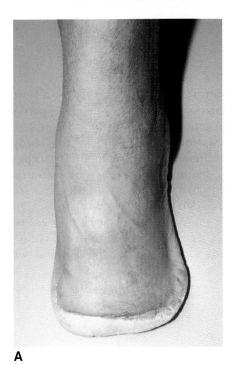
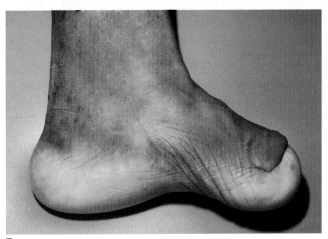

B

Figure 20-19 **Ideal transmetatarsal amputation. A,** Dorsal view. **B,** Medial view. Note placement of the distal plantar flap, overall length of the residual forefoot, maintenance of the medial arch, and absence of equinus deformity.

A

dorsiflexion is present, a concomitant percutaneous fractional lengthening of the Achilles tendon is indicated to effectively reduce distal peak pressures over the metatarsal shafts at the end of stance phase. A Kritter flow-through irrigation system is useful in removing wound detritus.[35] Before discharge, a well-padded total-contact cast is applied with the foot in a slightly dorsiflexed position to protect the wound and prevent equinus contracture. The cast is changed weekly until the wound is sound, usually at 6 weeks. At that time, a shoe with a stiff rocker sole and custom-molded insert with an integral filler, previously measured, is fitted. In the case of associated tibialis anterior weakness (drop foot), common in dia-

betic patients, a well-padded ankle-foot orthosis will be necessary.

Expected Functional Outcome

The work of McKittrick and associates, published in 1949, demonstrated what a high level of clinical acumen alone can achieve. Prior to the availability of any laboratory determinations of tissue perfusion, the authors obtained healing in 196 of 215 (91%) diabetic patients. Criteria for healing included gangrene limited to the toes, controlled infection, absence of dependent rubor, and a venous filling time of less than 25 seconds. They

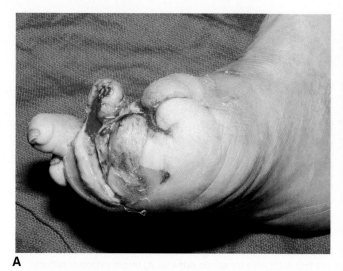

A

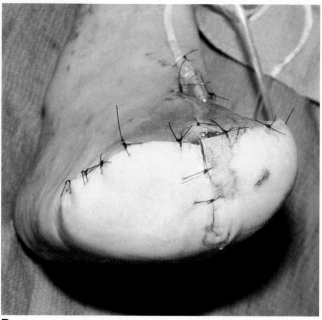

B

Figure 20–20   **A,** Foot of a 62-year-old diabetic male with a large forefoot defect following debridement for infection initiated by a penetrating ulcer beneath the second metatarsal head. **B,** Wide longitudinal excision of the ulcer required "T"-shaped closure of transmetatarsal amputation. Note the Kritter flow-through irrigation system. (*B, From Bowker JH, San Giovanni TP: Amputations and disarticulations. In Myerson M [ed]: Foot and Ankle Disorders. Philadelphia: WB Saunders, 2000, with permission.*)

found that palpable pedal pulses were not necessary and that the incision should not traverse an infected area. A satisfactory outcome in walking function was reported in 78% of patients.[36] The shoe should be fitted with a stiff rocker sole to avoid distal ulcers from a flexible shoe sole wrapping around the end of the residual foot. A distal filler will also be needed to maintain the shape of the toebox. Some patients may choose a custom-made short shoe, but because of the uncompensated shortened forefoot lever arm, this will result in an unequal drop-off gait. Another option for a short transmetatarsal amputation is an ankle-foot orthosis with an anterior shell to provide improved stability and balance. A variety of supramalleolar prostheses for this level have also been successfully fitted.

Tarsometatarsal (Lisfranc) Disarticulation

Disarticulation at the tarsometatarsal joints was described for trauma cases by Lisfranc in 1815.[37] It can also be used in cases of foot infection in carefully selected diabetic patients with the caveat that failure to control the infection at this level will risk the failure of a Syme ankle disarticulation. The Lisfranc procedure results in a major loss of forefoot lever length; therefore, it is important to preserve the tendon insertions of the peroneus brevis, peroneus longus, and tibialis anterior muscles to maintain a muscle-balanced residual foot. Careful dissection will spare the proximal insertions of the peroneus longus and tibialis anterior tendons on the medial cuneiform bone. The distal insertions of these tendons on the first metatarsal base can be reattached to the medial

cuneiform for reinforcement. Leaving a portion of the fifth metatarsal base will preserve the peroneus brevis tendon insertion. The above muscles will continue to provide eversion and inversion of the residual foot as well as counteracting the force of the triceps surae (gastrosoleus), helping to prevent equinus contracture (Fig. 20-21). The first, third, and fourth metatarsals can be disarticulated, but the "keystone" base of the second metatarsal should be left in place to preserve the proximal transverse arch. The occurrence of equinus contracture can also be minimized by doing a percutaneous fractional heel cord lengthening followed by casting with the foot in a slightly dorsiflexed position. Another method that the author uses in lieu of heel cord lengthening is cast immobilization of the residual foot in ankle dorsiflexion for 3 to 4 weeks to allow myostatic contracture of the ankle dorsiflexors while the triceps surae undergoes atrophy.

Expected Functional Outcome

Tarsometatarsal disarticulation represents a significant loss of forefoot length with a corresponding decrease in barefoot walking function. To restore fairly effective late stance phase walking function, an intimately fitted fixed-ankle prosthesis or orthosis is required, which is then placed into a shoe with a rigid rocker bottom.

Midtarsal (Chopart) Disarticulation

This disarticulation is through the talonavicular and calcaneocuboid joints, leaving only the hindfoot (talus and

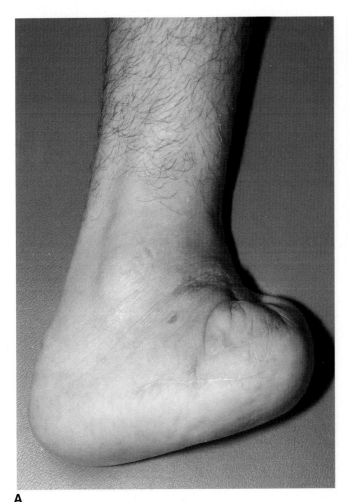

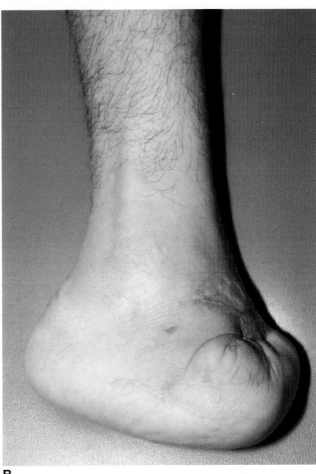

Figure 20–21   Lateral views of a foot with Lisfranc disarticulation, demonstrating the range of ankle motion available with preservation of midfoot insertions of extrinsic muscles. **A,** Maximum active dorsiflexion. **B,** Maximum active plantar flexion. *(From Bowker JH, San Giovanni TP: Amputations and disarticulations. In Myerson M [ed]: Foot and Ankle Disorders. Philadelphia: WB Saunders, 2000, with permission.)*

calcaneus). It can be used only occasionally in diabetic foot infections because of the proximity to the heel pad, as was discussed in the section on tarsometatarsal disarticulation. Loss of dorsiflexors and myostatic contracture of the unopposed tricep surae (gastrosoleus) combine to make equinus deformity inevitable unless dorsiflexion is restored to this extremely short residual foot by reattachment of the tibialis anterior tendon to the talar head. This can be done either by passing it through a drill hole in the head or by suturing it to a groove in the head.[38] Rather than lengthening the Achilles tendon to help maintain functional balance between dorsiflexors and triceps surae, the author has found it more effective to remove 2 to 3 cm of the tendon just proximal to the calcaneus. This is easily done through a separate longitudinal incision medial to the tendon, leaving the tendon sheath in place to allow rapid reconstitution at its new length. A well-padded total contact cast is applied with the ankle in slight dorsiflexion. This is worn for about 6 weeks with changes as necessary for wound evaluation. In addition to preventing equinus contracture of the

ankle, this method allows secure healing of the tibialis anterior tendon to the talus (Fig. 20-22). Excision of the sharp anteroinferior corner of the calcaneus is also recommended to remove a potentially problematic bony prominence.

The author has treated several cases of equinus contracture following Chopart disarticulation in which the anterior tibial tendon had not been surgically attached to the talus. Active dorsiflexion with restoration of heel pad weight-bearing was obtained by partial Achilles tendon excision and cast immobilization as described above. This simple salvage procedure, recommended by Burgess, avoids revision to a Syme or higher level.[39]

Expected Functional Outcome

Although midtarsal disarticulation does allow direct end-bearing, it provides no rollover function. With preservation of full limb length and a stable heel pad, the amputee can walk without a prosthesis for short distances. This is in contrast to the Syme ankle disarticulation, in

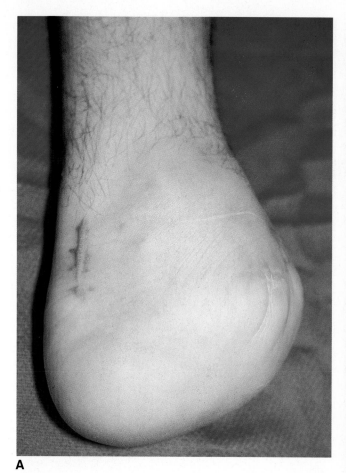
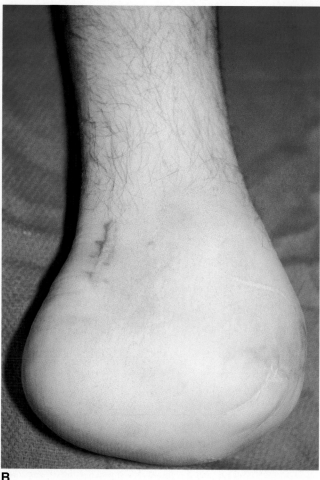

Figure 20-22   Medial views of foot with Chopart disarticulation. The patient presented with distal stump pain while walking in prosthesis secondary to severe equinus deformity. Photographs taken 3 weeks after excision of 2 cm of Achilles tendon to restore heel pad to a plantigrade position. Note short medial incision. **A,** Maximum active dorsiflexion. **B,** Maximum active plantar flexion. *(From Bowker JH, San Giovanni TP : Amputations and disarticulations. In Myerson M [ed]: Foot and Ankle Disorders. Philadelphia: WB Saunders, 2000, with permission.)*

which a prosthesis is essential to both heel pad stability and limb-length equality. Nonetheless, a close-fitting rigid ankle prosthesis or orthosis and a shoe with a rigid rocker sole are required to permit good late stance phase gait following a midtarsal disarticulation.

Syme Ankle Disarticulation

In 1843, James Syme, Professor of Surgery at the University of Edinburgh, succinctly described his operation as "disarticulation through the ankle joint with preservation of the heel flap to permit weight-bearing on the end of the stump."[40] Because the heel pad is salvaged, it can be considered a type of partial foot ablation. Its main indication is the inability to salvage a more distal functional level in an infected and/or dysvascular foot with an adequate posterior tibial artery, the main source of blood supply to the heel pad (Fig. 20-23). As was noted above, it is also indicated if an infection is too close to the heel pad to risk failure of a Syme by attempting a Lisfranc or Chopart disarticulation. Syme ankle disarticulation can also be a

reasonable choice in selected cases of severe neuroarthropathic destruction of the ankle joint. It offers these patients a much more rapid return to weight-bearing status than does ankle arthrodesis because it requires no fusion or fibrous ankylosis of bones (Fig. 20-24). At times, the Syme procedure can also be used to salvage end-weight-bearing when an unstable failed arthrodesis of a Charcot ankle cannot be controlled orthotically.

Contraindications include inadequate posterior tibial blood flow, infection of the heel pad, or ascending lymphangitis uncontrolled by systemic antibiotics.[20] A low serum albumin due to diabetic neuropathy or malnutrition as well as decreased immunocompetence reflected in a low total lymphocyte count can also seriously impede healing.[19,21] Uncompensated congestive heart failure will also impair healing by keeping wound tissues edematous. A past history of poor compliance with treatment regimens or overt psychosis should alert the surgeon to the likelihood of failure of the procedure.

This operation must be meticulously done to preserve the posterior tibial neurovascular structures and the

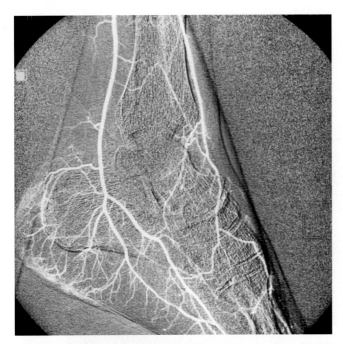

Figure 20–23   Angiogram demonstrating extensive blood flow to heel pad provided by intact posterior tibial artery. *(Courtesy of Professor Georg Neff, Berlin.)*

integrity of the fat-filled fibrous chambers of the heel pad, which provide shock absorption on heel contact. These points are thoroughly discussed and well illustrated in the classic article by R. I. Harris.[41] Wagner modified Harris's traditional method, which included removing 1 cm of the distal tibia, by merely cutting the malleoli flush with the tibial plafond and then narrowing them to match the width of the metaphyseal flare. He recommended that the procedure be done in two stages to reduce the chance of recurrent infection.[20] In the absence of infection directly adjacent to the heel pad, however, both stages can be safely combined.[42,43] If infection is close to the heel pad, however, the wound should be left open for 7 to 10 days to determine whether drainage and antibiotics have controlled the infection. If closure is then clearly indicated, the tibia will need to be shortened about 1 cm to accommodate interval shrinkage of the heel pad flap. Conversely, if infection has not been controlled, a long transtibial amputation is done without further delay.

Closure must be snug but not tight, with the heel pad accurately centered under the tibia by suturing the plantar fascia to the anterior tibial cortex through drill holes (Fig. 20-25). An alternative method, recommended by Smith and associates, is to neutralize the pull of the triceps surae on the heel pad by suturing the Achilles tendon to the posterior tibial cortex through drill holes.[44] Closed wound irrigation, using a modified Foley catheter or Shirley drain inserted through a lateral stab wound, is continued for 3 days (Fig. 20-26). Immediately after removal of the catheter, a carefully molded cast is applied, holding the heel pad centered and slightly

forward. The cast is changed weekly for 4 to 5 weeks to accommodate volume reduction; after this time, a temporary prosthesis is applied, consisting of a cast with a walking heel (Fig. 20-27). This is changed whenever it becomes loose, but at least every 2 weeks, until limb volume has stabilized. A definitive prosthesis is then fabricated and applied by the prosthetist.

Expected Functional Outcome

Because the Syme ankle disarticulation preserves heel pad weight-bearing along normal proprioceptive pathways, minimal prosthetic gait training is required. This level is also more energy efficient than the transtibial level.[45] The stump is remarkably activity tolerant, even if insensate, provided that an intimately fitted socket firmly holds the heel pad directly under the tibia (Fig. 20-28). This position must be maintained by timely replacement of the prosthesis as the inevitable calf atrophy occurs over time. Although the prosthesis is more difficult to contour cosmetically in its distal half compared to its transtibial counterpart, the patient's ability to comfortably engage in a wide variety of activities should lead to much wider use of this procedure than is occurring at present.

Transtibial Amputation

Despite the obvious functional advantages of partial foot ablations and the desire of the progressive amputation surgeon to conserve all possible length, at times it is impossible to salvage any portion of the foot. After determination that the foot cannot be saved and that the knee joint is usable, a choice must be made regarding the length to be retained, preferably by a surgeon with a definite bias toward preservation of locomotor function. The priorities at this juncture are to save as much tibial length as possible and to provide early prosthetic fitting. The shortest useful transtibial amputation must include the tibial tubercle to preserve knee extension by the quadriceps with flexion provided by the semimembranosus and biceps femoris. Stable, comfortable prosthetic socket fitting at this very high level is markedly enhanced by removal of the fibular head and neck and high transection of the peroneal nerve[46] (Fig. 20-29). To ensure that the inevitable peroneal neuroma will be proximal to the knee, gentle traction is applied to the nerve with the knee flexed and the hip extended, allowing maximum length to be excised.

Beyond universal acceptance of this shortest possible functional transtibial level, no agreement has been reached regarding the best length for optimum prosthetic function. Several amputation surgeons have strongly endorsed as distal a site as possible compatible with healing and good prosthetic function.[47-49] This conservative position is supported by a study showing that

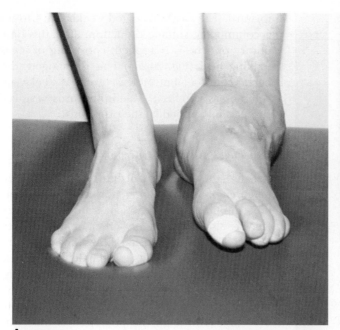

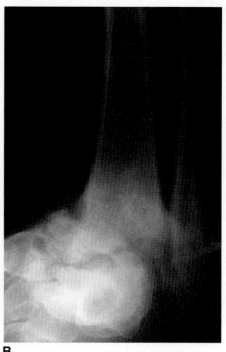

B

Figure 20–24 **A,** Note the severe medial displacement of the left foot of a 32-year-old female with type 1 diabetes 1 year after undisplaced bimalleolar fracture of ankle treated in a cast for 6 weeks. She was insensate to just below the knees. A pressure ulcer was produced over the lateral malleolus from a misguided attempt to control this irreducible, increasing deformity with ankle-foot orthosis. **B,** AP radiograph showing medial displacement of the left foot with dissolution of the ankle and subtalar joints. **C,** Appearance of Syme ankle disarticulation 8 years after surgery. The patient was actively wearing her prosthesis 14 to 16 hours daily.

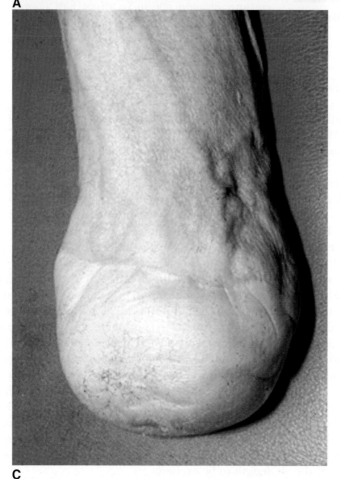

C

transtibial amputees with longer stumps require less energy to walk.[50] Prosthetic fitting is enhanced by the use of a myofasciocutaneous flap with myodesis to the anterior tibial cortex. Most patients with diabetic wet gangrene who have good perfusion will heal at the junction of the proximal two thirds and distal one third of the leg. Even in dysvascular cases, healing can usually be achieved at the midleg level. In a patient with dry gangrene of the entire foot, however, there might be no palpable pulse even at the groin. If the limb below the knee

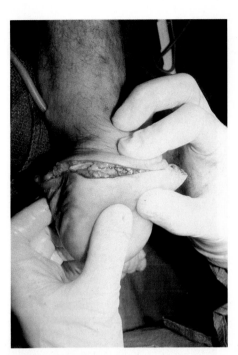

Figure 20–25   Syme procedure. Prior to closure, flap length is carefully checked. If redundant, skin can be removed from proximal flap. If the closure is too snug, the tibia will need to be appropriately shortened, most accurately with a broad hand saw. *(From Bowker JH, San Giovanni TP: Amputations and disarticulations, In Myerson M [ed]: Foot and Ankle Disorders. Philadelphia: WB Saunders, 2000, with permission.)*

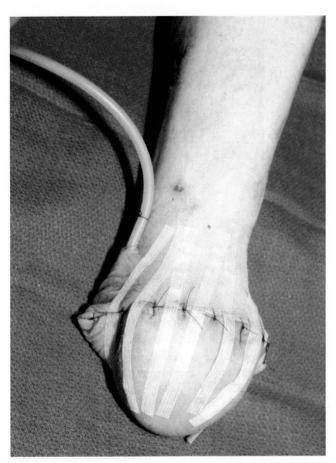

Figure 20–26   Syme procedure. Note the modified Foley catheter for closed wound irrigation exiting through lateral stab wound. Note that "dog-ears" have not been trimmed, avoiding further loss of perfusion by narrowing of heel pad pedicle. *(From Bowker JH, San Giovanni TP: Amputations and disarticulations. In Myerson M [ed]: Foot and Ankle Disorders. Philadelphia: WB Saunders, 2000, with permission.)*

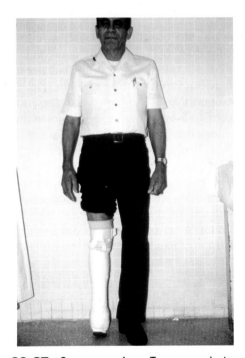

Figure 20–27   Syme procedure. Temporary plaster of Paris prosthesis applied by surgeon after a series of four or five nonweight-bearing casts, changed weekly. This weight-bearing cast-prosthesis is changed every 10 to 14 days until no further atrophy occurs. Measurement for definitive prosthesis is done at that time, and a final cast-prosthesis is applied. It is important that the patient is never without external support for the heel pad until the definitive prosthesis is fitted.

is warm, transcutaneous oxygen mapping of the skin will help to assess healing potential. If skin perfusion is found to be poor, even with an oxygen challenge, a vascular surgeon should determine whether proximal bypass or recanalization is feasible. Even when patches of gangrenous tissue are present distal to the knee at the time of a successful bypass, a short transtibial amputation can often be fashioned by using nonstandard flaps.

A major challenge to preservation of the knee joint occurs when a massive foot abscess has spread proximally along tissue planes into the crural compartment. Even with extension into the proximal leg, the knee joint might not yet be involved, and if sufficient vascularity can be demonstrated, there is no need to amputate above the infection (i.e., at the transfemoral level). Instead, an emergent open ankle disarticulation or a very low supramalleolar amputation is done. Each crural compartment, in turn, is then manually stripped from proximal to distal while the cross-section at the ankle is observed closely for expressed pus. Involved compartments are then incised

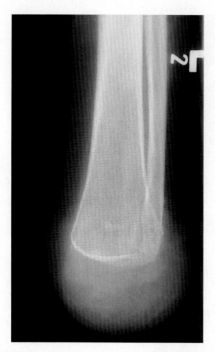

Figure 20–28   **Syme procedure.** Anteroposterior radiograph of a Syme stump. Note the thickness of heel pad and its central position under the tibia, providing excellent end-weight-bearing within the prosthetic socket.

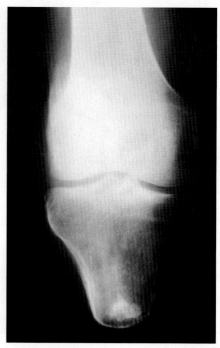

Figure 20–29   Anteroposterior radiograph of a very short right transtibial amputation following removal of fibula and shortening of peroneal nerve, showing a smooth lateral tibial contour, allowing intimate, comfortable socket fit. *(From Bowker JH, Goldberg B, Poonekar PD: Transtibial amputation: Surgical procedures and immediate postsurgical management. In Bowker JH, Michael JW [eds]: Atlas of Limb Prosthetics, 2nd ed. St. Louis: Mosby Year Book, 1992, with permission.)*

longitudinally, beginning distally and extending proximally to the limit of involvement. These may include the anterior and lateral compartments as well as the deep and superficial posterior compartments. If all compartments must be opened, the required anterolateral and posteromedial incisions must be spaced sufficiently apart to avoid too narrow an anterior flap. All infected and necrotic tissue is thoroughly excised. The thigh tourniquet is then deflated, hemostasis us achieved, and the wounds are firmly packed. Beginning the next day, the wounds are lightly packed thrice daily with wet-to-dry saline gauze dressings. After 10 to 14 days, the wounds should be well granulated and ready for reexcision and myodesis closure at the long transtibial level with a posterior myofasciocutaneous flap (Fig. 20-30).

Knee Disarticulation

Whenever the knee joint cannot be salvaged, knee disarticulation should be strongly considered as the next best level for prosthetic function, rather than transfemoral amputation. It is a simpler, less shocking procedure with minimal blood loss and rapid postoperative recovery because virtually no muscle tissue is transected. The prosthetic advantages include end-weight-bearing along normal proprioceptive pathways as well as a strong muscle-balanced lever arm with the thigh in a normally adducted position. Prosthetic suspension is enhanced by the metaphyseal flare of the distal femur. Even if the patient is permanently bed- and chair-bound, there are

advantages over the transfemoral level, including greater bed mobility due to retention of good kneeling and turning abilities as well as better sitting balance and easier transfers between various sitting surfaces (Fig. 20-31). To provide a superior soft tissue envelope, the author advocates the use of a long posterior myofasciocutaneous flap, which includes the gastrocnemius bellies[51] (Fig. 20-32). This method, first reported by Klaes and Eigler, allows comfortable direct end-weight-bearing.[52] Strong hip extension is restored by reattaching the biceps femoris and semimembranosus tendons and the iliotibial band to the remnants of the knee capsular structures. The patellar tendon is sewn to the cruciate stumps between the condyles to maintain proper quadriceps muscle tension.[51]

Transfemoral Amputation

Following transfemoral amputation, only about 25% of patients become functional prosthesis users because the excess energy expenditure is 65% or more, far beyond what many diabetic patients can safely generate due to cardiovascular disease.[50,53] On the basis of cadaver studies, Gottschalk calculated that up to 70% of hip adduction power and considerable hip extension power are lost with the division of the adductor magnus muscle related to its large cross-sectional area and distal attachment at the adductor tubercle (Fig. 20-33). The resulting muscular imbalance between hip abductors and adductors as well as flexors and extensors leads to a lurching prosthetic gait due to a relatively abducted and flexed position of the residual limb that cannot be adequately compensated for in the prosthetic socket. The increased lateral translation of the body's center of gravity during gait is one of the major causes of excess energy expenditure at this level. On the basis of these findings, Gottschalk developed a vastly improved technique for transfemoral amputation that preserves adductor magnus power.[54]

Following division of the femur 10 to 12 cm above the knee joint, the sterile tourniquet is removed prior to setting muscle tensions. With the femur held in maximum adduction and extension by an assistant, the adductor magnus tendon is attached under tension through drill holes to the distal-lateral cortex of the femur[55] (Fig. 20-34). The quadriceps muscle, which had been detached from the superior pole of the patella, is centered over the end of the femur and attached to posterior femoral drill holes, thus providing an excellent distal end pad (Fig. 20-35). The hamstrings and the iliotibial band are firmly reattached to assist in hip extension.

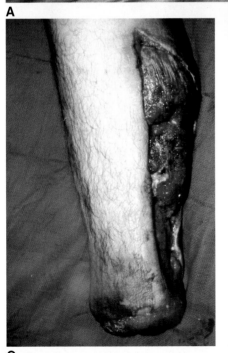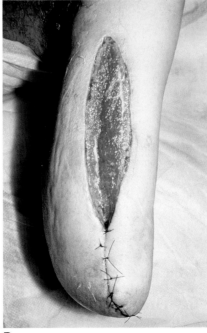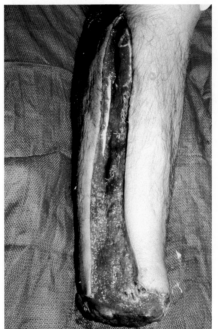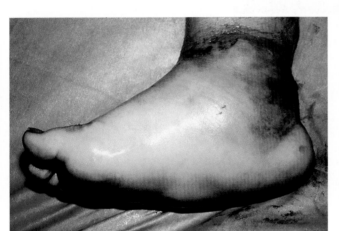

A
B
C
D

Figure 20–30 **A,** Severely abscessed right foot of a 43-year-old type 1 diabetic man prior to supramalleolar amputation and wide debridement of ascending infection of all crural compartments. Anterior (**B**) and posterior (**C**) compartment wounds were well granulated at 17 days and ready for excision and closure. Anterior wound (**D**) was closed distally.

Illustration continued on following page.

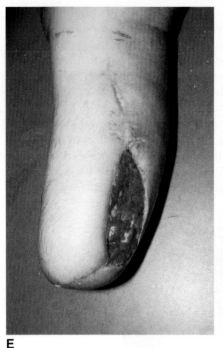

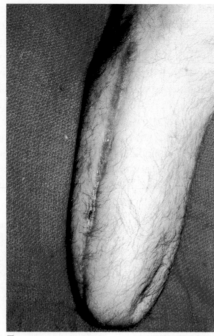

E

F

Figure 20–30, cont'd Posterior wound **(E)** was closed proximally. Wounds in D and E are pictured 3 weeks postoperatively. Residual wounds healed by secondary intention. Only enough distal bone was removed to effect myodesis closure. **F,** Lateral view 3 months after initial open amputation; the limb is ready for fitting of prosthesis. *(**A, B, D,** and **F** from Bowker JH, Goldberg B, Poonekar PD: Transtibial amputation: Surgical procedures and immediate postsurgical management. In Bowker JH, Michael JW [eds]: Atlas of Limb Prosthetics, 2nd ed. St. Louis: Mosby Year Book, 1992, with permission.)*

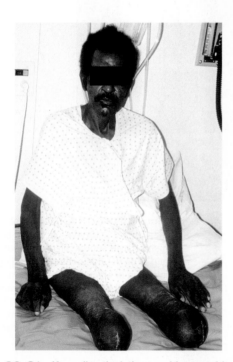

Figure 20–31 Knee disarticulation provides a stable platform for sitting and a strong lever arm to assist in transfers, in contrast to transfemoral amputation.

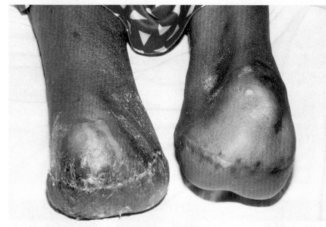

Figure 20–32 Bilateral knee disarticulations in a senile, bed-bound nursing home patient using posterior myofasciocutaneous flap of Klaes and Eigler. The left disarticulation is mature; the right one is recent.

Postoperative Management of Amputations

Primary closure is usually possible after amputation for ischemia. In some cases of low-grade foot infection, if the wound had little or no initial purulence and is visually clean following debridement (i.e., there is no compromised tissue or residual pus), a primary loose closure can

be done. If the wound has sufficient volume, it can be closed over a Kritter flow-through irrigation system.[35] A 14-gauge polyethylene venous catheter is passed into the depths of the wound from an adjacent site by means of its integral needle. The needle is then discarded, and the catheter is sutured to the skin and connected to a bag of normal saline. The fluid exits the wound between widely spaced simple skin sutures at the rate of 1 liter per day for 3 days (Fig. 20-36). The fluid containing residual wound detritus is collected in an absorbent dressing (Fig. 20-37). The outer layers of the dressing are changed every 4 to 5 hours.[56] After removal of the system on the third day, the surgeon gently compresses the edges of the wound. If any signs of purulence are present, the sutures are removed, and wound packing is commenced. If patients have been carefully selected, however, residual infection should be uncommon. The chief advantage is primary healing, usually within 3 weeks. The need for secondary closure or healing by secondary intention over several months, often augmented by skin graft, is avoided.

The management of open amputations or disarticulations resulting from significant infection is quite straightforward. Moderately wet saline gauze dressings, gently packed into all recesses of the wound, are appropriate in most cases. The advantages of this method are low cost and ease of execution. Requiring only clean technique, it is easily taught to the patient and family members before discharge. The dressing is changed every 8 hours, which is sufficient time for the gauze to adhere to the wound surface and debride detritus with each change. If the wound is producing excessive fluid, the gauze may be used dry until this ceases. Conversely, if the wound is too dry or if a vital tendon or joint capsule is exposed, a wet-to-wet method is useful. Four hours after each dressing change, the dressing is rewetted exteriorly with saline to prevent critical tissues from drying. Alternatively, one

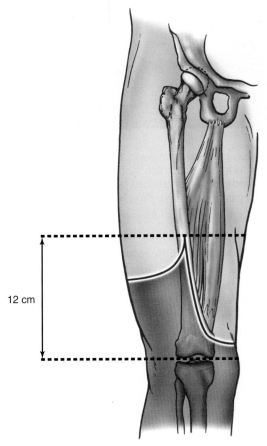

Figure 20–33   Schematic of transfemoral amputation with adductor magnus myodesis. Note the long medial flap, which allows easy access to the adductor magnus tendon. Also note that division of the femur is just proximal to the adductor canal. *(Redrawn from Gottschalk F: Transfemoral amputation: Surgical procedures. In Bowker JH, Michael JW [eds]: Atlas of Limb Prosthetics, 2nd ed. St. Louis: Mosby Year Book, 1992.)*

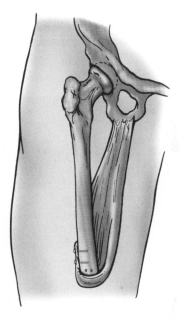

Figure 20–34   Schematic showing attachment of the adductor magnus tendon to the lateral cortex of femur. *(Redrawn from Gottschalk F: Transfemoral amputation: Surgical procedures. In Bowker JH, Michael JW [eds]: Atlas of Limb Prosthetics, 2nd ed. St. Louis: Mosby Year Book, 1992.)*

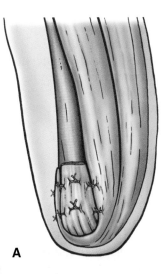

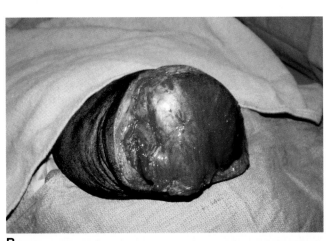

Figure 20–35   **A,** Schematic of myoplastic attachment of the quadriceps over the adductor magnus. Note that the adductor magnus tendon is sutured to the lateral cortex of the femur. **B,** Intraoperative photograph of quadriceps muscle myoplasty over the end of the femur prior to wound closure. *(**A** redrawn from Gottschalk F: Transfemoral amputation: Surgical procedures. In Bowker JH, Michael JW [eds]: Atlas of Limb Prosthetics, 2nd ed. St. Louis: Mosby Year Book, 1992.)*

A   **B**

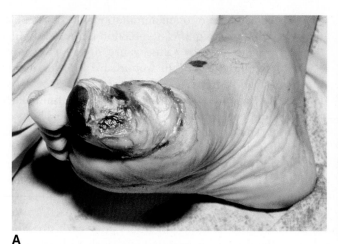

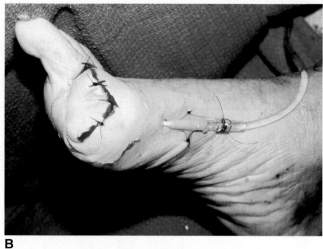

A

B

Figure 20–36 **A,** Wet gangrene of the right great toe in a diabetic man. The phalanges were infected, but some lateral skin was salvageable. Forefoot perfusion was adequate. **B,** Closure of MTP disarticulation with a lateral toe flap. Note the widely spaced sutures, which allow egress of irrigation fluid from the wound. Also note the catheter sutured to skin as described by Kritter. *(From Bowker JH: The choice between limb salvage and amputation: Infection. In Bowker JH, Michael JW [eds]: Atlas of Limb Prosthetics, 2nd ed. St. Louis: Mosby Year Book, 1992, with permission.)*

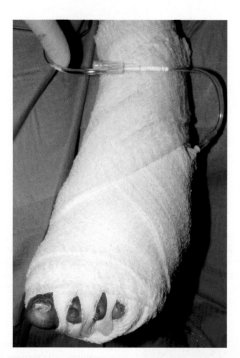

Figure 20–37 Kritter flow-through irrigation system installed in a second-ray amputation wound at the conclusion of surgery. Note the bulky bandage used to absorb irrigation fluid; the outer of three rolls is replaced every few hours. *(From Bowker JH: The choice between limb salvage and amputation: Infection. In Bowker JH, Michael JW [eds]: Atlas of Limb Prosthetics, 2nd ed. St. Louis: Mosby Year Book, 1992, with permission.)*

may use any of a number of occlusive dressings on the market to retain wound moisture. Repeated exposure of the wound surface to povidone-iodine or hydrogen peroxide can be cytotoxic to granulation tissue and is not recommended.[57,58] If *Pseudomonas* colonization occurs, as evidenced by a greenish tinge to the wound, dressings

moistened with a 0.25% solution of acetic acid can be used for a few days to suppress it. Duration must be limited because the bactericidal activity of the solution is exceeded by its fibroblast toxicity.[59] Soaks or whirlpool treatments are not indicated, as they will produce maceration of the wound.

Every 24 to 48 hours, the surgeon should manually strip the wound from proximal to distal to locate previously undetected pockets of infection, which may require further debridement. Preoperative and postoperative nutritional support must include sufficient caloric intake to compensate for a poor initial serum albumin level as well as the catabolic effect of infection and bed rest. Multivitamins as well as additional iron, zinc, and vitamin C provide essential elements for collagen formation in wound healing.[60,61] Oral hyperalimentation in patients with diabetes mellitus will require appropriate adjustments of hypoglycemic medication to prevent iatrogenic hyperglycemia. Before discharging the patient to outpatient status, the surgeon should observe formation of granulation tissue throughout the depths of the wound. The diabetologist who is consulted to assist with preoperative control of plasma glucose levels can provide the patient with a management program that will continue to assist in wound healing by decreasing tissue glycation.

The most important aspect of postoperative management in these cases is patient compliance with the program. This includes avoidance of direct weight-bearing on the wound until it is sound enough for suture removal, adequate nutrition, prohibition of vasoconstrictors such as nicotine and caffeine, and tight control of plasma glucose levels. With open ablations, it is often possible to allow protected weight-bearing using heel-bearing weight-relief shoes. The foot should be kept elevated whenever the patient is not walking, to reduce the negative effect of edema on wound healing. During the first few weeks, the wound should be evaluated weekly. In the case of closed wounds, the partial weight-bearing casts can be removed 3 weeks postoperatively, and ankle and subtalar motion should be resumed.

Summary

Amputations and disarticulations within the foot offer important advantages over more proximal levels, including direct weight-bearing with proprioceptive feedback along normal neural pathways. The degree to which full walking function can be restored prosthetically or orthotically is relative to the loss of forefoot lever length and associated muscles. Retention of even the hindfoot, however, provides for much greater independence and energy conservation than higher levels such as transtibial or transfemoral amputations. This is especially important for elderly patients with limited cardiovascular reserve. In addition, amputation levels within the foot result in the least alteration of body image and often require only shoe modifications or a limited orthosis or prosthesis.

With convergent advances in nutrition, plasma glucose control, wound healing, measurement of tissue oxygenation, and antibiotic therapy, as well as improvements in vascular reconstruction, amputation surgery, and prosthetics, today's surgeons have the opportunity to consider the foot rather than the tibia or femur as the site of election for amputations as a result of infectious and/or ischemic conditions of the foot in diabetic patients. This chapter may act as a reliable guide to both beginning and experienced team members as they face the daunting task of providing the most conservative treatment possible to diabetic patients facing minor or major loss of tissue of the lower limb. For further exploration of this challenging and rewarding but often-neglected area of care, the reader is referred to the third edition of *The Atlas of Amputations and Limb Deficiencies: Surgical, Prosthetic and Rehabilitation Principles,* published by the American Academy of Orthopaedic Surgeons in 2004.[62]

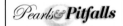

PEARLS

- Prohibit further weight-bearing on any infected foot.
- Probe all ulcers to determine whether the underlying bone is involved.
- Immediate decompression of a foot abscess prior to definitive surgical debridement will limit proximal spread of infection, helping to save critical limb length.
- Always evaluate tissue oxygen perfusion to the foot prior to definitive surgery; if perfusion is questionable, consult an interested vascular surgeon.
- Longitudinal rather than transverse amputation within the foot should be the goal whenever possible to enhance balance, gait, and shoe fitting.
- Retention of even the hindfoot can preserve independence in transfers and household ambulation without a prosthesis.
- When the foot cannot be salvaged, make every attempt to save the knee joint because a transtibial amputation is the most proximal level at which near-normal walking with a prosthesis can be expected.
- Always regard any amputation as reconstructive surgery, the first step in returning the patient to the highest possible functional status.
- Teach amputee patients how to protect their intact foot and residual limb from injury.

PITFALLS

- Diabetic patients who are noncompliant with care of their diabetes for any reason can frustrate the best efforts of the treatment team.
- When elective foot surgery is done in patients who continue to smoke cigarettes, their wounds will often fail to heal.
- Failure to correct muscular imbalance between ankle dorsiflexors and plantar flexors during hindfoot disarticulation will lead to equinus deformity and skin ulceration.
- Noncompliant patients often fail to follow postoperative protocols in hindfoot or Syme procedures, resulting in failure.

References

1. Bowker JH: Partial foot amputations and disarticulations Foot Ankle Clin North North Am 2:153–170, 1997.
2. Bowker JH: Transtibial amputation: Surgical management. In Smith, DG, Michael JW, Bowker JH (eds): Atlas of Amputation and Limb Deficiencies: Surgical, Prosthetic and Rehabilitation Principles, 3rd ed. Rosemont, IL: American Academy of Orthopaedic Surgeons, 2004, pp 481–501.
3. Bowker JH: Questions to ask your amputation team members before surgery. In First Step: A Guide for Adapting to Limb Loss, 2nd ed. Knoxville, TN: Amputee Coalition of America, 2001, pp 10–11.
4. McCollum PT, Walker MA: Major limb amputation for end-stage peripheral vascular disease. Level selection and alternative options. In Bowker JH, Michael JW (eds): Atlas of Limb Prosthetics: Surgical, Prosthetic and Rehabilitation Principles, 2nd ed. St Louis: Mosby Year Book, 1992, pp 25–38.
5. Livingston R, Jacobs RI, Karmody A: Plantar abscess in the diabetic patient. Foot Ankle 5:205–213, 1985.
6. Cianci P, Hunt TK: Adjunctive hyperbaric oxygen therapy in treatment of diabetic foot wounds. In Bowker JH, Pfeifer MA (eds): Levin and O'Neal's The Diabetic Foot, 6th ed. St. Louis: Mosby Year Book, 2001, pp 404–421.
7. Pecoraro RE: The nonhealing diabetic ulcer: A major cause for limb loss. Prog Clin Biol Res 365:27–43, 1991.
8. McCollum P, Spence VA, Walker WF, et al: Oxygen-induced changes in the skin as measured by transcutaneous oximetry. Br J Surg 73:882–885, 1986.
9. Matos LA, Nunez AA: Enhancement of healing in selected problem wounds. In Kindwall EP (ed): Hyperbaric Medicine Practice, 2nd ed. Flagstaff, AZ: Best Publishing, 2004, pp 813–850.
10. Sheffield PJ: Tissue oxygen measurements. In Davis JC, Hunt TK (eds): Problem Wounds: The Role of Oxygen. New York: Elsevier, 1988, pp 17–51.
11. Harward TRB, Volay R, Golbranson F, et al: Oxygen inhalation: Induced transcutaneous PO_2 changes as a predictor of amputation level. J Vasc Surg 21:220–227, 1985.
12. Wattel F, Mathieu D, Coget JM, et al: Hyperbaric oxygen in chronic vascular wound management. Angiology 41:59–65, 1990.
13. Beach KW, Strandness DE Jr: Arteriosclerosis obliterans and associated risk factors in insulin dependent diabetes. Diabetes 29:882–888, 1980.
14. Kannel WB: Cigarette smoking and peripheral arterial disease. Prim Cardiovasc 12:13, 1986.
15. Ricci MA, Fleishman C, Gerstein N: The effects of cigarette smoking and smoking cessation aids on transcutaneous oxygen levels. J Vasc Med Biol 4:256,1993.

16. Lind J, Kramhoff M, Bodker S: The influence of smoking on complications after primary amputations of the lower extremity. Clin Orthop 267:211–217, 1991.

17. Karanfilian RG, Lynch TG, Zirul VT, et al: The value of laser-Doppler velocimetry and transcutaneous oxygen tension determination in predicting healing of ischemic forefoot ulcerations and amputations in diabetics. J Vasc Surg 5:511–516, 1986.

18. McCollum PT, Raza Z: Vascular disease: Limb salvage versus amputation. In Smith DG, Michael JW, Bowker JH (eds): Atlas of Amputations and Limb Deficiencies: Surgical, Prosthetic and Rehabilitation Principles, 3rd ed. Rosemont, IL: American Academy of Orthopaedic Surgeons, 2004, pp 31–45.

19. Dickhaut SC, DeLee JC, Page CP: Nutritional status: Importance in predicting wound healing after amputation. J Bone Joint Surg 66A:71–75, 1984.

20. Wagner FW Jr: The Syme ankle disarticulation: Surgical procedures. In Bowker JH, Michael JW (eds): Atlas of Limb Prosthetics: Surgical, Prosthetic and Rehabilitation Principles, 2nd ed. St. Louis: Mosby Year Book, 1992, p 413.

21. Pinzur MS, Smith D, Osterman H: Syme ankle disarticulation in peripheral vascular disease and diabetic infection: The one-stage versus two-stage procedure. Foot Ankle Int 16:124–127, 1993.

22. Yue DK, Swanson B, McLennan S, et al: Abnormalities of granulation tissue and collagen formation in experimental diabetes, uraemia and malnutrition. Diabet Med 3:221–226,1986.

23. Yue DK, McLennan S, Marsh M, et al: Effects of experimental diabetes, uremia and malnutrition on wound healing. Diabetes 36:295–299, 1987.

24. Fahey TJ III, Sadaty A, Jones WG II, et al: Diabetes impairs the late inflammatory response to wound healing. J Surg Res 50:308–313, 1991.

25. Schaffer MR, Tantry U, Efron PA, et al: Diabetes-impaired healing and reduced wound nitric oxide synthesis, a possible pathophysiologic correlation. Surgery 121:513–519, 1997.

26. Diabetes Control and Complications Trial Research Group: The effect of intensive treatment of diabetes on the development and progression of complications in insulin-dependent diabetes mellitus. N Engl J Med 329:683–689, 1993.

27. Grayson MI, Gibbons GW, Balogh K, et al: Probing to bone in infected pedal ulcers: A clinical sign of underlying osteomyelitis in diabetic patients. JAMA 273:721–723, 1995.

28. Grayson ML: Diabetic foot infections: Antimicrobial therapy. Infect Dis Clin North Am 9:143–161, 1995.

29. Lipsky BA: Evidence-based antibiotic therapy of diabetic foot infections. FEMS Immunol Med Microbiol 26:267–276, 1999.

30. Lipsky BA, Berendt AR: Principles and practice of antibiotic therapy of diabetic foot infections. Diabetes Metab Res Rev 16(suppl 1):S42–S46, 2000.

31. Grodinsky M: A study of fascial spaces of the feet. Surg Gynecol Obstet 49:737–751, 1929.

32. Loeffler RD Jr, Ballard A: Plantar fascial spaces of the foot and a proposed surgical approach. Foot Ankle 1:11–15, 1980.

33. Wagner FW Jr: Partial-foot amputations: Surgical procedures. In Bowker JH, Michael JW (eds): Atlas of Limb Prosthetics: Surgical, Prosthetic and Rehabilitation Principles, 2nd ed. St. Louis, Mosby Year Book,1992, pp 389–401.

34. Mann RA, Poppen NK, O'Konski M: Amputation of the great toe: A clinical and biomechanical study. Clin Orthop 225:192–205, 1998.

35. Kritter AE: A technique for salvage of the infected diabetic foot. Orthop Clin North Am 1973; 4:21–30.

36. McKittrick LS, McKittrick JB, Risley TS: Transmetatarsal amputation for infection or gangrene in patients with diabetes mellitus. Ann Surg 130:826–835, 1949.

37. Lisfranc J: Nouvelle méthode opératoire pour l'amputation du pied dans son articulation tarsometatarsienne: Methode précédée des nombreuses modifications qúa subies celle de Chopart. Paris, France: Gabon, 1815.

38. Letts M, Pyper A: The modified Chopart's amputation. Clin Orthop 256:44, 1990.

39. Burgess EM: Prevention and correction of fixed equinus deformity in mid-foot amputations. Bull Prosthet Res 10:45, 1966.

40. Syme J: On amputation at the ankle joint. London Edinb Month J Med Science 2:93, 1843.

41. Harris RI: Syme's amputation: The technical details essential for success. J Bone Joint Surg 38B:614–632, 1956.

42. Bowker JH, Bui VT, Redman S, et al: Syme amputation in diabetic dysvascular patients. Orthop Trans 12:767–768, 1988.

43. Baumgartner R: Forefoot and hindfoot amputations. In Surgical Techniques in Orthopaedics and Traumatology. Paris: Elsevier, SAS, Editions Scientifiques et Médicales, 55-700-C-10, 2001, pp 4–5.

44. Smith DG, Sangeorzan BG, Hansen ST, Burgess EM: Achilles tendon tenodesis to prevent heel pad migration in the Syme's amputation. Foot Ankle 15:14–17, 1994.

45. Waters RL, Perry J, Antonelli D, Hislop H: Energy cost of walking of amputees: The influence of level of amputation. J Bone Joint Surg Am 58:42– 46, 1976.

46. Spira A, Steinbach T: Fibulectomy and resection of the peroneal nerve for "short tibial stumps." Acta Orthop Scand 44:589, 1973.

47. McCollough NC III, Harris AR, Hampton FL: Below-knee amputation. In Atlas of Limb Prosthetics. St. Louis: Mosby Year Book, 1981, pp 341–368.

48. Epps CH Jr: Amputation of the lower limb. In Evarts MC (ed): Surgery of the Musculoskeletal System, 2nd ed. New York: Churchill Livingstone, 1990, pp 5121–5161.

49. Moore TJ: Amputations of the lower extremities. In Chapman MW (ed): Operative Orthopaedics, 2nd ed. Philadelphia: JB Lippincott, 1993, pp 2443–2455.

50. Gonzales EG, Corcoran PJ, Reyes RL: Energy expenditure in below-knee amputees: Correlation with stump length. Arch Phys Med Rehabil 55:111–119, 1974.

51. Bowker JH, San Giovanni TP, Pinzur MS: North American experience with knee disarticulation with use of a posterior myofasciocutaneous flap: Healing rate and functional results in seventy-seven patients. J Bone Joint Surg Am 82:1571–1574, 2000.

52. Klaes W, Eigler F: Eine neue Technik der transgenikulären Amputation. Chirurg 56:735–740, 1985.

53. Bowker JH: Transtibial (below-knee) amputation: Report of ISPO Consensus Conference on Amputation Surgery. Copenhagen, International Society for Prosthetics and Orthotics, 1992, p 10.

54. Gottschalk F: Transfemoral amputation: Biomechanics and surgery. Clin Orthop 36l:15–22, 1999.

55. Gottschalk F: Transfemoral amputation: Surgical management. In Smith DG, Michael JW, and Bowker JH (eds): Atlas of Amputations and Limb Deficiencies: Surgical, Prosthetic and Rehabilitation Principles, 3rd ed. Rosemont, IL: American Academy of Orthopaedic Surgeons, 2004, pp 533–540.

56. Bowker JH: Ankle disarticulation and variants: Surgical management. In Smith DG, Michael JW, and Bowker JH (eds): Atlas of Amputations and Limb Deficiencies: Surgical, Prosthetic and Rehabilitation Principles, 3rd ed. Rosemont, IL: American Academy of Orthopaedic Surgeons, 2004, pp 445–446.

57. Rodeheaver G, Bellamy W, Kody M, et al: Bactericidal activity and toxicity of iodine-containing solutions in wounds. Arch Surg 117: 181–186, 1982.

58. Oberg MS, Lindsey D: Do not put hydrogen peroxide or povidone-iodine into wounds! [editorial]. Am J Dis Child 141:27–29,1987.

59. Lineaweaver W, Howard R, Soucy D, et al: Topical antimicrobial toxicity. Arch Surg 120:267–270, 1985.

60. Sieggreen MY: Healing of physical wounds. Nurs Clin North Am 22:439–447, 1987.

61. Stotts MA, Washington DF: Nutrition: A critical component of wound healing. AACN Clin Issues 1:585–594, 1990.

62. Smith DG, Michael JW, Bowker JH (eds): Atlas of Amputations and Limb Deficiencies: Surgical, Prosthetic and Rehabilitation Principles, 3rd ed. Rosemont, IL: American Academy of Orthopaedic Surgeons, 2004.

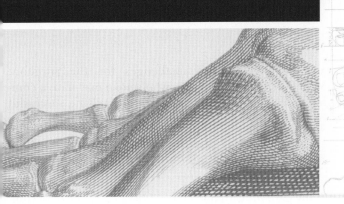

LOWER-LIMB ARTERIAL RECONSTRUCTION IN PATIENTS WITH DIABETES MELLITUS: PRINCIPLES OF TREATMENT

ALLEN D. HAMDAN AND FRANK B. POMPOSELLI, JR. ■

Introduction

Foot problems remain the most common reason for hospitalization of patients with diabetes mellitus.[1,2] Approximately 20% of the 12 million to 15 million people with diabetes in the United States can expect to be hospitalized for treatment of a foot complication at least once during their lifetime, accounting for an annual health care cost in excess of one billion dollars.[3] The primary pathologic mechanisms of neuropathy and ischemia set the stage for pressure necrosis, ulceration, and polymicrobial infection, which, if improperly treated, ultimately lead to gangrene and amputation.[4] Understanding the complex interplay of neuropathy, ischemia, and infection on an individual patient with a foot complication, as well as simultaneously effecting proper treatment, is essential to foot salvage. While this chapter focuses on the treatment of ischemia due to arterial insufficiency, it is important to remember that ischemia is accompanied by infection in approximately 50% of patients in our experience[5] and that most, if not all, patients will have peripheral neuropathy present as well. Although correction of ischemia, often by bypass grafting or endovascular intervention, is crucial, the vascular surgeon must account for the complex pathobiology of the diabetic foot to ultimately be successful.

Vascular Disease in Diabetic Patients

A detailed discussion of vascular disease in diabetic patients can be found elsewhere in this book. The most important principle in treating foot ischemia in patients with diabetes is recognizing that the cause of their presenting symptoms is macrovascular occlusion of the leg arteries due to atherosclerosis. In the past, many clinicians incorrectly assumed that gangrene, nonhealing ulcers, and incomplete healing of minor amputations or other foot procedures were due to microvascular occlusion of the arterioles, so-called small vessel disease.[6] This concept, although erroneous and subsequently refuted in several studies,[7-11] unfortunately persists to this day. In the minds of many clinicians and their patients, this has resulted in a pessimistic attitude toward treatment of ischemia that all too often leads to an unnecessary limb amputation without an attempt at arterial reconstruction. This attitude and approach are antiquated and inappropriate and must be discouraged in the strongest terms. In the authors' opinion, rejection of the small vessel theory alone could decrease the 40-fold increased risk of major limb amputation that a person with diabetes faces during his or her lifetime compared to nondiabetic counterparts.

Atherosclerosis in Diabetes

Although histologically similar to disease in nondiabetic patients, atherosclerosis in the patient with diabetes has certain clinically relevant differences. Previous studies have confirmed that diabetes mellitus is a strong independent risk factor for atherosclerotic coronary,[12,13] cerebrovascular,[14] and peripheral vascular disease.[14] Patients with diabetes face a higher likelihood of cardiovascular mortality. In addition, generalized atherosclerosis is more prevalent and progresses more rapidly in diabetic patients. Diabetic patients tend to seek help for manifestations of their disease up to a decade earlier than nondiabetic patients do. In patients with ischemic symptoms of the lower limb, gangrene and tissue loss are more likely to be present compared to nondiabetic patients. Diabetic patients with coronary atherosclerosis are more likely to have so-called silent ischemia, that is, absence of typical anginal symptoms or pain with myocardial infarction, particularly in those with significant polyneuropathy.[15]

These findings suggest that arterial reconstruction in this group carries a higher risk of adverse outcome, particularly myocardial infarction and/or death. Although both Lee[16] and Eagle[17] have listed diabetes mellitus as an independent risk factor for adverse cardiac outcomes in patients undergoing major surgery, our personal experience in the last two decades has refuted this position. By employing multivariate analysis in a study of over 6500 major vascular procedures of all types, including carotid endarterectomy, aortic aneurysm repair, and lower-limb bypass, diabetes mellitus did not predict increased perioperative cardiac morbidity or mortality.[18]

In a separate outcome study composed exclusively of nearly 800 lower-limb bypass procedures in diabetic patients, followed for a minimum of 5 years, the hospital mortality rate was 1%, and long-term graft patency, limb salvage, and patient survival rates were comparable to or better than those for nondiabetic patients treated over the same period.[19] In our opinion, careful perioperative management, including an aggressive approach toward invasive cardiac monitoring in the early postoperative period, has been responsible for the low cardiac morbidity and mortality rate in these high-risk patients.

From the vascular surgeons' perspective, the most important difference in lower-limb atherosclerosis in diabetic patients is the location of the occlusive lesions.[8,10] In patients without diabetes, typically smokers, atherosclerosis most commonly involves the infrarenal aorta, iliac arteries. and superficial femoral artery with relative sparing of the more distal arteries. In patients with diabetes. however, the most significant occlusive lesions occur in the crural arteries distal to the knee, that is, the anterior tibial, peroneal, and/or posterior tibial arteries, sparing the arteries of the foot (Fig. 21-1). This pattern of occlusive disease, known as "tibial artery disease," requires a different approach to vascular reconstruction

and presents special challenges for the surgeon. Moreover, diabetic patients who smoke may have a combination of both patterns of disease, making successful revascularization more complex.

Patient Selection

Many patients with diabetes will have evidence of peripheral vascular disease manifested by absence of palpable leg or foot pulses with either minimal or no symptoms. In these patients, their disease is well compensated, and no surgical treatment is necessary. However, education about vascular disease and reduction of associated risk factors, particularly cessation of smoking, tight plasma glucose control, and management of their dyslipidemia is critical. Regular follow-up examinations, usually at a 6- to 12-month interval, are reasonable. In addition, routine visits to a foot and ankle specialist and pedorthist regarding foot care and proper shoeing can be of benefit. Some clinicians will obtain baseline noninvasive arterial testing at this point, although this is not mandatory. Many patients have associated coronary and carotid atherosclerosis, which may also be asymptomatic. Although routine screening for disease in these vessels in the absence of symptoms, purely based on evidence of lower-limb atherosclerosis, might be appropriate in some patients, it is probably not cost-effective as a routine in all such patients.

In patients who present with typical symptoms mandating treatment, several factors must be taken into consideration. Certain patients might not be appropriate for arterial reconstruction such as those who are nonambulatory or bedridden and have no likelihood of successful rehabilitation. Similarly, patients with severe flexion contractures of the knee or hip are poor candidates. Patients with terminal cancer or similar lethal comorbidities with a very short life expectancy do poorly with vascular reconstruction and are probably better served by primary amputation. Individuals with an unsalvageable foot due to extensive necrotizing infection likewise require primary amputation. However, in patients who present with infection complicating ischemia, proper control of spreading sepsis must be accomplished prior to arterial reconstruction. Broad-spectrum intravenous antibiotic coverage of gram-positive, gram-negative, and anaerobic organisms should be started immediately after cultures are taken, since most infections in diabetic patients are polymicrobial.[1,20] Once culture data are available, antibiotic therapy can be appropriately adjusted. In addition, patients with abscess formation, septic arthritis, necrotizing fasciitis, and so on should undergo prompt incision, drainage, and debridement, including open toe, ray, or partial forefoot amputation[21] as indicated (Fig. 21-2).

In our series of pedal bypasses, secondary infection was present at the time of presentation in over 50% of

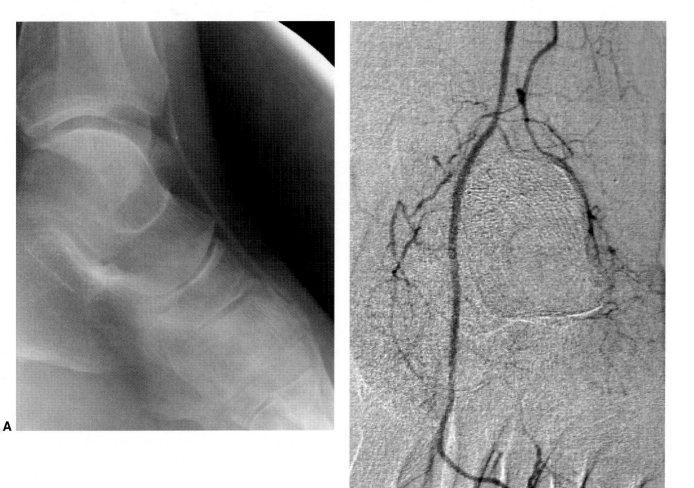

Figure 21-1   **A,** Lateral view of the foot (nonsubtraction) of a diabetic patient with severe tibial artery occlusive disease. This patient had no patent tibial vessels to which bypass could be performed. Note the location and patency of the dorsal pedis artery, which is an excellent target artery for bypass. **B,** Anteroposterior view of the same foot. The widely patent dorsalis pedis artery is well visualized and can be seen feeding the pedal arch. It is mandatory to obtain both lateral and anteroposterior angiographic views of the foot in evaluating the pedal vasculature.

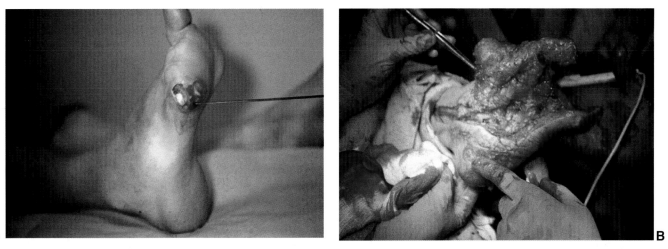

Figure 21-2   **A,** One of the simplest and most reliable tests for bone involvement is probing of the wound or ulcer directly to bone. Appropriate drainage and then revascularization can be undertaken. **B,** This case illustrates how aggressive clinicians might need to be in foot infections that present late. This patient ultimately had a bypass and healed a transmetatarsal amputation.

patients.[22] Infection places an increased metabolic demand on already ischemic tissues and may accelerate and exacerbate tissue necrosis. Since many diabetic patients have a blunted neurogenic inflammatory response, typical signs of inflammation might be absent or diminished. It is therefore imperative that all ulcers be carefully probed and inspected and that superficial eschar and callus be removed to look for potential deep space abscesses, which are not readily apparent from visual inspection of the foot. The need to control spreading infection might delay vascular surgery for several days, but waiting longer than necessary to sterilize wounds is inappropriate and can result in further tissue necrosis. It is important to look for signs of resolving infection, including reduction of fever and diminishment of cellulitis and lymphangitis, particularly in areas of potential surgical incisions. The return of glycemic control, which is probably the most sensitive indicator of improvement, should also be expected. During this period, which rarely extends beyond 4 or 5 days, contrast arteriography and other presurgical evaluations such as testing for coronary disease when necessary can be performed so that vascular surgery can be undertaken without unnecessary delay. One caveat is that dry eschars without any signs of infection in the face of ischemia should be debrided only if there is a plan for arterial reconstruction. Debriding a dry plantar eschar without first restoring pulsatile flow to the foot can lead to a deeper ulcer.

Occasionally, there are patients in whom infection cannot be totally eradicated prior to bypass. Until arterial blood flow has been adequately restored, some will have such severe ischemia as to make it impossible to deliver an adequate concentration of antibiotics to the infected tissues. It is also important in these patients to continue antibiotic coverage for several days following arterial reconstructive surgery. Occasionally, patients will seem to have worsening of their infection after revascularization due to the enhanced inflammatory response that may occur once arterial blood flow has been restored. These individuals might require one or more subsequent debridements to fully remove infected and necrotic tissue.

It is also important to realize that age alone is not a contraindication to arterial reconstruction. We have successfully performed these procedures in selected patients over the age of 90 years. In selecting patients for arterial reconstruction, their functional and physiologic status is far more important than chronological age. In fact, a limb-salvaging arterial reconstruction might mean the difference for an elderly patient between continued independent living and the need for permanent custodial nursing home care. We evaluated our results with arterial reconstruction in a cohort of patients 80 years of age or older at the time of arterial reconstruction, evaluating both the rate of success of the initial procedure and two important quality-of-life outcomes: the ability to ambulate and whether or not they returned to their own residence following surgery. At 1 year post-operatively, the vast majority (more than 80%) was still ambulatory and residing in their homes either alone or with relatives.[23]

Patients with limb ischemia who present with signs and symptoms of coronary disease such as worsening angina, recent congestive heart failure, or recent myocardial infarction need to have stabilization of their cardiac disease prior to arterial reconstruction. Occasionally, angioplasty or even coronary artery bypass grafting might be required prior to lower-limb surgery, although in our experience, this has been unusual. Moreover, routine noninvasive cardiac evaluation of all patients has proved both costly and unnecessary. Since virtually all diabetic patients with lower-limb ischemia have occult coronary disease,[24] screening tests such as dipyridamole-thallium imaging are almost always abnormal to some degree. Attempting to quantify the degree of abnormality with such testing has occasionally proved useful in stratifying patients who are at excessive risk for perioperative cardiac morbidity or mortality; however, most such patients with severely abnormal scans usually have obvious clinical signs or symptoms as well.[25] As a result, we rely mostly on the patient's clinical presentation and electrocardiogram in determining when further evaluation is needed and use imaging studies selectively in patients with unclear or atypical symptoms. In asymptomatic patients who are reasonably active with no acute changes on an electrocardiogram, no further studies are generally undertaken. Recently, we reviewed approximately 300 patients with diabetes mellitus undergoing lower-limb bypass surgery. Routine extensive cardiac workup did not improve outcomes and often delayed revascularization.[26]

We have found that careful monitoring of our patients using several techniques has significantly reduced perioperative cardiac morbidity and mortality. These include frequent use of invasive perioperative cardiac monitoring, including pulmonary arterial catheters and transesophageal echocardiogram, along with anesthesia management by personnel who are accustomed to treating patients with ischemic heart disease as well as managing patients in a specialized, subacute, monitored unit in the early postoperative period. Moreover, in a prospective randomized trial, the type of anesthesia that was given (i.e., spinal, epidural, or general endotracheal) did not affect the incidence of perioperative cardiac complications[27] or graft thrombosis,[28] contradicting an often held opinion that regional anesthesia should be used in these patients.

Patients presenting with renal failure pose special challenges. When acute renal insufficiency occurs, most commonly following contrast arteriography, surgery is delayed until renal function stabilizes or returns to normal. Most such patients will demonstrate a transient rise in serum creatinine without overt symptoms. It is rare that such patients will become anuric or require hemodialysis. Withholding contrast arteriography in patients with diabetes and compromised renal function is therefore generally inappropriate and unnecessary. If there are severe concerns about renal function, magnetic resonance angiography can sometimes provide adequate images to plan arterial reconstruction[29] or allow for more limited and selective contrast arteriography, such as of the tibial/pedal vessels alone.

Patients with chronic, dialysis-dependent renal failure can safely undergo arterial reconstruction. Many such patients have severe, advanced atherosclerosis and have target arteries that are often heavily calcified. Gangrene and tissue loss frequently are present, and the healing response in such patients is poor, even with restoration of arterial blood flow. Some such patients will require amputation even with patent arterial bypass grafts. Studies have demonstrated that although adequate, graft patency and limb salvage rates in these patients are lower than in those without chronic renal failure.[30–33] Our own study, of 146 patients with end-stage renal disease undergoing arterial reconstructive procedures for critical limb ischemia, demonstrated graft patency and limb salvage of 68% and 80%, respectively, at 3 years. Their perioperative mortality rate was reasonably low (3%), but long-term survival was poor with only 18% alive after 3 years. These results underscore the importance of clinical judgment in considering arterial bypass for limb ischemia in the dialysis patient. Until further studies clarifying the role of bypass surgery in this patient population are available, treatment plans must be individualized with the realization that for some patients, primary amputation could be the best option.[34]

It is also a common misconception that amputation is a "lesser" intervention from a cardiac stress standpoint than is bypass. Nothing could be farther from the truth. In our bypass patients, mortality is approximately 1%, while in patients undergoing transtibial amputation, it is 5.7% and rises to 16.5% for transfemoral amputations. Clearly, this overstates the point, since patients undergoing amputation are often closer to the end stage of their disease process than are those having bypass surgery.[35]

Evaluation and Diagnostic Studies

Patients requiring surgical intervention for lower-limb arterial insufficiency usually present with severely disabling intermittent claudication or signs and symptoms of limb-threatening ischemia. Intermittent claudication is pain, cramping, or a sensation of severe fatigue in the muscles of the leg that occurs with walking and is promptly relieved by rest. It should be reproducible with similar activities, causing many patients to adjust their lifestyle to minimize or eliminate any significant walking. The location of discomfort can give hints to the site of the occlusion; patients with aortoiliac atherosclerosis will often complain of buttock and thigh pain, while patients with femoral disease will typically have calf discomfort,

although patients with aortoiliac occlusive disease can have calf claudication as their only presenting symptom. Patients with tibial arterial occlusive disease will also have calf claudication and might also complain of foot discomfort or numbness with walking. Nocturnal muscle cramping, which is a common complaint among patients with diabetes, is not a typical symptom of vascular disease, even though it may involve the calf muscles and should not be mistaken for intermittent claudication. Studies on the natural history of claudication have demonstrated that progression to limb-threatening ischemia is uncommon.[36,37] Therefore, most patients with intermittent claudication do not require surgical intervention. Many respond to conservative treatment measures such as cessation of tobacco use, correction of risk factors for atherosclerosis, weight reduction when necessary, and an exercise program involving walking.[38] Additionally, two medications—pentoxifilline 400 mg orally three times daily or cilostazol 100 mg orally twice daily—are approved for the treatment of intermittent claudication due to atherosclerosis.[39–41] Both drugs are generally well tolerated but need to be taken for several weeks before an improvement in walking distance can be appreciated. In the authors' experience, however, pentoxifilline is rarely effective in relieving claudication symptoms. Although cilostazol has proven more effective, side effects, including headache and diarrhea, are occasionally problematic, and it is contraindicated in patients with a history of congestive heart failure. Our treatment strategy for claudication begins by discussing its cause with the patient and reassuring the patient that its course is usually benign. The need for smoking cessation, weight loss when appropriate, and lifestyle changes to reduce risk factors is strongly emphasized. Usually, an exercise program involving walking will be our first step in treatment, with cilostazol added if walking alone proves ineffective or if patients cannot or will not exercise. Interventions, including angioplasty or surgery, are reserved for those with very limited functional capacity, those who are unable to work owing to their symptoms, or those who have not responded to more conservative treatment. In the authors' experience, patient noncompliance is the most common reason for failure of conservative treatment measures. Many patients cannot or will not exercise, and others find the degree of improvement with conservative measures inadequate. With technologic improvements in lower-limb angioplasty and stenting, we have tended to offer this less invasive option to patients with lifestyle-limiting claudication more readily than we would have previously offered bypass surgery when it was the only available treatment.

Most diabetic patients who are referred for vascular intervention, however, have limb-threatening ischemic problems, which, if not promptly treated, are likely to ultimately result in amputation. The most common presenting problem is a nonhealing ulcer with or without associated gangrene and infection. Patients may initially develop an ulcer as a result of neuropathy, which will then fail to heal in spite of proper treatment due to associated arterial insufficiency, the so-called neuroischemic ulcer. Some patients are referred after a minor surgical procedure in the foot that fails to heal owing to ischemia. Patients can also present with ischemic rest pain with or without associated tissue loss. Ischemic rest pain typically occurs in the distal foot, particularly the toes. It is exacerbated by recumbency and relieved by dependency. Patients often give a history of noticing pain, numbness, or paresthesias when retiring for bed, which is then relieved by placing the foot in a dependent position. Often, dependency of the foot is not recognized as the cause of relief, which instead might be ascribed to maneuvers such as walking and stamping the involved foot on the floor or getting up and taking an oral analgesic medication. It is important but occasionally difficult to differentiate rest pain from painful diabetic neuropathy, which may also be subjectively worse at night. Neuropathic patients with severe foot ischemia may also present without rest pain owing to the complete loss of sensation.

After a detailed pulse examination, noninvasive studies by the vascular laboratory[42–43] are particularly useful in patients presenting with foot pain for which the etiology is unclear, being due to either ischemia or painful diabetic neuropathy. Patients with severe ischemia will usually have ankle brachial indices of less than 0.4. In patients with diabetes mellitus, however, care must be taken in interpreting ankle pressures, since many patients will have artifactually elevated pressures due to calcification of the arterial wall that makes these stiffened vessels difficult to compress with a blood pressure cuff.[44] In fact, approximately 10% of patients will have noncompressible vessels, making the ankle brachial index incalculable. Pulse volume recordings are useful in these patients, since they are unaffected by calcification of vessels. Severely abnormal waveforms at the ankle or forefoot suggest severe ischemia (Fig. 21-3). Some centers have found toe pressures[44] and transcutaneous oxygen measurements[45,46] also to be useful in these patients, although we do not routinely use these two modalities in our practice. Noninvasive arterial testing with exercise[42,44] is also useful in patients with claudication who present with palpable distal pulses. Baseline studies are taken and then repeated with exercise, usually by walking on a treadmill at an elevation of 10 degrees, until symptoms are reproduced. A subsequent reduction in arterial pressures or worsening of pulse volume waveforms suggests proximal stenotic lesions. Those individuals with muscular pain during walking who have normal

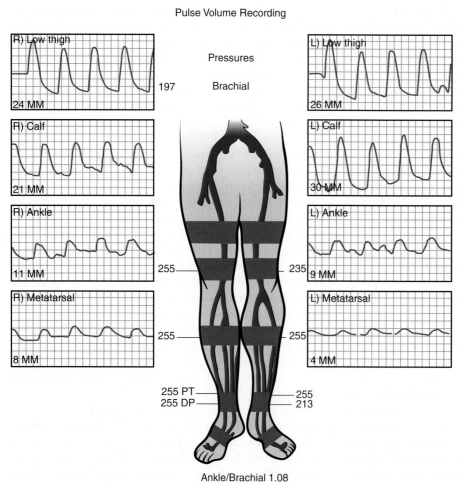

Figure 21–3 Pulse volume recordings from a diabetic patient who was noted to have elevated segmental pressures and ankle-brachial indices. This patient clearly has "dampening" of the waveforms in both limbs beginning at the level of the ankle. This decrease in amplitude of the tracing suggests that an occlusive vascular lesion exists between the calf and ankle. The results of this test, however, are merely qualitative and do not quantify the extent of vascular disease present.

Pulse Volume Recording

R) Low thigh 24 MM
R) Calf 21 MM
R) Ankle 11 MM
R) Metatarsal 8 MM

Pressures
Brachial 197

L) Low thigh 26 MM
L) Calf 30 MM
L) Ankle 9 MM
L) Metatarsal 4 MM

255
255

235
255

255 PT
255 DP

255
213

Ankle/Brachial 1.08
Index

waveforms before and after exercise may have another cause for their symptoms, such as spinal stenosis, so-called pseudoclaudication. Following vascular surgery, noninvasive testing can be used to quantify the degree of improvement in distal circulation. Arterial reconstructions with vein grafts are susceptible to the development of neointimal hyperplasia, which can lead to stenosis and, ultimately, graft thrombosis. Ultrasound evaluation of vein grafts with color flow duplex scanning is useful in detecting stenoses due to neointimal hyperplasia.[47] If found, significant stenoses can often be repaired by vein patch angioplasty, percutaneous angioplasty, or interposition grafts, thus averting graft thrombosis.[48]

Noninvasive testing, however, adds little to the evaluation of patients who present with obvious signs of foot ischemia and absent foot pulses. For most patients, a careful history and physical examination will detect significant arterial insufficiency. The most important feature of the physical examination is the status of the foot pulses. If the posterior tibial and dorsalis pedis artery pulses are impalpable in patients presenting with typical signs and symptoms of ischemia, no further noninvasive testing is necessary, and contrast arteriography should be performed straightaway.

The ultimate goal of lower-limb vascular reconstruction is the restoration of perfusion pressure in the distal circulation through bypassing all major occlusions and, if possible, reestablishing a palpable foot pulse. The outflow target artery, that is, the point of the distal anastomosis, should be relatively free of occlusive disease and demonstrate unimpeded flow to the arteries of the foot. Generally, the most proximal artery distal to the occlusion meeting these two criteria is chosen. To make these determinations, we perform a comprehensive contrast arteriogram of the entire lower-limb circulation, extending from the infrarenal aorta to the base of the toes. It is crucial to visualize the entire tibial and foot circulation, since the former is the most common location of the most significant occlusive lesions and the latter is an important potential site for placement of the distal anastomosis of the bypass graft. Iliac artery atherosclerosis accompanies more distal lower-limb disease in approximately 10% to 20% of patients with diabetes. When significant, balloon angioplasty of iliac lesions, with or without placement of a stent, is almost always possible and will improve arterial inflow for bypass. Moreover, this can be performed at the same time as the diagnostic arteriogram. For many years, our preference has been to exclusively use intra-arterial digital subtraction arteriography[49] to evaluate the lower-limb arterial circulation. With currently available equipment, it is possible to obtain a complete survey from the infrarenal aorta to the base of the toes with approximately 100 mL of contrast, which is half the amount required for conventional arteriography. Although conventional arteriography can provide excellent views of the arterial anatomy, we have found cases in which it failed to demonstrate a

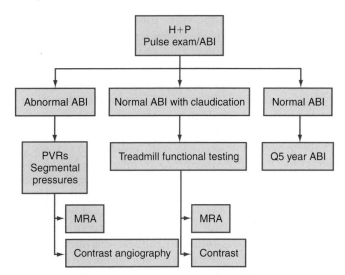

Figure 21–4 Algorithm for assessing peripheral vascular disease in the diabetic patient (based on recommendations laid out in the 2003 ADA Consensus Statement [Peripheral Arterial Disease in People with Diabetes, American Diabetes Association Consensus Statement, Diabetes Care, 26(12):3333–3341, Dec 2003]).

suitable outflow vessel that was subsequently seen by the digital subtraction method.

As was previously discussed, acute renal failure following contrast arteriography is a concern in diabetic patients, especially those with preexisting renal insufficiency. The most important factor in the prevention of renal failure in these patients has been the use of hydration prior to obtaining the angiogram.[24] Recent data suggest that sodium bicarbonate infusion prior to contrast exposure might be even more effective than normal saline hydration[50] while N-acetylcysteine treatment preceding and following contrast exposure has also been shown to help prevent contrast nephropathy.[51] Thus, when appropriately used, arteriography should never be withheld due to fear of exacerbating renal insufficiency. When renal function does worsen, it is usually asymptomatic and transient, with creatinine levels commonly returning to normal levels within a few days,[11] after which arterial reconstructive surgery can be undertaken. For patients with more severe renal dysfunction, magnetic resonance arteriography can provide images of the distal circulation that are adequate to plan the arterial reconstruction. Although some centers feel that this technique is superior to contrast arteriography,[29] we have found that intra-arterial digital subtraction arteriography continues to provide the best-quality images and reserve magnetic resonance arteriography for patients in whom the administration of contrast is potentially harmful or contraindicated (Fig. 21-4).

Vascular Reconstruction

One of the most important developments in vascular surgery has been the demonstration that autogenous saphenous vein, as opposed to prosthetic graft material, gives the best short- and long-term results for distal bypass. In a large multicenter, prospective, randomized clinical trial, 6-year patency of saphenous vein grafts was more than four times that of prosthetic grafts.[52]

For more than 50 years, the standard procedure performed for lower-limb arterial revascularization has been the reversed saphenous vein bypass.[53] An inherent problem with reversing the vein, which is necessary to overcome the impediment of flow past its valves, is the size discrepancy between the arteries and veins where they are connected. Vein grafts that are less than 4 mm in diameter at the distal end can thrombose when connected directly to the much larger common femoral artery at the groin, owing to the size discrepancy. For many years, some vascular surgeons would routinely discard saphenous veins that were smaller than 4 mm distally in order to prevent this cause of early thrombosis when performing a bypass with a reversed saphenous vein. Methods were developed to render the valves incompetent in order to allow the vein to be used nonreversed or "in situ." However, no procedure was widely accepted until the late 1970s, when Leather and associates[54] described a new technique using a modified Mills valvulotome that cut the valves atraumatically and quickly. Vascular surgeons enthusiastically embraced the Leather technique and began reporting improved results with the in situ bypass.[55–57] This led some to conclude that the in situ bypass possesses some inherent biologic superiority to the reversed saphenous vein graft.[58] However, evidence to support this concept is lacking.[59] Moreover, when in situ bypasses are compared to more contemporary series of reversed saphenous vein bypasses, no superiority is evident.[60] In our experience, we have frequently used both procedures and have observed essentially identical results with the two vein configurations.[61] Nevertheless, the in situ technique is an important advance in lower-limb reconstructive surgery and continues to be used widely by most vascular surgeons.

In the 1980s, Ascer and associates[62] reported the first series of bypass grafts with inflow taken from the popliteal artery. They showed results equivalent to those of the traditional approach of taking inflow from the common femoral artery. These outcomes have been confirmed by other groups,[63] including our own.[64] This procedure has proved to be another important advance in arterial reconstruction for patients with diabetes. Because atherosclerotic occlusive disease often spares the superficial femoral artery in diabetic patients, the popliteal artery can be readily used as a source of inflow for a distal vein graft. Doing so shortens the operative procedure and avoids potentially troublesome wound complications, which often accompany thigh and groin dissections. Short vein grafts are also advantageous in patients who have a limited quantity of adequate saphenous vein. Theoretically, shorter vein grafts should also have higher flow rates and possibly better long-term

patency. Our recent experience with extremely distal arterial reconstructions has shown that popliteal artery inflow is possible in about 60% of diabetic patients undergoing vascular reconstruction in the lower limb.[61]

When the saphenous vein is unavailable owing to previous harvesting or vein stripping, alternative sources of conduit must be sought. Although some surgeons will use a prosthetic graft in these circumstances, alternative vein grafts, including contralateral saphenous vein, arm vein, or lesser saphenous vein, can be used. We have generally not harvested the contralateral saphenous vein in diabetic patients who have distal pulses in that limb because our experience has shown that in patients with a missing ipsilateral saphenous vein, the likelihood of requiring arterial reconstruction in the opposite limb approaches 40% at 3 years following the first operation.[65] Moreover, in our tertiary care practice, many such patients do not have adequate available contralateral saphenous vein due to its use for other vascular procedures or because of venous disease. When saphenous vein is unavailable, our vein conduit of choice has been arm vein. Our results with arm vein grafts have been improved by examining the vein with the angioscope[66] to exclude segments with strictures or recanalization from trauma induced by previous venipuncture and thrombosis. Using the angioscope in this way to upgrade the quality of arm vein grafts has significantly improved our results and further reduced the number of patients requiring prosthetic conduits.[67] One potential disadvantage of arm vein grafts is their limited length, although the use of popliteal artery inflow makes the use of shorter arm vein grafts possible in many patients. Moreover, the use of composite grafts made of various segments of arm vein, including the cephalic-basilic vein loop graft,[68] can provide enough conduit length to reach from the groin to the distal tibial and even foot vessels in many patients. Our results with over 500 arm vein grafts have been reported.[69] Patency and limb salvage rates were 57.5% and 71.5%, respectively, at 5 years. These results were inferior to those with de novo reconstructions done with saphenous vein but significantly better than those reported with prosthetic conduits.

A review of our arteriograms, imaging the entire lower-limb circulation, has demonstrated that in 10% of cases a foot vessel, usually the dorsalis pedis artery, is the only suitable outflow. In another 15% of patients, the dorsalis pedis artery will appear to be a better-quality outflow target vessel than other patent but diseased tibial vessels. As a result, we began performing bypasses to the dorsalis pedis artery approximately 13 years ago in situations in which no other bypass option existed and in which we believed that the patient was definitely facing amputation as the only alternative. Early results proved gratifying enough that we standardized our indications and technique to encompass all patients in whom we thought the dorsalis pedis artery was the best bypass option even if more proximal outflow target arteries

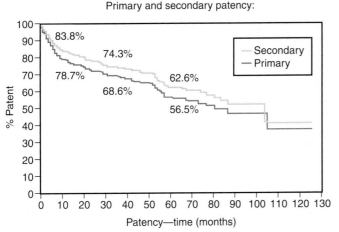

Figure 21-5   **A,** Patency rates of bypass to dorsalis pedis artery in over 1000 patients. **B,** Limb salvage after pedal bypass is excellent and durable.

were present.[70] Our experience with vein bypass grafts to the dorsalis pedis artery exceeds 1000 procedures with follow-up extending beyond 10 years. The long-term patency rate (5 years) was 63% with a limb salvage rate of 78%; however, the patient survival rate was less than 50%[71] (Fig. 21-5).

Approximately 60% of patients requiring pedal bypass will present with some degree of foot infection, raising concerns about placing an arterial graft in such close proximity. This has not proved hazardous provided that active, spreading sepsis is controlled prior to surgery.[5] Our results have compared favorably with other reports of pedal level arterial reconstruction[72–76] and are comparable to or better than results now routinely reported for popliteal and tibial artery reconstructions. In advanced cases of distal ischemia, patients might have no patent outflow vessel other than tarsal or plantar branches of the dorsalis pedis or distal posterior tibial artery. These arteries are small and often calcified, making bypass procedures technically challenging. However,

even with these "extreme" distal bypasses, limb salvage has been nearly 70% at 5 years.[77]

Distal arterial reconstructions present special technical challenges for the vascular surgeon and require meticulous attention to detail. The target arteries are usually small (1.0 to 2.0 mm in diameter) and are often calcified owing to medial calcinosis. Since long-term success requires the use of venous conduit, harvesting an adequate vein is essential and can often present problems, particularly when the ipsilateral saphenous vein is not available. In the early days of distal bypass surgery, many procedures were unsuccessful, resulting in amputation. Technical improvements in arteriography, surgical instruments, and sutures as well as techniques such as the in situ bypass have significantly improved the outcome of distal arterial bypass, with outstanding results often reported in more contemporary series. Again, these advances have proved to be especially beneficial to patients with diabetes mellitus, since their occlusive disease almost always requires a bypass to this level. In particular, the development and application of bypasses to the dorsalis pedis artery have had a direct effect, in our own experience, on the likelihood of amputation in patients with diabetes presenting with limb-threatening ischemia. Since its inception, pedal bypass has resulted in a significant decline in all amputations performed for ischemia.[78] Currently, bypasses to the dorsalis pedis artery constitute approximately 25% of all lower-limb arterial reconstructions in our diabetic patients.

Evaluation of Bypass Grafting

There are a number of different methods to evaluate bypass grafts intraoperatively. The previous gold standard was completion angiography. This is time consuming, exposes the patient to contrast, and can be misleading, sometimes mandating reexploration of an anastomosis only to find spasm of the distal vessel. Duplex evaluation can also be done and is very accurate but can be too sensitive to any minor problems. We prefer to do angioscopy of the vein conduit and then evaluate the distal anastomoses by palpating the pulse as well as listening for a triphasic signal with a continuous wave Doppler instrument.

Our postoperative protocol, which is similar to those across the country, involves an office visit and physical examination about 2 weeks after bypass, at which time the staples are removed. The first duplex scan is done sometime in the 6-week to 3-month range. For the first year, we continue with office visits and duplex examinations every 3 months. If there are no abnormalities on the duplex scan for the first 12 months, we perform one every 6 months during the next year. From the third year on, annual examinations are sufficient. The timing in this protocol takes into account the fact that most intimal hyperplasia in the graft occurs during the first 18 months postoperatively. After that, stenoses can develop within the graft or in the inflow or outflow artery.

The duplex examination involves color flow, gray scale, and peak systolic velocities at both anastomoses, at proximal and distal arteries, and at multiple points within the graft. The findings of concern are a peak velocity ratio of greater than 3, called a "step-up," and a velocity at any location greater than 250 cm/sec or less than 40 cm/sec. The caveats are that at the proximal anastomosis, the velocity may be elevated in the case of a small graft going into a large artery and that in very distal vessels (the dorsalis pedis artery or distal posterior tibial artery), velocities can be less than 40 cm/sec and still support a graft indefinitely. If there is concern, we would proceed to angiogram, and if the lesion is fairly focal, we would favor angioplasty. If the lesion is extensive, we would do either a vein patch or a jump graft. It is crucial to fix these stenoses before the vein graft occludes and is filled with clot, often necessitating complete replacement. The protocol is modified for so-called high-risk

grafts, such as an arm vein, spliced vein, or sclerotic vein, or if a new abnormality is detected. In these cases, more frequent examinations may be conducted until the abnormality resolves by vessel remodeling or worsens, necessitating an angiogram. We do not favor operation based on duplex scan alone because a high-grade midgraft lesion can mask a stenosis at the distal anastomosis.

It is important to remember, however, that foot artery bypass is not the only procedure applicable to patients with diabetes. In general, the goal of treatment is to restore maximal arterial flow to the foot, since this provides the best chance for healing. The diagnostic preoperative arteriogram is the key piece of information necessary in planning an appropriate surgical procedure. If a bypass to the popliteal or proximal tibial artery will restore maximal arterial flow with palpable foot pulses, a bypass need not extend to the level of the foot. Since the quality of the venous conduit is the most important determinant of long-term success, the basic rule is to use the shortest length of high-quality venous conduit necessary to achieve this goal. Each operation must be individualized on the basis of the patient's available venous conduit and arterial anatomy as demonstrated on the preoperative arteriogram.

Successful arterial reconstruction with restoration of maximal arterial flow does not end a vascular surgeon's responsibility for the patient. Often, significant wounds and/or ulcerations may still be present on the foot. Devising an appropriate treatment plan to close the wounds and heal the foot is the ultimate goal. Until the skin envelope is intact, the patient is still susceptible to infection, even with excellent arterial circulation. The methods involved in healing open wounds and ulcerations in the diabetic foot after restoration of arterial flow are complex and extend beyond the purview of this chapter. A variety of treatment methods is used, individualized according to the patient's clinical circumstances. While many small ulcers can be left to heal by secondary intention, some might require toe or partial forefoot amputations, especially when associated with gangrene and chronic osteomyelitis. For larger wounds, split-thickness skin grafts are used when the area involved is nonweight-bearing. For patients with complex wounds of the weight-bearing surfaces, particularly the heel, or when bone or tendons need to be covered, more sophisticated plastic surgical reconstructions involving local rotational flaps and even free tissue transfers have occasionally been employed in our practice. Proper application of these procedures requires the expertise of plastic surgeons in conjunction with foot and ankle surgeons to be successfully carried out.

Intensive medical therapy including tight control of plasma glucose may result in lower rates of infection and other serious perioperative complications. A prospective, randomized, controlled study of 1548 diabetic patients receiving mechanical ventilation in a surgical intensive care unit was done.[79] The treatment group received intensive insulin therapy with their plasma glucose level maintained between 80 and 110 mg/dL, while the control group received standard insulin management. At 12 months, the mortality rate was reduced from 8% in the control group to 4.6% in those who received intensive plasma glucose control ($p = .04$). This effect was most dramatic in patients who remained in the intensive care unit for longer than 5 days, with 20% mortality for the control group versus 11% for those receiving intensive therapy ($p = .005$). The beneficial effects were also seen in the reduction of infection and sepsis, renal failure requiring dialysis, and intensive care unit stay. Although the use of this intensive insulin protocol has not been studied in patients outside of the intensive care unit, it is likely that a similar clinical effect would be seen in diabetic patients undergoing lower-limb arterial reconstruction, in which the incidence of wound infection can range as high as 40%. At our institution, we are currently randomizing patients undergoing major vascular surgery to a similar intensive versus standard insulin management.

In addition to maintaining very strict plasma glucose control, our perioperative management plan includes the following measures designed to decrease cardiac and neurovascular complications and improve early graft patency:

- In the absence of contraindications, all patients, if not currently taking them, are started on atorvastatin, aspirin, and a β-blocker.
- Statin dosing is generally optimized as an outpatient.
- Aspirin, 325 mg, is given daily unless the patient is taking other anticoagulants, in which case the dose is reduced to 81 mg daily.
- Subcutaneous unfractionated heparin is administered every 8 hours until discharge.
- β-blockers are initiated preoperatively, with the goal of reducing heart rates to less than 70 preoperatively and less than 80 postoperatively.
- Hematocrit is kept above 26%.
- Intravenous fluid replacement is limited, and fluid overload is rapidly treated with intravenous diuretics.
- Patients are transferred to a special monitored "stepdown" nursing unit for 48 hours after surgery. This unit can accept patients with pulmonary artery catheters and radial arterial lines, which are used liberally, especially in patients with known uncorrected ischemic cardiovascular disease, a history of congestive heart failure, depressed myocardial function, and chronic renal failure.

Arterial Bypass in Young Type 1 Diabetic Patients

Young patients with type 1 diabetes mellitus may develop ischemic foot complications from premature atherosclerosis. In contradistinction to older patients, atherosclerosis in this group is rapidly progressive and associated with a worse prognosis.[1,4–10] When younger patients undergo revascularization they have been found to be at increased risk for perioperative complications,[1] have an increased rate of multiple revascularization procedures, and have more frequent progression to amputation. All patients under 40 years of age undergoing infrainguinal revascularization at our institution from 1990 to 2000, were reviewed. Fifty-one patients who underwent 76 lower-limb revascularizations were identified. Type 1 diabetes mellitus was very prevalent, afflicting over 94%. During the follow-up period, 11.8% of patients required additional ipsilateral revascularization, 31.3% needed a contralateral bypass graft, and a major amputation was ultimately necessary in 23.5%. The success rate for secondary procedures was marginal when compared to those of the primary procedures. The primary patency rate, secondary patency rate, and limb salvage rates were 66.7%, 62.5%, and 77.8%, respectively, at 1 year and 44.4%, 41.7%, and 64.8%, respectively, at 5 years. The long-term survival rate was 75% at 5 years.[80] The results were inferior to those of our older patients in whom the graft patency and limb salvage rates approach 70% and 80%, respectively, at 5 years. The worse outcomes might be due to a more aggressive and rapidly progressive form of atherosclerosis or might be consequent to the relatively high incidence of dialysis-dependent renal failure in these patients. As in most patients on chronic hemodialysis, the observed results were inferior to those in more "typical" patients, and attempts to salvage failed reconstructions were rarely successful. These facts must be discussed frankly with the patient prior to initiating therapy, and treatment must be individualized on the basis of the clinical situation, with the realization that for some patients, amputation might be the best initial treatment.

Endovascular Therapy

Vein bypass grafts for critical lower-limb ischemia are considered the gold standard based on their safety and efficacy. Perioperative mortality in contemporary series ranges from 1% to 5% and limb salvage approaches 80% at 5 years for many patients. Although these results are excellent, they do not reflect the high cost of recovery required for many patients who achieve this outcome. Wound morbidity is common, ranging from 10% to 40%. Limb swelling, delayed healing of ischemic wounds, and the need for further procedures may delay full recovery for many months. Early graft thrombosis, while uncommon, often results in amputation even with subsequent attempts to salvage the graft. For patients with inadequate saphenous veins requiring alternative vein conduits, bypass procedures are technically more difficult and have worse outcomes. In a study evaluating quality-of-life measures in our patients undergoing arterial bypass for limb salvage, fewer than 50% reported feeling that they were back to normal 6 months after surgery. In a similar study, only 15% of patients achieved the "ideal" outcome of a patent graft with no need for revision, no wound complications, and a healed foot following bypass.[81] These observations are especially sobering when we consider the fact that 50% of patients survive less than 5 years after their limb salvage procedure.

It is in this context that endoluminal therapies have been proposed for diabetic patients with critical limb ischemia. In the past, this treatment was limited mostly to angioplasty and stenting of iliac arteries to improve arterial inflow in preparation for a more distal bypass. The development of small-diameter balloons, stents, and steerable guidewires has made tibial and pedal angioplasty feasible, with a high likelihood of early technical success. Several authors have reported remarkably good immediate and short-term results, although most report a heterogeneous patient population with only small numbers of diabetic patients. In the best-reported series, technical success was achieved in 90% with limb salvage at 1 year of 80% to 90%. The likelihood of technical success is dependent on the extent of the occlusive lesions. In our own unpublished results of 105 tibial angioplasties, technical success was 100% for short, focal stenoses but decreased to 75% for long occlusions. The patency rate at 1 year was only 40%, but the limb salvage rate was 75%.

Only one randomized, multicenter, prospective trial has compared angioplasty to bypass for critical limb ischemia. At 2 years' follow-up, mortality, limb salvage, and survival rates were identical. Although the costs for bypass were higher, the angioplasty group required reintervention more frequently. Surprisingly, functional outcomes and quality-of-life measures were identical for both groups. In a post hoc analysis of patients who survived beyond 2 years, limb salvage and survival rates were higher for patients who underwent bypass. In spite of its shortcomings, the BASIL study validates the use of tibial angioplasty for critical limb ischemia, especially for patients with strong contraindications to surgery or anesthesia and with an anticipated life expectancy of less than 2 years.[82] For healthier patients with available venous conduit, primary bypass remains the best option, owing to less need for intervention and better long-term limb salvage and survival.

Summary

This chapter has reviewed the principles of evaluation, diagnosis, and treatment of arterial disease in patients with lower-limb ischemia in diabetes mellitus. Rejection of the small vessel hypothesis coupled with an understanding of the unique pattern of atherosclerotic occlusive disease in the lower limbs of patients with diabetes is key to effecting proper treatment. Recognizing the interplay of neuropathy and infection with ischemia and providing proper treatment for them as well as for arterial insufficiency are essential to ultimate success. A thorough understanding of the pathophysiology of ischemia and a carefully planned approach, including the prompt control of infection when present, a high-quality digital subtraction arteriogram, and distal arterial reconstruction or a catheter-based intervention to maximize foot perfusion, should lead to rates of limb salvage in patients with diabetes that equal or exceed those achieved in nondiabetic patients with lower-limb ischemia.

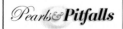

Pearls

1. In the presence of ischemia with tissue loss, restore pulsatile flow to the foot whenever possible.
2. Drain foot infections as soon as identified. This might require open toe or ray amputations involving several trips to the operating suite.
3. Increasing insulin requirements might be the only sign of a major foot infection, and return to normal plasma glucose levels is a key factor in determining when infection has been controlled.
4. Lack of a palpable foot pulse is abnormal regardless of how "good" the Doppler sounds are.
5. A policy of using only autogenous bypass grafts with ultrasound graft surveillance will provide the best results.

Pitfalls

1. A typical neuropathic location of an ulcer alone does not preclude ischemia as a major contributor.
2. Drain infections before revascularization, but do not debride dry eschars until revascularization has been completed.
3. Ankle-brachial indices can be falsely elevated or normal even in severe ischemia.
4. Ischemic wounds or ulcers will not granulate with wound care alone, whereas well-drained and vascularized ones may.
5. Revascularization is a crucial component of foot salvage, but the responsibility of the vascular surgeon does not end until the foot is healed.

References

1. Gibbons GW, Eliopoulos GM: Infection of the diabetic foot. In Kozak G (ed): Management of Diabetic Foot Problems. Philadelphia: WB Saunders, 1984.
2. Edmonds ME: The diabetic foot: pathophysiology and treatment. Clin Endocrinol Metab 15:889–916, 1986.
3. Grunfeld C: Diabetic foot ulcers: Etiology, treatment, and prevention. Adv Intern Med 37:103–32, 1992.
4. Levin M: The diabetic foot: Pathophysiology, evaluation and treatment. In Levin ME, O'Neal LW (eds): The Diabetic Foot. 2nd ed. St. Louis: Mosby Year Book, 1977.
5. Tannenbaum GA, Pomposelli FB Jr, Marcaccio EJ, et al: Safety of vein bypass grafting to the dorsal pedal artery in diabetic patients with foot infections. J Vasc Surg 15:982–988; discussion 989–990, 1992.
6. Goldenberg S, Alex M, Joshi RA, Blumenthal HT: Nonatheromatous peripheral vascular disease of the lower extremity in diabetes mellitus. Diabetes 8:261–273, 1959.

7. Barner HB, Kaiser GC, Willman VL: Blood flow in the diabetic leg. Circulation 43:391–394, 1971.
8. Conrad MC: Large and small artery occlusion in diabetics and nondiabetics with severe vascular disease. Circulation 36:83–91, 1967.
9. Irwin ST, Gilmore J, McGrann S, et al: Blood flow in diabetics with foot lesions due to "small vessel disease." Br J Surg 75:1201120–6, 1988.
10. LoGerfo FW, Coffman JD: Current concepts. Vascular and microvascular disease of the foot in diabetes: Implications for foot care. N Engl J Med 311:1615–1619, 1984.
11. Strandness DE PR, Gibbons GE: Combined clinical and pathological study of diabetic and nondiabetic peripheral arterial disease. Diabetes 13:366–372, 1964.
12. Kannel WB, McGee DL: Diabetes and cardiovascular disease: The Framingham study. JAMA 241:2035–2038, 1979.
13. Smith JW, Marcus FI, Serokman R: Prognosis of patients with diabetes mellitus after acute myocardial infarction. Am J Cardiol 54:718–721, 1984.
14. Petersen CM: Influence of diabetes on vascular disease and its complications. In Moore WS (ed): Vascular Surgery: A Comprehensive Review, 5th ed. Philadelphia: WB Saunders, 1998.
15. Zarich S, Waxman S, Freeman RT, et al: Effect of autonomic nervous system dysfunction on the circadian pattern of myocardial ischemia in diabetes mellitus [see comments]. J Am Coll Cardiol 24:956–962, 1994.
16. Lee TH, Marcantonio ER, Mangione CM, et al: Derivation and prospective validation of a simple index for prediction of cardiac risk of major noncardiac surgery. Circulation 100:1043–1049, 1999.
17. Eagle KA, Coley CM, Newell JB, et al: Combining clinical and thallium data optimizes preoperative assessment of cardiac risk before major vascular surgery. Ann Intern Med 110:859–866, 1989.
18. Hamdan AD, Saltzberg SS, Sheahan M, et al: Lack of association of diabetes with increased post-operative mortality and cardiac morbidity: results of 6565 major vascular operations. Arch Surg 137:417–421, 2002.
19. Akbari CM, Pomposelli FB Jr, Gibbons GW, et al: Lower extremity revascularization in diabetes: Late observations. Arch Surg 135:452–6, 2000.
20. Grayson ML, Gibbons GW, Habershaw GM, et al: Use of ampicillin/sulbactam versus imipenem/cilastatin in the treatment of limb-threatening foot infections in diabetic patients [published erratum appears in Clin Infect Dis 19:820, 1994]. Clin Infect Dis 18:683–693, 1994.
21. Gibbons GW: The diabetic foot: amputations and drainage of infection. J Vasc Surg 5:791–793, 1987.
22. Pomposelli FB Jr, Marcaccio EJ, Gibbons GW, et al: Dorsalis pedis arterial bypass: Durable limb salvage for foot ischemia in patients with diabetes mellitus. J Vasc Surg 21:375–384, 1995.
23. Pomposelli FB, Jr, Arora S, Gibbons GW, et al: Lower extremity arterial reconstruction in the very elderly: Successful outcome preserves not only the limb but also residential status and ambulatory function. J Vasc Surg 28:215–225, 1998.
24. Nesto RW: Screening for asymptomatic coronary artery disease in diabetes [editorial; comment]. Diabetes Care 22:1393–1395, 1999.
25. Zarich SW, Cohen MC, Lane SE, et al: Routine perioperative dipyridamole 201Tl imaging in diabetic patients undergoing vascular surgery. Diabetes Care 19:355–360, 1996.
26. Monahan TS, Shrikhande GV, Pomposelli FB, et al: Pre-operative cardiac evaluation does not improve or predict peri-operative or late survival in asymptomatic diabetic patients undergoing elective infrainguinal arterial reconstruction. J Vasc Surg 41:38–45; discussion 45, 2005.
27. Bode RH Jr, Lewis KP, Zarich SW, et al: Cardiac outcome after peripheral vascular surgery: Comparison of general and regional anesthesia [see comments]. Anesthesiology 84:3–13, 1996.
28. Pierce ET, Pomposelli FB Jr, Stanley GD, et al: Anesthesia type does not influence early graft patency or limb salvage rates of lower extremity arterial bypass. J Vasc Surg 25:226–232; discussion 232–233, 1997.
29. Carpenter JP, Baum RA, Holland GA, Barker CF: Peripheral vascular surgery with magnetic resonance angiography as the sole preoperative imaging modality. J Vasc Surg 20:861–869; discussion 869–871, 1994.
30. Lumsden AB, Besman A, Jaffe M, et al: Infrainguinal revascularization in end-stage renal disease. Ann Vasc Surg 8:107–112, 1994.
31. Carsten CG 3rd, Taylor SM, Langan EM 3rd, Crane MM: Factors associated with limb loss despite a patent infrainguinal bypass graft. Am Surg 64:33–37; discussion 37–38, 1998.
32. Johnson BL, Glickman MH, Bandyk DF, Esses GE: Failure of foot salvage in patients with end-stage renal disease after surgical revascularization. J Vasc Surg 22:280–285; discussion 285–286, 1995.
33. Korn P, Hoenig SJ, Skillman JJ, Kent KC: Is lower extremity revascularization worthwhile in patients with end-stage renal disease? Surgery 128:472–479, 2000.
34. Ramdev P, Rayan SS, Sheahan M, et al: A decade experience with infrainguinal revascularization in a dialysis-dependent patient population. J Vasc Surg 36:969–974, 2002.
35. Aulivola B, Hile CN, Hamdan AD, et al: Major lower extremity amputation: Outcome of modern series. Arch Surg 139:395–399; discussion 399, 2004.
36. Dormandy J, Heeck L, Vig S: The natural history of claudication: risk to life and limb. Semin Vasc Surg 12:123–137, 1999.
37. McDermott MM, McCarthy W: Intermittent claudication: The natural history. Surg Clin North Am 75:581–591, 1995.
38. Hertzer NR: The natural history of peripheral vascular disease: Implications for its management. Circulation 83:I12–I19, 1991.
39. Dawson DL, Cutler BS, Hiatt WR, et al: A comparison of cilostazol and pentoxifylline for treating intermittent claudication. Am J Med 109:523–530, 2000.
40. Dawson DL, Cutler BS, Meissner MH, Strandness DE Jr: Cilostazol has beneficial effects in treatment of intermittent claudication: Results from a multicenter, randomized, prospective, double-blind trial. Circulation 98:678–686, 1998.
41. Gillings DB: Pentoxifylline and intermittent claudication: Review of clinical trials and cost-effectiveness analyses. J Cardiovasc Pharmacol 25:S44–S50, 1995.
42. Gahtan V: The noninvasive vascular laboratory. Surg Clin North Am 78:507–518, 1998.
43. Raines J, Traad E: Noninvasive evaluation of peripheral vascular disease. Med Clin North Am 64:283–304, 1980.
44. Weitz JI, Byrne J, Claggett GP, et al: Diagnosis and treatment of chronic arterial insufficiency of the lower extremities: A critical review [published erratum appears in Circulation 29;102:1074, 2000]. Circulation 94:3026–3049, 1996.
45. White RA, Nolan L, Harley D, et al: Noninvasive evaluation of peripheral vascular disease using transcutaneous oxygen tension. Am J Surg 144:68–75, 1982.
46. Hauser CJ, Klein SR, Mehringer CM, et al: Superiority of transcutaneous oximetry in noninvasive vascular diagnosis in patients with diabetes. Arch Surg 119:690–694, 1984 .
47. Bandyk DF, Seabrook GR, Moldenhauer P, et al: Hemodynamics of vein graft stenosis. J Vasc Surg 8:688–695, 1988.
48. Cohen JR, Mannick JA, Couch NP, Whittemore AD: Recognition and management of impending vein-graft failure: Importance for long-term patency. Arch Surg 121:758–759, 1986.
49. Blakeman BM, Littooy FN, Baker WH: Intra-arterial digital subtraction angiography as a method to study peripheral vascular disease. J Vasc Surg 4:168–173, 1986.
50. Merten GJ, Burgess WP, Gray LV, et al: Prevention of contrast-induced nephropathy with sodium bicarbonate. JAMA 29119):2328–2334, 2004.
51. Birck R, Krzossk S, Markowitz F, et al: Acetylcysteine for prevention of contrast nephropathy: Meta-analysis. Lancet 362:598–603, 2003.
52. Veith FJ, Gupta SK, Ascer E, et al: Six-year prospective multicenter randomized comparison of autologous saphenous vein and expanded polytetrafluoroethylene grafts in infrainguinal arterial reconstructions. J Vasc Surg 3:104–114, 1986.
53. Kunlin J: Le traitement de l'arterite obliterante par la greffe veinuse: Arch Mal Coeur Vaiss 42:371, 1949.
54. Leather RP, Powers SR, Karmody AM: A reappraisal of the in situ saphenous vein arterial bypass: Its use in limb salvage. Surgery 86:453–461, 1979.
55. Buchbinder D, Rolins DL, Verta MJ, et al: Early experience with in situ saphenous vein bypass for distal arterial reconstruction. Surgery 99:350–357, 1986.
56. Hurley JJ, Auer AI, Binnington HB, et al: Comparison of initial limb salvage in 98 consecutive patients with either reversed autogenous or in situ vein bypass graft procedures. Am J Surg 150:777–781, 1985.
57. Strayhorn EC, Wohlgemuth S, Deuel M, et al: Early experience utilizing the in situ saphenous vein technique in 54 patients. J Cardiovasc Surg (Torino) 29:161–165, 1988.

58. Bush HL Jr, Corey CA, Nabseth DC: Distal in situ saphenous vein grafts for limb salvage. Increased operative blood flow and postoperative patency. Am J Surg 145:542–548, 1983.

59. Cambria RP, Megerman J, Brewster DC, et al: The evolution of morphologic and biomechanical changes in reversed and in-situ vein grafts. Ann Surg 205:167–174, 1987.

60. Taylor LM Jr, Edwards JM, Porter JM: Present status of reversed vein bypass grafting: Five-year results of a modern series. J Vasc Surg 11:193–205; discussion 205–206, 1990.

61. Pomposelli FB Jr, Jepsen SJ, Gibbons GW, et al: A flexible approach to infrapopliteal vein grafts in patients with diabetes mellitus. Arch Surg 126:724–727; discussion 727–729, 1991.

62. Ascer E, Veith FJ, Gupta SK, et al: Short vein grafts: A superior option for arterial reconstructions to poor or compromised outflow tracts? J Vasc Surg 7:370–378, 1988.

63. Cantelmo NL, Snow JR, Menzoian JO, LoGerfo FW: Successful vein bypass in patients with an ischemic limb and a palpable popliteal pulse. Arch Surg 121:217–220, 1986.

64. Stonebridge PA, Tsoukas AI, Pomposelli FB Jr, et al: Popliteal-to-distal bypass grafts for limb salvage in diabetics. Eur J Vasc Surg 5:265–269, 1991.

65. Holzenbein TJ, Pomposelli FB Jr, Miller A, et al: Results of a policy with arm veins used as the first alternative to an unavailable ipsilateral greater saphenous vein for infrainguinal bypass. J Vasc Surg 23:130–140, 1996.

66. Miller A, Campbell DR, Gibbons GW, et al: Routine intraoperative angioscopy in lower extremity revascularization. Arch Surg 124:604–8, 1989.

67. Stonebridge PA, Miller A, Tsoukas A, et al: Angioscopy of arm vein infrainguinal bypass grafts. Ann Vasc Surg 5:170–175, 1991.

68. Balshi JD, Cantelmo NL, Menzoian JO, LoGerfo FW: The use of arm veins for infrainguinal bypass in end-stage peripheral vascular disease. Arch Surg 124:1078–1081, 1989.

69. Faries PL, Arora S, Pomposelli FB Jr, et al: The use of arm vein in lower-extremity revascularization: Results of 520 procedures performed in eight years. J Vasc Surg 31:50–59, 2000.

70. Pomposelli FB Jr, Jepsen SJ, Gibbons GW, et al: Efficacy of the dorsal pedal bypass for limb salvage in diabetic patients: Short-term observations [see comments]. J Vasc Surg 11:745–751; discussion 751–752, 1990.

71. Pomposelli FB, Kansal N, Hamdan AD, et al: A decade of experience with dorsalis pedis artery bypass: Analysis of outcome in more than 1000 cases. J Vasc Surg 37:307–315, 2003.

72. Andros G, Harris RW, Salles-Cunha SX, et al: Bypass grafts to the ankle and foot. J Vasc Surg 7:785–794, 1988.

73. Darling RC 3rd, Chang BB, Shah DM, Leather RP: Choice of peroneal or dorsalis pedis artery bypass for limb salvage. Semin Vasc Surg 10:17–22, 1997.

74. Levine AW, Davis RC, Gingery RO, Anderegg DD: In situ bypass to the dorsalis pedis and tibial arteries at the ankle. Ann Vasc Surg 3:205–209, 1989.

75. Shanik DG, Auer AI, Hershey FB: Vein bypass to the dorsalis pedis artery for limb ischemia. Ir Med J 75:54–56, 1982.

76. Shieber W, Parks C: Dorsalis pedis artery in bypass grafting. Am J Surg 128:752–755, 1974.

77. Hughes K, Domenig CM, Hamdan AD, et al: Bypass to plantar and tarsal arteries: An acceptable approach to limb salvage. J Vasc Surg 40:1149–1157, 2004.

78. LoGerfo FW, Gibbons GW, Pomposelli FB Jr, et al: Trends in the care of the diabetic foot: Expanded role of arterial reconstruction. Arch Surg 127:617–620; discussion 620–621, 1992.

79. Van den Berge G, Wouters P, Weekers F, et al: Intensive insulin therapy in critically ill patients. N Engl J Med 345:1359–1367, 2001.

80. Saltzberg SS, Pomposelli FB, Belfield AK, et al: Outcome of lower extremity revascularization in patients younger than 40 years in a predominantly diabetic population. J Vasc Surg 38:1056–1059, 2003.

81. Nicoloff AD, Taylor LM, McLafferty RB, et al: Patient recovery after infrainguinal bypass grafting for limb salvage. J Vasc Surg 27:256–263; discussion 264–266, 1998.

82. BASIL trial participants: Bypass versus angioplasty in severe ischaemia of the leg (BASIL): Multicentre, randomised controlled trial. Lancet 366:1925–1934, 2005.

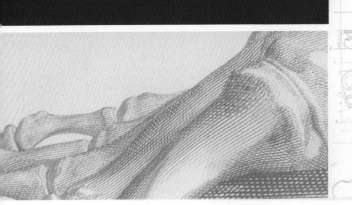

PLASTIC SURGICAL RECONSTRUCTION OF THE DIABETIC FOOT

JEFFREY M. PITCHER AND WILLIAM A. WOODEN ■

The field of plastic and reconstructive surgery emphasizes, as its primary goal, the restoration of form and function. The diabetic patient represents a significant challenge to the medical profession because of the progressive, unrelenting impact that diabetes mellitus has on the body as a whole. When the impact of diabetes mellitus on the lower limb is specifically addressed, the fight is certainly one of limb salvage. The plastic surgeon is often faced with difficult wound-healing challenges that require intricate reconstructive solutions that are complicated by the relentless physiologic impact of diabetes mellitus. As a result, the field has developed an extensive understanding of wound healing from metabolic and surgical standpoints and can provide significant support in the team management of the diabetic patient.

The human foot is composed of very complex and interdependent structures that support the body during standing, climbing, and ambulation. The foot's unique weight-bearing property as well as its necessary sensibility enables ambulation. Anatomically, the foot is similar to the hand; however, the foot is under a significantly greater mechanical load, which must be accounted for in assessing and planning functional reconstruction. The ability of the foot to support these significant forces depends on the unique and intricate anatomic interaction that exists between the soft tissue envelope, the musculotendinous structures, and the bony support of the foot. When breakdown or destruction of any of these

structures occurs, significant disability results. Approximately 20% of all hospitalized diabetic patients are admitted with foot-related problems.[1] Similarly, between 50% and 80% of lower-limb amputations are performed in the diabetic population.[2] Obviously, the most efficacious and cost-effective long-term management of the diabetic foot should involve ulcer prevention. Evidence indicates that four significant factors are responsible for diabetic foot ulceration: (1) poor blood supply secondary to infrapopliteal vascular disease present within the lower limb, (2) pressure points on the plantar surface secondary to orthopedic deformities (e.g., Charcot joint deformity) with or without concomitant hyperkeratosis at points of chronic trauma (Fig. 22-1), (3) neuropathic conditions resulting in decreased sensibility leading to repeated unrecognized foot trauma (Fig. 22-2), and (4) poor plasma glucose control, which may allow rapid progression of cellulitis or soft tissue infection (Fig. 22-3).

Prevention of foot ulceration may be addressed in four specific categories: (1) prevention of and vigilant attention to early signs of skin breakdown, pressure, or hyperkeratosis, particularly on the plantar and lateral aspects of the foot; (2) absolute glucose control; (3) optimization of macrovascular blood flow in the infrapopliteal region with appropriate medical treatment (i.e., alteration of red cell fluidity with pentoxyphylline) and perhaps surgical treatment of atherosclerotic occlusive disease; and (4) decompression of pedal sensory nerves in properly selected candidates to improve plantar sensation.

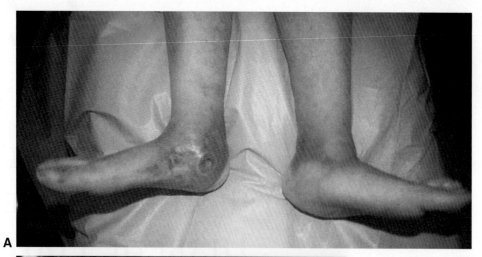

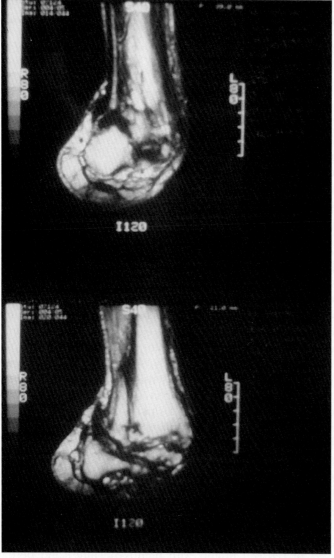

Figure 22–1 **A,** Example of Charcot deformity of the right and left ankles resulting from severe, progressive neuropathic changes and repetitive trauma. **B,** Magnetic resonance imaging scan of patient's right foot and ankle showing advanced radiographic changes.

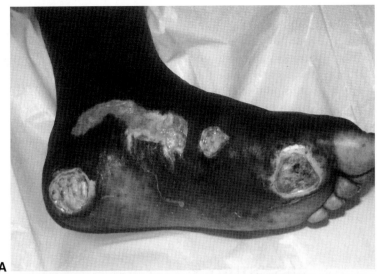

Figure 22-2 **A,** Classic example of neurotrophic ulcer formation at the heel, medial arch, and first metatarsal with hammertoe deformity and early Charcot changes. **B,** Neurotrophic ulcer overlying the fifth metatarsal head with chronic epidermal and dermal changes and necrotic base.

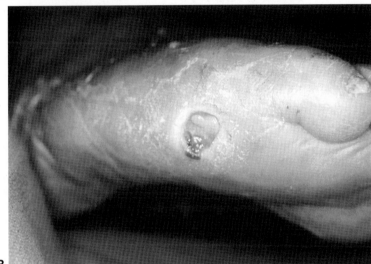

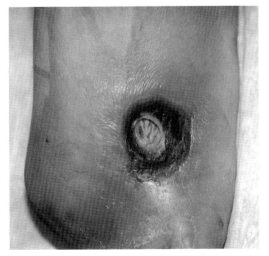

Figure 22-3 Necrotic dorsal foot wound in an insulin-dependent diabetic patient with surrounding necrosis, cellulitis, and necrotic wound base. Tissue cultures revealed both a polymicrobial flora and *Aspergillus*.

To be maximally effective and to ensure patient compliance, prevention mandates education of both patients and physicians about the importance of a multidisciplinary strategy.

Despite the most comprehensive and aggressive modes of prevention, either primary or secondary ulceration of the foot will be encountered. In these instances, plastic surgical reconstruction of the skin surface might be necessary and can be divided into distinct treatment categories. First, wound care basics, which are not particularly different for the diabetic foot ulcer than for the nondiabetic patient, must be instituted (Table 22-1). Thereafter, skin grafts, limited amputation, or local flaps can be used for discrete areas that do not heal primarily. For larger or more difficult locations, more anatomically distant rotational flaps or free tissue transfer might be necessary to provide adequate coverage. Ultimately, the goal of all reconstruction is to provide the opportunity for painless bipedal ambulation.

TABLE 22-1   Minimal Clinical Assessment

General
    Complete history
    Complete physical
Wound specific
    Infection
        Tissue culture–specific treatment
    Vascularity
        Need for revascularization
    Oxygenation
        Need for revascularization
        Need for hyperbaric oxygen therapy
    Metabolic assessment
        Glucose control
        Nutritional assessment
        Other factors (e.g., hypothyroidism)
    Need for surgical treatment
        Debridement
        Revascularization
        Flap reconstruction
        Amputation
    Orthotic or orthopedic
        Unloading of the wound
    Dressing
        Wound specific

When a clinician is faced with a new ulceration in the diabetic foot, several questions need to be initially addressed, such as: What is the foot's neuralgic and vascular status? This requires evaluation of sensory and motor function as well as both arterial and venous systems, because compromise in either system could be partially or solely responsible for foot ulceration. Arterial pulse examination, although necessary, is notoriously inconsistent for predicting wound healing if used as the sole modality of evaluation. Likewise, the ankle-brachial indices are also frequently misleading, as 30% of diabetic patients have noncompressible arterial walls, which falsely elevate results.[3] Therefore, noninvasive Doppler duplex scanning or arterial angiography and more recently magnetic resonant imaging angiography is often needed to elucidate specific flow abnormalities and anatomic lesions in the lower limb. These studies are key to planning and assessing the viability of reconstruction and salvage of the affected limb. Although each study is more reliable for predicting the likelihood of wound healing than is pulse examination, neither study is an absolute indicator of success or failure. Transcutaneous oxygen mapping has also been used as a parameter of healing. $TcPO_2$ readings of 25 mm Hg or less indicate wounds that are much less likely to heal,[4] whereas $TcPO_2$ less than 10 mm Hg equates to frank ischemia.[1] Duplex evaluation of the foot's venous drainage can also be useful in identifying patients with concomitant venous hypertension; however, this information is no absolute predictor for outcome. Early vascular assessment should be made before wide debridement of the wound to assess the likelihood of healing. If foot vascularity is poor, amputation need not be the only treatment alternative; vascular reconstructive efforts should be exhausted first. Since expeditious return to ambulation is the goal, only evidence of failed arterial reconstruction, nonrecon-

structible bypasses, gangrenous lesions, or significant soft tissue necrosis from infection should overwhelmingly prohibit salvage of the foot or any portion thereof. Other factors such as the patient's overall health, the neuralgic status of the limb, the patient's home and environmental status, and the patient's acceptance of the cost and risk of reconstructive surgery versus amputation must be considered. Revascularization should also be considered to ensure survival of a foot that is reconstructed with any of the options: skin grafts, local flaps, or free tissue transfer. It is important to understand and monitor for segmental ischemia. In diabetic patients with disease distal to the infrapopliteal region, lower-limb revascularization might not ensure survival of the leg or the entirety of the foot.

CASE STUDY 1

Figures 22-4A and 22-4B demonstrate the difficulty of wound management and the importance of revascularization. The patient is a middle-aged, insulin-dependent diabetic female who presented with a dorsal lateral foot wound. On initial assessment, she was thought to have reasonable vascularity to the foot and leg. The wound was treated with debridement, culture-specific antibiotics, and local wound care. The wound improved and was thought to be suitable for split-thickness skin grafting, which was done and failed. The patient was then referred to plastic surgery for reassessment. More detailed investigation revealed that the patient's arterial inflow was inadequate, and she subsequently underwent revascularization. This procedure restored flow to her foot, but note in Figure 22-4 that she still exhibited poor healing of her bypass incisions. Ultimately, the patient did well, but the scenario demonstrates the importance of a complete vascular evaluation in all diabetic patients, even if the wound seems minor.

Wound Management

The basic principles of wound management in the diabetic foot are not dissimilar to those in the nondiabetic foot. These include detailed wound evaluation of not only skin and soft tissue structures but also of the bony elements. Both neurologic function and vascular status of the foot must be thoroughly catalogued; then the full wound evaluation is put in the context of the patient's overall condition and performance status. All of these factors determine not only the patient's initial wound-healing performance, but also his or her ultimate outcome, and thereby dictate treatment planning.

For individuals with obvious cellulitis, elevation of the foot and appropriate tissue culture–directed antibiotic therapy are mandatory. For patients with suspected cavities of loculated infected materials, aggressive exploration, drainage, and requisite debridement of all necrotic debris are performed (Fig. 22-5). Often, the diabetic patient masquerades gross purulence and necrosis within

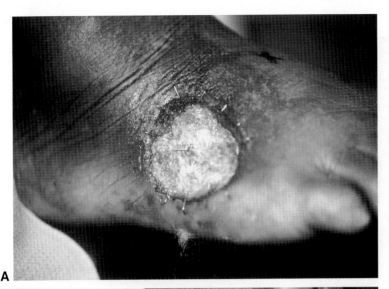

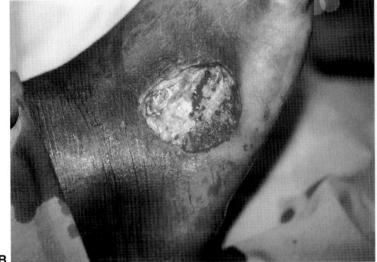

Figure 22–4   A, Failed initial skin graft prior to revascularization. **B,** Same wound following debridement at time of revascularization. Note the well-perfused wound base.

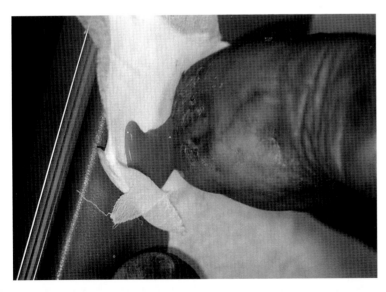

Figure 22–5   Small heel ulcer in an insulin-dependent diabetic patient with minimal clinical symptomatology but advanced plantar abscess and gross purulent drainage.

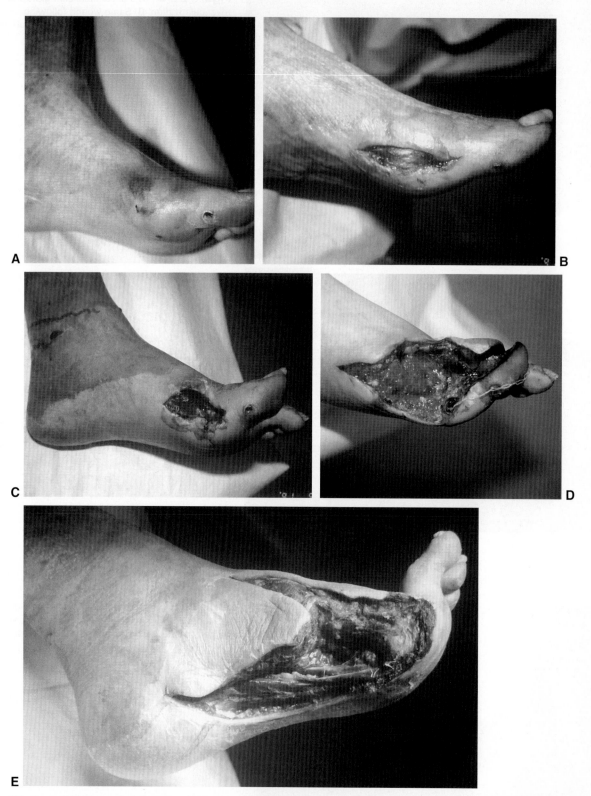

Figure 22–6   **A,** Middle-aged white male with long-standing insulin-dependent diabetes mellitus presenting with a small trophic ulcer over the first metatarsal head and signs of early infection surrounding the metatarsal head presenting for incision and drainage. **B,** Initial incision and drainage identifying involvement of the first metatarsal phalangeal joint and surrounding soft tissues. **C,** Progressive necrosis despite aggressive antibiotic therapy and debridement. **D,** Continued necrosis despite bony resection and systemic antibiotic therapy and serial debridement. **E,** Continued necrosis as a result of poor perfusion and hypovascularity.

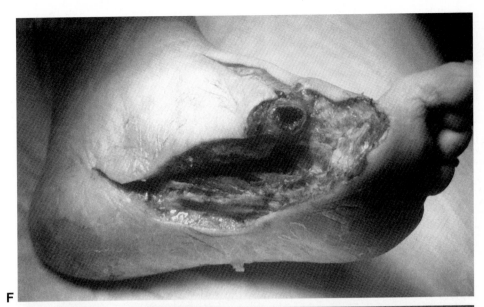

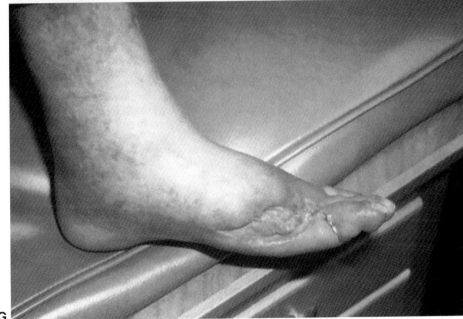

Figure 22-6, cont'd **F,** Early signs of wound stabilization. **G,** Healed wound following continued local wound care and subsequent split-thickness skin graft.

the deeper spaces of the foot; therefore, a high index of suspicion should be present in the early evaluation to prevent significant and often rapid progression of an infectious process. Sometimes, aspiration with an 18-gauge needle can unveil a subfascial abscess.[3] Following the drainage of purulent material and debridement of necrotic tissue, open wound packing with whirlpool or pulse irrigation lavage can facilitate clearing of the infection. Multiple debridements as well as amputations might be necessary prior to entertaining wound coverage options (Fig. 22-6). Of particular note, debridement of devitalized osteomyelitic bone segments might also be necessary. Accurate diagnosis of true osteomyelitis is frequently difficult in these situations, as surrounding soft tissues might be heavily contaminated.

Soft Tissue Reconstruction

Within plastic surgical literature, foot reconstruction has been classified according to a number of criteria. One of the more prevalent schemas is to divide the foot into anatomic areas for reconstruction.[5] The four regions that are most commonly described are (1) the heel and the midplantar region (Fig. 22-7); (2) the distal plantar region (Fig. 22-8); (3) the malleolar, Achilles tendon, and non-weight-bearing posterior heel area (Fig. 22-9); and (4) the dorsum (Fig. 22-10). The needs of each region vary and therefore dictate specific solutions to satisfy coverage needs.

The weight-bearing plantar surface is without question the most challenging area, as it ideally requires a

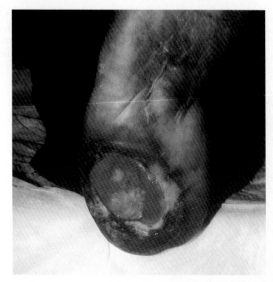

Figure 22–7   Classic long-standing trophic heel ulcer with neuropathic, Charcot changes.

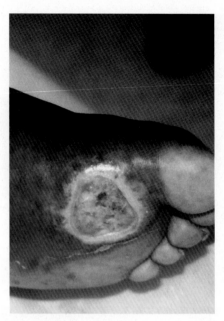

Figure 22–8   Classic neuropathic changes and first metatarsal head ulceration.

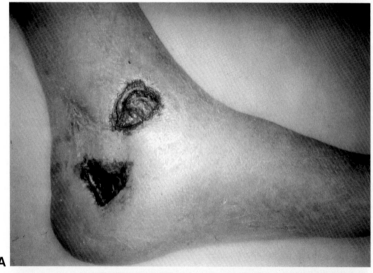

Figure 22–9   **A,** Subacute medial malleolus and ankle wounds of long-standing duration. **B,** Acute lateral malleolus and dorsal foot wound secondary to minor trauma and secondary infection.

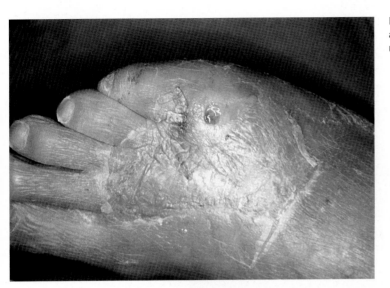

Figure 22–10 Dorsal foot ulceration secondary to and associated with deep infection of the fifth toe and metatarsophalangeal joint.

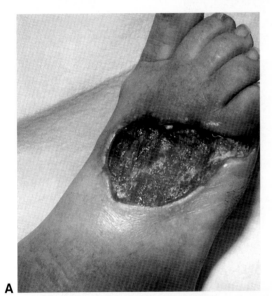

A

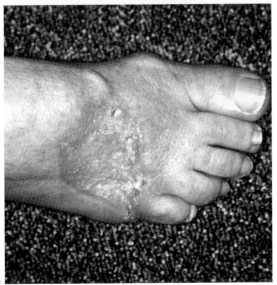

B

Figure 22–11 A, Complex dorsal foot wound following serial debridement, antibiotic therapy, and local wound care. **B,** Healed wound following split-thickness skin graft.

sensate surface that will tolerate the trauma of weight-bearing as well as providing a stable surface for the sheer forces related to ambulation. Ideally, that stable surface should be glabrous skin, which is difficult to recruit barring the plantar surface of the foot or palm of the hand. Conversely, the dorsal foot does not require the durability of the plantar foot, and coverage need not require sensation to allow for safe ambulation. Therefore, skin grafts, either full-thickness or split-thickness, can work well in this location (Figs. 22-11 and 22-12).

Local Flaps

A number of local skin and muscle flaps are available within the foot itself, many flaps being ideal for small defects. Local flaps have been shown to a have a high success rate of defect healing, resulting in a substantial percent of patients recovering the ability to ambulate.[6] While providing like tissue for a foot defect, local flaps are limited by their arc of rotation and sometimes by the vascular anatomy of the foot. Consequently, poor arterial inflow or collateral circulation between the anterior tibial, posterior tibial, and peroneal arteries may compromise the surgeon's ability to perform any of the local flaps. In addition, they are often inadequate for larger defects. Despite the above-mentioned limitations, the following local flaps have been successfully used to close foot wounds:[3,7,8]

1. Local random flaps such as the V-Y flap or rotational skin flap
2. The medial plantar artery flap (Fig. 22-13)
3. The lateral calcaneal artery flap (Fig. 22-14)
4. The superior malleolar artery flap
5. The medial calcaneal artery flap (Fig. 22-15)
6. The extensor digitorum brevis muscle flaps off of the lateral tarsal artery (Fig. 22-16)

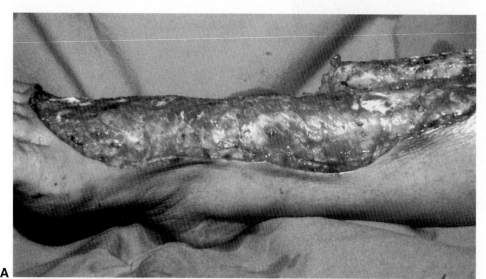

A

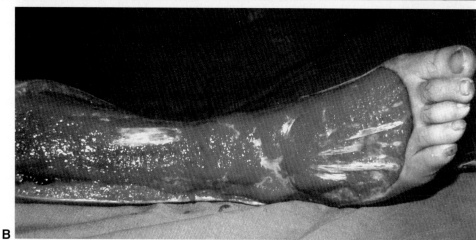

B

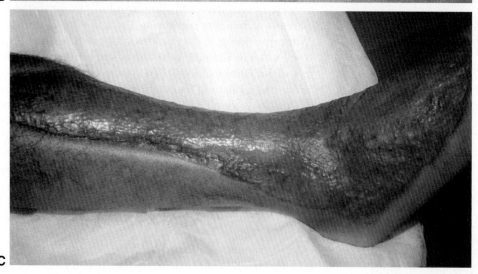

C

Figure 22–12   **A,** Complex dorsal foot and leg wound in an insulin-dependent diabetic patient following a local trauma and soft tissue infection. **B,** Same wound following antibiotics and aggressive local wound management. **C,** Wound following successful split-thickness skin grafting.

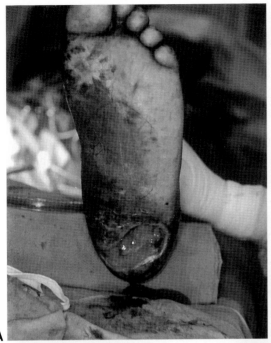

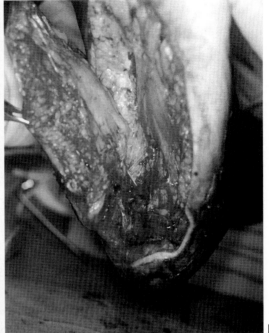

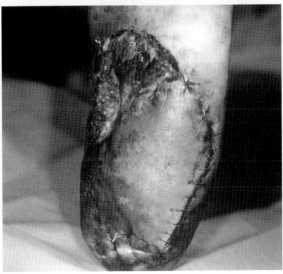

Figure 22-13   **A,** Stable but chronic heel ulcer in a long-standing insulin-dependent diabetic patient with prior first metatarsal head ulcer now healed and epithelialized for reconstruction using medial plantar artery flap and split-thickness skin grafting to the instep of foot. **B,** Medial plantar flap elevated. **C,** Flap insert with split-thickness graft to instep.

7. The abductor hallucis muscle flap
8. The abductor digiti minimi muscle flaps (lateral malleolar defects) (Fig. 22-17)
9. The flexor digiti minimi/flexor digitorum brevis muscle flaps (proximal small toe metatarsal defects) (Fig. 22-18)
10. The toe fillet flap (particularly useful in plantar defects on the weight-bearing heads of the metatarsophalangeal joints)

Free Tissue Transfer

After adequate wound debridement has been accomplished and no evidence of infection is present, free tissue transfer might be necessary for patients who have defects that are too large for skin graft or local flap coverage but who have adequate arterial inflow. Also, free tissue might be indicated for wounds with exposed tendons or bony structures or in which a durable yet pliable skin surface is otherwise not available. Free tissue transfer allows one the ability to resurface essentially any size defect in the foot. This freedom allows for aggressive resection of scarred cicatricial skin as well as infected or necrotic soft tissue when appropriate. However, free tissue transfer should be reserved for patients in whom lesser local plantar flaps or skin grafts are not suitable, as the expenditure of patient and physician time as well as the delay in ultimate unaided ambulation is greater in the free tissue transfer reconstruction than in local flap reconstruction.[9]

There are basically two types of free flap options for the foot: the fasciocutaneous flap (free radial forearm flap, free lateral arm flap, free tensor fascia latae flap)

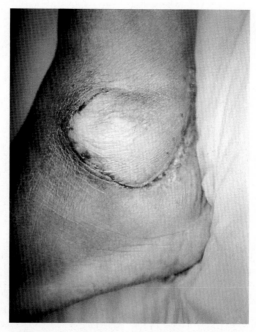

Figure 22–14   Lateral malleolar ulcer closed with rotation flap and skin graft to cover defect.

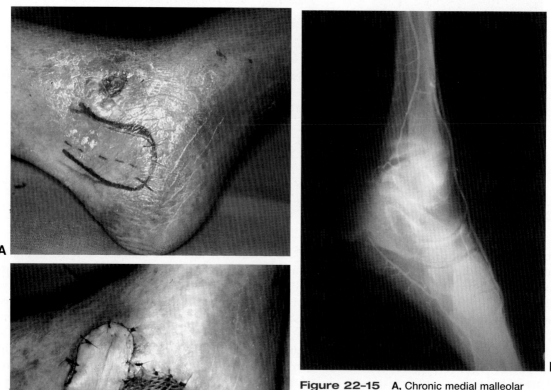

Figure 22–15   **A,** Chronic medial malleolar ulcer. **B,** Arteriogram demonstrated by medial calcaneal artery. **C,** Local flap based on medial calcaneal artery and split-thickness skin graft to donor site.

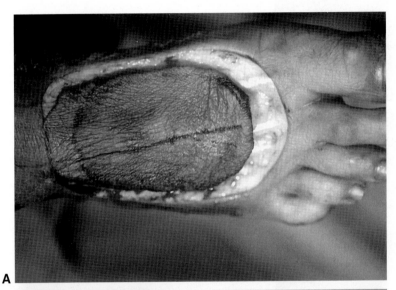

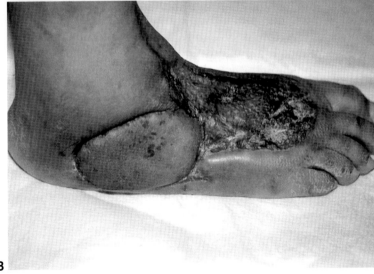

Figure 22–16   **A,** Dorsalis pedis artery flap for coverage of a complex lateral ankle with open ankle joint secondary to *Cryptosporidium* infection. **B,** Healed flap and donor site skin graft.

A

B

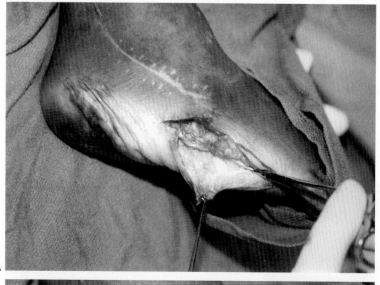

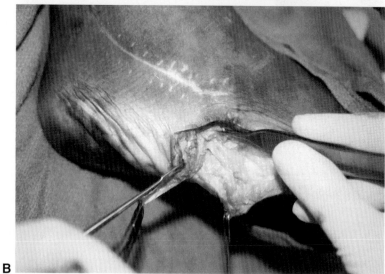

A

B

Figure 22–17   **A** and **B,** Elevation and dissection of an adductor digiti minimi muscular flap being elevated for reconstruction of a proximal lateral foot ulcer.

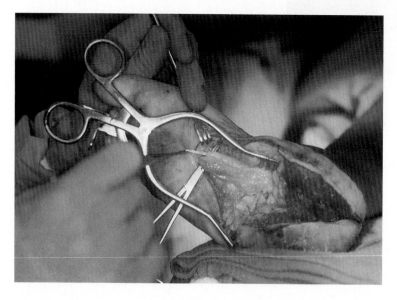

Figure 22–18   Elevation and demonstration of a flexor digiti brevis muscular flap for reconstruction of a proximal heel ulceration.

TABLE 22-2 Advantages and Disadvantages of Various Types of Pretissue Transfer

Flap Type	Advantages	Disadvantages
Fasciocutaneous Flaps		
Radial forearm	Easily accessible, long vascular pedicle; potential for providing sensation using dorsal sensory branch of radial nerve; relatively thin and pliable	Potential arm morbidity, may require radial artery reconstruction; limited by prior radial artery cannulation or injury
Scapular/parascapular	Relatively large flap(s) potentially for multiple components, including muscle and/or bone on a single large vascular pedicle	Potential need to reposition during operative procedure; donor site morbidity, shoulder stiffness, wide scars; potential requirement for secondary skin grafting
Lateral arm flap	Relatively accessible with reasonable pedicle length; potential for providing sensation	Potentially bulky; creates relatively large visible donor site
Anterior lateral thigh	Easily accessible, long vascular pedicle; relatively thin and pliable	Requires a degree of familiarity, for affective harvest may be impacted by femoral vascular disease or prior vascular procedures
Muscle Flaps		
Serratus muscular flap	Can be harvested in multiple segments depending on size of defect; pedicle is consistent, relatively reliable, and large	Creates a degree of shoulder and scapular weakness; dissection can be difficult at times along the thoracodorsal nerve
Latissimus dorsi flap	Large relatively straightforward dissection; good vascular pedicle length	Potentially bulky, creates relatively large donor site with degree of shoulder girdle weakness
Rectus abdominis flap	Easily accessible, reliable vascular pedicle and anatomy	Potential abdominal wall weakness and secondary hernia formation; potential for atherosclerotic involvement of vascular pedicle
Gracilis muscle flap	Generally accessible minimal donor site morbidity; fairly reliable vascular pedicle	Short vascular pedicle that can sometimes be affected by atherosclerotic disease

and the muscle flap with overlying skin graft (free rectus abdominis muscle flap, free gracilis muscle flap, free latissimus dorsi flap, free serratus anterior flap, free vastus lateralis). Many variables are analyzed before the type of free tissue transfer is chosen. The size of the defect, of course, is one major factor. The need for muscle bulk or fill versus the need for thin pliable resurfacing is contemplated. Also, the surgeon must evaluate the recipient blood vessels and the length of the donor vessels to determine the mechanical feasibility of the microvascular anastamosis. Finally, the impact or functional loss of the donor tissue is taken into account. Table 22-2 outlines the most commonly used free flaps for lower-limb reconstruction and their specifications.[10] Not only has evaluation of free tissue transfer reported excellent flap survival rates, but also patients afterward are capable of ambulation.[11-13] It should be noted that free tissue transfer, though often the only viable reconstructive solution, is a difficult and costly option that requires a dedicated patient and surgical team. It often requires an extensive hospitalization for recovery and rehabilitation. Therefore, strict patient selection and screening are warranted.

CASE STUDY 2

This case demonstrates the clinical complexity that is often encountered in the diabetic patient. The patient is a middle-aged insulin-dependent diabetic man with a long history of poor glucose control and prior foot ulcers. He suffered an acute silent myocardial infarction requiring emergent cardiac bypass. The postoperative period was quite complicated, accentuated by early mediastinitis requiring serial debridements and flap reconstruction. During this period, he developed a limb-threatening heel ulcer that exposed his calcaneus and Achilles tendons. After stabilization from cardiac, metabolic, nutritional, and wound standpoints, he underwent complete vascular assessment, which demonstrated good arterial inflow and venous outflow. The plastic surgery department was consulted, and it was decided that no local options were available for durable wound coverage; hence, free tissue transfer was chosen. Potential flap selections included radial forearm, scapular fasciocutaneous, rectus abdominis, and latissimus dorsi free flaps. Owing to the superior quality of muscle in general to cover bony prominences and clear bacteria, the rectus abdominis muscle free flap was chosen with an overlying skin graft. Arteriography was performed, and the posterior tibial vessels were chosen as recipient sites. The anastomosis was carried out in end-to-side fashion, allowing for continued foot perfusion. The case is outlined in Figure 22-19.

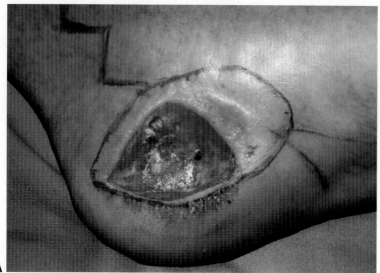

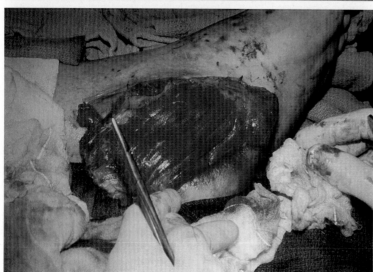

Figure 22–19 **A,** Complex heel wound following revascularization and local wound care. **B,** Flap following vascular repair prior to skin graft.

Other Adjuncts

Other important adjuncts in the fight to heal diabetic wounds come into play either preoperatively or postoperatively. A rather new modality for wound healing is subatmospheric, negative-pressure treatment for wounds with impaired healing. Now widely available is the Vacuum Assisted Wound closure device, currently marketed by KCI Corporation. This therapy concept was pioneered at Bowman Gray University and applies a vacuum (negative pressure) to a wound. This system has been shown to augment the formation of healthy granulation tissue in an open wound bed in a carefully selected group of patients.[14] Orthotic devices also provide valuable support and protection to the healing wound. In some patients, a total non-weight-bearing patellar tibial brace with contralateral custom orthotic shoe lift allows patients to maintain a moderate degree of mobility while still providing non-weight-bearing status to the limb (Fig. 22-20).

Summary

Although there are numerous adjuncts to wound healing, the critical factors remain as follows:

1. Control of infection both locally and systemically
2. Control of metabolic factors such as glucose control, nutrition, concurrent illnesses, and medications such as steroids
3. An educated, compliant, cooperative patient with the ability to participate in his or her assessment and care and fully educated and accepting of the risks and benefits of the options. The patient and family must be fully engaged.
4. A care team that includes the full spectrum of medical and nonmedical support
5. Mechanical unloading of the limb
6. Appropriate and complete debridement and drainage
7. Vascular perfusion or reperfusion of the limb

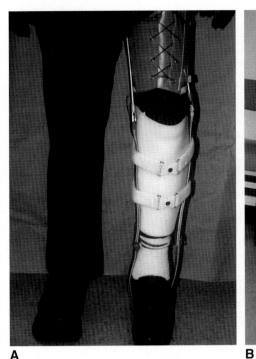 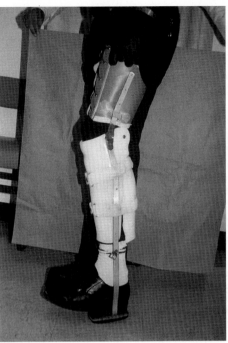

Figure 22-20 **A** and **B**, Anterior and lateral photograph of the full non-weight-bearing patellar tibial brace with contralateral orthotic shoe with sole lift, allowing secondary healing of weight-bearing foot ulcers in the postoperative period following reconstruction.

A   **B**

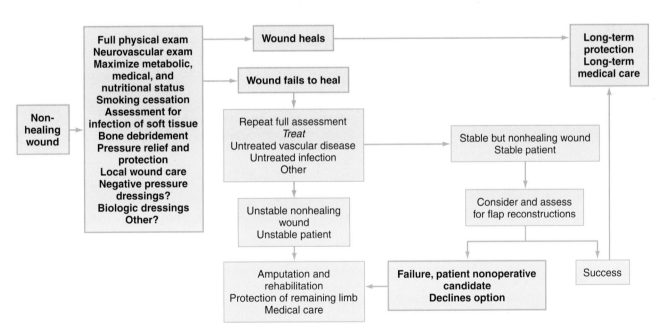

Figure 22-21 Algorithm to salvage the lower limb.

8. A reconstructive team that is capable of supporting and providing the complex options such that a full assessment and the full spectrum of options can be offered

Without perfusion, tissues cannot be oxygenated or nourished, infections will not be cleared, and tissues will not heal and therefore will not be eligible for reconstruction. A consistent, thorough vascular assessment is critical to salvage of a limb in the diabetic patient. Any plastic surgical reconstructive efforts, be they flaps or grafts, can provide an important adjunct to the salvage and maintenance of a limb; however, without perfusion, the limb is ultimately lost. Figure 22-21 provides a broad conceptual algorithm through which lower-limb salvage can be pursued. The threatened limb (i.e., one that demonstrates severe claudication, rest pain, significant tissue loss, dependent rubor, or deep infection) requires intervention from a medical as well as a surgical standpoint. Revascularization alone does not take the place of local adjuncts, medical management, and metabolic correction but proceeds rapidly in concert with the other interventions. Unfortunately, despite all our efforts, some wounds still fail to heal, owing to factors as yet unknown to us. Thus continues the great challenge within the art and practice of medicine.

References

1. Attinger CE: Foot and ankle preservation. In Aston SJ, Beasley RW, Thorne CMH (eds): Grabb and Smith's Plastic Surgery, 5th ed. Philadelphia, Lippincott-Raven, 1997, pp 1059–1075.
2. Banis JC, Derr JW, Richardson JD: A rational approach to ischemia and ischemic-diabetic foot reconstruction. In Jurkiewicz MJ, Culbertson JH (eds): Operative Techniques in Plastic and Reconstructive Surgery-Foot Reconstruction, vol 4. Philadelphia, WB Saunders, 1997, pp 217–235.
3. Parker JA, Searles JM: Local flaps for forefoot and midfoot reconstruction. In Jurkiewicz MJ, Culbertson JH (eds): Operative Techniques in Plastic and Reconstructive Surgery-Foot Reconstruction, vol 4. Philadelphia, WB Saunders, 1997, pp 148–157.
4. Rhodes G, Skudder P: Salvage of ischemic diabetic feet: Roles of transcutaneous O_2 mapping and multiple configurations of in situ bypass. Am J Surg 152:165–169, 1986.
5. Hidalgo DA, Shaw WW: Reconstruction of foot injuries. Clin Plast Surg 13:663–680, 1986.
6. Blume PA, Attinger CE: Single-stage surgical treatment of nonifected diabetic foot ulcers. Plast Reconstr Surg 109(2):601–609, 2002.
7. Heinz TR: Local flaps for hind foot reconstruction. In Jurkiewicz MJ, Culbertson JH (eds): Operative Techniques in Plastic and Reconstructive Surgery-Foot Reconstruction, vol. 4. Philadelphia, WB Saunders, 1997, pp 157–164.
8. Saltz R, Hochberg J, Given KS: Muscle and musculocutaneous flaps of the foot. Clin Plast Surg 18:627–638, 1991.
9. Levin LS: The reconstructive ladder: An orthoplastic approach. Orthop Clin Am 24:393–409, 1993.
10. Germann G, Erdmann D: Foot reconstruction with microvascular flaps. In Jurkiewicz MJ, Culbertson JH (eds): Operative Techniques in Plastic and Reconstructive Surgery-Foot Reconstruction, vol 4. Philadelphia, WB Saunders, 1997, pp 172–182.
11. Rainer C, Ninkovic, M: Microsurgical management of the diabetic foot. J Reconstr Microsurg 19(8):543–553, 2003.
12. Verhelle NA, Heymans O: Combined reconstruction of the diabetic foot including revascularization and free-tissue transfer. J Reconstr Microsurg 20(7):511–7, 2004.
13. Hong J: Reconstruction of the diabetic foot using the anterolateral thigh perforator flap. Plast Reconstr Surg 117(5):1599–1608, 2006.
14. Morykwas MJ, Argenta LC: Use of negative pressure to increase the rate of granulation tissue formation in chronic open wounds. Paper presented at the annual meeting of the Federation of American Society for Experimental Biology, March 28–April 1, 1993, New Orleans.

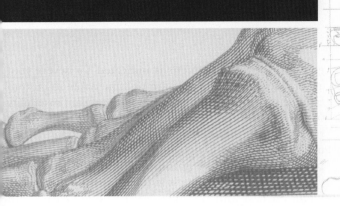

CHARCOT NEUROARTHROPATHY OF THE FOOT: SURGICAL ASPECTS

JEFFREY E. JOHNSON AND ANDREW BRIAN THOMSON ■

Nonsurgical treatment utilizing total-contact casting (TCC) followed by appropriate bracing and footwear is the gold standard for treatment of the majority of foot and ankle neuropathic (Charcot) fractures and dislocations. However, surgical treatment is indicated for chronic recurrent ulceration, joint instability, or, in some cases, pain that has failed nonoperative treatment. Selected acute fractures may also have operative indications. The goals of operative treatment are to preserve functional activity with the aid of appropriate footwear or bracing and to prevent amputation. These goals are achieved through restoration of the contour or alignment of the affected foot and ankle segment. Despite the potential for significant operative complications, the overall success rate of limb salvage reconstruction is approximately 80% to 90%.[1-4]

Charcot neuroarthropathy is a noninfective, destructive bone and joint fracture and/or dislocation associated with peripheral neuropathy. Diabetes is the most common cause for these deformity-causing fractures in the United States, with neuropathic arthropathy estimated to occur in 0.1% to 0.5% of patients with diabetes mellitus.[5,6] Approximately 30% of people with diabetes over age 40 have some degree of peripheral neuropathy.[7] As of November 2005, there were an estimated 20.4 million diabetic patients in the United States. Because of improvements in diabetes care, these patients are living longer. Therefore, neuropathic arthropathy, a late effect

of peripheral neuropathy of the foot and ankle, will continue to be a major clinical problem.

The etiology and pathophysiology of neuropathic bone and joint destruction are still poorly understood. Several risk factors for the development of Charcot neuroarthropathy have been defined: history of retinopathy, nephropathy, previous foot ulcer, diminished vibratory sensation and deep tendon reflexes, and loss of protective sensation as measured with the Semmes-Weinstein 5.07 monofilament.[8] The stages of bone and joint destruction followed by fracture healing and remodeling were described by Eichenholtz in 1966.[9] The Eichenholtz classification is temporally based on the characteristic clinical and radiographic changes that occur with neuropathic joint destruction or fracture over time.[10] These changes progress from the stage of development (acute dissolution) through the stage of coalescence (healing) to the stage of reconstruction (resolution). The timing and selection of a surgical procedure in a neuropathic patient should be made with a thorough understanding of the natural history and the temporal stage of the patient's neuroarthropathic process. Several authors have classified the characteristic patterns of neuropathic bone and joint destruction.[11-14] Fracture patterns are associated with a deficiency in peripheral bone mineral density, while dislocations usually occur in patients with normal bone mineral density.[15] An understanding of these patterns is helpful in making a diagnosis of a

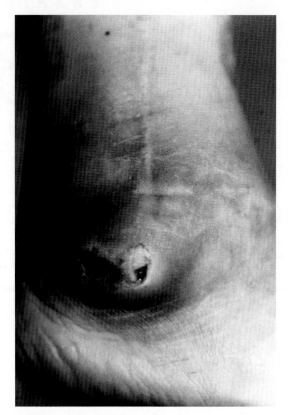

Figure 23-1 Right Charcot ankle fracture dislocation following open reduction and internal fixation of a bimalleolar ankle fraction. The resulting varus deformity caused recurrent ulceration over the distal fibula despite bracing.

Charcot foot in cases of occult neuropathy and in planning operative or nonoperative treatment.

Foot and ankle deformities from a neuropathic fracture or dislocation cause difficulty with shoe fit and marked alteration in weight-bearing loads, all leading to an increased propensity for ulceration in high-pressure areas (Fig. 23-1). Ulceration occurs in up to 40% of patients with Charcot neuroarthropathy, with an incidence of 17% annually.[16] These ulcers may become a portal of entry for bacteria, resulting in superficial or deep infection. Deformity may also be associated with joint instability, which is accentuated by weight-bearing, especially with hindfoot or ankle involvement. These changes result in loss of a plantigrade foot position and development of progressive varus, valgus, equinus, or calcaneus deformity. Charcot neuroarthropathy of the foot has significant effects on quality of life with SF-36 scores in diabetic patients with foot ulcers and Charcot foot arthropathy comparable to those in patients with lower-limb amputations.[17]

Treatment Recommendations

Nonoperative management is still indicated for the vast majority of Charcot foot and ankle deformities. However, recently published studies of Charcot cohorts have reported surgical intervention in 28% to 60% of patients.[18–21] In general, surgical treatment is indicated for severe foot and ankle deformities that are not amenable to custom bracing or custom footwear, such as significant instability of the hindfoot and ankle. Other indications include recurrent ulceration and selected acute fractures. A markedly unstable Charcot joint may be associated with pain; however, unlike painful osteoarthritis, a painful Charcot joint is rarely the sole reason for operative treatment. Success with nonoperative treatment varies with the site of involvement. Most neuropathic calcaneal fractures can be successfully managed nonoperatively, while 33% to 40% of midtarsal neuroarthropathy and 50% of transverse tarsal and forefoot neuroarthropathy might ultimately require surgical treatment for recurrent ulceration, instability, or infection.[19,22]

Goals of Surgical Treatment

The goal of surgical treatment for the Charcot foot and ankle is the restoration of their stability and alignment so that footwear and bracing are possible. For most patients with a deformity severe enough to require operative treatment, a partial foot or transtibial amputation is usually the only other treatment option. Two large series of Charcot neuroarthropathy have shown similar rates of amputation. Pinzur and colleagues reported a 9% amputation rate over a 10-year interval.[20] Saltzman and colleagues reported an annual incidence of amputation of 3%, although no patients in this series who had realignment or stabilization of their Charcot deformity went on to amputation.[21] Therefore, an additional goal of operative treatment is to prevent amputation of a limb that is destined to develop recurrent ulceration.

Patients with a significant deformity from neuropathic arthropathy will require specialized footwear with custom total-contact inserts (foot orthoses) and, in some cases, custom bracing to prevent recurrent ulceration and progressive deformity, whether or not they have surgery. Therefore, the treatment decision is not between operative treatment or prescription footwear and bracing but rather between operative treatment followed by prescription footwear and bracing or prescription footwear and bracing alone. Operative treatment is indicated primarily to make these patients better candidates for safe shoe and brace wear. Although some patients with a solid realignment arthrodesis may eventually be weaned from their ankle-foot orthosis (AFO), it is an unrealistic goal for many patients and can lead to recurrent ulceration or stress fractures of the tibia.[23,24]

Timing of Operative Treatment

Once the acute dissolution phase (Eichenholtz's stage I of development) has begun, regional bone demineralization (which hinders rigid internal fixation) and swelling make surgical management of the fracture difficult, leading to a higher rate of fixation failure, recurrent deformity, and infection. Operative treatment of the Charcot foot is usually done in the quiescent, resolution phase of the fracture (Eichenholtz's stage of reconstruction) after casting, footwear, and bracing have failed. This traditional approach is now being tested. A recent series involving midfoot arthrodesis via an open reduction with internal fixation in patients with Charcot arthropathy in the stage of development reported no immediate or long-term complications, challenging the traditional approach of avoiding operative treatment in this phase.[25] Acute fractures in neuropathic patients may be openly reduced and fixed if treatment is performed early, before significant neuropathic fracture inflammation occurs, while bone stock is still sufficient for rigid fixation. Surgery is generally recommended in the acute phase if the displacement of the fracture or dislocation is severe enough to produce significant deformity and/or soft tissue compromise. In the midfoot, the deformity should be manually reducible preoperatively, since an extensive dissection to reduce the deformity when the foot is acutely swollen can increase the chance of a wound complication.[26,27] Many patients do not present for treatment early enough for this approach to be utilized.

Foot ulcers in association with significant bony deformity, especially of the ankle and hindfoot, are treated, if possible, with TCC until the ulcer is healed so that the incision for the reconstructive procedure can be made through intact skin to reduce the possibility of postoperative infection.[1] If underlying osteomyelitis is suspected in association with the neuropathic fracture, nuclear imaging with a combined technetium-99m bone scan and indium-111 white blood cell scan utilizing the dual-window technique is helpful in making this determination.[28,29] Recently, PET scans have also been shown to have utility in the differentiation of chronic osteomyelitis from inflammation.[30,31] If osteomyelitis is present, appropriate debridement is done, and antibiotics are administered until resolution of the infection and wound healing occur. At this time, the decision regarding operative versus nonoperative treatment for the bony deformity can be made.

Reconstructive Procedures for Neuropathic Deformity

There are two types of procedures for treatment of severe neuropathic deformities. For the patient with a stable forefoot or midfoot bony deformity, an ostectomy (bumpectomy) is often satisfactory to prevent primary or recurrent ulceration and relieve severe shoe-fitting problems. Severe deformities associated with instability, especially in the hindfoot and ankle, require realignment and stabilization by arthrodesis to provide long-term correction.

Ostectomy

The midfoot is the most common location for neuropathic destruction, ranging from 53% to 73% of cases, the apex of a rocker-bottom foot deformity being a frequent source of recurrent ulceration.[19,22,32] The most common operative procedure for a neuropathic deformity of the midfoot is removal of a bony prominence on the medial, lateral, or plantar aspect that is creating recurrent ulceration and difficulty with the fitting of footwear. As was noted above, the first step in the operative treatment of any neuropathic deformity is to obtain closure of the overlying ulcer by TCC so that the incision to remove the bony prominence can be made through intact skin. An alternative technique is excision of the ulcer through a plantar longitudinal elliptical incision made directly over the prominence.[2] However, this technique exposes a significant amount of underlying cancellous bone to the open ulcer with the potential for bacterial colonization of the underlying bone.

The author's preferred method (Fig. 23-2) is to first obtain ulcer closure with TCC and then make an incision through intact skin on the medial or lateral border of the foot, whichever is closest to the bony prominence.[11,33] The skin incision is made down to the bony prominence as a full-thickness flap. A periosteal elevator is used to separate the overlying soft tissues from the protuberant bone. A small power saw or an osteotome is used to resect the bony prominence, which is then rasped to provide a smooth, broad, weight-bearing surface. Major tendon attachments such as those of the peroneus brevis, anterior tibial, and posterior tibial muscles and the Achilles tendon should be respected and reattached firmly to bone if they are detached. Resection of a large medial midfoot prominence, especially if it involves the medial cuneiform, should include reattachment of the anterior tibial tendon through drill holes in the remaining bone. Many patients have a coexistent triceps surae (gastrosoleus) contracture requiring a percutaneous Achilles tendon lengthening at the time of plantar ostectomy to achieve a plantigrade foot.[27] Achilles tendon lengthening has also been shown to decrease the recurrence rate of plantar forefoot ulcers in patients with diabetes and peripheral neuropathy.[34]

The skin is closed over a suction drain, which is left in place for 24 hours, and a compression splint is applied. The following day, a total-contact cast is applied to stabilize the soft tissues, promote wound healing, and allow the patient limited weight-bearing. It is important to avoid excessive bone resection, especially in the midfoot, where removal of the plantar ligaments can cause progression of the rocker-bottom deformity. Plantar midfoot ostectomy is more successful when the neuropathic deformity is stable, without sagittal or transverse plane instability.[2] Also, complication rates are reported to be higher in ostectomies of the lateral column than in those of the medial column.[35] The sutures are removed once the incision has

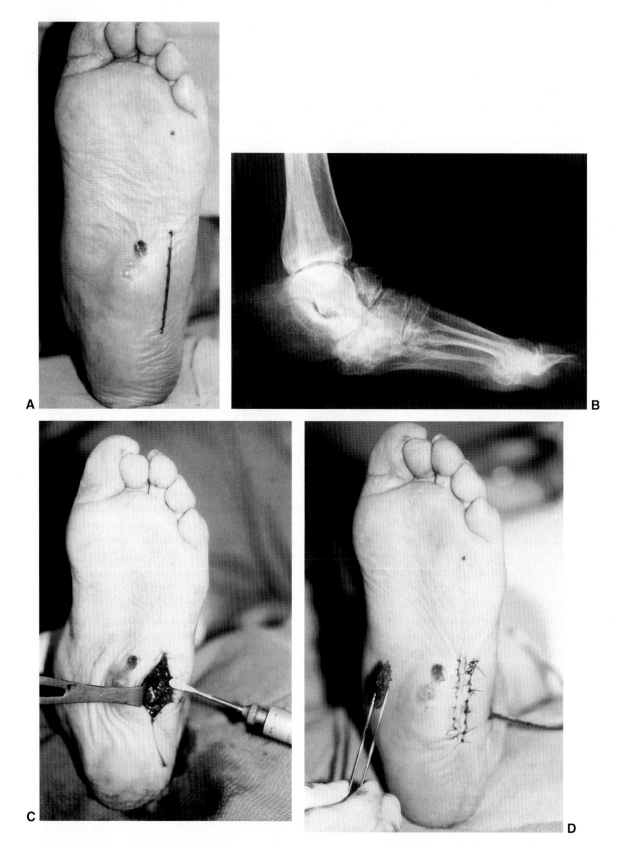

Figure 23–2   **A,** Plantar view demonstrating chronic recurrent plantar ulcer beneath rocker-bottom deformity. The ulcer was healed with total-contact casting prior to exostectomy. Note that the incision for resection of plantar prominence is on the plantar-lateral border of foot. **B,** Lateral radiograph demonstrating neuropathic midfoot rocker-bottom deformity with large plantar prominence. Note the equinus position of the hindfoot secondary to Achilles contracture. **C,** Intraoperative rasp is used to smooth the bone surface after the prominence has been osteotomized. Percutaneous Achilles tendon lengthening was also performed. **D,** Postoperative photograph following plantar ostectomy demonstrating the amount of bone resected. The patient has remained healed in a double-upright calf lacer ankle-foot orthosis attached to an in-depth shoe with a custom total-contact insert.

healed, usually 2 to 3 weeks after the procedure. A mold for a total-contact insert is made at one of the cast changes so that once healing has occurred, the appropriate footwear and custom insert will be ready for dispensing at the time of final cast removal.

Realignment and Arthrodesis

Severe Charcot foot and ankle deformity or instability is treated with realignment of the involved joint and stabilization by arthrodesis. For most patients who are considered for this treatment, bracing and footwear have failed, and amputation is the only other reasonable option for treatment (Fig. 23-3). The goal of operative treatment is to restore and augment the alignment and stability of the foot to allow ambulation with appropriate bracing and footwear, not as a substitute for these devices.

Contraindications to arthrodesis include the following:

1. Current soft tissue or bone infection (Arthrodesis with internal fixation may be performed as a staged procedure after the infection has been treated, all osteomyelitic bone has been resected, and the soft tissues have healed.)
2. Uncontrolled diabetes or malnutrition
3. Refusal to cease smoking permanently
4. Significant peripheral vascular disease
5. Insufficient bone stock to obtain rigid fixation
6. Inability to comply with the prolonged nonweight-bearing postoperative regimen due to psychosocial problems, significant upper-limb weakness precluding proper off-loading, or massive obesity

Realignment and Arthrodesis Technique

Hindfoot-Tibiotalocalcaneal Arthrodesis

Preoperatively, TCC is used until the acute phase of the Charcot fracture process has subsided and the skin is intact. Extensile longitudinal incisions are utilized with full-thickness skin flaps to bone. If mild to moderate deformity is limited to the ankle and subtalar joints, a posterior approach for tibiotalocalcaneal fusion may be used.[36] For correction of a severe deformity, exposure may be enhanced by medial and lateral ankle incisions as needed (see Fig. 23-3). Sufficient bone is resected to allow correction of the deformity and apposition of stable bleeding bone surfaces to promote successful fusion. Achilles tendon contractures are addressed with percutaneous lengthening, especially when performing a midfoot or hindfoot arthrodesis. Autologous bone graft is utilized to fill any defects and to provide both an intra-articular and an extra-articular arthrodesis when possible. Morselized pieces of resected tibia and fibula may also be used when bone graft is needed primarily for extra-articular application. Appropriate clinical alignment of the hindfoot must be achieved, with the hindfoot in slight valgus (5 to 10 degrees) so that the weight-bearing axis of the heel falls just lateral to the tibial crest. Slight external rotation should approximate that of the opposite limb. Sagittal alignment should be neutral plantigrade. Adequate alignment of the foot in all planes should help to lower the risk of postoperative ulceration.[3] Screws, large threaded Steinmann pins, compression blade plates, and custom intramedullary rods are used in whatever combination is deemed necessary to provide adequate rigid internal fixation (Figs. 23-3 to 23-6). External fixation, especially with small wire circular fixators, may be used when there is an open wound or when bone loss precludes satisfactory internal fixation. Stress fractures were reported in 28% of a series of patients in whom a blade plate was utilized for fixation of a tibiotalocalcaneal arthrodesis. This was prior to the authors' use of a bivalved AFO for additional support after union was achieved.[37] In a recent series utilizing long, retrograde intramedullary nails extending to the proximal tibia, no stress fractures were seen.[24]

Midfoot

The tarsometatarsal joints may be approached through two or three longitudinal incisions. If a corrective osteotomy is required owing to significant deformity or if plantar plating is planned, the first tarsometatarsal joint may be approached through a dorsomedial incision between the tibialis anterior and posterior tibial tendons. This is more useful if a corrective osteotomy is required owing to significant deformity or if plantar plating is planned. An alternative approach, useful for treatment of acute dislocation, is by a dorsomedial incision between the tibialis anterior and extensor hallucis longus tendons. Additional longitudinal incisions may be placed between the bases of the second and third metatarsals or over the fifth metatarsocuboid joint. It is best to have at least a 4-cm skin bridge between incisions. If one is concerned about the soft tissue status in, for example, the treatment of acute Charcot midfoot, minimally invasive percutaneous reduction techniques may be employed by using large bone reduction forceps and/or percutaneously placed Steinmann pins as joysticks for reduction (Fig. 23-7). Fixation options include cannulated 4.0-mm or 4.5-mm screws, a cannulated 6.5-mm screw placed axially in the medial column, or plating with 1/3 tubular plates placed on the plantar (tension) side of the medial column. Plating of the plantar aspect of the medial column of the midfoot has been advocated to enhance the rigidity of midfoot arthrodeses.[38,39] Plating may also prove useful in cases in which the naviculocuneiform and metatarsocuneiform joints must be stabilized.[26,39]

The ulcerated foot with midfoot rocker-bottom deformity with or without osteomyelitis presents a unique treatment challenge. Internal fixation in the presence of ulceration and/or osteomyelitis is not advisable, with a 25% rate of deep infection reported.[1] The author's

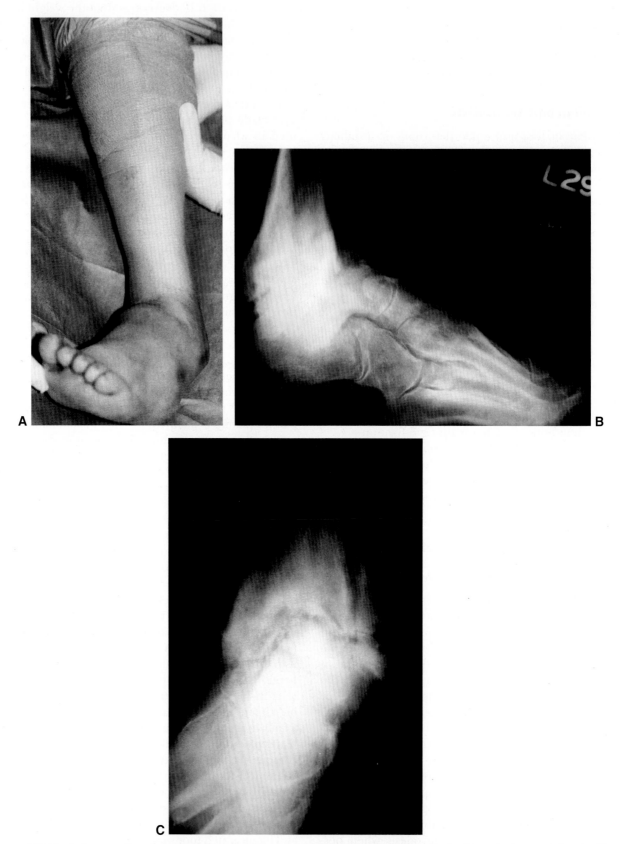

Figure 23–3   **A,** Preoperative photograph of neuropathic arthropathy of the ankle and hindfoot with marked varus deformity. Note prominence of the lateral malleolus with impending skin breakdown. **B,** Lateral radiograph of the same patient demonstrating neuropathic fracture dislocation of the hindfoot with dissolution of the body of the talus. **C,** Anteroposterior radiograph demonstrating varus angulation of the tibiotalocalcaneal joints.

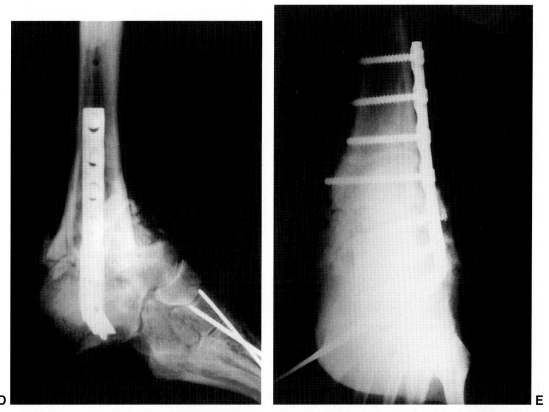

Figure 23–3, cont'd   D, Lateral radiograph following open reduction and tibiotalocalcaneal arthrodesis through lateral and medial incisions. Note the Steinmann pin fixation of the first metatarsal dorsiflexion osteotomy for correction of fixed forefoot valgus. **E,** Anteroposterior radiograph demonstrating a 4.5-mm titanium blade plate fixation of tibiotalocalcaneal fusion.

preferred method of treatment is obtaining ulcer closure with TCC prior to surgical intervention with corrective osteotomy and internal fixation. However, external fixation is gaining acceptance in this clinical scenario and provides another treatment alternative. Debridement of the ulceration and infected bony prominence and administration of culture-specific antibiotics may be followed by subsequent corrective osteotomy and external fixation with a thin-wire Ilizarov-type fixator or a traditional frame (Fig. 23-8). External fixation can provide adequate stability, but positioning the foot and ankle is more difficult with an external fixator. These patients may be converted from external fixation to TCC at approximately 2 to 3 months, once the ulceration has healed.[40,41] Farber and colleagues reported that all 11 ulcerated feet with Charcot deformity that were treated with external fixation ultimately achieved a braceable or shoeable foot that was ulcer-free. The average time until fixator removal was 57 days, followed by TCC.[41] On occasion, pin site problems may force early removal of the fixator, leading to nonunion or malunion.

Postoperative Care

Long-term immobilization is critical in obtaining bony union. In general, the immobilization period for an arthrodesis in a neuropathic patient is doubled in comparison to the postoperative regimen for nonneuropathic patients. The postoperative regimen includes 3 months in a nonweight-bearing TCC followed by 1 to 2 months in a weight-bearing one. The limb is then placed into a bivalved AFO with a rocker sole plate until footwear and definitive bracing are possible. Bracing is continued for 12 to 18 months postoperatively, similar to the treatment of a neuropathic fracture. For midfoot fusions, if swelling is minimal and the arthrodesis is solid, a depth rocker-soled shoe may be used. For hindfoot and ankle involvement, the shoe is attached to either a double upright calf lacer or a patellar-tendon-bearing AFO (Fig. 23-9). A custom molded polypropylene AFO, consisting of a posterior shell and an anterior shell ending proximal to the ankle, may be utilized inside a shoe with a rocker sole if the foot deformity is not severe (Fig. 23-6F and Fig. 23-10). When there is significant residual deformity in the foot after surgery, it is preferable to use whatever customized shoe and foot orthosis combination is necessary to accommodate the deformity and then to have this shoe attached to a double-upright AFO (see Fig. 23-9) because a custom molded polypropylene AFO takes up space within the shoe and therefore will not allow as much accommodation for severe deformities of the foot, possibly resulting in recurrent ulceration.

Postoperative casting, followed by bracing, is required following midfoot, hindfoot, and ankle fusions for at least 12 to 18 months to allow complete healing and a return to full weight-bearing. Ankle, hindfoot, and midfoot fusions at the talonavicular joint level are prone to either recurrent Charcot changes at adjacent joints or stress fractures and should be protected by bracing indefinitely.[10] Midfoot fusions distal to the talonavicular joint level may remain stable in a depth shoe with a total-contact insert, an extended steel shank, and rocker soles. The question of whether to wean a patient from the AFO at 12 to 18 months following arthrodesis depends on mul-

tiple factors, including the location of the arthrodesis, the union and stability of the arthrodesis site, the patient's reliability, and the patient's activity level. Hindfoot arthrodeses involving the tibiotalocalcaneal joints in active patients are prone to distal tibial stress fractures (Fig. 23-11). These fractures are usually minimally displaced and will heal with 6 to 12 weeks of TCC. Bracing is needed for strenuous weight-bearing activities to prevent fractures due to the stresses placed on the tibia from the foot acting as a long, rigid lever arm.[10,23,,37]

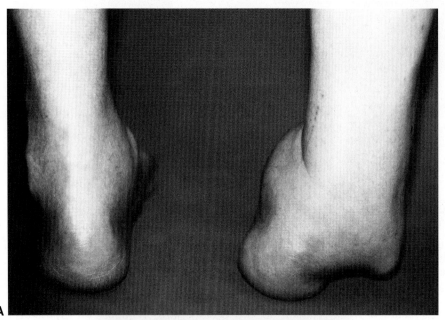

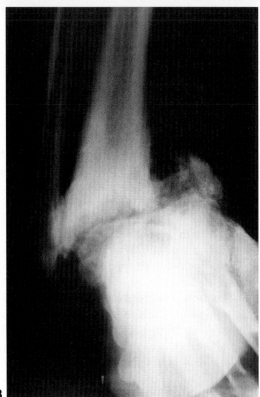

Figure 23–4   A, Posterior view of a 65-year-old male with insulin-dependent diabetes mellitus and severe peripheral neuropathy with progressive right hindfoot varus following ankle injury. **B,** Anteroposterior radiograph of the same patient demonstrating an old fracture-dislocation of tibiotalar joint and marked varus angulation.

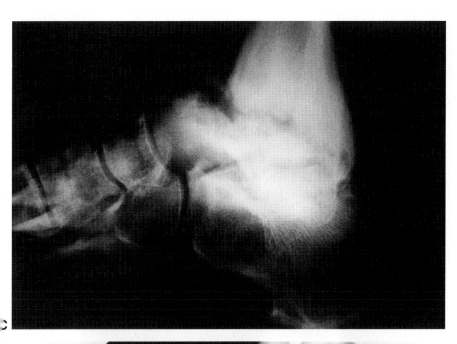

Figure 23–4, cont'd   C, Lateral radiograph of ankle demonstrating collapse of talar body and destruction of ankle and subtalar joints. **D,** Intraoperative lateral fluoroscopic image of the same patient demonstrating removal of the talar neck and body with retention of talar head to maintain length of the medial column of the foot. Note that the distal tibia has been osteotomized and "mortised" into the anterior portion of the calcaneus. A guide pin has been placed from the plantar aspect of the calcaneus up the medullary canal of the distal tibia in preparation for insertion of the interlocking intramedullary rod.

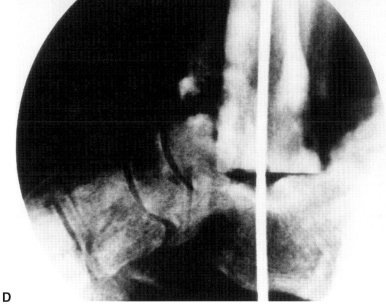

D

Illustration continued on following page.

Results of Charcot Reconstruction

The reported bony union rates of foot and ankle fusions for neuropathic deformity range from 50% to 100%.[1-4,18,24,37,42,43] However, the goal of achieving a stable, braceable, and shoeable foot is obtainable in 80% to 100% of patients following the initial operative procedure regardless of whether a solid arthrodesis or a stable nonunion (fibrous union) is obtained.[1,3,4,24,25,27,28,37,42] Complications that can lead to failure of the procedure requiring a repeat procedure include deep wound infection, unstable nonunion, and malunion. Although earlier reports expressed caution in performing arthrodeses for neuropathic arthropathy,[44,45] modern techniques of internal fixation and prolonged immobilization have significantly improved the union rate and decreased complications. The satisfaction rate for these procedures is high, in large part because pain is not a major factor.[1,2,3,37,43,46] Most patients are grateful if they can avoid amputation and be restored to walking status in an appropriate shoe or brace.

Charcot Reconstruction: Triumph of Technique over Reason?

Because of the technical difficulty in managing these patients, the potential complications, and the prolonged treatment time required, some practitioners favor

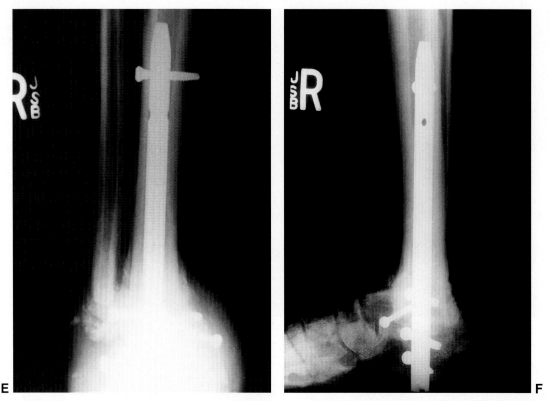

Figure 23–4, cont'd   E, Postoperative anteroposterior radiograph demonstrating corrected alignment of the ankle joint with the interlocking screws placed lateral to medial. **F,** Lateral radiograph at 6 months postoperatively. Note the plantigrade position of the foot with the appropriate calcaneal pitch angle. The talar neck has fused to the anterior tibia.

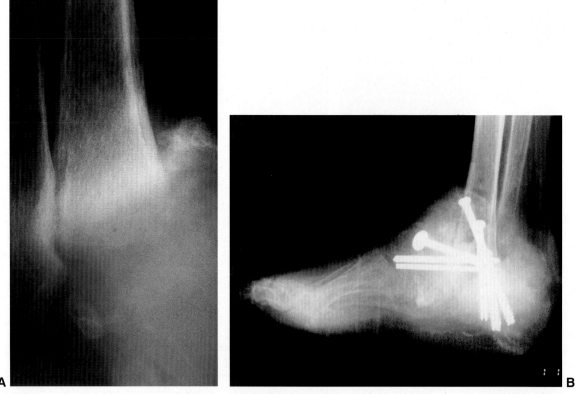

Figure 23–5   A, Anteroposterior radiograph of a 72-year-old female with kidney-pancreas transplant and progressive hindfoot varus deformity from neuropathic arthropathy of the hindfoot. **B,** Postoperative lateral radiograph demonstrating realignment and arthrodesis utilizing multiple cannulated cancellous screws augmented with threaded Steinmann pins.

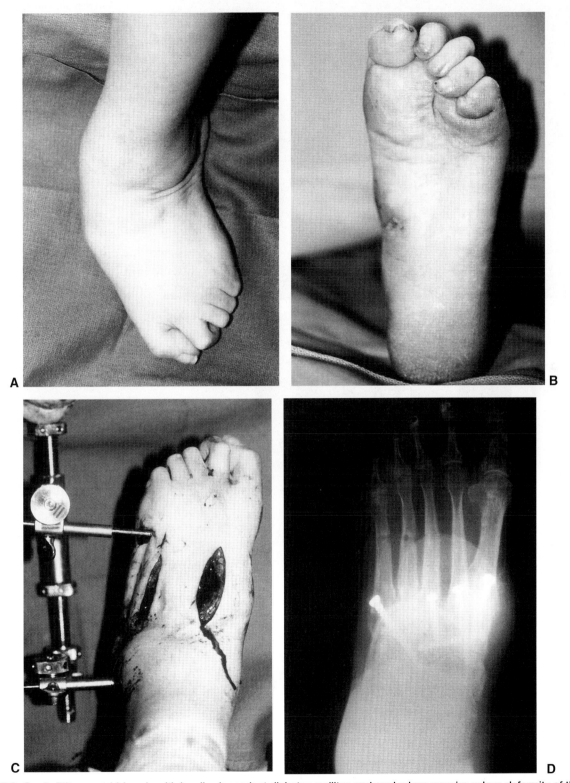

Figure 23–6   **A,** Fifty-year-old female with insulin-dependent diabetes mellitus and marked progressive valgus deformity of the left foot with recurrent plantar medial midfoot ulceration despite custom footwear. **B,** Plantar view demonstrating a pressure area beneath the medial midfoot and severe claw toe deformities. **C,** Intraoperative photograph of the same patient demonstrating the use of the femoral distractor to assist in correction of the deformity. After the tarsometatarsal joints were denuded of their cartilage, a Schanz pin was placed in the calcaneus and the fourth metatarsal. Distraction on the lateral side of the foot corrected the severe forefoot abduction until the internal fixation was placed. **D,** Anteroposterior radiograph demonstrating screw fixation of the arthrodesis across all five tarsometatarsal joints.

Illustration continued on following page.

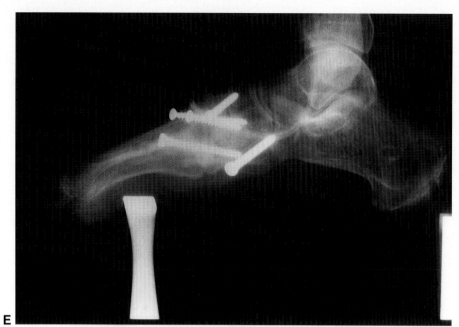

Figure 23–6, cont'd   E, Lateral radiograph demonstrating restoration of the medial longitudinal arch following arthrodesis. F, Six months postoperatively, demonstrating correction of midfoot and forefoot deformity. Note the posterior shell ankle-foot orthosis is used for 12 to 18 months postoperatively.

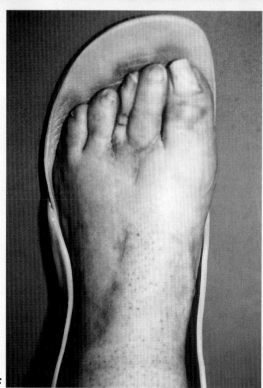

F

amputation rather than reconstruction for the unbraceable neuropathic deformity. Previous studies on energy expenditure and amputation level demonstrate that the more distal the level of amputation, the less energy expenditure is required for walking.[47,48] Therefore, it would seem logical that the Charcot reconstruction arthrodesis patient would have less energy expenditure with walking and have a higher functional level than would an amputee, especially a patient with limited cardiovascular reserve. Although it has not been studied prospectively, there is a trend for lower amputation rates in patients who have had realignment arthrodeses of their Charcot deformities.[21] Perhaps the most compelling reason for limb salvage is the long-term uncertainty about the status of the other foot. Peripheral vascular disease or an ulcer leading to a deep wound infection may occur in the contralateral foot, necessitating an amputation in the future. Reconstruction instead of amputation for the "salvageable" neuropathic deformity might avoid creating a future bilateral amputee.

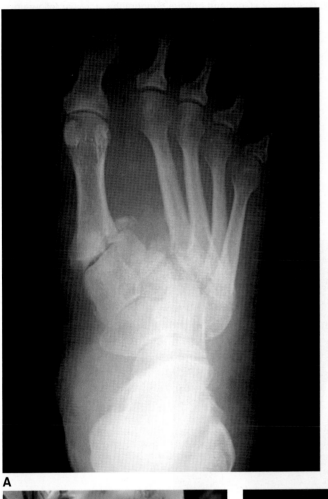

A

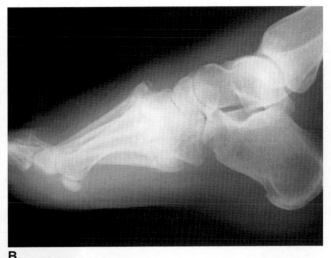

B

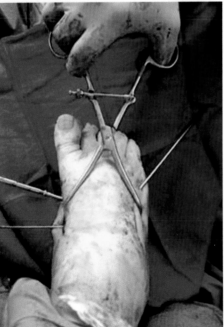

C

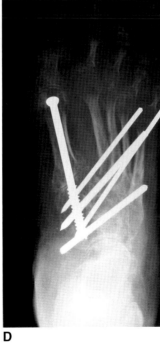

D

Figure 23–7   A, B, Anteroposterior and lateral radiographs of a 54-year-old female with type 2 diabetes mellitus 2 weeks after she sustained a twisting injury to right foot. **C,** Intraoperative percutaneous/minimally invasive reduction techniques. **D,** Anteroposterior radiograph at 5 months postoperative when Steinmann pins were removed.

Illustration continued on following page.

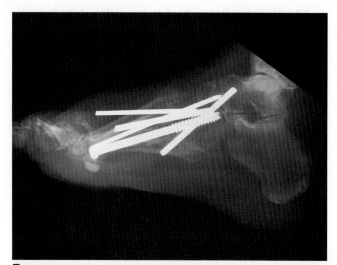

Figure 23–7,cont'd **E,** Lateral radiograph at 5 months postoperative when Steinmann pins were removed. **F, G,** Anteroposterior and oblique radiographs at 2-year follow-up.

E

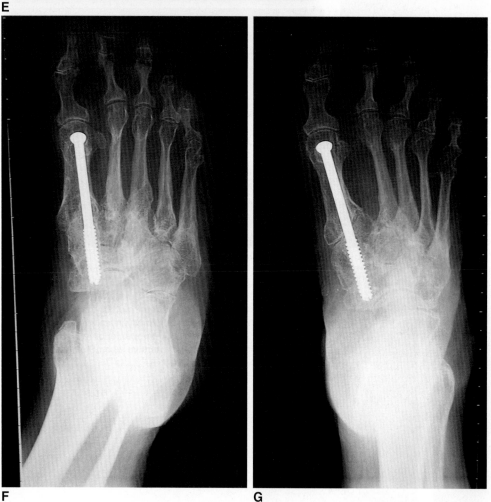

F   G

Prevention of Charcot Deformity by Specific Methods of Acute Fracture Management in Patients with Neuropathic Arthropathy

The most important factor in successful management of an acute fracture and prevention of late deformity in a neuropathic patient is to recognize the fact that the patient indeed has significant peripheral neuropathy. A series of small nylon monofilaments (Semmes-Weinstein type) can be used to determine the severity and location of the sensory neuropathy.[49] If monofilament testing shows loss of protective sensation (level 5.07/10 g or greater), it is important to alter the typical treatment regimen to help prevent subsequent Charcot joint destruction. It is also important to warn the patient about the potential risk of Charcot joint involvement

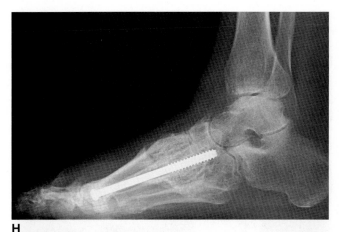

H

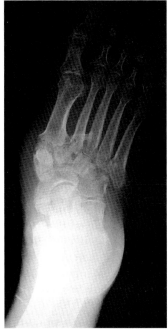

J

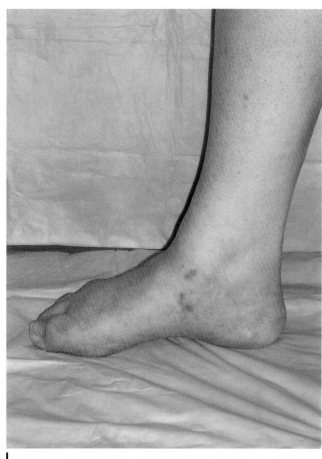

I

Figure 23–7,cont'd   H, I, J, Clinical photographs at 2-year follow-up. The patient is ambulating in depth shoes with total-contact insert and is brace-free.

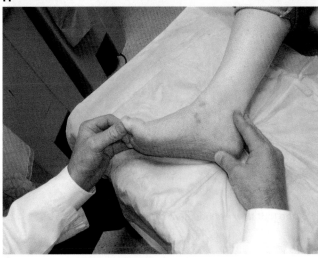

A

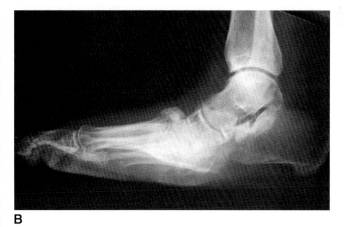

B

Figure 23–8   A, B, Anteroposterior and lateral radiographs of a 60-year-old patient with type 2 diabetes who had a tarsometatarsal neuropathic fracture-dislocation and now has a rocker-bottom deformity, forefoot abduction, and chronic plantar-lateral midfoot ulceration.

Illustration continued on following page.

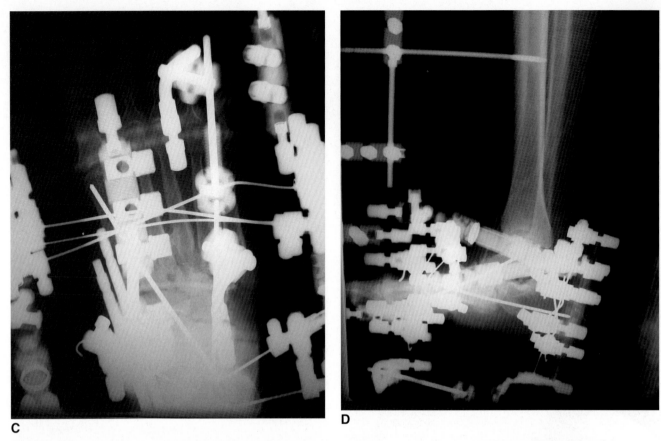

C   D

Figure 23–8, cont'd   C, D, Anteroposterior and lateral radiographs of the foot after debridement of the ulcer and midfoot
osteotomy with application of a thin-wire external fixator.

whether operative or nonoperative treatment of the fracture is undertaken.

The first step in acute fracture management is to differentiate an acute neuropathic fracture (Eichenholtz's
stage I of development) from an acute fracture in a
patient who has a significant peripheral neuropathy. This
distinction can often be made by the patient's history.
For example, the patient who suffers a relatively minor
injury such as an ankle or foot "sprain" followed by
several days or weeks of erythema and swelling who then
presents with a displaced fracture would usually be
treated for an acute neuropathic injury with TCC. In
contrast, the patient with a significant diabetic peripheral neuropathy who sustains an acute displaced fracture
as a result of significant trauma might be treated with the
same operative or nonoperative fracture management
principles as the nonneuropathic patient, if seen acutely.
The caveat is that a higher rate of complications should
be anticipated, and therefore a prolonged postoperative
period of nonweight-bearing and TCC immobilization,
followed by bracing, is indicated in the neuropathic
patient. Routine postoperative fracture management
with early range of motion, limited weight-bearing, and
removable prefabricated walking braces can result in
failure of fixation prior to fracture healing (Fig. 23-12).
Acute fractures of the ankle, talus, and midfoot may be
treated with the established indications for open reduction and internal fixation, assuming that the patient is

medically fit, vascular status is adequate, there is minimal
swelling, and the skin is in good condition. Patients who
have already entered the acute dissolution phase with
early demineralization and soft tissue inflammation are
poorer candidates for operative treatment of their acute
fractures.

Management of Unstable Ankle Fractures in the Neuropathic Patient

Ankle fractures are encountered by a wide spectrum of
providers. Appropriate clinical management can reduce
the possibility of severe disability or deformity. When
compared to healthy patients with an ankle fracture, diabetic patients have increased in-hospital mortality, postoperative complications, length of stay, and total hospital
charges.[50] Complications of treating ankle fractures in
diabetic patients have ranged from 32% to 64%, with
amputation rates ranging from 10% to 42%.[51-58] However,
poor results have not been limited to operative treatment of ankle fractures in neuropathic patients. In one
series, a 66% incidence of infection occurred in diabetic
patients whose ankle fractures were treated with casting
alone.[52] Closed management has also been reported to
have an incidence of malunion of up to 70%.[56] Overall,
results of open or closed treatment of open ankle fractures in diabetic patients have been disastrous, with deep

infec-

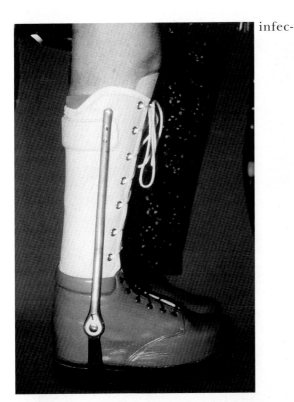

Figure 23–9 Double-upright modified calf lacer ankle-foot orthosis attached to an in-depth shoe with an extended steel shank and a rocker sole. This style of ankle-foot orthosis is utilized when there is significant foot deformity that requires specialized footwear for accommodation.

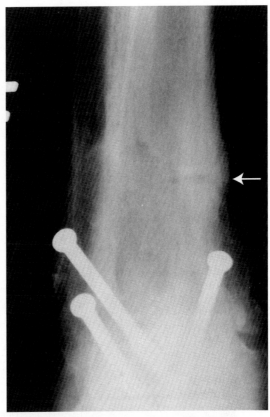

Figure 23–11 Anteroposterior radiograph following tibiotalocalcaneal arthrodesis with cannulated screws. Note the cortical lucency proximal to the arthrodesis site (*arrow*) indicating a tibial stress fracture. The fracture occurred while the patient was walking without her brace or in-depth shoe with rocker sole. The fracture was treated with 8 weeks of TCC followed by resumption of brace use.

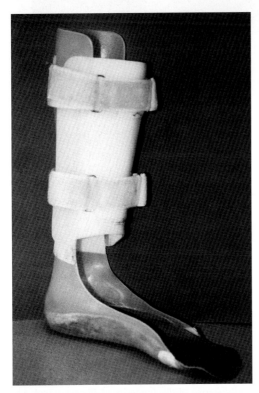

Figure 23–10 Two-piece polypropylene clamshell type ankle-foot orthosis used for immobilization of an Eichenholtz stage II or III neuropathic fracture or following hindfoot arthrodesis of a neuropathic deformity.

tion in 64%, amputations in 42%, and a mortality rate of up to 11%.[58] To address this problem, the author has developed a protocol for the treatment of unstable bimalleolar ankle fractures in the neuropathic patient.[53] Traditional ankle fracture internal fixation is augmented by the addition of one or two Steinmann pins across the ankle and subtalar joints[59] to prevent hardware failure, mortise displacement, and joint deformity (Fig. 23-13). The pins are cut off below the level of the plantar skin and removed in 6 to 10 weeks at a cast change.

It is important to approximately double the length of nonweight-bearing immobilization for a given fracture in neuropathic patients. Therefore, the typical ankle fracture would be kept nonweight-bearing for approximately 3 months, as opposed to 6 weeks. Casting would continue for approximately 4 to 5 months following injury, until the fracture demonstrated radiographic union and the patient was able to become fully ambulatory in a cast. Bracing the foot and ankle for hindfoot and ankle fractures would then be utilized for 1 year following the injury to prevent the late development of a Charcot joint. If the patient has a stable, well-aligned ankle and hindfoot after 12 to 18 months of acute fracture management and bracing, the patient may be weaned from the brace

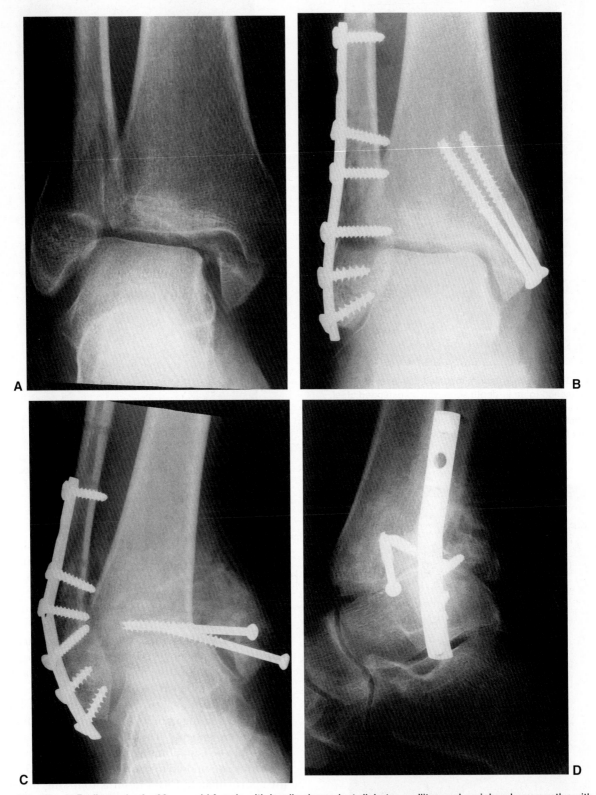

Figure 23-12   A, Radiograph of a 33-year-old female with insulin-dependent diabetes mellitus and peripheral neuropathy with loss of protective sensation and a bimalleolar right ankle fracture. **B,** Anteroposterior radiograph of the same patient following open reduction and rigid internal fixation of bimalleolar ankle fracture. The patient was placed in a prefabricated removable brace for postoperative immobilization. **C,** Touch weight-bearing was allowed, and this varus deformity was noted within 4 weeks postoperatively. Note the displacement of the medial malleolus and the bending of the fibular plate with varus angulation at the ankle joint. **D,** Lateral radiograph 4 weeks postoperatively, demonstrating posterior subluxation of the talar body and collapse of the posterior malleolus, which was not present on the initial inquiry radiographs.

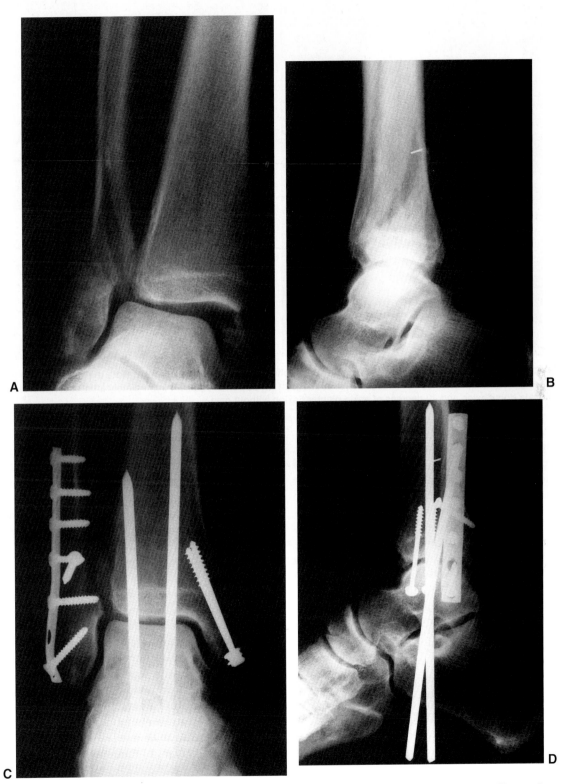

Figure 23–13   **A, B,** Mortise and lateral radiographs of a 58-year-old male with insulin-dependent diabetes mellitus and severe peripheral neuropathy with displaced bimalleolar right ankle fracture. **C,** Postoperative mortise view radiograph following open reduction and internal fixation of the bimalleolar ankle fracture and insertion of two smooth Steinmann pins across subtalar and ankle joints to enhance stability. **D,** Lateral radiograph following open reduction and internal fixation. Note that one of the pins engages the posterior cortex of the tibia, significantly improving pin fixation.

Illustration continued on following page.

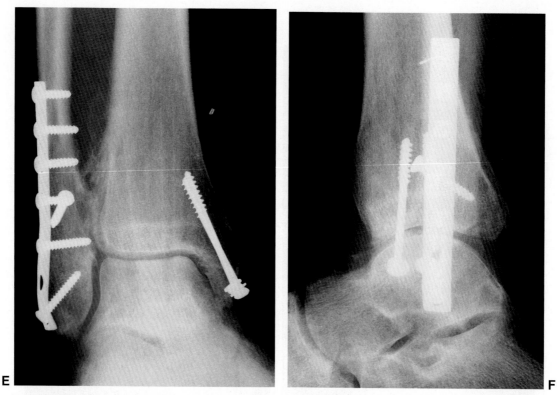

Figure 23–13, cont'd   E, F, Mortise view and lateral radiographs at 5 months postoperatively. Note the healing of the fracture without displacement or destruction of the ankle joint. Ankle range of motion on this patient immediately after cast removal was 5 degrees of ankle dorsiflexion and 40 degrees of ankle plantar flexion without pain.

into appropriate footwear. During the weaning period, patients are carefully monitored for the development of a Charcot joint. When this protocol was used, the major complication rate was 25% with 13% progressing to amputation. This represents an improved outcome compared to most historical controls.[53] This protocol for prolonged immobilization might be overtreatment for some patients who are not destined to progress to a Charcot joint. However, there are no known predictors of which fracture in a given neuropathic patient will progress to a Charcot joint. Therefore, it seems prudent to treat every patient with loss of protective sensation as if a Charcot joint will develop, in hopes of preventing severe deformity (Fig. 23-14).

Summary

Reconstruction of the Charcot foot and ankle is a valuable technique for the patient with a severe deformity who cannot be managed by appropriate footwear and bracing. The goals of surgery are to render the patient able to wear shoes and braces and to prevent amputation. Despite complications, the overall success rate is approximately 80%. Stability and appropriate alignment are more important than bony union in obtaining a successful result. Important operative techniques include meticulous handling of the soft tissues and rigid internal fixation with bone grafting. Prolonged immobilization is necessary with doubling of the standard periods for nonweight-bearing and weight-bearing casting and bracing. Limb salvage with realignment and arthrodesis of the severely deformed foot and ankle will in most cases prevent amputation and likely provide a more functional limb. When these operative indications and techniques are used, patient satisfaction following these procedures is high. Recognizing and understanding the reasons for the high rate of complications in the treatment of ankle and foot fractures in diabetic neuropathic patients make up an important factor in improving outcomes of these injuries.

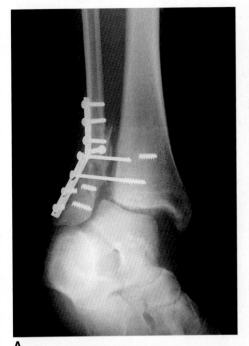

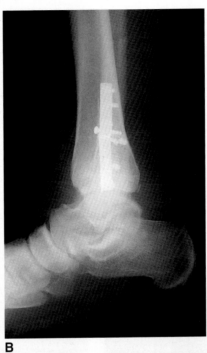

A

B

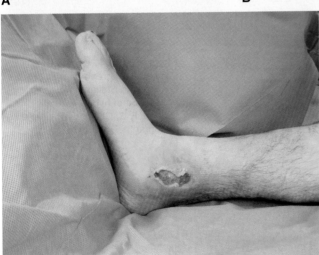

C

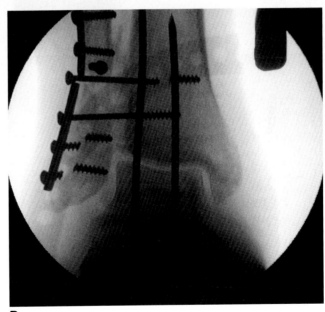

D

Figure 23–14 **A, B,** Mortise and lateral ankle radiographs of a 52-year-old male with type 2 diabetes mellitus at 3 months after ankle fracture fixation. He had begun aggressive physical therapy and was performing one-legged hopping. **C,** An open medial ankle wound precludes revision internal fixation. **D,** Intraoperative fluoroscopic mortise radiograph demonstrating closed reduction with placement of axial Steinmann pins and application of a small wire external fixator.

Illustration continued on following page.

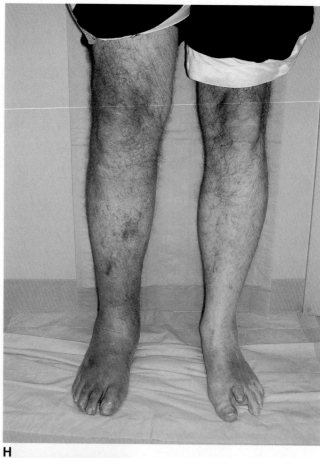

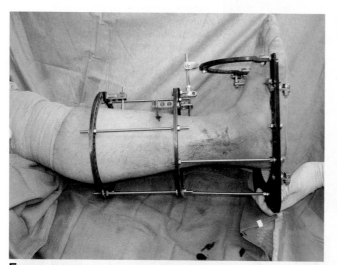

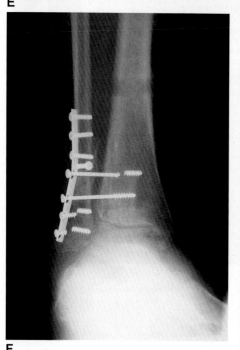

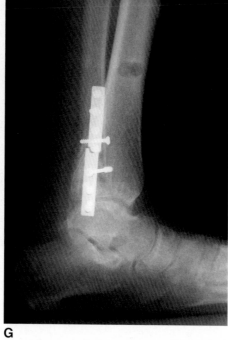

Figure 23–14, cont'd E, Clinical photograph after axial fixation with Steinmann pins and application of hybrid external fixation. **F, G,** Oblique and lateral radiographs 7 months after treatment of malunion/nonunion. Note that the fibular fracture has united. **H,** Clinical standing photograph 7 months after treatment of malunion/nonunion. The patient discontinued the molded polypropylene ankle-foot orthosis at one year post surgery and remains ambulating ulcer free with a stable ankle 2 years postoperatively.

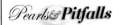

Pearls

- With both conservative and surgical management of neuropathic patients with acute ankle or foot fractures, double everything: fixation, duration of nonweight-bearing, duration of TCC, and vigilance for problems.
- Appropriate surgical indications include the following: selected acute fractures in neuropathic patients, deformities of the foot or ankle that are not amenable to management with custom bracing or custom footwear, deformity with significant instability, and recurrent ulceration due to deformity.
- Consider thin-wire and ring external fixators in correcting deformities in patients with active ulceration.
- Address equinus contracture with judicious use of proximal gastrocnemius and/or soleus lengthening or Achilles tendon lengthening.
- During the surgical approach, develop full-thickness flaps down to bone. Avoid unnecessary soft tissue dissection.

Pitfalls

- Failure to approach surgery on limbs in the Eichenholtz stage I of development of Charcot arthropathy with caution.
- Failure to follow appropriate postoperative management, including too little time in a total-contact cast, too short a nonweight-bearing period, and improper or ineffective orthotic or pedorthic management.
- Overlengthening of the Achilles tendon.
- Using internal fixation for reconstruction in the presence of ulcers.
- Failure to recognize the poor vascular status of a limb prior to surgical intervention.

References

1. Early JS, Hansen ST: Surgical reconstruction of the diabetic foot: A salvage approach to midfoot collapse. Foot Ankle Int 17:325–330, 1996.
2. Myerson MS, et al: Symposium: Neuroarthropathy of the foot. Contemp Orthop 26:43–64, 1993.
3. Papa J, Myerson M, Girard P: Salvage, with arthrodesis, in intractable diabetic neuropathic arthropathy of the foot and ankle. J Bone Joint Surg Am 75(7):1056–1066, 1993.
4. Sammarco GJ, Conti SF: Surgical treatment of neuroarthropathic foot deformity. Foot Ankle Int 19(2):102–109, 1998.
5. Johnson JT: Neuropathic fractures and joint injuries: Pathogenesis and rationale of prevention and treatment. J Bone Joint Surg Am 49(1):1–30, 1967.
6. Kristiansen B: Ankle and foot fractures in diabetics provoking neuropathic joint changes. Acta Orthop Scand 51(6):975–979, 1980.
7. National Institute of Diabetes and Digestive and Kidney Diseases: National Diabetes Statistics Fact Sheet: General Information and National Estimates on Diabetes in the United States, rev ed. Bethesda, MD: National Institutes of Health, 2005.
8. Foltz KD, Fallat LM, Schwartz S: Usefulness of a brief assessment battery for early detection of Charcot foot deformity in patients with diabetes. J Foot Ankle Surg 43(2):87–92, 2004.
9. Eichenholtz SN: Charcot Joints. Springfield, IL: Charles C. Thomas, 1966.
10. Johnson JE: Surgical reconstruction of the diabetic Charcot foot and ankle. Foot Ankle Clin 2:37–55, 1997.
11. Brodsky JW, Rouse AM: Exostectomy for symptomatic bony prominences in diabetic Charcot feet. Clin Orthop, 296:21–26, 1993.
12. Cofield RH: Diabetic neuroarthropathy in the foot: Patient characteristics and patterns of radiographic change. Foot Ankle 4:15, 1983.
13. Harris JR, Brand PW: Patterns of disentegration of the tarsus in the anaesthetic foot. J Bone Joint Surg, 48-B:4–16, 1966.
14. Sanders LJ, Frykberg RG: Diabetic neuropathic osteoarthropathy: The Charcot foot. In Frykberg RG (ed): The High Risk Foot in Diabetes Mellitus. New York: Churchill Livingstone, 1991.
15. Herbst SA, Jones KB, Saltzman CL: Pattern of diabetic neuropathic arthropathy associated with the peripheral bone mineral density. J Bone Joint Surg Br 86(3):378–383, 2004.
16. Larsen K, Fabrin J, Holstein, PE: Incidence and management of ulcers in diabetic Charcot feet. J Wound Care 10(8):323–328, 2001.
17. Willrich A, Pinzur M, McNeil M, et al: Health related quality of life, cognitive function, and depression in diabetic patients with foot ulcer or amputation: A preliminary study. Foot Ankle Int 26(2):128–134, 2005.
18. Pakarinen TK, Laine HJ, Honkonen SE, et al: Charcot arthropathy of the diabetic foot: Current concepts and review of 36 cases. Scand J Surg 91(2):195–201, 2002.
19. Pinzur M: Surgical versus accommodative treatment for Charcot arthropathy of the midfoot. Foot Ankle Int 25(8):545–549, 2004.
20. Pinzur MS: Benchmark analysis of diabetic patients with neuropathic (Charcot) foot deformity. Foot Ankle Int 20(9):564–567, 1999.
21. Saltzman CL, Hagy ML, Zimmerman B, et al: How effective is intensive nonoperative initial treatment of patients with diabetes and Charcot arthropathy of the feet? Clin Orthop Relat Res 435:185–190, 2005.
22. Schon LC, Easley ME, Weinfeld SB: Charcot neuroarthropathy of the foot and ankle. Clin Orthop Relat Res 349:116–131, 1998.
23. Mitchell JR, Johnson JE, Collier BD, Gould JS: Stress fracture of the tibia following extensive hindfoot and ankle arthrodesis: A report of three cases. Foot Ankle Int 16(7):445–448, 1995.
24. Pinzur MS, Noonan T: Ankle arthrodesis with a retrograde femoral nail for Charcot ankle arthropathy. Foot Ankle Int 26(7):545–549, 2005.
25. Simon SR, Tejwani SG, Wilson DL, et al: Arthrodesis as an early alternative to nonoperative management of Charcot arthropathy of the diabetic foot. J Bone Joint Surg Am 82-A(7):939–950, 2000.
26. Myerson MS, Edwards WH: Management of neuropathic fractures in the foot and ankle. J Am Acad Orthop Surg 7(1):8–18, 1999.
27. Myerson MS, Henderson MR, Saxby T, Short KW: Management of midfoot diabetic neuroarthropathy. Foot Ankle Int 15(5):233–241, 1994.
28. Johnson JE: Prospective study of bone, indium-111-labeled white blood cells, and gallium-67 scanning for the evaluation of osteomyelitis in the diabetic foot. Foot Ankle Int 17:10–16, 1996.
29. Schauwecker DS, Park HM, Burt RW, et al: Combined bone scintigraphy and indium-111 leukocyte scans in neuropathic foot disease. J Nucl Med 29(10):1651–1655, 1988.
30. Hopfner S, Krolak C, Kessler S, et al: Preoperative imaging of Charcot neuroarthropathy in diabetic patients: Comparison of ring PET, hybrid PET, and magnetic resonance imaging. Foot Ankle Int 25(12):890–895, 2004.
31. Termaat MF, Raijmakers PG, Scholten HJ, et al: The accuracy of diagnostic imaging for the assessment of chronic osteomyelitis: A systematic review and meta-analysis. J Bone Joint Surg Am 87(11):2464–2471, 2005.
32. Brodsky JW: The diabetic foot. In Mann RA, Coughlin MJ (eds): Surgery of the Foot and Ankle. St. Louis: Mosby, 1993.
33. Johnson JE: Operative treatment of neuropathic arthropathy of the foot and ankle. J Bone Joint Surg Am 80(11):1700–1709, 1998.
34. Mueller MJ, Sinacore DR, Hastings MK, et al: Effect of Achilles tendon lengthening on neuropathic plantar ulcers: A randomized clinical trial. J Bone Joint Surg Am 85-A(8):1436–1445, 2003.
35. Catanzariti AR, Mendicino R, Haverstock B: Ostectomy for diabetic neuroarthropathy involving the midfoot. J Foot Ankle Surg 39(5):291–300, 2000.
36. Russotti GM, Johnson KA, Cass JR: Tibiotalocalcaneal arthrodesis for arthritis and deformity of the hind part of the foot. J Bone Joint Surg Am 70(9):1304–1307, 1988.
37. Alvarez RG, Barbou, TM, Perkins TD: Tibiocalcaneal arthrodesis for nonbraceable neuropathic ankle deformity. Foot Ankle Int 15:354–359, 1994.
38. Marks RM, Parks BG, Schon LC: Midfoot fusion technique for neuroarthropathic feet: Biomechanical analysis and rationale. Foot Ankle Int 19(8):507–510, 1998.
39. Schon LC, Marks RM: The management of neuroarthropathic fracture: Dislocations in the diabetic patient. Orthop Clin North Am 26(2):375–392, 1995.

40. Cooper PS: Application of external fixators for management of Charcot deformities of the foot and ankle. Foot Ankle Clin 7(1):207–254, 2002.
41. Farber DC, Juliano PJ, Cavanagh PR, et al: Single stage correction with external fixation of the ulcerated foot in individuals with Charcot neuroarthropathy. Foot Ankle Int 23(2):130–134, 2002.
42. Stone NC, Daniels TR: Midfoot and hindfoot arthrodeses in diabetic Charcot arthropathy. Can J Surg, 43(6):449–455, 2000.
43. Tisdel CL, Marcus RE, Heiple KG: Triple arthrodesis for diabetic peritalar neuropathy. Foot Ankle Int 16:332–338, 1995.
44. Cleveland M: Surgical fusion of unstable ankle joints due to neuropathic disturbance. Am J Surg 43:580, 1939.
45. Stuart MJ, Morrey BF: Arthrodesis of the diabetic neuropathic ankle joint. Clin Orthop Relat Res 253:209–211, 1990.
46. Bono JV, Roger DJ: Surgical arthrodesis of the neuropathic foot: A salvage procedure. Clin Orthop 296:14–20, 1993.
47. Pinzur MS, Gold J, Schwartz D, Gross N: Energy demands for walking in dysvascular amputees as related to the level of amputation. Orthopedics 15(9):1033–1036; discussion 1036–1037, 1992.
48. Waters RL, Perry J, Antonelli D, Hislop H: Energy cost of walking of amputees: The influence of level of amputation. J Bone Joint Surg Am 58(1):42–46, 1976.
49. Mueller MJ: Identifying patients with diabetes mellitus who are at risk for lower-extremity complications: Use of Semmes-Weinstein monofilaments. Phys Ther 76(1):68–71, 1996.
50. Ganesh SP, Pietrobon R, Cecilio WA, et al: The impact of diabetes on patient outcomes after ankle fracture. J Bone Joint Surg Am 87(8):1712–1718, 2005.
51. Blotter RH, Connolly E, Wasan A, Chapman MW: Acute complications in the operative treatment of isolated ankle fractures in patients with diabetes mellitus. Foot Ankle Int 20(11):687–694, 1999.
52. Flynn JM, Rodriguez-del Rio F, Piza PA: Closed ankle fractures in the diabetic patient. Foot Ankle Int 21(4):311–319, 2000.
53. Jani MM, Ricci WM, Borrelli J Jr, et al: A protocol for treatment of unstable ankle fractures using transarticular fixation in patients with diabetes mellitus and loss of protective sensibility. Foot Ankle Int 24(11):838–844, 2003.
54. Jones KB, Maiers-Yelden KA, Marsh JL,. et al: Ankle fractures in patients with diabetes mellitus. J Bone Joint Surg Br 87(4):489–495, 2005.
55. Low CK, Tan SK: Infection in diabetic patients with ankle fractures. Ann Acad Med Singapore 24(3):353–355, 1995.
56. McCormack RG, Leith JM: Ankle fractures in diabetics: Complications of surgical management. J Bone Joint Surg Br 80(4):689–692, 1998.
57. Mendicino RW, Catanzariti AR, Saltrick KR, et al: Tibiotalocalcaneal arthrodesis with retrograde intramedullary nailing. J Foot Ankle Surg 43(2):82–86, 2004.
58. White CB, Turner NS, Lee GC, Haidukewych GJ: Open ankle fractures in patients with diabetes mellitus. Clin Orthop Relat Res 414:37–44, 2003.
59. Childress HM: Vertical transarticular-pin fixation for unstable ankle fractures. J Bone Joint Surg 47-A:1323–1334, 1965.

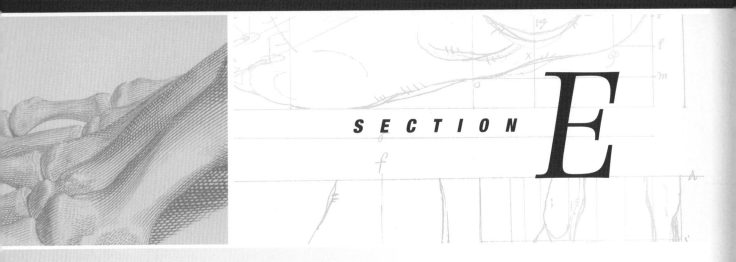

SECTION E

TEAM APPROACH

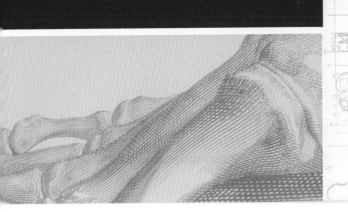

DIABETIC FOOT PROBLEMS AND THEIR MANAGEMENT AROUND THE WORLD

ANDREW J. M. BOULTON AND LORETTA VILEIKYTE ∎

"One day everything will be well—that is our hope.
Everything is fine today—that is our illusion."

— Voltaire

At the beginning of the 21st century, we are facing a global diabetes epidemic. The prevalence of diabetes is rising owing to a number of factors, including the increasing frequency of obesity, increasing physical inactivity, population growth, aging, and urbanization. The global prevalence of diabetes was estimated to be 2.8% in 2000 and is predicted to increase to 4.4% by 2030, meaning that there will be more than 366 million individuals with diabetes worldwide by that year.[1] These depressing statistics have immense consequences for the future incidence and prevalence of complications, including neuropathy, peripheral vascular disease, and diabetic foot problems. The vast majority of the increase in prevalence is accounted for by people with type 2 diabetes. Such individuals have usually had asymptomatic hyperglycemia for many years before diabetes is diagnosed; therefore, they frequently present with the complications of diabetes at diagnosis. This rapidly rising incidence of diabetes suggests that there will be a parallel increase in the frequency of diabetic foot problems, particularly in developing countries. The words of Voltaire quoted above aptly summarize the global situation with regard to the diagnosis and management of diabetic foot

problems. However, there have been a number of encouraging developments since the previous edition of this book was published. These have occurred partly as a result of the realization of the vast economic consequences of lower-limb diabetic complications. In 1998, Holzer and colleagues[2] studied a database of 7 million U.S. residents for health insurance; in 2 years, the total expenditure for treated diabetic foot ulcers was $16 million, an average of $4595 per ulcer episode. In 2001, the expenditure on diabetic foot ulceration and amputations was estimated to have cost U.S. health payers $10.9 billion.[3]

In the United Kingdom, diabetic patients are four times more likely to be admitted to hospital, and this figure rises 16 times for those with peripheral neuropathy.[4] U.K. estimates on cost, using the same methodology as the U.S. studies, were that 5% of the total national health service expenditure in 2001 (UK£ 3 billion) was attributable to diabetes. The total annual cost of diabetes-related foot complications was estimated to be UK£ 252 million.[5] The data from Sweden are equally depressing: In a careful study of the economics of treating foot ulcers, the cost of healing with hospitalization and surgery was $57,300 per case, compared with $8,500 per case for primary healing alone (1990 prices).[6] As Johnson and Williams pointed out,[7] though, many of these economic analyses failed to take account of the indirect costs, such as absence from work, disability benefits, and costs of home alterations.

Reassuringly, however, it has not only been health care economics that have resulted in increased awareness of foot problems. There has also been a steady rise in the volume of research and presentations in this area observed worldwide, resulting in a marked increase in the number of peer-reviewed publications on the topic of the diabetic foot. Taken as a percentage of all PubMed listed papers on diabetes, papers on the diabetic foot have increased from 0.7% between 1980 and 1988 to more than 2.7% in the last 6 years. During the same period, foot councils and study groups have been formed in the European and American Diabetes Associations, and the International Working Group on the Diabetic Foot has published its consensus. Symposia on the diabetic foot are frequently held at annual meetings of national and international societies, and developing countries such as Colombia and India have founded their own diabetic foot societies.

The year 2005 was a landmark year for the diabetic foot on a global basis. The International Diabetes Federation designated 2005 as the Year of the Diabetic Foot. Press conferences were held on every continent, with activities in many countries around the world. This culminated in a global press conference held in Brazil on World Diabetes Day (the birthday of Frederick Banting, discoverer of insulin) on November 14, 2005. Another "first" was that the international medical journal *The Lancet* dedicated almost an entire issue to the problems of the diabetic foot, containing reviews and original articles; the front cover (Fig. 24-1) carried the dramatic message that "Every 30 seconds a lower limb is lost somewhere in the world as a consequence of diabetes."[3]

Other developments include the formation of multinational groups specifically established to gather data and institute multinational studies and guidelines. Examples include the Lower Extremity Amputation group, which has a study in progress designed to compare the incidence of lower-limb amputation over time within and between communities across the world.[8] The International Working Group on the Diabetic Foot was established in 1997, and its guidelines on diagnosis and management issues were published in 1999. During the International Diabetes Federation's Year of the Diabetic Foot, the International Diabetes Federation and the International Working Group on the Diabetic Foot published a book entitled *Diabetes and Foot Care: Time to Act*.[9] Finally, strong evidence of increasing activity in the diabetic foot clinical and research areas is provided by the large number of national and multinational meetings being held solely on this topic. The Fifth International Meeting on the Diabetic Foot will be held in the Netherlands in 2007, and the Twelfth International Malvern Diabetic Foot meeting will be held in Malvern, United Kingdom, in

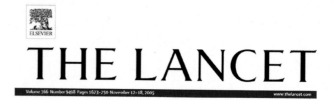

THE LANCET

Volume 366 Number 9498 Pages 1623-750 November 12-18, 2005   www.thelancet.com

"Every 30 seconds a lower limb is lost somewhere in the world as a consequence of diabetes."

See Review page 1719

Articles	Articles	Articles	Review	Review
SIDESTEP: ertapenem for diabetic foot infections *See page 1695*	Wound therapy after diabetic foot amputation *See page 1704*	Skin microcirculation and muscle metabolism of diabetic foot *See page 1711*	Treatment of diabetic foot ulcers *See page 1725*	Wound healing in diabetic foot *See page 1736*

Figure 24–1   The *Lancet* issue that coincided with World Diabetes Day, November 14, 2005. For the first time, virtually the whole issue of *The Lancet* was dedicated to the diabetic foot. *(Reprinted with permission from The Lancet 366:9498; 2005.)*

2008. A newer international meeting entitled "DF Con" (Diabetic Foot Conference) is now held annually in Los Angeles. Regular national meetings are also held in countries from every continent, including the Scandinavian countries, Belgium, the United States, Canada, Italy, and many others. Thus, reverting to Voltaire's words, it appears that whereas the illusion of good global foot care remains, we have reason to be hopeful that improvements will continue.

In approaching the vast topic of this chapter, it soon became apparent that no expert could possibly be all inclusive on global foot care. Whereas the risks and prevalence of foot problems vary according to geographic location, there is no diabetic population that is immune to neuropathy, vascular disease, ulceration, and amputation. Although published data on the epidemiologic aspects of foot problems are of variable quality, in Table 24-1 we have attempted to provide a global overview of the problem, with references taken from published articles or presentations at national meetings. We have also attempted to collect data from countries representing all the remaining continents, but again, the sources of data vary from regional experts to papers in peer-reviewed journals. In our defense, we believe that it is important to include information from as many countries as possible, even if published data are unavailable.

TABLE 24-1 Epidemiologic Data on Diabetic Foot Problems Worldwide, Indicating the Prevalence and Incidence of Foot Ulcers and Amputations in Diabetic Populations

Study and Country	N	Prevalence (%)		Incidence (%)		Risk Factors for Ulcers (%)	Note
		Ulcers	Amputation	Ulcers	Amputation		
Population-Based Studies							
Abbott et al., 2002 (UK)[18]	9,710	1.7	1.3	2.2	—	7	
Humphrey et al., 1996 (Nauru, Pacific Region)[54]	1,564	—	—	—	0.76	—	From estimated 7.6/1000 person-years
Kumar et al., 1994 (UK)[17]	811	1.4	—	—	—	41.6	Type 2 diabetes only
Manes et al., 2002[34] (Greece)	821	4.8	—	—	—		
Muller et al., 2002 (Netherlands)[19]	665	—	—	2.1	0.6	—	
Clinic-Based Studies							
Belhadj, 1998 (Algeria)[60]	865	11.9	6.7	—	—	58.4	
Pendsey, 1994 (India)[42]	11,300	3.6	—	—	—	—	
Urbancic-Rovan and Slak, 1998 (Slovenia)[38]	701	7.1	—	—	—	86.3	

N, total diabetic population.

Europe

Aside from North America, most information on research and clinical management of diabetic foot problems is available from Europe. Most European countries have participated in the implementation of the International Guidelines on Diabetic Foot care,[9] and many have established multidisciplinary foot clinics. Nonetheless, much disparity remains; for example, few eastern European countries have foot clinics or podiatry services. There have been collaborative ventures between European countries in the area of the diabetic foot. In one example, no major differences were observed in comparing risk factors for foot ulceration among large clinics in four countries, two in northern and two in southern Europe.[10] Therefore, it was concluded that similar strategies for the prevention of foot problems should be equally successful in all European countries.

United Kingdom

Many reports and publications on the diabetic foot have been produced in the United Kingdom over the years. It was Pryce, a surgeon working in Nottingham, who realized the importance of peripheral neuropathy in the pathogenesis of diabetic foot ulcers,[11] and it was almost 70 years ago in London that McKeown performed the first successful wedge or ray excision.[12] More recently, the first detailed reports on the potential success of the team approach and the combined diabetic foot clinic were reported.[13,14] Despite this, "Everything is fine today—that is our illusion" is sadly true.

Every resident is entitled to free health care from the National Health Service, and all have access to a general practitioner at the primary care level. Many type 2 diabetic patients are cared for by the general practitioner,

often with a practice nurse. Most, but certainly not all, practices can provide podiatry care. Onward referral to hospital diabetes clinics may occur, especially if there are complications. Moreover, specialist multidisciplinary diabetic foot clinics are increasingly common in the United Kingdom (population 56 million). Diabetes care is provided, with the annual review[15] being the cornerstone of management. Detailed guidelines have been published as part of the St. Vincent initiative.[16] Disturbing evidence as to the lack of chiropody (podiatry) care in certain districts of the United Kingdom was highlighted in this report.

A large population-based study from three districts in the United Kingdom confirm that 1.4% of type 2 diabetic patients had active foot ulcers and 5% had ever had ulcers.[17] More recently, a larger community-based U.K. study reported a 2% annual incidence of foot ulcers,[18] similar to a comparable primary-care population in the Netherlands[19] (see Table 24-1). Perhaps the most important message from the U.K. community-based study was that simple clinical tests predict those who are at risk of ulceration.[18] This finding has implications for screening strategies in developing countries. A composite clinical score with dichotomous variables (the modified neuropathy disability score) was the best predictor of risks. This score requires only a tuning fork, a pin, and a reflex hammer and no specialist equipment. Interesting data exist on foot ulcer risks for patients from ethnic minorities within the United Kingdom; South Asian and African-Caribbean patients seem to have a much reduced risk of foot ulcers.[20]

France

There is increasing interest in diabetic foot problems in France, where most type 2 diabetic patients are cared for by general practitioners, as in the United Kingdom.

Moreover, there are no podiatrists in France, although local nail care is provided by pedicurists. In a country with a population of approximately 60 million, it is estimated that there are only about 15 multidisciplinary diabetic foot clinics. With an increasing realization of the problem, however, there have been recent efforts to improve the knowledge of diabetic foot problems among health care professionals.[21] Studies from Grenoble have also estimated the cost of diabetic foot care in that center.[22] The average cost of a hospital admission for a foot ulcer in 1997 was Fr103,718, (US $17,000), including direct and indirect costs. These varied from Fr55,500 (US $8770) for a Wagner grade 1 lesion up to Fr175,700 (US $28,800) for a gangrenous grade 4 foot.[22] The establishment of a team approach in a Paris clinic has been shown to be beneficial, with a 33% reduction in hospital inpatients' length of stay and, with regard to the St. Vincent Initiative, a significant 50% reduction of major amputations.[23]

Germany

As in other European countries, diabetes care is mainly based on a primary care model for type 2 diabetes. Because of current funding difficulties, referral from primary care to either outpatient specialist or hospital clinics is regulated. In the largest country in Europe (population: approximately 80 million), there are about 150 multidisciplinary diabetic foot clinics, which are equally divided between primary and secondary care. Since the previous edition of this book, podiatry has developed as a profession in Germany with 2 years' training, and podiatry treatment is now reimbursed, but only for people with diabetes. There are also well-trained orthopedic shoe makers who receive public reimbursement for custom-made diabetic shoes. The German Diabetes Association has established a working group on the provision of foot care across the country, and there is a diabetic foot special interest group that has regular meetings every year for those who are interested in these problems. Recently, data were published of a survey across 351 general practices in Germany.[24] According to this study, the number of patients with active ulcers was somewhat lower than that in other European countries (1%), but 1.5% had already undergone some level of amputation. Despite setting up a patient education program, Trautner and colleagues were unable to demonstrate any change in the incidence of amputations over an 8-year period in the city of Leverkusen.[25]

Italy

There are a number of major centers with a particular interest and excellence in diabetic foot care in Italy, but as in other countries, large rural areas have no specific foot services. Podiatry services are not routinely available, but there are a number of good footwear suppliers. Indeed, one of the first randomized studies to demonstrate the efficacy of therapeutic footwear in reducing recurrent ulcers was performed in Rome.[26] Two more recent studies suggest an improvement in ulcer and amputation rates in Italy. Anichini and colleagues have demonstrated a 20% reduction in hospital admissions for diabetic foot problems 5 years after implementation of the International Consensus Group on the Diabetic Foot Guidelines.[27] This was achieved through population screening and the establishment of a prevention program. Similarly, Faglia and colleagues demonstrated a reduction in the incidence of new ulcers and major amputation, which they attributed to the widespread use of intensive education and training together with the use of therapeutic shoes.[28]

Benelux Countries

The Netherlands, unlike many other European countries, have a well-developed network of podiatrists, all of whom undergo a 3-year training degree course. Bakker and colleagues reviewed the role of podiatrists and diabetic foot care and found, in a national survey, that in 32% of hospitals a podiatrist was specifically available for the care of diabetic patients.[29] Six years after the original report of Bakker and colleagues, the number of hospitals with both podiatrists and a diabetic foot clinic has more than doubled, and this might explain the significant reduction of amputations recently reported from the Netherlands by van Houtum and colleagues.[30] Although Belgium does not have such a well-developed podiatry program, a national training program in diabetic foot care for all doctors treating diabetic patients (including general practitioners) was established in 1997, and a well-attended course was conducted in 1998. This is led by the group from Antwerp, the same group that previously participated in the European Study of Risk Factors for Foot Ulcers, which demonstrated no major differences between northern and southern European clinics.[10]

Scandinavia

In comparison with other European countries, standards of screening and educational foot care are generally high in all Scandinavian countries, with qualified podiatrists available throughout the area. Multidisciplinary diabetic foot clinics have been established in many other cities across the four countries, and a number of important studies have been published by diabetic foot experts in Scandinavia, who have also demonstrated significant reductions in amputation rates.[6,31,32] Many Scandinavian studies have emphasized the costs of diabetic foot care and amputations.[3] In a cost-utility analysis based on the Markov model, it was suggested that if intensive prevention could reduce the incidence of foot ulcers and amputations by 25%, the simulated preventive strategy would be cost effective and save money in all patients with diabetes mellitus except those without specific risk factors.[33]

Other Western European Countries

Austria, with a population of approximately 8 million, has no fully trained podiatrists, but at least 10 foot clinics have been established in recent years. There is no structured diabetic foot service in Greece, whose population is approximately 10 million. There are a number of overseas trained podiatrists in Greece, and a multidisciplinary diabetic foot service was established in Athens in 1998 and one in Thessalonica several years later. In a recent study from the latter center, the prevalence of foot ulcers was reported to be 4.8% (see Table 24-1).[34] Structured foot care programs have now been established in some Spanish cities, including Madrid and Barcelona. In a community-based study in the Barcelona region, however, a high prevalence of diabetic foot problems was reported, with 10% of 2595 type 2 diabetic patients identified as being affected.[35] Much work on the team approach and the importance of patient education has originated in Geneva, Switzerland, where a structured educational program for footwear has been established for many years. As Peter-Reisch and colleagues demonstrated in a presentation, reulceration rates can be significantly reduced by regular foot clinic attendance and medical supervision.[36]

Eastern Europe

Problems in diabetic foot care still exist in former Soviet countries, although progress is being made, as is indicated by a large, very oversubscribed meeting held in Moscow in spring 2005. Multidisciplinary foot clinics now exist in large cities in a number of countries, including Russia, Ukraine, Byelorussia, and Georgia. Of the former Soviet countries, however, the Baltic states probably have the best foot care system. More than seven foot clinics are now operational in Lithuania. The establishment of a multidisciplinary foot care team, with provision of appropriate footwear when needed, resulted in a 48% reduction of recurrent ulcers over 2 years.[37] Former Warsaw Pact countries are developing organized foot care programs in many cities; however, major difficulties remain in the former Yugoslavia. Organized foot care programs are being established in Slovenia (population 2 million), Bosnia (4 million), and Macedonia (2 million), but reliable data were not available for Serbia (10 million), Croatia (4 million), or Montenegro (1 million). Most progress has been made in Slovenia; some form of foot care is available in 15 centers, four having specialized diabetic foot clinics. During a period of 16 months, over

700 patients were screened in Ljubljana; 9% had a history of foot ulcers, and only 14% had healthy feet.[38] Foot clinics are also being established in many other countries, including Bulgaria, the Czech Republic, Slovakia, Poland, and Hungary.

Asia

Considering the vast population of this continent, there are sparse data on diabetic foot problems from this part of the world. As was done for Europe, some countries will be discussed in individual sections, but for many others, reliable information was unavailable.

China

China is the world's most populous country. The prevalence of diabetes rose from 0.5% to 2.5% in the adult population between 1991 and 1995, when it was estimated that 15 million Chinese had diabetes and that a further 18 million had impaired glucose tolerance.[3] By 2000, it was believed that 21 million people had diabetes, and again, this is predicted to rise to 42 million by 2030, representing a greater than 100% increase in prevalence over 30 years.[1] Until recently, most diabetic patients lived in rural communities with access to a three-tier health care system. At the first level, people with diabetes are cared for by village physicians, who received less than a year's training after junior high school. Physicians in district health centers and county hospitals, in contrast, had full medical school training.[39] Realizing the challenge of providing appropriate care for over 20 million patients, the Ministry of Health has taken the first steps through the development of a national program for diabetes. With this background, it is not surprising that foot care problems are common in Chinese diabetic patients. There is no podiatry program for diabetic patients, and amputations are common. However, interest in the diabetic foot is increasing, and some centers have established multidisciplinary teams for foot care.[40] During the International Diabetes Federation's Year of the Diabetic Foot, 2005, a large, oversubscribed meeting was held in Beijing that brought together parties interested in the diabetic foot from all over China.

Japan

Although there are no major publications on the prevalence of foot problems in Japan, foot ulceration and amputations are increasingly being reported as significant problems, with multidisciplinary foot teams being established. Diabetic foot patients, when admitted to hospital, often come under the care of dermatologists or surgeons rather than diabetologists. There is no podiatry, but several study groups comprising diabetologists, surgeons, and nurses exist. One of the main centers in Tokyo has recently reported on the high incidence of vascular foot lesions in diabetic dialysis and predialysis patients.[41] Such patients are seen by the diabetic foot care team.

Philippines

Reports from the Philippines to the International Working Group on the Diabetic Foot[9] suggested that its main problems were too many transfemoral amputations, a lack of financial support, and a lack of education for people with diabetes on problems of foot care. Unfortunately, there are no data on amputation or ulceration rates from this country. A few years ago, two Australian podiatrists started an education and training program; subsequently, a few diabetic foot care centers have been set up. Physicians from one such center have now been traveling to other parts of the country, providing educational courses under the auspices of the Philippines Diabetic Association. Thus, it appears that much progress is being made in this country.

India

India, with a population greater than 1.1 billion, has the dubious distinction of having a larger number of people with diabetes than any other country in the world. It was estimated in 2000 that there were 32 million people with diabetes in India, a number that is predicted to increase to nearly 80 million by 2030.[1] Although there are no major differences in risk factors, the clinical features of diabetic foot problems do vary in developing countries because of regional factors.[42] The hallmark of diabetic foot problems in India is gross infection; major contributing factors for late presentation include the frequency of barefoot gait, attempts at home surgery, trust in faith healers, and often undetected diabetes. Certain atypical features peculiar to this part of the world include rodents (usually rats) nibbling at insensitive feet while the patients sleep on the floor, maggots feeding on open wounds, and red ants swarming inside dressings.

Sandal-induced ulcers (from the use of chappals, with a single thong between the hallux and the second toe) are frequent, as the result of pressure and shear from the thong. Pressure points also occur on the tips of the toes from the extra force exerted while trying to keep the sandals on.[43,44] Apart from a few specialist centers in major cities, care of the diabetic foot is not organized, a problem that is compounded by a lack of podiatrists and shoe fitters. A comparative study of centers in Germany, India, and Tanzania emphasized that foot ulcers in developing countries are much more likely to be of neuropathic origin[45] and therefore highly preventable.[46] The challenge facing the developing world, in which the greatest increases in the prevalence of type 2 diabetes over the next 20 years will be seen, is to establish simple screening and education programs for people with diabetes. Such programs in India could have a major impact on reducing foot ulcer and amputation rates, as well as leading to huge economic savings.[33]

Other Asian Countries

In Singapore, a number of hospitals have established diabetic foot services with the services of podiatrists, many of whom were trained in Australia. A survey of patients in a podiatry clinic showed that ulcer causation was related mainly to barefoot gait, sandals, and other inappropriate footwear.[47] A number of centers in Taiwan have established specialist diabetic foot clinics, and studies have been reported on the variable risk factors for high levels of amputation.[48] Other Asian countries with historical connections to European countries have benefited from educational visits and training by overseas experts. For example, teams of diabetologists, podiatrists, and surgeons from the Netherlands have visited Indonesia to assist in the formation of the diabetic foot service in Jakarta.

Australasia

Although this region covers a vast area, it has a relatively low population per square mile. The main nations are Australia and New Zealand, but there are also many others, including a large number of Pacific island communities. The prevalence of type 2 diabetes is generally high among the native populations of these areas, such as the Aborigines in Australia and the Maoris in New Zealand.

Australia

Australia has a well-developed health care system, and podiatrists are available in many centers. Until recently, however, there have been few multidisciplinary diabetic foot clinics. This problem is now being addressed by the establishment of a national diabetes foot care network under the auspices of the national diabetes strategy, which is endorsed by the Australian government. With funding from this source, the Sydney group has piloted this program at 14 sites, most of which have a doctor, a nurse, and a podiatrist. After training in Sydney, each team arranged teaching sessions and practical workshops for local physicians, surgeons, general practitioners, nurses, and podiatrists. More recently, this education and training program has included many rural outposts through the use of telemedicine.[49,50] A population-based study from Australia suggested that risk factors for foot ulceration might be lower than those in other Western countries,[51] but a subsequent report showed that foot screening is poor, with less than half of the diabetic population reporting a regular foot exam.[52]

New Zealand

As in Australia, there is a well-developed health care system in New Zealand. Although podiatrists are available, the level of service remains well below the recommended 0.5 full-time equivalent per 100,000 of the population.[53] One study reported on hospital discharges for diabetic foot disease over a 13-year period ending in 1993; during this time, the national number of discharges actually increased from 14 per 100,000 total population in 1980 to 26 per 100,000 in 1993.[53] Translated into costs for this country of 3.3 million people, it is equivalent to a total inpatient management cost for diabetic foot disease in 1993 of $7.7 million (U.S. dollars). Considerable efforts have been made in certain areas of New Zealand to improve the identification and management of diabetic foot disease. The Aotearoa get-checked program was instigated by the Ministry of Health in 2000 and has resulted in a growing trend toward early detection and screening of foot pathology. The provision of free annual checks, which includes foot care and "foot health weeks," which are run by podiatrists, also raises awareness of general foot care among the population.[9]

Other Australasian Countries

The prevalence of diabetes in Fiji is high, more than 10%. Until recently, the most common cause for surgical admission to one hospital was diabetic foot ulcers, and in a 3-month period before the establishment of a foot clinic, the number of diabetic amputations at the Suva Hospital was a staggering 39. Armed with such statistics and a grant from the Australian government in collaboration with the Fijian government, the diabetes center at a Sydney hospital established high-risk diabetic foot clinics in the three main centers of Fiji. The clinic in Suva now sees 155 patients per month with ulceration or infection, and the number of admissions has been reduced to three or four per month with a dramatic reduction in amputations (M. McGill, personal communication, 1998). Sadly, despite this considerable effort, recent evidence suggests that local staff have not been able to continue and expand this program.[9] Another Pacific island, Nauru, which once had the dubious distinction of having the highest national prevalence of diabetes in the world, has been the focus of a study of amputations in diabetes.[54] The incidence of first amputation in Nauru in type 2 diabetic patients was 7.6 per 1000 person-years (see Table 24-1), but a decrease was seen after the introduction of a national foot care health education and prevention campaign in 1992.[54]

Africa

Sub-Saharan Africa

Sub-Saharan Africa contains 33 of the 50 poorest countries in the world, and this region is predicted to experience the greatest rise in the prevalence of diabetes in the next 20 years.[1] Diabetic foot complications constitute an increasing public health problem and are a leading cause of admission, amputation, and mortality in diabetes patients.[55-57] Because neuropathy is the major underlying cause, these outcomes should be, in many cases, preventable.[45] A review of the epidemiology of diabetic foot problems in Africa highlighted not only the prevalence of neuropathy, but also the increasing frequency of peripheral vascular disease, presumably as a result of increasing urbanization.[55] Unhygienic conditions, poverty, frequently coexisting HIV infection, barefoot gait, low income, and many negative cultural practices often interact to compound the situation. Early diagnosis of foot lesions, education, and appropriate treatment of sepsis are essential to improve these depressing statistics.[58]

North Africa

For North Africa, data were available from Morocco and Algeria. In Morocco, with a population of 30 million, the prevalence of diabetes is high: 13% of the population over 30 years of age. In Casablanca, 67% of foot ulcer patients are male, 88% have type 2 diabetes, and 47% of lesions are shoe induced, with 15% secondary to traditional "healing" methods.[59] The authors of this study concluded that special education is required for patients with poor knowledge, especially those who rely on traditional healing methods. Last, a study from Algeria in 1996 reported on 865 patients from 14 centers[60] (see Table 24-1). Over half of the group had experienced foot problems, including 15.5% with symptomatic neuropathy, 12% with infected ulcers, and 6.7% who had already undergone amputation. There is clearly a major need for an educational program for diabetic foot care.

South and Central America

The prevalence of diabetes is high throughout this region. A recent study from Paraguay reported an age-standardized prevalence of 6.5% in the urban Hispanic population, with a further 11% with impaired glucose tolerance.[61] Similar prevalence rates of around 7% have been reported in Argentina, Brazil, Uruguay, and Venezuela. In northern Brazil, as in tropical areas of Asia and Africa, patients may have leprotic as well as diabetic neuropathy, both of which can contribute to foot complications.

Diabetic foot care in Brazil is well organized, an example of excellent cooperation between health care professionals and the Ministry of Health. With assistance from U.K. and U.S. centers, the "Save the Diabetic Foot—Brazil" project was initiated in 1992 in Brasilia, when the first multidisciplinary foot clinic was opened. By the end of 2005, over 60 clinics were in operation across the country,[62] and there is increasing evidence that they are having an effect on amputation rates. A further promising sign was the setting up of the Grupo Latinamericano de Estudos de Pe Diabetico in September 2004; it is hoped that this will provide a forum for the exchange of knowledge on foot care across the region. Farther north, multidisciplinary teams for wound care have been set up in Costa Rica that have had a major impact on diabetic foot care.[63]

North America

In the United States, diabetic foot complications are a major cause of hospital admission; up to the end of 2000, nearly 70% of all amputations were for people with diabetes.[46] Foot ulcers and amputations are more common in ethnic minority groups, especially Hispanic and Black people, who are less likely to have health insurance.[64,65] In the Caribbean, diabetes prevalence is approaching 20% in many islands, and the number of amputations in diabetic patients is among the highest in the world.[66] Indeed, in one hospital in Barbados, patients with diabetic foot lesions occupied 75% of all surgical beds.[67]

Summary

In this brief global tour, we have attempted to review the standards of foot care and to identify what research is progressing in the different parts of the world. There are many developments that encourage optimism for future improvement in diabetic foot care. However, it is important for readers who are based in Western countries to acknowledge that much of what is known as the management of the insensitive diabetic foot was derived from observations many years ago on the management of foot problems secondary to leprosy in countries such as India and Brazil. It was Dr. Milroy Paul, working in Ceylon (now Sri Lanka), for example, who first used walking below-knee plaster casts for his leprosy patients with foot ulcers over 60 years ago.[68] So successful was this treatment that it spread to other leprosy centers and later to diabetes clinics.[69] Therefore, it now behooves us to attempt to improve matters by disseminating, worldwide, the key areas of knowledge in the screening, education, and management of diabetic patients who are at risk of foot problems. The many activities highlighted during the Year of the Diabetic Foot, 2005, together with other international developments do provide optimism for the future. One notable example is the Step by Step program

(supported by the World Diabetes Foundation), which is a pilot educational project for India, Bangladesh, Sri Lanka, Nepal, and Tanzania. However, there is no room for complacency, and the high profile achieved by diabetic foot problems and amputations during 2005 must be maintained if we are going to continue our quest to reduce morbidity and mortality from the lower-limb complications of diabetes in the future.

ACKNOWLEDGMENTS

We wish to thank many friends and colleagues worldwide who have provided information for this chapter, but in particular we wish to thank J.-L. Richard, I. Got, G. Va-Han (France); H. Reike, M. Spraul (Germany); L. Uccioli (Italy); K. Bakker, W. van Houtum (Netherlands); I. Dumont, K. Van-Acker (Belgium); J. Apelqvist, K. Brismar (Sweden); T. Pieber (Austria); N. Tentolouris, D. Voyatzoglou, C. Manes (Greece); I. Gourieva (Russia); V. Dargis (Lithuania); A. Helds (Latvia); V. Urbancic-Rovan (Slovenia); X. Zhangrong (China); K. Hosokawa, S. Kono (Japan); M. T. P. Que (Philippines); C. V. Krishnaswami, S. Pendsey (India); M. McGill, J. E. Shaw (Australia); Z. G. Abbas (Tanzania), J.-C. Mbanya (Cameroon); Z. Slaoui (Morocco); O. Jaramillo (Costa Rica); P. Aschner (Colombia); and H. Pedrosa (Brazil).

References

1. Wild S, Roglic G, Green A, et al: Global prevalence of diabetes: Estimates for 2000 and projection for 2030. Diabetes Care 27: 1047–1053, 2004.
2. Holzer SE, Camerota A, Martens L, et al: Costs and duration of care for foot ulcers for people with diabetes. Clin Ther 20:169–181, 1998.
3. Boulton AJM, Vileikyte L, Ragnarson-Tennvall G., Apelqvist J: The global burden of diabetic foot disease. Lancet 366:1721–1726, 2005.
4. Greener M: Counting the cost of diabetes. Curr Opin Diabetes 10:4–6, 1996.
5. Gordois A, Scuffham P, Shearer A, Oglesky A: The healthcare costs of diabetic neuropathy in the UK. Diabetic Foot 6:62–73, 2003.
6. Apelqvist J, Ragnarson-Tennvall G, Persson U, Larsson J: Diabetic foot ulcers in a multi-disciplinary setting: An economic analysis of primary healing and healing with amputation. J Intern Med 235:463–471, 1994.
7. Johnson FN, Williams DRR: Economic aspects of diabetic neuropathy and related complications. In Boulton AJM (ed): Diabetic Neuropathy. Carnforth, UK: Marius Press, 1997, pp 77–96.
8. LEA Study Group: Comparing the incidence of lower extremity amputations across the world: The global lower extremity amputation study. Diabet Med 12:14–18, 1995.
9. International Diabetes 9 Federation: Diabetes and foot care: Time to Act. Brussels, IDF Publications, 2005, pp 1–198.
10. Veves A, Uccioli L, Manes C, et al: Comparison of risk factors for foot problems in diabetic patients attending teaching hospital outpatient clinics in four different European states. Diabet Med 11:709–711, 1994.
11. Pryce TD: A case of perforating ulcers of both feet associated with diabetic and ataxic symptoms. Lancet 2:11–12, 1887.
12. McKeown KC: The history of the diabetic foot. Diabet Med 12:19–23, 1995.
13. Edmonds ME, Blundell MP, Morris HE, et al: Improved survival of the diabetic foot: The role of a specialist foot clinic. Q J Med 232:763–771, 1986.
14. Thomson FJ, Veves A, Ashe H, et al: The team approach to diabetic foot care: The Manchester experience. Foot 1:75–82, 1991.
15. Boulton AJM: The annual review: Here to stay [editorial]. Diabet Med 9:887, 1992.

16. Edmonds ME, Boulton AJM, Buckenham J, et al: Report of the Diabetic Foot and Amputation Group. Diabet Med 13(suppl):S27–S42, 1996.

17. Kumar S, Ashe H, Parnell L, et al: The prevalence of foot ulceration and its correlates in type 2 diabetic patients: A population-based study. Diabet Med 11:480–484, 1994.

18. Abbott CA, Carrington AL, Carrington AL, et al: The North-West Diabetes Foot Care study: Incidence of, and risk factors for new diabetic foot ulcers in a community-based cohort. Diabetic Med 20:377–384, 2002.

19. Muller S, DeGraw WJ, van Gerwen WH, et al: Foot ulceration and lower-limb amputation in type 2 diabetic patients in Dutch primary care. Diabetes Care 25:570–574, 2002.

20. Abbott CA, Garrow AP, Carrington AL, et al: Foot ulcer risk is lower in South Asian and African-Caribbean compared to European diabetic patients in the UK. Diabetes Care 28:1869–1875, 2005.

21. Richard J-L, Merle-Dubourg D: Comment reconnaître en pratique courante le risque d'ulcération d'un pied chez le diabétique. J Plaies Cictrisation 7:80–82, 1997.

22. Carpentier B, Benhamou PY, Pradines S, et al: Le cout économique du pied diabétique: Étude analytique. Diabetes Metab 24(suppl 1): XXIV, 1998.

23. Heurtier A, Danan JP, Ha Van G, et al: Bilan d'une strategie thérapeutique pluridisciplinaire du pied diabétique dans une unité de podologie. Diabetes Metab 24(suppl 1):LXVI, 1998.

24. Muller U, Lindth C, Tschauner T, et al: Prevalence of diabetic foot syndrome in Germany 2002–2004. Diabetologia 48(suppl 1):A255, 2005.

25. Trautner C, Haastert B, Spraul M, et al: Unchanged incidence of lower-limb amputations in a German city 1990–1998. Diabetes Care 24: 855–859, 2001.

26. Uccioli L, Faglia E, Monticone G, et al: Manufactured shoes in the prevention of diabetic foot ulcers. Diabetes Care 18:1376–1378, 1995.

27. Anichini R, de Bellis I, Cerretini I, et al: The number of amputations as a quality marker of diabetic foot therapy: Results after 5 years implementation of disease management. Diabetologia 48(suppl 1):A254, 2005.

28. Faglia, E. Favales F, Morabito A: New ulceration, amputation and survival rate in diabetic subjects hospitalized for foot ulceration from 1990–1993: A 6.5 year follow-up. Diabetes Care 24:78–83, 2001.

29. Bakker K, van Houtum WH, Schaper NC: Diabetic foot care in the Netherlands: An evaluation. Pract Diabetes Int 15:41–42, 1998.

30. Van Houtum WH, Rauwerda JA, Ruward D, et al: Reduction in diabetes-related lower extremity amputations in the Netherlands 1991–2000. Diabetes Care 27:1042–1046, 2004.

31. Apelqvist J, Larsson J, Agardh CD: Long-term prognosis for diabetic patients with foot ulcers. J Intern Med 233:485–491, 1993.

32. Larsson J, Apelqvist J, Agardh CD, Sternstrom A: Decreasing incidence of major amputation in diabetic patients: A consequence of a multidisciplinary foot care team approach? Diabet Med 12:770–776, 1995.

33. Ragnarson-Tennvall G, Apelqvist J: Prevention of diabetes-related foot ulcers and amputations: A cost-utility analysis based on Markov model simulators. Diabetologia 44:2077–2078, 2001.

34. Manes C, Papazoglou N, Sassidon E, et al: Prevalence of diabetic neuropathy and foot ulceration: A population-based study. Wounds 14:11–15, 2002.

35. Gimbert RM, Mendez A, Llussa J, et al: Diabetic foot in primary health care: Catalan community-based study. Diabetologia 40(suppl 1):A467, 1997.

36. Peter-Reisch B, Assad J-PH, Reiber GE: Foot re-ulceration in diabetes: Which important markers for effective prevention? Diabetologia 40(suppl 1):A473, 1997.

37. Dargis V, Pantelejeva O, Jonushaite A, et al: Benefits of a multidisciplinary approach in the management of recurrent diabetic foot ulceration in Lithuania. Diabetes Care 22:1428–1431, 1999.

38. Urbancic-Rovan V, Slak M: Results of 16 months foot screening in Ljubljana, Slovenia. Paper presented at 7th National Meeting on Diabetic Foot, Malvern, UK, May 1998.

39. Tan MH, Freeman T, Mancuso L, et al: Diabetes care in China: Observation from project Hope. Pract Diabetes Int 15:38–40, 1998.

40. Zhangrong XU, Yuzheng W, Xiancong W, et al: Chronic diabetic complications and treatments in Chinese diabetic patients. Natl Med J China 77:119–122, 1997.

41. Hosokawa K, Atsumi Y, Mokubo A, et al: Vascular disease of the lower extremities in renal dysfunction patients. Diabetologia 40(suppl 1):A477, 1997.

42. Pendsey S: Epidemiolgical aspects of the diabetic foot. Int J Diabetes Dev Countries 2:37–38, 1994.

43. Pendsey S: The diabetic foot in India [editorial]. Int J Diabetes Dev Countries 14:35–36, 1994.

44. Pendsey S: The Diabetic Foot: Clinical Atlas. New Delhi, India: Jaynee Brothers, 2003.

45. Morbach S, Lutale JK, Viswanathan V, et al: Regional differences in risk factors and clinical presentation of diabetic foot lesions. Diabetic Med 21:91–95, 2004.

46. Boulton AJM, Vileikyte L, Kirsner RS: Neuropathic diabetic foot ulcers. N Engl J Med 351:48–55, 2004.

47. du Perez DC, Walsh J: Clinical observations of the distribution of foot ulcerations in Asian patients. Diabetologia 40(suppl 1):A466, 1997.

48. Hseih S-H, Chang H-Y, Chen J-F, et al: Risk factors for high level amputation in diabetic foot in Taiwan. Diabetologia 40(suppl 1):A473, 1997.

49. McGill M, Yue DK: Diabetic foot disease: A view from down under. Diabetic Foot 6:165, 2003.

50. McGill M, Nube V, Clingan T, et al: Diabetes amputation programme: A structured, systematic approach. Diabetic Foot 6:172–176, 2003

51. Tapp RJ, Shaw JE, de Courten MP, et al: Foot complications in type 2 diabetes in Australia: A population-based study. Diabetic Med 20:105–113, 2003.

52. Tapp RJ, Zimmett PZ, Harper CA, et al: Diabetes care in an Australian population: Frequency of screening for eye and foot complications in diabetes. Diabetes Care 27:688–693, 2004.

53. Payne CB, Scott RS: Hospital discharges for diabetic foot disease in New Zealand 1980–1993. Diabetes Res Clin Pract 39:69–74, 1998.

54. Humphrey ARG, Thoma K, Dowse GK, Zimmet PZ: Diabetes and non-traumatic lower extremity amputations: Incidence, risk factors and prevention—A 12 year follow-up study in Nauru. Diabetes Care 19:710–713, 1996.

55. Abbas ZG, Archibald LK. Epidemiology of the diabetic foot in Africa. Med Sci Monitor 11:RA262–270, 2005.

56. Kidmas AT, Nwadiaso CH, Igun GO: Lower limb amputation in Jos, Nigeria. East Africa Med J 81:427–429, 2005.

57. Tchakonte B, Ndip A, Aubry P, et al: The diabetic foot in Cameroon. Bull Soc Pathol Exot 98:94–98, 2005.

58. Abbas ZG, Gill GV, Archibald LK: The epidemiology of diabetic limb sepsis: An African perspective. Diabetic Med 19P:575–579, 2002.

59. Slaoui Z, Arabou MR: Evaluation des facteurs déclenchants des lésions de pied chez le diabétique. Diabetes Metab 24(suppl 1): LXVI, 1998.

60. Belhadj M: La place du pied diabétique. Diabetes Metab 24(suppl 1): LXVII, 1998.

61. Jiminez JT, Palacia SM, Canete F, et al: Prevalence of diabetes mellitus and associated risk factors in an adult urban population in Paraguay. Diabet Med 15:334–338, 1998.

62. Pedrosa HC, Leme LAP, Novaes C, et al: The diabetic foot in South America: Progress with the Brazilian 'Save the diabetic foot' project. Int Diab Monitor 16:10–16, 2004.

63. Jaramillo O, Elizondo J, Jones P, et al: Practical guidelines for developing a hospital-based wound and ostomy clinic. Wounds 9:94–102, 1997.

64. Lavery LA, Armstrong DG, Wunderlich RP, et al: Diabetic foot syndrome: Evaluation of the prevalence and incidence of foot pathology in Mexican Americans and non-Hispanic whites from a diabetes health management cohort. Diabetes Care 26:1435–1438, 2003.

65. Resnick HE, Valsania P, Philips CI: Diabetes mellitus and non-traumatic lower extremity amputation in black and white Americans. Arch Int Med 159:2470–2475, 1999.

66. Gulliford MC, Mahabir D: Diabetic foot disease in a Caribbean community. Diabet Res Clin Pract 56:35–40, 2002.

67. Walrond ER: The Caribbean experience with the management of the diabetic foot. West Ind Med J 50(suppl 1):24–26, 2001.

68. Brand PW: Insensitive Feet: Practical Handbook on Foot Problems in Leprosy. London: Leprosy Mission, 1981.

69. Boulton AJM: Diabetic foot ulceration: The leprosy connection. Pract Diabetes Dig 3:35–37, 1990.

ORGANIZATION AND OPERATION OF AN EDUCATION- AND RESEARCH-BASED DIABETIC FOOT CLINIC

JOHN H. BOWKER ∎

Introduction

The number of people with diabetes is increasing inexorably. It is estimated that by 2025, they will number 350 million worldwide, compared to 135 million in 1995. The feet of many of these people will be at risk of ulceration with the onset of sensory neuropathy. It has been found that in diabetic people, foot ulceration precedes 85% of nontraumatic amputations.[1,2] Most significantly, it has been estimated that 75% of these amputations could have been prevented by early identification and education of those who are at risk of ulceration. These services can be efficiently provided only by a team of caregivers with complementary skills who can work in an interdisciplinary, proactive manner with "preventive rehabilitation" as their common goal. This approach is necessary if the deplorable annual worldwide number of one million major lower-limb amputations due to diabetes is to be reduced.

Certain centers have clearly demonstrated that an integrated approach to diabetic foot care can be effective in dramatically altering the incidence of major amputations. For example, over a 4-year period, the Diabetes Treatment and Teaching Unit of the University Hospital of Geneva attained an 85% reduction in transtibial amputations. The unit's fiscal analysis revealed that the cost of preventing just five of these major amputations was equivalent to the combined annual salaries of the entire staff of 12.[3] The diabetic foot clinic team at King's College Hospital, London, during their first 3 years of operation, achieved healing rates of 86% of 238 neuropathic ulcers and 72% of 148 ischemic ulcers.[4]

It is clear from the preceding data that the need exists for education-based diabetic foot clinics in every community where people with diabetes reside. Unfortunately, even in the most developed regions, despite the availability of the personnel required to staff such clinics, diabetic foot care remains a fragmented process with little coordination and communication among caregivers. The standard medical model, in which patients are seen at separate times and venues by various physicians, surgeons, podiatrists, nurses, and others, perpetuates this fragmented, ineffective, and costly care of diabetic foot complications. An education-based diabetic foot clinic, in contrast, can be designed to provide an integrated, and thus inherently more cost-effective, approach to the management of these needy patients by recognizing the fact that no one specialist possesses all the skills needed to prevent lower-limb amputation.[5,6] Funding for these clinics will vary widely among locales and countries.

The clinic does not have to be associated with a large regional or university hospital; successful programs can be organized in any community by a local group of interested health professionals. Initially, all that is necessary is recognition of the need and a willingness to apply well-known principles of care to these patients. Next, the team members should visit a well-established diabetic foot care clinic as a group to see how it operates on a day-to-day basis.[7] If this is not feasible, one or more consultants

TABLE 25-1 Basic Equipment Needed for a Diabetic Foot Clinic

1. 10-g Semmes-Weinstein filaments
2. 128-Hz tuning fork
3. Glucose meter
4. Nonsterile latex gloves
5. Nail clipper
6. #15 scalpels
7. Rongeurs
8. Thumb forceps
9. Surgical scissors
10. Small straight or curved hemostats
11. Orange sticks
12. Cotton-tipped applicators
13. Preinked footprint sheets
14. Clear radiographic film and indelible markers
15. 15-cm rule
16. Digital camera
17. Dressing materials
18. Bandage scissors
19. Weight-relief shoes
20. Casting materials
21. Brannock shoe-measuring device
22. Radiographic equipment (readily accessible)

from that clinic could be brought in to meet with the team members for formal lectures and informal discussions. An excellent handbook on diabetic foot care, developed by the International Working Group on the Diabetic Foot, is highly recommended for review prior to organizing a clinic.[8] Entitled the *International Consensus on the Diabetic Foot/Practical Guidelines on the Management and Prevention of the Diabetic Foot*, it has been translated into 26 languages. It is available in both printed and CD-ROM formats from the International Diabetes Federation for a modest fee.*

Exactly how the clinic is organized and who staffs it can vary widely, as is amply demonstrated by the differing combinations of caregivers who successfully run such programs throughout the world (see Chapter 24). What is important is that the clinic have certain basic programmatic elements and essential equipment (Table 25-1) and that the specialists who are most often required be in regular attendance. Those who are needed less frequently should be available at short notice to provide their expertise as required. The clinic should meet regularly and frequently, with provision for prompt, effective self-referral both during and after regular clinic hours. In short, for such a program to be effective, its services must be readily accessible.

Clinic Organization

The Team

The clinic team has three objectives. The primary objective is the prevention of lower-limb amputation. A secondary objective, if limb loss is unavoidable, is to do

* www.idf.org/bookshop

the least disabling amputation possible (see Chapter 20). The tertiary objective, which applies to those who have lost part or all of one foot, is to prevent or greatly delay loss of the other limb. The immediate goals of the clinic team are (1) identification, evaluation, and correction or amelioration of factors that have led or might lead to ulceration and amputation; (2) triage of patients with acute problems into the proper treatment pathway; and (3) healing of both acute and chronic wounds. The long-term goal is breaking the cycle of recurrent ulceration, which often leads to major amputation, by providing a comprehensive approach to diabetic foot care.

The central figures on the team must be the patient together with responsible family members, domestic partners, or friends. Without their full cooperation in treatment, the team's work will be an exercise in futility. Most often, an internist or surgeon will head the team, the choice often being based on which person has the most interest and time available for this task. In an ideal situation, a complete physician roster, inclusive of the team leader, should include an internist specializing in diabetes, a foot and ankle surgeon, a vascular surgeon, a plastic surgeon, an ophthalmologist, a rehabilitation physician, and a dermatologist. As was noted above, not all physician members need to be present at all clinic meetings, but they should be readily available for consultation. The nurse-educator, by virtue of having a complete overview of clinic function, can perform as an effective team coordinator. Other essential nonphysician team members include the podiatrist, pedorthist, orthotist, prosthetist, dietitian, physical therapist, social worker, psychologist, and health administrator. Students and trainees in the appropriate disciplines should also participate in supervised patient care.

Basic Organization

There are many possible ways to organize the day-to-day operations of an interdisciplinary diabetic foot clinic. A format that works well for the author in a large county hospital with limited resources will be described as just one approach to managing a large number of patients. From its beginnings as a unified clinic in 1982, the program rapidly evolved into a two-tiered system, based on the acuity of the patient's foot condition. The first-tier, full-team clinic is held weekly for patients who are undergoing active treatment for either acute or chronic foot lesions. Many of them have, for a wide variety of social and economic reasons, presented late with severe problems such as infective (wet) gangrene, ischemic (dry) gangrene, or acute Charcot neuroarthropathy. Chronic ulcers, as well as all postoperative wounds, are also seen, usually by the operating surgeon. This clinic is also the venue for intake evaluation of new patients.

The second-tier clinic, termed the Patient-Family Education Clinic (PFEC), provides long-term preventive foot care and is managed by the same nurse-educator who attends the first-tier clinic. Patients are usually seen at bimonthly intervals. This clinic meets each week on the day before the full-team clinic, allowing easy and prompt referral within 24 hours for any acute problems that may arise. The goals of this clinic are maintenance of foot health by the provision of basic care such as nail and callus debridement and the prevention of initial or recurrent foot lesions through comprehensive education in self-care.[9,10] The teaching involves both the patient and family members. The term *family* is used in its broadest sense, including not only actual family members but also domestic partners and friends. Over time, the PFEC becomes an integral part of the diabetic patient's support network. Patients with acute events such as infective gangrene or sudden onset of limb ischemia are, of course, seen promptly in either clinic and triaged to the appropriate service. After hours or on nonclinic days, patients are counseled via the 24/7/365 hot line and, if deemed necessary, referred to the emergency department.

Only the interests and creativity of the clinic team members and their available resources limit clinical research opportunities inherent in the operation of an interdisciplinary diabetic foot clinic. Data collected and tracked soon become essential for both effective patient care and useful clinical research. Needed areas of research include longitudinal studies of ulcer risk levels, vasculopathy, and progressive foot and ankle deformities. Evaluation of the efficacy of new off-loading methods or devices compared to the gold standard of total-contact casting will continue to be essential.[11] Also of great interest are the effects of HbA1C-monitored patient adherence to serum glucose control, use of prescribed footwear, and abstinence from cigarette smoking in the long-term prevention of ulcer formation. The internist also has the opportunity for early discovery and management or appropriate referral of patients with the complications commonly associated with diabetes, such as neuropathy, retinopathy, nephropathy, hypertension, abnormal lipid profiles, and cardiovascular disease.

A variety of force-measuring devices can be used to identify areas of high pressure that are prone to ulceration and to document the preventive effect of pedorthic or limited surgical intervention. Gait analysis, following partial foot amputation at various levels, can be used to compare different orthotic, prosthetic, and footwear options to determine whether weight-bearing has been equalized between the feet rather than shifted toward the intact foot, thereby increasing forces on it (see Chapter 6). Energy consumption studies of people with partial foot amputations compared to those with transtibial and transfemoral amputations are also needed to determine the efficacy of various footwear options, orthoses, and prostheses in reducing cardiovascular stress. The potential for greatly increasing the power of any of the above studies by networking with multiple centers is enormous.

Essential Elements of the First-Tier (Acute Care) Program

Intake Evaluation

History

As in managing any other disease entity, a thorough, pertinent historical review serves to enhance the subsequent physical examination and more effectively guide the foot care of the individual diabetic patient. While obtaining facts regarding other disease processes is essential to holistic management, the majority of the questions will be specific to diabetes mellitus and complications related to the feet. The replies that are given will allow the historian to assess not only the presenting complaint but also the patient's concepts and knowledge of diabetes and the level of the patient's involvement in self-care.

The answers to the following basic questions will often lead to further lines of inquiry:

1. Time since onset of diabetes symptoms
2. Time since diagnosis of diabetes (often significantly less than answer to question 1)
3. Type of practitioner seen:
   a. Family physician
   b. General internist
   c. Endocrinologist
   d. General/vascular/orthopedic surgeon
   e. Ophthalmologist/optometrist
   f. Podiatrist
   g. Other
   h. None
4. Method of plasma glucose management:
   a. Diet only
   b. Diet and exercise
   c. Noninsulin agents only
   d. Noninsulin agents and insulin
   e. Insulin only
   f. None
5. Schedule of plasma glucose measurements:
   a. At home:
      i. How often?
      ii. Before breakfast?
      iii. Level?
   b. Doctor's office:
      i. Frequency?
      ii. Level?
      iii. Rarely or never
6. Frequency and type of follow-up care:
   a. Glycohemoglobin measurements:
      i. How often?
      ii. Latest percentage?
   b. Comprehensive lipid measurements
   c. Eye examinations:
      i. Yearly?
      ii. Laser treatment?

d. Kidney function tests:
   i. Dialysis?
e. Dietetic reviews
f. Blood pressure measurement
g. Cardiac evaluations
h. Foot examinations

7. Complications to date:
   a. Eyes
   b. Kidneys
   c. Feet
   d. Cardiac problems
   e. Peripheral vascular problems
   f. Neuropathic symptoms

8. Cigarette smoking history:
   a. Pack-years
   b. Current consumption
   c. Time of cessation
   d. Use of other tobacco products

9. Vocation/avocations:
   a. Hours on feet
   b. Exercise type and frequency

10. Type of footwear commonly used:
    a. High-fashion shoes (men and women)
    b. Narrow/pointed toebox
    c. High heels
    d. Walking shoes
    e. Sport shoes
    f. Prescribed diabetic (depth) shoes
    g. Work boots
    h. Sandals
    i. Slippers
    j. Barefoot/socks only
    k. Frequency and location

11. Footwear use:
    a. At all times
    b. Outside home only
    c. Work only
    d. Rarely or never

12. Details of presenting foot complaint:
    a. Time since onset
    b. Cause of problem
    c. Care sought/received to present

Foot Examination

It is essential that both feet be examined at every visit. Patients with profound neuropathy will frequently fail to note obvious abnormalities of one foot if the other happens to be of more immediate concern to them. To avoid missing any significant findings, the feet should be at a level that is readily accessible to the examiner's eyes and hands. First, observe the overall conformation of the feet and ankles and note common deformities such as clawed toes with secondarily depressed metatarsal heads; bunions; bunionettes; and plantar, medial, or malleolar masses secondary to Charcot neuroarthropathy.

Second, look for signs of acute and chronic shoe pressure over bony prominences, such as localized redness, hard corns over the dorsal aspect of the proximal interphalangeal joints, and web-space soft corns, often associated with web space maceration and ulcer formation. Third, examine the skin for dryness, fissures, and nail disease.

Fourth, check for signs of unequal plantar weight distribution, including calluses and ulcers, under prominent metatarsal heads or associated with midfoot and other bony masses secondary to Charcot neuroarthropathy. Areas of clinically significant callus formation and inflammatory "hot spots" will not be missed if the examiner lightly passes the hands over all foot surfaces. Because an ulcer may be fully developed beneath a visually intact callus or corn, which has not yet been elevated by underlying fluid pressure, the callus or corn should always be carefully shaved to assess this possibility. Ulcers can be visually deceiving in regard to their actual depth; therefore, they should be probed to determine whether they penetrate to the bone and/or joint beneath. This can be easily done with a sterile applicator or instrument. If bone is felt, one may safely assume that osteitis or osteomyelitis is present.[12]

Fifth, look for signs of neuropathic changes in the feet. Sensory neuropathy results in the loss of protective sensation and is detected by applying a 10-g Semmes-Weinstein filament to multiple sites on the foot (see Chapter 3). Joint proprioception should be tested at the level of the great toe, ankle, and knee. Motor neuropathy will be manifested by weakness of the ankle dorsiflexors as noted by manual resistance testing. Autonomic neuropathy results in dryness and fissuring of the skin and evidence of arteriovenous shunting in the feet. The latter can be deduced from the persistence of dorsal vein engorgement on elevation of the dependent foot. When a neuropathic patient presents with a swollen, warm foot or ankle and shows no signs of systemic illness, Charcot neuroarthropathy should always be the first diagnosis considered (see Chapter 12). Even if the initial radiographs are negative for fracture and/or dislocation, it is still the most likely diagnosis until disproved by serial radiographs. If the process appears to involve the forefoot or midfoot, weight-bearing radiographs of the foot in anteroposterior, lateral, and oblique views should be sufficient. Alternatively, if the ankle and/or hindfoot is affected, anteroposterior, lateral, and mortise views of the ankle, also weight-bearing, should be added.

Sixth, check for loss of functional range of motion of the great toe metatarsophalangeal joint and the ankle joint secondary to glycation of their capsules. Seventh, evaluate the arterial inflow to the feet. Lack of hair growth, coolness to touch, and dependent rubor of the feet followed by blanching on elevation should alert the examiner to the probability of arterial insufficiency. Although this can often be confirmed by palpation for the dorsalis pedis, posterior tibial, popliteal, and femoral pulses, more quantitative testing might be required (see Chapter 11). Eighth, the feet should also be examined with the patient standing, since their conformation can change remarkably on weight-bearing. The position of the toes should be observed for persistence of apparent clawing as well as height of the medial arch, noting whether there is a very high arch (cavus), a normal arch, an absence of arch (planovalgus), or a reversed arch (rocker bottom). Areas of increased plantar pressure can be easily documented in a semiquantitative manner with a standing or walking imprint obtained with a commercially available preinked sheet that can be placed into the patient record. Last, the patient walks away from, toward, and then back and forth in front of the examiner, who carefully notes signs of ataxia related to poor proprioceptive function or a drop foot or steppage gait secondary to weakness of the foot dorsiflexors. Careful correlation of the historical and examination data will allow the risk level for foot lesions to be estimated (see Chapter 28).

Shoe Examination

Because of their intimate interrelation, evaluation of the patient's shoes is as much an integral part of the intake evaluation as is examination of the feet. By correlating the findings on foot examination with those of shoe evaluation, the causation of skin lesions, such as excessive callus formation and ulcers, is often made quite apparent. To begin, evaluate the shoe design and fit, then note the materials (leather or plastic) from which the upper and counter are formed. Shake out the shoes to discover any foreign objects and then insert the hand into the shoe to find any irregularities, such as internally projecting seams, creases, or torn or worn lining material. Remove the inserts and examine them for impressions from plantar bony prominences. The wear patterns of the shoe can also be quite helpful. As examples, severe wear of the sole at the toe might indicate a drop-foot gait, while lateral shifting of the shoe upper and/or counter to the medial or lateral side, associated with abnormal wear of the sole, might indicate major malalignment of the foot and/or ankle.

If any skin breakdown has been noted during the examination, it should be carefully classified in regard to its depth and any signs of peripheral ischemia. Brodsky's classification of foot lesions is clinically relevant and easy to use (see Chapter 9). If a penetrating ulcer is confined to the distal forefoot or to a specific toe, coned-down anteroposterior, lateral, and oblique radiographs of those areas will be the most useful. In determining a plan of treatment, bone scans are rarely needed and can be misleading. Magnetic resonance imaging (T1 and T2 weighted), however, can be useful at times if indications of osteomyelitis are equivocal (see Chapter 10). If the lesion is associated with significant ischemia, further testing might be deemed necessary by the team's vascular surgeon (see Chapter 11).

Clinic Management of Acute Foot Problems

As was noted previously, care of wounds is an essential service provided by the acute care clinic. These include ulcers, debridement wounds, and partial foot amputations left open because of severe infection. Treatment of neuropathic ulcers that are not infected and do not involve bone consists of regular sharp debridement of overhanging callus and the use of weight relief or weight-redistributing shoes, orthoses, or total-contact casts (see Chapter 13). If the patient cannot or will not comply with the consistent use of patient-removable off-loading devices for any reason, a series of total-contact casts is recommended but only if the ulcer is Brodsky classification 1A. The cast is changed every 7 to 10 days for ulcer care and observation. In carefully selected cases, a wheelchair can be an acceptable off-loading device. If localized superficial infection is present, a punch biopsy culture should be taken, and broad-spectrum antibiotics should be prescribed.

Wounds resulting from major debridements or open partial foot amputations can be effectively treated with twice-daily absorbent, nonadhesive, and nonocclusive dressings such as normal saline-moistened gauze dressings. For home preparation of normal saline solution, see Table 25-2. If the dressings show a greenish tinge, indicating *Pseudomonas* colonization, a 1/4% acetic acid solution can be used, for a few days only, to suppress it; use of the solution must be limited because its fibroblast toxicity exceeds its bactericidal activity.[13] For home preparation of 1/4% acetic acid solution, see Table 25-2. At times, a copiously draining wound may benefit from a few days of dry gauze dressings. As soon as the drainage lessens, normal saline dressings can be started. The patients and/or family members are taught to change these dressings with clean, not sterile, technique, thus keeping the cost reasonable without compromising the

TABLE 25-2   Home Preparation of Wound Dressing Solutions

A. Normal saline solution
1. Wash teaspoon, measuring cup, glass jar, and lid in warm, soapy water. Rinse well in hot water.
2. Boil a pot of water for 20 minutes and allow to cool.
3. Pour 4 cups of boiled water into jar.
4. Add 2 teaspoons of salt.
5. Cap and store in refrigerator.
6. Make a new solution each week.

B. One-quarter percent (1/4%) acetic acid solution
1. Wash tablespoon, measuring cup, glass jar and lid in warm, soapy water. Rinse well in hot water.
2. Boil a pot of water for 20 minutes and allow to cool.
3. Pour 5 cups of boiled water into jar.
4. Add 4 tablespoons of white vinegar.
5. Cap and store in refrigerator.
6. Make a new solution each week.

result. Patients are warned to avoid the use of hydrogen peroxide and iodine solutions, alcohol, or other home remedies, which have been shown to inhibit wound healing.[14,15] These wounds must also be relieved of weight by the use of off-loading orthoses or shoes, sometimes augmented with the support of a walking frame. The progress of wound closure can be followed by photographs, measurements, or tracings on clear radiographic film, from which the wound area can be measured. Reviewing these evidences of healing with the patient can be helpful in securing compliance with wound care.

If reduction in wound volume is not proceeding as expected, the reasons must be sought. They may be physiologic, related to poor tissue oxygen perfusion secondary to peripheral vascular disease or anemia, poor nutrition,[16,17] renal disease, chronic hyperglycemia, or persistent infection, the latter possibly requiring surgical intervention. Behavioral factors that affect wound healing include failure to properly and/or consistently use off-loading devices or to regularly change dressings and take antibiotics and continued use of vasoconstrictors such as nicotine and caffeine. Noncompliance with overall diabetic management may be based on denial, depression, or displaced locus of control or a combination of these[18] (see Chapter 31).

In managing acute Charcot neuroarthropathy of the foot, a total-contact cast is applied immediately after satisfactory radiography. Minimal touch-down weight-bearing to assist balance with use of a walking frame is allowed for essential needs, with elevation of the foot while sitting. The initial cast will need to be changed in 1 week or less, owing to rapid reduction in edema. Thereafter, cast changes are done every 3 weeks or whenever the cast loosens, becomes wet, or is otherwise damaged. Radiographs are taken every 6 weeks until the skeletal structure of the foot is deemed to be stable and clinical signs of inflammatory activity such as localized excessive heat and swelling are totally gone. This interval can last up to 6 months, after which full weight-bearing in a cast is permitted. If there is no recurrence of inflammation over the next few weeks, a custom-made Charcot Restraint Orthotic Walker is fitted and used for up to 4 months. Thereafter, ready-made depth shoes with custom inserts and soles can be fitted, unless the foot is grossly deformed. In this case, both shoes and inserts should be custom-made. In regard to Charcot neuroarthropathy of the ankle, the author has seen patients with unstable ankle fracture-dislocations placed in an ankle-foot orthosis and told to bear full weight rather than being referred for surgical stabilization. It should be noted that an ankle-foot orthosis, no matter how well fitted, can neither prevent an unstable ankle deformity from increasing under full body weight nor reduce a fixed deformity. Since an ankle-foot orthosis utilizes a three-point pressure system, ulcers will inevitably occur in an insensate foot and ankle. The end result is often amputation of the foot. For a discussion of the surgical management of Charcot neuroarthropathy, see Chapter 23.

The frequency of visits to the acute care clinic is determined by the progress of wound healing and can range from weekly to monthly. Once healing is complete, the patient is referred to the PFEC for long-term foot health maintenance. If a new lesion develops or an old one recurs, the patient is referred back to the acute care clinic for management.

Essential Elements of the Second-Tier (Chronic Care) Program

There are several groups of patients who are referred to the PFEC for long-term care. The first category consists of patients without a history of foot lesions who have completed intake evaluation and have been fitted with protective shoes, often provided by Medicare or other third-party carriers with provision of proper documentation. Those with severe sensory neuropathy (i.e., lacking protective sensation), bony deformities, and evidence of peripheral vascular disease are seen every 3 months. Patients with severe sensory neuropathy but no foot deformities are seen every 6 months, and those with protective sensation are seen yearly following thorough counseling on foot care and footwear. The second category includes patients with severe sensory neuropathy with wounds that have healed either completely or to the point at which the wounds are expected to heal without further incident. These patients are seen every 1 to 3 months, partly depending on their demonstrated level of compliance. The third category consists of diabetic patients with major amputations, many of whom have continued to be active walkers with a prosthesis. The remaining foot is often visually intact but at a statistically increased risk of amputation, thus requiring regular preventive care along with the residual amputated limb, which may be insensate as well.

The main goal of foot health maintenance is met in the PFEC by providing several specific services. These include monitoring of foot condition by visual inspection and palpation, regular nail and callus trimming, careful shoe and insert inspection, and referral to the pedorthist for shoe modification or replacement as needed. Shoes and inserts are generally replaced on an annual basis. Patients are regularly questioned about compliance with diabetes management and eye care, with assistance provided in obtaining referrals to appropriate clinics.

One of the most important functions of the PFEC is the education of patients about specific preventive foot care measures. The style of instruction, including the terminology used, is tailored to the patient's ability to comprehend his or her disease process. It is also very important that the information given by all team members be consistent and be repeated as often as necessary to ensure comprehension. Most important, patients are taught never to walk barefoot and to remove their shoes for a visual foot examination twice daily, using a mirror if necessary. If retinopathy has impaired the patient's vision, family members are shown how to perform this essential task. At the same time, the feet should be palpated for areas of increased warmth, which can indicate inflammation from increased skin pressure or Charcot changes. Patients are encouraged to wear their protective shoes at all times, changing to another pair at midday or at least alternating shoes each day, since each pair may exert varying pressures on different areas of the feet. Patients are also advised to invert and shake out their shoes before putting them on to remove foreign bodies, such as small stones.

Patients are also taught to avoid thermal injury from home-heating sources such as floor furnace grids and fireplaces as well as from hot water bottles, heating pads, and hot baths. They are also advised to avoid walking directly on hot sand or paving at the beach or pool and to avoid sunburn and sharp objects in the water or on the beach by wearing commercially available water shoes. Contact with car heaters or transmission tunnels (in older automobiles) is also dangerous to the unwary on long automobile trips. Patients are warned to limit outdoor exposure in cold climates to avoid frostbite to an insensate limb. They are encouraged to avoid any form of "home surgery" and instead to come on a regular basis to the PFEC for nail and callus trimming. The destructive effect of salicylic acid–based callus removers is emphasized. The use of emollients on the feet to compensate for skin dryness is recommended, except between the toes, where it will cause maceration of the skin. Vegetable shortening is an inexpensive, effective substance for this purpose. Patients are encouraged to take shorter, slower steps and to avoid excessive walking to decrease weight-bearing trauma, which can lead to tissue inflammation and breakdown. Many helpful booklets on diabetic foot care are provided free of charge by manufacturers of insulin and other hypoglycemic agents for distribution to diabetic patients. They are useful in reinforcing the team members' instructions and as a rapid home reference for the patient and family (see Chapter 30).

As was noted above, among the chief reasons for poor patient compliance with clinic programs are the three "Ds": denial, depression, and displaced locus of control. The PFEC is the ideal place to address these issues in a gently repetitive, nonconfrontational manner. The result of this informal counseling should be the empowerment of the patient to assume responsibility for care of his or her feet as well as other aspects of diabetic management. If the patient proves resistant to instruction and informal counseling, referral to the team psychologist may be appropriate (see Chapter 31).

An additional feature of great value is the 24/7/365 telephone hotline. For assistance or advice outside of regular clinic hours, the patient should be given this specific number to report foot problems. If the person receiving the call judges the situation to be urgent, the patient is referred immediately to the emergency department. Otherwise, the patient is given some simple instructions regarding care and told to come in the very next morning for further evaluation. This method encourages the early reporting of foot problems and essentially avoids the dangerous delay in treatment that is common whenever patients without the benefit of pain use their own judgment in regard to when they should appear for evaluation and treatment.

Summary

Interdisciplinary diabetic foot clinics are needed in every community where people with diabetes reside. The composition of the treatment team will vary from locale to locale, depending on the interest and availability of the required personnel. The clinic does not have to be directly affiliated with a large regional or university hospital to be highly effective on the local level. The immediate goals of the clinic team are (1) identification and correction of factors that have led or might lead to

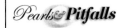

Pearls

- The need exists for an education-based diabetic foot clinic in every community where people with diabetes reside.
- An effective clinic program can be organized in any community by a local group of interested health professionals, which will vary in composition in different locales.
- *The International Consensus on the Diabetic Foot/Practical Guidelines on the Management and Prevention of the Diabetic Foot,* available through the International Diabetes Federation website (idf.org/bookshop), can serve as an effective guide to organizing a clinic.
- Both feet must be examined at each visit, as both are likely to be at risk from loss of protective sensation.
- Removal of callus from a bony prominence will reduce pressure over that area by about 30%.
- Foot ulceration precedes 85% of nontraumatic amputations in people with diabetes.
- Seventy-five percent of amputations in people with diabetes can be prevented by early identification and education of those at risk.
- Clinical research activities will tend to improve the quality of patient care over time.
- The long-term goal of a medically integrated clinic is to break the cycle of recurrent ulceration by providing a comprehensive approach to diabetic foot care.

Pitfalls

- Use of the traditional fragmented medical model is ineffective and costly in the treatment of diabetic foot complications.
- A clinic that does not include the patient and the patient's significant others as central members of the team has little chance of long-term success.
- Failure to remove callus can lead to missing an underlying ulcer.
- Failure to gently probe ulcers to their full depth can result in failure to diagnose osteomyelitis.

ulceration, (2) prompt treatment of acute problems, and (3) healing of wounds. The long-term goal is breaking the cycle of recurrent ulceration by providing a comprehensive approach to diabetic foot care. Finally, a well-organized diabetic foot clinic, providing consistent patient education as well as preventive and acute care for diabetic foot problems, can be expected to bring about a marked reduction in the need for major lower-limb amputations.

References

1. Larsson J, Agardh C, Apelquist J, Stenstrom A: Long-term prognosis after healed amputations in patients with diabetes. Clin Orthop 350:149–158, 1998.
2. Pecoraro RE, Reiber GE, Burgess EM: Pathways to diabetic foot amputation: Basis for prevention. Diabetes Care 13:513–521, 1990.
3. Assal JP, Muelhauser I, Pernet A, et al: Patient education as the basis for diabetes care in clinical practice and research. Diabetologia 28:602–613, 1985.
4. Edmonds ME, Blundell MP, Morris ME, et al: Improved survival of the diabetic foot: The role of a specialized foot clinic. Q J Med 232:763–771, 1986.
5. Edmonds M, Foster AVM: Diabetic foot clinic. In Levin ME, O'Neal LW, Bowker JH (eds): The Diabetic Foot, 5th ed. St. Louis: Mosby Year Book, 1993, p 603.
6. Spraul M, Chamberlain E, Schmid M: Education of the patient, the diabetic foot clinic: A team approach. In Bakker K, Nieuwenhvijzen Kruseman AC (eds): The Diabetic Foot. Amsterdam: Excerpta Medica, 1991, pp 150–161.
7. Blair VP III, Drury DA: Starting the diabetic foot center. In Levin ME, O'Neal LW (eds): The Diabetic Foot, 4th ed. St. Louis: Mosby Year Book, 1988.
8. International Consensus on the Diabetic Foot: International Working Group on the Diabetic Foot. Amsterdam, 1999.
9. Lemerman RD, Wade NP: A rehabilitation clinic for the client and family. Rehabil Nurs 9:21–23, 1984.
10. Wade NP, Lemerman RD, Mastrionni EJ: Rehabilitation care and education: Practical guidelines for preparing the patient to function at home. Rehabil Nurs 5:32–34, 1983.
11. Katz IA, Harlan A, Miranda-Palma B, et al: A randomized trial of two irremovable off-loading devices in the management of plantar neuropathic diabetic foot ulcers. Diabetes Care. 28:555–559, 2005.
12. Grayson JL, Gibbons GW, Balogh K, et al: Probing to bone in infected pedal ulcers: A clinical sign of underlying osteomyelitis in diabetic patients. JAMA 273:721–723, 1995.
13. Lineaweaver W, Howard R, Soucy D, et al: Topical antimicrobial toxicity. Arch Surg 120:267–270, 1985.
14. Rodeheaver G, Bellamy W, Kody M, et al: Bacterial activity and toxicity of iodine-containing solutions in wounds. Arch Surg 117:181–186, 1982.
15. Oberg MS, Lindsey D: Editorial: Do not put hydrogen peroxide or povidone iodine into wounds! Am J Dis Child 141:27–29, 1987.
16. Sieggreen MY: Healing of physical wounds. Nurs Clin North Am 22:439–447, 1987.
17. Stotts NA, Washington DF: Nutrition: A critical component of wound healing. AACN Clin Crit Care Nurs 1:585–594, 1990.
18. Bowker JH: An holistic approach to foot wound healing in diabetic persons with or without dysvascularity. Wounds 12(suppl B):72B–76B, 2000.

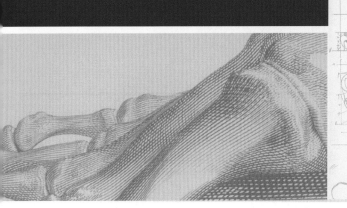

ROLE OF THE PODIATRIST IN THE CARE OF THE DIABETIC FOOT

LAWRENCE B. HARKLESS, V. KATHLEEN SATTERFIELD, ■

AND KENRICK J. DENNIS

Never do what a specialist can do better. Discover your own specialty.
Do not despair if your specialty appears to be more delicate,
a lesser thing. Make up in finesse what you lose in force.

— Jean Cocteau (1889–1963) French poet, novelist, and film director

Introduction

The specialty of podiatry has gone through profound changes over the past century. The podiatrist of the early 20th century was educated in two years and was skilled in palliative treatments of the foot. Having transitioned from chiropody, the fledgling field of podiatry slowly added more advanced modalities to its regimen but still remained heavily involved in the cutting of corns and calluses, debridement of troublesome toenails, padding, and strapping.

In recent years, the profession has moved toward uniform residency training by implementing the Comprehensive Podiatric Medical and Surgical 36 Month Program. Podiatrists can opt to follow their residency training with a fellowship in advanced surgery, sports medicine, research, or diabetic foot care. In a practice survey commissioned by the American Podiatric Medical Association in 2005, 96% of respondents had staff privileges at one or more hospitals.[1]

According to the Centers for Disease Control and Prevention, there were over 18.2 million people with diabetes mellitus in the United States in 2002, a startling 6.3 percent of the population.[2] It is estimated that 1.3 million people with diabetes are newly diagnosed each year. Diabetes is a complex process and requires the attention of a number of medical specialties. Pathologies associated with the disease are often manifested in the lower limb. In fact, diabetes mellitus remains the leading cause (>60%) of amputations unrelated to trauma in the United States,[3] with about 82,000 reported in 2000–2001. The number of hospital days associated with amputation, the costs to the health care system, and the impact on longevity are well documented.[4]

Since publication of the first edition of this text in 1973, foot care has gradually become recognized as a major issue in the management of diabetic individuals. A position statement issued by the American Diabetes Association in 1998 included the following: "Patients with a history of foot lesions, especially those with prior amputation, require preventive foot care and lifelong surveillance, preferably by a foot care specialist."[5] The podiatrist serves as an important resource for the mechanical and medical conditions affecting the foot, and the podiatric visit represents an ideal time to focus on the pedal manifestations of the disease. Ongoing education, aggressive follow-up, and thorough evaluation are all vital elements in reducing the morbidity and mortality from diabetic foot lesions. Too often, foot management does not occur in the primary care setting.[6] Harrington, in an analysis of diabetic foot ulcers using Medicare claims data for 1995–1996, found that 70% of patients had little or no follow-up after treatment of the acute problem.[7] To prevent the onset and recurrence of foot ulcers, it is important that patient management be biased toward regular preventive care rather than just emergency interventional care.

Multidisciplinary centers have been organized to provide comprehensive service for the patient with diabetes.[8–11] The team approach continues to develop and mature, gradually becoming more sophisticated and sensitive to the needs of the patient. In one recent outcome study, the joint clinical efforts of vascular surgeons and foot care specialists resulted in an 85% limb salvage rate.[12]

There are obviously many factors that play a role in diminishing the rate of amputation, but patient education and responsibility for self-care play significant roles. In addition, the mandate of "pay for performance" in many health care systems is requiring that practitioners utilize evidence-based medicine to maximize outcomes and minimize costs.[13]

Linking the Risk Factors

The clinical experience of podiatrists qualifies them to care for the lower limb throughout the progression of disease. Comprehensive knowledge of the patient's condition allows podiatrists to link the risk factors and select the best options for each patient to provide effective and economic outcomes in a timely manner. Management is based on the physical features of the diabetic wound, including its location, area and depth, character of margins and base, and involvement of deeper structures, as well as infection and the patient's position on the vascular risk spectrum.

The primary factors that are evaluated in establishing the patient's position on the vascular risk spectrum are as follows:

Macrovascular disease
Microvascular disease
Autonomic neuropathic complications
Metabolic syndrome
Family history
Duration of diabetes

The mind-set that can be achieved by first establishing the vascular risk factors for each patient in assessing the patient's immediate and long-range care needs might help to improve the outcome. The value of this approach is best illustrated by the following case study.

CASE STUDY

Several weeks prior to presenting himself to the emergency department of the senior author's hospital, an obese 36-year-old African American man with a 14-year history of type 2 diabetes had walked extensively in poorly fitting shoes on a summer outing. On admission, he had a fever of 101°F and expressed concern about an ulcer beneath the first metatarsophalangeal (MTP) joint of his left foot. Review of symptoms was significant for peripheral neuropathy, retinopathy, impotence, and gastroparesis. His diabetes was uncontrolled, evidenced by a hemoglobin A1C of 16.1%. Both parents were diabetic, his father having had renal failure and a transtibial amputation before succumbing to a myocardial infarction.

Physical findings included nonpalpable popliteal, dorsalis pedis, and posterior tibial pulses and pitting ankle edema on the left. With the use of the 10-g Semmes-Weinstein monofilament, protective sensation was noted to be absent in both feet. The full-thickness plantar ulceration beneath the first MTP of the left foot was 3 cm in diameter and had a fibrofatty, avascular base with serous drainage (Figs. 26-1A and 26-1B). Infection was found to track proximally along the flexor tendons. The history and clinical presentation placed the patient at the moderate-to-severe end of the vascular risk spectrum. The development of an ulcer was predictable because of chronic hyperglycemia, lost protective sensation combined with poor footwear, a high activity level, and denial.[14] Given these factors, the patient was at significant risk for major limb loss without immediate and aggressive intervention.

This patient had a complete vascular evaluation, both noninvasive and by arteriogram, indicating an occluded posterior tibial artery. He required a femoral to dorsalis pedis artery bypass graft with a concomitant open first ray amputation (Figs. 26-2 and 26-3). Because of his vascular disease and diabetes, he had difficulty healing, manifested by partial dehiscence of the wound, with eventual healing by secondary intention (Fig. 26-4). Further ulceration with osteomyelitis due to continued use of inadequate footwear required a transmetatarsal amputation, which healed (Fig. 26-5).

Evaluation of the Foot in Diabetic Patients

History-Taking

In evaluating the patient with diabetes, specific questions about vascular disease should be asked:

1. Where is the patient on the vascular risk spectrum; that is, does the patient have mild, moderate, or severe disease?
2. What evidence is there to support the presence of vascular disease by history and examination?
3. Macrovascular disease: Is there a history of coronary artery disease or stroke?
4. Microvascular disease: Is there a history of retinopathy, nephropathy, or neuropathy indicating advanced

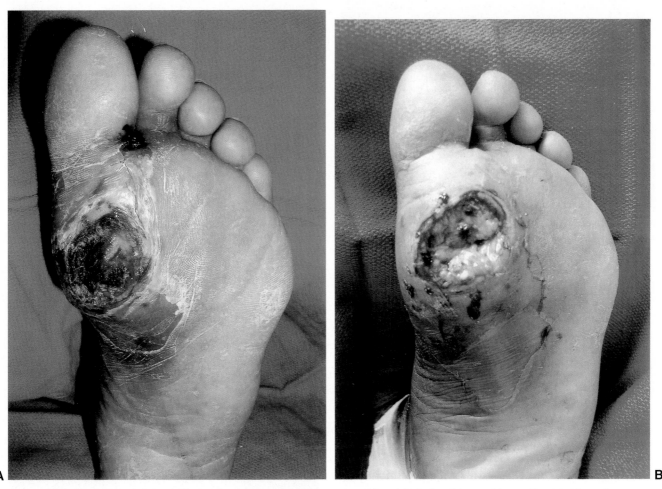

Figure 26-1   **A,** Infected ischemic ulcer beneath first metatarsal head. **B,** Ischemic wound base after debridement.

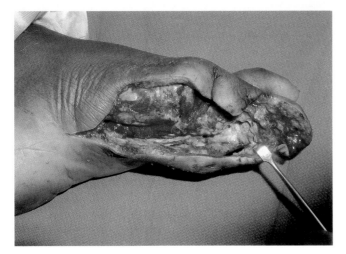

Figure 26-2   Wound three days after open partial first ray amputation and concomitant femoral to dorsalis pedis artery bypass.

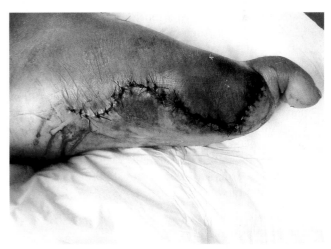

Figure 26-3   Wound closed with dorsal flap to cover plantar defect.

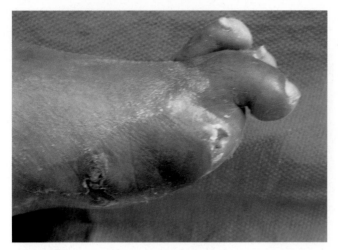

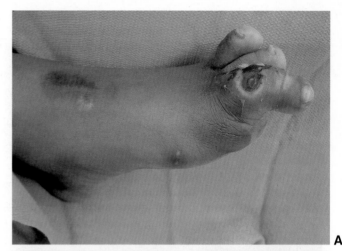

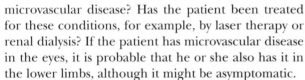

Figure 26-4 Partial dehiscence of wound 9 months postoperatively despite bypass surgery.

microvascular disease? Has the patient been treated for these conditions, for example, by laser therapy or renal dialysis? If the patient has microvascular disease in the eyes, it is probable that he or she also has it in the lower limbs, although it might be asymptomatic.

5. Autonomic neuropathic complications: Does the patient have a history of gastroparesis or impotence? These symptoms are related to autonomic neuropathy and depletion of nitric oxide, a condition that is prevalent in patients with long-standing diabetes, which causes impairment of smooth muscle vasodilation. This, in turn, leads to endothelial cell damage, causing capillary leakage with resultant difficulty in wound healing.[15]

6. Metabolic syndrome: Does the patient have a history of dyslipidemia (high triglycerides, low HDL cholesterol)? Is there a history of glucose intolerance or a history of obesity or hypertension?

7. Family history: Is there a familial history of diabetes? Did any of the affected family members have renal dysfunction, retinopathy, or lower-limb amputations? If the family has a history of diabetes with microvascular complications, there is the likelihood of the patient having similar problems due to genetic predisposition.

8. Duration of diabetes: Vascular complications are directly related to the duration of poorly controlled diabetes. Patients with diabetes over 10 years often have severe vascular disease with signs and symptoms in the foot and leg.

Physical Examination

The intimate relationship between neuropathy and vascular disease[16] forms the foundation for future foot complications. By recognizing early signs of diabetic peripheral neuropathy, such as plantar xerosis and contracture of the toes with associated corns and calluses, and then understanding the predictive nature of these

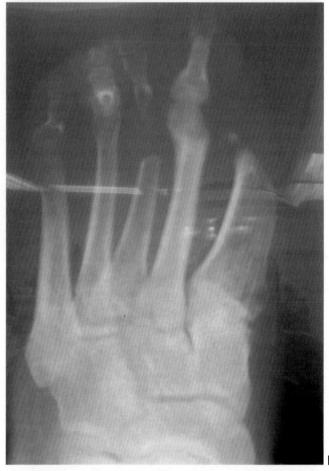

Figure 26-5 **A,** Ulcer over second proximal interphalangeal joint with osteomyelitis due to use of footwear with tight toebox. **B,** Radiograph showing bone loss of the second metatarsal head consistent with osteomyelitis. Note the previous partial third ray amputation.

findings, simple education and home self-care can be implemented.

Various other factors combined with the clinical presentation help to identify increased risk for diabetic foot disease. Factors such as duration of diabetes, medications, allergies, previous surgery, and any history of slow

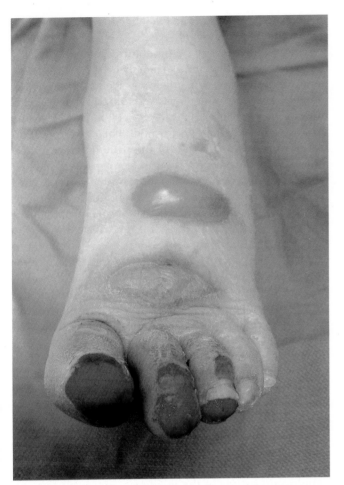

Figure 26–6 Thermal burns on the distal aspect of toes 1, 2, and 3 with bullae of the dorsal forefoot due to soaking in hot water.

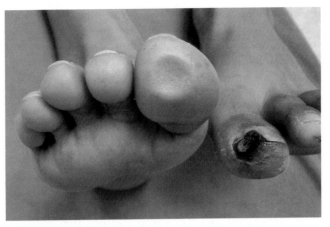

Figure 26–7 Subcutaneous tissue atrophy of right great toe ("baked potato toe") with ischemic ulcer of the contralateral hallux consistent with advanced vascular disease.

healing or slow recovery are relevant. Additional risk factors to assess are smoking, neuropathic sensations of cold, burning or numbness of the feet, previous infection or amputation, and average blood sugar levels monitored at home. Asking patients how they care for their feet can also give insight into present and future problems. Patients with or without retinopathy who shave their calluses with a razor, trim their nails with tin snips, or soak their feet in hot water need to be counseled immediately about the dangers of "bathroom surgery" and thermal injury (Fig. 26-6). Physical examination of the diabetic limb should be approached from a systems perspective: vascular, dermatologic, neurologic, and musculoskeletal/biomechanical. A relevant lower-limb examination should take no more than 5 to 10 minutes and requires little instrumentation.

Vascular Examination

Assessing the patient's history will provide an index of suspicion for vascular disease prior to the physical examination. Symptoms of vascular disease include cold feet, edema, blue toes, muscle cramps with activity or at rest,

and leg pain while in bed at night relieved by foot dependency. Patients with intermittent claudication complain of cramping in the legs that is reproducible by walking a certain distance. Relief is obtained with rest for 10 to 15 minutes. The symptoms are usually unilateral and may include the musculature of the foot, calf, thigh, and/or buttocks.

The vascular examination should include palpation of the femoral, popliteal, dorsalis pedis, and posterior tibial pulses in both limbs, noting any differences between the limbs. Capillary fill time should be assessed with the foot raised above the level of the heart. Foot pallor on elevation and rubor on dependency indicate poor vascular status. Subcutaneous atrophy of the distal toe is easily noted by squeezing the end of the toe, which feels quite similar to a baked potato, a poor prognostic sign (Fig. 26-7). The presence of small focal areas of distal gangrene may be due to microemboli. Sparse hair growth and skin atrophy are also clues to vascular disease of the foot and leg. The ability to notice these subtle pathologies and correlate them with the long-term prognosis is critical to reducing the morbidity associated with long-standing diabetes.[17] Nonpalpable pulses can sometimes be found by using a handheld Doppler flow unit. In patients with symptoms of arterial insufficiency, a vascular workup including both Doppler examination and an arteriogram might be indicated.[18,19]

Neurologic Examination

Diabetic patients may present with one or more of the following types of neuropathy: distal symmetric sensorimotor polyneuropathy, autonomic neuropathy, mononeuropathy multiplex, cranial neuropathy, radiculopathy, and plexopathy. Thus, diabetic neuropathy affects much more than the feet; in fact, it affects every major organ system of the body.[16,20] The differential diagnosis for peripheral neuropathy should always include alcoholism, malignancy, malnutrition, vitamin deficiencies, lead poisoning, spinal cord lesions, syphilis, and various medications. Diabetic peripheral neuropathy affects the sensory, autonomic, and motor nerves of the foot and leg. Sensory neuropathy may cause burning, tingling, heaviness, coldness, and numbness of the feet. With autonomic neuropathy, patients lose eccrine gland function, resulting in dryness and fissuring of the skin, creating portals for infection (Fig. 26-8). Motor neuropathy leads to changes in foot structure and gait patterns. Initially, the small intrinsic muscles of the foot begin to atrophy owing to a loss of motor innervation. The result is the loss of the stabilizing effect they provide on the long flexors and extensors of the toes, allowing them to markedly extend the MTP joints and flex the interphalangeal joints. The toes become contracted in this position, increasing the plantar prominence of the metatarsal heads (Fig. 26-9).

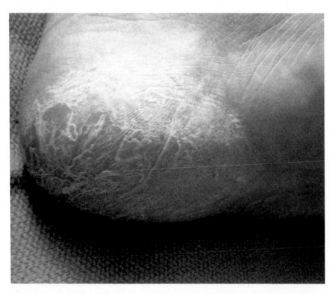

Figure 26–8   Plantar medial aspect of heel with xerosis and hyperkeratosis.

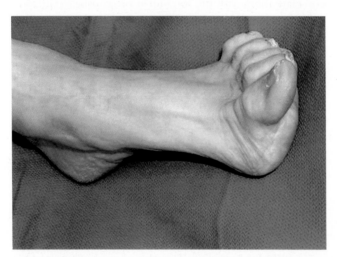

Figure 26–9   Intrinsic minus foot with prominent extensor tendons and claw toes with distal migration of the fat pad to the toe sulcus.

Neurologic testing of the diabetic limb should include evaluation of Achilles and patellar reflexes, protective sensation, and vibratory, temperature, and proprioceptive sensation. Instruments needed for these tests are a percussion hammer, a 10-g Semmes-Weinstein monofilament, a 128-Hz tuning fork or biothesiometer, and a thermal probe. Have the patient recline and close the eyes as these tests are performed. They are important to determine a level of risk for the patient and as a baseline to follow the progression of neuropathy. The 10-g Semmes-Weinstein monofilament probably represents the pressure threshold required to protect against ulceration.[20] In fact, the patient who cannot feel this filament on the skin is at increased risk for ulceration or injury.

A 128-Hz tuning fork provides an easy, qualitative evaluation of the patient's peripheral large afferent fiber function. The patient's ability to detect the vibration in the foot is compared to the examiner's ability to feel the vibration in his or her hand. The vibration perception threshold (VPT) can be measured by using a handheld biothesiometer placed on the pulp of the great toe. Voltage is increased until the patient perceives a vibration, which is recorded as the VPT voltage. The quantitative nature of the VPT is a major advantage for documenting the progression of neuropathy, since vibratory sensation is lost first in diabetic patients. Young reported that a VPT greater than 25 V carried a sevenfold risk of foot ulceration compared with a VPT less than 15 V.[21] Abbott and colleagues also demonstrated, in a multicenter study of the incidence and predictive risk factors for diabetic neuropathic foot ulcerations, that VPT and Michigan DPN scores for muscle strength and reflexes were significant predictors of foot ulceration.[22]

In a study designed to identify a practical neurologic screening test, Lavery and colleagues[23] found that a 10-g Semmes-Weinstein filament test, in which patients lacked perception at four out of ten sites on the foot, was 97% sensitive and 83% specific for identifying loss of protective sensation. The biothesiometer was 90% sensitive and 84% specific at a cutoff of 25 V. Overall, the best method for evaluating loss of protective sensation was a combination of these two modalities yielding a focused neuropathy symptom score, with 97% sensitivity and 86% specificity, emphasizing the usefulness of a thorough, multifactorial examination to accurately assess the patient's neurologic status. A handheld thermal probe is used to detect focal areas of inflammation ("hot spots") and to diagnose and follow the progress of Charcot neuroarthropathy. Joint proprioceptive function is considered impaired if the patient cannot detect passive movement of the first MTP or ankle joint.

Dermatologic Examination

The skin is the largest body organ and the primary barrier against infection. In people with diabetes, however, the skin is compromised by vascular, neurologic, and musculoskeletal disease. Assessment should include skin quality, turgor, texture, and hair growth (Fig. 26-10). Diabetic patients with arterial disease commonly have shiny atrophic skin on the dorsum of the foot. The nails, as skin appendages, must also be evaluated. Koilonychia (spoon-shaped nails), pitting of the nail plate, onycholysis, subungual hemorrhage, subungual ulceration secondary to onychomycosis, infected ingrown nails, and nail color changes are associated with diabetes mellitus[24] (Fig. 26-11). Chronic tinea pedis with its "moccasin" distribution and slightly erythematous superficial scaling and xerosis are other common findings. Dishydrotic eczema is often mistaken for tinea pedis. It presents with water-filled vesicles on a nonerythematous base and builds by desquamation (Fig. 26-12). This condition is commonly seen in diabetic patients with depression, anxiety, or other psychosocial problems.

Autonomic neuropathy has been implicated in several of the cutaneous findings in people with diabetes. With long-standing disease, the patient might complain of cold feet, pruritus associated with dry skin, and an occa-sional burning sensation. The most common manifesta-tion of autonomic neuropathy, however, is decreased or lost vasomotor function resulting in dryness of the pedal skin, although patients might complain of increased sweating in other areas of the body. The resultant thick-ening of the stratum corneum is followed by the forma-tion of brittle callosities on the feet, which, coupled with peripheral neuropathy, become areas of high pressure subject to ulceration. Caregivers must stress the impor-tance of adequate pedal hygiene and the use of mois-turizing emollients. Another consequence of autonomic neuropathy is loss of sympathetic control, which will result in vasodilation, arteriovenous shunting, and edema with prominent vessels and varicosities of the feet (Fig. 26-13).

Although callus formation is the body's mechanism to protect an area of skin that is subject to chronic irrita-tion, it can lead directly to skin ulcers in the insensate diabetic patient. The etiology of callus is bony deformity, resulting in abnormal biomechanical function. Repetitive pressure and shear in the neuropathic foot, along with neuropathy, have been consistently described as a factor in callus formation. It has also been stated that nonenzy-matic glycosylation results in alterations of the structural

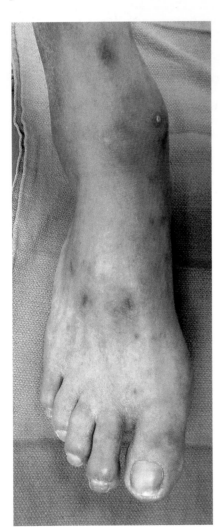

Figure 26-10 Foot of a type 2 diabetic male with atrophic hairless skin, pigmentary changes, pallor, and xerosis due to anhidrosis.

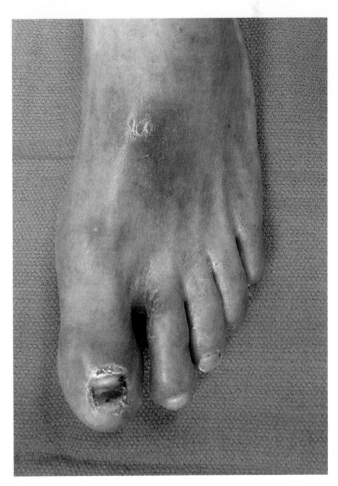

Figure 26-11 Absent hallux nail due to microtrauma with subungual hematoma.

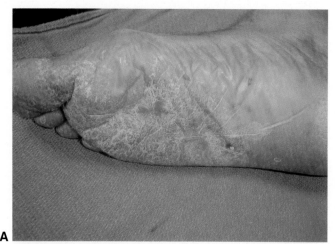

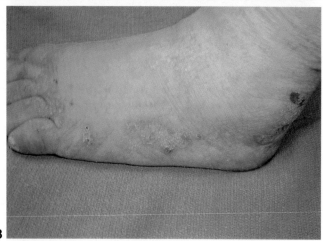

Figure 26–12　**A,** Dishydrotic eczema with xerosis, hyperkeratosis, and pruritic vesicles that are unresponsive to topical antifungal therapy. **B,** Same condition with scaling and vesicles on the lateral aspect of the foot and dorsal aspect of the toes.

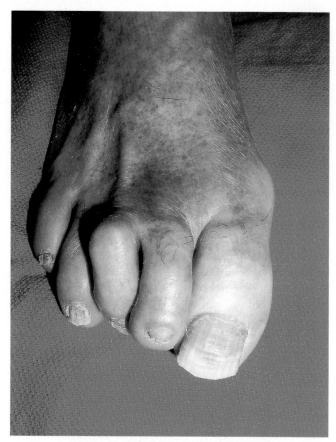

Figure 26–13　Prominent dorsal veins with hyperpigmented macular areas consistent with autonomic neuropathy and diabetic dermopathy.

stability of the skin, predisposing the diabetic person to increased callus formation. Although witnessed in patients with good glycemic control, keratin and collagen disturbances have been most commonly related to chronically elevated plasma glucose levels, resulting in skin that is inflexible and more resistant to collagenase digestion. According to Delbridge and colleagues,[25] glycosylated keratin builds up secondary to repetitive pressure and shear forces and is not removed from the superficial layers of the foot, resulting in hyperkeratosis and ultimate ulceration. They also described several steps in the development of a neuropathic ulcer in the diabetic foot. The initial hyperkeratotic lesion, with continued repetitive pressure and shear, will result in the breakdown of deeper tissues. Eventually, a cavity will form, fill with blood, and enlarge to the point at which it ruptures, revealing an ulcer. These usually develop beneath a callus that was unrecognized and untreated.

Several other dermatologic findings have been observed in diabetic patients, including paronychia, yellow nails, fungal nails, pigmented purpura, periun-

gual telangiectasias, and necrobiosis lipoidica diabeticorum. Some of these conditions have been attributed to poor plasma glucose control, nonenzymatic glycosylation, and/or the degree of vascular compromise. Yellowing of the skin, once attributed to carotenemia, is now thought to be due to glycosylation end products that become yellow. Purpura, on the other hand, is attributed to the extravasation of red blood cells from the superficial vascular plexus. These lesions are commonly referred to as "cayenne pepper spots" and consist of tan or orange patches on the skin. Purpura is commonly found in conjunction with diabetic dermopathy and is precipitated by lower-limb edema.

Diabetic dermopathy (shin spots) is considered the most common skin manifestation, found in up to 65% of diabetic patients. Lesions are usually bilateral, asymmetrical, circumscribed, atrophic, and hyperpigmented macules on the shins of affected individuals. The etiology of such lesions is unknown, although they have been closely associated with posttraumatic atrophy and postinflammatory hyperpigmentation in poorly vascularized skin. Because they have also been observed in nondiabetic individuals, it has been postulated that the presence of four or more lesions is more diagnostic of diabetic dermopathy. One study found that 14% of

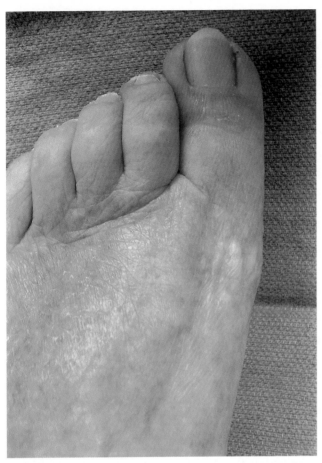

Figure 26–14   Ingrown great toenail with medial and lateral erythematous paronychia.

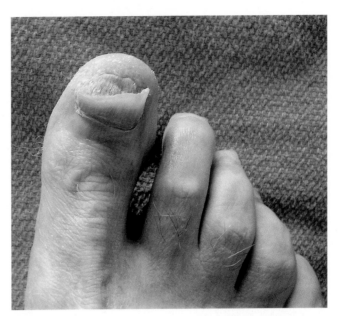

Figure 26–15   Onychomycosis with onycholysis.

diabetic patients and none of the nondiabetic persons were affected by multilesional dermopathy.

Paronychia has been attributed to several factors, including trauma, nail dystrophy, tight footwear, nail morphology, and improper nail debridement. Trauma and nail morphology being uncontrollable, one should be aware of the remaining factors and work toward preventing their progression. Should the diabetic patient present with a paronychia, the degree of the infection, noted by purulence and erythema, should be noted, as well as the duration of symptoms (Fig. 26-14). In the presence of adequate pedal pulses and capillary fill time, the offending border may be removed by partial matrixectomy. If vascular status is of concern, antibiotic therapy as well as a more conservative debridement of the border should be done, with close continued follow-up of the patient.

Onychomycosis, common in the general population, is also highly prevalent and a greater risk in the diabetic patient. Though the etiology of onychomycosis is unclear, it has been proposed that undetected subungual hemorrhage secondary to neuropathy acts as a nidus for fungal infection and results in thickened, hypertrophic nails. Other factors of concern are immunopathy and vasculopathy, which decrease the ability to fight off such infections. Invasion of the nailbed results in increased thickness of the nail and the accumulation of subungual debris, which can result in subungual ulceration from vertical footwear pressure or lifting of the nail (Fig. 26-15). For these reasons, adequate regular nail debridement is important in the care of the diabetic patient. With the high incidence of fungus-infected toenails, tinea pedis as well as interdigital tinea become associated risks. Common findings with such infections include vesicular lesions, areas of skin breakdown, and interdigital maceration, any of which may allow invasion of the subcutaneous layers by normal skin flora to produce a superimposed bacterial infection.

The importance of identifying a diabetic foot ulcer and then providing proper follow-up care was recognized clearly in a study that showed that Medicare expenditures for patients with diabetic foot ulcers were three times higher than those for Medicare patients in general: $15,309 versus $4,226.[7] Care for ulcers represented 24% of spending for the diabetic patient population. The fact that the majority of patients had little or no follow-up on a regular basis was the reason given for the discrepancy. Moreover, Ramsey demonstrated, in an HMO population of 8904 diabetic patients, that the estimated costs for a middle-aged patient with a new foot ulcer were $28,000 over a two-year period.

Eight questions should be answered to provide a thorough evaluation of a neuropathic ulcer.

1. *Where is the ulcer located?* There is a close relationship between an ulcer's location and its etiology. For example, ulcers located along the lateral or medial foot margins are secondary to constant low pressures (e.g., tight shoes), while those on the plantar aspect of the foot are caused by repetitive moderate pressures (e.g., prominent metatarsal head) (Fig. 26-16).

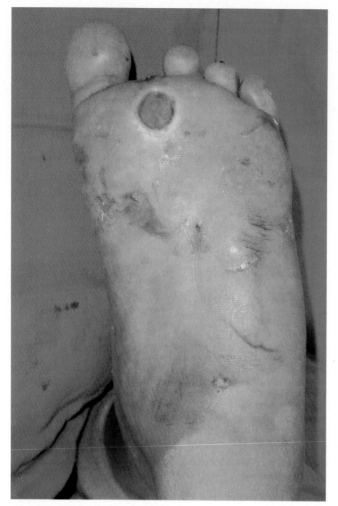

Figure 26–16 Ulcer beneath a prominent second metatarsal head after second toe amputation in a foot with functional equinus.

2. *How large is the ulcer?* This is a key factor in determining the duration of wound healing. The wound area and depth should be recorded at each visit to gauge healing progress.
3. *What do the wound margins look like?* If adequate debridement and off-loading have been implemented, the margins should be adherent to the underlying subcutaneous structures with a gentle slope upward toward normal epithelium. If a wound has been inadequately debrided and off-loaded, however, undermining of the leading edge will predominate. This phenomenon is due to the "edge-effect," which dictates that an interruption in any matrix (in this case, the dermal matrix) magnifies both shear and vertical stresses on the edges of that interruption. Shearing makes the wound larger by undermining, while increased vertical pressure makes the wound progressively deeper. This effect can be mitigated by regular, adequate debridement and off-loading techniques. Wound margins should be described as undermined, adherent, macerated, and/or viable versus necrotic.

4. *What does the wound base look like?* Descriptive terms include granular, fibrotic, and necrotic.
5. *Is there purulent drainage?* Note the odor of the wound.
6. *Are underlying structures involved in the depths of the ulcer?* Wound depth is by far the most commonly utilized descriptor in wound classification. The depth of the ulceration is categorized by the University of Texas Wound Classification System[26] according to the progressively deeper structures that are involved:
   Grade 0: No history of ulcer or an ulcer now completely epithelialized
   Grade 1: Superficial skin ulcer
   Grade 2: Ulcer deep to tendon and/or capsule
   Grade 3: Ulcer deep to bone
   Practitioners have long suspected that wounds that penetrate to bone are usually associated with osteomyelitis. Grayson and colleagues demonstrated that probing to bone is up to 66% sensitive and 85% specific in diagnosing osteomyelitis.[27]
7. *Is the ulcer infected?* The diabetic person might be unable to mount an adequate immune response to an infection. Therefore, white blood cell counts might not be elevated in over 50% of these patients.[28]
   Similarly, fever and other signs of infection are absent about 86% of the time.[5] This makes the diagnosis of infection difficult; however, one must watch for the five cardinal signs of infection: redness, heat, swelling, pain, and loss of function. Infection is loosely defined as the presence of cellulitis, often with associated purulence, or more than two of the cardinal signs of infection (Fig. 26-17).
8. *Is the ulcer ischemic?* An ulcer can be deemed ischemic on the basis of its necrotic appearance, its lack of a red granular base, or its behavior, that is, slow healing despite adequate local wound care and off-loading techniques. These findings warrant the use of noninvasive vascular studies and/or a vascular consultation for possible surgical intervention to optimize perfusion to enhance wound healing (Fig. 26-18).

Following a detailed diabetic foot examination, a clear description of risk that incorporates the salient findings from the history and physical examination is of paramount importance in developing a treatment plan designed to prevent lower-limb amputation. To effectively treat ulcers, it is helpful to have an established classification and risk system that allows the practitioner to predict outcomes based on ulcer characteristics and the patient's comorbidities. Using a proven protocol allows the medical and research communities to speak a common language. The University of Texas Wound Classification System fulfills these requirements. It was developed at the University of Texas Health Sciences Center at San Antonio by Armstrong and colleagues.[26] It is based on the evaluation and treatment, over a six-month period, of the foot lesions of 360 patients and has been validated[29] (Fig. 26-19). Moreover, treatment guidelines are designed to bring the patient from a high-risk category to the lowest-risk category possible for that individual. Categories 0 to 3 are risk factors for ulceration, and categories 4 to 6 are risk factors for amputation. Risk factors for development of ulceration include neuropathy, deformity or limited joint mobility, and a previous history of ulceration or amputation. Lavery and colleagues[23] evaluated 255 patients and found that those with category 1 neuropathy (loss of protective sensation) were at 1.7 times greater risk of ulceration. Patients in category 2, defined as neuropathy plus deformity, were at 12 times greater risk for ulceration. Patients in category 3 who had neuropathy plus deformity as well as a history of ulceration, Charcot neuroarthropathy, or amputation were at 36 times greater risk for ulceration. Clearly, all diabetic patients should be screened and placed in the relevant risk category and followed at appropriate intervals.

Musculoskeletal/Biomechanical Evaluation

Foot function is dynamic and cannot be thoroughly appreciated by a solely non-weight-bearing examination. One mandatory aspect of a complete lower-limb examination is the evaluation of the foot both in quiet standing and throughout the gait cycle. The foot must be able to accommodate many times the body's weight while converting rapidly from mobile adapter during weight acceptance to rigid lever for propulsion at the end of the stance phase of gait while efficiently dispersing both direct and shear loads.

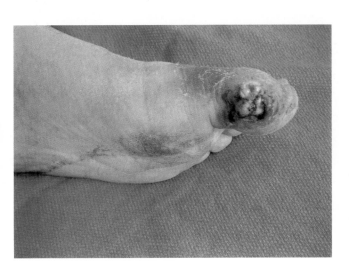

Figure 26–17 Neuropathic ulcer on the medial aspect of the hallux with purulence and dorsal cellulitis.

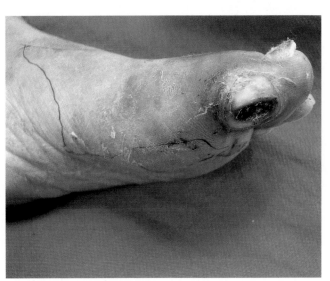

Figure 26–18 Ischemic ulcer on the plantar medial aspect of the hallux interphalangeal joint.

		GRADE/DEPTH "How deep is the wound?"			
		0	**I**	**II**	**III**
STAGE/COMORBIDITIES "Is the wound infected, ischemic, or both?"	**A**	Pre- or postulcerative lesion, completely epithelialized	Superficial wound, not involving tendon, capsule, or bone	Wound penetrating to tendon or capsule	Wound penetrating to bone or joint
	B	Pre- or postulcerative lesion completely epithelialized with infection	Superficial wound, not involving lesion, capsule, or bone, with infection	Wound penetrating to tendon or capsule, with infection	Wound penetrating to bone
	C	Pre- or postulcerative lesion, completely epithelialized with infection and ischemia	Superficial wound, not involving tendon, capsule, or bone, with ischemia	Wound penetrating to tendon or capsule, with ischemia	Wound penetrating to bone or joint, with ischemia
	D	Pre- or postulcerative lesion, completely epithelialized with infection and ischemia	Superficial wound, not involving tendon, capsule, or bone, with infection and ischemia	Wound penetrating to tendon or capsule, with infection and ischemia	Wound penetrating to bone or joint, with infection and ischemia

Figure 26–19 The University of Texas Classification System for Diabetic Foot Wounds.

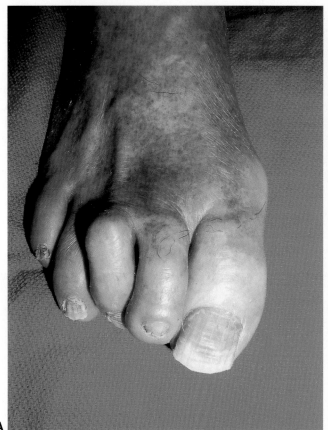

A

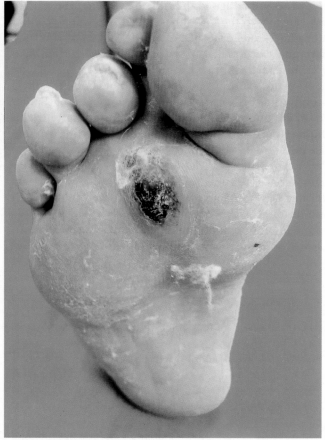

B

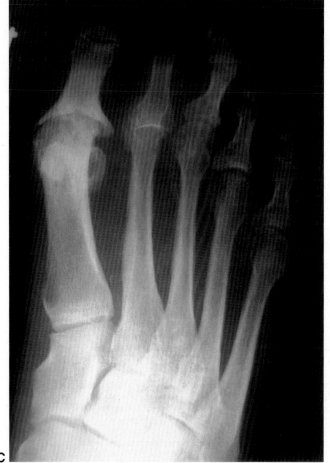

C

Figure 26–20   A, Rigid hammertoe deformity of the second and third toes with dorsal dislocation of the second and subluxation of the third MTP joints. **B,** Callus beneath the second metatarsal head with an old hemorrhage (preulcerative lesion). **C,** Radiograph of severely dislocated second and subluxated third MTP joints. Note degenerative arthritis of the first MTP joint.

During this phase of the clinical examination, it is essential to identify areas of pressure and increased friction. Changes in color such as erythema, bony prominences, hyperkeratosis, and complaints of localized pain are good indicators of problem areas. No matter the foot type, the potential for complications exist. The cavus foot, with its contracted toes and high arch, may have digital and metatarsal pressure areas, just as the rocker-bottom foot may show the changes of Charcot neuroarthropathy and midfoot ulceration. Range of motion, both active and passive, should be assessed, including the MTP joints, the midtarsal joints, and the subtalar and ankle joints. Manual muscle testing of all muscle groups should be performed.

Weight-bearing radiographs of both feet should be considered as a baseline if sensory neuropathy is present because the foot often has a significantly different shape during weight-bearing versus non-weight-bearing. Early collapse of the midtarsal and subtalar joints, for example, might be evident only on weight-bearing studies.

With each step during the stance phase of gait, bony prominences or shoe pressure can cause blood to be displaced from the adjacent soft tissues, creating a local area of transient ischemia. In the neurologically intact foot, this would normally cause pain, but in the neuropathic patient, this protective function is absent. Shear and pressure forces combine over these areas of high stress to initially produce hyperkeratosis. Continued stress eventually leads to ulceration. Pressure points may be created by long or plantarflexed metatarsals, prominent sesamoid bones, exostoses, contracted digits, and footwear (Figs. 26-20 and 26-21).

Of great concern in the overall assessment of the musculoskeletal function of the diabetic foot is the degree of flexibility versus rigidity of any joint deformities that are encountered. These findings have been extensively discussed by several authors, including Delbridge and colleagues,[25] Fernando and associates,[30] and Lavery and colleagues,[31] and have been attributed to joint stiffening secondary to nonenzymatic glycosylation of soft tissue structures. Lavery and colleagues noted that limited joint mobility can best be appreciated by assessing the range of motion of the first MTP joint. A finding of less than 50 degrees of passive dorsiflexion has been accepted as a criterion for increased risk of ulceration. One must also take into consideration the amount of motion at the other

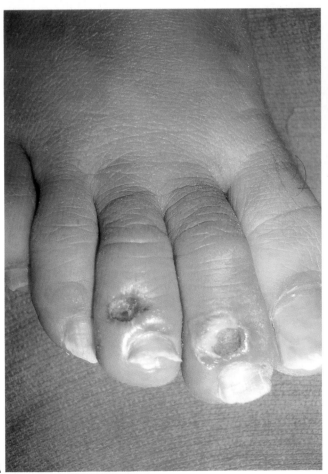

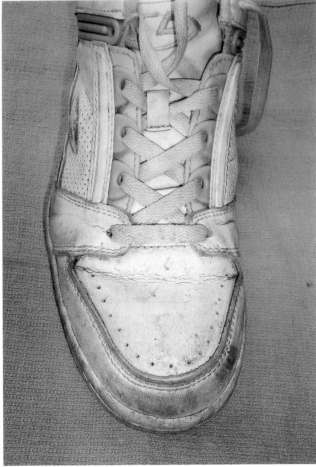

Figure 26–21   **A,** Ulcers over the dorsal aspect of the distal interphalangeal joints of the second and third toes due to pressure from the toebox. Shoes were not evaluated before treatment of a dorsal wound on the contralateral foot. **B,** Tennis shoe with tight toebox that caused digital ulcers.

MTP joints, subtalar joint, and ankle, since any limitation in these areas can result in increased pressures.

Off-Loading Principles

One of the areas where the foot specialist can be very effective in preventing initial or recurrent ulceration is in off-loading of areas of risk within appropriate shoes. Again, questioning the patient about footwear specifics is the foundation of proper treatment. The practitioner needs to know the following:

- What did the patient wear to the appointment?
- Is this typical of what the patient wears at home?
- Does the patient go barefoot or in socks at home? Examining the feet and socks for soiling or debris may reveal the answer.
- Has the patient been provided with prescription footwear and is it being worn? Examine the shoes for wear patterns. Too often, the patient will report that the prescription shoes are being saved for "special occasions" and they show no signs of wear. The patient must be persuaded that the shoes are similar to medication and must be used exactly as prescribed.

At the same time, one cannot be totally inflexible in dealing with the patient. The practitioner must take into consideration the patient's social, work, and personal needs when prescribing footwear. For instance, a patient who works as a laborer is not likely to wear prescription shoes during working hours. Besides appropriateness of style, care must be taken to utilize the materials and features that will most benefit the patient. Although these will be specific to the patient, certain features are universally important: a deep toebox to accommodate digital deformities, a sturdy heel counter to stabilize the foot, and adequate width and accommodation with insoles to protect pressure points, all of which can be incorporated in work boots for the laborer.

The same philosophy of protection using off-loading principles is applied during the treatment phase. An example is the use of the total contact cast. The biomechanics of the total contact cast are better understood now because of determination of plantar pressure and ground reaction forces in the device,[32] and with that knowledge comes the ability to better use this modality. Shaw and colleagues determined that the total contact cast is successful in treating forefoot ulcers on a dependable basis but that treatment of hindfoot ulcers is dependent on appropriate foam padding.[32]

Summary

The pedal manifestations of diabetes may be quite diverse, with multiple etiologic factors combining to complicate the clinical presentation. A thorough understanding of the pathogenesis of diabetic foot disease pro-

vides the basis for effective treatment. As was stated by Cavanagh, the key is linking all of the associated risk factors of structure, function, footwear, lifestyle, and activity level. These factors are dynamic, not static; therefore, constant reassessment is essential to prevention. This must be followed by systematic implementation to provide efficient and effective prevention and treatment. When knowledge and implementation meet, the podiatrist is afforded an exceptional opportunity to truly make a difference in the quality of life of the diabetic patient.

References

1. 2005 Podiatric Practice Survey. Available at www.apma.org.
2. Centers for Disease Control and Prevention: Available at www.CDC.org.
3. National Diabetes Fact Sheet: General Information and National Estimation of Diabetes in the United States. Atlanta, Centers for Disease Control and Prevention, 2005.
4. Izumi Y, Satterfield VK, Lee S, Harkless LB: Risk of amputation in diabetic patients stratified by limb and level of amputation: A 10 year observation. Diabetes Care 29:566–570, 2006.
5. American Diabetes Association: Foot care in patients with diabetes mellitus (position statement). Diabetes Care 21(suppl 1):554–555, 1998.
6. O'Brien KF, Chandramohan V, Nelson DA, et al: Effect of a physician-directed educational campaign on performance of proper diabetic foot exams in an outpatient setting. J Gen Intern Med 18:258–265, 2003.
7. Harrington C, Zagari MJ, Corea J, Klitenic J: Cost analysis of diabetic lower extremity ulcers. Diabetes Care 23:1333–1338, 2000.
8. Gottrup FA: A specialized wound-healing center concept: Importance of a multidisciplinary department structure and surgical treatment facilities in the treatment of chronic wounds. Am J Surg 187:38S–43S, 2004.
9. Larsson J, Apelqvist J, Agardh DD, Stenstrom A: Decreasing incidence of major amputation in diabetic patients: A consequence of a multidisciplinary foot care team approach? Diabet Med 12:770–776, 1995.
10. Thomson FJ, Veves A, Ashe H, et al: A team approach to diabetic foot care: The Manchester experience. Foot 2:75–92, 1991.
11. Armstrong DG, Harkless LB: Outcomes of preventative care in a diabetic foot specialty clinic. J Foot Ankle Surg 37:460–466, 1998.
12. van Gils CC, Wheeler LA, Mellstrom M, et al: Amputation prevention by vascular surgery and podiatry collaboration in high-risk diabetic and non-diabetic patients. Diabetes Care 22:678–683, 1999.
13. Grossbart SR: What's the return?: Assessing the effect of "pay for performance" initiatives on the quality of care delivery. Med Care Res Rev 63(1, suppl):29S–48S, 2006.
14. Cavanagh PR: What the practicing physician should know about diabetic foot mechanics. In Boulton AJM, Connor H, Cavanagh PR (eds): The Foot in Diabetes, 3rd ed. Chichester, UK, John Wiley and Sons, 2000, pp 37–39.
15. Pham H, et al: The role of endothelial function on the foot. Clin Podiatr Med Surg 15:85–94. 1998.
16. Boulton AJM: The pathogenesis of diabetic foot problems: An overview. Diabet Med 13:S12–S16. 1996.
17. de Heus-van Putten MA, Schaper NC, Bakker K: The clinical examination of the diabetic foot in daily practise. Diabet Med 13(suppl 1):S55–S57, 1996.
18. Schaper NC: Early atherogenesis in diabetes mellitus. Diabet Med 13:S17, 1996.
19. Takolander R, Rauweda JA: The use of non-invasive vascular assessment in diabetic patients with foot lesions. Diabet Med 24:S39–S42, 1996.
20. Ziegler D: Diagnosis and management of diabetic peripheral neuropathy. Diabet Med 13:S34–S38, 1996.
21. Young MJ: The prediction of diabetic neuropathic foot ulceration using vibration perception thresholds: A prospective study. Diabetes Care 17:557–560, 1999.

22. Abbott CA, Vileikyte L, et al: Multicenter study of the incidence of and predictive risk factors for diabetic neuropathic foot ulceration. Diabetes Care 21:1071–1075, 1998.

23. Lavery LA, Armstrong DG, et al: Choosing a practical screening instrument to identify patients at risk for diabetic foot ulceration. Arch Intern Med 159:157–162, 1998.

24. Herzberg A: Nail manifestations of systemic disease. In Clinics in Podiatric Medicine and Surgery. Philadelphia, WB Saunders, 1995, pp 314–317.

25. Delbridge L, Ellis CS, Robertson K, et al: Nonenzymatic glycosylation of keratin from the stratum corneum of the diabetic foot. Br J Dermatol 112:547–554, 1985.

26. Armstrong DG, Lavey LA, Harkless LB: Treatment based classification system for assessment and care of diabetic feet. J Am Podiatr Med Assoc 86:311–316, 1996.

27. Grayson ML, Balogh K, et al: Probing to bone in infected pedal ulcers: A clinical sign of underlying osteomyelitis in diabetic patients. J Am Podiatr Med Assoc 273:721–723, 1995.

28. Lavery LA, Armstrong DG, Quebedeaux TL, Walker SC: Puncture wounds: Normal laboratory values in the face of severe infection in diabetics and non-diabetics. Am J Med 101:521–525, 1996.

29. Armstrong DG, Lavery L, Harkless LB: Validation of a diabetic wound classification system. Diabetes Care 23:855–859, 1998.

30. Fernando DJS, Masson EA, Veves A, Boulton AJM: Relationship of limited joint mobility to abnormal foot pressure and diabetic foot ulceration. Diabetes Care 14:8–11, 1991.

31. Lavery LA, Armstrong DG, et al: Practical screening criteria for patients at high risk for diabetic foot ulceration. Arch Intern Med 158:157–162, 1998.

32. Shaw JE, Hsi WL, Ulbrecht JS, et al: The mechanism of plantar unloading in total contact casts: Implications for design and clinical use. Foot Ankle Int 18:809–817, 1997.

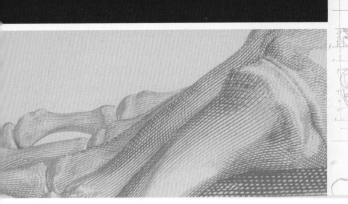

ROLE OF THE WOUND CARE NURSE

DOROTHY B. DOUGHTY ∎

Current data clearly demonstrate the importance of a comprehensive and multidisciplinary approach to management of the diabetic foot; such programs have documented ability to reduce the number of amputations and to reduce the cost of care.[1-5] Effective programs involve both culturally appropriate educational and outreach strategies and appropriate use of each professional's unique knowledge, skills, and frame of reference.[4,6,7] The wound care nurse has much to offer the diabetic foot care team, with particular skills in the areas of preventive foot care, wound management, patient education, and outreach. The specific roles and expertise of other health care professionals are addressed in separate chapters within this text; in this chapter, I will address the qualifications, skills, and role of the wound care nurse.

Qualifications of the Wound Care Nurse

The term *wound care nurse* is not an official title and can therefore be used by any nurse who considers herself or himself a wound specialist. The issue is further clouded by the fact that the title "nurse" is used to refer to professionals with significantly different educational backgrounds, including the licensed practical or licensed vocational nurse, who has graduated from a 12- to 18-month training program; the registered nurse, who may have graduated from a two-year associate degree program, a 3-year diploma program, or a 4-year baccalau-

reate program; and the advanced practice nurse (nurse-practitioner). All nursing education programs include some content related to wound care, but it is typically procedurally focused, limited in both depth and scope, and sometimes out of date. This means that the title "nurse" does not signify preparation for complex wound care, though it does signify basic knowledge regarding the various disease processes that predispose to skin and tissue breakdown as well as skill in clean versus sterile technique and in basic wound care procedures such as dressing changes and wound irrigations. All registered nurse programs also include significant content related to holistic health care, factors that affect patient and family compliance with established management plans, issues and strategies for effective patient and family education (including cultural and socioeconomic issues and strategies), and basic research principles.

While the title "nurse" is an umbrella term for practitioners with varied educational backgrounds and the title "wound care nurse" can be self-assumed, there are titles and certifications that do indicate knowledge and skill in the area of wound care. Formal education is available through postbaccalaureate certificate programs accredited by the Wound Ostomy Continence Nurses Society;[8] these programs provide intense didactic instruction as well as clinical preceptorship, and graduation signifies demonstration of acceptable knowledge and skill in the area of wound care. These programs are available in a variety of formats but typically involve at least 120 hours of full-time instruction in advanced wound care. The core curriculum for these programs is guided by accreditation requirements. All programs must demonstrate adequate scope and depth in the following areas:[8]

- Anatomy and physiology of the skin and soft tissues
- Etiologic factors for skin breakdown (with a focus on elimination or amelioration of these etiologic factors)
- Pathology of chronic wounds (to include lower-limb ulcerations and pressure ulcers)
- Critical assessment factors and techniques (to include primary vascular and sensorimotor assessment for the individual with a lower-limb ulceration)
- Systemic factors affecting wound repair, with a strong emphasis on nutritional requirements for repair and on tight glycemic control
- Principles governing outcomes-oriented topical therapy (and appropriate use of dressings and other topical agents)
- Indications for adjunctive therapies (e.g., growth factors, electrical stimulation, hyperbaric oxygen therapy, negative pressure wound therapy, and surgery)
- Current regulatory and reimbursement issues related to wound care

Many programs also include primary foot and nail care for the individual with a compromised lower limb (e.g., a patient with lower-limb arterial disease or diabetes mellitus).

Some of these accredited programs award graduate credits (the program is equivalent to a two- or three-semester-hour course); all award certificates signifying successful completion of the program. On graduation, these nurses have earned the title "wound care nurse"; they are then eligible for the national certification examination provided by the Wound Ostomy Continence Nursing Certification Board (WOCNCB).[9]

For the nurse who has not completed a formal certificate program, certification provides an alternative pathway for documentation and validation of his or her knowledge base. There are currently several nationally recognized certifications in wound care: The WOCNCB provides the CWCN (Certified Wound Care Nurse), CWON (Certified Wound Ostomy Nurse), and CWOCN (Certified Wound Ostomy Continence Nurse);[9] and the American Academy for Wound Management (AAWM) provides the CWS (Certified Wound Specialist).[10] The WOCNCB also offers a certification exam in basic foot and nail care, the Certified Foot Care Nurse (CFCN) examination; this examination does not focus on wound care but assesses knowledge of basic preventive foot and nail care.[9] Both the WOCNCB and the AAWM adhere to national standards for certifying bodies and have obtained recognition by national boards that certify valid certification programs; the WOCNCB is accredited by the National Commission for Certifying Agencies, and the AAWM is a full voting member of the National Association for Competency Assurance.[9,10]

Eligibility criteria for CWCN (or CWON or CWOCN) and CWS certification are outlined in Boxes 27-1 and 27-2. It must be emphasized that eligibility for certification simply denotes candidacy for the certification examination; certification itself requires a passing score on the examination. Certification obtained through the WOCNCB is valid for 5 years, and certification obtained through the AAWM is valid for 10 years; at that time, the certificant must recertify to maintain the credential. Recertification can be obtained by retesting or by documenting professional activities related to wound care that are indicative of current knowledge and practice.[9,10]

Anyone employing wound care nurses should be aware that CWCN (or CWON or CWOCN) and CWS are the only nationally recognized certifications in wound care for nurses and should carefully evaluate the credentials of applicants with other credentials or certifications. For example, some providers of continuing education in nursing provide posttests for their educational programs, and successful completion of the posttest leads to "certification"; however, these programs do not adhere to the criteria and guidelines required for a valid certification process.

In summary, a wound care nurse typically has at least a baccalaureate degree and has validated his or her

---

BOX 27-1   Eligibility Criteria for CWCN (CWON, CWOCN) Exam

- Current licensure as registered nurse
- Documentation of baccalaureate degree
- Documentation of *one* of the following:
  Successful completion of a postbaccalaureate course in wound care accredited by the WOCN Society
  Successful completion of a graduate program in nursing with documentation of at least 2 semester hours in wound care
  Completion of 50 contact hours and 1500 clinical hours in wound care over the previous 5 years

---

BOX 27-2   Eligibility Criteria for CWS Exam

- Nurses with a doctorate degree: Evidence of graduation from accredited university and documentation of 2 years postresidency clinical or research experience in wound care
- Nurses with a master's degree: Evidence of master's degree in nursing or related health care discipline and 2 years of documented clinical or research experience in wound care
- Nurses with a baccalaureate degree: Evidence of baccalaureate degree and 5 years of documented clinical or research experience in field of wound care
- Licensed nurses who do not have a baccalaureate degree: Five years of documented clinical or research experience in field of wound care
- All candidates must have three professional reference letters forwarded directly to AAWM that address wound care knowledge, skills, and expertise and must document the required years of experience

knowledge regarding wound care through satisfactory completion of an accredited certificate program and/or through satisfactory completion of the certification process. The prospective employer would therefore be well advised to look for the specific titles that bespeak completion of formal training and/or validation of knowledge and skills through a certification process; if the individual being considered has completed no formal training and is not certified in wound care, the employer should certainly look beyond the individual's self-assumed title and ask for explanations regarding preparation and education for the role of wound care nurse.

Services Provided by the Wound Care Nurse

The wound care nurse can contribute significantly to the prevention and management of diabetic foot wounds and to follow-up care designed to minimize the risk of recurrence; in some settings the wound care nurse has primary responsibility for screening assessment, preventive care, wound management, and initiation of referrals, while in other settings the role of the wound care nurse is defined by the needs of the multidisciplinary team in addition to the knowledge and skills of the nurse.

Whatever the setting, the wound care nurse is prepared to provide the following services in the areas of preventive care and education (Box 27-3) and holistic wound management (Box 27-4):[8]

Preventive Care and Education

The first goal of any comprehensive diabetic foot management program is ulcer prevention,[2,3,5,11] and the wound care nurse is in an excellent position to contribute to outreach, screening, and preventive care and education. Wound care nurses practice in a variety of health care settings and are frequently involved in health fairs, health education programs, and other outreach initiatives. Specific services provided by the wound care nurse include the following:

- Screening for indicators of ischemic disease: color and temperature of the limb and response to elevation and dependency; presence and quality of pulses; capillary refill and venous filling time; measurement of ankle-brachial and/or toe-brachial index; inspection of skin, hair, and nails for ischemic changes[2,12]
- Screening for indicators of sensorimotor neuropathy: response to monofilament testing, vibratory sense, position sense, range of motion, reflexes, gait, presence/absence of deformities, wear patterns in shoes, reports of neuropathic pain[2,13]
- Screening for indicators of autonomic neuropathy: hyperhidrosis or anhidrosis, Charcot deformity[2,13]
- Assessment of skin and nails: skin turgor and skin condition; hygiene status and hygiene routine; presence/absence of skin lesions, rashes, ulcers, corns, calluses; length, thickness, and color of nails; presence/absence of hypertrophic or excessively long nails, deformed nails, encurvated nails, "ingrown" nails, infected nails[8]
- Evaluation of factors affecting self-care: understanding of diabetes, management plan, and preventive foot care; current self-care behaviors to include adherence to dietary and medication guidelines, self-monitoring of blood glucose, and current foot care routines; visual acuity; manual dexterity; socioeconomic and cultural issues affecting adherence to management plan; appropriateness of current foot care routines (based on vascular and sensorimotor status)[8]
- Preventive foot and nail care, to include:[13]
  - Instruction in proper hygienic care (bathing guidelines, application of emollients to damp skin, importance of drying between toes, precautions to prevent injury for patient with sensory neuropathy)

BOX 27–3 Role of Wound Care Nurse in Preventive Care

- **Screening Assessment**
  Vascular assessment
  Sensorimotor assessment
  Autonomic function
  Status of skin and nails
  Self-care status
- **Preventive Foot and Nail Care**
  Instruction in hygienic care
  Clipping and debridement of nails
  Paring of corns and callouses
  Instruction/referrals for preventive foot care and proper footwear
  Referrals as indicated for complex foot conditions

BOX 27–4 Role of Wound Care Nurse in Holistic Wound Management

- Comprehensive assessment (vascular and sensorimotor status, etiologic factors, ulcer characteristics, pain associated with ulcer, systemic factors affecting healing, behavioral factors affecting healing, risk factors for further/recurrent injury)
- Measures to correct etiologic factors (e.g., referrals, assistance, and education regarding off-loading; referrals and education regarding measures to optimize perfusion, including smoking cessation)
- Systemic support measures (education regarding tight glycemic control, nutritional management, and edema control; recommendations regarding topical vitamin A for patient on high-dose steroids)
- Implementation/recommendations for principle-based topical therapy
- Serial evaluations of wound status/prompt identification and intervention for nonhealing wound
- Patient and family education

- ◆ Clipping of nails and debridement of hypertrophic nails with electric grinder
- ◆ Paring of corns and calluses and modification of footwear (referral to orthotist) to prevent recurrence
- ◆ Instruction in preventive foot care and proper footwear (individualized based on identified problems and on presence/absence of neuropathy and/or ischemia)
- ◆ Referrals as indicated for complex foot conditions
- Education regarding diabetes, impact of neuropathy and ischemia, measures to optimize glycemic control (individualized based on current knowledge level, patient and family concerns, social and cultural issues, and presence/absence of complications)[8]

Holistic Wound Care

Effective management of the patient with a foot ulcer requires thorough assessment of the ulcer and of the patient and a three-pronged approach to ulcer management: identification and correction of the specific etiologic factors; attention to systemic factors affecting wound healing; and principle-based topical therapy, with particular attention to early aggressive debridement, elimination of infection and control of bacterial burden and maintenance of a clean, moist, protected wound surface.[1–3,14,15] The wound care nurse is prepared to conduct or contribute to the initial assessment, to initiate or recommend appropriate management, and to request referrals as indicated for additional evaluation or for medical-surgical management. Specific interventions provided by the wound care nurse include the following:

- Assessment to include vascular and sensorimotor evaluation as outlined in section on prevention; determination of etiologic factors (e.g., painless trauma, abnormal weight-bearing, ischemia, prolonged pressure); ulcer characteristics (i.e., dimensions, depth, undermined or tunneled areas, status of wound bed/inflammatory versus proliferative stage in wound healing process, status of surrounding tissue, status of wound edges, volume and character of exudate, indicators of infection, including observation or palpation of bone in wound bed); pain associated with ulcer (baseline pain and procedural pain, severity, exacerbating and relieving factors); systemic factors affecting the healing process (e.g., perfusion, nutritional status, glucose control, current intake of steroids at doses of more than 30 mg/day); behavioral factors affecting the healing process (e.g., patient and family understanding of etiologic factors for ulcer; potential seriousness of ulcer; potential for adverse outcomes/amputation; principles and specifics of the management plan; patient and family/caregiver concerns, issues, and goals; ability to access and afford needed care; willingness and ability to comply with treatment plan); risk factors for further/recurrent injury[8,14,16,17]

- Measures to correct etiologic factors (i.e., instruction in principles and strategies for off-loading, with referrals as indicated for orthotics, contact casting or removable cast walker application, or alternative off-loading strategies; patient education on strategies to prevent painless trauma; referrals as indicated for vascular assessment/revascularization; patient instruction regarding measures to maximize perfusion, to include in-depth education and counseling regarding smoking cessation)[1,2,12,13,18]
- Systemic support measures (i.e., education regarding the importance of tight glucose control and instruction in specific strategies to promote normoglycemia; instruction regarding impact of nutritional status on wound healing and specific recommendations to ensure adequate intake of protein, calories, vitamins, and minerals; nutritionist referral as indicated; instruction in leg elevation or application of compressive wrap/stocking as indicated to control edema; recommendations for topical vitamin A for patient receiving high-dose steroids)[1,9,18,19]
- Implementation/recommendations for principle-based topical therapy (i.e., selection of appropriate wound-cleansing techniques and dressings/topical agents based on assessment of wound status and principles of moist wound healing; conservative sharp wound debridement or enzymatic debridement when indicated and ordered by the physician; $AgNO_3$ cauterization of hypertrophic granulation tissue or closed nonproliferative wound edges when indicated and ordered by the physician). The focus of topical therapy changes based on the stage of wound healing; during the inflammatory phase, the emphasis is on complete elimination of necrotic tissue, eradication of infection, and management of exudate, and during the proliferative phase, the emphasis shifts to maintenance of a moist and protected wound surface.[1,4,8,19–21] See Table 27-1 for principles of topical therapy and specific considerations for diabetic patients.
- Serial (weekly) evaluations of wound status to ensure continued progress in wound healing and to promptly identify any wound that is not progressing; consultation with other team members to determine reasons for failure to heal and to modify treatment accordingly; recommendations regarding active wound therapies for any wound that is refractory to standard management with no identifiable cause for failure to progress. (Active wound therapies are interventions and treatments that are designed to actively stimulate wound healing, such as topical application of growth factors, use of electrical stimulation, or hyperbaric oxygen therapy. See Table 27-2).[1,8,22,23]
- Patient and family education regarding principles and procedures for wound care, expected outcomes, indications of adverse outcomes and appropriate response (prompt reporting), and follow-up care to prevent recurrence[8]

TABLE 27-1   Principles of Topical Therapy and Considerations for Diabetic Patients

Principle	Considerations
• Debride all avascular tissue when the goal is wound healing or the wound is infected.	Debridement is contraindicated in dry, uninfected, ischemic wounds; should paint these wounds with povidone-iodine to keep them dry and must monitor closely for infection. When the wound is adequately perfused and the goal is repair, data support aggressive early debridement to establish a clean wound bed. (Surgical debridement is the best option for most patients.)
• Identify and treat infection promptly; control bioburden to prevent critical colonization (bacterial burden sufficient to interfere with healing but not sufficient to cause invasive infection). Critical colonization evidenced by sudden deterioration in quantity or quality of granulation tissue, increasing volumes of exudate, increasing pain, or failure to granulate/epithelialize with no apparent reason.	If osteomyelitis is suspected (visible or palpable bone or nonhealing tract), consult an orthopedist and/or infectious disease specialist for workup and management. For cellulitis (erythema and induration of surrounding tissue), provide systemic antibiotic therapy (ideally culture-based). Critical colonization: topical treatment with sustained-release iodine or silver frequently adequate to prevent or treat critical colonization.
• Lightly pack ("wick") any tracts or tunnels to eliminate all exudate and to prevent premature closure of narrow tracts.	Avoid overpacking tunnels or tracts, as this creates wound bed ischemia and creates a mechanical barrier to wound closure.
• Manage exudate effectively: The goal is to wick exudate away from wound surface and prevent "pooled" exudate while keeping wound surface moist. (Chronic wound fluid contains high levels of inflammatory mediators and is an impediment to wound repair, but a dry wound surface is also an impediment owing to impaired cell migration and increased risk of cell death.)	—Alginates, hydrofiber dressings, and foam dressings are effective absorbers and are appropriate for exudative wounds. —Gels and nonadherent dressings donate or trap moisture and are appropriate for dry wounds. Occlusive dressings such as hydrocolloids should be used with caution when the wound is infected (owing to potential for increased anaerobic activity).
• Maintain open proliferative wound edges. —Pare any callous surrounding wound. —Excise or cauterize any wound edges that are rolled and closed.	Epithelialization occurs only in the presence of an open advancing epithelial border.
• Protect the healing wound from trauma and bacterial invasion.	Consider the need for a cover dressing with a bacterial barrier. (Note that gauze provides no bacterial barrier and frequently causes trauma with removal and so is now considered a suboptimal dressing choice.)

TABLE 27-2   Advanced Wound Therapies

Therapy	Description and Indications
• Topical growth factors (e.g., Regranex)	Platelet-derived growth factors produced by recombinant DNA technology; supplied in gel form; indicated only for nonhealing but viable ulcer in which infection has been controlled, glucose levels are controlled, and patient is compliant with off-loading Applied daily and covered with appropriate dressing Requires prescription and is expensive
• Electrical stimulation	Use of high-voltage pulsed current to stimulate repair; multiple studies report positive outcomes in a variety of chronic wounds Typically administered by physical therapists
• Hyperbaric oxygen therapy	Administration of inhaled oxygen in a pressurized chamber; provides marked increase in amount of oxygen dissolved in the plasma (improves oxygenation in poorly perfused tissues) Indicated for wounds that are perfused but ischemic; not indicated for gangrenous wounds Also indicated for treatment of chronic refractory osteomyelitis
• Negative-pressure wound therapy	Wound bed lightly filled with porous foam or damp gauze; wound sealed on all sides with transparent adhesive drape; suction device applied and connected to negative suction Application of negative pressure effectively controls wound drainage and causes cell deformation that activates intracellular processes critical to healing Clinical outcomes: enhanced granulation and wound closure; reduced exudate Contraindicated in wound with poorly controlled bleeding and in necrotic wound

In addition to providing clinical services, the wound care nurse is prepared to educate other caregivers regarding etiologic or risk factors for breakdown, preventive strategies, and the principles and procedures involved in comprehensive wound management. Education is provided through in-service programs; one-on-one interactions; and updated policies, procedures, protocols, and algorithms for care. To promote optimal care, the wound care nurse must remain abreast of current research findings and product development in the area of wound care. In addition to serving as a research consumer and disseminator, the wound care nurse is prepared to contribute to the body of research by participating in clinical research studies.

The wound care nurse is also prepared to coordinate the various services needed to optimize wound healing and prevent recurrence and is able to interface with third-party payors to obtain appropriate reimbursement.

Role of the Wound Care Nurse

As was noted above, the specific role of the wound care nurse varies according to the setting as well as the availability and involvement of other health care professionals. In the acute care setting, the wound care nurse frequently has primary responsibility for topical therapy and shared responsibility for correction of etiologic factors and provision of systemic support for wound healing. In the home health setting, the wound care nurse may function either as the primary nurse or as a consultant to the primary nurse; in either case, the wound care nurse is responsible for providing or directing comprehensive assessment and holistic management, to include correction of etiologic factors, systemic support measures, appropriate topical therapy, and initiation of indicated referrals. In the outpatient setting, the wound care nurse typically functions as a member of a multidisciplinary team, with specific functions determined by the team member mix and needs. Alternatively, the wound care nurse may function as the primary caregiver/coordinator in a nurse-managed clinic with medical oversight; in this case, the role of the wound care nurse is to provide primary care and to initiate and coordinate appropriate referrals.

In many settings, the wound care nurse is assuming the role of the case manager. The wound care nurse is well equipped to assume this role, since he or she has a broad understanding of the care issues involved in both prevention and management of foot ulcers, is skilled in patient/family education and counseling, is familiar with the services provided by other team members, and is usually able to follow the patient through the various care settings (assuming compatibility with employment contract and demands). In addition, nurses have traditionally been responsible for coordinating the various services needed by patients and are therefore skilled in this role.

Benefits Provided by the Wound Care Nurse

The ability to improve outcomes and reduce costs is of critical importance in today's managed care environment. The wound care nurse is prepared to contribute significantly to each of these goals and to assist with the development of care maps or critical pathways that standardize this outcomes-oriented approach to care. Specific ways in which wound care nurses affect outcomes and costs include the following:

1. Immediate establishment of a comprehensive management plan based on thorough assessment of the patient's care needs. Prompt establishment of a comprehensive management plan minimizes the time to healing (or reduces the risk of ulceration) and thus minimizes the associated costs.
2. Ongoing monitoring of progress in healing (or in maintenance of intact skin status) and prompt intervention whenever there is a lack of progress or a regression in wound status or an increased risk of ulceration. This approach again minimizes the time to healing (or the risk of acute ulceration), which reduces the cost of care in addition to improving outcomes.
3. Appropriate referrals for further evaluation or adjunctive therapies. The wound care nurse can identify patients who require additional services and/or evaluation, which serves to maximize outcomes while ensuring appropriate resource utilization.
4. Cost-effective use of supplies. The wound care nurse is extremely knowledgeable with regard to the many products available for wound management; this permits the nurse to select products for topical therapy that are therapeutically appropriate yet cost-effective, taking into consideration the cost of the dressing, the frequency of dressing change, additional supplies required, and potential impact on time to healing.
5. Improved patient compliance resulting from a team approach in which the patient and family are recognized as team members who are integral to success of the management plan, and a strong emphasis on patient education and counseling. Wound care nurses are prepared to address psychosocial issues that interfere with patient compliance, and to initiate patient-provider contracts when indicated to promote compliance.
6. Communication with third-party payers to explain the rationale for recommended therapies from both outcomes and cost perspectives, thus promoting reimbursement for appropriate care.

Studies in the home care setting have supported the value of the wound care nurse in management of chronic wounds. Patients who were managed by wound care nurses had a significantly greater healing rate and a significantly lower cost of care, despite use of "more expensive" products.[24,25]

Summary

Management of the diabetic foot is a complex challenge that is most effectively handled by a multidisciplinary team. The wound care nurse is a critical component of this team. He or she is prepared to assist with preventive care as well as with effective management of the ulcerated foot. Specific services provided by the wound care nurse include screening assessments and individualized preventive education and counseling, comprehensive wound assessment and establishment of a holistic management plan; patient and caregiver education; dissemination of current research; coordination of needed services; and communication with third-party payers to optimize reimbursement. The importance of these services is underscored by studies documenting significantly higher healing rates and reduced care costs when a wound care nurse is involved in the care of patients with chronic wounds.

References

1. Cavanagh R, Lipsky B, Bradbury A, Botek G: Treatment for diabetic foot ulcers. Lancet 366:1725–1733, 2005.
2. Frykberg R: A summary of guidelines for managing the diabetic foot. Adv Skin Wound Care 18(4):209–214, 2005.
3. Giurini JM, Lyons TE: Diabetic foot complications: Diagnosis and management. Int J Lower Extremity Wounds 4(3):171–182, 2005.
4. Gottrup F: Management of the diabetic foot: Surgical and organizational aspects. Horm Metab Res 37:69–75, 2005.
5. Rauner M, Heidenberger K, Pesendorfer E: Model-based evaluation of diabetic foot prevention strategies in Austria. Health Care Manage Sci 8(4):253–265, 2005.
6. Reiber G, Raugi G: Preventing foot ulcers and amputations in diabetes. Lancet 366:1676–1677, 2005.
7. Watson J, Obersteller E, Rennie L, Whitbread C: Diabetic foot care: Developing culturally appropriate educational tools for aboriginal and Torres Strait Islander peoples in the Northern Territory, Australia. Aust J Rural Health 9:121–126, 2001.
8. Wound Ostomy Continence Nurses Society: Accreditation Policy and Procedure Manual and Curriculum Blueprint. Mt. Laurel, NJ: WOCN, 2005.
9. Wound Ostomy Continence Nursing Certification Board: www.wocncb.org. Accessed March 8, 2006.
10. American Academy of Wound Management: www.aawm.org. Accessed March 8, 2006.
11. Wieman TJ. Principles of management: The diabetic foot. Am J Surg 190(2):195–199, 2005.
12. Sieggreen M, Kline R: Vascular ulcers. In Baranoski S, Ayello E (eds): Wound Care Essentials: Practice Principles. Philadelphia: Lippincott, Williams, and Wilkins, 2004, pp 271–310.
13. Lavery L, Baranoski S, Ayello E: Diabetic foot ulcers. In Baranoski S, Ayello E (eds): Wound Care Essentials: Practice Principles. Philadelphia: Lippincott, Williams, and Wilkins, 2004, pp 311–332.
14. Grey J, Enoch S, Harding K: Wound assessment. BMJ 332(7536): 285–288, 2006.
15. Rolstad B, Ovington L, Harris A: Principles of wound management. In Bryant R (ed): Acute and Chronic Wounds: Nursing Management (2nd ed). St. Louis: Mosby, 2000, pp 85–124.
16. Baranoski S, Ayello E: Wound assessment. In Baranoski S, Ayello E (eds): Wound Care Essentials: Practice Principles. Philadelphia: Lippincott, Williams, and Wilkins, 2004, pp 79–90.
17. Anstead G: Steroids, retionoids, and wound healing. Adv Wound Care 11:277–285, 1998.
18. Edmonds M, Foster AVM: Diabetic foot ulcers. BMJ 332(7538): 407–410, 2006.
19. Waldrop J, Doughty D: Wound healing physiology. In Bryant R (ed): Acute and Chronic Wounds: Nursing Management (2nd ed). St. Louis: Mosby, 2000, pp 17–40.
20. Baranoski S, Ayello E: Wound treatment options. In Baranoski S and Ayello E, eds: Wound Care Essentials: Practice Principles. Philadelphia: Lippincott, Williams, and Wilkins, 2004, pp 127–156.
21. Ovington L: Wound care products: How to choose. Home Healthcare Nurse 9(4):224–231, 2001.
22. Broussard C, Mendez-Eastman S, Frantz R: Adjuvant wound therapies. In Bryant R (ed): Acute and Chronic Wounds: Nursing Management (2nd ed). St. Louis: Mosby, 2000, pp 431–454.
23. Cooper D: Assessment, measurement, and evaluation: Their pivotal roles in wound healing. In Bryant R (ed). Acute and Chronic Wounds: Nursing Management (2nd ed). St. Louis: Mosby, 2000, pp 51–84.
24. Arnold N, Weir R: Retrospective analysis of healing in wounds cared for by ET nurses versus staff nurses in a home setting. J Wound Ostomy Continence Nurs 21:156–160, 1994.
25. Robinson SM: Advancing home care nursing practice with an ET clinical nurse specialist. Home Healthcare Nurse 14:269–274, 1996.

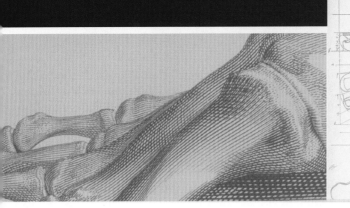

PEDORTHIC CARE OF THE DIABETIC FOOT: CORRELATION WITH RISK CATEGORY

DENNIS J. JANISSE AND WILLIAM COLEMAN ∎

The human foot evolved over millennia as our fore-bears walked barefoot on the ground. As a result, the multiple bones and articulations of the human foot enable it to adapt to many different walking surfaces. Slight variances in foot structure and function are rarely a problem when the foot meets the uneven and sloping features of unmodified natural surfaces because, with every step, a different part of the plantar surface meets the ground at varying angles. The majority of foot problems that are encountered in industrialized countries are the direct consequence of walking on hard concrete and blacktop surfaces combined with poor footwear choices. Since the foot contacts these uniform surfaces in exactly the same orientation with every step, small differences in skeletal alignment, general foot angulation, and available joint motion can have devastating consequences as the foot repeatedly strikes these unyielding surfaces thousands of times daily. Add peripheral neuropathy and the finding by Veves and colleagues that 39% of all patients with diabetic neuropathy have higher than normal pressures under their feet, and the frequent results are foot ulceration and Charcot fractures rather than the foot pain and stress fractures that are seen in nondiabetic individuals with normal sensation.[1]

Burden of the Problem

As sensation is lost, the wearing of dress shoes becomes a risk for both men and women. Many dress shoes are too tight, particularly around the toes. This is a far more common problem with women than with men because women wear dress shoes much more frequently than men do and for many different types of occasions. Frey has reported that 88% of women in the United States wear shoes that are an average of 1.2 cm narrower than their feet.[2] Several studies have reported on the increase of pressure under the metatarsal heads when high-heeled shoes are worn. Snow correlated the pressure increase to heel height.[3] A 1.9-cm heel resulted in a 22% higher pressure, a 5-cm heel led to a 57% higher pressure, and an 8.3-cm heel increased the pressure by 76%. Also, when a high-heeled shoe is worn, the pressure under the forefoot shifts from the central metatarsal heads to the first metatarsal head.[4]

Plantar-flexed metatarsals, hallux limitus, clawed toes, equinus deformity, forefoot varus, and ligament glycosylation are all conditions that produce limited joint mobility in the foot and ankle. Glycosylation refers to changes in the structure of collagen associated with chronic hyperglycemia, which make it less elastic. These problems are rarely detected by the general medical community despite being major contributing factors in the pathway toward amputation of the neuropathic limb. Owing to glycosylation of joint ligaments and capsules, the range of motion of the major joints of the foot can become reduced.[5] This has been established as a contributing factor to higher pressures under the feet of people with diabetes. The early recognition of these problems and the ability to adapt footwear for them are key elements in reducing the incidence of over 90,000 diabetic lower-limb amputations annually. Clawed toes are a common finding in neuropathic patients because as denervation progresses, the toes contract as the result of paralysis of the intrinsic foot muscles.[6] Studies have shown that after the toes claw, pressure under the metatarsal heads increases, while pressures are reduced under the toes.[7,8]

In most cases, foot care for diabetic patients begins with treatment of their first injury. In an ideal situation, however, the possibility of the first foot injury should have been anticipated. The most successful diabetic foot programs worldwide always include an aggressive program of injury prevention. To this end, all medical practitioners treating people with diabetes need to inspect their patients' feet regularly. All diabetic patients need education on injury prevention, footwear selection, and foot self-inspection. As soon as vascular or neuropathic changes due to diabetes are noted in the feet, people who sell, modify, or construct medically indicated shoes need to be included as contributing consultants.

In a study of patient compliance reported from Germany in 1993, 51 previously ulcerated patients who were compliant with regular foot clinic visits and consistently used their prescribed footwear were free of recurrent ulcers after 20 months. Thirty-eight percent of the patients who were not compliant with visits or footwear reulcerated. After 40 months, 54% of the compliant patients had reulcerated, whereas 100% of the noncompliant patients had developed another open wound. The authors attributed most of the new foot ulcers of the compliant patients to failure of the footwear materials to maintain the original levels of protection, concluding that footwear needs to be renewed every 2 years.[9]

Role of the Certified Pedorthist

With the exclusive and proper use of appropriate footwear and instruction related to foot care, most diabetic patients can expect to avoid a skin wound on their feet. Convincing the diabetic patient to consistently wear appropriate footwear, however, particularly when that person has never had a foot injury, continues to be a difficult problem. Few medical practitioners have sufficient training in the applications and prescription of protective footwear; most shoe modifications are recommended as the result of trial-and-error experience and training based on the empiric findings of shoemakers of previous generations. Fortunately, there are now objective, experimentally derived data to support pedorthic shoe therapy.[10]

Diabetic patients with peripheral neuropathy need an expert shoe professional to assist them with shoe selection and fitting and should always inform shoe fitters of their disease. A person with insensitive feet can no longer trust the "feel" of a shoe to determine proper fit. To obtain the same "feel" on feet that have lost sensation,

the diabetic often selects a smaller-sized shoe. The National Shoe Retailers Association estimates that, unfortunately, only 5% of all people who sell shoes have any significant training or experience in fitting footwear.[11]

In the United States, the role of footwear consultant is frequently filled by the certified pedorthist. Pedorthics encompasses the design, manufacture, fit, and modification of shoes and foot orthoses to alleviate problems caused by disease, overuse, or injury.[12] Pedorthists fit and dispense footwear according to a physician's prescription. A board-certified pedorthist is trained in foot anatomy as well as the construction of shoes and foot orthoses. To achieve certification, a candidate's qualifications have been tested and accepted by the American Board for Certification in Orthotics, Prosthetics, and Pedorthics (ABC). To maintain certification, certified pedorthists are required to participate in a continuing education program under ABC auspices.[12] The certified pedorthist designation is intended to provide the prescribing physician and consumer with the assurance of competence in dispensing prescription footwear. Both the ABC and the Pedorthic Footwear Association work to establish and maintain standards and provide educational opportunities for individuals involved in the practice of pedorthics.

Footwear for Injury Prevention

Shoes have their greatest utility as a means of injury prevention. They are not typically regarded as a reliable part of wound or fracture management, and if they are used for this purpose in lieu of off-loading techniques, the time needed to heal will usually be prolonged.[13] Even if a shoe is perfectly fitted to the foot and relieves stress on an open ulcer, the patient will remove the shoe at home. Many people with diabetes need to urinate in the middle of the night, but when they walk to and from the bathroom, they seldom wear their protective shoes. One unguarded step on an insensitive foot with an ulceration, fracture, or infection can be devastating to that foot.[13] In short, a person with an insensitive foot should never walk on an open foot wound or fracture. If the patient with a neuropathic ulcer or fracture must walk, then casts or splints are a more effective means of protection than shoes.[14]

Frequently, diabetic patients cannot afford medically indicated footwear. Many third-party reimbursement systems do not cover shoes intended for the prevention of injury to the feet of a diabetic. As of May 1993, people at risk from complications related to diabetes and covered by the U.S. Medicare program are entitled to reimbursement for up to 80% of the allowable amount for a pair of therapeutic shoes and up to three pairs of foot orthoses per year. This is known as the Therapeutic Shoes for Persons with Diabetes program. To obtain the shoes and foot orthoses, the patient must be referred to a Medicare-participating provider. A study conducted to evaluate the cost of this provision found that this benefit increased the possibility that a person with diabetes would obtain and use prescribed footwear.[15]

As the risk of ulceration rises, so does the need for more frequent foot examination. With deformity or previous ulceration, these vulnerable areas need further footwear modifications to limit stress. Also, as the risk increases, the patient needs ever-increasing levels of education to encourage the exclusive wear of protective footwear and the prompt identification of possible sites of injury. In a survey of patients with diabetes at Kings College Hospital, London, the recurrence rate of ulceration was 26% among those using prescribed footwear and 83% among those who returned to using their previous footwear.[16]

Assisting people with diabetes in preventing ulcerations can be very frustrating. Diabetic patients with sensory neuropathy may develop psychological problems such as denial that interfere with successful injury prevention or management.[17] Despite careful patient education and examination, a single careless action on the part of a neuropathic person often results in foot injury. Over a 4-year period, King's College Diabetic Foot Clinic staff reported 86 preventable foot injuries among people with diabetes who had received education on foot care.[18] These injuries resulted from wearing inappropriate footwear, picking at skin, or walking barefoot.

Education is essential at every visit for evaluation of the feet, but the educator must be careful not to overwhelm the patient with information. Each patient should be educated in accordance to his or her risk of developing a foot problem and level of understanding. As the risk increases, foot care education should become more extensive. To ensure that every patient obtains complete instructions, this form of education can be provided on videotape. The patient should view the tape, then have any questions answered by clinic personnel. If a specific behavior is required, it should be rehearsed by the patient under supervision of the clinic staff.

Footwear Basics for the Medical Professional

Unless the medical team has a footwear professional present during every examination of the feet of a person with diabetes, the team members should educate themselves on some basic principles of footwear. For example, they should be capable of making a preliminary determination as to the appropriateness of the fit and function of footwear that the patient wears to the clinic. To begin, the number and letter assigned by the manufacturer as the size for a particular shoe can be used only as a general guideline for fitting a particular foot.[19] This is because shoes that are of the same numbered/lettered size vary greatly in length and width owing to differences in shoe lasts, the wooden or plastic forms over which shoes are constructed. Therefore, shoes for an insensitive patient should never be purchased just by asking for a specific length and width.

Ideally, when neuropathy is present, footwear should be selected by an educated and experienced fitter in a facility that has an inventory of footwear of many different shapes, styles, lengths, and widths. Correct shoe fit is best determined by a professional, such as a certified pedorthist, who has the knowledge to objectively determine whether the shoe fits without any input from the patient because when neuropathy is present, the previous experience of the patient is unreliable owing to the absence of protective sensation. Prescription footwear is made over a variety of last shapes; examples include the combination last, which has a narrower heel than the standard last; the inflare last, which provides more medial forefoot surface area; and the in-depth last, which is shaped to allow extra volume for the foot inside the shoe and provides enough room for a generic insert (insole) or a custom orthosis.

Specific parts of the shoe upper also affect shoe fit. Terms that are useful in describing the upper are (1) *counter*, the part of the shoe extending around the heel; (2) *toebox*, the part that covers the toe area; (3) *vamp*, the part that covers the instep; and (4) *throat*, the part at the bottom of the laces. These, along with other important parts of a shoe, are illustrated in Figure 28-1. The counter controls the heel and determines heel fit. Strong counters are necessary to adequately control the foot inside the shoe.[20,21] A shoe that has a high and rounded or oblique toebox provides the best fit by allowing the toes to fit and move comfortably inside the shoe. A shoe with a tapered toebox or a pointed toe is inappropriate for the diabetic foot, because it applies pressure to the toes and forces them into an unnatural posture, leading to calluses, ulcers, and eventual deformity.[16,20] As with the toebox, the vamp should be high enough to prevent pressure on the instep. A shoe with either lacing or a hook-and-loop closure is best for the diabetic foot because these systems provide the adjustability that is needed to accommodate for edema or deformities while preventing the shoe from slipping off. Of the two types of throat openings, the Blucher is preferred over the Balmoral because the Blucher allows for greater adjustability and easier entry and is more compliant to foot shape[19,21,22] (Fig. 28-2).

Once a properly shaped shoe has been found, the next step is to determine the appropriate size. There are three essential measurements in determining shoe size: overall foot length (heel to toe), arch length (heel to ball), and width. The correct size is the one that accommodates the first metatarsophalangeal joint (i.e., the widest part of the foot) in the widest part of the shoe; it is for this reason that shoes must be fit by arch length rather than by overall foot length.[19,21,22] Feet can have the same overall foot length but require different size shoes because of the difference in arch length (Fig. 28-3).

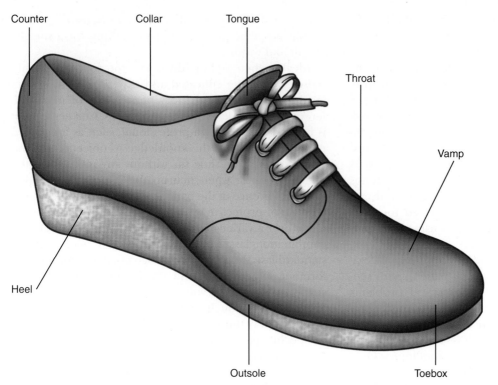

Figure 28–1 Parts of a shoe.

Counter

Collar

Tongue

Throat

Vamp

Heel

Outsole

Toebox

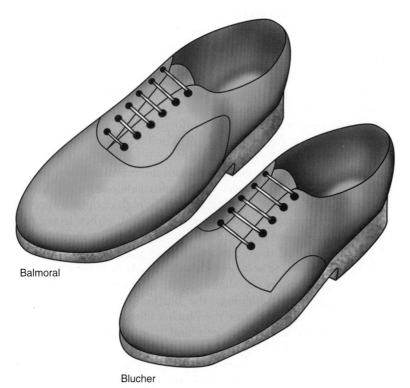

Figure 28–2 The two types of throat openings. **Left,** Balmoral. **Right,** Blucher. (Redrawn from Rossi WA, Tennant R: Professional Shoe Fitting. New York: National Shoe Retailers Association, 1984, with permission.)

Balmoral

Blucher

Guidelines for Proper Shoe Fit

The following is a set of guidelines that can be used to achieve correct shoe fit:[11,19,21,22]

1. Measure both feet with an appropriate measuring device. The Brannock measuring device is the most complete tool, although there are other devices, such as the Ritz stick. Each foot should be measured when both weight-bearing and non-weight-bearing. The three main measurements are heel to toe, heel to ball, and width. Pedorthic Footwear Association members measured the feet of 6800 adults in 1983. They found that 70% of all the people surveyed had one foot longer than the other. In 25% of the subjects, the difference was a whole size or greater.[11]

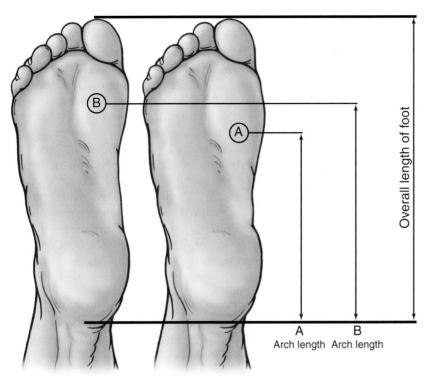

Figure 28–3 Overall foot length versus arch length. These feet have the same overall foot length, but the foot on the left would require a larger size shoe because it has a longer arch length. (Redrawn from Rossi WA, Tennant R: Professional Shoe Fitting. New York: National Shoe Retailers Association, 1984, with permission.)

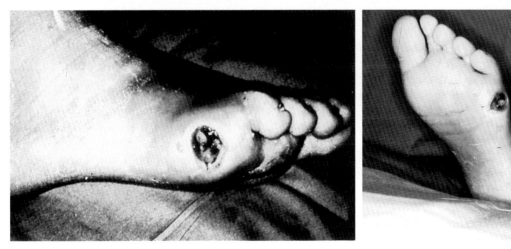

Figure 28–4 The ulcerations were on the feet of patients whose shoes were too tight.

2. Remember that shoe sizes are not standard; they vary from manufacturer to manufacturer and often even among styles produced by the same manufacturer. This is why it is essential to have shoes fit by a certified pedorthist or other trained shoe-fitting professional. A good shoe fitter will have an intimate knowledge of how each shoe fits and how each style's sizing scale corresponds to that of the Brannock device.

3. Pay close attention to shape. The outline of the shoe sole should be roughly the same shape as an outline made of the foot. Pay particular attention to fit around the fifth (little) toe. Too much pressure on the side of this toe leads to many corns over or between the toe and is a frequent cause of ulceration.

4. Check for the proper position of the first metatarsophalangeal joint. It should sit comfortably in the pocket of the widest part of the shoe.

5. Check for the correct toe length. Allow 3/8 to 1/2 inch between the end of the shoe and the longest toe; generally speaking, the allowance should be the width of the patient's thumb.

6. Check for the proper width, allowing adequate room across the ball of the foot. When a shoe is too tight, ulcers usually develop medial to the first metatarsal head and lateral to the fifth metatarsal head (Fig. 28-4). The ulceration is due to pressure ischemia, as a result of tension within the leather that applies the greatest stress in areas of smallest circumference.[23]

Skin breakdown is also related to the length of time an ill-fitting shoe is worn. For damage to occur, pressure from a shoe that is too tight must be maintained for hours with no relief. A diabetic patient should be taught to change shoes at midday and perhaps again in the evening. By doing this, pressures are not allowed to remain in one place on the foot for an excessive period of time.

7. Look for a snug fit around the heel of the foot, particularly where the top of the upper meets the heel. When the heel sits well forward away from the back of the shoe, it does not mean that the shoe is too long for the person's foot. It just means that the foot is sliding forward in the shoe. The vamp, the part of the shoe over the instep, needs to hold the heel back against the counter of the shoe. In pump-style shoes and many loafer styles, the heel of the shoe is held in place by jamming the toes and metatarsal heads into the toe of the shoe. After buying many pump-style shoes over the years, most women choose shoes that are too short for their feet. Pumps do not have a vamp covering the instep to hold the heel back in the shoe. As a result, the patient is left with the impression that slipping of a standard depth shoe at the back is attributable to excessive shoe length. Proper fit over the instep can be achieved by an appropriately high vamp, preferably with laces to allow adjustability.

8. Fit shoes on both feet while the patient is weight-bearing. If the feet measure differently, the larger foot should be accurately fit. In the majority of cases, insert adjustments can be made to get the other shoe to fit the smaller foot.[24]

Treatment Recommendations

Depth Shoes

The majority of diabetic footwear prescriptions begin with the depth shoe. It is generally a Blucher-style oxford or athletic shoe with an additional 1/4 to 1/2 inch of depth throughout the shoe (Fig. 28-5). This provides the extra volume needed to accommodate severe deformities or edema. It also provides room to accommodate any foot orthosis or brace that may be used. The additional depth is also useful in accommodating deformities associated with the diabetic foot, such as hammertoes and clawed toes, as well as moderate medial, plantar, or lateral bony prominences resulting from Charcot deformities.[7,25]

Other features common to depth shoes that are especially useful in the care of the diabetic foot include their lightweight, shock-absorbing soles and strong counters (heel reinforcement). Depth shoes are made with a variety of upper materials, including deerskin, which, though a softer leather than cowhide, can quickly stretch out of shape, resulting in a much looser fit. Cowhide, which is frequently stiffer on initial fit, is more durable and will maintain a fit for a much longer period of time. Some depth shoes have a heat-moldable lining material that allows the upper to be molded to the individual foot; this is especially useful for severe deformities. Shoe uppers can also be constructed of a stretchable, elasticized fabric. A new type of depth shoe is shaped wider in the midfoot area to accommodate a Charcot deformity. Depth shoes come in a wide range of shapes and sizes to accommodate almost any foot except those with severe skeletal distortion. As more manufacturers become involved in the production of depth shoes, the shoes' appearance has steadily improved.

Postoperative Shoe

This shoe is generally open-toed, with uppers made of canvas or nylon mesh; the upper may be padded for additional comfort (Fig. 28-6). It has a wide forefoot opening with either hook-and-loop straps or lace closures and can accommodate extreme swelling and the bulkiest dressings. The postoperative shoe is most often manufactured with a more rigid sole made of a very firm crepe or lightweight polyurethane. This is particularly helpful for allowing ambulation while limiting the range of motion.

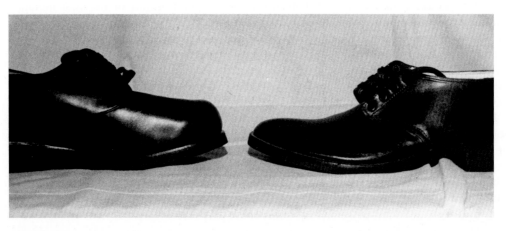

Figure 28–5 **Right,** A conventional oxford shoe. **Left,** A shoe with extra vertical depth.

Controlled Ankle Motion Device

For the patient who can be mobile but must maintain a fixed ankle position or limit ankle motion, the controlled ankle motion device can provide the necessary stability and support while allowing a comfortable, relatively natural gait pattern. This appliance is essentially a postoperative shoe to which medial-lateral uprights and a posterior Achilles plate have been added (Fig. 28-7). The foot and ankle are held in place with wide hook-and-loop straps, and the ankle joint may be held in a fixed position or be allowed to move within a limited range. A cushioned liner provides pressure relief, and a rocker sole allows a more natural walking gait. A total-contact orthosis inside a controlled ankle motion device can be used for wound healing as an alternative to total-contact casting, allowing the patient easier access to view, dress, and bathe the wound.[24]

External Modifications of Depth Shoes

The exterior of the shoe can be modified in a variety of ways.[26] Some of these are described in the following subsections.

Rocker Sole

The rocker sole is one of the most commonly prescribed shoe modifications. As its name suggests, its basic function is to literally rock the foot from midstance to toe off without bending the shoe or foot (Figs. 28-8 and 28-9). However, the actual shape of a rocker sole varies according to the patient's specific foot problems and the desired effect of the rocker sole. In general, the biomechanical effects of a rocker sole are (1) compensation for limited ankle joint dorsiflexion by transferring the motion to the bottom of the shoe sole[26,27] and (2) relief of pressure under a metatarsal head or toe.[10,26,28] As the patient transfers his or her weight to the forefoot, there is less pressure because rather than pressing the forefoot against a solid walking surface, the shoe sole rolls away from the foot. Two terms are relevant to a discussion of rocker soles: the *midstance*, or the portion of the rocker sole that is in contact with the floor when in a standing position, and the *apex*, or the most forward part of the rocker sole in the standing position. It is important to note that the apex must be placed behind any area for which pressure relief is desired. For example, a rocker sole that is designed to relieve pressure on the metatarsal heads must be made with the apex behind the metatarsal heads. In general, rocker soles are custom-made for each

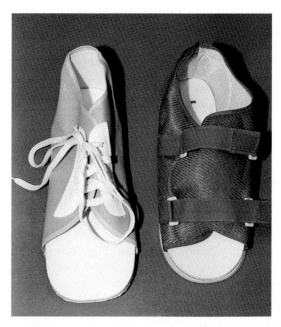

Figure 28-6   Postoperative shoes. **Left,** Canvas upper with lace closure. **Right,** Nylon mesh upper with Velcro closure.

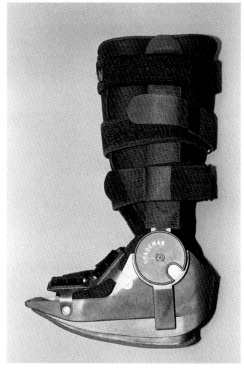

Figure 28-7   Controlled ankle motion device.

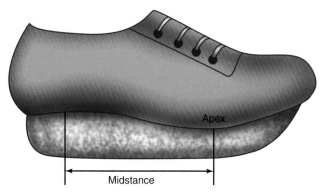

Figure 28-8   Rocker sole, illustrating midstance and apex.

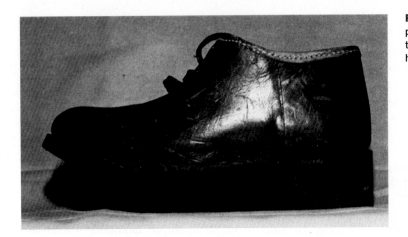

Figure 28-9   The rocker-style sole is rigid, and as a person walks, the shoe rotates over a ridge (fulcrum) in the sole, which is located posterior to the metatarsal heads.

patient; however, the following basic types of rocker soles can be identified.

Mild Rocker Sole

This most widely used and basic of rocker soles has a mild rocker curvature at both the heel and the toe (Fig. 28-10A). It can relieve metatarsal pressure and may assist gait by increasing propulsion and reducing the amount of energy expended in walking. It is appropriate for the foot that is not at risk and is found on most off-the-shelf walking and running shoes. The other types of rocker soles are essentially variations of this basic, mild rocker sole.

Heel-to-Toe Rocker Sole

This type of rocker sole is shaped with a more severe angle at both the heel and the toe (Fig. 28-10B). It is intended to aid propulsion at toe off, decrease heel-strike forces on the calcaneus, and reduce the need for ankle motion. The heel-to-toe rocker sole may be indicated for patients with a fixed clawed toe or rigid hammertoe, midfoot amputation, or calcaneal ulcers.

Toe-Only Rocker Sole

As the name suggests, the toe-only rocker sole has a rocker angle only at the toe, with the midstance extending to the back end of the sole (Fig. 28-10C). The purposes of this rocker sole are to increase weight-bearing proximal to the metatarsal heads, provide a stable midstance, and reduce the need for toe dorsiflexion on toe off. Indications for the toe-only rocker sole include hallux rigidus; callus or ulcer on the distal portion of a clawed toe, hammertoe, or mallet toe; and metatarsal ulcers.

Severe Angle Rocker Sole

This type of rocker sole is similar to the toe-only type but has a much more severe angle than that found on the toe-only rocker sole (Fig. 28-10D). The purpose of the

severe rocker angle is to eliminate weight-bearing forces anterior to the metatarsal heads. It is indicated for extreme relief of ulcerated metatarsal heads.

Negative Heel Rocker Sole

Shaped with a rocker angle at the toe and a negative heel, this type of rocker sole results in the patient's heel being at the same height or lower than the ball of the foot when in a standing position (Fig. 28-10E). The purpose of the negative heel rocker sole is to accommodate a foot that is fixed in dorsiflexion.

Double Rocker Sole

This type of rocker sole actually consists of two shorter rocker soles with two short midstances. It is used to treat midfoot pathology. While an unmodified shoe and shoes with the other types of rocker soles actually increase pressure under the midfoot when compared to walking barefoot, the double rocker sole does not.[10] This modification can be used to off-load midfoot bony prominences associated with a Charcot foot deformity (Fig. 28-10F).

Stabilization

A second type of external shoe modification involves the addition of material to the medial or lateral portion of the shoe to stabilize some part of the foot.

Flare

A flare is an extension to the heel of the shoe, the sole, or both (Fig. 28-11). Flares can be medial or lateral, and their purpose is to stabilize a hindfoot, midfoot, or forefoot instability. For example, a medial heel flare might be used to support a foot with a fixed valgus heel deformity.

Stabilizer

A stabilizer is an extension added to the side of the shoe, including both the sole and upper (Fig. 28-12). Made

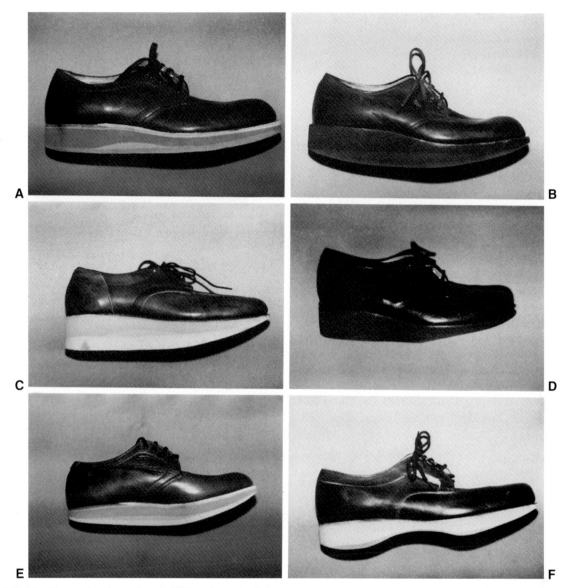

Figure 28–10   Types of rocker soles. **A,** Mild rocker sole; **B,** heel-to-toe rocker sole; **C,** toe-only rocker sole; **D,** severe angle rocker sole; **E,** negative heel rocker sole; **F,** double rocker sole.

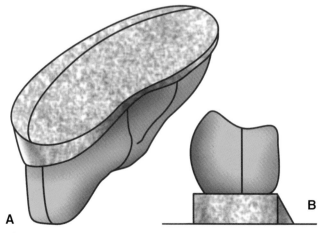

Figure 28–11   Lateral flare. **A,** Plantar view. **B,** Posterior view.

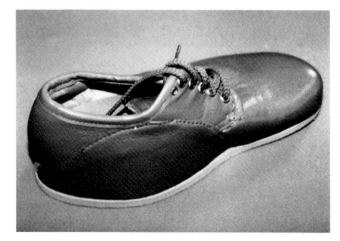

Figure 28–12   Medial stabilizer.

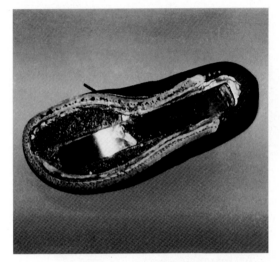

Figure 28–13   Extended steel shank.

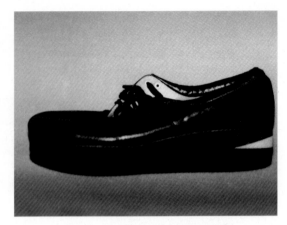

Figure 28–14   Cushion heel.

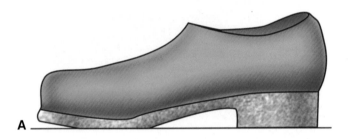

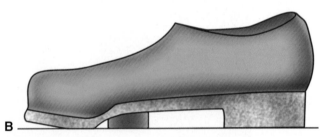

Figure 28–15   **A,** A conventional shaped shoe. **B,** A properly constructed metatarsal bar may relieve stresses in the region of the metatarsal heads. These shoes are not recommended for insensitive feet.

from rigid foam or crepe, it provides more extensive stabilization than a flare and is used for a hindfoot or midfoot with severe medial or lateral instability, for example, a medially collapsed Charcot foot. Before the stabilizer is added, the patient must wear the shoe for a few weeks until it is "broken in" (i.e., has taken on the shape of the deformed foot). Adding a stabilizer to a new shoe can lead to serious skin breakdown in the diabetic foot.

Extended Steel Shank

An extended steel shank is a strip of spring steel inserted between the layers of the sole, extending from the heel to the toe of the shoe (Fig. 28-13). New, lighter-weight carbon fiber materials are also available for this modification. It is most commonly used in combination with a rocker sole and helps to maintain the shape and effectiveness of the rocker sole. An extended steel shank can also prevent the shoe from bending, limit toe and midfoot motion, aid propulsion on toe off, and strengthen the entire shoe. It is indicated for hallux limitus or rigidus or limited ankle motion. It is also a useful tool for replacing the toe-off lever arm that is lost to amputation of the great toe and/or forefoot.

Cushion Heel

A cushion heel consists of a wedge of shock-absorbing material layered into the heel of the shoe (Fig. 28-14). Its purpose is to provide a maximum amount of shock absorption under the heel (in addition to that provided by a total-contact orthosis) while maintaining a stable stance. It is indicated for calcaneal ulcers or for a rigid ankle and hindfoot as a result of Charcot deformity.

Custom Foot Orthoses

Well-molded custom foot orthoses are usually required within depth shoes to adequately distribute forces around

foot deformities. If a pedorthist or orthotist wants to redistribute plantar forces with foot orthoses, the means of doing so fall into four general categories:

1. Pressure under one part of the foot can be relieved by increasing the pressure (elevating the insole) on an adjacent part. Metatarsal pads, buildups such as metatarsal bars, and depressions in the insole are included in this group (Fig. 28-15). The placement of these modifications is crucial to the success of the offloading. Incorrect placement could have negative results, ranging from simply being ineffective to actually causing an ulcer. Optimal placement can be verified with in-shoe plantar-pressure–reading devices.
2. Pressure under one part of the foot can also be reduced by exactly molding an insole (foot orthosis) to the plantar shape, thus giving the orthosis a total-contact effect. Since pressure is equal to force (body

weight) divided by the area (amount of foot in contact with the insole), exact molding reduces pressure under every part of the foot by increasing the area of contact.

3. The effects of pressure can be spread over time. Soft materials take time to compress. This compression slows the foot as it presses down into the insole. Thicker foam insoles are more effective than thinner insoles of the same material, but as the material used becomes thicker, the foot may begin to develop blisters due to rubbing up and down (shearing) against the side of the shoe.

4. In theory, dynamic functional foot orthoses can reduce the pressure in one part of the foot by altering internal motions of the bones within the foot. If properly constructed, they can successfully control the effects of mild to moderate pronatory deformities. Excessive pronation results in localized forces under one or two metatarsal heads and, in some cases, the first toe.[27] Effective control of pronation reduces these localized pressures by allowing all metatarsal heads to share the force of each step. It should be noted that a functional orthosis should be used with extreme caution, if at all, in treating an insensate foot. An orthosis should not be molded under the toe portion of an insensitive foot, since the foot elongates with pronation, and the toes must be able to slide forward freely without passing over ridges which could result in distal toe ulceration.

Material Selection

A great variety of insole materials are available from medical suppliers. Softer polyethylene materials help to cushion the foot but cannot fully replace all capabilities of human soft tissues. These materials are easily molded and trimmed. Unfortunately, this is often the only reason they are selected for insole construction when they are really best suited as a temporary or trial device.[29] When used as the only material in the construction of an orthosis, the softest polyethylene materials, such as #1 Plastazote, will not hold their molded shape for a long time. Repetitive compression and decompression break down the cellular structure, causing the orthosis eventually to "bottom out."

The current preference in insole design for long-term wear is a lamination of different materials or a single firm material. By combining materials in one insole, the pedorthist can take advantage of the good properties of one material and minimize its weaknesses by using a second material with different mechanical characteristics (Figs. 28-16 and 28-17). Rigid materials generally hold their shape for longer periods of time and are not as easily deformed by walking on them. In addition to the fact that rigid materials provide little or no cushioning, another problem with them is that the technician fabricating the device needs to have a very high level of expertise to prevent injuring the insensate foot.

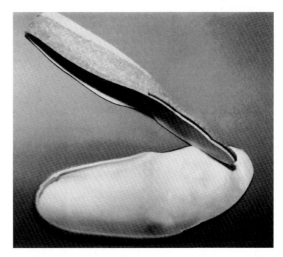

Figure 28–16   Multiple-layer total-contact orthosis. This total-contact orthosis has a polyethylene foam shell, a middle layer of micropore rubber, and cork posting.

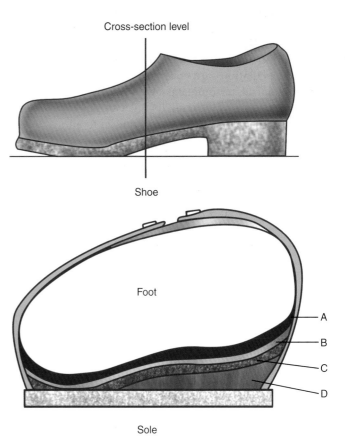

Figure 28–17   This cross section shows layers of different materials in one type of laminated orthotic device. Layer A is nylon-covered PPT or Spenco. Layer B is Pelite. Layer C is Subortholene (JMS Berkshire Resource, Inc., Clifton, NJ). Layer D is neoprene crepe. The nylon covering reduces shear stress, and the underlying foam allows for cushioning. The Pelite molds well to the shape of the positive model and is then reinforced by the rigid Subortholene. The neoprene crepe provides a firm support for the other materials.

A laminated insole of Plastazote, cork, polyurethane foam, and leather was used in a study in Germany.[9] Patients who routinely wore the molded foot orthoses greatly reduced their chance of developing foot ulceration when compared to people who returned to non-molded footwear occasionally. This study reinforces the concept that a properly made insole must be worn all the time. A person with sensory neuropathy must not even occasionally wear shoes that are not especially designed to protect their feet.

Whenever possible, it is preferable to utilize the person's own soft tissue structures as a cushion. Human soft tissues have viscoelastic properties that provide more effective injury protection than do any synthetic materials. A viscous material performs like the shock absorber on a car, while an elastic material performs like the spring. The shock absorber controls the speed with which the spring can be compressed. The various degrees of elastic protection provided by synthetic foam materials depend on their degree of firmness (durometer).

Managing Partial Foot Amputations and Disarticulations

Prescription footwear for several types of amputations and disarticulations are covered in this section: toe, ray, transmetatarsal, tarsometatarsal (Lisfranc), and midtarsal (Chopart). Although the pedorthic care for each type is different, several objectives are common to all:

1. *Provide shoe filler.* Unless the amputation is extensive and a custom-made or shortened shoe is used, some type of shoe filler is needed for the portion of the foot that has been amputated. In most cases, the filler can be incorporated into the orthosis.
2. *Equalize weight-bearing.* Amputation of a portion of the foot will often result in uneven patterns of weight-bearing on the remaining foot. Just as with the intact diabetic foot, any areas of excessive pressure must be eliminated, and even distribution of weight-bearing must be maintained.
3. *Protect and accommodate the remaining portion of the foot.* Because the occurrence of an amputation implies severe foot problems, special care must be taken to protect and accommodate the remaining portion of an at-risk foot. The presence of skin grafts, scar tissue, or any postsurgical complications must also be taken into consideration when one is providing prescription footwear for a partial foot.
4. *Improve the gait.* When part of the foot has been amputated, a natural gait pattern is no longer possible. The addition of an appropriate type of rocker sole can often improve the gait pattern after an amputation.

The proper shoe for a partial foot is determined by the extent of the amputation. If the metatarsal heads remain intact, shoe size does not change. Only when one

or more metatarsal heads have been removed can the patient be fit with a shorter (i.e., smaller size) shoe.

Toe and Ray Amputations

Objectives

The first three of the objectives stated above are the most relevant to toe and ray amputations; depending on the extent of the amputation, gait might not be significantly affected. A shoe filler can help to minimize drifting of the remaining toes, which is particularly important after a great toe amputation. In the case of a ray amputation, especially the first ray, the removal of one or more metatarsal heads results in increased pressure on the remaining heads; it is therefore important to maintain even distribution of weight-bearing to protect the remaining metatarsal heads.[10]

Shoes

As was indicated earlier, shoe size after a toe amputation does not change because the metatarsal heads remain intact. Even after a ray amputation, in which one or more metatarsals have been removed, a well-constructed shoe filler can usually allow the patient to wear a full-length shoe. Other important shoe features include a strong medial counter for stability, especially if the first ray has been removed, and a soft, moldable upper to protect and accommodate the remaining foot.

External Shoe Modifications

Many shoes for toe and ray amputations do not require external modifications. However, possible modifications include a rocker sole with an extended steel shank to improve gait and protect remaining metatarsal heads and a flare for additional stability, especially if more than one ray has been removed.

Orthoses

After removal of one or more toes, the remaining toes have a tendency to drift out of position. The use of an orthosis with a filler will help to maintain the position of the remaining toes; it can also equalize weight-bearing, thereby eliminating excessive pressure on the remaining toes and metatarsals.

Transmetatarsal Amputation

Objectives

The shoe filler that is provided to fill the void left by the amputated portion of the forefoot, in conjunction with a stiffened rocker sole, will help to prevent creasing of the shoe at the point of amputation, avoiding breakdown and eventual collapse of the shoe. A filler can also help to control the remaining foot inside the shoe, decrease soft tissue shear at its distal end, and often eliminate the need for a costly, less cosmetically appealing custom-made shoe. Equalizing weight-bearing is especially important after a transmetatarsal amputation.

Shoes

A shoe with a Blucher opening and a long medial counter can best control the remaining foot and help to decrease soft tissue shear. The upper should be made of a soft, moldable leather to accommodate and protect the remaining foot. A custom-made shoe is generally not necessary for a transmetatarsal amputation because enough of the foot remains to keep a shoe on with the aid of a filler; however, a smaller size shoe might be appropriate if the patient finds it cosmetically acceptable.

External Shoe Modifications

An extended steel shank in conjunction with an appropriate rocker sole can reduce pressure and impact shock while aiding propulsion and reducing the amount of shoe distortion. The use of a cushion heel will further minimize impact shock. Medial and lateral flares may be added to stabilize and control the amputated foot and decrease shear.

Orthoses

An orthosis with a filler will help to stabilize or restrict joint motion, accommodate bony prominences and deformities, decrease shear and shoe distortion, and equalize weight-bearing. Socks are now available that are especially made for use following a transmetatarsal amputation, which may also be helpful in protecting and accommodating the remaining foot.

Tarsometatarsal and Midtarsal Disarticulations

Objectives

In addition to the objectives already listed, pedorthic care for a tarsometatarsal or midtarsal disarticulation should be concerned with containing the remaining foot inside the shoe and preventing equinus contracture.

Shoes

A high-top shoe is best because it can most effectively contain the foot in the shoe and provide the control necessary to prevent equinus contracture. A strong counter can also aid in providing control while improving medial and lateral stability. A wedge sole will provide a broader base of support, and a shorter shoe size will decrease the resistance to rollover on toe off and aid in propulsion.

For the smaller remaining foot, a custom-made shoe will best meet the treatment objectives by providing total accommodation of the foot.

External Shoe Modifications

An extended steel shank and an appropriate rocker sole are needed to decrease shock impact, decrease shoe distortion, and aid in propulsion. A medial or lateral flare can improve stability and weight-bearing. Because a smaller area must assume the weight that would normally be spread out over the entire foot, the use of a cushion heel will improve gait by reducing shock at heel strike.

Orthoses

An orthosis with any necessary filler will give maximum accommodation and protection of the remaining foot while stabilizing or restricting joint motion. An orthosis will also lessen shear, reduce shoe distortion, and equalize weight-bearing. Further protection of the remaining foot is made possible with the use of a custom-made sock.

As an alternative to incorporating the shoe filler into the foot orthosis, a Chopart filler boot with a built-in shoe filler may be used. This orthotic device is made of leather, laces up the ankle, and resembles a high-top boot without a sole. Made to fit inside the patient's shoe, it offers additional control and helps to maintain medial and lateral stability without the need for a high-top shoe.

Writing Footwear Prescriptions

Ideally, the foot care of a person with diabetes is managed by a specialist with extensive training in foot anatomy, function, and pathology. In these situations, the prescribing physician provides a very extensive background in formal education and clinic experience regarding both the ideal foot and the subtle pathological variances found in each individual's foot. To achieve the best protection for the insensate patient, the specialist physician must include these insights with the prescription so that the footwear specialist can incorporate them in the prescribed footwear. Since the physician rarely has the expertise to manufacture, or even recommend, specific materials for a custom orthosis, this knowledge must come from the fabricator of the orthoses. The physician, however, is obligated to communicate the goals for foot protection he or she wishes to achieve. The fabricator must then inform the physician how he or she plans to achieve those goals. The more information the pedorthist has, the more likely he or she is to obtain third-party reimbursements. Though the prescribing physician does not often evaluate the performance of an orthotic device, in a case involving insensate limbs, it should be a matter of routine clinical practice. Verbal communication between physician and fabricator would be ideal. If this is not possible, the physician or assistant should include the following in the written prescription:[27,30]

1. *Complete diagnosis.* Include primary and secondary diagnoses. A history of recent ulceration or fracture should be communicated. Any particular anatomic or functional observations should be identified, such as forefoot varus, plantar-flexed metatarsal, or limited subtalar joint range of motion.
2. *Desired effect.* The physician should convey the goals to be achieved by the new orthosis and footwear. These may include "relieve pressure under a metatarsal head," "post the forefoot varus," "stabilize the midtarsal joint," or "reinforce the lateral counter."
3. *Other factors that may have to be considered.* These would include factors such as using a boot rather than a low-quarter shoe or making room for an ankle-foot orthosis that is being made at a different facility.

Risk Categorization

The risk categories presented here can all be included within grade 0 (intact skin) of the ulcer classification system described by Wagner.[6]

Risk Category 0

Category 0 (Table 28-1) risk includes all patients who have been diagnosed as having diabetes who retain protective levels of sensation. Sensory systems within the foot and vascular supply to the foot, however, can be lost during any stage of the disease. Since this loss can be so gradual that it is not noticed by the patient, a periodic objective evaluation of sensation should be done to help prevent tissue damage. A standardized record of foot risk factors should be maintained for the duration of the patient's life (Table 28-2).

Risk Category 1

Although patients in category 1 have not had foot ulcers, they have lost protective levels of sensation, placing them at a higher risk of injury. The repetitive stress of walking can, by itself, result in damage to their feet. Veves and colleagues reported that 39% of all patients with diabetic neuropathy had higher than normal pressures under their feet.[1] For most patients, the inability to feel the Semmes-Weinstein monofilament that bends with a pressure of 10 g (5.07) would place them in this category.

Risk Category 2

Patients in category 2 have lost sensation and also have a deformity in their foot but have not yet had ulcers. Deformity results in the concentration of stress in that small area of the foot. The added stress usually occurs in a part of the foot that is not accustomed to additional pressure, resulting in injury. Surgical correction of a deformity can result in moving a diabetic patient to a lower risk category.

Risk Category 3

People in category 3 not only have lost sensation but also have a history of previous foot ulceration. The skin and underlying soft tissues are more easily reinjured in areas where previous damage has occurred.

TABLE 28-1   Risk and Management Categories

Risk	Management
Category 0 Protective sensation present No history of plantar ulcer May have foot deformity Has a disease which could lead to insensitivity	Foot clinic once Patient education to include proper shoe style selection
Category 1 Protective sensation absent No history of plantar ulceration No foot deformity	Foot clinic every 6 months Review all footwear the patient wears Add soft insoles—Spenco,* nylon-covered PPT[†]
Category 2 Protective sensation absent No history of plantar ulcer Foot deformity present	Foot clinic every 3–4 months Custom-molded orthotic devices are usually necessary Prescription footwear often required
Category 3 Protective sensation absent History of foot ulceration and/or vascular laboratory findings indicate significant vascular disease	Foot clinic every 1–2 months Custom orthotic devices are necessary Prescription shoes are often required

* Spenco Medical Corporation, Waco, TX.
[†] Professional Protective Technology, Deer Park, NY.

TABLE 28-2 **Insensitive Foot Examination***

Examination	Justification
General	Inspect for possible ulceration, areas of inflammation, or other skin changes related to vascular disease
Sensory	Test vibratory sensation and perform a quantifiable sensory test to determine level of protective sensation
Temperature	With no sensation, a localized skin temperature increase > 2°C in a localized area indicates an area of inflammation
Shoes	Identify the characteristics of the footwear that because of wear or style pose a threat to the feet
Muscle	Diseases that result in sensory loss can also lead to muscle paralysis; in the feet, intrinsic paralysis is the most frequent early involvement and results in clawed toe deformities

* Patient education for self-examination should be provided to expand or reinforce the patient's active participation in his or her own care on every visit.

Patient Management by Risk Category

Management Category 0

Patients in risk category 0 need education on footwear selection. The feet of patients in this group could lose sensation before their next visit. These patients should begin to wear only shoes that will pose no threat to their feet if loss of sensation develops. Since insensitivity or vascular disease can occur at any time, the peripheral sensory and circulatory status of each diabetic should be reevaluated each year.

Management Category 1

Patients in risk category 1 exhibit loss of protective sensation. Since the only internal system providing protection has been lost, external behavioral changes have to be taught. People in this category need more complete information on common foot problems, such as callus formation, redness, and swelling.

A multidisciplinary clinic for the management of diabetic feet should have a reliable means of determining the pressures under a person's foot as the person walks. Ideally, the device would have the ability to record these pressures within the shoe as a person walks. People with insensate feet often experience higher pressures under their feet than normally sensate people do.[1] There seems to be a threshold of pressure that can increase a person's risk from walking. The actual threshold has not yet been definitively established. Owing to glycosylation of tissues around the joint, the range of motion of the major joints of the foot can become reduced. This has been established as a contributing factor that results in higher pressures under the feet of people with diabetes.

Patients with sensory loss in their feet should never walk barefoot or in socks alone. After stepping on a sharp object, the person with an insensitive foot will keep walking as though the foot was not injured. This often results in added injury, delayed healing, or abscess formation. Pressures are reduced under the feet when the person wears most forms of low-heeled footwear as compared to walking barefoot or in socks. Patients with insensitive feet need to maintain vigilance for possible dangerous circumstances at all times. Occasionally, injuries occur because of objects that have fallen into the shoe since it was last worn. Before a shoe is put on, the inside should be inspected for foreign objects by the patient, then turned upside down and shaken to be sure nothing is inside.

As a person walks, the bottom of the foot is subjected to repetitive stress. To minimize the effects of this stress, people in category 1 should have soft insoles made of materials such as microcellular rubber or polyurethane foam in all shoes they wear. These materials are available in precut insoles or in sheets of material that can be cut to the proper size. A nylon covering helps to minimize shear force between the insole and the foot, and the soft cushion helps to reduce vertical (normal) force. Being at a higher risk of injury, people in this category need to visit their foot care physician more frequently than those in category 0. A visit every 6 months can help to detect developing problems such as clawed toe deformity.

Management Category 2

Deformity in the foot sometimes requires custom footwear to accommodate the shape. Many custom shoes are made from a plaster model of the foot that is sent to a manufacturer for last construction and shoe fabrication. This process creates a communication gap between the foot care providers and the shoe fabricators. The person who actually sees the foot needs to inform the shoemaker of any special observation that might need to be considered in the construction of the shoe. For example, a shoemaker who sees a unique bulge on the plaster model of a foot does not know whether that bulge represents soft tissue that can be compressed or a rigid bony deformity requiring that the upper of the shoe be molded around it. This communication gap often results in less than ideal footwear. Most of the patients in category 2 do not require custom footwear. Depth footwear appropriately fit and modified by a prescription shoe fitter will provide the necessary accommodations for most common deformities, such as clawed toes. People in this category need to visit a foot specialist at least every 4 months and probably more often until the problem foot is fully protected by shoes or the deformity is corrected by surgery.

Management Category 3

Patients in category 3 have insensate feet that have previously ulcerated. Ulcers occur most frequently at the location of previous ulcers. Scarring makes tissues less strong and flexible and more likely to break down, particularly as the result of shear, a force that is applied parallel to the skin surface. Soft tissues withstand shear by one layer of tissue gliding over adjacent tissues. Scar binds tissue layers together and prevents this gliding action. With this greater degree of susceptibility, these patients need a higher level of protection within their footwear.

Also in category 3 are patients with significant peripheral vascular disease. These patients have tissues that are more friable and that, once injured, have a much more difficult time healing. Often, when peripheral vascular disease and neuropathy coexist, the injury occurs in a manner typical of neuropathic lesions but requires much more protection and time to heal because of poor tissue perfusion. These patients need the most intense efforts of the medical community, often requiring visits every few weeks or more often.

Case Studies

The following case studies illustrate the broad range of pedorthic care for the diabetic foot.

CASE STUDIES

CASE 1: PLANTAR ULCER

A 45-year-old man, 6 feet tall and weighing 225 pounds, with size 14 feet and a 20-year history of type 1 diabetes, had pes cavus feet with very little remaining fatty tissue, impaired sensation, and a history of numerous ulcers associated with severe callusing under the metatarsal heads. The pes cavus foot, it should be noted, does not absorb shock well; it puts extreme weight-bearing on the metatarsal heads, which are already at risk because of the lack of fatty tissue and impaired sensation.

His original prescription was for depth shoes and custom foot orthoses with a viscoelastic polymer added under the metatarsal heads to provide pressure relief. Callus buildup improved somewhat but remained problematic under the first and fourth metatarsal heads. Addition of toe-only rocker soles provided further relief, but hemorrhaging under the first metatarsal calluses continued. After consultation with the prescribing physician, it was decided that the orthosis should be modified by adding extreme posting proximal to the metatarsal heads to transfer the excessive plantar pressure from the first and fourth metatarsal heads to the second and third. The callus has virtually disappeared since the patient began wearing the new orthosis.

CASE 2: COMPLEX PLANTAR ULCER

A 55-year-old, overweight man (5 feet 6½ inches tall, weighing 225 pounds) had a 15-year history of type 2 diabetes. His vascular insufficiency had been improved with a vein bypass, but peripheral neuropathy had resulted in a completely insensate foot.

Visual examination revealed a severe calcaneal ulcer stretching from the plantar to the posterior part of the heel. Radiologic examination revealed soft tissue involvement only.

The ulcer was treated with total-contact casting, which successfully closed the ulcer except for a small area that subsequently healed while the patient used a custom Plastazote sandal. Maintaining this healed area was especially challenging, owing to the very large skin deficit and a considerable amount of scar tissue, which left the heel extremely susceptible to breakdown.

The prescription called for a heat-moldable shoe to provide maximum accommodation for this at-risk foot. The shoe was modified with a heel-to-toe rocker sole and—very important—a cushion heel to absorb considerable shock on heel strike. With the cushion heel and rocker sole, there was virtually no weight-bearing on the postulcer heel area; significant weight-bearing began at a position that was distal to the heel. A triple-layer orthosis served to further protect and accommodate the heel deficit as well as other minor plantar prominences. The shell was made of soft Plastazote, and the deficit area of the heel was filled and supported with a low-density viscoelastic polymer. After 2 years, the patient has had no recurrence of ulceration or tissue breakdown.

CASE 3: DORSAL ULCER

A 66-year-old woman with a 19-year history of type 2 diabetes had a chronic dorsal ulcer on her second toe. Her insensate foot had collapsed medially, and she had a dynamic hammertoe deformity, that is, the deformity worsened when she walked.

Her first prescription was for a heat-moldable shoe and orthosis. The shoe was stretched as much as possible over the second toe in an attempt to eliminate pressure from the shoe upper, but even after repeated attempts to further stretch the upper, reulceration of the toe occurred. The patient was treated in between shoe-stretching attempts with a custom Plastazote sandal with no pressure on the toes, resulting in rapid healing. The final solution was to remove all of the moldable lining material from the shoe in the area over the hammertoe. The remaining deerskin was extremely soft and even more stretchable without the lining material. For the past 4 years, there has been no recurrence of the ulcer. This case illustrates the importance of evaluating the foot dynamically. In most cases, the initial stretching of the shoe would probably have been successful, but this patient's toe position changed so dramatically while walking that normal stretching was ineffective in relieving dorsal pressure.

CASE 4: RAY AMPUTATION

A 51-year-old man with a 32-year history of type 1 diabetes had peripheral neuropathy resulting in completely insensate feet and a history of metatarsal ulcers. He had a persistent plantar ulcer under the first metatarsal head of his left foot. His physician requested trying to close the ulcer in-shoe so that the man could continue to work. This was done by using in-depth steel-toed boots, rocker soles, and a triple-layer orthosis with extensive relief of the first metatarsal head. The ulcer had nearly closed when a sudden infection occurred. The bone infection was so severe that the first toe and a portion of the first metatarsal had to be amputated. The foot was closed dorsally and medially with a skin graft, but the skin on the plantar surface remained intact and was therefore not especially difficult to maintain.

The new prescription made use of the patient's previous oblique-toed depth shoes. The rocker sole was modified to provide a small amount of heel rock and considerably more rock on the toe. An extended steel shank was also added. The new triple-layer orthosis had a soft toe filler added to maintain the position of the lesser toes. Supportive material was added under the remaining first metatarsal so that it would bear some weight and therefore balance overall weight-bearing on the foot. This also served to eliminate excessive plantar pressure on the second through fifth metatarsal heads, thereby minimizing the chances of future callusing and ulceration.

CASE 5: TRANSMETATARSAL AMPUTATION

A 37-year-old man with a 15-year history of type 1 diabetes was a heavy user of alcohol and was otherwise noncompliant. He had twice frozen his insensate feet, resulting in bilateral transmetatarsal amputations. His plantar skin was in good condition.

The choice of prescription footwear was made easy by the patient's desire to return to work. High-top work shoes with added rocker soles controlled his remaining feet well, but a smaller size was used because of the lack of metatarsal heads. An orthosis made with a combination of medium and firm density materials served to protect and balance the remaining foot and provide the necessary toe filler.

CASE 6: MIDTARSAL (CHOPART) DISARTICULATION

A 70-year-old man had a 25-year history of type 2 diabetes. An infection occurred 2 years previously in his right foot, resulting in a midtarsal disarticulation. The original prescription called for depth shoes of the same size on both feet and orthoses. The use of the same-size shoe on the amputated foot caused gait problems owing to its length, creating the potential for breakdown in the distal portion of the partial foot.

The prescription was reevaluated, and the decision was made to use a custom-made shoe with a triple-layer orthosis and a rocker sole. A custom sock was also fabricated for the amputated foot. Although the patient was initially concerned about the appearance of different-sized shoes, he was willing to give the shorter custom-made shoe a try. He found the comfort, protection, and ease of gait so much improved that acceptance came easily. He is now wearing his second pair.

CASE 7: CHARCOT FOOT (CONVENTIONAL IN-DEPTH SHOE)

A 66-year-old woman with a 20-year history of type 2 diabetes had impaired sensation and a history of ulceration on the medial plantar aspects of her feet. She had bilateral medially collapsed Charcot foot deformities. The patient had been wearing standard cowhide depth shoes, which were hard to break in and caused callusing and discomfort until they were "deformed" enough to conform to the shape of her feet.

Her prescription included triple-layer orthoses with Plastazote shells that molded well to the entire plantar surfaces of her feet; the orthoses therefore had an increased midfoot width to accommodate her medially collapsed midfeet. Viscoelastic polymer was added to the orthoses under the bony prominences. Thermal-moldable shoes were used because of their soft, accommodating uppers, which were molded for some hammertoe deformities that were also present. The soles of the shoes were cut lengthwise through both outsoles and

insoles and split apart to accommodate her deformed feet, that is, making shoe shape match foot shape. A double rocker sole with an extended steel shank was also added to each shoe. This patient was extremely satisfied with the "split-sole" modification because her entire foot was contained within each shoe. Previously, she had always felt that the medial aspect was falling either out of the shoe or off the side of the shoe.

CASE 8: CHARCOT FOOT (CUSTOM-MADE SHOE)

A 66-year-old man, 5 feet 9 inches tall, weighing 280 pounds, had an 18-year history of type 2 diabetes. He had a severely deformed left foot and ankle because of Charcot destruction. The foot was very large, with extremely prominent medial displacement and hallux varus. In the past, he had experienced plantar ulceration on the medial prominence. A plastic patellar-tendon–bearing orthosis had apparently contributed to the ulceration problem, because the foot was quite mobile and moved within the orthosis. The Charcot foot was stabilized with the use of total-contact casting. The physician followed this with the use of a patellar-tendon–bearing orthosis attached to a shoe for 6 months. The brace was then removed, and the patient now needs only a custom-made shoe.

A conventional shoe would simply not be possible for this foot, even with extensive modifications. A custom-made shoe was therefore prescribed. It was able to accommodate the extensive deformities and was made with a padded collar because of the large size of the patient's legs. The orthosis was extended quite high on the medial aspect of the foot for maximum protection. Hook-and-loop closures were added because the patient cannot reach his feet to tie laces. The shoe was made as a high-top to offer added ankle support. This prescription has been highly successful for the past 3 years.

Summary

If clinical programs of injury prevention for insensitive feet are going to be successful, medical professionals will have to insist that people who fit and modify medically indicated footwear are knowledgeable, professional, and precise in their work. Shoes are the primary means of protecting insensitive feet. The responsibility to ensure proper shoe applications must rest with the physician. Several publications have emphasized the need to develop multidisciplinary teams under the direction of a physician to adequately manage the many foot problems of people with diabetes.[11,15,31,32] The best data for developing programs to benefit patients with diabetic foot problems and reducing amputation rates have come from physicians who have brought together diabetic foot care teams.

The primary day-to-day management of the vast majority of people with diabetes must be under the supervision of medical professionals who are familiar with the pathology and mechanics of the foot. Because foot problems can develop quickly and unexpectedly in the diabetic patient, the team must be readily available. Medical as well as surgical expertise is needed on the team to make comprehensive diabetic foot care as seamless as possible. But just as important to the team is the shoe and orthotic expert. These individuals provide the protective devices that provide the first line of defense against foot injury. Physicians who accept the responsibility for the foot care of diabetic patients should be familiar with every aspect of shoe modification for therapeutic use. They should also accept the fact that the patient with an insensitive foot will need life-long assistance to prevent tissue damage.

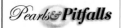

Pearls

- The team approach reinforces the importance of therapeutic footwear for the diabetic foot.
- Shoes can be resoled and orthoses can be recovered to increase their lifespan and help reduce out-of-pocket expense to the patient.
- Shoe modifications, although very helpful, are often overlooked.
- A gradual break-in schedule for new shoes and orthoses can prevent many problems, especially when the patient is transitioning from a cast to a shoe.

Pitfalls

- Poor communication between the patient and the treatment team, especially in regard to comprehension of the direction and goals of the treatment plan, is a major deterrent to success.
- Follow-up is crucial because patients who fall through the cracks are likely to develop major problems.
- A lack of family support is often detrimental to the success of a conservative foot care plan.
- Having little or no insurance coverage can deter the patient from obtaining therapeutic footwear. The importance of these modalities therefore needs to be stressed and confirmed by the entire team to the patient and family.

References

1. Veves A, Murray HJ, Young MJ, et al: The risk of foot ulceration in diabetic patients with high foot pressure: A prospective study. Diabetologia 35:660–663, 1992.
2. Frey C, Thompson F, Smith J, et al: American Orthopedic Foot and Ankle Society: Women's shoe survey. Foot Ankle 14:78–81, 1993.
3. Snow RE, Williams KR, Holmes GB: The effects of wearing high heeled shoes on pedal pressure in women. Foot Ankle 13:85–92, 1992.
4. Corrigan JP, Moore DP, Stephens MM: Effect of heel height on forefoot loading. Foot Ankle 14:148–152, 1993.
5. Fernando DJS, Hutchison A, Veves A, et al: Relationship of limited joint mobility to abnormal foot pressures and diabetic foot ulceration. Diabetes Care 14:8, 1991.
6. Wagner FW Jr: A classification and treatment program for diabetic, neuropathic, and dysvascular foot problems. AAOS Instuctional Course Lecture, Vol 28. St. Louis: CV Mosby, 1979.
7. Ctercteko GC, Dhanendran MK, Hutton WC, et al: Vertical forces acting on the feet of diabetic patients with neuropathic ulceration. Br J Surg 68:608–614, 1981.
8. Stokes IAF, Faris IB, Hutton WC: The neuropathic ulcer and loads on the foot in diabetic patients. Acta Orthop Scand 46:839–847, 1975.
9. Chantelau E, Haage P: An audit of cushioned diabetic footwear: Relation to patient compliance. Diabet Med 10:114–116, 1993.
10. Janisse D, Brown D, Wertsch J, Harris G: Effects of rocker soles on plantar pressures and lower extremity biomechanics. Arch Phys Med Rehabil 85:81–86, 2004.
11. American Orthopaedic Foot and Ankle Society, National Shoe Retailers Association, Pedorthic Footwear Association: Shoe Fit: What You Need to Know. Columbia, MD: Pedorthic Footwear Association, 1997.
12. Pedorthic Footwear Association: Pedorthic Reference Guide. Columbia, MD: Pedorthic Footwear Association, 1996.
13. Cavanagh PR, Ulbrecht JS: Biomechanics of the foot in diabetes mellitus. In Levin ME, O'Neal LW, Bowker JH (eds): The Diabetic Foot, 5th ed. St. Louis: Mosby-Year Book, 1993, pp 199–232.
14. Edmonds ME, Watkins PJ: Management of the diabetic foot. In Dyck PJ, Thomas PK, Asbury AK, et al (eds): Diabetic Neuropathy. Philadelphia: WB Saunders, 1987.
15. Wooldridge J, Moreno L: Evaluation of the costs to Medicare of covering therapeutic shoes for diabetic patients. Diabetes Care 17:541–547, 1994.
16. Edmonds ME, Blundell MP, Morris ME, et al: Improved survival of the diabetic foot: The role of a specialised foot clinic. Q J Med 232:163–171, 1986.
17. Assal JP, Muhlhauser I, Pernat A, et al: Patient education as the basis for diabetic foot care in clinical practice. Diabetologia 28:602, 1985.
18. Foster AVM, Snowden S, Grenfell A, et al: Reduction of gangrene and amputations in diabetic renal transplant patients: The role of a special foot clinic. Diabet Med 12:632–635, 1995.
19. Rossi WA, Tennant R: Professional Shoe Fitting. New York: National Shoe Retailers Association, 1984.
20. Coleman WC: Footwear in a management program for injury prevention. In Levin ME, O'Neal LW, Bowker JH (eds): The Diabetic Foot, 5th ed. St. Louis: Mosby-Year Book, 1993, pp 531–547.
21. Janisse DJ: The art and science of fitting shoes. Foot Ankle 13:257–262, 1992.
22. Janisse DJ: The shoe in rehabilitation of the foot and ankle. In Sammarco GJ (ed): Rehabilitation of the Foot and Ankle. St. Louis: Mosby-Year Book, 1995.
23. Brand PW: The insensitive foot (including leprosy). In Jahss MH (ed): Disorders of the Foot and Ankle, 2nd ed. Philadelphia: WB Saunders, 1991, pp 1266–1286.
24. Baumhauer JF, et al: A comparison study of plantar foot pressures in a standardized shoe, total contact cast, and prefabricated pneumatic walking brace. Foot Ankle Int 18:26–33, 1997.
25. Bergtholdt HT: Thermography on insensitive limbs. In Uematsu S (ed): Medical Thermography: Theory and Clinical Applications. Los Angeles: Brentwood, 1976.
26. Janisse DJ: The role of the pedorthist in the prevention and management of diabetic foot ulcers. Ostomy Wound Manage 40:54–65, 1994.
27. Ullman BC, Brncick M: Orthotic and pedorthic management of the diabetic foot. In Sammarco GJ (ed): The Foot in Diabetes. Philadelphia: Lea & Febiger, 1991, pp 207–225.
28. Nawoczenski DA, Birke JA, Coleman WC: Effect of rocker sole design on plantar forefoot pressures. J Am Podiatr Med Assoc 78:455–460, 1998.
29. Enna CD, Brand PW, Reed JP Jr, et al: The orthotic care of the denervated foot in Hansen's disease. Orthot Pros 30:33, 1976.
30. Janisse DJ: Footwear prescriptions. Foot Ankle Int 18:526–527, 1997.
31. Hobgood E: Conservative therapy of foot abnormalities, infections and vascular insufficiency. In Davidson JK (ed): Clinical Diabetes Mellitus. New York: Thieme, 1986, pp 599–610.
32. Schaff PS, Cavanagh PR: Shoes for the insensitive foot: The effect of a "rocker bottom" shoe modification on plantar pressure distribution. Foot Ankle 11:129–140, 1990.

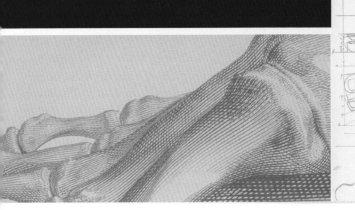

REHABILITATION OF THE DIABETIC AMPUTEE

ROBERT S. GAILEY, CURTIS R. CLARK, AND IGNACIO A. GAUNAURD ■

Approximately 115,000 to 135,000 lower-limb amputations are performed in the United States annually.[1] An estimated 70% to 90% of these are the result of peripheral vascular disease, the greater percentage (45% to 83%) of peripheral vascular disease–related amputations being related to diabetes mellitus.[2,3] The Centers for Disease Control and Prevention estimated that in 2002, about 82,000 nontraumatic amputations were performed in people with diabetes.[4] Patients with diabetes are 15 times more likely to undergo a second amputation than the general population.[5-7] Gordois and colleagues estimated that the annual cost in dollars in 2001 of amputation of the toes, foot, and/or leg attributable to diabetes was about 2 billion dollars.[8] The rate of new amputation after 1, 3, and 5 years has been suggested to be 14%, 30%, and 49%, respectively.[9] The mortality rate 1, 3, and 5 years after the first amputation was found to be 15%, 38%, and 68%, respectively.[9]

Metabolic Cost of Amputee Ambulation

Conservation of effort is one of the most important concerns of the amputee and, as a result, can have a tremendous impact on the successful return to premorbid lifestyle. If the physical effort of ambulation is too great, there is a good chance that the person will be reluctant to complete the course of rehabilitation and will then become sedentary. For this reason, an overview of the physiologic energy requirements for prosthetic ambulation becomes worthwhile.

For amputees in general, the metabolic cost of ambulation is increased, while overall walking velocity is decreased.[10] This issue becomes one of concern for diabetic amputees, who typically have decreased cardiopulmonary capacity and additional comorbid conditions that further affect their overall physical health. Declining abilities such as memory, attention span, concentration, and organizational and cognitive skills create additional impediments to successful prosthetic management.[11]

Summarizing the past two decades of relevant publications provides the following generalizations concerning the metabolic cost of ambulation for the amputee. The greater the loss of limb length, the greater the energy the amputee will have to expend while walking at a substantially lower velocity.[12,13] Two exceptions to this principle should be noted. The first involves the patient with a knee disarticulation, who has a significantly higher O_2 cost (mL/kg·meter) than does either the transtibial amputee (TTA) or the transfemoral amputee (TFA). However, the speed of walking of the person with a knee disarticulation falls between the two levels, being slightly faster than that of the TFA but slower than that of the TTA.[13]

The relationship between people with Syme ankle disarticulation and TTAs is the second exception to the generalization about ambulation efficiency. People with ankle disarticulation appear to walk faster than TTAs;

however, both groups expend the same amount of energy.[14] Interestingly, there does appear to be a significant reduction in the rate of oxygen consumption (ml/kg·min) between a short TTA (<20% of total tibial length) and a standard TTA (20% to 40% of tibial length).[15] The long TTA (>40% of tibial length) does not appear to have been investigated with respect to the standard TTA or the person with ankle disarticulation. In general, these findings appear to emphasize the long-standing philosophy, first expressed by Nathan Smith in 1825, that "as a general rule, you should save all the stump you can."[16] In effect, it appears that the greater the residual limb length, the more likely it is that there will be a lower energy expenditure and/or a greater potential for increased ambulation velocity.

Aside from residual limb length, the cause of amputation—vascular or nonvascular—is directly related to the oxygen cost and speed of ambulation (Table 29-1). Vascular amputees will adopt a comfortable walking speed that will enable them to reach their desired destination without undue exertion. Keeping in mind that most diabetic amputees also suffer from significant deconditioning from inactivity, ambulation is often reserved for short distances or areas that are difficult to access with a wheelchair.

Because approximately one third of diabetic amputees will lose the contralateral limb within 3 years of the primary amputation, it is important to note the increased metabolic cost incurred by the bilateral amputee compared to the unilateral amputee. Unfortunately, most available data are from studies performed on relatively small cohorts (see Table 29-1). The key to ambulation success for the diabetic bilateral amputee is the preservation of at least one anatomic knee.[17] The likelihood of ambulation as a bilateral TFA is very remote in this population, not only because of the physiologic limitations,[18] but also because the time required for the process of prosthetic fitting and gait rehabilitation becomes overwhelming. For the bilateral vascular amputee, use of a wheelchair becomes a considerably more efficient form of mobility, reducing energy cost and increasing velocity.[19,20]

It is important to note that for nonamputees using crutches, either of the underarm or forearm type, with a three-point gait, the energy cost compared to normal walking approximately doubles.[21] Similarly, Pagliarulo and colleagues demonstrated that for TTAs who have no vascular disease, the energy rate rose significantly from a mean of 15.5 mL O_2/kg/min with a prosthesis to 22.3 mL O_2/kg/min when ambulating with crutches only.[22] This suggests that the amputee should be encouraged to use the prosthesis even if an assistive device is required.

It should be mentioned that particular components of the prosthesis itself have not been shown to reduce the energy cost of ambulation. Numerous authors have demonstrated that there is no metabolic cost difference between dynamic and nondynamic response foot-ankle assemblies.[15,23,24] Although the ability to vary cadence with fluid-controlled prosthetic knee units is a possibility, conservation of energy has yet to be established. Even though there may exist a possibility for socket designs to influence energy cost, this has been demonstrated only at a higher walking speed (2.5 mph) with traumatic TFAs and not at a slower speed (1.75 mph) with vascular amputees.[25] It had long been assumed that any reduction in the weight of the prosthesis would have a direct effect on the energy cost to the wearer. However, when additional weight of up to 2 pounds for TTAs[26] and 3 pounds for TFAs[27–29] was applied to the shank of an average prosthesis, there was no appreciable influence on the metabolic cost during ambulation. Therefore, the addition of components that will improve the function and durability of the prosthesis might be of more importance than the overall mass of the prosthesis.

No one entity might be responsible for reducing the metabolic cost of ambulation for the amputee. Diabetic and vascular amputees, in most instances, will walk more slowly while exerting a greater effort to cover the same distances as their nonamputee counterparts. Collectively, the surgery, prosthetic fitting, and therapy can make a difference. Surgery should be skillfully designed to preserve limb length and anatomic joints whenever possible. A satisfactory overall prosthetic fitting will help to ensure that the amputee will accept the limb and wear it regularly. Finally, the proper strength, endurance, and prosthetic gait-training programs should lead to maximal use

TABLE 29-1   Energy Expenditure of Unilateral and Bilateral Vascular Amputees

Vascular Amputee	Speed (m/min)	O₂ Rate (mL/kg·min)	O₂ Cost (mL/kg·m)	Pulse (beats/min)
Unilateral				
TF	36	10.8	0.28	126
TT	45	9.4	0.20	105
AD	54	9.2	0.17	108
Bilateral				
TT/TT	40	11.6	0.31	113
AD/AD	62	12.8	0.21	99
Nonamputee				
Adults (20–59 years)	80	12.1	0.15	99

TF, transfemoral; TT, transtibial; AD, ankle disarticulation.
Data from Bowker JH, Michael JW: Atlas of Limb Prosthetics (2nd ed.) St Louis: Mosby Year-Book 1992. Waters RL, Perry J, Antonelli D, Hislop H: The energy cost of walking of amputees: Influence of level amputation. J Bone Joint Surg 58(A):42–46, 1976.

of the prosthesis by reducing the amputee's efforts with daily activities.

The importance of being a physically fit prosthetic ambulator cannot be overstated. A properly fitting prosthesis that is worn daily will provide the opportunity for greater mobility and probably increase the activity level over that of amputees who do not wear a prosthesis. Several authors have suggested that an amputee's level of activity is not dictated by the level of amputation, cause of amputation, number of limbs amputated, or age.[30–32] In fact, the most important predictor of postamputation activity appears to be the level of activity prior to the amputation. If the amputee was involved and motivated before amputation, chances are the person will continue to remain so after amputation. If the person was sedentary and noncompliant before the loss of limb, unfortunately the prospects for change are not strong.

Immediate Postsurgical Treatment

Generally, the goals of postoperative treatment for the new amputee are to reduce edema, promote wound healing, prevent loss of joint motion, increase cardiovascular endurance, and improve strength. Functional skills must also be introduced as early as possible to promote independence in bed mobility, transfers, and ambulation techniques. Prevention of further injury may be addressed with education in the self-care of the residual and sound limbs. Moreover, each member of the rehabilitation team should be aware of the need to assist the patient with the psychological adjustment to limb loss.

Acute Bedside Amputee Assessment

The amputee's initial postsurgical assessment has many significant components. The first step is to obtain the baseline information necessary to determine the goals of rehabilitation and formulate a treatment plan. However, to help restore the amputee to his or her premorbid lifestyle with a positive attitude, the rehabilitation team must view amputation surgery as a reconstructive procedure, not a destructive one. Action must also be taken to prevent further injury. This requires that the amputee be immediately taught how to effectively care for the healing residual limb and be instructed in functional skills, protection of the sound limb, and avoidance of physical deconditioning, all in preparation for prosthetic training.

Throughout the short time the amputee is seen on an inpatient basis, the rehabilitation team must focus on endorsing the total rehabilitation process from the acute stages to completion of prosthetic training. Educating the person can reduce the anxiety of not knowing what lies ahead and enhance compliance as the amputee is made aware of the entire process, including the value of each step. The inclusion of amputee support groups or peer visitors can be a tremendous asset when they are well informed and hold views that are consistent with those of the rehabilitation team. The Amputee Coalition of America, a nonprofit organization, has developed a National Peer Network, which maintains a database of certified peer visitors nationwide who are available to provide encouragement and information and serve as role models for those who have recently lost a limb.[33]

Postoperative Dressings

Postoperative dressing selection will vary according to the level of amputation, surgical technique, healing requirements, patient compliance, and physician's preference. The five major types are soft dressings, semirigid/rigid dressings, immediate postoperative prostheses (IPOPs), removable rigid dressings, and prefabricated pneumatic prostheses. Soft dressings are most often used for vascular patients when regular dressing changes are required and alternative wound environments are to be used. The disadvantage of soft dressings is that patients frequently decrease their bed mobility, as they are more hesitant to move the painful operated limb, increasing the risk of cardiopulmonary complications.[34,35] Also, patients tend to hold their residual limbs in a constant flexed position, encouraging the development of joint contractures. A semirigid or rigid dressing applied to a TTA will help to control edema, reduce healing time,[34] provide protection and support to the wound, and assist in preventing a knee flexion contracture while offering the amputee greater confidence with bed mobility.

IPOPs are often not prescribed for people with amputations secondary to vascular disease because of the increased risk of damage to the soft tissue from weight-bearing forces during the period of postsurgical healing. However, if the amputee is a candidate, an IPOP, besides offering the aforementioned benefits, will allow the amputee limited weight-bearing on the residual limb with an assistive device. Furthermore, it affords the amputee the physiologic and psychological advantages of walking on two limbs. To date, there has been no evidence that IPOPs lead to an increased number of falls or injuries to the healing residual limb. In fact, additional support to the amputated limb, in the case of the amputee with a neuropathic sound limb, can potentially reduce foot pressures, improve balance, and reduce the effort of ambulation with an assistive device.

Removable rigid dressings originally were fabricated from plaster and suspended with a variety of supracondylar cuff systems. They may now consist of a prefabricated copolymer plastic shell with a soft lining with, in some instances, the provision for attaching a pylon and foot to create an IPOP. The removable rigid dressing provides the protection and other benefits of the classic rigid dressing with the option of removal for wound inspection or bathing. Additionally, socks may be added to tighten the system for progressive shrinkage of the residuum. This has been shown to shorten the time to ambulatory discharge from hospital with a temporary prosthesis.[36]

The prefabricated pneumatic prosthesis enhances the IPOP properties of early weight-bearing and residual limb protection by lining the socket with an air-bag system. This device is lightweight, reduces edema by providing more uniform compression of the residual limb, and can be easily removed to inspect the wound.[34] It has been demonstrated to decrease postoperative complications and the likelihood of future higher-level revisions.[37] Another method of reducing the risk of knee contractures and protecting the postsurgical wound is the use of a knee immobilizer. A standard soft knee immobilizer with Velcro closure is applied postoperatively and worn for 2 to 6 weeks or until the amputee is casted for the temporary prosthesis. It must be stressed that the effectiveness of any device that can be removed by the patient is largely dependent on the patient's compliance with its proper and consistent use.

Positioning

While in a supine position, the TFA should place a pillow along the lateral aspect of the residual limb to maintain neutral rotation with no abduction. If the prone position is tolerable during the day or evening, a pillow is placed under the residual limb to maintain hip extension. TTAs should avoid knee flexion for prolonged periods of time. A residual limb board will help to maintain knee extension when in a wheelchair. All amputees must be made aware that continual sitting in a wheelchair can lead to limited hip extension, negatively affecting prosthetic ambulation.

Bed Mobility

The importance of good bed mobility extends beyond simple positional adjustments for comfort or getting into and out of bed. The patient must acquire bed mobility skills to maintain correct bed positioning in order to both prevent joint contractures and avoid excessive friction of the sheets against the suture line or frail skin. Regardless of age, each patient should be taught a safe and efficient manner in which to roll, come to sitting, or adjust his or her bed position. If the patient is unable to perform the skills necessary to maintain proper positioning, a family member or caregiver must be taught how to provide assistance.

Transfers

Once bed mobility has been mastered, the patient is taught to transfer from the bed to a chair or wheelchair, progressing to more advanced transfer skills such as to a toilet, tub, and car seat. For TTAs using an immediate postoperative or temporary prosthesis, weight-bearing

through the prosthesis can assist the patient in transfers while providing additional safety. In contrast, for TTAs who are not walking candidates, a lightweight transfer prosthesis may allow more independent transfers. This prosthesis is typically fit when the residual limb is healed and the patient is ready for training. Bilateral amputees who are not fitted with an initial prosthesis transfer in a "head-on" manner, in which the patient slides forward from the wheelchair onto the desired surface by lifting the body and pushing forward with both hands. Early assessment by the rehabilitation team of a patient's ability to make transfers is an essential part of planning discharge from an acute care setting. Many elderly amputees can be discharged to home if they are able to complete transfers either independently or with limited help. If moderate to maximum assistance is needed for transfers, a facility that offers skilled physical assistance is often required until the amputee becomes more independent.[38]

Amputee Mobility

Wheelchair Propulsion

The primary means of mobility for a large majority of vascular amputees, either temporarily or permanently, will be a wheelchair. The energy conservation of wheelchair use over prosthetic ambulation is considerable with some levels of amputation.[19,20] Therefore, wheelchair skills should be taught to most amputees as an integral part of their rehabilitation program. Bilateral and older amputees might require greater use of a wheelchair, while unilateral and younger amputees will be more likely to utilize other assistive devices when not ambulating with their prosthesis. Because of the loss of body weight anteriorly, the amputee will be prone to tipping backwards while in a standard wheelchair, especially when ascending ramps or curbs. To prevent this, amputee wheel adapters are installed that set the wheels back approximately 2 inches, thus moving the center of mass (COM) anteriorly. An alternative method is to add antitippers in place of, or in addition to, amputee wheel adapters. TTAs will also require an elevating leg rest or residual limb board designed to maintain the knee in extension, thus preventing prolonged knee flexion and reducing the dependent position of the limb in order to minimize edema formation. Finally, it is recommended that the wheelchair be fitted with removable armrests to enable ease of transfer to or from either side of the chair.

Ambulation with Assistive Devices

All amputees will need an assistive device for times when they choose not to wear their prosthesis or occasions when they are unable to wear their prosthesis secondary to edema, skin irritation, or poor prosthetic fit. Moreover, at the end of the day, when in the comfort of their home, some amputees prefer the freedom of not wearing a prosthesis and instead will rely on their assistive device for household mobility. Safety is the primary factor in selecting the appropriate assistive device; however, mobility is an important secondary consideration that cannot be overlooked. The criteria for selection should include (1) the ability for unsupported standing balance, (2) the degree of upper-limb and sound-limb strength, (3) coordination and skill with the assistive device, and (4) cognition (mental status). A walker is chosen when an amputee has poor to fair balance, strength, and coordination. If balance and strength are good to normal, Lofstrand (Canadian) crutches may be used for ambulation with or without a prosthesis. A cane may be selected to ensure safety when balance is questionable while ambulating with a prosthesis. The TFA will hold the cane in the hand opposite the prosthesis to help balance the pelvis during single-limb support on the prosthetic side. Some patients who have difficulty ambulating on one limb with a walking frame or crutches because of obesity, blindness, or generalized weakness can still be successful ambulators when additional support is provided by a prosthesis.

Residual Limb Care

Education

Educating the amputee about self-care and a home exercise program is critical to the ultimate outcome of the rehabilitation process. The most difficult task is ensuring retention and compliance. The use of an itemized checklist that the amputee may take home can assist in achieving a positive outcome by providing both the patient and the clinician with a format that will help avoid overlooking important items. This checklist, designed specifically for the diabetic amputee, provides the clinician with a systematic method of educating the amputee and should always be offered as a home guide to the patient (Table 29-2).

Phantom Sensation, Phantom Pain, and Residual Limb Pain

Some of the most common and least understood phenomena experienced by amputees are phantom sensation, phantom pain, and residual limb pain.[39] The International Association for the Study of Pain categorizes phantom limb pain as a subtype of chronic pain.[40] It is estimated that 85% of amputees will experience one or all three forms of sensation or pain at one time or another.[41] During the first year after amputation, the majority of amputees will have the greatest number of episodes, with a significant decrease in intensity and duration as time after amputation increases. The amputee

eventually becomes familiar with the unique manner in which their phantom sensation or pain will present with respect to onset, type of sensation, duration, intensity, and effect of treatment.

Before the 1960s, many amputees were reluctant to describe their phantom sensation or pain for fear that they would lose their physician's confidence. However, current literature suggests that these phenomena and their symptoms are independent of age, sex, race, cause of amputation, health status, or psychological profile.[39] As a result, the suggestion that particular personalities or "types" of patients are more prone to complain of phantom sensation or pain is no longer an accepted theory. Moreover, many practitioners are now adopting the regular practice of discussing the occurrence of phantom sensation or pain prior to or immediately after amputation to reassure the amputee that these feelings are totally normal and expected. Unfortunately, there are still no universally accepted explanations of the cause(s) of a phantom sensation or pain. Multiple theories exist, but their review is beyond the scope of this chapter. Clinically, the ability to compare and contrast the three forms of adverse sensation is presumably of more importance and will be briefly presented.

Phantom Sensation

Phantom sensation is defined as a nonpainful awareness that gives form to a body part with specific dimensions, weight, or range of motion. Phantom sensation is more frequently described than is phantom pain. Jensen and colleagues identified three categories of phantom sensation: (1) kinesthetic sensations that give rise to impressions of postural changes, length, and volume of the residual limb; (2) kinetic sensations described as the perception of willed, spontaneous, or associated movements; and (3) exteroceptive sensations such as touch, temperature, pressure, and other more commonly experienced sensations that are not painful in nature (wetness, itching, fatigue, and generalized discomfort).[42] Researchers have estimated that virtually all[43] or a very high percentage of amputees (80%)[41] experience phantom limb sensation, the frequency and duration of the sensation declining with time.[44]

Phantom Pain

Phantom pain is a noxious sensation experienced within the nonexistent amputated portion of the limb. Phantom pain differs from phantom sensation in that perceived sensations are indeed painful in nature and that most postural impressions place the limb in unnatural positions such as with the foot backwards or the leg twisted. Researchers have been able to define the characteristics of phantom pain in terms of onset, frequency, duration, intensity, and quality. The onset of phantom pain is early, typically just a few days following amputation,[41,44,45] and

TABLE 29-2   Physical Therapy Diabetic Amputee Limb Care Checklist

Topic Item	Date Completed
Skin Inspection Education	
Daily inspection of skin with mirror for difficult-to-see areas	
Attention to bony prominences, between toes, and scars	
Attention to problem areas	
Skin Care	
Daily cleansing techniques with mild, unscented soap	
Application of moisturizer	
Avoid hot water	
Minimize exposure to perspiration and wet weather	
Minimize exposure to extreme heat and cold	
Foot Care	
Toe deformity care (lamb's wool between toes)	
Clean, dry socks without elastic bands	
Extra-depth shoes with custom molded inserts	
Appropriate house slippers or shoes worn at all times in the home	
Never walk barefoot, especially on beaches, on hot surfaces, or at night in the home	
Assistance with nail and callus trimming (if patient is independent, have them use nail file for nails and pumice stone for corns and calluses; NO sharp implements)	
Friction Reduction	
Bed mobility, avoid excessive sound limb use	
Posture and positioning	
Transfer techniques	
Equal weight-bearing during standing and ambulation	
Ambulation turning techniques; avoid pivoting on sound foot	
Appropriate shoe wear with socks	
Residual Limb	
Skin inspection (same as above)	
Skin care (same as above)	
Positioning	
Prosthetic Care	
Sock regulation (correct ply, sock application, and maintain dry sock wear)	
Prosthetic wear schedule (discuss procedure if skin lesions appear)	
Daily socket cleansing	
Compression Therapy	
Wrapping or shrinker application techniques	
Precautionary signs (pain and swelling)	
Phantom Sensation and Pain	
Awareness and desensitization	
Support Group Participation	
Contact person and phone number	
Footwear	
Suggest purchase of two or three pairs of proper shoes for daily rotation of shoes	
Change shoes with perspiration or when wet and soiled.	
Methods of assessment to insure proper fit of shoes	
Inspect the inside of shoes daily for foreign objects.	
Inspect for excessive wear (sole wear, split in leather, holes, etc.)	
Wear dry cotton or wool socks without elastic bands.	
Wound Care	
Always follow prescribed treatment from your health care professional.	
Ensure that the dressing always remains dry and clean.	
Check for drainage of the wound into the sock or shoe; if this occurs, have the dressing changed.	
Take all prescribed medications and never alter the dosage without consulting your physician.	

Date item understood or mastered by amputee is signified in the "Date Completed" column.
Adapted from Clark and Gailey. From One Step Ahead: an integrated approach to lower extremity prosthetics and amputee rehabilitation. Course workbook. Advanced Rehabilitation Therapy, Inc., 1996. Used by permission.

is typically provoked by emotional stress, exposure to cold, and local irritation. Phantom limb pain tends to be intermittent or episodic, with only a few individuals reporting constant pain.[44–49] Phantom pain intensity is typically described as moderate in nature and has been described as dull aching, burning, knife-like stabbing, sticking, squeezing, electrical shocks, or the feeling that the limb is being pulled off.[50] Traumatic amputees may complain of pain that replicates the painful sensation experienced during the trauma. Long-standing pain from limb pathology prior to amputation may persist in the form of phantom pain after amputation.

Residual Limb Pain

Residual limb pain arises from a specific anatomic structure that can be identified within the residual limb. Some of the more common causes include an improperly fitting prosthesis, neuromas entrapped in scar, bone spurs, abnormal soft tissues, sympathetic pain, referred pain (radiculopathy, joint pain, myofascial pain), and residual limb changes (skin thinning, muscle atrophy, changes in blood flow, and insufficient nutrition).[39]

A wide variety of treatments for amputees who experience phantom sensation or pain has been used without consistent success. Sherman's survey of 8000 amputees found that only 7% benefited from their treatments and that there was no uniformity to the type of treatment.[50] It is important for the clinician to assure the amputee that phantom pain and sensation are very common and are experienced by most amputees for some time after amputation. The clinician must accurately assess the nature of the pain or sensation and then be open to trying a variety of therapies. Unfortunately, most treatments are not successful for any length of time. The most effective treatment, which should always be encouraged by the rehabilitation team, is the use of the prosthesis.

Desensitization

Postsurgically, many amputees experience skin hypersensitivity as a result of disruption of the neuromuscular system and associated edema. As wound compression techniques reduce edema, progressive desensitization of the residual limb frequently becomes necessary to assist in restoring normal sensation. The concept of this technique is to gradually introduce stronger stimuli to reduce the hyperirritability of the limb. Initially, for example, a soft material such as cotton cloth or lamb's wool is rubbed around the residual limb, gradually followed by coarser materials such as corduroy. The amputee should progress as quickly as possible to tapping with the hand, massage, and eventually, when the suture line is healed, applying pressure through the residual limb during transfers, mobility skills, and exercise. These measures will help to expedite the ability to wear the prosthesis.

Residual Limb Compression Methods

The early use of rigid or semirigid dressings, compression wrapping, or a shrinker sock can have a number of potentially positive effects for the residual limb: (1) decreased edema, (2) increased circulation, (3) assistance in proper shaping, (4) provision of skin protection, (5) reduction of redundant tissue, (6) decreased phantom limb sensation and/or pain, and (7) desensitization of the residual limb. Rigid dressings applied with the knee in extension will prevent knee flexion contractures and aid in greater confidence with early bed mobility by protecting the

wound from trauma.[35] In the case of transfemoral residual limbs, there may be some value in counteracting hip flexion/abduction contracture forces with specific compression wrapping techniques.

Controversy does exist around the use of traditional compression wrapping versus the use of residual limb shrinker socks. Currently, many institutions prefer commercial shrinkers for their ease of donning. Advocates of compression wrapping state that it provides more control over pressure gradients and tissue shaping.[51] Condie and colleagues found that both TTAs and TFAs using a shrinker sock within 10 days after amputation had a significantly reduced time from amputation to prosthetic casting compared to amputees using wrapping methods.[52] Moreover, even shorter times to prosthetic casting have been observed with TTAs receiving semirigid and rigid dressings.[51,52]

Many teams prefer to wait until the sutures or staples have been removed before using a shrinker sock. In the case of diabetic amputees, this period can often be as long as 21 days. In this case, compression therapy can begin at the conclusion of surgery with a wrap or a rigid dressing and progress to a shrinker after the suture line has healed. This is a controversial area, and each rehabilitation team should determine the best course for its respective clients. All compression techniques must be performed correctly and in a consistent manner to prevent constriction of circulation with distal edema and poor residual limb shaping. Patient compliance is considered essential to an effective compression program. All wrappings or shrinker socks must be routinely checked and reapplied, if necessary, several times per day. Furthermore, the application of a nylon sheath over the residual limb prior to wrapping or donning a shrinker sock can reduce shear forces to the skin and provide additional comfort.

Long-Term Limb Management for the Diabetic Amputee

Sound Limb Issues

In planning a treatment program for the diabetic amputee, long-term management of the sound limb plays an important role. Preservation of the sound but neuropathic limb, in many cases, permits continued bipedal ambulation and delays further medical complications that can reduce the quality of life. A major problem is that the sound limb routinely compensates for the new amputee's inability to maintain equal weight distribution between limbs, resulting in altered gait mechanics with two effects on the nonamputated limb. The first is the alteration of forces on the weight-bearing surfaces of the foot; the second is the change in ground reaction forces passing upward through the skeletal structures of the limb. Increased forces placed on the intact limb can be of considerable concern during ambulation, since the foot has most often lost protective sensation and is therefore vulnerable to soft tissue injury brought about by the altered biomechanics.

The overall gait pattern of the neuropathic diabetic is tentative as a result of feeling insecure during standing and walking.[53] This conservative walking style is characteristically the product of poor proprioception, diminished sensory information, and an overall lack of stability resulting in a reduction of velocity and stride length with an altered displacement of forces.[54] Nonamputee diabetic persons with peripheral neuropathy demonstrate alterations in foot biomechanics that can increase peak foot pressures, facilitating foot injuries or ulceration, and it is believed that most of these ulcers develop during walking.[55–57] In some cases, a shuffling gait is adopted that, while reducing peak foot pressures by distributing applied forces over a greater area, will cause increased fatigue from this inefficient gait pattern.[5]

Fifty percent of diabetic nonamputees will develop contralateral foot infections, putting them at risk of amputation within 2 years.[58,59] Therefore, the clinician working with a diabetic amputee must be alerted to the potential of complications that can arise with the nonamputated foot. The term *sound limb* can be very misleading. In fact, it is probably just a twist of fate that one foot became infected before the other and thus only a matter of time before problems begin to arise with the contralateral limb if the patient does not take extreme care. The odds are certainly working against the patient, especially if any deformity of the contralateral foot is present as the amputee learns to use a prosthesis.

Because the diabetic amputee with neuropathy will often avoid full weight-bearing through the prosthesis, the contralateral limb must accept a greater proportion of body weight. Specifically, there is an increase of ground reaction forces at anatomic heel contact, comparatively decreased midstance time, and rapid and significantly increased ground reaction forces during terminal stance as the foot rolls over the metatarsal heads.[60,61] In the case of great toe amputation, as with so many diabetic patients, peak foot pressures become significantly higher under the first metatarsal head, lesser metatarsal heads, and toes.[6] Unfortunately, if not closely monitored, this can lead to ulceration and infection or possible amputation.

Serroussi and colleagues demonstrated that the amputee's intact ankle works about 33% more than a normal ankle does during terminal stance.[62] The increased work of the sound limb during terminal stance might be a compensatory mechanism for the lack of push-off by the prosthetic foot or might provide additional stability needed during double support as the prosthetic limb enters stance phase. Additionally, the intact limb has a significantly longer period of stance phase support than the prosthetic limb,[63] with greater hip extensor work during early stance[60,62] further com-

pounding the forces placed on the plantar surface of the sound foot. Moreover, it has been shown that the loss of subtalar joint motion in an insensate foot can result in higher foot pressures and has the potential to lead to ulceration in the nonamputee diabetic.[64,65] Consequently, it is important for clinicians to be aware that the increased work at the hip and ankle coupled with potentially limited ankle joint mobility of the sound limb can have a tremendous impact on the ground reaction forces exerted on the plantar surface of the intact forefoot during the stance phase of gait. The combination of additional vertical and shear forces placed on the intact foot and the increased possibility of disproportionate weight-bearing can result in skin ulcers and/or Charcot joint degeneration in the diabetic amputee. Therefore, rehabilitation must include educational measures designed to reduce the risks of skin ulceration and additional degeneration of the sound limb.

The loss of a limb and its replacement with a prosthetic device clearly affect gait biomechanics in most diabetic amputees. There are deviations from normal gait kinematics that add increased vertical and shear forces to preexisting diminished sensation, devascularization, scar tissue, and any foot and/or ankle deformity. Collectively, this represents a dire combination not only for the limb, but also for the patient's general health. This is manifested by the 50% increased incidence of amputation in the same or contralateral limb within 4 years after the primary amputation.[58,66–68] Without hesitation, the patient should be made aware of these impending dangers as rehabilitation is begun. Accordingly, care of the remaining foot becomes even more critical after amputation for the diabetic because the chance of achieving functional ambulation as a bilateral amputee will decline.

Residual Limb Issues

Every diabetic patient should be instructed to visually inspect the residual limb as well as the sound foot on a daily basis or after any strenuous activity. The residual limb is inspected to reveal inflamed or abraded areas that would indicate abnormal pressure or shear from the socket. Inspection of the sound limb has greater importance after amputation, since additional axial and shear forces, as described above, will be experienced by the foot in compensation for prosthetic weight-bearing adjustment. More frequent inspection of both limbs should be performed in the initial months of prosthetic training. A hand mirror can be used to view the posterior residual limb and plantar foot. Reddened areas should be monitored very closely as potential sites for abrasions. Amputees with visual impairment should seek the assistance of a family member for daily inspections. If a skin abrasion occurs, the amputee must understand that in almost all cases, the prosthesis should not be worn until healing occurs. Occasionally, a protective barrier can be used to avert further insult to the integrity of the tissue while permitting continued use of the prosthesis. In all cases, however, any lesion of the skin should be reported and followed clinically to avoid further complications.

With regard to the residual limb, the amputee must understand that the care of skin and scar tissue is extremely important to prevent breakdown during prosthetic rehabilitation. This routine preventive care is essential for two reasons: because the healing time of skin lesions is usually increased for the diabetic population and because inability to wear the prosthesis during skin healing will delay prosthetic rehabilitation and lead to further deconditioning. Therefore, the patient must be orientated to the proper fit of the socket and be taught the difference between weight-bearing and pressure-sensitive areas.

Prosthetic Management

Prescription of prosthetic components has become a very complex and subjective topic. There are literally hundreds of combinations of components in considering suspension devices, socket designs, knee systems, and foot-ankle assemblies. Suspension methods have advanced considerably from straps, cuffs, and simple suction to include roll-on sleeve designs, more complex suction approaches, and a wide variety of liner/suspension combinations. Socket designs have expanded tremendously to improve muscular function, suspension methods, and comfort. Knee units have become lighter, with improved durability, better performance, and greater stability. Lighter-weight foot-ankle assemblies with more dynamic foot keels have provided amputees with greater mobility on varied terrain and have improved performance during higher-level activities. Rotators, shock absorbers, and more versatile coupling systems offer additional options with improved overall comfort and function of the finished prosthesis. Most of these advances have been the result of introducing a wider variety of materials to the field of prosthetics. The prosthetic technology revolution was instigated by amputee clients who were no longer complacently accepting outdated technology and by the concerted efforts of prosthetists and manufacturers worldwide.

To adequately cover the subject of prosthetic components in this chapter would be impossible, while reducing the information to its most basic level would be an injustice to the developments within the profession. Fortunately, there is an excellent current resource that explains in detail specific components, their designs, and their functions.[14] For these reasons, the information presented here will be directed toward the components that affect the protection of the skin and toward the management of the residual limb and prosthetic gait training and are designed to prevent further injury of the residual and intact limbs, especially in regard to the diabetic/dysvascular amputee.

Some might argue that even though many advances have been made in the field of prosthetics, the latest technology is focused on the younger, more active traumatic amputee and not the older diabetic/dysvascular amputee. However, the geriatric population has benefited tremendously from advances first utilized by younger traumatic amputees and as a result now enjoys more comfortable and better-functioning prosthetic devices. Currently, the prescription of newer prosthetic designs is, in many cases, just as appropriate for the older amputee as for their younger counterparts. The selection of more sophisticated components for senior amputees, however, must be based solely on improvement of their function.

Socket Care

The socket should be cleaned daily to promote good skin hygiene and to prevent deterioration of prosthetic materials. As a rule, plastic laminate, copolymer plastic, and silicone materials are cleaned with a mild soap on a damp cloth, while foam materials are cleansed with rubbing alcohol. After use of the cleansing agent, a clean damp cloth should be used to wipe away any residue. To ensure the maximum life and safety of the prosthesis, patients are reminded that its routine maintenance should be performed by their prosthetist.

Sock Regulation and Suspension Sleeve Use

Sock regulation is of extreme importance to ensure a properly fitting socket. The patient should carry extra socks at all times to add if "pistoning" occurs or for a change of socks in case of extreme perspiration. The correct number of sock plies is emphasized to prevent excessive pressures from damaging skin or underlying soft tissues. A thin nylon sheath covering the residual limb will assist in reducing friction at the residual limb/socket interface. Socks are available in assorted plies or thicknesses, permitting the patient to obtain the desired fit within the socket. Socks should be applied wrinkle-free with the seam horizontal and on the outside to prevent additional irritation to the skin. Many suppliers now offer seamless socks to eliminate this problem.

Recently, the use of silicone suspension sleeves and gel liners has gained widespread acceptance and use. Some of the benefits of suspension sleeves are reduced pistoning, better management of unstable limb volume, improved cosmetic appearance, and, in some cases, easier donning of the prosthesis for those with impaired hand function. Frequently, gel liners can be used for suspension in addition to their primary function of reducing shear forces over scarred areas and bony prominences.

Internal suspension sleeves and roll-on liners are widely accepted, but some amputees have problems with skin reactions from the material used because some silicones and gels are not medical grade and therefore not hypoallergenic. Fortunately, a wide variety of materials is available if a problem becomes evident. For example, a nylon sheath can be used next to the skin beneath the sleeve or liner. Internal sleeves and roll-on liners are also categorized according to thickness or ply, and most sleeves allow the use of socks to adjust for volume changes. Lake and Supan found, through a survey of suspension sleeve users, that the low to moderately active amputee and the older diabetic/dysvascular amputee reported a lower incidence of perspiration, heat rash, and folliculitis; the latter amputees also have less trouble with contact dermatitis and residual limb soreness.[69] Although these differences were not statistically significant, they are worth noting. Another interesting finding was that the longer the amputee used a silicone suspension sleeve, the greater was the likelihood of dermatologic problems. In light of this study, it appears that silicone suction sleeves offer the diabetic/dysvascular amputee a better alternative to traditional suspension, with less risk of problems, than the younger traumatic amputee, who tends to wear the prosthesis for longer periods of time each day.[10]

Physical Conditioning in Preparation for a Prosthesis

General Conditioning

Encouraging activity as soon as possible after amputation surgery helps to speed recovery in several ways. First, it offsets the negative effects of immobility by promoting joint movement, muscle activity, and increased circulation. Second, the patient will begin to reestablish his or her independence, which might have been perceived as threatened by loss of the limb. Finally, the psychological advantage derived from activity and independence will affect the patient's motivational status throughout the rehabilitation process. Often, decreased general conditioning and cardiovascular endurance contribute to difficulties in learning functional activities, including prosthetic gait training. Regardless of age or physical condition, a progressive general exercise prescription can be designed for every patient. This begins immediately after surgery, continues throughout the preprosthetic period, and is incorporated into the amputee's daily routine thereafter.

The list of possible general strengthening/endurance exercise activities is vast: cuff weights in bed, dynamic stump exercises, resistive band exercises, wheelchair propulsion for a predetermined distance, ambulation with an assistive device prior to fitting of the prosthesis, lower- or upper-limb ergonometry, wheelchair aerobics, swimming, aquatic therapy, lower- and upper-body strengthening at the local fitness center, and any sport or recreational activity of interest. The amputee should select one or more of these activities and begin participation to tolerance, progressing to a minimum of 30 minutes of moderate activity 5 or more days a week or 20 to 60 minutes of vigorous activity 3 or more days a week.[70] The advantages of participation extend well beyond improving the chances of ambulating well with a prosthesis. The individual has the opportunity to experience and enjoy activities probably not thought possible. If difficulties are experienced, the amputee is still within an environment in which assistance can be readily obtained, either from the therapist or from a fellow amputee who has mastered a particular activity.

Prevention of decreased joint range of motion (ROM) is a major concern for all involved. Limited ROM can often result in difficulties with prosthetic fit, gait deviations, or the ability to ambulate with a prosthesis altogether. The best way to prevent loss of ROM is to remain active and ensure full ROM of affected joints. A daily stretching program, as part of general fitness, can be of substantial benefit in preparation for a prosthesis. Eisert and Tester first described dynamic stump exercises in 1954.[71] Since then, their antigravity exercises have been the most favored method of strengthening the residual limb. Dynamic stump exercises require little in the way of equipment; a towel roll and a step stool are the only requirements. These exercises offer additional benefits aside from strengthening, such as desensitization, bed mobility, and joint ROM. Incorporating isometric contractions at the peak of the isotonic movement will help to maximize strength increases.[72] All amputees should also consider performing abdominal and back extensor strengthening exercises to maintain trunk strength, decrease the possible risk of back pain, and assist in the reduction of gait deviations associated with the trunk. The strengthening of the trunk and pelvic musculature can best be achieved by stabilization or dynamic closed kinetic chain exercises performed with a Swiss ball or some other compliant surface in conjunction with other strengthening exercises.[73]

Amputees who have access to a wellness center with isotonic equipment can take advantage of the benefits derived from these forms of strengthening with just a few modifications in body positioning on the weight machines. A major advantage to participating at a supervised exercise facility is that the amputee is creating a healthy exercise habit. But more important, participating in an aerobic and resistant exercise program, known as circuit training, can significantly improve the health of a diabetic. Studies have demonstrated that an 8- to 16-week circuit training program implemented by individuals with type 2 diabetes mellitus increases muscular strength, peak oxygen uptake, and high-density lipoprotein levels.

The program also decreases HbA1C and fasting serum glucose levels, insulin sensitivity, and percent of body fat.[74-81] If the diabetic amputee is introduced to the benefits of regular exercise during rehabilitation and makes it a lifelong practice, the secondary rewards that are achieved can reduce a variety of complications associated with inactivity.

Prosthetic Gait Training

The need to know the specific gait-training protocol or treatments is probably not necessary for the majority of clinicians, with the exception of the physical therapist. There is a need nonetheless for the members of the rehabilitation team who are involved in assessing gait, primarily the physician and the prosthetist, to understand the specific limitations or deviations that could have an adverse affect on the residual and sound limbs. The following are selected deviations that are commonly observed in amputees, their effect on gait, and corrective measures. If deviations are not rectified, there exists a greater opportunity for the amputee to fall short of reaching his or her full ambulatory potential, regardless of age.

Standing Balance

With the loss of a limb, the decrease in body weight will alter the body's COM. To maintain the single-limb balance necessary during stance without the prosthesis and ambulating with an assistive device or single-limb hopping, the amputee will shift the COM over his or her base of support (BOS), which is the foot of the sound limb. However, the amputee must learn to maintain the COM, and thus the body's weight, equally over the prosthesis and the sound limb to maintain the COM at midline during bipedal standing and ambulation activities. Various types of proprioceptive and visual feedback can be employed to promote the amputee's ability to maximize the displacement of the COM over the BOS. The amputee must learn to displace the COM in all directions to maintain balance during dynamic activities such as walking.

Furthermore, with the nonamputee neuropathic diabetic, Courtemanche illustrated nicely that a deterioration of the peripheral sensory system could produce gait and balance problems because of increasing attentional demands for postural tasks.[82] The diabetic neuropathic patient feels less safe during standing and walking; as a result, fear of falling and the associated lack of confidence alter postural control and gait behavior.[83,84] The neuropathic amputee must be permitted early in gait training to reorganize his or her postural strategies and adapt to the prosthetic limb in the pseudostatic task of standing prior to accepting the overwhelming dynamic act of walking. If the amputee is prematurely forced into an insecure walking setting, the amputee's fear will frequently curtail progress and might result in failure to reach their ambulation potential.

Single-Limb Standing Balance

Weight acceptance onto the prosthesis is one of the most difficult challenges facing the amputee. Without the ability to maintain full single-limb weight-bearing and balance on the prosthesis for an adequate amount of time (0.5 second minimum), the amputee may exhibit a number of gait deviations, including (1) decreased stance time on the prosthetic side resulting in a faster step with the intact limb, which will then strike the floor at an accelerated speed, thus increasing shear and direct forces; (2) a shortened stride length on the sound side; or (3) lateral trunk bending over the prosthetic limb. More important for the diabetic/dysvascular amputee, as his or her confidence in balancing over the prosthetic limb increases, the forces placed on the sound limb will decrease as the weight is shared between the limbs.

The amputee's ability to control sound limb advancement during walking is directly related to the ability to control prosthetic limb stance. The following are three learned tasks that will help the amputee to achieve adequate balance over the prosthetic limb. The first is muscular control of the residual limb sufficient to maintain balance over the prosthesis. The second is utilizing the available sensation at the residual limb/socket interface, such as proprioception, to control the prosthesis. Simultaneously, the amputee must also begin to appreciate the amount of force or pressure that must be experienced at the residual limb/socket interface to achieve a functional gait pattern. For most, this pressure is far greater than they imagined. Third, the amputee must envision the prosthetic foot and its relationship to the ground and therefore develop a sense of where the body weight is in relationship to the prosthetic foot.[72]

Gait-Training Skills

Prosthetic developments over the last two decades have resulted in limbs that closely replicate the mechanics of the human leg. Therefore, the goal of gait training should be restoration of function to the remaining joints of the amputated limb. Prosthetic gait training should not alter the amputee's gait mechanics for the prosthesis; instead, the mechanics of the prosthesis should be designed around the amputee's individual gait. For the majority of amputees, if pelvic and trunk movements can be returned to their premorbid level of function, the ability of the prosthetic limb to provide stability during the stance phase and to advance naturally during the swing phase of gait should require very little effort. However, understanding the role of the pelvis and trunk in controlling COM over BOS and thus providing balance with functional movement patterns is essential. The pelvis and the body's COM move as a unit in four directional manners: vertical displacement, lateral shift, horizontal tilt, and transverse rotation. Each of these motions can directly affect the amputee's gait, resulting in gait deviations with a concomitant rise in energy consumption during ambulation. If restoration of function to the remaining joints of the amputated limb is one goal of gait training, then pelvic motions play a decisive role in determining the final outcome of an individual's gait pattern.

Vertical Displacement

Vertical displacement is simply the rhythmic upward and downward motion of the body's COM, with the knee flexing 10 to 15 degrees during loading response[12] and extending during midstance. The TTA retains the ability to flex and extend the knee during the stance phase of gait. The TFA, unfortunately, is at a disadvantage, as the knee must remain in extension throughout the entire stance phase to avoid buckling (collapsing). Some theoretical evidence suggests that stance phase knee flexion does not appreciably alter the amount of vertical displacement during normal walking.[85]

Lateral Shift

During lateral shift, the pelvis moves from side to side approximately 5 cm. The amount of lateral shift is determined by the width of the BOS, which is 5 to 10 cm, depending on the individual's height.[12] Because amputees have to spend an inordinate amount of time standing on the sound limb, as when they are on crutches, hopping without the prosthesis, or standing in a relaxed manner, they are adept at maintaining COM over the sound limb and therefore have a habit of crossing the midline with the sound foot. Often, adequate space is not available for the prosthetic limb to follow a natural line of progression. The result is an abducted or circumducted gait with an increase in lateral displacement of the pelvis toward the prosthetic side. Most frequently, this is observed in TFAs; however, this altered BOS may also be seen with TTAs.

The consequence of this deviation was discussed above; however, the importance of reducing the torsional forces to the joints of the limb must not be ignored. By simply reestablishing the position of the sound limb during initial contact and throughout the stance phase, improved balance with less stress to the sound foot and limb can be achieved.

Horizontal Tilt

Horizontal tilt of the pelvis is normal up to 5 degrees. Weak hip abductor muscles, specifically the gluteus medius, have been identified as the primary cause of excessive pelvic tilt. Maintenance of the residual femur in adduction via the socket theoretically places the gluteus medius at its optimal length/tension ratio. However, if the limb is in an abducted position in the socket, the muscle is placed in a compromised position and is unable to function properly. The result is a compensatory gait, in which the trunk leans laterally over the prosthetic limb in an attempt to maintain the body's COM over the BOS.

TFAs also walk with a slightly abducted gait, using the prosthesis as a strut, thus decreasing the need for muscular effort to control the pelvis. Because the gluteus medius and gluteus minimus are intact, greater pelvic stability should be possible, since only the tensor fascia latae is lost in TFAs, although adductor power is frequently greatly diminished. However, many amputees of all levels have difficulty maintaining their pelvis in a horizontal position. Therefore, effective gait training should include educating the hip musculature to contract at a more rapid rate to control for sway. For the neuropathic diabetic amputee who already has a significant loss of sensory feedback from the intact limb, this form of training undoubtedly has even greater significance.

Transverse Rotation

Transverse rotation of the pelvis occurs around the body's longitudinal axis approximately 5 to 10 degrees to either side.[12] This rotation assists in shifting the body's COM from one limb to the other, as well as providing adequate step length. In addition, it helps to initiate the 30 degrees of knee flexion of the trailing limb that is seen during toe off, which is necessary to achieve 60 degrees of knee flexion during the acceleration phase of swing. Knee flexion during toe off is also augmented by plantar flexion of the foot, horizontal tilt of the pelvis, and gravity. No prosthetic foot provides active plantar flexion during terminal stance, and since horizontal tilt greater than 5 degrees is abnormal, restoration of transverse rotation of the pelvis becomes of great importance in order to obtain sufficient knee flexion. Another benefit to the restoration of pelvic rotation is the chance that the work and plantar peak pressures produced by the contralateral ankle and foot could be reduced. For the insensate foot, prone to ulceration, this could be of great value not only in reducing pressures, but also in reducing the effort required to walk.

There is a wide variety of training techniques that the physical therapist can use to restore normal pelvic and lower-limb biomechanics. Resistive gait-training methods assist in facilitating appropriate movements, strength, and timing. Normalization of trunk, pelvic, and limb biomechanics should, however, be taught to the amputee in a systematic way.[72] First, independent movements of the various joint and muscle groups are developed. Second, these independent movements are incorporated into the functional movement patterns of the gait cycle. Finally, all component movement patterns are integrated to produce a smooth normalized gait.[72]

Maintenance of equal stride length might not be immediately forthcoming, as many amputees have a tendency to take a longer step with the prosthetic limb than with the sound limb.[60] When adequate weight-bearing through the prosthetic limb has been achieved, the amputee will have the ability to maintain equal stride length. One technique to promote equality in stride length is to have the amputee take longer steps with the sound limb and slightly shorter steps with the prosthetic limb. This principle also applies in increasing cadence.

Normal cadence is considered to be 90 to 120 steps per minute, or 2.5 to 3.0 miles per hour.[86] Arm swing, which is the result of trunk rotation in opposition to pelvic rotation, provides balance, momentum, and symmetry of gait and is directly influenced by the speed of ambulation.[87] As the speed of walking increases, so does the amplitude of arm swing, thus permitting a more efficient gait. Amputees who walk at slower speeds will demonstrate a diminished arm swing, especially on the prosthetic side. Restoring trunk rotation and arm swing is easily accomplished by utilizing a variety of gait-training techniques, such as manually guiding the trunk as the amputee ambulates.

Both amputees who will be independent ambulators and those who will require an assistive device can benefit to varying degrees from the above systematic rehabilitation program. Most patients can progress to the point of ambulating outside the parallel bars. At that time, the amputee must practice walking with the chosen assistive device, maintaining pelvic rotation, adequate BOS, equal stance time, and equal stride length, all of which can have a direct influence on the energy cost of walking. Trunk rotation will be absent with amputees who use a walker as an assistive device; however, those who ambulate with crutches or a cane should be able to incorporate trunk rotation into their gait pattern.

Considering the special needs of every individual patient, the therapist should design a customized program to meet the needs of each amputee. In many cases, the amputation will be only one of many comorbidities for which the patient is being treated. The clinician or patient must not internalize frustration over the delays in prosthetic rehabilitation that occur while adequate time for urgent treatment of other, more serious conditions is allowed. However, the amount of physical deconditioning that can occur during this time can be devastating. For this reason, the clinician must keep focused on the amputee's overall progress and realize that the amputation may be a life-saving procedure because of other anatomic system failures. Once the health status of the patient improves, then and only then can a successful prosthetic rehabilitation program begin.

Summary

It is important for the clinician to remember that age can influence the amputee's ability to ambulate with a prosthesis, just as age influences the gait of nonamputee ambulators. This is not to say that age alone dictates an amputee's capabilities. On the contrary, level of activity prior to amputation has a greater influence on rehabilitation outcome than does age, level of amputation, or number of limbs involved.[30,32,88–91] Therefore, it is wrong

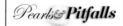

Pearls

- In general, the greater the length of residual limb maintained during amputation surgery, the less the metabolic cost of walking, with the potential for decreased rehabilitation time.
- Proper bed positioning and bed mobility training are imperative to prevent hip and/or knee flexion contractures, ulcer formation, and deconditioning in the diabetic amputee.
- Core stability exercises, focusing primarily on pelvic and trunk musculature, may improve sitting and standing posture, dynamic balance, and ambulation with a prosthesis.
- Well-designed rehabilitation and prosthetic interventions may increase overall function, prosthesis use, and social integration.
- Functional activities such as sit to stand, transfers, and household ambulation are the minimal skills required that allow diabetic amputees to return home by decreasing their need for assistance from family members and helping to maintain acceptable levels of independence.
- Circuit training, combining aerobic and resistance exercises, can produce demonstrable increases in muscular strength, peak oxygen uptake, and high-density lipoprotein levels. It has also been shown to decrease HbA1C levels, fasting serum glucose levels, insulin resistance, and percent of body fat.
- Regular clinic visits, patient education, and proper footwear can reduce the incidence of amputation of the diabetic/dysvascular amputee's sound foot.
- Functional outcomes are largely dependent on the patient's activity level prior to amputation.

Pitfalls

- Complications associated with advanced diabetes, deconditioning prior to amputation, long periods of inactivity, and delays in prosthetic fitting can limit the amputee's potential to be a successful prosthetic ambulator.
- Lack of collaboration among the surgeon, prosthetist, and physical therapist in planning the surgical, prosthetic, and therapeutic interventions can negatively affect the functional outcome of the diabetic amputee.
- An inappropriate postoperative dressing for the diabetic amputee can decrease bed mobility, increase the risk of cardiopulmonary complications and soft tissue damage, and fail to prevent flexion contractures at either the hip or the knee.
- Following amputation, the sound limb becomes vulnerable to soft tissue injuries due to the increased forces placed on it. Educating the diabetic amputee to distribute weight equally through both lower limbs thus becomes a vital aspect of their prosthetic rehabilitation.
- Clinicians can easily fall prey to discriminating against the older diabetic amputee regarding the prescription of appropriate prosthetic componentry. The geriatric amputee can often benefit greatly from the same prosthetic components prescribed for the young traumatic amputee, with a focus on improving function.
- Failure to provide adequate prosthetic gait training for the diabetic amputee can lead to chronic issues such as postural changes, gait abnormalities, and fear of falling, which will impede the diabetic amputee's ambulation and overall functional potential.

to predetermine the outcome of the amputee based only on the information found in a chart. An individual's motivation and character play a far greater role in determining the final result.

Since the diabetic/dysvascular amputee may have the same rehabilitation potential as the nondysvascular amputee of the same age, preconceived bias must be eliminated prior to the clinician's initial assessment. The key to improving quality of life and preventing further injury is to protect the intact foot and limb by teaching the amputee to become reliant on the prosthetic limb. The rehabilitation team must stress the need for compliance with the program and further emphasize the need for participation in follow-up foot and postamputation clinics and health care appointments. The process of prosthetic gait training must include the same gait principles that are taught to other amputees, with recognition that the comorbidities associated with the diabetic patient may result in some delays during convalescence, requiring variations in the progression of treatment. The key to success with the diabetic amputee is teamwork, which includes a meaningful educational program for the patient and family. If the diabetic amputee is willing to participate fully in his or her own rehabilitation program, the potential for once again being a productive member of society will increase tremendously.

References

1. U.S. Department of Health and Human Services: Vital and Health Statistics: Detail Diagnosis and Procedures. Hyattsville, MD: Public Health Service, Centers for Disease Control, National Center for Health Statistics, 1993.
2. American Diabetes Association: 1991 Fact Sheet on Diabetes. Alexandria, VA: American Diabetes Association, 1991.
3. Armstrong DG, Lavery LA, Harkless LB, Van Houtum WH: Amputation and re-amputation of the diabetic foot. J Amer Pod Med Assoc 87:255–259, 1997.
4. Centers for Disease Control and Prevention: National Diabetes Fact Sheet: United States, 2005. http://www.cdc.gov/diabetes/pubs/factsheet.htm. Accessed February 10, 2006.
5. Lavery LA: Epidemiology and prevention of diabetic foot disease. In Frykberg RG (ed): The High Risk Foot in Diabetes Mellitus. New York: Churchill Livingstone, 1991.
6. Lavery LA, Lavery DC, Quebedeax TL: Increased foot pressures after great toe amputation in diabetes. Diabetes Care 18:1460–1462, 1995.
7. Most RS, Sinnock P: The epidemiology of lower extremity amputations in diabetic individuals. Diabetes Care 6:87–91, 1983.
8. Gordois A, Scuffham P, Shearer A, et al: The health care costs of diabetic peripheral neuropathy in the US. Diabetes Care 26:1790–1795, 2003.
9. Larsson J, Agadh CD, Apelqvist J, Stenström A: Long term prognosis after healed amputation in patients with diabetes. Clin Orthopaed Rel Res 350:149–157, 1998.
10. Pinzur MS, Gottschalk F, Smith D, et al: Functional outcome of below-knee amputation in peripheral vascular insufficiency: A multi-center review. Clin Orthop 286:247–249, 1993.
11. Pinzur MS, Gold J, Schwartz D, et al: Energy demands for walking in dysvascular amputees as a result of the level of amputation. Orthopedics 15:1033–1036, 1992.
12. Perry J: Gait Analysis: Normal and Pathological Function. Thorofare, NJ: SLACK, 1992.
13. Waters RL, Perry J, Antonelli D, Hislop H: The energy cost of walking of amputees: Influence of level amputation. J Bone Joint Surg 58(A):42–46, 1976.
14. Smith DG, Michael JW, Bowker JH: Atlas of Amputations and Limb Deficiencies, 3rd ed. Rosemont, IL: American Academy of Orthopaedic Surgeons, 2004.
15. Gailey RS, Wenger MA, Raya M, et al: Energy expenditure of transtibial amputees during ambulation at self-selected pace. Prosthet Orthot Int 18:84–91, 1994.
16. Sanders GT: Lower Limb Amputation: A Guide to Rehabilitation. Philadelphia: FA Davis, 1986.
17. Volpicelli LJ, Chambers RB, Wagner FW Jr: Ambulation levels of bilateral lower-extremity amputees: Analysis of one hundred and three cases. J Bone Joint Surg Am 65:599–605, 1983.
18. Hoffman MD, Sheldahl LM, Buley KJ, Sandford PR: Physiological comparison of walking among bilateral above-knee amputee and able-bodied subjects, and a model to account for the differences in metabolic cost. Arch Phys Med Rehabil 78:385–392, 1997.
19. DuBow LL, Witt PL, Kadaba MP, Reyes R, Cochran V et al: Oxygen consumption of elderly persons with bilateral below knee amputations: Ambulation vs. wheelchair propulsion. Arch Phys Med Rehabil 64:255–259, 1983.
20. Malone JM, Snyder M, Anderson G, et al: Prevention of amputation by diabetic education. Am J Surg 158:520–523, 1989.
21. Fisher SV, Patterson RP: Energy cost of ambulation with crutches. Arch Phys Med Rehabil 62:250–256, 1981.
22. Pagliarulo MA, Waters R, Hislop HJ: Energy cost of walking of below-knee amputees having no vascular disease. Phys Ther 59:538–543, 1979.
23. Lehmann JF, Price R, Boswell-Bessette S, et al: Comprehensive analysis of energy storing prosthetic feet: Flex foot and Seattle foot versus standard SACH foot. Arch Phys Med Rehabil 74:1225–1231, 1993.
24. Perry J, Shanfield S: Efficiency of dynamic elastic response prosthetic feet. J Rehabil Res Dev 30:137–143, 1993.
25. Gailey R, Lawrence D, Burditt C, et al: Comparison of metabolic cost during ambulation between the contoured adducted trochanteric-controlled alignment method and the quadrilateral socket. Prosthet Orthot Int 17:95–106, 1993.
26. Gailey R, Nash M., Atchley T, et al: The effects of prosthesis weight on metabolic cost of ambulation in non-vascular trans-tibial amputees. Prosthet Orthot Int 21:9–15, 1997.
27. Czerniecki JM, Gitter A, Weaver K: Effect of alterations in prosthetic shank mass on the metabolic costs of ambulation in above-knee amputees. Am J Phys Med Rehabil 73:348–52, 1994.
28. Gitter A, Czerniecki J, Meinders M: Effect of prosthetic mass on swing phase work during above-knee amputee ambulation. Am J Phys Med Rehabil 76:114–121, 1997.
29. Gitter A, Czerniecki J, Weaver K: A reassessment of center-of-mass dynamics as a determinate of the metabolic inefficiency of above-knee amputee ambulation. Am J Phys Med Rehabil 74:332–338, 1995.
30. Brodzka WK, Thornhill HL, Zarapkar SE, et al: Long term function of persons with atherosclerotic bilateral below-knee amputation living in the inner city. Arch Phys Med Rehab 71:898–900, 1990.
31. Gailey RS: Recreational pursuits of elders with amputation. Topics Geriatric Rehab 8:39–58, 1992.
32. Medhat A, Huber PM, Medhat MA: Factors that influence the level of activities in persons with lower extremity amputation. Rehab Nursing 13:13–18, 1990.
33. Amputee Coalition of America: You Don't Have to Deal with Amputation Alone: Special Report on the ACA's National Peer Network. http://www.amputee-coalition.org/inmotion/nov-de04/deal_alone.html. Accessed February 10, 2006.
34. Smith DG, McFarland LV, Sangeorzan BJ, et al: Postoperative dressing and management strategies for transtibial amputation: Critical review. J Rehabil Res Dev 40:213–224, 2003.
35. Burgess EM: Immediate postsurgical prosthetic fitting: A system of amputee management. Phys Ther 51:139–143, 1971.
36. Wu Y, Keagy RD, Krick HJ, et al: An innovative removable rigid dressing technique for below-the-knee amputation. J Bone Joint Surg 61:724–729, 1979.
37. Schon LC, Short KW, Soupiou O, J et al: Benefits of early prosthetic management of transtibial amputees: A prospective clinical study of a prefabricated prosthesis. Foot Ankle Int 23:509–514, 2002.
38. Gailey RS, Clark CR: Physical therapy. In Smith DG, Michael JW, Bowker JH: Atlas of Amputation and Limb Deficiencies: Surgical, Prosthetic, and Rehabilitation Principles, 3rd ed. Rosemont, IL: American Academy of Orthopaedic Surgeon, 2004, pp 589–619.

39. Davis RW: Phantom sensation, phantom pain, and stump pain. Arch Phys Med Rehab 74:79–91, 1993.

40. Gard SA, Childress DS: The effect of pelvic list on the vertical displacement of the trunk during walking. Gait Posture 5:233–238, 1997.

41. Jensen TS, Krebs B, Nielsen J, Rasmussen P: Phantom limb, phantom pain and stump pain in amputees during the first 6 months following limb amputation. Pain 17:243–256, 1983.

42. Jensen TS, Krebs B, Nielsen J, Rasmussen P: Non-painful phantom limb phenomena in amputees: Incidence, clinical characteristics and temporal course. Acta Neurol Scand 70:407–414, 1984.

43. Loeser JD: Pain after amputation: Phantom limb pain and stump pain. In Bonica J (ed): The Management of Pain. London: Churchill Livingstone, 1994, pp 224–256.

44. Smith DG, Ehde DM, Legro MW, et al: Phantom limb, residual limb, and back pain after lower extremity amputations. Clin Orthop 361:29–38, 1999.

45. Sherman RA: Phantom Pain. New York: Plenum Press, 1997, p 264.

46. Jensen MP, Turne JA, Romano JM, Karoly P: Coping with chronic pain: A critical review of the literature. Pain 47:249–283, 1991.

47. Jensen TS, Krebs B, Nielsen J, Rasmussen P: Immediate and long term phantom pain in amputees: Incidence, clinical characteristics, and relationship to pre-ambulation limb pain. Pain 83–95, 1984.

48. Wartan SW, Hamann W, Wedley JR, McColl I: Phantom pain and sensation among British veteran amputees. Br J Anaesth 78:652–659, 1997.

49. Gallagher P, Allen D, Maclachlan M: Phantom limb pain and residual limb pain following lower limb amputation: A descriptive analysis. Disabil Rehabil 23:522–530, 2001.

50. Sherman RA: Stump and phantom limb pain. Neurol Clin 7:249–264, 1989.

51. May BJ: Stump bandaging of the lower extremity amputee. Phys Ther 44:808, 1964.

52. Condie E, Jones D, Treweek S, Scott H: A one-year national survey of patients having a lower limb amputation. Physiotherapy 82:14–20, 1996.

53. Cavanagh PR, Derr JA, Ulbrecht JS, et al: Problems with gait and posture in neuropathic patients with insulin dependent diabetes mellitus. Diabet Med 9:469–474, 1992.

54. Mueller MJ, Sinacore DR, Hoogstrate S, Daly L: Hip and ankle walking strategies: Effect on peak plantar pressures and implications for neuropathic ulceration. Arch Phys Med Rehabil 75:1196–1200, 1994.

55. Katoulis EC, Ebdon-Parry H, Vileikyte L, et al: Gait abnormalities in diabetic neuropathy. Diabetes Care 20:1904–1907, 1997.

56. Brand PW: The diabetic foot. In Ellenberg M, Rifkin H (eds): Diabetes Mellitus: Theory and Practice, 3rd ed. Hyde Park, NY: Medical Examination Publishing, 1983, pp 829–849.

57. Mueller MJ, Diamond JE, Delitto A, Sinacore DR: Insensitivity, limited joint mobility, and plantar ulcers in patients with diabetes mellitus. Phys Ther 69:453–462, 1989.

58. Ecker ML, Jacobs BS: Lower extremity amputations in diabetic patients. Diabetes 19:189–195, 1970.

59. Goldner MG: The fate of the second leg in the diabetic amputee. Diabetes 9:100, 1960.

60. Jaegers SMHJ, Arendzen JH, de Jongh HJ: Prosthetic gait of unilateral transfemoral amputees: A kinematic study. Arch Phys Med Rehabil 76:736–743, 1995.

61. Mueller MJ, Minor SD, Sahrmann SA, et al: Differences in gait characteristics of patients with diabetes and peripheral neuropathy compared with age-matched controls. Phys Ther 74:299–313, 1994.

62. Seroussi RE, Gitter A, Czerniecki JM, Weaver K: Mechanical work adaptations of above-knee amputee ambulation. Arch Phys Med Rehabil 77:1209–1214, 1996.

63. Jaegers SMHJ, Arendzen JH, de Jongh HJ: An electromyographic study of the hip muscles of transfemoral amputees in walking. Clin Orthop Rel Res 328:119–128, 1996.

64. Delbridge L, Perry P, Marr S, et al: Limited joint mobility in the diabetic foot: Relationship to neuropathic ulceration. Diabetic Med 5:333–337, 1988.

65. Fernando DJS, Masson EA, Veves A, Boulton AJM: Relationship of limited joint mobility to abnormal foot pressures and diabetic foot ulceration. Diabetes Care 14:8–11, 1991.

66. Kucan JO, Robson MC: Diabetic foot infections: Fate of the contralateral foot. Plast Reconstr Surg 77:439–441, 1986.

67. McCollough NC, Jennings JJ, Sarmiento A: Bilateral below-the-knee amputation in patients over fifty years of age. J Bone Joint Surg 54:1217–1223, 1972.

68. Whitehouse FW, Jurgensen C, Block MA: The later life of the diabetic amputee: Another look at fate of the second leg. Diabetes 17:520–521, 1968.

69. Lake C, Supan TJ: The incidence of dermatological problems in the silicone suspension sleeve user. JPO 9:97–104, 1997.

70. Centers for Disease Control and Prevention: Overweight and Obesity: Resource Guide for Nutrition and Physical Activity Intervention to Prevent Obesity and Other Chronic Diseases. http://www.cdc.gov/nccdphp/dnpa/obesity/resource_guide.htm. Accessed February 13, 2006.

71. Eisert O, Tester OW: Dynamic exercises for lower extremity amputees. Arch Phys Med Rehab 33:695–704, 1954.

72. Gailey RS, Gailey AM: Prosthetic Gait Training for Lower Extremity Amputees. Miami, FL: Advanced Rehabilitation Therapy, 1989.

73. Gailey RS, Gailey AM, Sandelbach SJ: Home Exercise Guide for Lower Extremity Amputees. Miami, FL: Advanced Rehabilitation Therapy, 1995.

74. Maiorana A, O'Driscoll G, Goodman C, et al: Combined aerobic and resistance exercise improves glycemic control and fitness in type 2 diabetes. Diabetes Res Clin Pract 56:115–123, 2002.

75. Eriksson JG: Exercise and the treatment of type 2 diabetes mellitus: An update. Sports Med 27:381–391, 1999.

76. Dunstan DW, Puddey IB, Beilin LJ, et al: Effects of a short-term circuit weight training program on glycemic control in NIDDM. Diabetes Res Clin Pract 40:53–61, 1998.

77. Dunstan DW, Daly RM, Owen N, et al: High-intensity resistance training improves glycemic control in older patients with type 2 diabetes. Diabetes Care 10:1729–1736, 2002.

78. Cauza E, Hanusch-Enserer U, Strasser B, et al: The relative benefits of endurance and strength training on the metabolic factors and muscle function of people with type 2 diabetes mellitus. Arch Phys Med Rehabil 86:1527–1532, 2005.

79. Mosher PE, Nash MS, Perry AC, et al: Aerobic circuit exercise training: Effect on adolescents with well-controlled insulin-dependent diabetes mellitus. Arch Phys Med Rehabil 79:652–657, 1998.

80. Ibanez J, Izquierdo M, Arguelles I, et al: Twice-weekly progressive resistance training decreases abdominal fat and improves insulin sensitivity in older men with type 2 diabetes. Diabetes Care 3:662–667, 2005.

81. Castaneda C, Layne JE, Munoz-Orians L, et al: A randomized controlled trial of resistance exercise training to improve glycemic control in older adults with type 2 diabetes. Diabetes Care 12:2335–2341, 2002.

82. Courtemanche R, Teasdale N, Boucher P, et al: Gait problems in diabetic neuropathic patients. Arch Phys Med Rehabil 77:849–855, 1996.

83. Alexander NB: Postural control in older adults. J Am Geriatr Soc 42:93–108, 1994.

84. Tinetti ME, Powell L: Fear of falling and low self-efficacy: A case of dependence in elderly persons. J Gerontol 48(special issue):35–38, 1993.

85. Gard SA, Childress DS: The influence of stance phase knee flexion on the vertical displacement of the trunk during normal walking. Arch Phys Med Rehabil 80:26–32, 1999.

86. Smidt G (ed): Clinics in Physical Therapy: Gait in Rehabilitation. New York: Churchill Livingstone, 1990, p 312.

87. Peizer E, Wright DW, Mason C: Human locomotion. Bull Prosthet Res 10:48–105, 1969.

88. Chan KM, Tan ES: Use of lower limb prosthesis among elderly amputees. Ann Acad Med 19:811–816, 1990.

89. Nissen SJ, Newman WP: Factors influencing reintegration to normal living after amputation. Arch Phys Med Rehab 73:548–551, 1992.

90. Pinzur MS, Littooy F, Daniels J, et al: Multi-disciplinary assessment and late function in dysvascular amputees. Clin Orthop 281:239–243, 1992.

91. Walker CRC, Ingram MG, Hullen MG, et al: Lower limb amputation following injury: A survey of long-term functional outcome. Injury 25:387–392, 1994.

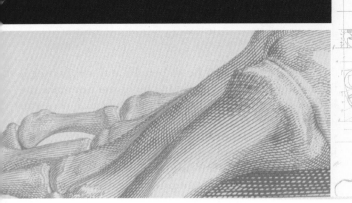

LOWER-LIMB SELF-MANAGEMENT EDUCATION

LINDA HAAS ■

A goal of Healthy People 2010 is to reduce lower-limb amputations in people with diabetes from 4.1 per 1000 persons to 1.8 per 1000 persons, a 57% decrease.[1] While treatments of ulcers and revascularization of dysvascular limbs may help to reach this goal, a critical component of amputation reduction is teaching the people with diabetes how to care for their feet and prevent the trauma that frequently leads to amputation[2] and to care for trauma when it occurs. The education of patients, their caregivers when indicated, and health care professionals to reduce risk factors for lower-limb morbidity and prevent limb loss is an important strategy in diabetes management. Appropriate diabetes self-management education and preventive care have been shown to reduce lower-limb complications.[3–10] This important knowledge must be transferred to patients with diabetes—or their caregivers if they are unable to care for themselves—since they are the only ones who can incorporate this knowledge into self-care behaviors. Clinicians who are convinced that foot care is a critical component of diabetes regimens can help patients to change their attitudes and ultimately their foot self-care behaviors.

Historical Perspective

Barth and colleagues compared the results of a comprehensive program of foot care education with a conventional program.[3] This study found that an intensive foot care education program resulted in greater knowledge and compliance and a lower frequency of foot problems in the experimental group compared to the conventional group.

Del Aguila and colleagues documented that clinicians were more likely to prescribe preventive foot care behaviors when they were aware of patients' high risk for lower-limb amputation, as evidenced by a history of a foot ulcer.[11] The authors recommended that physicians, in addition to patients, receive periodic education and reinforcement to modify care delivered to individuals who are at high risk for lower-limb complications.

In a randomized controlled trial, Litzelman and colleagues showed that educating a group of patients and a group of clinicians in proper foot care reduced foot problems in comparison with a group of patients and providers who were not equally educated.[12] Patients, clinicians, and systems interventions were studied for 1 year. The patient educational intervention was effective in increasing self-care activities such as bathing and foot and shoe inspection and in eliminating soaking. The clinician educational intervention led to providers who were more likely to document pulses, dry or cracked skin, calluses, and ulcers. There were fewer minor and serious foot lesions in the intervention group, and these patients were three times more likely to report appropriate foot care behaviors and to have foot examinations during office visits.

Assal and colleagues showed that education and training of patients with diabetes markedly decreased lower-limb amputations: 12 times fewer transtibial amputations, reduction by half of below-knee amputations, and a fourfold decrease in toe amputations.[13] Larson and colleagues found a 78% long-term decrease in the incidence of major amputations following implementation of a multidisciplinary program for prevention, education, and treatment of diabetic foot ulcers.[14] Malone and colleagues, in a prospective, randomized, controlled trial, evaluated the influence of education on the incidence of lower-limb complications in diabetes patients. Although there were no significant differences in medical management or risk factors between the two groups, the ulceration and amputation rates were three times higher in the group that did not receive the educational intervention.[7]

Thus, it appears that diabetic foot care self-management education activities and programs have been shown in some settings to improve foot care behaviors and decrease lower-limb morbidities. However, despite the long-standing role of foot care education in diabetes management, randomized controlled trials evaluating its effects are sparse.[15]

Treatment Recommendations: Diabetes Foot Care Education

Theoretical Models

Foot care education is more than imparting information; the ultimate goal is behavior change by assisting patients to acquire the skills, knowledge, and attitudes to manage their diabetes optimally, including caring for their lower limbs.[16] For many patients, simply acquiring the appropriate knowledge will be enough for them to practice good foot care hygiene and select appropriate footwear. For others, the educational process will have to include assistance so that patients can see and reach their feet or assistance in identifying resources, such as family members, support systems, or community resources to assist in lower-limb care.

Several approaches have been used in diabetes self-management education. These include patient empowerment, the health belief model, social cognitive theory, reasoned action and planned behavior, and the transtheoretical model.[16] Patient empowerment encourages patients to take control of their diabetes and their lives, increases their choices, and influences their ability to influence their environment, including individuals. It uses a five-step behavior change model.[17] The five steps of the empowerment self-directed behavior change model are as follows:

1. Define the problem.
2. Identify feelings related to the problem.
3. Identify the long-tem goal.
4. Identify short-term behavior change goals.
5. Implement and evaluate the plan.

The health belief model posits that behavior change will occur if the patient feels vulnerable, believes the perceived condition or illness to be serious, believes that changing behavior will be of benefit and will outweigh the barriers, has confidence that he or she can make the behavior change, and believes that external cues can assist in making behavior changes.[18] Tan has shown that subjects who felt more vulnerable and believed that diabetes was serious and who had fewer barriers were more apt to do preventive self-care. Scollon-Koliopoulos used this model successfully to improve foot self-care through African American churches.[19] This study included identification of perceived risk, video instruction in foot care, instruction in how to use a monofilament, and provision of educational materials.

Social-cognitive theory posits there is a continual interaction of the person, his or her behavior, and the environment, which exerts external forces on the individual. In addition, social-cognitive theory involves the knowledge and skills to do the behavior, the expectations regarding the behavior and the use of the experiences of others to acquire the desired behavior. Other constructs of social-cognitive theory include reinforcements for self and others that encourage or discourage the behavior and self-efficacy and how confident the person is that he or she can do the behavior.[18] There have been no published studies using social-cognitive theory in foot self-care. The combined model of the theory of reasoned action and theory of planned behavior posits that people have attitudes and beliefs toward behaviors and that people are influenced by how others view the behavior and how well people can perform the behavior, that is, have the knowledge and skills.[18] There have been no published studies of this combined model on foot care in people with diabetes.

The transtheoretical model uses stages of change as a major construct. These six distinct changes are precontemplation, contemplation, preparation, action, maintenance, and termination.[20] This model views behavior change as a process, and identification of a person's readiness to change and tailoring interventions to where the individual is in the process are important components of the education process. Motivational interviewing is a technique, rather than a model, and is used in several models. The goals of this technique are to identify and resolve ambivalence and to motivate behavior change.[16] Motivational interviewing involves reflective listening, expressing empathy, exploring discrepancies or ambivalence, and rolling with resistance; that is, do not argue or try to force behaviors and supporting self-efficacy. In applying educational theories to behavior change, it is often helpful to determine a patient's conviction that a behavior is important and confidence that he or she can do the behavior. Using a scale of 0 to 10, the patient can be asked what his or her conviction level is. If the answer is a four, the question "Why a 4 and not a 0?" will give information as to why the person thinks change is important. The question "What would help this behavior be a 6 or 7?" will help to identify barriers. Using the same scale can help to identify a person's self-efficacy or confidence that he or she can make the change. "How confident are you that you can examine your feet daily?" is one such question. Using the 0 to 10 scale, an answer of 4 or 5 will help to identify why someone thinks he or she can do the task. Asking what would help the person to get to a higher number will help to identify barriers and allows the interviewer or health care provider to find or supply resources to help the patient.

Diabetes self-management foot care education must involve the person with diabetes in all phases of the education process. Doing so may enhance patients' ability to carry out the plan for safe foot care.[21] With mutual planning, the individual with diabetes will help to set the goals. This mutual goal determination is important because patients or their caregivers are the ones who will implement the indicated behavior changes. For people with diabetes to assume the therapeutic role, they must have the knowledge they need and want. Clinicians can help patients to see the need for this knowledge, promote motivation to learn about lower-limb self-care, teach foot care self-management principles, and assist in identification of resources. Clinicians can also demonstrate the importance of foot care by examining patients' feet frequently and asking about self-care behaviors and problems.

Adult Education

Before delineation of the aspects of foot care self-management education, it may be appropriate to review the principles of adult learning, as the majority of people with diabetes are adults, particularly those with current or potential foot problems. These principles, which should be utilized in development of educational plans, are that adults do the following[22]:

- *Assume responsibility for lifelong learning and continually learn and apply new concepts and skills.* The clinician can point out how new knowledge and skills can be applied and incorporated into patients' activities of daily living.
- *Build on previously acquired experience and knowledge.* Pointing out how adults have learned previous skills is helpful and encourages them to apply prior successes to current challenges.
- *Have already formulated major life and learning goals.* The educational assessment can identify these goals. Then family, work, and leisure goals can be incorporated into the self-care management plan to create a win-win situation.
- *Translate new information into practical applications.* Adults are problem oriented rather than theory oriented. Adult learners, for the most part, want to know how to use information. If an adult patient with diabetes is supposed to select shoes on the basis of particular criteria, the patient wants to know exactly what the criteria are and how the task is best accomplished within his or her frame of reference.

- *Want to see a need for learning.* Adults want to know why they should make changes, how health care interventions will affect their everyday lives, and how to make the interventions work. Therefore, the educational focus should be on necessary knowledge rather than on academic facts that might be interesting but not necessary.
- *Analyze new knowledge.* Adults will continually evaluate new knowledge in terms of who is making the recommendation, what they themselves already know (or think they know), what others say (including friends and relatives), and what they are willing to do. This principle causes adults to pose the same question to several health care providers. Therefore, to establish credibility, clinicians should be consistent in their information. When scientific evidence is not established, it is helpful to tell patients that there is no one right answer to their question but that several approaches may be acceptable. Then providers can help patients to select the intervention that best fits their needs and lifestyles.

The Diabetes Self-Management Educational Process

Diabetes foot care education is an individualized, planned process that includes assessment, planning, the actual teaching, and evaluation.[23] It is more than handing out a preprinted foot care pamphlet. It is a continuous process, determined by the patient's physical, emotional, and social status, which is, in turn, determined by the educational assessment.

Assessment

The principles of an educational assessment are similar to those of a physical assessment. Determining educational readiness and determining the most efficacious educational approaches are the primary goals of educational assessment for a particular patient or group of patients.[24] Areas to explore in doing an educational assessment of an adult include the following:

- *Usual health practices.* Specifically for diabetes foot care, by asking questions such as how they examine their feet and how often, what types of footwear they use, where and how they buy their shoes, the amount and type of exercise they do, and type of shoes worn during exercise, clinicians can identify educational areas on which to focus.
- *Health beliefs.* It is important to assess whether patients believe that they can make a difference in their health status and who they believe is responsible for their health (e.g., health care providers, their spouses [external control], a higher power, fate [chance control], or themselves [internal control]).[18] Knowing

patients' health beliefs can help clinicians to determine whether to use collaborative or authoritarian educational approaches.

- *Present knowledge level and abilities (especially problem-solving abilities)*. Assessment for foot care self-management education should include patients' current knowledge of diabetes and its effect on the lower limbs, current foot care behaviors, beliefs, attitudes, and ability to solve problems.[17]
- *Attitudes toward health in general and diabetes specifically*. Patients' feelings and concerns about their susceptibility to the consequences of diabetes should be explored, as well as any negative impacts of diabetes on their lives. Assessment should include whether patients believe that following recommendations can make a difference and whether they believe that the benefits of self-care offset the personal and financial costs. Affirmative answers to these questions indicate that the patient will most likely be receptive to education. Negative answers, on the other hand, indicate that work that is more preliminary needs to be done. Often, clinicians will have to develop rapport with patients to assist them to believe that they can make a difference and that what they do for their own self-care will be beneficial.
- *Functional status*. Employment status; independence in activities of daily living; visual, auditory, mobility, and hand-eye coordination abilities; and tremors are important functional areas to assess.[25–30] If there are difficulties in any of these areas, the clinician might need to identify resources such as family, friends, or visiting nurses.
- *Cognitive ability*. Assessment should include the patients' ability to understand and remember directions and any short-term memory loss or confusion.[27,31]
- *Educational level*. Although educational level is not a surrogate measure for intelligence,[32] it often indicates the types of educational materials and approaches that might be most appropriate and may be an indicator of reading level.
- *Literacy level*. Whether patients spend their time watching TV or videos or reading, what types of material they read, and familiarity with computers can help to determine if educational interventions should include video, written materials, or computer-assisted materials.
- *Current self-care practices, particularly of the lower limbs*. Do they soak feet? What type of shoes are worn?
- *History of, or current, substance abuse.*
- *Access to and use of health care resources.*
- *Social supports, including need for and availability of caregivers.*
- *Environmental factors*. These might include occupation, financial resources, and physical surroundings, as these can affect patients' abilities to perform adequate lower-limb hygiene.

Identification of the Foot at Risk

Not all patients with diabetes need the same foot self-care education. To be efficient with providers' and patients' time, it is reasonable to identify patients' risk for lower-limb morbidity. Self-management education for those who are at low risk can focus on preventive measures, whereas education for those who are at high risk will be more intensive. Screening refers to the application of a test, procedure, or examination to people who are asymptomatic to classify them regarding their likelihood of having a particular disease or outcome. The screening procedure itself does not diagnose the outcome but indicates those who are at high risk. Thus, in addition to an educational assessment, patients should be screened to determine their risk for lower-limb morbidity.

History

A study at the Veterans Affairs Puget Sound Health Care System, Seattle Division, used a backwards stepwise logistic regression model to identify risk factors to predict ulceration of the lower limb.[33] The variables that predicted foot ulceration were the following:

- A1C
- Impaired vision
- History of amputation
- Sensory neuropathy (inability to perceive the 5.07 Semmes-Weinstein monofilament)
- Tinea pedis
- Onychomycosis

These predictors of foot ulceration can be obtained by questioning patients and a brief examination. Patients who have had a foot ulceration or amputation can be categorized as "high risk," and no further screening questions or examinations are necessary.

Physical Examination of the Foot

Patients understand the importance of diabetic foot care better when it is demonstrated by a provider who examines their feet carefully at least annually and asks about foot problems at every visit. A standardized assessment form that lists the specific screening activities to be done, foot risk categories, and the recommended interventions facilitates implementation and documentation of this activity.

Along with questions about a history of foot ulceration, peripheral vascular disease, or amputation, a foot risk-screening visit includes questions about limb changes since the last visit, such as intermittent claudication and symptoms of neuropathy. The presence or absence of current foot ulceration should be recorded.

Since a foot inspection includes the tops, bottoms, and sides of each foot and between the toes, patients' abilities to do this self-care behavior should be assessed. A vision examination with a handheld or wall-mounted Snellen chart will give clues as to whether patients can see their feet well enough for a visual inspection. Vision worse than 20/40 in both eyes might be inadequate. If vision is poor, manual inspections may substitute for visual inspections. If visual or mobility impairment makes it difficult for patients to reach their feet, a mirror, magnifying glass, or magnifying mirror can be used. Alternatively, family members, neighbors, or other care-givers might need to assist with daily limb inspection.

Patients should demonstrate the ability to reach their feet for foot care and manual inspection. Thomson showed that in three groups of elderly patients (mean age: 76 years), two groups of whom had diabetes, only 14% could remove 0.5-cm red dots that had been placed on their plantar surfaces over the first and fifth metatarsal heads.[34] Limited joint mobility has been shown to be associated with development of foot ulcers.[26] This lack of joint mobility can significantly limit patients' abilities to perform lower-limb self-care. Other barriers can be obesity, which can cause the inability to see or reach the feet; neuropathy (autonomic, motor, and sensory); peripheral vascular disease; homelessness; and the presence of alcohol and drug abuse.

Sensory Examination

In the clinical setting, sensory examination with a 5.07 Semmes-Weinstein monofilament is the single most practical measure of neuropathy.[35,36] After demonstrating the procedure in an area of intact sensation, such as the arm, the examiner tests the most common sites of potential ulceration: the plantar surface of the great toe and the first, third, and fifth metatarsal heads.[37] Patients should be instructed to say when they feel something or raise their hand when they feel something. When the plastic wire bends to a C shape, 10 g of pressure is being applied. Insensitivity is the inability to feel this monofilament at any site on either foot. The 5.07 Semmes-Weinstein monofilament is an accurate and easily used discriminator between those with protective sensation and those without.[33,38]

Peripheral Vascular Disease

Boyko showed that the probability of peripheral vascular disease can be obtained from knowledge of patients' age, history of vascular disease, venous filling time, and palpation of lower-limb pulses.[39] Palpation of the dorsalis pedis and posterior tibialis pulses should be recorded as present or absent. Determination of the ankle-arm index should be made in patients without palpable pulses or those who are otherwise suspected of having peripheral vascular disease. Venous filling time is determined after identification of a prominent pedal vein. Examiners assist patients to elevate their legs to 45 degrees for

1 minute. Patients are then asked to sit up and hang their legs over the side of the examining table. The time in seconds until the veins bulge above the skin level is recorded. The time to reappearance of the veins can be recorded, or results can be classified as normal (20 seconds) or abnormal (>20 seconds).

Structural Deformities

Structural deformities include the presence or absence of prominent metatarsal heads, hammertoes or clawed toes, Charcot foot deformity (collapse of the foot arch), bony prominences (exostosis), hallux valgus (bunion), hallux limitus (also called hallux rigidus, stiff great toe joint with limited range of motion), and corns and calluses. Corns and callused areas are signs of increased pressure.

Footwear

Shoes and socks should be examined to determine fit and condition and to assess style. In addition, the ability of the patient to put his or her socks and shoes on should be assessed.

Skin Abnormalities

Skin abnormalities include excessive dryness and macerated intertriginous areas, indicating severe tinea pedis (athlete's foot fungus). Nail deformities such as fungal dystrophy (thickened and deformed toenails) or ingrown toenails should be noted. The way the nails are trimmed should also be noted.

After the examination, the foot risk category is determined, and a plan for foot care education and annual foot examinations is made for low-risk patients. High-risk patients will require more frequent foot examinations by clinicians and more detailed self-management education emphasizing daily inspection, protective footwear, and the need to report foot problems promptly.

Planning

Educational plans for adults are most effective when the patient participates in the planning process.[40] The elements of an effective teaching plan for knowledge and skills acquisition include measurable behavioral objectives, selection of appropriate content, teaching materials and instructional methods, and a plan to evaluate learning and skills. The actual educational process should take place in a comfortable, well-lit, relaxed environment. When feasible, several short sessions, each session focused on a specific topic, are more effective than one long session during which everything is covered.

The educational plan is developed with the principles of adult education in mind. Patients should be asked what they want to learn about diabetic foot care. It is reasonable for clinicians to set educational goals and objectives, but patients should be asked whether the goals and objectives are acceptable. Providers need to be flexible and open to change. If the clinician's goal is to teach foot self-care according to guidelines and the patient wants to learn how to select shoes for hiking, the session could be ineffective and lead to frustration for both teacher and learner.

Once goals have been set, measurable objectives should be delineated, with the patient's input. Objectives can be related to any aspect of the management plan, but they must be specific, measurable, and time limited.[41,42] For example, a goal might be to ensure that a patient with insensate feet who plans to start a walking program protects his or her feet. Objectives under that goal might be as follows:

- The patient describes how to purchase and break in the appropriate shoes.
- The patient states the appropriate type of socks to wear.
- The patient identifies appropriate surfaces for a walking program.
- The patient demonstrates how to examine his or her feet after exercise and describes what reddened areas or blisters indicate.
- The patient has the name and telephone number of the person to call at the earliest sign of foot problems.

The plan must be feasible and achievable within a reasonable time. Although prevention of amputation is the ultimate goal of foot care self-management education, the educational session focuses on behaviors that lead to short-term goals and objectives. The focus should be on keeping the skin soft by application of emollients or daily foot inspection, rather than on never having a lower-limb amputation. Written contracts can help patients to adhere to the self-care process.[43]

When the behavioral objectives have been determined, the appropriate presentation methods are identified, since people learn in different ways.[44] Most people are visual learners; they learn best by seeing. These people will say, "I see what you are saying." However, some people learn better by hearing and others by touching. People who are auditory learners might say things such as "I hear what you are saying," while kinesthetic learners use the word "feel" frequently. Thus, in a group situation, it is advisable to use different methods, such as lecture, slides, videos, demonstrations, return demonstrations, problem solving, handouts, repetition, and feedback. Both individual and group sessions should be as interactive as possible.

Teaching Methodology

Teaching involves imparting information and ensuring that learners have acquired the required knowledge or skills and are able to apply these concepts. The teaching content is based on the identified objectives. Principles involved in teaching a skill, such as toenail trimming, involve determining and facilitating readiness to learn, modeling (demonstrating) the desired task, having active participation by patients (return demonstration), and giving feedback as to the appropriateness of the learners' techniques. When learning new psychomotor skills, people have better retention if the procedural steps are verbalized as they are performed. This can be evaluated in a return demonstration. The return demonstration should be repeated until safe behavior is demonstrated. Feedback enables patients to know how they are doing and is often motivating.

Repetition facilitates learning. Therefore, material should be repeated, preferably in different ways or by using different analogies or examples to make the same point. Material should be presented in a positive manner, stressing what patients can do to protect their feet, rather than with a threatening attitude, stressing that if they do not do these things, they will lose a limb. It is important to repeat the most critical facts learners need to know at the end of the session.

Written Educational Materials

Written educational materials give patients tangible reminders of what to do to prevent lower-limb problems, when to do it, and what to do if problems occur. The written educational materials should be appropriate in terms of ethnicity, age, and reading level for each patient.[18,32,45] Twenty percent of adults in the United States have reading skills below the fifth-grade level, and the average reading level in the United States is about eighth grade,[32,46] although it may be even lower in the elderly.[47] Unfortunately, the majority of health education materials are written at higher than a ninth-grade reading level.[46] Therefore, a selection of patient education materials should be available for different patient groups. Illustrations in handouts or take-home materials should be of the type to which patients can relate. For example, written materials for patients with type 2 diabetes starting an exercise program should not use a picture of children playing at school recess as an illustration. To personalize the information, providers should review all handouts with patients and highlight principles to emphasize, or cross out irrelevant items. Patients need practical and realistic information provided with a "can do" attitude.

Teaching Content

There are several essentials of foot self-care education for people with diabetes.

Inspection

Patients with neuropathy should be instructed how to perform daily visual or manual foot inspection. Patients without neuropathy will be likely to perceive injuries to their feet, but daily foot inspection is a good habit for everyone with diabetes. It does not have to be a burden but can consist of a brief examination of the feet in good light when drying them after a shower or bath, when putting on socks or skin lotion, or before going to bed.

The feet and interdigital areas should be inspected daily. Patients should be instructed to look for cuts, blisters, bruises, and anything unusual. A magnifying glass, mirror, or magnifying mirror may be helpful. After the daily foot inspection has been explained and demonstrated, patients, families, or other caregivers should perform a return demonstration and verbalize what they will look for.

Daily Hygiene

Patients should be instructed to wash and dry their feet thoroughly, especially between the toes. Patients should be instructed to check the bathwater temperature with their forearms, elbows, or a bath thermometer to prevent burns. Routine soaking is not recommended, as it can cause dry skin. Emollients such as lanolin or hand lotion should be applied to dry skin but not between the toes, where the excess moisture may cause maceration. A few strands of lamb's wool may be wound between the toes to separate overlapping or contacting toes and help to prevent maceration.

Toenails

Patients should be instructed to cut or file their toenails keeping to the contour of the toe. All sharp or jagged edges should be smoothed with a file or emery board. If patients have poor vision or difficulty reaching their feet, other resources such as family members, nurses, or podiatrists should be identified to trim patients' toenails.

Self-Treatment of Abnormal Conditions

Patients should be instructed never to use chemicals, sharp instruments, or razor blades on their feet. Flaky fungal debris can be loosened with a soft nailbrush during regular bathing. Patients or family members should be instructed to gently buff corns or calluses with a pumice stone or towel after bathing and to apply a moisturizer while the skin is damp to help soften corns or calluses.

Footwear

Patients should be instructed to wear socks that do not have seams or holes and should be instructed that socks with holes should be discarded rather than mended. Patients with sweaty feet should be instructed to wear well-fitting soft cotton or wool socks that will absorb moisture and to avoid a warm, moist environment, in which fungus can thrive. Socks with extra padding can provide comfort and added protection for high-risk patients.

Since the most common cause of foot trauma has been shown to be related to shoes,[2,6,38,48,49] shoe selection and maintenance is a critical component of foot self-care education. Patients should be instructed to purchase shoes in the middle of the day. Patients with sensory neuropathy should be instructed to have shoes fitted by a professional, if possible. If these patients must buy shoes "off the rack," the shapes of their feet can be traced on a piece of paper. Then, when buying shoes, patients can be sure that these shapes fit the shoes being purchased.

Patients should be instructed to wear athletic shoes[50] or oxford-type shoes with adjustable vamps, made from leather or canvas. Instruction should also include that new shoes should fit well around the heel so that the heel does not move around in the shoe, which can cause blisters. Patients should also be instructed that when purchasing new shoes, they should stand upright in the shoes to be sure that the heel counter is firm and the ball width, the widest part of the shoe, corresponds to the metatarsal heads. Since manufacturers' sizes are only guidelines and are variable, patients with insensate feet should be instructed not to buy shoes by size alone.

Shoes must provide adequate toe room. Therefore, patients should learn that the adequacy of the toebox is related to the style of the shoe rather than the size. They should wear shoes that have an adequate toebox, to accommodate their forefeet and toes, and yet fit well at the heel. Shoes with extra depth might be needed. The shoe length should be approximately an inch longer than the longest toe. If clawed toes or hammertoes are present, extra depth or custom shoes might be indicated. In addition, people with severe foot deformities might need custom molded footwear.[51] Energy-absorbing insoles can distribute weight-bearing forces equally over the plantar surfaces. Since Medicare will cover 80% of the cost of therapeutic shoes and orthotics for enrollees with Medicare Part B, the educational process might need to include assisting patients to access this benefit.[52]

Shoes should be broken in gradually, worn only 1 or 2 hours a day for the first week. Patients should be instructed to examine their feet after removing the shoes and to look for reddened areas, which can indicate increased pressure. Patients should also be instructed to switch to another pair of shoes at least once during the day for pressure relief. If this is not possible, they should remove their shoes for 10 to 15 minutes every 2 to 3 hours to limit repetitive local pressures.

Patients with any limb insensitivity should be instructed to examine their shoes before putting them on and to feel inside the shoes for torn or loose linings, cracks, pebbles, nails, or other objects or irregularities that might irritate the skin. Patients should be instructed to develop the habit of shaking out their shoes before putting them on to find "lost" objects.

Patients with insensate feet should be instructed never to go barefoot (except in the shower or bed) to avoid trauma, puncture wounds, and burns from hot sand or pavement. Patients with diabetes and neuropathy should not apply external heat to their feet. If their feet are cold, socks can be worn to bed.

When to Seek Assistance

It is important that patients know and can state when, how, and whom to contact regarding limb problems. Patients should be instructed to report the following: any breaks in the skin or discoloration that does not begin healing after 2 to 3 days, swelling of the limbs, abnormal shapes, burns, frostbite, or obvious infection. Patients should be given a specific name and telephone number or the telephone number of the emergency room or contact. They should be encouraged to call with any problems or concerns they have regarding their lower limbs.

Exercise/Increased Activity

Exercise is an important modality in the management of diabetes. However, before beginning an exercise program, the patient with diabetes should undergo a medical evaluation to screen for the presence of conditions that could be worsened by exercise.[53] The medical history and physical examination should focus on the signs and symptoms of cardiovascular, cerebrovascular, and peripheral vascular disease and peripheral sensory neuropathy. For patients who are planning to participate in low-intensity forms of exercise, such as walking, the clinician may use his or her judgment in deciding whether diagnostic studies are necessary. The vast majority of people with diabetes in good metabolic control and without complications can participate in exercise if they are careful to avoid hypoglycemia during periods of increased activity.

A standard recommendation for all exercise sessions is to include proper warm-up and cool-down periods. A warm-up consists of 5 to 10 minutes of aerobic activity at a low-intensity level followed by gently stretching for another 5 to 10 minutes. A cool-down period of another 5 to 10 minutes of low-intensity activity should follow the high-activity exercise period.[54]

Patients who are starting moderate to high-intensity exercise programs might need graded exercise testing, especially if they are elderly, have a long history of diabetes, have additional risk factors for cardiovascular disease, or have established complications of diabetes. Patients with known coronary artery disease should undergo a supervised evaluation of the ischemic response to exercise, ischemic threshold, and propensity to arrhythmia during exercise.

Autonomic neuropathy can limit patients' exercise capacity and increase the risk of adverse cardiovascular events during exercise. Hypotension and hypertension after vigorous exercise are more likely to develop in patients with autonomic neuropathy, particularly when they are starting a new exercise program. Because these individuals often have difficulty with thermoregulation, they should avoid exercise in hot or cold environments and should be vigilant about adequate hydration.

When patients have active proliferative diabetic retinopathy, strenuous activity can precipitate vitreous hemorrhage or retinal detachment. These individuals should avoid anaerobic exercise and exercise that involves straining, jarring, or Valsalva-like maneuvers.[55]

Patients with peripheral arterial disease often self-limit their walking owing to intermittent claudication. After an evaluation for lower-limb blood flow, a supervised walking program might be recommended as a treatment for intermittent claudication. Patients with peripheral neuropathy and loss of protective sensation to their feet should limit or avoid repetitive weight-bearing exercises such as jogging, prolonged walking, treadmills, and stair step exercises. Patients with sensory peripheral neuropathy must be cautioned to avoid hot sand and pavement around pools and sport courts. These surfaces can be too hot for neuropathic feet even when shoes are worn if the shoes are thin-soled, as are many sandals and moccasins.

The presence of an active foot ulcer is an absolute contraindication for weight-bearing exercise. Even patients who have a healed ulcer must take special precautions when exercising to prevent a recurrence. Special shoes and padded socks appropriate to the particular activity are important for injury prevention. Patients with healed ulcers or with severe foot deformities can participate in non-weight-bearing exercising such as swimming, bicycling, rowing, and upper body exercises.

In spite of these cautions, exercise programs are beneficial for patients with diabetes. Several long-term studies have demonstrated the positive effects of regular exercise on carbohydrate metabolism and insulin sensitivity. Exercise also has the potential to decrease cardiovascular risk factors and is associated with improvements in dyslipidemia, hypertension, and obesity.[56–61]

Evaluation

Evaluation of the educational process is necessary to ensure that the goals and objectives were met. Providers and patients evaluate the education session and process by referring back to the goals and objectives.[62] If the goals are met, praise and feedback are very encouraging for patients and can encourage them to set and achieve farther-reaching goals and objectives. If goals were not met, the feasibility of the objectives should be reassessed, and another educational plan should be developed. Occasionally, posttests are used to evaluate knowledge. If used, posttest questions should relate to the learning objectives. The most important evaluation relates to behavior change. These behaviors include incorporation of foot care management into patients' daily lives, practicing good lower-limb hygiene, and obtaining and wearing adequate footwear. Clinicians can question patients at subsequent visits to determine whether the patients are changing their behaviors.

Another evaluation method is problem-solving questions. Patients can be asked what they would do in particular situations. For example, "What would you do if you notice a blister after your exercise?" or "What foot problems would you call me about?"

Summary

Most patients with diabetes are fearful of lower-limb amputations, and sensitivity must be used to present accurate information to encourage behavior changes while avoiding scaring the patient. The most important lower-limb self-care concepts for patients to understand and incorporate into their diabetes self-management regimens are proper foot inspection and foot care, selection and safe use of footwear, and when and how to contact a health care provider.

Teaching and learning about lower-limb self-care are not easy tasks. Foot care self-management education is a complex, ongoing process. Every office visit should be an opportunity for self-management education. Families and support systems should be included whenever possible, since family and social support have been shown to increase adherence.[63,64] Lower-limb self-management education involves giving people with diabetes the knowledge to make intelligent choices about their behavior and the changes they can and will make to improve their chances of delaying or avoiding the devastating lower-limb complications of diabetes.

References

1. Centers for Disease Control and Prevention, National Institutes of Health: Healthy People 2010: 5 Diabetes. Available at http://www.healthypeople.gov/Document/HTML/Volume1/05Diabetes.htm#_Toc494509739.
2. Pecoraro RE, Reiber GE, Burgess EM: Pathways to diabetic limb amputation: Basis for prevention. Diabetes Care 13:513–521, 1990.
3. Barth R, Campbell LV, Allen S, et al: Intensive education improves knowledge, compliance, and foot problems in Type 2 diabetes. Diabet Med 8:111–117, 1991.
4. Corbett CF: A randomized pilot study of improving foot care in home health patients with diabetes. Diabetes Educator 29:273–282, 2003.
5. Deakin TA, Cade JE, Williams R, Greenwood DC: Structured patient education:the diabetes X-PERT Programme makes a difference. Diabet Med 23:944–954, 2006.
6. Donohoe ME, Fletton JA, Hook A, et al: Improving foot care for people with diabetes mellitus: A randomized controlled trial of an integrated care approach. Diabet Med 17, 2000.
7. Malone JM, Snyder M, Anderson G, et al: Prevention of amputation by diabetic education. Am J Surg 158:520–524, 1989.
8. Valk GD: Patient education for preventing diabetic foot ulceration. Cochrane Rev Abstr 2006.
9. Viswanathan V, Madhaven S, Rajasekar S, et al: Amputation prevention initiative in south India: Positive impact of foot care education. Diabetes Care 28:1019–1021, 2005.
10. Ward A, Metz L, Oddone EZ, Edelman D: Foot education improves knowledge and satisfaction among patents at high risk for diabetic foot ulcer. Diabetes Educator 25:560–567, 1999.
11. Del Aguila MA, Reiber GE, Koepsell TD: How does provider and patient awareness of high-risk status for lower-extremity amputation influence foot care practice? Diabetes Care 17:1050–1054, 1994.
12. Litzelman DK, Slemenda CW, Langefeld CD, et al: Reduction of lower extremity clinical abnormalities in patients with non-insulin-dependent diabetes mellitus: A randomized, controlled trial. Ann Intern Med 119:36–41, 1993.
13. Assal JP, Peter-Riesch B, Vaucher J: The cost of training a diabetic patient: Effects on prevention of amputation. Diabetes Metab 19:491–495, 1993.
14. Larson J, Apelqvist J, Agardh CD, Stenstrom A: Decreasing incidence of major amputation in diabetic patients: A consequence of a multidisciplinary foot care team approach? Diabet Med 12:770–776, 1995.
15. Valk GD, Kriegsman DM, Assendelft WJ: Patient education for preventing foot ulceration: A systematic review. Endocrinol Metab Clin North Am 31:633–658, 2002.
16. Andersen RE, Funnell MM, Tang TS: Self-management of health. In Mensing C (ed): The Art and Science of Diabetes Self-Management Education: A Desk Reference for Healthcare Professionals. Chicago, American Association of Diabetes Educators, 2006, pp 43–58.
17. Funnell MM, Anderson RM: Professional development: Patient empowerment: A look back, a look ahead. Diabetes Educator 29:454–464, 2003.
18. Glantz K, Rimer BK, Lewis FM: Health Behavior and Health Education: Theory, Research and Practice, 3rd ed. San Francisco, Jossey-Bass, 2003.
19. Scollan-Kiliopoulos M: Theory-guided intervention for preventing diabetes-related amputations in African Americans. J Vasc Nurs 22:126–133, 2004.
20. Prochaska JO: Health behavior change research: A consortium approach to collaborative science. Ann Behav Med 29(suppl):4–6, 2005.
21. Duchin S, Brown SA: Patients should participate in designing diabetes educational content. Patient Educ Couns 16:255–267, 1990.
22. Knowles MS: The Adult Learner: A Neglected Species. Houston, TX, Gulf Publishing, 1990.
23. Pichert JW, Schlundt DG: Assessment: Gathering information and facilitating engagement. In Mensing C (ed): The Art and Science of Diabetes Self-management Education: A Desk Reference for Healthcare Professionals. Chicago, The American Association of Diabetes Educators, 2006, pp 578–595.
24. American Association of Diabetes Educators: The Scope of Practice, Standards of Practice and Standards of Professional Performance for Diabetes Educators. Chicago, The American Association of Diabetes Educators, 2005.
25. Egede LE: Diabetes, major depression, and functional disability among U.S. adults. Diabetes Care 27:421–428, 2004.
26. Fernando DJS, Masson EA, Veves A, Boulton AJM: Relationship of limited joint mobility to abnormal foot pressures and diabetic foot ulceration. Diabetes Care 14:8–11, 1991.
27. Jagger C, Spiers N, Arthur A: The role of sensory and cognitive function in the onset of activity restriction in older people. Disabil Rehabil 27:22–28, 2005.
28. Jerant AF, von Friederichs-Fitzwater MM, Moore M: Patients' perceived barriers to active self-management of chronic conditions. Patient Educ Couns 57:300–307, 2005.
29. Kamper AM, Stott DJ, Hyland M, et al: Predictors of functional decline in elderly people with vascular risk factors or disease. Age Ageing 34:450–455, 2005.
30. Salive ME, Guralnik JM, Glynn RJ, et al: Association of visual impairment with mobility and physical function. J Am Geriatr Soc 42:287–292, 1994.
31. Fontbonne A, Berr C, Ducimetiere P, Alperovitch A: Changes in cognitive abilities over a 4-year period are unfavorably affected in elderly diabetic subjects: Results of the Epidemiology of Vascular Aging Study. Diabetes Care 24:366–370, 2001.

32. Doak CC, Doak LG, Root JH: Teaching Patients with Low Literacy Skills. Philadelphia, JB Lippincott, 1996.
33. Boyko EJ, Ahroni JH, Cohen V, et al: Prediction of diabetic foot ulcer occurrence using commonly available clinical information. Diabetes Care 29:1202–1207, 2006.
34. Thomson FJ, Masson EA: Can elderly diabetic patients co-operate with routine foot care? Age Ageing 21:333–337, 1992.
35. Holewski JJ, Stess RM, Graf PM, Grunfeld C: Aesthesiometry: Quantification of cutaneous pressure sensation in diabetic peripheral neuropathy. J Rehabil Res Devel 25:1–10, 1988.
36. Rith-Najarian SJ, Reiber GE: Prevention of foot problems in persons with diabetes. J Fam Pract 20:S30–S39, 2000.
37. Dorgan MB, Birke JA, Moretto JA, et al: Performing foot screening for diabetic patients. Am J Nurs 95(11):32–36, 1995.
38. Abbott CA, Carrington AL, Ashe H, et al: The North-West Diabetes Foot Care Study: Incidence of, and risk factors for new diabetic foot ulceration in a community-based patient cohort. Diabet Med 19:377–384, 2002.
39. Boyko EJ, Ahroni JH, Davignon D, et al: Diagnostic utility of the history and physical examination for peripheral vascular disease among patients with diabetes mellitus. J Clin Epidemiol 50:659–668, 1997.
40. Van Korff M, Gruman J, Schaefer J, et al: Collaborative management of chronic illness. Ann Intern Med 127:1097–1002, 1997.
41. Lorig KR, A. S, Ritter P: Outcome measures for Health Education and Other Health Care Interventions. Thousand Oaks, CA, Sage, 1996.
42. Lorig KR, Sobel DS, Ritter PL, et al: Effect of a self-management program on patients with chronic disease. Effective Clin Pract 4:256–262, 2001.
43. Redman BK: The Practice of Patient Education. St. Louis, Mosby 2001.
44. Moss VA: Assessing learning abilities, readiness for education. Semin Perioper Nurs 3:113–120, 1994.
45. Schillinger D, Grumbach K, Piette JD, et al: Association of health literacy with diabetes outcomes. JAMA 288:475–482, 2002.
46. Dollahite J, Thompson C, McNew R: Readability of printed sources of diet and health information. Patient Educ Couns 27:123–134, 1996.
47. Ryan CM: Diabetes, aging and cognitive decline. Neurobiol Aging 26S:S21–S25, 2005.
48. Basu S, Hadley J, Tan R, et al: Is there enough information about foot care among patients with diabetes? Int J Lower Extremity Wounds 3:64–68, 2004.
49. Lawrence A: Foot care education in renal patients with diabetes. EDTNA/ERCA J Renal Care 30:153–156, 2004.
50. Perry JE, Ulbrecht JS, Derr JA, Cavanagh PR: The use of running shoes to reduce plantar pressures in patients who have diabetes. J Bone Joint Surg 77A:1819–1828, 1995.
51. Chantelau E, Kushner T, Spraul M: How effective is cushioned therapeutic footwear in protecting diabetic feet?: A clinical study. Diabet Med 7:335–339, 1990.
52. Clements DA, Myers RJ: 2005 Guide to Social Security and Medicare. Louisville, KY, Marsh & McLennan, 2004.
53. American Diabetes Association: Standards of medical care in diabetes: 2006. Diabetes Care 29(suppl 1):S4–S42, 2006.
54. Kirk AF, Mutrie N, Macintyre PD, Fisher MB: Promoting and maintaining physical activity in people with type 2 diabetes. Am J Prev Med 27:289–296, 2004.
55. Aiello LM, Cavallerno J, Aiello LP, Bursell SE: Retinopathy. In Ruderman NB, Devlin JT (eds): The Health Professional's Guide to Diabetes and Exercise. Alexandria, VA, American Diabetes Association, 1995.
56. Barnett A, Smith B, Lord SR, et al: Community-based group exercises improves balance and reduces falls in at-risk older people: A randomised controlled trial. Age Ageing 32:407–414, 2003.
57. Gregg EW, Beckles GL, Williamson DF, et al: Diabetes and physical disability among older U.S. adults. Diabetes Care 23:1272–1277, 2000.
58. The Diabetes Prevention Program Group: Reduction in the incidence of type 2 diabetes with lifestyle intervention or metformin. N Engl J Med 346:393–402, 2002.
59. Leveille SG, Wagner EH, Davis CL, et al: Preventing disability and managing chronic illness in frail older adults: A randomized trial of a community-based partnership with primary care. J Am Geriatr Soc 46:1191–1198, 1998.
60. Lord SR, Castell S, Corcoran J, et al: The effect of group exercise on physical functioning on falls in frail older people living in retirement villages: A randomized, controlled trial. J Am Geriatr Soc 51:1685–1692, 2003.
61. Skelton DA, Beyer N: Exercise and injury prevention in older people. Scand J Med Sci Sports 13:77–85, 2003.
62. Mulcahy K, Maryniuk MD, Peeples M: Diabetes self-management education core outcomes measures. Diabetes Educator 29:768–788, 2003.
63. Dunbar-Joseph J, Dwyer K, Dunning EJ: Compliance with antihypertensive regimen: A review of the research in the 1980s. Ann Behav Med 13:31–39, 1991.
64. Langa KM, Vijans S, Hayward RA, et al: Informal caregiving for diabetes and diabetic complications among elderly Americans. J Gerontol B Psychol Sci Soc Sci 57:S177–S186, 2002.

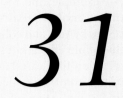

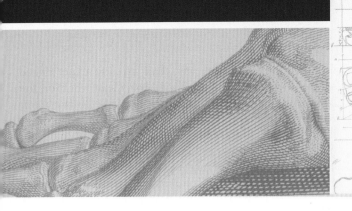

CHAPTER

31

PSYCHOSOCIAL ASPECTS OF DIABETIC FOOT COMPLICATIONS

LORETTA VILEIKYTE AND JEFFREY S. GONZALEZ ■

F oot ulceration is an increasing problem worldwide (see Chapter 24) with over 80% of amputations preceded by foot ulcers[1] and little evidence of reduction in amputation rates in people with diabetes.[2] There is therefore a need to better understand the psychosocial factors involved in the development of diabetic foot ulcers and the ways in which foot ulceration influences an individual's functioning and quality of life (QoL).

Until recently, psychosocial research in diabetes focused almost exclusively on self-care behaviors and the burdens associated with management of glycemia, to the near total neglect of the effects of chronic complications such as diabetic neuropathy and foot ulceration. There has now been some progress in this area, as evidenced by the emergence of patient-centered and theory-based methods to identify psychological factors that influence adherence to foot self-care, emotional status, and QoL of patients suffering from diabetic foot complications. In response to a steady increase in publications in this field over the past 5 years, this chapter on psychosocial aspects is an extensive revision and update of this subject since the previous edition of *The Diabetic Foot*. It summarizes the key findings from recently conducted and ongoing studies into how patients adapt to diabetic foot complications by focusing on two areas: the role of psychological factors in guiding adherence to preventive foot self-care and foot ulcer treatment and the impact of diabetic foot ulceration on an individual's emotional state and QoL.

The chapter opens with an overview of the earlier educational and behavioral studies in this area, highlighting the limitations of previous research, which include poor methodologic quality and the lack of a theory-driven, patient-centered approach in studying adherence to foot self-care. Subsequently, it introduces a novel approach to the study of psychological factors influencing adherence behaviors and demonstrates how patients' lay beliefs about foot complications combine with medical information and foot ulcer experience in shaping adherence to foot self-care. Next, studies linking diabetic foot ulceration to depressive symptoms are reviewed. Finally, by comparing and contrasting the generic (nonspecific to foot ulceration) approach to QoL assessment with patient-centered, foot problem–focused investigations, this chapter describes the ways in which foot ulceration affects an individual's functioning and QoL.

Review of Educational and Behavioral Studies of Foot Ulcer Prevention

Three systematic reviews of educational and behavioral studies have been conducted to evaluate the role of patients' foot care education in the prevention of foot ulceration.[3–5] The reviewers were unanimous in their main conclusion, that is, owing to the poor methodologic quality of the studies, the available evidence is "generally unsatisfactory," is "inconclusive," or "needs confirmation."

For example, the results of the eight randomized controlled trials[6-13] that were selected for the most recent review by Valk and colleagues,[5] though conflicting, suggest that while education seems to have a short-term positive effect on foot care knowledge and behaviors, whether it can prevent foot ulceration and amputations remains uncertain. Most of these studies were insufficiently powered to detect clinically important effects of patient education on the hard end points (foot ulceration and amputation) and had inadequate follow-up to assess the potential for prevention of foot complications. Moreover, the eligibility criteria with regard to risk for foot ulceration were adequately described in only one of the randomized controlled trials,[9] and monitoring of adherence to the intervention and outcomes was largely unacceptable (only three studies assessed both adherence to foot care and ulceration/amputation rates).[8,12,13]

One of the most commonly cited studies, conducted by Litzelman and colleagues,[12] introduced a system of reminders and assessed the effect of this intervention on the prevalence of risk factors for lower-limb amputation in type 2 diabetic subjects. This 12-month intervention was multifaceted and aimed at both the patient and the health care provider. Patients received foot care education and entered into a behavioral contract for foot self-care, which was reinforced through telephone and postcard reminders. In addition, the file folders for intervention patients had special identifiers that prompted health care providers to (1) ask that patients remove his or her footwear, (2) perform foot examinations, (3) provide foot care education, and (4) refer to specialist care (podiatric, vascular, and/or orthopedic) when appropriate. It is an important study, as it demonstrated that foot self-care and professional foot care matter in reducing foot ulcer rates: Patients who received the intervention were more likely to report appropriate foot self-care behaviors than control patients and were less likely to have serious foot lesions. However, it is unknown whether these behaviors were retained or faded out after the intervention ended. It is conceivable that the behavioral change might not have been sustained, as it was not intrapersonally generated, that is, it was not determined by a patient's understanding and beliefs about foot complications but rather was imposed by researchers.

The other commonly cited study, that of Malone and colleagues,[9] randomized diabetic patients presenting with severe foot complications (foot infection, ulceration, or prior amputation) into those receiving basic foot care education and those with no education. A brief 1-hour education session consisted of fear-inducing communication (review of slides depicting infected diabetic feet and amputated diabetic limbs) and the provision of a simple set of instructions for patients regarding foot self-care. After 2 years' follow-up, the ulceration and amputation rates were three times lower in the intervention group than in the control group. Because this study

included only patients who had already experienced severe foot complications, it is not clear whether the behavioral change took place in response to the intervention or whether it was the development of a foot ulcer that affected foot self-care, as it is known that foot ulcer experience is predictive of better foot self-care.[14] Thus, while education might well be more effective in this group, generalization to patients who have never experienced diabetic foot complications remains questionable.

It is important to note that all the aforementioned trials were designed to provide patients with an action plan, that is, a list of preventive foot self-care behaviors and/or enhancement of their behavioral skills, but none of the studies attempted to understand the psychological factors that might be implicated in patients' foot care routines. This, at least in part, could explain why the behavioral change was short-lived[10,13] or not achieved.[8,11]

Previous Studies of Psychological Factors Affecting Foot Self-Care

Earlier reports examining psychological factors underlying adherence to foot self-care are sparse and mainly restricted to published abstracts.[15,16] Vileikyte and colleagues,[15] using the Health Belief Model,[17] investigated the perceived severity of and vulnerability to foot complications and perceived barriers to and benefits of foot care. Intriguingly, despite the fact that the researchers explained the results of the tests, patients who were diagnosed as having neuropathy and no evidence of peripheral vascular disease perceived themselves as being significantly more vulnerable to gangrene of the feet (a vascular complication) than to foot ulceration (a consequence of having neuropathy). Although this was an interesting finding, the researchers were unable to explain, within the Health Belief Model framework, why neuropathic patients rated their vulnerability to vascular complications as significantly greater than their vulnerability to foot ulceration. This may be due to the limitations of the Health Belief Model outlined by Leventhal and Nerenz.[18] Although the Health Belief Model provides global evaluations of vulnerability to health threats, it lacks content and thus explanatory power for how vulnerability judgments are made.

The study of McKay and colleagues[16] tested the role of personality traits in predicting a series of relatively independent self-management behaviors (diet, exercise, blood glucose testing, and foot care) in a sample of 221 users of an Internet-based diabetes support system. They found that the conscientiousness score was an independent predictor of adherence to foot care. However, this observation needs to be treated with caution because it was made in a highly self-selected group of patients. Additionally, as there is evidence to suggest that personality traits predict health care actions through patients' representations or understanding and beliefs about their illness,[19] the role of personality might have been more fully understood if assessed by introducing the patients' interpretation of foot complications as a factor potentially linking conscientiousness to foot self-care. Nevertheless, it is an interesting finding and supports a belief commonly held by practitioners that a patient's personality influences adherence to treatment recommendations.

Several other reports, though not explicitly assessing the psychological factors that influence adherence to foot care, point to the possibility that such factors are at play when patients make behavioral decisions about preventive foot self-care. When comparing the two groups of high-risk neuropathic patients, that is, those with and without foot ulcer history, Vileikyte[20] reported that although both groups had sufficient knowledge regarding preventive foot care, scores for self-reported foot care practice were significantly higher in patients who had experienced a foot ulcer than in those with no ulcer history. It could be speculated that the development of a foot ulcer resulted in reappraisal of the health threat, making it more relevant to the self and therefore more threatening, resulting in better foot care practice. Similarly, Breuer[21] showed that adherence to protective footwear was significantly higher in patients who perceived the health status of their feet as less favorable than in those who perceived the health status of their feet more favorably. These observations indicate that patients' behavioral decisions are influenced by their representation of the health threat and point to the need for an examination of how diabetic patients who are at high physical risk for developing an insensate foot ulcer understand and control their foot ulcer risks.

The Commonsense Model of Illness Behavior

The commonsense model (CSM) of illness behavior provides a framework for exploring how people give meaning to the diagnosis and symptoms associated with chronic illness and make decisions to take specific actions in response to them.[22] The CSM postulates that patients process health-threatening information by constructing commonsense disease models or understanding about illness in terms of symptoms and diagnostic labels, antecedent conditions that are believed to cause illness, expected duration, possibility of cure or prevention, and anticipated impact of illness. Two types of information are integrated when patients construct commonsense views of their health status: verbal information from other people—including physicians, other patients. and family members—and concrete experience of symptoms and physical dysfunction.

Guided by the CSM, studies of patient adherence to treatment for chronic conditions such as hypertension and congestive heart failure indicate that inconsistencies between information provided by practitioners and the patients' commonsense interpretation of medical diagnoses and symptom experience result in nonadherence to treatment recommendations.[23,24] Baumann and Leventhal, for example, showed that people with hypertension tend to believe that they can tell when their blood pressure is elevated and use symptoms as indicators as to whether or not to take antihypertensive medication.[25] More recently, Horowitz and colleagues demonstrated that patients with chronic heart failure perceive it to be an acute medical condition and, as a result, do not manage symptoms on a regular basis, thus failing to prevent exacerbations.[24] In the area of diabetes, Hampson and colleagues have demonstrated that personal models or perception of diabetes and its symptoms predicted adherence to dietary recommendations and levels of physical activity.[25]

The main concept of the CSM can be further illustrated by the clinical example of a patient with painful neuropathy and no evidence of peripheral vascular disease (Fig. 31-1). His commonsense understanding or "folk" model that the painful sensations in his feet were caused by poor circulation led him to set as a goal the improvement of the blood supply to his feet; he therefore decided to cut the toebox off his shoes, thereby enabling him to wiggle his toes, which he believed would improve the circulation. As his actions alleviated pain, thus confirming his "diagnosis" of poor circulation, he continued to engage in potentially damaging behaviors (wearing open-toed shoes). From the medical perspective, his symptoms could be described as allodynia, which improved when the nonnoxious stimulus, that is, the pressure from the shoes, was removed, which then, of course, exposed his toes to potential injury. This clinical case demonstrates that patients respond to foot complications by constructing their own images or models that are inconsistent with the biomedical processes underlying the disease.

In the context of diabetic foot complications, it is therefore important to determine whether the patients' understanding and perception of neuropathy capture the features of this medical disorder that are critical for their participation in foot self-care. For example, do patients understand the nature of their risks, that is, that the absence of symptoms does not indicate that the feet are healthy? Do they understand how neuropathy may result in foot ulceration and why, for example, it is important to have their feet measured when buying shoes or why regular removal of callus reduces their risk for foot ulceration? Thus, uncovering the patients' representations of diabetic foot complications and understanding how they merge lay beliefs with information from practitioners can hold the key to understanding patients' participation in foot self-care.

Commonsense Model

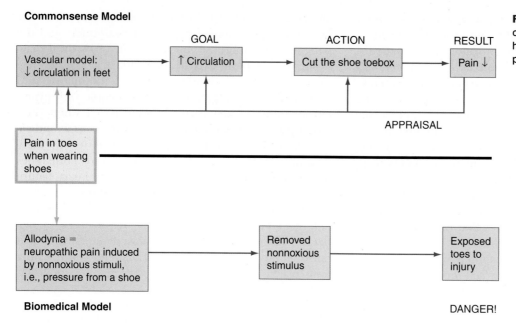

Figure 31–1 Patient's commonsense model versus health care provider's model of painful neuropathy.

Patient's Commonsense Model (Interpretation) of Diabetic Foot Complications and Foot Self-Care

The combination of the CSM with clinical experience and evidence from interviews with patients who are at high risk for foot ulceration informed the development of the Neuropathy Psychosocial Inventory, an instrument that assesses patients' representations of neuropathy and foot ulceration.[26] A large U.K. and U.S. study employed the Neuropathy Psychosocial Inventory to describe the ways in which the patients' folk beliefs combine with medical information in predicting engagement in preventive foot self-care.[14] It also examined the role of foot ulceration in shaping their beliefs about diabetic foot complications and foot self-care behaviors (Fig. 31-2). The results of this prospective study indicate that the majority of patients who have been diagnosed with diabetic neuropathy believe that the development of a foot ulcer will be accompanied by pain. Additionally, patients anticipate that foot damage from diabetes would be vascular and that vascular damage should be reflected in poor circulation manifested as "cold feet." These lay beliefs falsely reassure patients that their feet are healthy, leading to a failure to engage in preventive foot self-care, thereby resulting in behaviors practiced by individuals with intact sensation in the feet (see Fig. 31-2; pink arrows). In contrast, patients who accurately interpret the health care provider's diagnosis of neuropathy and realize that it is possible to have a serious medical condition even if the feet are warm and asymptomatic report higher levels of preventive foot self-care (see Fig. 31-2; purple arrows). Furthermore, our results showed that ulcer causal beliefs are among the strongest predictors

of preventive foot self-care. That is, patients who have a coherent picture of how various neuropathic risk factors can lead to foot ulceration are more likely to engage in foot self-care actions that reduce the impact of these risk factors. Having had a foot ulcer motivates actions to avoid risks and prevent recurrence (see Fig. 31-2; red arrows). It teaches patients that lay beliefs, such as "good circulation means healthy feet," are inaccurate and that pain is not a necessary feature of foot ulcers. Moreover, a foot ulcer experience facilitates better understanding of how such ulcers occur. This could simply be a reflection of the learning by experience process; for example, an individual who develops a painless foot ulcer while wearing a new pair of shoes realizes that footwear, in combination with reduced feeling in the feet, can result in ulceration. As Del Aguila and colleagues demonstrated, it is also possible that practitioners are more likely to provide information about the health threats when confronted with a patient who actually has a foot ulcer than when they are dealing with a patient who has the risk factors alone.[27] It is most likely, however, that foot ulcer experience interacts with medical information processing in shaping patients' perceptions about diabetic foot complications. Experience of a foot ulcer and accompanying health worry are likely to result in increased attention to medical information. Interestingly, beliefs about the nature of neuropathy were independent of foot ulcer history, suggesting that foot ulcer experience is not sufficient to teach patients that neuropathy is a core problem underlying diabetic foot complications and requires additional explanation by the health care provider.

Contrary to the belief, commonly held by clinicians, that their patients ignore the risks because the patients are using denial as a protective mechanism to avoid being

Interpretation of medical information:

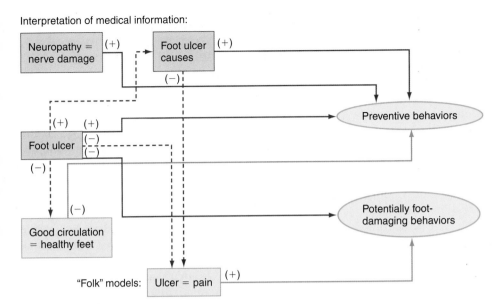

Figure 31–2   The role of foot ulceration in shaping patients' beliefs about diabetic foot complications and foot self-care behaviors.

emotionally overwhelmed, the results of the current study did not find evidence for curvilinearity; higher levels of fear of amputation were associated with better foot self-care. It is important to note that it is not the intensity of fear but the source of fear or the nature of beliefs underlying emotion that is critical. For example, while fear of complications might lead to seeking medical care by someone with poorly controlled diabetes on oral hypoglycemics alone, fear can sometimes result in avoidance behaviors if it is the potential treatment (e.g., insulin injections) that is feared. Moreover, while the specific emotion of worry about foot ulcers and amputation appears to motivate preventive actions, generalized (nonspecific, not related to illness) anxiety does not seem to affect foot self-care actions. These observations are consistent with increasing research evidence that emotional responses that are attached to specific aspects of illness (fear of threatening outcomes such as cancer or AIDS) are important predictors of health care behaviors in contrast to the weak and inconsistent relationships between illness behaviors and measures of generalized distress.[28,29] Finally, of the five personality traits (neuroticism, conscientiousness, intellect, extraversion, and agreeableness) and personality-like characteristics (hostility), only conscientiousness was significantly associated with better foot self-care. It appears that conscientiousness is linked to foot self-care actions both directly and indirectly, that is, through more accurate understanding about neuropathy and foot ulceration. These findings strongly suggest that patients' commonsense beliefs about foot complications are important determinants of a lack of foot self-care and that the health care provider's ability to identify these misperceptions and correct them, by communicating clear and consistent messages about the nature of neuropathy, is pivotal for ensuring effective patient foot self-care.

Furthermore, loss of pain sensation not only affects adherence to preventive foot self-care, but also results in a lack of adherence to prescribed foot ulcer treatment (e.g., wearing an ulcer-off-loading device to reduce mechanical stress) and contributes significantly to nonhealing of foot ulcers.[30] Whereas people with foot lesions in the absence of neuropathy avoid walking on such wounds because of pain, patients with insensitive feet continue to walk on plantar ulcers. This prolongs the patients' physical and psychosocial dysfunction, including restrictions on activities of daily living and associated emotional distress.[31]

Foot Ulceration and Depression: Is There a Link?

Depressive symptoms are known to be more common in people with diabetes than in the general population[32] and are associated with a range of negative outcomes, including nonadherence to treatment,[33] poor glycemic control,[34] diminished function, and increased health care costs.[35,36] A growing body of evidence suggests that depression is associated with the long-term complications of diabetes,[37,38] although the relationship between diabetic foot complications and depression is less clear.

Recently, Vileikyte and colleagues have investigated, both cross-sectionally[39] and prospectively,[40] the relationship between depressive symptoms and neuropathy-specific somatic experiences, including pain, unsteadiness, reduced feeling in the feet, and foot ulceration. The results of this study have demonstrated that while neuropathic symptoms, in particular unsteadiness, were the strongest independent predictors of depression, no association was found between diabetic foot ulcers and depressive symptoms. Similarly, Ismail and colleagues examined the role of depression in recurrence and healing of foot ulcers over an 18-month period in patients presenting with the first foot ulcer episode and showed that depression is not predictive of foot ulcer recurrence or healing.[41] Furthermore, Willrich and colleagues, using the Zung self-rating depression scale and the Short Form-36 (SF-36) questionnaire, demonstrated that while foot ulcers and Charcot neuroarthropathy have a negative effect on patients' physical and mental functioning, the negative effect on functioning does not seem to be associated with clinical depression.[42] Moreover, Lin and colleagues examined the relationship between depression and various diabetes self-care activities and found that depression was associated with poorer exercise, diet, and medication adherence but not with preventive foot self-care.[43]

It therefore appears that while foot ulcer–specific emotional responses are prominent and include fear of potential consequences and anger directed at health care providers as a result of a perceived lack of timely and clear explanation about foot complications,[44] no evidence for an association between foot ulceration and depressive symptoms has been found. The lack of a link between foot ulceration and depression is somewhat unexpected, in view of the evidence that foot ulcers are associated with severe restrictions in mobility, loss of work time, and other disruptions in activities of daily living. A possible explanation as to why foot ulcers are not associated with depression could be that neuropathic diabetic foot ulcers are typically painless, thereby intruding little on an individual's consciousness and causing minimal emotional distress. Also, the levels of physical disruption caused by foot ulceration might not reach those needed to produce depression, as it is well established that depressed affect is a function of prolonged restrictions in activities of daily living.[45] It is also possible that patients who are affected by foot ulceration receive sufficient social (family and medical) support, which might act as a buffer against depression. Additionally, other psychological variables, such as a perceived lack of treatment control and chronicity of illness, that are known to be important determinants of depression might not be sufficiently pronounced to cause depression in patients who are experiencing foot ulceration; that is, although foot ulcers are difficult to treat and do take a long time to heal, they are usually curable and thus of limited duration. It is important to remember, however, that even though foot ulceration is not associated with depressive symptoms, other experiences of neuropathy, such as pain and, in particular, unsteadiness, are important predictors of depression in this group of patients. Therefore, people with diabetic neuropathy have an increased risk of depressive symptoms; they should be carefully monitored to determine whether they are depressed and provided with treatment or referral as necessary.

Diabetic Foot Ulceration and Quality of Life: Studies That Employed a Generic (Nonspecific to Foot Ulcer) Experience Approach

Studies on the effects of foot ulceration on patients' physical and psychosocial functioning and QoL made clear that foot ulcers can be a source of severe disability, which, in turn, has a negative impact on QoL. One of the first studies in this area was conducted in Manchester, England, by Carrington and associates.[46] Using a battery of self-report psychological instruments, the investigators compared the psychological status of diabetic people with chronic foot ulcers or unilateral lower-limb amputations with that of diabetic control subjects with no history of foot ulceration. Psychological assessment included the Psychosocial Adjustment to Illness Scale, the Hospital Anxiety and Depression scale, a foot questionnaire specifically designed to assess the attitudes and feelings that people with diabetes have toward their feet, and a QoL ladder. The study reported that patients with chronic foot ulcers or unilateral amputations had poorer psychosocial adjustment to diabetes than did the control subjects. Specifically, these two groups had made significantly poorer psychosocial adjustments to their situations in the domains of domestic and social environment and reported poorer overall QoL. In addition, foot ulcer patients reported significant problems with their employment and more psychological stress than did the control subjects. Interestingly, no significant differences in psychosocial adjustment were observed between the ulcer group and the amputee group. This could in part be due to patient selection bias, as the authors of this paper pointed out; while all subjects with foot ulceration had recurrent, nonhealing foot ulcers of at least 3 months' duration, all but one of the amputee patients had a transtibial amputation and were mobile with no ulcers on the remaining foot at the time of the interview. It was therefore concluded that future studies should include patients with varying amputation levels, that is, minor (e.g., toe) and major (transtibial/transfemoral) and varying duration of foot ulceration.

A study from Sweden by Ragnarson-Tennvall and Apelqvist compared the health status of 457 diabetic patients divided into three groups: those with current foot ulcers, those with primary healed ulcers, and those who had undergone minor or major amputations.[31] The researchers used a five-item generic measure of health status, the EQ-5D. Each item of this instrument assesses a separate health-related dimension: mobility, self-care, usual activities, pain/discomfort, and anxiety/depression; the response choices are no problems, some problems, and severe problems. A single numeric index of health status was then generated from the five dimensions. In addition, this instrument contains a visual analog scale by which patients are asked to rate their present health on a scale from 0 to 100. The results of this study demonstrated that subjects with current ulcers had a poorer health status than did patients who had healed primarily without any amputation and those who had undergone a minor amputation. Patients who had undergone a major amputation had a poorer health status than did either those who healed primarily and those who had undergone a minor amputation. Interestingly, this study also failed to demonstrate significant differences between the current foot ulcer and major amputation groups, as did the study by Carrington and colleagues.[46] This could indicate either that the two groups do not differ in terms of their health status or that the generic questionnaires are not sensitive enough to pick up subtle differences between these groups.

The results of the following reports cast further doubt as to the appropriateness of generic questionnaires in examining the health status of patients with foot ulceration, especially in the domain of mental functioning. A study by Meijer and colleagues, using the SF-36, compared the health status and mobility between diabetic patients with either past or present foot ulceration and diabetic individuals without a history of foot ulcers.[47] The results of the study demonstrated that the presence or history of foot ulceration has a negative impact on physical (physical role, physical functioning, and mobility) but not mental functioning. Similar results were obtained by Ahroni and colleagues, who demonstrated prospectively that the development of neuropathic complications, including foot ulceration and amputation, were associated with a decline in four out of eight SF-36 scales representing physical functioning (general health, physical functioning, physical role, and vitality).[48] Most recently, Nabuurs-Franssen and colleagues, using the SF-36, prospectively evaluated the effect of a foot ulcer on QoL of patients and their caregivers and demonstrated that healing of a foot ulcer resulted in marked improvement in QoL, while a persistent foot ulcer was associated with a progressive decline in QoL. Intriguingly, having a nonhealing foot ulcer did not affect the patients' emotional functioning, while it appeared to inflict a severe emotional burden on their caregivers.[49]

In contrast, a recent study that compared the performance of the generic SF-12 and a neuropathy and foot ulcer–specific questionnaire, the NeuroQoL (described below), demonstrated that while the mental functioning scale from the SF-12 was not associated with foot ulcer presence, a foot problem–specific emotional burden scale from the NeuroQoL showed a strong association with the presence of foot ulceration and was the most important link between foot ulceration and reduced QoL.[50] These findings point to the importance of using condition-specific questionnaires in studying the effects of foot ulceration on an individual's health status and QoL.

Diabetic Foot Ulceration and Quality of Life: Addressing the Patient's Perspective

Because the above studies used generic questionnaires, the content of which was imposed by investigators and did not originate with patients affected by foot ulcers, the findings left a gap between foot ulceration as abstractly defined and the patient's experience of foot ulceration, which is essential for framing effective interventions. It is increasingly recognized that QoL, rather than being a mere rating of health status, is actually a uniquely personal experience, representing the way in which individuals perceive and react to their health status.[51] This recognition emphasizes the importance of addressing the patient's perspective rather than the researcher's views in measuring QoL. In an attempt to overcome these shortcomings, several questionnaires assessing QoL from the perspective of an individual affected by foot ulceration were recently developed. Examples include the Diabetic Foot Ulcer Scale (DFS)[52] and the Neuropathy and Foot Ulcer-specific Quality of Life instrument (NeuroQoL).[50] A series of interviews with foot ulcer patients and their caregivers were conducted to elicit life domains affected by foot ulceration that are important to an individual's QoL. These interviews demonstrated that the loss of mobility caused by nonweight-bearing treatment is central to foot ulcer experience. It results in severe restrictions in activities of daily living, including daily tasks, leisure activities, and employment. Brod, for example, reported that approximately half of the interviewed patients had either retired early or lost time from work, and career opportunities were sometimes missed.[53] Moreover, limited mobility causes problems with social and interpersonal relationships, including perceptions of diminished value of the self due to inability to perform social and family roles.

A recent study employed the NeuroQoL to investigate the impact of diabetic neuropathy (symptoms and foot ulceration) on individuals' QoL.[50] Findings from this investigation were largely consistent with the main themes that emerged from qualitative studies. Patients experiencing neuropathic symptoms (pain, lost or reduced feeling in the feet, and unsteadiness) and foot ulcers reported severe restrictions in daily activities (e.g., leisure, paid work, and daily tasks), problems with interpersonal relationships and changes in self-perception (e.g., being treated differently from other people). This study demonstrated that among the psychosocial variables, changes in self-perception as a result of foot complications have the most devastating effects on an individual's QoL.

Summary

Diabetic foot ulceration is a source of severe physical dysfunction, emotional distress, and poor quality of life.

While foot ulceration is not predictive of depressive symptoms, it is a source of ulcer-specific emotional responses, which either facilitate (fear of potential consequences) or inhibit (anger at health care providers) preventive foot self-care actions. Patients respond to diabetic foot complications by creating their own models or understanding about this medical disorder, which are largely inconsistent with the practitioner's or biomedical view, resulting in a lack of foot self-care. The health care provider's ability to understand and share the patients' commonsense perspective is therefore central to effective health care provider-patient communication and should potentially lead to better foot self-care and fewer foot ulcers and lower-limb amputations.

References

1. Pecoraro R, Reiber GE, Burgess EM: Pathways to diabetic limb amputation. Diabetes Care 13:513–521, 1990.
2. Trautner C, Haastert B, Spraul M, et al: Unchanged incidence of lower-limb amputations in a German city, 1990–1998. Diabetes Care 24:855–859, 2001.
3. Mason J, O'Keefe CO, Hutchinson A, et al: A systematic review of foot ulcers in patients with type 2 diabetes mellitus II: Treatment. Diabetic Med 16:889–909, 1999.
4. Majid M, Cullum N, O'Meara S, et al: Systematic reviews of wound care management: Diabetic foot ulceration. Health Technol Assess (Rockv) 21:113–238, 2000.
5. Valk GD, Kriegsman DM, Assendelft WJJ: Patient education for preventing diabetic patient ulceration: A systematic review. Endocrinol Metab Clin N Am 31:633–658, 2002.
6. Mazzuca SA, Moorman NH, Wheeler ML: The diabetes education study: A controlled trial of the effects of diabetes patient education. Diabetes Care 9:1–10, 1986.
7. Rettig BA, Shrauge DG, Recker RR: A randomized study of the effects of a home diabetes education program. Diabetes Care 9:173–178, 1986.
8. Bloomgarden ZT, Karmally W, Metzger MJ: Randomized controlled trial of diabetic patient education: Improved knowledge without improved metabolic status. Diabetes Care 10:263–272, 1997.
9. Malone JM, Snyder M, Anderson G, et al: Prevention of amputation by diabetic education. Am J Surg 158:520–523, 1989.
10. Barth R, Campbell LV, Allen S, et al: Intensive education improve knowledge, compliance, and foot problems in type 2 diabetes. Diabetic Med 8:111–117, 1991.
11. Kruger S, Guthrie D: Foot care: Knowledge retention and self-practices. Diabetes Educ 18:487–490, 1992.
12. Litzelman DK, Slemenda CW, Langefeld CD, et al: Reduction of lower extremity clinical abnormalities in patients with non-insulin-dependent diabetes mellitus. Ann Intern Med 119:36–41, 1993.
13. Ronnemaa T, Hamalainen H, Toikka T: Evaluation of the impact of podiatrist care in the primary prevention of foot problems in diabetic subjects. Diabetes Care 20:1833–1837, 1997.
14. Vileikyte L, Gonzalez JS, Leventhal H, et al: The role of patients' representations of diabetic foot complications in guiding foot self-care: A longitudinal study. Diabetes (suppl 1), 2006.
15. Vileikyte L, Shaw JE, Boulton AJM: Diabetic foot: patients' perceptions of risks and barriers to foot care may be the final determinants of ulceration [abstract]. Diabetes 46(suppl 1):A147, 1997.
16. McKay HG, Boles SM, Glasgow RE: Personality (conscientiousness) and environmental (barriers) factors related to diabetes self-management and quality of life. Diabetes 47(suppl 1):A44, 1998.
17. Rosenstock IM: The health belief model and preventive health behavior. Health Educ Monogr 2:354–386, 1974.
18. Leventhal H, Nerenz D: The assessment of illness cognition. In P. Karoly (ed): Measurement Strategies in Health. NewYork: John Wiley & Sons, 1985, pp 517–554.
19. Skinner TC, Hampson SE, Fife-Schaw C: Personality, personal model beliefs, and self-care in adolescents and young adults with type 1 diabetes. Health Psychol 21:61–70, 2002.
20. Vileikyte L: Psychological aspects of diabetic peripheral neuropathy. Diabetes Rev 7:387–394, 1999.
21. Breuer U: Diabetic patients' compliance with bespoke footwear after healing of neuropathic foot ulcers. Diabete Metab 20:415–419, 1994.
22. Leventhal H, Meyer D, Nerenz D: The common sense representation of illness danger. In Rachman S (ed): Contributions to medical psychology, vol 2. New York: Pergamon, 1980, pp 7–30.
23. Baumann LJ, Leventhal H: I can tell when my blood pressure is up, can't I? Health Psychol 4:203–218, 1985.
24. Horowitz CR, Stephanie BR, Leventhal H: A story of maladies, misconceptions and mishaps: Effective management of heart failure. Soc Sci Med 58:631–643, 2004.
25. Hampson SE, Glasgow RE, Foster LS: Personal models of diabetes among older adults: Relationship to self-management and other variables. Diabetes Educ 4:300–307, 1995.
26. Vileikyte L, Rubin RR, Leventhal H, et al: The Neuropathy Psychosocial Inventory: A novel approach to identify factors associated with foot care adherence. Diabetes (suppl 1) 2002.
27. Del Aguila MA, Reiber GE, Koepsell TD: How does provider and patient awareness of high risk status for lower extremity amputation influence foot-care practice? Diabetes Care 17:1050–1054, 1994.
28. Diefenbach MA, Miller SM, Daly MB: Specific worry about breast cancer predicts mammography use in women at risk for breast and ovarian cancer. Health Psychol 18:532– 536, 1999.
29. Mora P, Robitaille C, Leventhal H et al : Trait negative affect relates to prior weak symptoms, but not to reports of illness episodes, illness symptoms and care seeking. Psychosom Med 4:436–449, 2002.
30. Boulton AJM, Armstrong DG: Clinical trials in plantar neuropathic diabetic foot ulcers: Time for a paradigm shift? Diabetes Care 26:2689–2690, 2003.
31. Ragnarson Tennvall G, Apelqvist J: Health-related quality of life in patients with diabetes mellitus and foot ulcers. J Diab Compl 14:235–241, 2000.
32. Anderson RJ, Freedland KE, Clouse RE, Lustman PJ: The prevalence of comorbid depression in adults with diabetes: A meta-analysis. Diabetes Care 24:1069–1078, 2001.
33. DiMatteo MR, Lepper HS, Croghan TW: Depression is a risk factor for non-compliance with medical treatment: Meta-analysis of the effects of anxiety and depression on patient adherence. Arch Intern Med 160:2101–2107, 2000.
34. Lustman PJ, Anderson RJ, Freedland KE, et al: Depression and poor glycemic control: A meta-analytic review of the literature. Diabetes Care 23:934–942, 2000.
35. Ciechanowski PS, Katon WJ, Russo JE: Depression and diabetes: Impact of depressive symptoms on adherence, function, and costs. Arch Intern Med 160:3278–3285, 2000.
36. Egede LE, Zheng D, Simpson K: Comorbid depression is associated with increased health care use and expenditures in individuals with diabetes. Diabetes Care 25:464–470, 2002.
37. Peyrot M, Rubin RR: Levels and risks of depression and anxiety symptomatology among diabetic adults. Diabetes Care 20:585–590, 1997.
38. de Groot M, Anderson R, Freedland KE, et al: Association of depression and diabetes complications: A meta-analysis. Psychosom Med 63:619–630, 2001.
39. Vileikyte L, Leventhal H, Gonzalez JS, et al: Diabetic peripheral neuropathy and depression: The association revisited. Diabetes Care 28:2378–2383, 2005.
40. Vileikyte L, Gonzalez JS, Leventhal H, et al: Predictors of depression in subjects with diabetic peripheral neuropathy: A longitudinal study. Ann Behav Med 11(suppl 1):P62, 2004.
41. Ismail K, Winkley K, Chalder T, Edmonds ME: Is depression associated with a worse prognosis following the first onset of a diabetic foot ulcer? Diabetes (suppl 1) P1969, 2005.
42. Willrich A, Pinzur M, McNeil M, et al: Health related quality of life, cognitive function, and depression in diabetic patients with foot ulcer or amputation: A preliminary study. Foot Ankle Int 26:128–134, 2005.
43. Lin EH, Katon W, Von Korff M, et al: Relationship of depression and diabetes self-care, medication adherence, and preventive care. Diabetes Care 26:2154–2160, 2004.

44. Vileikyte L, Rubin RR, Leventhal H: Psychological aspects of diabetic neuropathic foot complications: An overview. Diabetes Metab Res Rev 20(suppl 1):S13–S18, 2004.

45. Williamson GM: The central role of restricted normal activities in adjustment to illness and disability: A model of depressed affect. Rehabil Psychol 43:327–347, 1998.

46. Carrington AL, Mawdsley SK, Morley M, et al: Psychological status of diabetic people with or without lower limb disability. Diab Res Clin Pract 32:19–25, 1996.

47. Meijer JW, Trip J, Jaegers SM, et al: Quality of life in patients with diabetic foot ulcers. Disabil Rehabil 23:336–340, 2001.

48. Ahroni JH, Boyko EJ: Responsiveness of the SF-36 among veterans with diabetes mellitus. J Diab Compl 14:31–39, 2000.

49. Nabuurs-Franssen MH, Huijberts MSP, Nieuwenhuijzen Kruseman AC, et al: Health-related quality of life of diabetic foot ulcer patients and their caregivers. Diabetologia 48:1906–1910, 2005.

50. Vileikyte L, Peyrot M, Bundy EC, et al: The development and validation of a neuropathy and foot ulcer specific quality of life instrument. Diabetes Care 26:2549–2555, 2003.

51. Gill TM, Feinstein AR: A critical appraisal of the quality of quality-of-life measurements. JAMA 272:619–625, 1994.

52. Abetz L, Sutton M, Brady L, et al: The Diabetic Foot Ulcer Scale (DFS): A quality of life instrument for use in clinical trials. Pract Diab Int 19:167–175, 2002.

53. Brod M: Quality of life issues in patients with diabetes and lower extremity ulcers: Patients and care givers. Qual Life Res 7:365–372, 1997.

REIMBURSEMENT AND MEDICAL–LEGAL ASPECTS

DIAGNOSTIC AND PROCEDURAL CODING

WALTER J. PEDOWITZ ∎

To be reimbursed for your work in the care of the diabetic patient, you must document what you have done on the forms you send to the insurance companies. This includes the ICD-9-CM (diagnosis) and CPT (procedural) codes. If you do something and do not document it on both the form and the medical record, you will be underpaid for your efforts and be subject to costly insurance audits. Since only the physician who encounters the patient truly understands the details of what was done, we strongly urge that you do your own coding. You evaluated the patient, did the procedure, and/or performed the service, and this puts you in the best position to select the correct codes. People who are not familiar with the procedure or service might unbundle codes or underrepresent your efforts, often leading to poor reimbursement. Also, if you do not code correctly the first time, reimbursement will be excessively prolonged. As anyone in practice must realize, accurate coding is not always black and white. In many cases, there are different ways to code the same scenario. You want to pick the one code that is not only accurate but also reflects the level of work you did for the diabetic patient. In this regard, it must be remembered that care of these patients is always more difficult and complex and involves greater risk than care of the usual foot and ankle patient.

To accurately code, you need two books, which change yearly or even undergo several updates during each year. You must have the most recent Current Procedural Terminology (CPT) and the latest version of the International Classification of Diseases (ICD-9-CM) with all the updates as well as an Explanation of Benefits (EOBs) from all the insurance carriers with which you participate. Most of what is contained in this chapter is based on Centers for Medicare and Medicaid Services (CMS) rules. Non-Medicare payers have their own payment policies and should be contacted for their individual guidelines.

ICD-9-CM Diagnosis Coding

This compendium is prepared by the World Health Organization and must be the source of your information. The ICD-9 terminology is old-fashioned, lacking many common medical terms, and the index is incomplete. The ICD-10 is currently being prepared, and its rules will be similar. The diagnosis must be as accurate as possible, since communication with third-party payers is of the utmost importance.

At the time you see the patient you can code only what you know to be correct, even if it is only a symptom. For example, suppose a type 2 diabetic presents with a red, hot, swollen foot and ankle. Your differential diagnosis is infection or Charcot arthropathy. Do not code "Rule out Charcot foot" or "Rule out infection." Code *Effusion of joint* (719.07) or *Pain in joint* (719.47), *Arthralgia of ankle and foot*. When the specific diagnosis is proven, change to the proper ICD code, such as *Neurogenic arthropathy* (713.5).

Code to the highest available level of specificity. ICD 250 is the code for diabetes. But if you know that the patient has neurologic findings, code *Diabetes with neurological manifestations* (250.6). It is required that you always code to the fifth digit. From the ICD-9-CM Book (as of 2006), 250 *Diabetes Mellitus* excludes *gestational diabetes* (648.8), *hyperglycemia NOS* (Not Otherwise Specified) (790.6), *neonatal diabetes mellitus* (775.1), *nonclinical diabetes* (790.2), and *diabetes complicating pregnancy, childbirth, or the puerperium* (648.0).

The fourth-digit categories used with 250 are as follows:

250.0 Diabetes mellitus without mention of complication
Diabetes mellitus without mention of complication or manifestation classifiable to 250.1–250.9
Diabetes (mellitus) NOS
250.1 Diabetes with ketoacidosis
Diabetic: acidosis (without mention of coma)
          ketosis (without mention of coma)
250.2 Diabetes with hyperosmolarity
Hyperosmolar (nonketotic) coma
250.3 Diabetes with other coma
Diabetic coma (with ketoacidosis)
Diabetic hypoglycemic coma
Insulin coma NOS

EXCLUDES diabetes with hyperosmolar coma (250.2X)

250.4 Diabetes with renal manifestations
Use additional code to identify manifestation, as:
diabetic: nephropathy NOS (583.81)
        nephrosis (581.81)
        intercapillary glomerulosclerosis (581.81)
        Kimmelstiel-Wilson syndrome (581.81)
250.5 Diabetes with ophthalmic manifestations
Use additional code to identify manifestation, as
diabetic: blindness (369.00–369.9)
        cataract (366.41)
        glaucoma (365.44)
        macular edema (362.07)
        retinal edema (362.07)
        retinopathy (362.01–362.07)
250.6 Diabetes with neurological manifestations
Use additional code to identify manifestation, as
diabetic: amyotrophy (358.1)
        gastroparalysis (536.3)
        gastroparesis (536.3)
        mononeuropathy (354.0–355.9)
        neurogenic arthropathy (713.5)
        peripheral autonomic neuropathy (337.1)
        polyneuropathy (357.2)
250.7 Diabetes with peripheral circulatory disorders
Use additional code to identify manifestation, as
diabetic: gangrene (785.4)
        peripheral angiopathy (443.81)
250.8 Diabetes with other specified manifestations
Diabetic hypoglycemia
Hypoglycemic shock
Use additional code to identify manifestation, as
    any associated ulceration (707.10–707.9)
    diabetic bone changes (731.8)
Use additional E code to identify cause, if drug-induced.

The fifth digit categories used with 250 are:
0 type 2 or unspecified type, not stated as uncontrolled
  Fifth digit 0 is used for type 2 patients, even if the patient requires insulin
  Use additional code, if applicable, for associated long-term (current) insulin—use V58.67
1 type I [juvenile type], not stated as uncontrolled
2 type 2 or unspecified type, uncontrolled
  Fifth digit 2 is for use for type 2 patients, even if the patient requires insulin
  Use additional code, if applicable, for associated long-term (current) insulin—use V58.67
3 type I [juvenile type], uncontrolled
Source: ICD-9-CM diagnosis book.

Use the alphabetic index to locate the area where the code will be. Although the index is incomplete and usually does not have the fifth digits, it does direct you to the correct section of the tabular list. Always use the tabular list to select the definitive code and to obtain directions for using the fifth-digit classification for that category. When the problem is complex and involves multiple diagnoses, first list the diagnosis that is responsible for the initial procedure or encounter and then list the diagnoses for the comorbidities. You will be treating a complication of diabetes and should code for it. But the inclusion of the major disease code as a comorbidity adds to the complexity. Code only active diagnoses, avoiding conditions that no longer exist. If the diagnosis changes after the operation or during the course of treatment, change to the new diagnosis. Do not continue to use the old one.

You must have an appropriate diagnosis for each procedure that is billed. If a postoperative complication occurs and needs treatment, this now becomes the initial diagnosis, for example, postoperative infection (998.5). Evaluation of the diabetic patient in the office or hospital always brings additional burdens. What can initially be considered a simple musculoskeletal problem always brings with it the tasks of evaluating an immunosuppressed patient, usually with comorbidities, who is on complicated multiple medication schedules and whose neuropathy will confuse the validity of the history. As a concerned physician, you will evaluate this, but if it is not documented in the record, reimbursement will be denied.

Evaluation and Management (E&M) Coding

The extent of history taking, physical examination, and medical decision making is the key component in determining the level of E&M code reported. With a new patient or consultation, all three levels must be equal to report the appropriate code, while in the follow-up visit, two out of three of these areas must be covered in order to report the highest code. In the musculoskeletal examination, the body is divided into six areas: (1) head and neck; (2) spine, ribs, and pelvis; (3) right upper extremity; (4) left upper extremity; (5) right lower extremity; and (6) left lower extremity. To qualify for a level 4 or 5 E&M examination, four of the six areas must be evaluated. With the diabetic foot, you are evaluating a lower-limb problem that often requires diminished or non-weight-bearing. Can the patient use crutches or a walker? Is a wheelchair or bed rest required? You must also evaluate the functional capacity of the upper limbs and the torso. Although you do this, it is rarely documented. If it is documented, you can more easily qualify for an upper-level examination.

The diabetic foot patient is frequently frail and may return often as a follow-up patient with a new problem. Statistically, this is most often coded as a level 3. A level 4 examination requires a detailed or comprehensive history, a detailed or comprehensive examination, and a medical decision of straightforward or low complexity. Obtaining two out of three is made easier owing to the nature of the disease with its inherent increased complexity.

You can base your E&M coding on time if the following criteria are met:

- Over 50% of the time used for E&M is spent counseling and coordinating care.
- The total time with family and/or patient is documented.
- The total time counseling and/or coordinating is documented.
- The nature and/or content of the counseling and/or coordination of care is documented.

Consultations

A consultation is a request by another health care provider for your advice as to evaluation and management of a medical problem that falls in your area of expertise. This is signified by an oral or written request by the original physician or acknowledgement by the patient that the request was made. Documentation of the request must be reflected in the office record. You must communicate your findings to the requesting physician in a letter. If the requesting physician initially asks you to assume the care of the patient, this is not a consultation. The place of service will change the type of coding you do for the encounter.

Office Consultations: 99241–99245
Initial Inpatient Consultations:
    99251–99255

After the initial consultation, you may assume the further care of the patient, coded as follow-up care. If you decide that the patient requires surgery within 24 hours of the consultation, you must add the -57 modifier (deci-

sion for surgery) to protect the consultation reimbursement. If you are called to see a patient by the emergency room (ER) doctor to offer your opinion, this is coded as an outpatient consultation. If you ask the patient to meet you in the ER for an evaluation, this is an outpatient visit. ER codes are for emergency room doctors only. According to current convention, a patient is a new patient if you or a member of your group has not seen the patient in the last 3 years. If the time duration is less, the patient is a follow-up patient. However, if the requesting physician asks for a consultation for a new problem, the time duration is moot, and it can be coded as a new consultation. Although there are CPT codes for time spent on the telephone with the patient, federal programs such as Medicaid and Medicare prohibit billing for them. Third-party carrier rules vary, but they rarely pay for phone time.

Modifiers of CPT Codes

It happens to everyone sooner or later. A new or old diabetic patient appears in your office giving a history of having just returned from a (pick one) tropical isle, ski slope, mountain trek, or medieval village and explains in excruciating detail that he or she (pick one) crashed a scooter, caught an edge, followed the wrong trail, or tripped on the quaint old cobblestoned street. The story will also differ in the quality of the personal lament, the size of the cast in place, and how quickly you can return the patient to normal life. The problem you face is: How do I code this encounter?

Since you are all now attuned to my pleas for personal coding to ensure reimbursement, you will go to the CPT book, look for the appropriate modifier, and code the visit. The CPT book reveals a choice:

- Modifier -54: Surgical care only
- Modifier -55: Postoperative management only
- New patient E&M codes (99201–99205)
- Established Patient E&M codes (99211–99215)
- Outpatient consultations E&M codes (99241–99245)

It would seem logical to use the -55 modifier (postoperative management only), but that would be wrong. You can use the -55 modifier only if the operative surgeon used the -54 modifier (surgical care only), which is highly unlikely. To be properly reimbursed, use a code that describes your visit. Is this a new patient or a follow-up visit (seen in your office within the last 3 years)? It is a consultation if a health care provider requested that the patient consult you. Remember to bill for replacement casts, including the casting material, and send a consultation letter if appropriate. You can bill fully for all subsequent surgery, as you are not affected by the other surgeon's global period. A list with explanations of all modifiers is found at the end of this chapter.

Surgical Coding

Standard surgical coding is applicable to the diabetic patient. Just code from the CPT book with a related ICD code giving the diagnosis justifying the procedure. However, scenarios occur repeatedly that may be coded in several different ways. Again, remember that the diabetic patient requires much more postoperative care than almost any other type of patient. Diabetic patients often present with gangrenous toe tips or deep ulcers with exposed bony prominences. The otherwise healthy patient could be brought to the operating room (OR) with the procedure coded either *Amputation, toe* (28825); *interphalangeal joint* or *Partial excision (craterization, saucer-ization, sequestrectomy or diaphysectomy) tarsal or metatarsal bone for osteomyelitis* (28122). Both of these codes carry a 90-day global period. In a diabetic case, however, it is better to use the debridement codes 11040–11044 with a maximum global period of 10 days. The Relative Value Unit (RVU) of the original procedure is less, but the intense postoperative management, codable after a maximum of 10 days, should help to create appropriate value for the intense effort.

Postoperative problems are much more common in diabetic foot patients. A metatarsal head removal or toe amputation often leads to a transmetatarsal amputation later in the global period. In turn, a transmetatarsal amputation might require later conversion to a transtibial amputation. Since this often happens in the global period, the patient's return to the operating room is mistakenly accompanied by a -78 modifier (*Return to the Operating Room for a Related Procedure During the Postoperative Period*). The 78 lowers the subsequent procedure's value. The proper modifier is -58 (*Staged or Related Procedure or Service by the Same Physician During the Postoperative Period*). The -78 modifier implies that a complication took place, while the -58 modifier acknowledges that the cause of the additional surgery is the underlying disease state and was not unexpected. The same -58 modifier would apply to serial debridements in the operating room. A contrary example would be a return to the operating room 2 to 3 days later because of continued postoperative bleeding requiring a -78 modifier. As a part of surgery for diabetic infection, you might elect to implant antibiotic beads. Code 11981 covers the insertion of a nonbiodegradable drug delivery implant, and 11983 covers the removal and reinsertion of such an implant.

Surgery today commonly involves the application of xenogenic implants such as:

- Oasis acellular xenogenic implant (15400, 15401)
- Graft Jacket and Integra acellular dermal replacement (15170–15176)
- Apligraft (15340, 15341)
- Gamma Graft (15300–15321) (allograft skin application).

New materials receive approval all the time, and you must keep alert to the updates. These codes are new for 2006.

Outpatient Debridement

Serial debridement of the diabetic foot is very common in the outpatient setting, often two to three times a week. Reimbursement is based on both medical necessity and documentation of the service. Initially, with necrotic tissue present, debridement will be frequent. As the wound becomes cleaner, frequency will decrease. Debridement coding depends on the extent of needed debridement, not on the size, classification, or actual depth of the wound. A number of Medicare carriers have local coverage determination policies on ulcer treatment. They may limit the number of ulcers that can be coded at one time. Claims that exceed local policy numbers may be deemed "not reasonable and necessary." With debridement of multiple ulcers, a -59 modifier should be added to each subsequent code to indicate a separate site.

Superficial debridement codes 11040, 11041, and 11042 have zero global days, so frequent use is not a problem. If it is done on the same day as a significant separately identifiable E&M code (usually level 3 or higher), a -25 modifier must be appended to the evaluation code. Codes 11043 and 11044 additionally involve muscle and then bone. They both have a 10-day global period and are less frequently done on an outpatient basis. Supplies and wound dressings, according to CMS, are not reimbursable in the office setting. However, if supplies are dispensed for home use and you are a Durable Medical Equipment Regional Carrier (DMERC) provider, payment should be expected. Representative supplies include Amerigel, Promogram, and Polymem, all of which have Health Care Common Procedure Coding System (HCPCS) "A" codes assigned to them. Documentation for reimbursement should include type of wound, location, drainage, date, and depth of wound. 707.1–707.9 with the appropriate fifth digit are the ICD codes for ulcers.

Surgical Grafting

Bone, cartilage, tendon, or skin grafting often accompanies surgery of the foot and ankle in the diabetic patient and has always been confusing to code. In addition, CPT seems to modify the rules on a frequent basis, further confusing the issue. In general, if the code states "includes obtaining the graft," the graft cannot be coded. If the code states "with autograft" but does not include the words "including obtaining the graft," the graft can be coded separately.

Examples:

28305: Osteotomy tarsal bones, other than calcaneus or talus with autograft includes obtaining graft. (In this case, the graft is not coded.)

28307: Osteotomy, first metatarsal, with or without lengthening, shortening, or angular correction, with autograft. (In this case, obtaining the graft from a separate site is coded.)

A grafting code can be added to any procedure as long as you document the necessity and take the graft from a separate site. Only grafts that are taken from a separate site through a separate incision can be coded. The harvesting of local graft material through the same incision to use in the operation is not coded. The -59 modifier is added to the graft code to indicate the separate site. Allografts (except in the spine) cannot be coded.

With bone grafts, there is a code for a small graft (20900) and a code for a large graft (20902). At the AAOS coding committee, we have accepted the standard that anything larger than a Russe bone graft for the carpal navicular is a large graft. All of the stand-alone graft codes for our purpose are 20900–20926. A small circle with a line across it (∅) indicates that the codes are -51 modifier exempt. They should not be halved in value as an additional procedure (indicated by the -51 modifier). Be careful, because the insurance companies play fast and loose with this rule.

The following are answers to frequently asked questions:

- As part of a subtalar arthrodesis, you take a bone graft from the distal tibia or through a separate incision in the heel. These grafts are coded.
- As part of an ankle arthrodesis, the distal fibula is removed and morselized as an on-lay bone graft. The removal of the distal fibula is part of the surgical approach and is not coded. Because the bone graft is from local material, it is not coded.
- To fill a defect of the talus, an osteocartilagenous graft is taken from the condyles of the knee. This graft is coded. In a similar situation, a graft is taken from a different part of the talus through the same incision. This graft is not coded.
- To fill a defect on the dorsum of the foot after removal of the metatarsocuboid joints, a peroneus tertius graft is obtained through a separate incision. This is coded (20924-59). In contrast, if local extensor muscle and tendon are used to fill the defect from an arthroplasty at the metatarsophalangeal joint, this graft is not coded.

Casting

Casting is an important part of diabetic foot care. Total-contact casting (TCC) is used in the treatment of plantar mal Perforans (ulcer) and Charcot arthropathy. The total-contact cast (29445) has a much higher value than a routine short leg walking cast (29425) because of the associated neuropathy and the patient's inability to be a cooperative assistant in the casting. A trained office assistant is needed to hold the foot in neutral, and meticulous care is needed to avoid wrinkles or gaps in the materials, which are likely to cause localized skin pressure.

The frequency of TTC is based on medical necessity and needs to be supported in the patient record. If you cast the patient in your office. you should use the HCPCS or CMS Q codes to be reimbursed for the casting material. Although CMS is discussing this issue, Medicare will not reimburse for casting supplies if the diagnosis does not include fracture or dislocation (a part of Charcot foot but not of plantar mal perforans). Often, the TCC is applied after debridement of a plantar ulcer. The debridement is a CPT procedure, and all procedural coding includes the initial dressing or cast. However, the debridement codes are in the integumentary section. In these cases the AMA says you can code for both the debridement and the cast at the same encounter.

Injections

In the past, inserting a needle into the soft tissues or joints of diabetic patients was done with trepidation because of the potential metabolic effect of steroids on diabetic control and fear of causing infection or other tissue damage. Today, with the close cooperation of our internal medicine colleagues, injections and arthrocentesis have become standard parts of our armamentarium for care of the diabetic foot. It should be emphasized, however, that improper coding of injections is a major source of revenue loss.

In a foot and ankle practice, the physician will use four major injection codes:

20550: *Injection, tendon sheath, ligament, trigger points, or ganglion cyst*
Examples: injection of the plantar fascia, a painful ligament, the area around a Morton's neuroma, or a ganglion cyst.
20600: *Arthrocentesis, aspiration and/or injection; small joint, bursa, or ganglion cyst*
Examples: injections into small joints: interphalangeal, proximal interphalangeal, metatarsophalangeal, cuneiform, and midtarsal.
20605: *Arthrocentesis, aspiration and/or injection; intermediate joint, or ganglion cyst*
Examples: injections into the subtalar or ankle joint.
64450: *Injection, anesthetic agent; other peripheral nerve or branch*
This code has an RVU of 2.76 and is used for diagnostic nerve blocks of the sural, posterior tibial, superficial peroneal, and other nerves about the foot and ankle.

All of these injection codes have 000 global service days.

Multiple injections of the same foot require a -51 modifier. If the same type of injection is given in the opposite foot, a -50 modifier is used. A -25 modifier is attached to a significant E&M code that is done in addition to the CPT code. Although it is not officially written down, it has been my experience (and that of many consultants) that Medicare and other third-party carriers do not consider any visit below level 3 to be significant.

The physician must also be sure to code for the injectable materials. The codes for these materials are located in the HCPCS National Level 11 coding book, which each office should have. Medicare sets the fees once a year. Most the injectables are located in the J category (e.g., prednisolone 80 mg: J1690). Check the strength of the material and bill accordingly. Injectables have varying dose codes. For example, for Depomedrol (methylprednisolone), the codes are 20 mg: J1020, 40 mg: J1030, 80 mg: J1040. With HCFA, the fee is set, but if you find that other insurers are reimbursing less than your actual cost, confront them with your invoice.

Noninvasive Vascular Testing

Vascular assessment is a critical part of our daily practice routine. Patients with diabetes, peripheral vascular disease, or trauma must have their circulatory status documented on the chart. Indeed, how many of us would take a patient to surgery without assessing vascular competency? When in doubt, many of us send the patient to an outside vascular laboratory for testing. However, there is an increasing trend to perform these tests in one's own office for convenience and possible increased reimbursement, but are these tests reimbursable, are there guidelines, and what kind of equipment do you need? Medicare requires the production of a "two dimensional image with spectral analysis and color flow" or a "plethysmographic recording that allows for quantitative analysis." There are hand-held models that do this. Hard copies of the above tests, which allow for interpretation of the Doppler studies, will be reimbursed using CPT code 93922. This code is not valid for a cursory study performed with a hand-held machine that is not bidirectional and lacks a waveform printout. The state of Washington will pay only for a test from a certified vascular laboratory, although the same test will be reimbursed in the New York metropolitan area. Check with your carrier.

The test cannot be done merely for screening purposes. Carriers will reimburse for arterial Dopplers only when there are signs or symptoms of impending limb ischemia in an individual who is a possible candidate for an invasive therapeutic procedure. The following conditions qualify:

1. Claudication of such severity that it interferes with occupation or lifestyle
2. Rest pain, usually associated with absent pulses, that becomes increasingly severe with elevation and diminishes with dependency
3. Tissue loss, gangrene, or pregangrenous changes of the limb or ischemic ulceration occurring in the absence of pulses
4. Aneurysmal disease
5. Evidence of thromboembolic events
6. Blunt or penetrating trauma (including complications of diagnostic or therapeutic procedures)
7. Follow-up of vascular grafts

Alternatively, if the patient does not meet the above criteria but would still like the test, you can perform it after the patient signs an Advance Beneficiary Notice (ABN) agreeing to the fact that his or her insurance does not pay for it and that the patient is financially responsible. In summary, the medical record must include support for the study. The record must include a hard copy of the bidirectional waveform. There must be a written interpretation or analysis, including a conclusion, in the record. It must also be documented how the information will be used in the context of this patient's care.

Routine Foot Care and Nail Debridement

The Office of the Inspector General (OIG) recently studied the appropriateness of Medicare payments for nail debridement, which is the single largest paid podiatric service. The OIG found that about one in every four claims did not include documentation of medical need for nail debridement in beneficiaries' medical records and that more than half of these inappropriate payments included other related inappropriate payments. This section explains the requirements for payment of Medicare claims for foot and nail services, including information about Routine Foot Care Exclusion, Exceptions to Routine Foot Care Exclusion, Class Findings, Billing Instructions, Required Claim Information, and documentation on file.

Routine Foot Care Exclusion

Except as noted in the "Exceptions to Routine Foot Care Exclusion" section, routine foot care is excluded from coverage. Services that are normally considered routine and therefore not covered by Medicare include:

1. The cutting or removal of corns and calluses
2. The trimming, cutting, clipping, or debriding of nails
3. Other hygienic and preventive maintenance care such as cleaning and soaking the foot, use of skin creams to maintain skin tone of either ambulatory or bedfast patients, and any other service performed in the

absence of localized illness, injury, or symptoms involving the foot

Exceptions to Routine Foot Care Exclusion

- Services performed as a necessary and integral part of otherwise covered services such as diagnosis and treatment of ulcers, wounds, infections, and fractures.
- The presence of a systemic condition such as metabolic, neurologic, or peripheral vascular disease that may require scrupulous foot care by a professional.

Certain procedures that are otherwise considered routine may be covered when systemic conditions, demonstrated through physical and/or clinical findings, result in severe circulatory embarrassment or areas of diminished sensation in the legs or feet and may pose a hazard if performed by a nonprofessional person on patients with such systemic conditions. In the case of patients with systemic conditions such as diabetes mellitus, chronic thrombophlebitis, and peripheral neuropathies involving the feet, associated with malnutrition and vitamin deficiency, carcinoma, diabetes mellitus, drugs and toxins, multiple sclerosis, and uremia, the patient must also be under the active care of a doctor of medicine or doctor of osteopathy who documents the condition in the patient's medical record.

Services performed for diabetic patients with a documented diagnosis of peripheral neuropathy and loss of protective sensation (LOPS) and no other physical and/or clinical findings sufficient to allow a presumption of coverage as noted in the Medicare Carriers Manual can receive an evaluation and treatment of the feet no more often than every 6 months as long as the patient has not seen a foot care specialist for some other reason in the interim. LOPS shall be diagnosed by sensory testing with the 5.07 monofilament using established guidelines, such as those developed by the National Institute of Diabetes and Digestive and Kidney Diseases. Five sites should be tested on the plantar surface of each foot, according to these guidelines.

4. Treatment of warts, including plantar warts, may be covered. Coverage is to the same extent as services provided for in treatment of warts located elsewhere on the body.

Treatment of mycotic nails for an ambulatory patient is covered only when the physician attending a patient's mycotic condition documents in the medical record that (1) there is clinical evidence of mycosis of the toenail and (2) the patient has marked limitation of ambulation, pain, or secondary infection resulting from the thickening and dystrophy of the infected toenail plate. Treatment of mycotic nails for a nonambulatory patient is covered only when the physician attending a patient's mycotic condition documents in the medical record that (1) there is clinical

evidence of mycosis of the toenail and (2) the patient suffers from pain or secondary infection resulting from the thickening and dystrophy of the infected toenail plate.

Note: Active care is defined as treatment and/or evaluation of the complicating disease process during the 6-month period prior to rendition of the routine care or the patient had come under such care shortly after the services were furnished, usually as the result of a referral.

Class Findings

A presumption of coverage may be made by Medicare when the claim or other evidence available discloses certain physical and/or clinical findings that are consistent with the diagnosis and indicative of severe peripheral involvement. For the purposes of applying this presumption, the following findings are pertinent:

Class A Findings
    Nontraumatic amputation of foot or integral skeleton portion thereof
Class B Findings
    Absent posterior tibial pulse
    Advanced trophic changes; three of the following are required:
        hair growth (decrease or absence)
        nail changes (thickening)
        pigmentary changes (discoloration)
        skin texture (thin, shiny)
        skin color (rubor or redness)
    Absent dorsalis pedis pulse
Class C Findings
    Claudication
    Temperature changes
    Edema
    Paresthesia
    Burning

Billing Instructions

The following are the main CPT codes for billing of foot and nail care services (additional codes can be found in the HCPCS/CPT code book):

11719: Trimming of nondystrophic nails, any number
11720: Debridement of nail(s) by any method(s); one to five
11721: Debridement of nail(s) by any method(s); six or more
11730: Avulsion of nail plate, partial or complete, simple; single
11732: Avulsion of nail plate, partial or complete, simple; each additional nail plate (list separately in addition to code for primary procedure).

An Advanced Beneficiary Notice (ABN) should be given to the patient when the physician has good reason to believe that the foot procedure might not be covered by CMS or the third-party carrier. It allows the patient the opportunity to make an informed decision whether or not to allow the physician to perform a procedure for which the patient might be personally financially responsible. If the patient is not presented with the ABN in these situations, subsequent billing of the patient when the procedure is denied could be unlawful (July 31, 2002 CMS transmittal AB-02-114).

Example: A Medicare-qualified at-risk diabetic patient insists on having routine foot care performed every 30 days, but Medicare does not allow reimbursement of such qualified services at treatment intervals of less than 61 days. While CMS carriers have the right, given the appropriate circumstances, to bypass the edit and reimburse qualified foot services on a more frequent basis, the likelihood of this occurring is remote at best. Because qualified routine foot care is a benefit of the Medicare program, a claim of "in between covered services" would need to be submitted to Medicare, and the patient would need to be informed via the reading and signing of an ABN that if Medicare does not reimburse the service, the patient agrees to be financially liable for the service. A complete list of ABN requirements is available in §1862 of the Social Security Act (Codingline Print October 2002).

Required Claim Information

Program Memorandums AB-02-096 dated July 17, 2002, and AB-02-109 dated July 31, 2002, published in the September 2002 Medicare Advisory, contain claim and billing instructions for peripheral neuropathy. For information on completing the CMS-1500 form, see the "Medicare Made Easy" publication (or other carrier-specific guides) from your local CMS carrier. All the above information is from the Medicare website.

Nonmedical Necessity Coverage and Payment Rules for Shoes

Therapeutic shoes, inserts, and/or modifications to therapeutic shoes are covered if the following criteria are met:

The patient has diabetes mellitus (ICD-9-CM diagnosis codes 250.00–250.93); and
The patient has one or more of the following conditions:
Previous amputation of the other foot, or part of either foot, or
History of previous foot ulceration of either foot, or
History of preulcerative calluses of either foot, or
Peripheral neuropathy with evidence of callus formation of either foot, or
Foot deformity of either foot, or
Poor circulation in either foot; and
The certifying physician who is managing the patient's systemic diabetic condition has certified that indica-

tions (1) and (2) are met and that the physician is treating the patient under a comprehensive plan of care for his or her diabetes and that the patient needs diabetic shoes.

If criterion 1, 2, or 3 is not met, the therapeutic shoes, inserts, and/or modifications to therapeutic shoes will be denied as noncovered. When codes are billed without a KX modifier (see the Documentation section of the accompanying Local Coverage Determination), they will also be denied as noncovered.

For patients who meet the coverage criteria, coverage is limited to one of the following within one calendar year (January–December):

- One pair of custom molded shoes (A5501) (which includes inserts provided with these shoes) and two additional pairs of inserts (K0628 or K0629) or
- One pair of depth shoes (A5500) and three pairs of inserts (K0628 or K0629) (not including the noncustomized removable inserts that are provided with such shoes).

Quantities of shoes and/or inserts greater than those listed above will be denied as noncovered.

Modifiers of CPT Codes

The CPT system contains thirty-one modifiers. General guidelines for using modifiers appear in the form of questions to be considered. If the answer to any of the following is yes, then it is appropriate to use the applicable modifier.

- Will the modifier add more information regarding the anatomic site of the procedure?
- Will the modifier help to eliminate the appearance of duplicate billing?
- Would a modifier help to eliminate the appearance of unbundling?

All modifiers are listed in Appendix A of the CPT book. CPT modifiers and their definitions are explained below.

-21 Prolonged Evaluation and Management (E&M) Services

This modifier reports services that take more time or are greater than the highest level E&M code in a particular category. This modifier is used with codes such as 99205, 99215, 99223, 99233, 99245, 99255, and so on.

-22 Unusual Procedural Services

The Unusual Procedural Services modifier has conceptually distinct uses in CPT. Its primary purpose is to denote circumstances for which a procedure or service required an "unusual" amount of time or effort to perform. As such, a higher fee is charged. A word of caution regarding the use of the unusual service modifier: Its use implies that the procedure or service was demonstrably more time-consuming or difficult to perform. When using the modifier, you must also send a special report to the insurance carrier that describes the unusual nature of the service and justifies the additional charge. Even when it is justified, it can be difficult, at best, to obtain higher-than-normal reimbursement from the majority of payers.

Consider a surgical procedure that typically requires 1 to 2 hours to perform. Reimbursement from payers will be the same whether the procedure takes 1 or 2 hours. Why? It is because reimbursement averages out across patients over time. The use of the unusual services modifier would not be appropriate if the procedure took 2 hours, just as use of the reduced service modifier would not be appropriate if the procedure took 1 hour. However, use of the unusual services modifier would be more appropriate for the above hypothetical surgery if the operation was very difficult and required 3 hours to perform because the patient was obese.

-23 Unusual Anesthesia

Under some circumstances, general anesthesia is given when normally either a local or no anesthesia is provided. The use of this modifier is generally restricted to anesthesiologists.

-24 Unrelated Evaluation and Management Service by the Same Physician During a Postoperative Period

This modifier allows the physician to report that a service was performed during a postoperative or global period for a reason(s) unrelated to the original procedure. Modifier -24 should be billed with an E&M code. Do not use this modifier with a surgical code. The diagnosis code that is used must support the service.

Example: A patient who is being followed by her orthopedic surgeon for postoperative care following a transmetatarsal amputation comes in for an additional visit because she has developed acute gout. The gout is unrelated to the amputation and necessitated an additional visit over and above her regular amputation checkups. The E&M code for the visit is billed to the insurance carrier with a -24 modifier, and the diagnosis code used is 274.0 (*Gout*).

-25 Significant Separately Identifiable Evaluation and Management Service by the Same Physician on the Same Day of the Procedure or Other Service

This modifier indicates that on the day a procedure or service identified by a CPT code was performed, the patient's condition required a significant, separately identifiable E&M service above and beyond the usual preoperative and postoperative care associated with the procedure that was performed. Assign the proper E&M code and amount as appropriate for the service rendered.

The E&M service may be prompted by the symptom or condition for which the procedure and/or service was provided. As such, different diagnoses are not required for reporting of the E&M services on the same date. This circumstance may be reported by adding the modifier -25 to the appropriate level of E&M service. Note: This modifier is not used to report an E&M service that resulted in a decision to perform surgery.

Modifier -25 should be appended only to E&M service codes within the range of 92002–92014 and 99201–99499.

-26 Professional Component

Many listed procedures consist of both technical and professional components. Technical components include such things as equipment, technician time, and supplies that are used in the performance of a procedure. The professional component refers to the physician's time, skill, and judgment in interpreting the results of tests and procedures.

Example: Consider the simple foot radiograph described in code 73630. If the radiograph of the patient's foot is taken in the physician's office utilizing both the physician's equipment and staff, the charge for the procedure will include the use of the equipment, film, chemicals, and staff time as well as the physician's time to interpret the radiograph. As such, the charge for code 73630 will include both the technical and professional components. In contrast, suppose that the physician does not have radiographic equipment and refers the patient to a local hospital for the image to be taken. When the hospital, in turn, sends the radiograph to a radiologist for interpretation, the radiologist will bill the patient for interpreting the radiograph only and use the -26 modifier as shown below.

73630-26 Interpretation, three view foot radiographs

By the use of this modifier, the radiologist can restrict his or her charge to the professional component, that is, the interpretation.

-27 Multiple Outpatient Hospital E&M Encounters on the Same Date

For hospital outpatient reporting purposes, utilization of hospital resources related to separate and district E&M encounters performed in multiple outpatient hospital settings on the same date may be reported by adding the modifier -27 to each appropriate level outpatient and/or emergency room E&M code(s). This modifier provides a means of reporting circumstances involving evaluation and management services provided by physician(s) in more than one (multiple) outpatient hospital settings(s). Modifier -27 should be appended only to E&M service codes within the range of 92002–92014 and 99201–99499.

-32 Mandated Services

Mandated services are those requested by an insurance carrier, peer review organization, utilizations review panel, Health Maintenance Organization (HMO), Preferred Provider Organization (PPO), or other entity. Typically, the request is for a second or third opinion regarding a patient's illness or treatment. When mandated services are requested, the physician performing the service is usually required to accept assignment from the payer, and in turn, the payer reimburses the doctor 100% of the payer's allowable fee for the service. An example of a mandated service would be an extended additional opinion consultation. This would be reported as 99274-32. The -32 modifier is used to alert the payer's claim processors that the service was mandated and should receive special handling.

-47 Anesthesia by Surgeon

In general, this is not paid for by CMS or third-party carriers.

-50 Bilateral Procedures

The bilateral modifier is restricted to surgical procedures only (CPT codes 10040–69990). It is not required for radiology procedure codes or diagnostic procedure codes. Procedures are assumed to be unilateral unless they either are always performed bilaterally or are otherwise noted in CPT. The most commonly accepted method of reporting bilateral procedures is to list the procedure twice and add the -50 modifier to the second procedure.

Example: A metatarsal osteotomy is performed on a patient's left and right foot:

Metatarsal osteotomy second ray 28308, right, Metatarsal osteotomy second ray 28308 left - 50

Note that the words *right* and *left* have been added to clarify that the procedures were indeed performed bilaterally. Also, it is common for physicians to report their full charge for each procedure and let the payer reduce the amount paid for the second, or bilateral, procedure. Some payers accept an alternative method of billing bilateral procedures. This method involves listing the procedure once and adding the -50 modifier. Check your local carrier rules.

28308-50 Metatarsal osteotomy, bilateral

If this method is used, place a "2" in the "UNITS" column of the claim form so that the payer is aware that two procedures were performed. The charge reported on the claim for the procedures is typically twice that of what the physician charges for performing one of the procedures. Bilateral procedures are identical procedures (i.e., you use the same CPT code) performed on the same anatomic site but on opposite sides of the body. Furthermore, in most instances, each procedure must be performed through its own separate incision to qualify for bilateral. Note: Modifier -50 does not apply to radiology procedures.

-51 Multiple Procedures

This modifier has traditionally been used to identify multiple surgical procedures performed on a patient during the same operative session. It is applicable when unrelated procedures are performed during the same operative session or when multiple related procedures are performed and there is no single inclusive code available. List the major procedure or service (most revenue intensive) first on the HCFA-1500 claim form, then attach modifier -51 to each applicable secondary procedure code.

Example: The repair of a metatarsal fracture and the repair of a foot laceration would be coded as

23500 Treatment, closed, metatarsal fracture without manipulation
12005-51 Simple closure foot wound

Note that the higher charge procedure (fracture treatment in this case) is listed first and that the multiple procedure modifier is added to the lesser or secondary service. If three procedures had been performed, the services would be ranked from highest to lowest charge on the claim form, and the -51 modifier would be added to all but the first (highest-charge) procedure.

-52 Reduced Services

Just as the unusual services modifier (-22) is used to denote abnormally difficult or time-consuming procedures, the reduced service modifier -52 or 09952 signifies the opposite: that a procedure was reduced or eliminated in part.

Example: The physician does a transmetatarsal amputation but does not do a primary suture of the skin flap so that he can continue cleansing the wound for a time prior to secondary closure of the wound. The proper way to report the procedure would be 28805-52. At a later date, the physician would code for the appropriate wound closure procedure, 15920-52. Many coders mistakenly use the -52 modifier to reduce a charge for a patient who is indigent. The -52 modifier should not be used for this purpose because a Medicare recipient is not medically indigent. Effective January 1, 1999, a new modifier, -73, replaced modifier -52 for reporting discontinued services. Modifier -52 still applies to radiology services for reduced but not terminated procedures.

-53 Discontinued Procedure

This modifier indicated that the physician elected to terminate a surgical or diagnostic procedure—a surgical procedure had been started but, because of extenuating or threatening circumstances, was discontinued. Modifier -53 is not used to report elective cancellation of a procedure prior to the anesthesia induction and/or surgical preparation in the operating suite. Effective January 1, 1999, a new modifier, -74, replaced modifier -53 for reporting these discontinued services. Modifier -53 is no longer an acceptable modifier for hospital reporting, including radiology procedures.

-54 Surgical Care Only

When one physician performs a surgical procedure and another physician provides preoperative and/or postoperative management, surgical services may be identified.

-55 Postoperative Management Only

When one physician performs the surgical procedure and another physician performs the postoperative care and evaluation, the postoperative component may be identified by adding the modifier -55 to the usual procedure number.

-56 Preoperative Management Only

When only one physician performs the preoperative care and evaluation and another physician performs the surgical procedure, the preoperative component may be identified by addition of the modifier -56 to the usual procedure number.

-57 Decision for Surgery

Modifier -57 identifies an evaluation and management service that results in the initial decision to perform surgery. Even though modifier -57 is included in the guidelines for evaluation and management, surgery, and medicine services, it should be reported only with E&M codes. It is to be used in circumstances in which a major surgery is performed within less than 24 hours of the initial evaluation.

Medicare has said that modifier -57 should be used only with major surgical procedures. These are defined as procedures having a preoperative period of 1 day and a postoperative period of 90 days. Many commercial carriers have also adopted this ruling.

Example: A patient presents to the emergency room complaining of acute lower leg pain. She is evaluated by an orthopedic surgeon, who determines that she has a serious limb-threatening abscessed foot. He immediately transfers her to the operating suite and performs an incision and drainage. The services would be coded as follows:

99204-57 Emergency room E&M outpatient service
28002 Incision and drainage foot below fascia

-58 Staged or Related Procedure or Service by the Same Physician During the Postoperative Period

There are many ways to use modifier -58: for a surgery planned in stages; for a staged procedure, such as serial debridements of an infected diabetic foot (11040); for debridement of skin, muscle, and bone in the original global period; to report a more extensive procedure performed during the postoperative period of a less extensive procedure, such as amputation of toes (28805).

Example: 28805-58 Transmetatarsal amputation during the global period for worsening diabetic foot infection that had already involved amputation of several toes.

-59 Distinct Procedural Service

Modifier -59 allows the physician to indicate that a procedure or service was distinct or independent from other services performed on the same day.

Modifier -59 is appropriate for procedures or services that are not normally reported together but are appropriate under the circumstances. CPT states that modifier -59 may represent a different session or patient encounter, different site or organ system, separate incision or excision, separate lesion, or separate injury (or area of injury in extensive injuries) not ordinarily encountered or performed on the same date by the same physician. A -59 modifier is also used to break a Corrupt Coding Initiative (CCI) edit.

Example: A Charcot foot is being reconstructed. A tarsometatarsal fusion is done, but a tendo-Achilles lengthening is also needed because of gastrosoleus contracture. To be recognized as being independent of other procedures, a -59 modifier is added to the tendon-lengthening code.

28730 Tarsometatarsal fusion multiple or transverse
27685-59 Lengthening or shortening of tendon

-62 Two Surgeons

This modifier has two distinct uses: First, it is reported when the two physicians are acting as cosurgeons. That is, each surgeon is acting as a primary surgeon performing a different aspect of a complex procedure. Third-party payers often allow 60% of their prevailing reimbursement to each surgeon in such cases. Second, the -62 modifier may be used when two primary surgeons, usually in different specialties, perform different procedures on a patient during the same operative session.

Example: A vascular surgeon corrects a proximal vascular blockage while another surgeon debrides necrotic tissue in the diabetic foot under the same anesthesia.

Each surgeon should list their CPT code(s) with the addition of the -62 modifier, thus denoting that the services were performed during the same operative session. Use of the two surgeons modifier is important in such circumstances; it helps to ensure that the payer understands that two surgeons were involved in performing the procedure and that double-billing is not taking place. Owing to increasing third-party payment restrictions, it may be helpful to send a special report with the claim that clearly and simply explains and justifies the need for two primary surgeons. Some payers might assume that the procedure(s) can be performed by a primary surgeon and an assistant rather than by two primary surgeons.

-66 Surgical Team

Certain complex surgical procedures require the skills of more than two surgeons. As with the "62" modifier, the physicians who are performing the surgery usually have different skills or specialties. Each member of the team would add the -66 modifier to the procedures he or she performed as part of the surgical team. As with the two surgeons situation, it may be necessary to communicate the need for the team of surgeons to the insurance company. This is especially true in cases in which the need for the team might not be immediately obvious to the claims processor.

-73 Discontinued Outpatient Hospital/Ambulatory Surgery Center Procedure Prior to the Administration of Anesthesia

Because of extenuating circumstances or those that threaten the patient's well-being, the physician may cancel a surgical or diagnostic procedure subsequent to the patient's surgical preparation (including sedation, when provided, and being taken to the room where the procedure is to be performed) but prior to the administration of anesthesia (local, regional block(s), or general). Under these circumstances, the intended service for which the patient has been prepared but which is then canceled can be reported by its usual CPT procedure code with the addition of this modifier.

-74 Discontinued Outpatient Hospital/Ambulatory Surgery Center Procedure After Administration of Anesthesia

Because of extenuating circumstances or those that threaten the patient's well-being, the physician may terminate a surgical or diagnostic procedure after the administration of anesthesia or after the procedure was started (incision made, intubation started, scope inserted, etc). The elective cancellation of a service prior to the administration of anesthesia and/or surgical preparation of the patient should not be reported. For physician reporting of a discontinued procedure, see modifier -53.

-76 Repeat Procedure by Same Physician During the Postoperative Period

-77 Repeat Procedure by Another Physician During the Postoperative Period

These two modifiers are to be used when the procedure has been repeated subsequent to the original service. You need to submit these modifiers because without them, the insurance company might think that you accidentally double-billed for the service.

Example: A diabetic patient is brought to the hospital with a trimalleolar fracture. Three days after surgery, the patient begins physical therapy, falls, and completely disrupts the fracture. The surgeon must perform the same repair again. Would you use the repeat procedure modifier for the second repair? Yes, assuming that the same procedure code was being reported. If a different physician performed the second repair, he or she would use the -77 modifier. It might be necessary to send a special report with the claim explaining why the procedure needed to be repeated. This is appropriate in cases in which the need for the repeat might not be clear to the carrier.

-78 Return to the Operating Room for a Related Procedure During the Postoperative Period

Modifier -78 reports related procedures performed in the operating room within the assigned postoperative period of a surgical procedure. This modifier is often utilized when the patient develops a complication that requires a return trip to the operating room for intervention.

Example: A patient's operative site bleeds after an initial surgery and requires a return to the operating room to stop the bleeding; that is, the same procedure is not repeated. Thus, a different code, 35860 (*exploration for postoperative hemorrhage, thrombosis or infection; extremity*), would be reported with the -78 modifier appended. Since the same procedure is not repeated, modifier -76 would not be appropriate to use.

-79 Unrelated Procedure or Service by the Same Physician During the Postoperative Period

Modifier -79 notifies payers that the procedure was performed during the postoperative period of another procedure but is not related to that surgery. The diagnostic codes must document the medical necessity of the service, so the ICD-9-CM codes are usually different for this service from those reported with the initial procedure.

Example: A patient has an open reduction internal fixation of a tarsal bone fracture 28465 and goes home. The incision and fracture heal well. However, the patient develops acute renal failure a week after being home and is hospitalized. The patient does not respond to medical treatment of the renal failure. Hemodialysis is indicated, and a second physician (a general surgeon) inserts a cannula for hemodialysis (36810). The services of the second surgeon are reported as 36810-79 because this service is unrelated to the open reduction internal fixation performed during the previous hospitalization. If the -79 modifier is not appended to this procedure, the third-party payer might assume that this service is related to the fracture fixation (i.e., the computer program used by the third-party payer might not be able to distinguish that this service is not related to the previous surgery and may automatically reject this claim). Providing documentation to indicate that the service is unrelated to the first procedure may be helpful to avoid having to clear up a problem retrospectively.

-80 Assistant Surgeon

If an assistant surgeon assists a primary surgeon and is present for the entire operation or a substantial portion of the operation, then the assisting physician reports the same surgical procedure as the operating surgeon. The operating surgeon does not append a modifier to the procedure that he reports. The assistant surgeon reports the same CPT code as the primary surgeon, with modifier -80 appended.

Example: To report a triple arthrodesis, the primary surgeon codes 28715, and the assistant surgeon reports 28715-80. The individual operative report submitted by each surgeon should indicate the distinct service provided by each surgeon.

-81 Minimum Assistant Surgeon

At times, while a primary surgeon might plan to perform a surgical procedure alone, circumstances may arise during an operation that require the services of an assistant surgeon for a relatively short time. In this instance, the second surgeon provides minimal assistance, for which the second surgeon reported the surgical procedure code with the -81 modifier appended.

-82 Assistant Surgeon (Where Qualified Resident Surgeon Not Available)

The prerequisite for using the -82 modifier is the unavailability of a qualified resident surgeon. In certain programs (e.g., teaching hospitals), the physician who is acting as the assistant surgeon is usually a qualified resident surgeon. However, there may be times (e.g., during rotational changes) when a qualified resident surgeon is not available and another surgeon assists in the operation. In these instances, report the services of the nonresident-assistant surgeon with the -82 modifier appended to the appropriate code. This indicates that another staff surgeon is assisting the operating surgeon instead of a qualified resident surgeon.

-90 Reference (Outside) Laboratory

When the physician bills the patient for laboratory work that was performed by an outside or ("reference") laboratory, add the -90 or 09990 modifier to the laboratory procedure codes. Physicians should never bill Medicare or Medicaid patients for laboratory work done outside their office.

Example: An internist performs an examination of a patient and, as part of the examination, orders a complete blood count. A staff member performs the venipuncture, but since the doctor does not perform in-office laboratory testing, he has an arrangement with a laboratory to bill him for the testing procedure, and, in turn, he bills the patient. The physician reports the appropriate E&M code, the venipuncture (36415), and 85024-90 for the CBC performed by the outside laboratory.

-91 Repeat Clinical Diagnostic Laboratory Test

This modifier may be appended to a laboratory test code to indicate that a test was performed several times on the same day for the same patient and that it was necessary to obtain multiple results in the course of treatment. Modifier -91 is not intended to be used when laboratory tests are rerun to confirm initial results due to testing problems encountered with specimens or equipment or for any other reason when a normal, one-time, reportable result is all that is required. Modifier -91 may not be used when there are other code(s) to describe a series of test results (e.g., glucose tolerance tests, evocative/suppression testing).

-99 Multiple Modifiers

If two or more different modifiers are added to the same procedure, a third modifier, the -99 or 09999, can be added to alert the carrier to the fact that two or more modifiers are associated with the procedure.

Example: To report for the physician who assisted on a bilateral deep incision and drainage of the feet (28005), you would code as shown below. Since the procedure is bilateral, you must list each procedure separately. In this case, each procedure will list the assistant surgeon modifier (-82), and the second, bilateral procedure requires the use of the -50 modifier. Since there are two modifiers on the second procedure, the -99 modifier is listed: 19182-82 (for the first procedure), 19182-99 (-99 for multiple modifiers on second procedure), or 19182-50/82.

Most carriers require that you have a charge for each line used on the claim form. Thus, you may want to string the modifiers together on the same line on the claim form. You can do this by putting the -99 modifier next to the code in the procedure column and listing the other modifiers in the procedure description column.

In conclusion, the information contained in this chapter should provide you with the basics of both CPT and ICD-9 coding and give insight into how they can be applied to the management of diabetic foot problems.

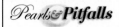

Pearls

- To obtain reimbursement that reflects the extra effort required for care of the diabetic foot, always do your own coding.
- Double-check forms for accuracy; a simple misplaced number will delay reimbursement interminably.
- Precode surgery the day you book it, and mail the forms the day you do the surgery.

Pitfalls

- Never code by analogy. If you do not see the appropriate code, use the code for unlisted procedures.
- Failure to keep current on EOBs (Explanations of Benefits) can result in major revenue loss.

Using out-of-date coding manuals will lead to denial of payment.

Suggested Readings

All modifier information from VHA Health Information Management Department of Veterans Affairs 10 Handbook for Coding Guidelines V2.0, April 26, 2002 Attachment A

CPT 2006 Current procedure technology AMA Press

Codingline Print
Editors Richard Horseman DPM and Harry Goldsmith DPM CopyCraft Printers, Lubbock, Texas

AAOS Guide to CPT Coding
AAOS Press, 1998

CODEX Coding Program
AAOS, 2005

Empire Medicare Website: *www.empiremedicare.com*

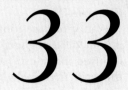

MEDICAL–LEGAL ASPECTS OF TREATING DIABETIC FOOT PROBLEMS

STEVEN Y. LEINICKE AND SHELLEY H. LEINICKE ∎

The purpose of this chapter is to assist physicians in understanding the medical-legal aspects of diabetic foot treatment so that they may reduce the risk of medical malpractice (negligence) claims and improve their chances of defending against any medical malpractice lawsuit that might be brought.

The legal elements of a negligence action are outlined in this chapter, and the risks for potential liability exposure are analyzed. General information is provided regarding the plaintiff patient's burden of proof and issues relating to the presentation of evidence at trial. Recommendations are made for a strategy to reduce potential liability exposure and to defend against medical malpractice claims and lawsuits. Seventeen representative reported legal decisions are summarized.

Elements of a Negligence Claim or Suit

In general, claims of negligence must allege (1) that a duty of care exists; (2) that a breach of that duty occurred; (3) that the breach of duty was a proximate cause of loss, injury, or damages; and (4) the amount of damages sustained. In a medical negligence action, the specific allegations that a patient must prove are (1) that the physician had a duty to provide care and treatment to the patient as a result of an existing doctor/patient relationship, (2) that the physician breached a commonly accepted or recognized standard of medical practice in

providing such care, (3) that the breach of care (or negligence) was the direct, proximate cause of injury to the patient, and (4) the precise scope of the injury caused by the negligent care. While each of these elements is separate and distinct, they are interrelated and must all be established before a patient can prevail in the claim.

Negligence is generally defined as the failure to use reasonable care. In a medical malpractice case, reasonable care is generally described as that degree or level of care and treatment that a reasonably careful, prudent physician of the same or similar medical specialty would provide to the patient under the same or similar circumstances. "In the early stages of a foot disease, the etiology of which may be obscured by the pervasive effects of a chronic disease like diabetes, treatment modalities are frequently a 'judgment call' on the part of the clinician or surgeon. Nonetheless, treatment of diabetic foot disease is subject to some rather well defined standards."[1] Defendant physicians may not successfully rely on a defense that they exercised their best medical judgment where such judgment is "predicated on cursory clinical examinations, inadequate and improper diagnostic testing procedures and equipment, and failure to give due regard to the patient's history, symptoms and complaints at each visit. ... Only if [the patient] had received the benefit of the acceptable standard of diagnostic care for a diabetic patient exhibiting [these] symptoms, and provided treatment in accordance with the basic standards ... would there be no liability by the defendant for a mere mistake in judgment in making a faulty diagnosis."[2]

A jury, or occasionally a judge, acts as the trier of fact in a medical negligence lawsuit. The factual issues to be resolved include (1) the true facts of the case based on the evidence, including such matters as the patient's condition at the time of the initial visit, the patient's past medical history, the medical history and complaints that were relayed to the health care provider, the accuracy of the medical records, and the details of the care and treatment provided;[3] (2) what is the applicable standard of care; (3) whether the physician met the applicable standard of care; (4) whether any failure of the physician to meet the standard of care (deviation) caused any injury or damage to the patient; and (5) the nature and extent of any damages that were caused by the negligence or deviation from the applicable standard of medical care, including determining what damages may have been preexisting, unavoidable no matter what course of treatment was provided, and/or were caused by either the patient or other health care providers.[4] "Medical care for foot pain and possible infection that would meet acceptable standards for a patient in good health, may be grossly deficient where the patient is a known diabetic with possible concomitant vascular and nerve complications of diabetes affecting his legs and feet, particularly when these conditions may be exacerbated by smoking."[5]

In cases in which more than one health care provider is joined in the lawsuit, a different standard of care may be applicable to each one, especially if different medical specialties are involved. Generally, a medical expert must practice in the same specialty as the defendant physician.[6] For example, a podiatrist usually cannot testify as an expert against a family practitioner.[7] However, in many instances, a physician who attempts to treat a medical condition such as diabetes may be held to the standard of care that is applicable to diabetes specialists.[8] Therefore, a general practice physician who elects to treat a patient's diabetic foot without referral to, or consult from, a specialist in the field may be held to the same standard of care as the specialist.

A jury or judge who listens to the facts of a case in a trial is asked to decide the applicable standard of care relevant to the particular set of facts of the case and whether the defendant health care provider met the standard of care or fell below it.[9] In most cases, the standard of care is determined by listening to expert witnesses for both sides of the case express their differing opinions and explanations of the appropriate standard of care and whether the defendant health care provider met or deviated from it. In some instances, the attorneys may use textbooks, medical journal articles, research studies, and/or other publications in an attempt to challenge or cross-examine an expert's opinion as to the applicable and appropriate standard of care.[10] Generally, however, such materials may not be affirmatively presented by the expert to support or bolster his or her testimony and opinions during direct examination of the expert.[11]

In a medical negligence lawsuit, it is not enough for a patient to prove only that a defendant health care provider acted negligently or below the standards of accepted medical practice. A patient must also present evidence and prove that the health care provider's negligence actually caused harm to the patient within a reasonable degree of medical probability. "Causation may be established by facts and circumstances which, in the light of ordinary experience, reasonably suggest that the defendant's [physician's] negligence operated to produce the injury. It is also not necessary that only one conclusion follow from the evidence. However, where from the proven facts the nonexistence of the fact to be inferred appears to be just as probable as its existence, then the conclusion that the fact exists is a matter of speculation, surmise, and conjecture, and the trier of fact cannot be allowed to draw it."[12] "The proof must establish causal connection beyond the point of conjecture. It must show more than a possibility."[13] "Proximate cause is not established where the causal connection is contingent, speculative, or merely possible."[14] "Liability in a medical malpractice suit cannot be made to turn upon speculation or conjecture. The proof must establish causal connection beyond the point of conjecture. Again, it must show more than a possibility. Accordingly, while a 'fair summary' is something less than all the evidence necessary to establish causation at trial, even a fair summary must contain sufficiently specific information to demonstrate causation beyond mere conjecture."[15]

Not only must a patient who pursues a medical negligence claim plead and prove that the physician failed to meet the standards of accepted medical practice and that this negligence caused damage to the patient, the patient must also establish the nature of the damages that were directly and proximately caused by the substandard care. In a typical medical malpractice lawsuit, the physician will generally attempt to present evidence and argue not only that the care and treatment of the patient met the applicable standards of good medical practice and that no injury was suffered as a result of this care, but also that any health care problems currently suffered by the patient had different causes. These other causes may include (1) the patient's failure to follow medical advice and/or specifically acting against medical advice, (2) the ongoing and progressive nature of the patient's physical condition despite the appropriate care and medical treatment by the physician, or (3) actions or inactions of other health care providers.

Many medical negligence cases involving care and treatment of the diabetic foot include a claim for damages resulting from limb amputation. When the trier of fact is quantifying the damage award for a claim of medical negligence involving amputation of a limb, considerations include "plaintiff's extent of recovery and general physical and mental condition before and after the amputation, including past and future physical pain, suffering and mental anguish (including any future residual psychological or emotional problems having their genesis in or exacerbated by the amputation); the nature of and extent of the amputation ...; plaintiff's life expectancy at the time of the amputation; occupational status at the time of the amputation and loss of earnings or profits; impairment of vocational skill or employability; impairment of avocational skills and enjoyment of life; disfigurement resulting from the amputation; past and future medical expenses, including those for future complications; cost of prostheses and the expenses for future replacements; and any other losses or special damages flowing from the injury."[16]

General Aspects of the Successful Defense of a Medical Negligence Claim

The four key elements to successful defense of a medical negligence claim require the physician to establish (1) the skill, experience, training, and competence of the physician; (2) that the physician is caring, compassionate, deliberate, and thoughtful; (3) the reasonable treatment plan that was developed for the medical management of the patient; and (4) that the physician acted reasonably and aggressively to execute the treatment plan. To present an effective defense, each of these elements must be carefully explained to the jury through the testimony of the defendant physician and the defense experts. Failure to address any one element may cause the jury to reject the physician's entire defense.

During trial, the physician must detail for the jury his or her past education, training, and experience in the diagnosis and treatment of diabetes, diabetic foot wounds, and related medical conditions so that the jury will understand and trust the physician's explanations and reasons for the care and treatment that was provided to the plaintiff patient. If the physician lacks sufficient training and experience in the treatment of the diabetic foot, then it is critical to show that (1) timely referrals were made to appropriate specialists and (2) there was reasonable follow-up with the patient and with the consulting specialists.

The jury's perception of a physician's dedication to and interest in his or her patients is equally important. Jurors expect physicians and other health care providers to be friendly, open, candid, frank, calm, honest, authoritative yet humble, and assertive but not argumentative. When a jury sees a physician who is focused on patients' well-being, is committed to providing high-quality care and treatment, and acts in a patient's best interest, the jury will generally infer that the physician brought those same qualities and attention to the care of the plaintiff patient, too. A jury will be less inclined to accept the testimony of a patient's expert who criticizes the judgment and actions of the defendant physician if that physician

is liked and trusted by the jury. A defendant physician who combines an excellent background of education and experience with a likeable demeanor during trial provides a good foundation for convincing the jury of the propriety of their care of the plaintiff patient.

The physician must be able to clearly explain the plan of medical management that was developed and followed for the plaintiff patient as well as the medical reasoning behind the particular treatment decisions and judgment. This explanation is typically made by using the patient's medical records, the physician's own independent recollections of the interactions with the patient and/or other health care providers, and the physician's standard practices and procedures for treating similar patients under the same or similar conditions.

Finally, the jury must be convinced that the defendant physician used his or her best efforts to aggressively treat the plaintiff patient. This is especially true in diabetic foot wound cases because patients and their experts commonly allege that more aggressive treatment would have prevented more serious medical conditions such as septicemia or osteomyelitis and/or avoided the need for more severe treatment such as limb amputation so as to improve the patient's final outcome.

Medical Negligence Actions Arising from or Related to Diabetic Foot Wounds

The challenges and problems in the medical management of diabetes and the diabetic foot occur in several different settings, including (1) medical office,[17] (2) hospital, (3) home health care, (4) nursing home,[18] (5) rehabilitation facility, (6) community health center,[19] or (7) prison.[20] One or more facilities or settings may be involved in any particular claim.[21] Each setting presents both common and unique risks of potential legal liability exposure to the health care provider.

These risks generally can be identified as (1) failure in timely diagnosis, (2) failure of appropriate treatment, (3) failure of timely referral to consulting specialist(s), (4) failure to hospitalize the patient for more aggressive treatment, (5) failure to prevent development or progression of diabetic foot wounds, and (6) failure to prevent the general diabetic condition and diabetic foot from affecting other medical conditions. These scenarios are discussed more fully below in case studies of particular medical malpractice lawsuits.

Summaries of Selected Cases Alleging Medical Negligence in the Treatment of the Diabetic Foot

1. The patient alleged that negligence of the defendant caused "fractures of her left and right legs, fracture of her left arm, multiple Stage II, III, and IV decubitis

ulcers, uncontrolled diabetes, sepsis, gangrene, above the knee left leg amputation, medication overdose, internal bleeding, and her eventual death."[22] The case focuses on procedural issues relating to amendment of pleadings.

2. The patient, a type 1 [juvenile-onset] diabetic, filed suit following the partial amputation of his left foot, claiming that the physician had negligently treated an ulcer on the sole of the foot. The patient alleged that the physician deviated from the acceptable standard of care by failing to hospitalize, failing to timely prescribe intravenous antibiotics, and failing to monitor his diabetic condition. The patient ultimately underwent transtibial amputations of both legs. The patient had been hospitalized on prior occasions for uncontrolled blood sugars and suffered from neuropathy, particularly in his feet. The foot ulcer, for which the patient had been receiving treatment from a podiatrist, was first brought to the physician's attention when the patient was hospitalized for surgical repair of an inguinal hernia. The ulcer was treated conservatively, followed by surgical debridement and intravenous antibiotic treatment during a five-week hospital course. When the wound failed to heal completely, the patient consulted a physician at the Mayo Clinic, where a bone infection was discovered. The foot was partially amputated, but the patient continued to develop ulcers on the stump, followed by ulcers on the right foot as well, ultimately necessitating the transtibial amputations. At trial, it was the patient's burden to overcome substantial evidence indicating that his injuries were caused by subsequent treatment by intervening doctors and/or by the progressive nature of the diabetes. Testimony was presented that the transtibial amputations were neither uncommon nor necessarily the result of medical negligence when a patient's diabetes is complicated by neuropathic limbs. The jury returned a verdict for the physician based on evidence that the patient did not lose his legs as a proximate result of any negligence by the physician.[23]

3. A patient developed a severe blister on his left foot and was treated by basketball team physicians. The condition worsened, and an emergency room physician diagnosed untreated diabetes. Within a short time, the patient underwent a transtibial amputation of the left leg and a partial amputation of the right foot. The case discusses what constitutes a triggering event for the statute of limitations under Ohio law.[24]

4. A wrongful death lawsuit against a nursing facility alleged medical negligence in failing to properly treat the decedent's diabetes. The jury awarded $385,000 for aggravation of preexisting conditions, $1,060,000 for pain and suffering, and $55,172 for medical expenses. The decision focuses on the propriety of evidentiary rulings by the trial court and whether the jury award was supported by the evidence.[25]

5. A diabetic patient/prisoner alleged that the failure of prison physicians to perform appropriate tests and properly diagnose a foot infection resulted in amputation of several toes. The patient's medical history included "tuberculosis, eye trouble, high blood pressure, arthritis, in addition to a prior amputation."[26] The patient's expert, a podiatrist, opined that there were multiple breaches of the standard of care, including (1) failure to take a radiograph of the area (though agreeing that the ability to detect osteomyelitis by radiography depends on the extent of the infection), (2) failure to obtain an anaerobic bacterial culture, (3) failure to prescribe antibiotics for a minimum of 5 to 10 days and up to 6 weeks if osteomyelitis was diagnosed, (4) not switching antibiotics, (5) performing wound debridement under nonsterile conditions, (6) using ointment rather than Betadine to heal the infection, (7) failure to timely perform debridement, (8) improperly instructing the patient to soak his foot at the same time the toe was being debrided, and (9) failure to closely supervise the patient's blood sugar level. The defense presented expert testimony that criticisms expressed by the patient's expert were flawed because they assumed that the patient had osteomyelitis at the time of the initial visit before he was released from incarceration. The treating doctor testified that he ordered an aerobic culture for the gangrenous toe at the initial examination and prescribed Keflex. The antibiotic was not changed because the culture indicated sensitivity to the medication. Radiographs were deemed unnecessary because there was no redness or swelling in the foot, indicating that the condition had not progressed. The patient was referred to a general surgeon. Debridement was performed, and Betadine hydrotherapy and Betadine ointment were prescribed, to which the patient responded. The foot healed and had no sign of infection for 3 months, when reddening of the toes then reoccurred. The doctor said that this was a recurrent problem rather than a persistent one. The court held that the podiatrist was not competent to render expert opinions as to the standard of care to be followed by a family practitioner.

6. A patient had begun treatment for a diabetic foot infection when peripheral vascular disease was discovered. Periodic debridement and wet soaks were recommended, as well as antibiotic treatment and expectant autoamputation of the toes. The patient subsequently developed dry gangrene in the right foot and an ulcer on the left foot that later developed dry gangrene. The patient underwent bilateral transtibial amputations. The patient attempted to allege breach of oral contract or warranty of result, claiming that the physician had assured him that if he underwent the prescribed course of treatment, including the expectant autoamputation of the toes,

he would not lose his legs. The court said that "in the absence of a special contract in writing, a health care provider is neither a warrantor nor a guarantor of a cure"[27] according to Section 606 of Pennsylvania's Health Care Services Malpractice Act.

7. A patient "underwent surgical amputation of her left leg below the knee, due to the defendant internist's malpractice in treating a diabetic foot ulcer."[28] The jury verdict was reduced to $300,000 for past pain and suffering, $114,750 for past lost earnings, and $73,100 for future lost earnings.

8. A diabetic man was injured at work when a metal pipe hit his left second toe. Two days later, he visited his long-standing personal physician, who found the toe swollen with pus under the nail. Foot soaks, keeping the toe dry, and oral Keflex were prescribed. A urinalysis was ordered but not a culture to determine whether the infection was sensitive to Keflex. The next patient contact was 1 month later when the patient presented at an emergency room with the toe severely swollen and discolored. Radiographs, a culture study, continuation of Keflex, and hospital admission were ordered. A bilateral arteriogram showed poor blood flow in both ankles and feet but no blockage of the femoral arteries. Gangrene of the toe did not respond to conservative treatment, the patient was referred to a surgeon, and the toe was amputated five days later. The patient developed a posthospitalization septicemic infection that required a left transtibial amputation 1 month later. Three months later, the patient developed an ulcer on the right heel that required a transtibial amputation a few months later. Despite expert testimony for the patient that "aggressive efforts were necessary to treat a diabetic foot infection in order to avoid the possibility of gangrene, leading to amputation,"[29] and, within reasonable medical probability, amputation could have been avoided if the treating physician had met the standard of care, the jury determined that the personal physician was not negligent and that the surgeon's actions were not the proximate cause of any injury to the patient.

9. A patient with a long history of diabetes and vascular disease sued three physicians, a medical center, and a plastic surgery center following development of an ulcer on his heel that ultimately required a transtibial amputation. Patient presented an expert opinion that if an arteriogram had been done, there was a possibility that the patient "may have had bypassable lesions and that amputation may have been avoided."[30] The court dismissed the suit because the expert's report failed to provide sufficient "information linking the defendants' alleged inaction (failure to do an arteriogram) and the [patient's] injury (the amputation.)"[31] The court explained that it could not infer from the expert's "statements that bypassable lesions were the only proper diagnosis. In fact, [the expert]

seems to suggest that not all lesions are 'bypassable.' We can not infer from [the expert's] statements that discovery of bypassable lesions would have prevented amputation. In fact, [the expert] does not state that [the patient] would have been a candidate for a bypass procedure had an arteriogram been done, or that [the patient's] amputation would have been avoided. At most, [the expert] concludes that amputation 'may have been avoided.' [The expert's] report does not link the defendants' purported breach of the standard of care to [the patient's] amputation."[32]

10. The patient alleged that negligent care and treatment of diabetic foot ulcers required a foot amputation and later a transtibial amputation. The jury determined that both the patient and one health care provider were each 50% at fault. A $49,140 verdict was entered in favor of patient, which represented 50% of the total damages, less $15,000 that had already been paid in a settlement with a podiatrist.[33]

11. This case focuses on what constitutes a single "medical incident" under a medical malpractice insurance policy. In 1972, a physician failed to diagnose hypertension in a 32-year-old man and therefore failed to prescribe appropriate medication and monitoring. Diabetes mellitus was diagnosed in 1986 and was likely exacerbated by the continual failure to treat the patient's hypertension. The doctor was "also clearly negligent in treating the diabetes. He failed to inform [the patient] of the gravity of his condition and the need for medication, proper diet, and monitoring; he failed to schedule regular visits; he failed to conduct regular tests of [the patient's] fasting blood sugar (FBS) levels; he failed to prescribe medication in the proper dosages; he failed to treat [the patient's] condition aggressively despite consistently high FBS levels; he failed to schedule other appropriate tests, such as a hemoglobin A1C test; and, he failed to refer [the patient] to a specialist, despite evidence that his condition was not being effectively controlled."[34] Owing to the negligent treatment, the patient became susceptible to peripheral vascular disease and peripheral neuropathy. In 1998, the physician failed to aggressively treat a left foot infection, failing to (1) order appropriate antibiotics, (2) schedule timely follow-up visits, (3) order radiographs, (4) refer the patient to a specialist, and (5) timely hospitalize the patient for IV drugs. The patient then underwent three amputations, including a transtibial amputation. The court determined that under the terms and conditions of the particular insurance policy in issue, two acts of medical negligence had occurred, and the patient was therefore entitled to an additional $100,000 recovery for the second incident of negligence.

12. The administrator of the patient's estate sued a nursing home, alleging that negligent failure to diagnose and treat diabetes led to bilateral transtibial

amputations and the patient's subsequent death. The case discusses expert qualification and disclosure requirements under New York State law.[35]

13. A board-certified family practice physician treated a patient for 5 to 6 years for obesity, diabetes, and hypertension. The patient then appeared with a complaint of a sore on his foot that began when he wore tennis shoes to exercise. Physical examination showed a "large, ulcerated, foul-smelling wound on the plantar surface of the right foot."[36] A diabetic foot ulcer was diagnosed, and antibiotics and soaks were prescribed. When there was little improvement 4 days later, the patient was referred to a surgeon for debridement. The patient was told to use wet-to-dry dressings. The wound continued not to heal, and 2 months later, a two-stage surgical debridement was scheduled. Wet-to-dry dressings were again prescribed. In error, potassium hydroxide (a solution used for wet mounts during vaginal examinations) was used in the dressing instead of normal saline solution because of the similarity of the bottles. The suit against the physician alleged (1) failure to supervise employees in dispensing of solutions, (2) failure to establish adequate precautions to distinguish between solutions, and (3) negligently treating the open sore with a caustic solution. The evidence established that the physician was not present when the dressing was changed, that the physician had properly instructed the nurse on the procedure and supplies required for the dressing change, and that the nurse was employed by someone other than the physician.

14. A podiatrist scraped a piece of skin underneath the third toe while cutting a diabetic patient's toenails. The patient consulted a second podiatrist when the toe became red and swollen. Cellulitis was diagnosed, and the patient was instructed to use Betadine soaks followed by Bacitracin ointment. A wound culture was performed on a subsequent visit, along with a radiograph that was reported to show "no radiographic evidence of osteomyelitis but if that is a clinical concern, bone scan is advised."[37] Approximately 5 weeks later, the patient complained of a sore on her right lower leg that was warm to touch. Within 4 weeks, the patient was hospitalized for a diabetic septic foot, for which a button toe amputation of the third toe was performed. The opinion of the patient's podiatric expert was sufficient to establish that the treating podiatrist had departed from accepted standards of care and was the proximate cause of the patient's injuries. The expert's report stated that on the patient's first visit, there was an inadequate history; a failure to order radiographs, CBS, or blood sugar; and failure to evaluate her neurologic status. The expert further opined that the "conservative treatment of [the patient's] infected toe, in light of her diabetic condition, fell below the

applicable standard of care."[38] He also questioned a delay in performing debridement and stated that the podiatrist failed to evaluate properly the [patient's] presenting condition, and therefore underestimated the severity of the infection."[39]

15. The patient "suffered from numerous health problems, including, but not limited to, hypertension, possible coronary artery disease, asthma, and insulin-dependent diabetes, which once resulted in ketoacidosis."[40] The patient injured his foot when he hit it on a steel bed. A licensed practical nurse examined the foot within 30 minutes, cleaned the wound with saline, applied ointment, and covered it with gauze. A physician examined the patient the following day and claimed that he saw "no swelling, no redness, and no physical wound," though he conceded that "he could not recall whether he looked between the toes" on the patient's foot.[41] The physician failed to examine the patient on other dates or to order treatment or referral. Following a lengthy series of visits, the patient underwent amputation of several toes. The court ruled that there were questions of fact as to whether the physician acted with deliberate indifference to the patient's condition. The court said that "refusal to treat chronic pain, delay in prescribing pain medication, or erroneous treatment based on a substantial departure from accepted medical judgment may evidence deliberate indifference."[42] The court also said that "neither medical malpractice nor reasonable medical judgment that leads to a bad result amounts to deliberate indifference."[43] The doctor admitted that "wound care in diabetics is especially important and wounds must be treated aggressively because wounds in diabetics take a long time to heal. [The physician] explained that a diabetic with a cut, wound, or ulcer on his foot should be treated with antibiotics, if necessary, or provided topical treatment, such as cleaning and dressing."[44]

16. A former client sued his attorney for legal malpractice for failing to timely pursue a medical negligence lawsuit. The attorney prevailed at trial because the client failed to establish that he would have prevailed in the medical malpractice action. The former client/patient was "morbidly obese, partially blind, and in end-stage renal failure resulting from insulin-dependent diabetes."[45] The patient developed an infected foot after he stepped on a piece of glass. A clinic disinfected and bandaged the wound and told the patient to apply Bacitracin. Dialysis clinic personnel periodically asked about the wound but did not provide further care for it. The patient then saw a podiatrist, who ordered home health wound care. The patient was later hospitalized for a gangrenous foot that led to amputation of most of the left leg. Hyperbaric treatment that was provided to try to speed healing of the surgical site caused a hearing impairment. The court said that the patient

and his spouse "did not raise more than of a [sic] scintilla of evidence to prove that they would have prevailed in the medical negligence suit against the dialysis clinic. Accordingly, they failed to establish that [former counsel] committed legal malpractice by failing to bring a medical negligence claim against the clinic."[46]

17. A 52-year-old former prisoner suffered a transtibial amputation of the right leg and recovered $500,000. While previously incarcerated, the patient had been treated by the medical staff for diabetes mellitus and developed a bacterial infection in his right foot. The suit alleged that the bacterial infection resulted either from an abrasion caused by improperly fitting institutional boots or from an athlete's foot fissure. The facility asserted that the infection was "blood-borne and gangrene was primarily the result of complications incident to his diabetic condition (diabetic neuropathy, microangiopathy and other vascular insufficiency)."[47] The facility also argued that the diabetic complications were aggravated by the patient's "heavy cigarette smoking, [his] prior history of intravenous narcotic drug use, alcoholism, and by trauma to his right foot when he fell out of bed."[48] The case contains a particularly detailed recitation of the patient's history, the experts' opinions as to the quality and efficacy of the medical care, and the patient's medical course.

Summary

A determination of liability requires proof of both negligence and its causation of damages. Four elements must be pleaded and proven to recover in a negligence lawsuit: (1) duty of care, (2) breach of that duty, (3) that the breach is a proximate cause of injury or damages, and (4) the nature and extent of damages sustained. The trier of fact resolves (1) the true facts of the case, (2) the applicable standard of care, (3) whether the defendant physician met this standard, (4) whether any failure to meet the standard of care caused injury or damage to the patient, and (5) the nature and extent of those damages. Generally, a medical expert must practice in the same specialty as the defendant physician. Authoritative literature generally may not be used to bolster an expert's opinion.

Successful defense of a medical negligence claim requires that the physician prove (1) the skill, experience, training, and competence of the physician; (2) that the physician is caring, compassionate, deliberate, and thoughtful; (3) that a reasonable treatment plan was developed to medically manage the patient; and (4) that the physician acted reasonably and aggressively to execute the treatment plan. The jury must be convinced that the defendant physician used his or her best efforts to aggressively treat the plaintiff patient.

Endnotes

1. Williams v. United States, 747 F.Supp. 967, 969 (S.D. N.Y. 1990).
2. Id. at 1009.
3. "'Good medical care implies that you don't send a person from one hospital to another or one facility to another without any history at all.' 'A good history is usually more valuable in diagnosis than the physical examination, or even than extensive laboratory studies.'" Id. at 996.
4. See, e.g., id. at 985.
5. Id.
6. Cleckley v. State of Illinois, 1994 WL 906660 (Ill. Ct. Cl.).
7. "A family practitioner is 'a doctor regularly called by a family in time of medical need.' As such [the physician is] expected to furnish a variety of medical services to regular patients." Medical Malpractice Joint Underwriting Association of Rhode Island v. Lyons, 2004 WL 3190049 at *6 (R.I. Super.).
8. The treatment of diabetic foot wounds often presents a variety of problems and typically may involve the medical specialties of endocrinology, vascular surgery, general surgery, and/or infectious diseases. Carter v. Azaran, 332 Ill. App.3d 948, 774 N.E.2d 400 (Ill. 1st DCA 2002); Williams, 747 F.Supp. 967.
9. Williams, 747 F.Supp. at 1010.
10. Cleckley, 1994 WL 906660.
11. Donshik v. Sherman, 861 So.2d 53 (Fla. 3rd DCA 2004); Medina v. Variety Children's Hospital, 438 So.2d 138 (Fla. 2nd DCA 1983); Williams, 747 F.Supp. at 986, 990.
12. Carter, 774 N.E.2d at 412 (internal cites omitted).
13. Hutchinson v. Montemayor, 144 S.W.3d 614, 618 (Tex. App. 2004).
14. Cleckley, 1994 WL 906660 at *13.
15. Hutchinson, 144 S.W.3d at 618 (internal cites omitted).
16. Williams, 747 F.Supp. at 1011.
17. Hutchinson, 144 S.W.3d 614; Medical Malpractice Joint Underwriting Association of Rhode Island, 2004 WL 3190049.
18. Carter, 774 N.E.2d 400; Muniz v. Our Lady of Mercy Medical Center, 2003 WL 21436132 (N.Y. Sup.).
19. Nickerson v. Lee, 42 Mass. App. Ct. 106, 674 N.E.2d 1111 (Mass. App. 1996); Williams v. Briscoe, 137 S.W.3d 120 (Tex. App. 2004); Williams, 747 F.Supp. 967.
20. Cleckley, 1994 WL 906660; Spencer v. Sheahan, 158 F.Supp.2d 837 (N.D. Ill. 2001).
21. Bishop v. Baz, 215 Ill. App.3d 976, 575 N.E.2d 947 (Ill. 3rd DCA 1991); Flora v. Moses, 727 A.2d 596 (Pa. Super. 1998); Howard v. St. Luke's Hospital, 1986 WL 7516 (Ohio App. 8 Dist.); Neff v. Wenzl, 2002 WL 31414447 (Neb. App.).
22. Acevedo v. Augustana Lutheran Home, 7 Misc.3d 1005(A), 2004 WL 3261175 at **1 (N.Y. Sup.).
23. Bishop, 575 N.E.2d 947.
24. Boop v. Moyer, 1998 WL 405036 (Ohio App. 9 Dist.).
25. Carter, 774 N.E.2d 400.
26. Cleckley, 1994 WL 906660 at *13.
27. Flora, 727 A.2d at 598.
28. Free v. Nassau Queens Medical Group, P.C., 242 A.D.2d 668, 668 (N.Y. S.Ct. 1997).
29. Howard, 1986 WL 7516, at *2.
30. Hutchinson, 144 S.W.3d at 617.
31. Id.
32. Id.
33. Marshall v. Firster, 2000 WL 1466196 (Ohio App. 11 Dist.).
34. Medical Malpractice Joint Underwriting Association of Rhode Island, 2004 WL 3190049 at *1.
35. Muniz, 2003 WL 21436132.
36. Neff, 2002 WL 31414447 at *1.
37. Nickerson, 674 N.E.2d at 1113.
38. Id. at 1114.
39. Id. at 1115.
40. Spencer v. Sheahan, 158 F.Supp.2d at 839.
41. Id. at 840.
42. Id. at 848.
43. Id.
44. Id. at 849.
45. Williams v. Briscoe, 137 S.W.3d at 122.
46. Id. at 126.
47. Williams, 747 F.Supp. at 968.
48. Id.

APPENDIX I: PATIENTS' INSTRUCTIONS FOR THE CARE OF THE DIABETIC FOOT

Marvin E. Levin, MD and Lawrence W. O'Neal, MD, FACS

1. Inspect your feet daily for blisters, cuts, scratches, and reddened areas. The use of a mirror can aid you in seeing the bottoms of the feet or you can have a family member check your feet, top and bottom. Always check between the toes.
2. Wash your feet daily. Dry carefully, especially between the toes.
3. Avoid extreme temperatures. Test water with hand or elbow before bathing.
4. If your feet feel cold at night, wear socks. Do not apply a hot water bottle, electric blanket, or heating pad.
5. Do not walk barefoot on hot surfaces such as sandy beaches or on the cement around swimming pools. Wear protective footwear when swimming in the sea, lakes, rivers or pools. The bottom of pools may be rough, causing foot abrasions.
6. Do not walk barefoot.
7. Do not cut corns. Do not use chemical agents for removal of corns and calluses. Do not use corn plasters. Do not use strong antiseptic solutions on your feet. Do not use callus files. Do not do "bathroom surgery." If, for example, you have an ingrown toenail, see your medical foot care specialist.
8. Do not use adhesive tape on your feet.
9. Inspect the inside of your shoes daily for foreign objects, nail points, torn linings, and rough areas.
10. If your vision is impaired, have a family member inspect your feet daily, trim nails, and buff down calluses.
11. Do not soak your feet unless specifically instructed.
12. For dry skin, use a very thin coat of a lubricating oil or cream. Apply after bathing. Do not put the oil or cream between toes. Consult a physician for type of lubricant and detailed instructions.
13. Wear properly fitting stockings. Do not wear mended stockings. Avoid stockings with seams or heavy elastic tops. Change stockings daily. Do not wear garters.
14. Shoes should be comfortable at the time of purchase. Purchase shoes in the afternoon when feet tend to be the largest. Do not depend on them to stretch. Shoes should be made of leather. Running or walking shoes may be worn after checking with the physician.
15. Inform your shoe salesperson that you are diabetic.
16. Do not wear shoes without socks or stockings.
17. Do not wear sandals with thongs between the toes.
18. Ask about therapeutic shoes if you have a foot deformity, such as bunions or claw toes, or if you have had a previous ulcer.
19. Take special precautions in wintertime. Wear wool socks and protective footgear, such as fleece-lined boots.
20. Cut nails straight across or follow the curve of the nail. Do not cut nails too short. If you have neuropathy, impaired vision, or difficulty reaching your nails, have your medical foot care specialist trim them.
21. Do not cut corns and calluses. Follow special instructions from your physician or foot care specialist. If your nails are thick or difficult to cut, have a family member, physician, or medical foot care specialist trim them.
22. See your physician regularly and be sure that your feet, including areas between the toes, are examined at each visit.
23. Do not smoke.
24. Notify your physician or medical foot care specialist at once should you develop a blister or sore on your foot or if your foot becomes swollen, red, or painful.
25. Be sure to inform your medical foot care specialist that you are diabetic.

APPENDIX II: USEFUL WEBSITES

Advanced Rehabilitation Therapy
Information on prosthetic rehabilitation
- *http://www.advancedrehabtherapy.com*

American Academy of Family Physicians
Resources for patients with neuropathy
- *http://familydoctor.org/050.xml*

American Board for Certification in Orthotics and Prosthetics
Information on prostheses
- *http://www.oandpcare.org*

American Diabetes Association
Standards of Medical Care for Patients with Diabetes Mellitus
Clinical practice recommendations
Technical review on foot problems in diabetic patients
- *http://www.diabetes.org*
- *http://www.diabetes.org/for-health-professionals-and-scientists/cpr.jsp*
- *http://care.diabetesjournals.org/cgi/content/extract/29/suppl 1/s4*

American Orthopaedic Foot and Ankle Society
Advice on foot care for diabetic patients
- *http://www.aofas.org*

American Pain Foundation
Information on painful diabetic neuropathy
- *http://www.painfoundation.org*

American Podiatric Medical Association
Diabetic foot information
- *http://www.apma.org/s*
- *http://www.apma/index.asp*

Amputation Surgery Education Center
Techniques of amputation surgery
- *http://www.ampsurg.org*

Amputee Coalition of America
Support and education resource for diabetic/dysvascular amputees
- *http://www.amputee-coalition.org*

Centers for Disease Control and Prevention
National Diabetes Fact Sheet
National Diabetes Surveillance System
- *http://www.cdc.gov/diabetes/pubs/factsheet 05.htm*
- *http://www.cdc.gov/diabetes/statistics/index.htm*

The Diabetic Foot
General source for diabetic foot care; well-illustrated
- *http://www.diabeticfoot.org.uk*

Diabetic-Foot.com.au
Diabetic foot information and resources
- *http://www.diabetic-foot.com.au*

Empire Medicare Services
Medicare coding for diabetic foot care (northeast US)
- *http://www.empiremedicare.com*

Foot in Diabetes
Assistance in development of diabetic foot care teams
- *http://www.footindiabetes.org*

International Working Group on the Diabetic Foot
International Consensus on the Diabetic Foot
Practical Guidelines on the Management and Prevention of the Diabetic Foot
- *http://www.diabetic-foot-consensus.com/index.php*
- *http://www.idf.org/bookshop* (to purchase)

MedEd Online
Information on education of diabetic persons regarding foot care
- *http://www.mededonline.org*

Michigan Neuropathy Screening Instrument (MNSI)
Description and use of this neuropathy screening tool
- *http://www.med.umich.edu/mdrtc/survey/index.html#mnsi*

National Baromedical Services, Inc.
Sources for hyperbaric oxygen treatment of diabetic foot lesions
- *http://www.baromedical.com*

National Hansen's Disease Programs
Total contact casting technique, illustrated
- *http://bphc.hrsa.gov/nhdp/CASTING_PT.htm*

National Institutes of Health
Sites on neuropathy and diabetes
- *http://diabetes.niddk.nih.gov/dm/pubs/neuropathies*
- *http://www.nih.gov/disorders/diabetic/diabetes/htm*

Pedorthic Footwear Association
Pedorthic management of the diabetic foot
- *http://www.pedorthics.org*

Society for Vascular Surgery
Vascular surgery information
- *http://www.vascularweb.org*

Undersea and Hyperbaric Medicine Society
General information on the role of hyperbaric oxygen treatment of insensate foot lesions
- *http://www.uhms.org*

Department of Health and Human Services, Bureau of Primary Health Care, National Hansen's Disease Program Website
Description of federal programs for treatment of the insensate foot
- *http://www.hrsa.gov/hansens/publications.htm*

Wound Healing Research Unit at Cardiff University
Information regarding ongoing research programs in wound healing at this center
- *http://www.whru.co.uk*

Note: Page numbers followed by b refer to boxed materials; page numbers followed by f refer to figures; page numbers followed by t refer to tables.